W9-BVD-418

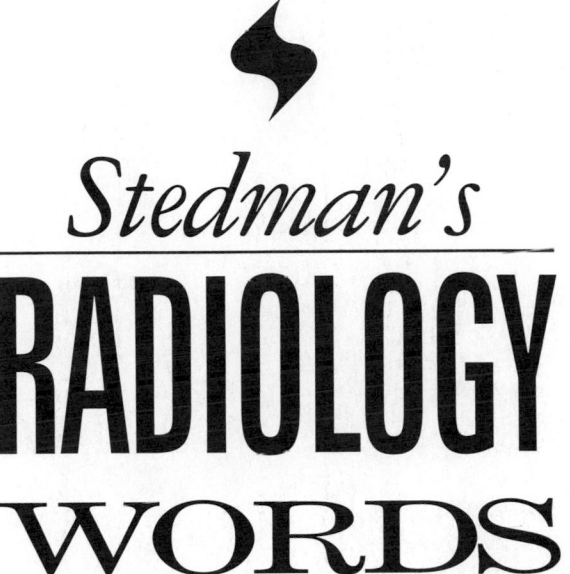

Stedman's
RADIOLOGY
WORDS

INCLUDES
NUCLEAR MEDICINE
& OTHER IMAGING

FIFTH EDITION

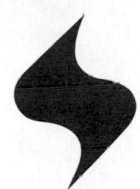

Stedman's

RADIOLOGY

WORDS

INCLUDES
NUCLEAR MEDICINE
& OTHER IMAGING

FIFTH EDITION

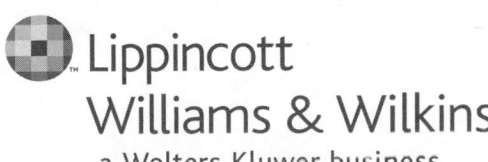

Lippincott
Williams & Wilkins
a Wolters Kluwer business

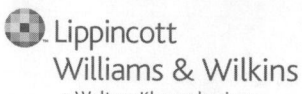
Lippincott
Williams & Wilkins
a Wolters Kluwer business

Publisher: Julie K. Stegman
Senior Product Manager: Eric Branger
Associate Managing Editor: Cecilia González
Typesetter: Kristi Lukens
Manufacturing Coordinator: Dana Jackson
Printer & Binder: Malloy Litho, Inc.

Copyright © 2006 Lippincott Williams & Wilkins
351 West Camden Street
Baltimore, Maryland 21201-2436

All rights reserved. This book is protected by copyright. No part of this book may be repro-
duced in any form or by any means, including photocopying, or utilized by any information
storage and retrieval system without written permission from the copyright owner.

Printed in the United States of America

Fifth Edition, 2006

Library of Congress Cataloging-in-Publication Data
Stedman's radiology words: includes nuclear medicine & other imaging.— 5th ed.
    p. ; cm. ˆ (Stedman's word books)
    Includes bibliographical references.

    ISBN13: 978-0-7817-7073-6
    ISBN10: 0-7817-7073-4
    1. Radiology—Terminology. 2. Radiography, Medical—Terminology.
    3. Diagnosis, Radioscopic—Terminology. 4. Diagnostic imaging
    —Terminology. 5. Radioisotope scanning—Terminology. I. Stedman,
    Thomas Lathrop, 1853–1938. II. Title: Radiology words. III. Series.
    [DNLM: 1. Diagnostic Imaging—Terminology—English. WN 15 S812 2006]
    RC78.A3S74 2006
    616.07'57014—dc22

                                                                2006001172

                                                    10 09 08 07 06
                                                    2 3 4 5 6 7 8 9 10

Contents

Acknowledgments

An important part of our editorial process is the involvement of medical language specialists and other health professionals — as advisors, reviewers, and/or editors.

We extend special thanks to Raymond Lukens and Sue Dickinson for editing the manuscript and for helping to resolve many difficult questions. We are grateful to the members of our Editorial Advisory Board, who were instrumental in the development of this reference: Norma Braunstein; Janell DeMello, MLS; Cheryl Klopcic; Patricia O'Brien-Giglia, CMT; and Vicki Runnels. They shared their valuable judgment, insight, and perspective.

Our appreciation goes to the following reviewers who helped to enhance the A-to-Z content for this edition: Ellen Atwood, Sue Bartolucci, Shemah Fletcher, Robin Koza, and Heather Little.

We also extend our gratitude to Janet West for revising and developing the appendices; to Sue Dickinson and Andrea DiChiaro's for their assistance with the anatomical illustrations; and to Jo-Ann Clarke for her contributions to the Sample Reports appendix. Thanks also go to Jeanne Bock for performing the final prepublication review.

As always, Barb Ferretti played an integral role in the process by reviewing the content files for format, updating the manuscript, and providing a final quality check.

As with all our *Stedman's* word references, this resource incorporates the suggestions and expertise of our many contacts in the medical community. Thanks to all of our advisory board participants, reviewers, and editors; AAMT meeting attendees; and others who have written to us with requests and comments — keep talking, and we'll keep listening.

Editor's Preface

Grateful thanks to the extraordinary staff of Lippincott Williams & Wilkins and Stedman's for helping prepare this fifth edition of *Stedman's Radiology Words*, including Heather Rybacki, Eric Branger, Tiffany Piper, and Cecilia González. Stedman's staff is committed to meeting the needs of medical transcriptionists and all others involved with medical terminology and language.

Radiology continues to evolve more rapidly than many other medical disciplines: new technologies, tests, equipment, and procedures all must be described, discussed, and transcribed using an ever-evolving vocabulary that often incorporates terminology from other medical specialties.

Stedman's radiology lexicon has grown so much over the past few years that this newest edition is a formidable word book. We believe you will find this newest edition of *Stedman's Radiology Words* to be a useful and comprehensive compilation of the latest terms being used. As with the previous edition, we tried to limit words with only tangential bearings on radiology, nuclear medicine, and other imaging. Although other specialty terms (e.g., from anatomy, surgery, and oncology) are included in this edition as they relate to radiology and medical imaging, we ask the reader to refer to word books related to other specific disciplines for more comprehensive coverage in those areas.

In addition to the inclusion of many of the most up-to-date new terminology related to radiology, nuclear medicine, and other imaging, we have compiled two new appendices — one of common breast imaging terms and the other of common radiographic imaging techniques. The appendix section also includes anatomical illustrations; contrast media, imaging agents, and related substances; common radiation oncology terms; and sample reports, which will all be of great assistance to the user.

A special thanks to our loyal users for your continuing support of the word book line.

Raymond Lukens

Publisher's Preface

Stedman's Radiology Words, Fifth Edition offers an up-to-date, authoritative reference for the wordsmiths of the healthcare professions — medical transcriptionists, medical editors and copyeditors, health information management personnel, court reporters, medical coders, and the many other users and producers of medical documentation.

With the rapid rate of technological advancement, we realized the need to develop a comprehensive reference that reflects the changes that have taken place within radiology, nuclear medicine, and imaging since the publication of the previous edition. With this revised edition, we have focused on incorporating new developments in technology, including thorough coverage of the equipment and contrast materials used in imaging today, as well as techniques, procedures, tests, and phrases.

Stedman's Radiology Words, Fifth Edition provides users with tens of thousands of words and phrases encompassing various aspects of imaging and nuclear medicine, including: diagnostic, therapeutic, and interventional radiology; abdominal, chest, gastrointestinal, genitourinary, and skeletal imaging; CT, MRI, PET, and SPECT imaging; mammography, ultrasonography, x-ray, neuroradiology, roentgenology, investigational radiology, radiographics, and radiologic technology terminology; as well as various contrast materials. Users will also find terms for diagnostic and therapeutic procedures, new techniques, and equipment names, plus abbreviations with their expansions. The appendix sections provide labeled anatomical illustrations, contrast media and other related materials, sample reports, and common terms by procedure.

This compilation of more than 110,000 entries, fully cross-indexed for quick access, includes over 2,400 more terms than the previous edition. The extensive A-to-Z list was developed from manufacturers' literature, scientific reports, books, journals, CDs, and Web sites (please see list of References on page xvii).

We at Lippincott Williams & Wilkins strive to provide you with the most up-to-date and accurate word references available. Your use of this word book will prompt new editions, which we will publish as often as updates and revisions justify. We welcome your suggestions for improvements, changes, corrections, and additions — whatever will make this *Stedman's* product more useful to you. Please complete the postage-paid card in this book, or contact us by email at stedmans@lww.com.

Explanatory Notes

Medical transcription is an art as well as a science. Both approaches are needed to correctly interpret the dictation of a physician, whose language is a product of education, training, and experience. This variety in medical language means that there are several acceptable ways to express certain terms, including jargon and word parlance. *Stedman's Radiology Words, Fifth Edition,* seeks to reflect current usage of medical language and provides variant spellings and phrasings for many terms. These elements, in addition to complete cross-indexing, make *Stedman's Radiology Words, Fifth Edition,* a valuable resource for determining the validity of terms as they are encountered.

Alphabetical Organization

Alphabetization of main entries is letter by letter as spelled, ignoring punctuation, spaces, prefixed numbers, Greek letters, or other characters. For example:

HWP
    hydrops
    hydropyonephrosis
    5-hydroxyindoleacetic acid (5-HIAA)
    Hypaque
    hypoxia-ischemia

In subentry alphabetization, the abbreviated singular form or the spelled-out plural form of the noun main entry word is ignored.

Format and Style

All main entries are in **boldface** to expedite locating a sought-after term, to enhance distinction between main entries and subentries, and to relieve the textual density of the pages.

Irregular plurals and variant spellings are shown on the same line as the singular or preferred form of the word. For example:

index, indices, indexes
mammoplasty, mammaplasty

Hyphenation

As a rule of style, multiple eponyms (e.g., Alibert-Bazin syndrome) are hyphenated. Also, hyphens have been added between a manufacturer and one or more eponyms (e.g., Vital-Metzenbaum dissecting scissors). Please note, however, that in many cases, hyphenation is a question of style, not of accuracy, and thus is a matter of choice.

Possessives

Possessive forms have been dropped in this reference for the sake of consistency and of conformance with the guidelines of the American Medical Association (AMA), American Association for Medical Transcription (AAMT), and other professional groups. Please note, however, that in many cases retaining the possessive, like hyphenating, is a question of style, not of accuracy, and thus is a matter of choice. To form the possessive of a word in the singular, add an apostrophe and an "s" to the end of the word, and to form the possessive of a word in the plural, add only an apostrophe.

Cross-indexing

The word list is in an index-like main entry–subentry format that contains two combined alphabetical listings:

(1) A *noun* main entry–subentry organization, which is typical of the A-to-Z section of medical dictionaries like *Stedman's*:

arachnoiditis
  adhesive a.
  cystic a.

pancreatography
  endoscopic retrograde p.
  intraoperative p.

(2) An *adjective* main entry–subentry organization, which lists words and phrases as they are actually written and spoken. The main entries are the adjectives or modifiers in a multiword term. The subentries are the nouns around which the terms are constructed and to which the adjectives or modifiers pertain:

cardiovascular
  c. accident
  c. anomaly

polycystic
  p. ovarian disease (PCOD)
  p. ovary syndrome (PCOS)

This format provides the user with more than one way to locate and identify a multiword term. For example:

gradient
  diastolic g.

diastolic
  d. gradient

assessment
  sonographic a.

sonographic
  s. assessment

It also allows the user to see together all terms that contain a particular descriptor, as well as all types, kinds, or variations of a noun entity. For example:

compliance
  craniospinal c.
  lung c.
  c. matching stent (CMS)
  reduced pulmonary c.

sensitivity
  contrast s.
  C sign s.
  s. encoding (SENSE)

Wherever possible, abbreviations are separately defined and cross-referenced. For example:

BI-RADS
  Breast Imaging Reporting and Data System

Breast
  B. Imaging Reporting and Data System (BI-RADS)

system
  Breast Imaging Reporting and Data S. (BI-RADS)

To avoid duplication, phrases that include commonly used imaging abbreviations, such as MRI, are only listed with the abbreviated phrase. For example, "cine magnetic resonance imaging" will be listed as "cine MRI." At the main entry for "magnetic resonance imaging," you will be referred to the abbreviated phrase for additional listings, as indicated below:

imaging (*See* image, MRI)
   magnetic resonance i. (MRI)

Multiple Descriptors

Often, a single medical term can be referred to in many different ways, creating a number of synonyms in medical language. For example, Alzheimer disease and Alzheimer disorder can be used interchangeably and mean the same thing. To avoid duplication and thus making this book even larger, terms that can take multiple descriptors are listed only once in the manuscript; similar listings can be found at the main entry:

syndrome (See disease, phenomenon)

References

In addition to the lists of our MT Editorial Advisory Board members (from their daily transcription work), we used the following resources in the development of *Stedman's Radiology Words, Fifth Edition*.

Books

Barkovich, A. James. Pediatric Neuroimaging, 4th Edition. Baltimore: Lippincott Williams & Wilkins, 2005.

Baum, Stanley and Michael J. Pentecost. Abrams' Angiography: Interventional Radiology, 2nd Edition. Baltimore: Lippincott Williams & Wilkins, 2005.

Brandao, Lara A. and Romeu C. Domingues. MR Spectroscopy of the Brain. Baltimore: Lippincott Williams & Wilkins, 2003.

Cardenosa, Gilda. Breast Imaging (The Core Curriculum). Baltimore: Lippincott Williams & Wilkins, 2003.

Castillo, Mauricio. Neuroradiology (The Core Curriculum). Baltimore: Lippincott Williams & Wilkins, 2002.

Chew, Felix S. and Mitchell J. Kline. Musculoskeletal Imaging (The Core Curriculum). Baltimore: Lippincott Williams & Wilkins, 2003.

Erkonen, William E. and Wilbur L. Smith. Radiology 101: The Basics and Fundamentals of Imaging, 2nd Edition. Baltimore: Lippincott Williams & Wilkins, 2004.

Greenspan, Adam. Orthopedic Imaging: A Practical Approach, 4th Edition. Baltimore: Lippincott Williams & Wilkins, 2004.

Hashemi, Ray H., William G. Bradley Jr., and Christopher J. Lisanti. MRI: The Basics, 2nd Edition. Baltimore: Lippincott Williams & Wilkins, 2003.

Health Professions Institute. Radiology Imaging Words and Phrases, 2nd Edition. Modesto, CA: Health Professions Institute, 2005.

Health Professions Institute. Vera Pyle's Current Medical Terminology: A Health Professions Institute Publication, 9th Edition. Modesto, CA: Health Professions Institute, 2003.

Kazerooni, Ella A. and Barry H. Gross. Cardiopulmonary Imaging (The Core Curriculum). Baltimore: Lippincott Williams & Wilkins, 2003.

Torres, Lillian S., Terriann Linn-Watson Norcutt, and Andrea Guillen Dutton. Basic Medical Techniques and Patient Care in Imaging Technology, 6th Edition. Baltimore: Lippincott Williams & Wilkins, 2003.

Von Schulthess, Gustav K. and Gustav Konrad Von Schulthess. Clinical Molecular Anatomic Imaging: Pet, Pet/Ct, and Spect/Ct, Revised Edition. Baltimore: Lippincott Williams & Wilkins, 2003.

Yochum, Terry R. and Lindsay J. Rowe. Essentials of Skeletal Radiology, 3rd Edition. Baltimore: Lippincott Williams & Wilkins, 2004.

Images

Agur, A. M. R. and M. J. Lee. Grant's Atlas of Anatomy, 10th Edition. Baltimore: Lippincott Williams & Wilkins, 1999.

Bennett, J. Bethesda, MD, National Institutes of Health.

Brant, W. E. and C. A. Helms. Fundamentals of Diagnostic Radiology, 2nd Edition. Baltimore: Williams & Wilkins, 1999.

Daffner, R. H. Clinical Radiology: The Essentials, 2nd Edition. Baltimore: Williams & Wilkins, 1998.

Erkonen, W. E. and W. L. Smith. Radiology 101: Basics and Fundamentals of Imaging. Philadelphia: Lippincott Williams & Wilkins, 1998.

Hardy, Neil O. In Stedman's Medical Dictionary, 28th Edition. Baltimore: Lippincott Williams & Wilkins, 2006.

MediClip Human Anatomy 1-3, CD-ROM. Baltimore: Lippincott Williams & Wilkins.

Mission Hospital Regional Medical Center, Mission Viejo, CA.

Senkarik, Mikki. In Stedman's Medical Dictionary, 27th Edition. Baltimore: Lippincott Williams & Wilkins, 2000.

Westheimer, R. and S. Lopater. Human Sexuality: A Psychosocial Perspective. Baltimore: Lippincott Williams & Wilkins, 2002.

Journals

Journal of Computer Assisted Tomography. Lippincott Williams & Wilkins, 2003, 2005.

Journal of Vascular and Interventional Radiology. Society of Interventional Radiology, 2005.

The Latest Word (Cardiology/Infertility, Geriatrics/Dementia, and Radiology). WB Saunders Co., 2003, 2004.

Let's Talk Terms (Radiology), Journal of the American Association of Medical Transcriptionists. Lippincott Williams & Wilkins, 2003, 2004.

Topics in Magnetic Resonance Imaging. Lippincott Williams & Wilkins, 2002, 2004, 2005.

The Radiologist. Lippincott Williams & Wilkins, 2002, 2003.

Web Sites

www.bracco.com

www.ezem.com

www.fda.gov

www.mtdesk.com

www.neurophysics.com

www.hpisum.com/perspectives

Newsletters

Medquist

A
>A level of esophagus
>A point
>A ring of esophagus
>A scan

AA
>acetabular anteversion
>anaplastic astrocytoma
>ascending aorta

AAA
>abdominal aortic aneurysm

AAI
>ankle-arm index
>atrial inhibited
>axial acetabular index
>>AAI rate-responsive mode

AAL
>anterior axillary line

AAOS
>American Academy of Orthopaedic Surgeons
>>AAOS acetabular abnormalities classification

Aaron sign

AAS
>acute abdominal series

AASA
>acetabular sector angle

A1-A5 segment of anterior cerebral artery

AB
>ankle-brachial

ab
>>ab externo laser sclerotomy
>>ab interno laser sclerotomy

abandonment
>>mode a.

abapical pole

ABBI
>advanced breast biopsy instrumentation
>>ABBI system

Abbokinase

Abbott artery

abbreviated injury scale (AIS)

ABC
>aneurysmal bone cyst
>aortic-brachiocephalic
>argon beam coagulator

abciximab

abdomen
>>distended a.
>>flat plate of a.
>>gasless a.

abdominal
>>a. abscess

a. adenopathy
a. adhesion
a. air collection
a. aorta
a. aorta thrombosis
a. aortic aneurysm (AAA)
a. aortic artery
a. aortic coarctation
a. aortic plexus
a. aortography
a. apron
a. blunt trauma
a. canal
a. carcinosis
a. cavity
a. circumference (AC)
a. collection of fluid
a. compression cylinder
a. content
a. CT scan
a. distention
a. ectopic pregnancy
a. fat
a. fibromatosis
a. fissure
a. fistula
a. fluid wave
a. gas
a. girth
a. great vessel
a. heart
a. hemorrhage
a. heterotaxia
a. hysterectomy
a. inflammation
a. irradiation
a. kidney
a. left ventricular assist device (ALVAD)
a. lymph node
a. muscle deficiency syndrome
a. paracentesis
a. pseudotumor
a. raphe
a. ring
a. roentgenography
a. sac
a. series
a. situs inversus
a. situs solitus
a. sonography
a. space
a. splenosis
a. stoma
a. ultrasound

abdominal *(continued)*
    a. vascular accident
    a. vertebra
    a. view
    a. visceral arteriography
    a. viscus
    a. wall calcification
    a. wall defect
    a. wall desmoid tumor
    a. wall hernia
abdominogenital
abdominopelvic
    a. actinomycosis
    a. cavity
    a. mass
    a. viscus
abdominoscrotal
abdominothoracic
abdominovaginal
abdominovesical
abducens
**abducted and externally rotated
(ABER)**
abduction
    a. fracture
    a. position
    a. stress test
abduction-external
    a.-e. rotation fracture
    a.-e. rotation position
abductor
    a. digiti quinti (ADQ)
    a. digiti quinti muscle
    a. digiti quinti tendon
    a. hallucis muscle
    a. hallucis tendon
    a. pollicis brevis (APB)
    a. pollicis brevis muscle
    a. pollicis brevis tendon
    a. pollicis longus (APL)
    a. pollicis longus tendon
abductovalgus
    hallux a.
abductus
    pes a.
ABE
   anatomy-based extraction
ABER
   abducted and externally rotated
    ABER position
aberrant
    a. artery
    a. band
    a. bone marrow
    a. bundle
    a. ganglion
    a. intrahepatic bile duct
    a. origin
    a. pancreas

    a. papilla
    a. right subclavian artery
    a. spleen
    a. tissue
    a. umbilical stomach
    a. vascular channel
    a. venous drainage
    a. vessel
aberration
    chromatid-type a.
    intersegmental a.
    intraventricular a.
    ventricular a.
ABI
   ankle-brachial index
ability
    cardiac pumping a.
Ablatherm HIFU system
ablation
    6-a., 14-ablation scheme
    acetic acid injectable for tumor a.
    Amazr radiofrequency catheter a.
    ethanol a.
    image-guided radiofrequency
     tumor a.
    image-guided tumor a.
    laser thermal a. (LTA)
    laser uterosacral nerve a. (LUNA)
    microwave a.
    microwave endometrial a. (MEA)
    MRI-guided laser thermal a.
    percutaneous chemical a.
    percutaneous radiofrequency
     catheter a.
    radioactive iodine a.
    radiofrequency a. (RFA)
    radiofrequency catheter a. (RFCA)
    radiofrequency thermal a.
    radiopharmaceutical a.
    saline-enhanced radiofrequency
     tissue a.
    small-volume tissue a.
    soft tissue a.
    stereotactic a.
    thermal a.
    total a.
    transaortic radiofrequency a.
    transapical endocardial a.
    transcatheter a.
    transseptal radiofrequency a.
    transurethral needle a. (TUNA)
    tumor a.
    ultrasound-guided percutaneous
     interstitial laser a.
    Urolase fiber laser a.
ablative laser therapy
abluminal
**AbMap electrophysiologic imaging
system**

abnormal
a. adherence of placenta
a. bright signal
a. cisterna magna
a. dimensions of cardiac chamber
a. ejection fraction response
a. esophageal fold
a. esophageal peristalsis
a. heart chamber dimension
a. lung opacity
a. lung pattern
a. ossification
a. peristaltic esophagus
a. placental size
a. position of foot
a. small bowel fold
a. tissue
a. tracer accumulation
a. tracking
a. tubular function
a. umbilical cord attachment

abnormality
accumulation a.
arch of aorta a.
bony a.
bulbar a.
calyceal a.
cardiopulmonary a.
congenital a.
congruent signal intensity a.
definitive a.
drug-induced brain a.
dyskinetic segmental wall
   motion a.
facial a.
fetal a.
focal limb a.
focal metabolic a.
focal wall motion a.
focal white matter signal a.
functional a.
gestational sac a.
global wall motion a.
gray matter a.
gyral a.
high-signal a.
hyperkinetic segmental wall
   motion a.
hypokinetic segmental wall
   motion a.
ileocecal valve a.
interstitial a.

intracranial vascular a.
labeling a.
left ventricular regional wall
   motion a.
limb reduction a.
mesenchymal a.
microcirculation a.
migration a.
mucosal a.
obstructive a.
osseous a.
paraspinal a.
perfusion a.
placentation a.
pulmonary interstitial a.
regional perfusion a.
restrictive a.
reticular a.
rostrocaudal extent signal a.
screening-detected a.
segmental bronchus perfusion a.
snowman a.
soft tissue a.
spinal cord injury without
   radiographic a. (SCIWORA)
stellate a.
structural a.
subsegmental perfusion a.
torsion a.
tracer a.
ultrastructural a.
urachal a.
vascular a.
vertebral border a.
vertebral endplate a.
vessel wall a.
wall motion a. (WMA)
white matter a.
abnormally thin skull
aborad
aboral direction
abortive neurofibromatosis
above
a. diaphragm (AD)
a. elbow (AE)
above-knee amputation (AKA)
above-selected threshold (AST)
ABPA
allergic bronchopulmonary aspergillosis
ABR
artery bronchus ratio
Abrahams sign

NOTES

Abrams biopsy needle
abrasion
    cortical a.
    subperiosteal cortical a.
abrasor
Abrikosov tumor
abruption
    placental a.
abrupt vessel closure
abscess
    abdominal a.
    actinomycotic brain a.
    acute a.
    amebic a.
    anaerobic lung a.
    anular a.
    aortic anulus a.
    appendiceal a.
    Aspergillus cerebral a.
    atheromatous a.
    bilateral iliopsoas a.
    bone a.
    brain a.
    breast a.
    Brodie metaphysial a.
    cerebral a.
    chronic breast a.
    cold breast a.
    cold spine a.
    collar-button a.
    crypt a.
    cuff a.
    daughter a.
    deep interloop a.
    deep pelvic a.
    diverticular a.
    a. drainage catheter
    echinococcal a.
    encapsulated brain a.
    enteroperitoneal a.
    epidural a.
    extradural a.
    a. formation
    frontal a.
    gallbladder wall a.
    growth plate a.
    hepatic a.
    horseshoe a.
    iliac fossa a.
    iliopsoas a.
    interloop a.
    intermesenteric a.
    intersphincteric a.
    intraabdominal a.
    intradural a.
    intrahepatic a.
    intramesenteric a.
    intraosseous a.
    intraperitoneal a.

    intrascrotal a.
    ischiorectal a.
    kidney a.
    lacunar a.
    lesser sac a.
    liver a.
    lung a.
    mediastinal a.
    metaphysial a.
    midpalmar a.
    Nocardia brain a.
    orbital a.
    ovarian a.
    Paget a.
    pancreatic a.
    paracolic a.
    parapharyngeal a.
    pararectal a.
    pararenal a.
    paraspinal a.
    parotid a.
    partial pericardial a.
    pelvic a.
    perianal a.
    periappendiceal a.
    pericecal a.
    pericholecystic a.
    pericolic a.
    pericolonic a.
    perihepatic a.
    perinephric a.
    perinephritic a.
    perirectal a.
    perirenal a.
    peritoneal a.
    pharyngeal a.
    phlegmonous a.
    postchemoembolization liver a.
    Pott a.
    premasseteric space a.
    prostate a.
    psoas a.
    pulmonary a.
    pulp a.
    pulpal a.
    pyogenic brain a.
    pyogenic liver a.
    renal a.
    retropharyngeal a.
    scrotal a.
    soft tissue a.
    space of Retzius a.
    spinal epidural a. (SEA)
    splenic a.
    sternal a.
    subaponeurotic a.
    subdiaphragmatic a.
    subdural a.
    subgaleal a.

subhepatic a.
subperiosteal a.
subphrenic a.
subungual a.
testicular a.
thecal a.
thenar space a.
thyroid a.
tuboovarian a.
ventral epidural a.
walled-off a.

Abscession drainage catheter
abscessogram
abscissa
abscission needle
absconsio
abscopal effect
absence
congenital pericardial a.
a. of haustral marking
a. of innominate line
limb a.
a. of outer end of clavicle
partial pericardial a.
a. of primary peristalsis
a. seizure
a. of spleen
a. of uptake
a. of vascular marking

absent
a. aortic knob
a. bow-tie sign
a. bronchial cartilage
a. diaphragm sign
a. greater sphenoid wing
a. kidney
a. kidney outline
a. lower esophageal sphincter
  relaxation
a. peripheral vein
a. peristalsis
a. radiotracer uptake
a. runoff
a. valve
a. ventricle

absolute
a. artery dimension
a. blood flow
a. curative resection
a. dose intensity (ADI)
a. efficiency
a. emission probability

a. granulocyte count
a. linearity
a. noncurative resection
absolute-peak efficiency calibration
absorbance
absorbed
a. dose (AD)
a. dose range
a. fraction
absorbent
a. gland
a. vessel
absorptiometer
single-energy x-ray a. (SXA)
absorptiometry
dual-energy x-ray a. (DEXA,
  DXA)
dual-photon a. (DPA)
morphometric x-ray a.
single-photon a. (SPA)
absorption
a. atelectasis
bone radiation a.
broad-beam a.
a. cavity
a. coefficient
electromagnetic a.
external a.
interstitial a.
laser energy a.
a. line
photoelectric a.
radiofrequency a.
radioiron oral a.
a. of radionuclide
ratio of photoelectric to
  Compton a.
a. spectrophotometer
a. unsharpness
a. x-ray spectrum
abut
abutment
abutting
AC
abdominal circumference
acromioclavicular
alcoholic cirrhosis
anterior commissure
aortic closure
AC 3 plate reader
ACA
anterior cerebral artery

NOTES

ACAD
  atherosclerotic carotid artery disease
acalculia
acalculous cholecystitis
acallosal
acanthiomeatal line
acanthocytosis
acantholysis
acanthopelvis
acanthopelyx, acanthopelvis
acanthosis
  glycogenic a.
  a. nigricans
acanthotic
acardia
ACAT
  automated computed axial tomography
ACBE
  air-contrast barium enema
accelerated
  a. atherosclerosis
  a. fractionation
  a. particle
  a. peristalsis
  a. phase
  a. phase gain
  a. silicosis
acceleration
  fetal growth a.
  flow a.
  growth a.
  a. index (AI)
  a. map
  a. time (AT)
accelerator
  alpha particle a.
  dedicated linear a.
  dual-energy linear a.
  electron linear a.
  a. factor
  high-energy bent-beam linear a.
  linear a. (LINAC)
  a. mass spectrometry (AMS)
  Microtron a.
  modified linear a.
  particle a.
  Philips linear a.
  racetrack microtron a.
  Siemens Mevatron 74 linear a.
  University of Florida linear a.
  Varian a.
Accel stopcock
accentuation
  a. of marking
  paramagnetic enhancement a.
access
  arterial a.
  central venous a.
  E^{3}xtreme A.

femoral a.
intravenous a. (IVAC)
jugular venous a.
a. loop
a. set
accessory
  a. adhesion molecule
  a. atlantoaxial ligament
  a. atrium
  BabyFace 3D surface rendering a.
  a. blood supply
  a. breast
  a. canal
  a. cephalic vein
  a. communicating tendon
  a. cusp
  a. diaphragm
  a. digit
  extravasation detection a.
  a. fissure
  a. hemiazygos vein
  a. hemidiaphragm
  a. hepatic duct
  a. hepatic vein
  a. lobe
  a. lymph node
  a. middle cerebral artery
  a. multangular bone
  a. muscle
  a. nasal cartilage
  a. navicular bone
  a. nerve
  a. organ
  a. ossicle
  a. ossification center
  a. pancreas
  a. pancreatic duct
  a. placenta
  a. process
  a. right renal artery
  a. right uterine artery
  a. saphenous vein
  a. sesamoid bone
  a. sign colon
  a. sinus
  a. spleen
  a. thyroid gland
  a. tubercle
  a. ureteral bud
  a. vertebral vein
accident
  abdominal vascular a.
  cardiovascular a. (CVA)
  cerebrovascular a. (CVA)
accidental
  a. correction
  a. intradural injection
accompanying vein

accordion
- a. fold
- a. sign
- a. vertebra

accordion-shaped pleat

accreta
- placenta a.

Accuclot D-dimer assay

Accucore II biopsy needle

accuDEXA
- a. bone densitometer
- a. bone mineral density assessment system

AccuLase excimer laser

AccuLength arthroplasty measuring system

Acculink stent

accumulation
- a. abnormality
- abnormal tracer a.
- dependent extracellular fluid a.
- fluid a.
- a. of gas
- intratumoral a.
- nonspecific a.
- parenchymal tracer a.
- a. phase
- radiotracer a.
- residual urine a.
- Thorotrast a.
- tracer a.

Accunet distal protection device

AccuProbe

accuracy calibrator

AccuView computer workstation

Accu-Vu sizing catheter

ACD
- annihilation coincidence detection
- anterior capsular distance

ACE
- angiotensin-converting enzyme
- ACE inhibition renography
- ACE inhibition scintigraphy

acervuloma

acetabular
- a. anteversion (AA)
- a. bone
- a. cavity
- a. cup
- a. depth
- a. depth-to-femoral head diameter (AD/FHD)
- a. fossa
- a. head index (AHI)
- a. index
- a. labrum
- a. line
- a. posterior wall fracture
- a. protrusion
- a. reconstruction plate
- a. residual dysplasia
- a. rim fracture
- a. roof
- a. sector angle (AASA)
- a. shell
- a. teardrop figure

acetabular-prosthetic interface

acetabulum, pl. acetabula
- cartilaginous a.
- deep-shelled a.
- os a.
- Y-shaped a.

acetazolamide
- a. challenge brain SPECT imaging
- a. dual-isotope image
- a. renography
- a. vasodilator test

acetazolamide-enhanced SPECT

acetic acid injectable for tumor ablation

acetrizoate
- A. contrast agent
- meglumine a.
- a. sodium

acetylated

acetylation

acetylator

acetylsalicylic acid

ACF
- anterior cervical fusion

ACG
- angiocardiogram
- angiocardiography
- apexcardiogram
- apex cardiogram

achalasia
- cricopharyngeal a.
- a. of esophagus
- megaesophagus of a.
- primary a.
- secondary a.
- ureteral a.
- vigorous a.

acheiria

NOTES

achievable
as low as reasonably a. (ALARA)
Achiever balloon dilatation catheter
Achilles
A. bursa
A. densitometer
A. tendon
A. tendon rupture
A. tendon shortening
A. tendon xanthoma
acholangic biliary cirrhosis
achondrogenesis
achondroplasia
achondroplastic dwarfism
achoresis
acid
acetylsalicylic a.
ametriodinic a.
amidotrizoic a.
benzoic a.
chenodeoxycholic a.
deoxyribonucleic a. (DNA)
diethylenetriaminepentaacetic a.
(DTPA)
dimer captosuccinic a. (DMSA)
dimethyl iminodiacetic a. (DIDA)
dimethylsuccinic a.
ethylenediaminetetramethylene
phosphonic a. (EDTMP)
^{18}F-fluoro-6-thia-heptadecanoic a.
(FTHA)
^{18}F-labeled fatty a.
flavone acetic a. (FAA)
free fatty a. (FFA)
gadolinium diethylenetriamine-penta-
acetic a. (Grl-DTPA)
gadolinium diethylenetriamine
pentaacetic a. (Gd-DTPA)
gadolinium ethoxybenzyl
diethylenetriamine pentaacetic a.
(Gd-EOB-DTPA)
gadolinium
tetraazacyclododecanetetraacetic a.
(Gd-DOTA)
gadopentetic a.
gadoxetic a.
gamma-aminobutyric a. (GABA)
glucoheptonate a. (GHA)
hepatoiminodiacetic a. (HIDA)
homovanillic a. (HVA)
hydroxyethylidene-1,1-
diphosphonic a. (HEDP)
5-hydroxyindoleacetic a. (5-HIAA)
^{123}I heptadecanoic a.
iobenzamic a.
iocarmic a.
iocetamic a.
iodine-123 iodophenyl
pentadecanoic a. (IPPA)

iodoalphionic a.
iodopanoic a.
iodophenyl pentadecanoic a. (IPPA)
iopanoic a.
iothalamic a.
ioxaglic a.
long-chain fatty a.
low-dose folic a.
meclofenamic a.
mefenamic a.
metrizoic a.
mycophenolic a.
nonesterified fatty a. (NEFA)
okadaic a.
ophenoxic a.
palmitic a.
paraaminobenzoic a.
paraaminohippuric a.
paraaminosalicylic a. (PAS)
para-isopropyl-iminodiacetic a.
(PIPIDA)
a. peptic ulcer
phenoxyacetic a.
polylactic a. (PLA)
a. reflux
ribonucleic a. (RNA)
^{99m}Tc-labeled iminodiacetic a.
technetium-99m diethylenetriamine
pentaacetic a. (^{99m}Tc-DTPA)
technetium-99m
dimercaptosuccinic a. (^{99m}Tc-
DMSA)
tetraazacyclododecanetetraacetic a.
(DOTA)
trichloroacetic a.
triiodobenzoic a.
(V)-dimer captosuccinic a. (DMSA)
acidophilic
a. adenoma
a. pituitary tumor
acid-Schiff
periodic a.-S.
acid-Schiff-positive
acinar
a. adenocarcinoma
a. collapse
a. nodule
a. pancreatic cell carcinoma
a. pattern
a. sarcoidosis
a. tuberculosis
acinarization
acinic
a. cell adenocarcinoma
a. cell carcinoma
a. cell tumor
acinous adenoma
acinus, pl. **acini**

ACIS
>automated cellular imaging system

ACIST contrast delivery injection system

Ackerman criteria for osteomyelitis

Ackrad balloon-bearing catheter

ACL
>anterior cruciate ligament

aclasis
>>diaphysial a.
>>tarsoepiphysial a.

ACM
>automated cardiac flow measurement
>ACM ultrasound

ACoA, AcomA
>anterior communicating artery

Acoma portable x-ray machine

acoprosis

acoustic
>>a. artifact
>>a. canal
>>a. crest
>>a. cyst
>>a. enhancement
>>a. gel
>>a. imaging
>>a. impedance
>>a. interface
>>a. lens
>>a. meatus
>>a. nerve
>>a. nerve sheath tumor
>>a. neuroma
>>a. papilla
>>a. penetration
>>a. pressure
>>a. pressure amplitude
>>a. quantification
>>a. reflection method
>>a. response technology
>>a. schwannoma
>>a. shadow
>>a. standoff
>>a. trauma
>>a. tubercle
>>a. velocity
>>a. vesicle
>>a. wave
>>a. window

acousticofacial
>>a. crest
>>a. ganglion

AC-PC
>anterior commissure-posterior commissure
>>AC-PC line
>>AC-PC plane
>>AC-PC referenced MR imaging

ACPL
>antibody-conjugated paramagnetic liposome

AcQsim CT simulator

acquired
>>a. acroosteolysis
>>a. adult Fanconi syndrome
>>a. aortic valve stenosis
>>a. atelectasis
>>a. bronchiectasis
>>a. cystic kidney disease
>>a. epidermoid
>>a. fragility
>>a. hepatic cyst
>>a. hepatocerebral degeneration
>>a. hydrocephalus
>>a. immunity
>>a. immunodeficiency syndrome (AIDS)
>>a. intestinal lymphangiectasis
>>a. left ventricle aneurysm
>>a. megacolon
>>a. mitral stenosis
>>a. occupational lung disease
>>a. porencephaly
>>a. radiation resistance
>>a. renal cystic disease
>>a. spinal stenosis
>>a. tracheobronchomalacia
>>a. unilateral hyperlucent lung
>>a. urethral diverticulum

acquisition
>alternated delay a. (ADA)
>biphasic a.
>cine a.
>combined dynamic 2D and bolus-chase 3D a.'s
>continuous volumetric a.
>data a.
>3D fast low-angle shot a.
>2D fast spin-echo a.
>3D fast spin-echo a.
>3D FLASH a.
>double-helix a.
>dynamic a.
>electronic picture a.

NOTES

acquisition *(continued)*
   elliptic centric a.
   fast spin-echo a.
   first-pass a.
   FLASH a.
   generalized autocalibrating partially parallel a. (GRAPPA)
   gradient a.
   image a.
   interleaved image a.
   long axis a.
   a. matrix
   multigated a. (MUGA)
   multiple gated a. (MUGA)
   multiple overlapping thin-slab a. (MOTSA)
   multiple slice a.
   multiple thin slab a. (MTSA)
   multisection multirepetition a.
   multislice a.
   off-axis rotational a.
   a. optimization
   polarity-altered spectral-selective a.
   primary digital a.
   reduced a.
   segmented k-space data a.
   sequential image a.
   short axis a.
   signal a.
   simultaneous multislice a.
   4-slice a.
   small-voxel a.
   spirometric a.
   a. technique
   thin-slab coronal a.
   a. time
   T1-weighted a.
   volume a.
   volumetric a.
   whole-brain a.
   a. window

ACR
   American College of Radiology
   ACR rate
   ACR teleradiology standard

acrania
Acrel ganglion
acridine orange
acrocephalosyndactyly,
  acrocephalosyndactylia
   Pfeiffer a.
   Saethre-Chotzen a.
acrodermatitis enteropathica
acrodysostosis
acrofacial
acrokeratosis
acromegaly
acromelia

acromelic
   a. dwarfism
   a. dysplasia
acromesomelic dysplasia
acromial
   a. angle
   a. articular surface
   a. bone
   a. slope
   a. spur
acromiale
   os a.
acromicria
acromioclavicular (AC)
   a. articulation
   a. injury classification
   a. joint
   a. joint disc
   a. joint separation
   a. ligament
   a. space
acromiocoracoid ligament
acromiohumeral
   a. distance
   a. interval (AHI)
acromion
   cupping of a.
   hooked a.
   a. process
acromutilation
acroosteolysis
   acquired a.
acroosteosclerosis
acropachy
   thyroid a.
acropachyderma
acroparesthesia
acropectorovertebral dysplasia
acrosomal vesicle
acrosyndactyly
acrylic
   a. microsphere
   a. syringe shield
ACS
   Advanced Cardiovascular Systems
   American Cancer Society
   ACS balloon catheter
   ACS Concorde catheter
   ACS Endura coronary dilation catheter
   ACS OTW Photon coronary dilatation catheter
   ACS RX Comet coronary dilatation catheter
   ACS Tourguide II guiding catheter
ACS-grade pyridine
ACS-NT
   Gyroscan ACS-NT

act
    Mammography Quality
      Standards A. (MQSA)
    Needlestick Safety and
      Prevention A.
ACTH
    adrenocorticotropic hormone
ACTH-producing tumor
actinic
    a. granuloma
    a. keratosis
    a. ray
    a. reticuloid
actinic keratosis
actinium emanation
actinomycetes
    thermophilic a.
actinomycosis
    abdominopelvic a.
    retroperitoneal a.
actinomycotic brain abscess
action
    phase-specific a.
    a. space
Activase
    Cathflo A.
activated
    a. atom
    a. partial thromboplastin time
    a. voxel cluster
activation
    a. analysis
    compensatory cortical a.
    a. factor
    a. pattern
    PMC a.
    premotor coret a.
    region of a.
activation-induced uncoupling of
  cerebral oxygen
activation-sequence mapping
activator
    alteplase recombinant tissue
      plasminogen a.
    recombinant tissue plasminogen a.
    tissue plasminogen a. (tPA)
    tissue-type plasminogen a.
active
    a. acquired immunity
    a. biplanar MR imaging guidance
    a. congestion
    a. duodenal ulcer

    a. emptying fraction
    a. hyperemia
    a. infiltrate
    a. mode
    a. MRI stent (AMRIS)
    a. needle tip
    a. osteomyelitis
    a. parenchymal disease
    a. precordium
    a. shielding
    a. shimming
activity
    a. assessment
    background a.
    biliary excretion bowel a.
    blood pool a.
    body background a.
    bone morphogenetic a.
    brain a.
    colonic a.
    cortical a.
    cross-over of a.
    decreased a.
    dihydropyrimidine dehydrogenase a.
    electrical a.
    extrapulmonary a.
    increased tracer a.
    lung-heart ratio of thallium 201 a.
    mast cell-enhancing a.
    normalized to plasma a.
    osseous a.
    osteoblastic a.
    peak parenchymal a.
    peristaltic a.
    physiologic high a.
    problematic abdominal a.
    radiotracer a.
    reflux a.
    retained cortical a. (RCA)
    scatter a.
    slow-wave a.
    specific a.
    time-to-peak a.
    tracer a.
    ventricular ectopic a. (VEA)
actocardiotocograph monitor
actuator
    linear a.
AcuNav ultrasound catheter
acupuncture laser
Acuson
    A. 128 apparatus

NOTES

Acuson *(continued)*
   A. computed sonography
   A. 128 Doppler ultrasound
   A. 128EP imager
   A. 128EP scanner
   A. linear array transducer
   A. 5-MHz linear array
   A. Sequoia 512 scanner
   A. transvaginal sonography
   A. V5M monitor
   A. V5M multiplane transesophageal echocardiographic transducer
   A. XP 10 scanner
   A. 128XP transducer
   A. 128XP ultrasound system

acute
   a. abdominal obstruction
   a. abdominal series (AAS)
   a. abscess
   a. alveolar hypoperfusion
   a. alveolar infiltrate
   a. aortic pathology
   a. atelectasis
   a. avulsion fracture
   a. berylliosis
   a. central cord syndrome
   a. cerebellar hemispheric lesion
   a. cerebral infarct imaging
   a. cerebrovascular insufficiency
   a. chest syndrome
   a. cholecystitis
   a. compartment syndrome
   a. compression triad
   a. coronary insufficiency
   a. cortical necrosis
   a. diffuse bacterial nephritis
   a. diffuse interstitial fibrosis
   a. disseminated encephalomyelitis (ADEM)
   a. diverticulitis
   a. eosinophilic pneumonia
   a. erosive gastritis (AEG)
   a. esophagitis
   a. extrinsic allergic alveolitis
   a. focal bacterial nephritis
   a. focal bacterial pyelonephritis
   a. glomerulonephritis
   a. heart failure
   a. hematogenous osteomyelitis (AHO)
   a. hemodynamic overload
   a. hemorrhagic leukoencephalitis
   a. hepatitis
   a. hydrocephalus
   a. hydronephrosis
   a. interstitial lung edema
   a. interstitial nephritis (AIN)
   a. interstitial pneumonia (AIP)
   a. interstitial pneumonitis

   a. intramural hematoma
   a. ischemic brain infarct
   a. juvenile cirrhosis
   a. lethal carditis
   a. lymphoblastic lymphoma
   a. lymphocytic leukemia
   a. marginal branch
   a. mediastinal widening
   a. mesenteric ischemia (AMI)
   a. myelofibrosis
   a. myeloid leukemia
   a. myocardial infarct
   a. native kidney tubular necrosis
   a. nonhemorrhagic infarct
   a. nonsuppurative ascending cholangitis
   a. obstructive cholangitis
   a. on chronic fracture
   a. pancreatitis
   a. peptic ulcer
   a. phase of inflammation
   a. pleurisy
   a. posttraumatic myelopathy
   a. pulmonary edema
   a. radiation injury
   a. radiation pneumonitis
   a. radiation syndrome (ARS)
   a. renal failure (ARF)
   a. renal infarct
   a. renal transplant tubular necrosis
   a. renal vein thrombosis
   a. respiratory distress syndrome (ARDS)
   a. respiratory failure (ARF)
   a. retroviral syndrome
   a. sclerosing hyaline necrosis (ASHN)
   a. silicoproteinosis
   a. sinusitis
   a. splenic tumor
   a. sprain
   a. stretch injury
   a. subarachnoid hemorrhage
   a. subdural hematoma
   a. suppurative ascending cholangitis
   a. suppurative pyelonephritis
   a. suppurative sialadenitis
   a. suppurative thyroiditis
   a. testicular torsion
   a. thoracic aortic injury
   a. thromboembolic pulmonary arterial hypertension
   a. transverse myelitis
   a. traumatic aortic injury (ATAI)
   a. tubular necrosis (ATN)
   a. vertebral collapse
AcuTect imaging agent
acutely symptomatic scrotum

ACV
    adaptive cardio volume
        ACV reconstruction
acyanotic congenital heart disease
acyl CoA oxidase deficiency
AD
    above diaphragm
    absorbed dose
    Alzheimer disease
    aortic diameter
ADA
    alternated delay acquisition
ADAC MCD Vertex Plus MCD gamma camera
adactyly, adactylia
adamantinoma of long bone
adamantinomatous craniopharyngioma
Adamkiewicz
    arteria radicularis magna of A.
    A. artery
Adams-Stokes syndrome
adapted standard mammography unit
adapter
    ventricle impedance a.
    VIA 7991 ventricle impedance a.
adaptic detector configuration
adaptive
    a. cardiac volume reconstruction
    a. cardio volume (ACV)
    a. carpus
    a. correction
    a. focusing technology (AFT)
    a. hyperplasia
    a. hypertrophy
adaptor
    Tuohy-Borst a.
ADC
    apparent diffusion coefficient
    ADC decline
    ADC map
    ADC quantization error
ADCav value
Addison
    A. disease
    A. point
add-on
    A.-O. Bucky direct x-ray detector
    A.-O. Bucky image acquisition system
    A.-O. Bucky radiographer detector image

    a.-o. stereotactic unit
    a.-o. technique
adducted thumb
adduction
    a. fracture
    a. frame
    a. to neutral
    a. position
    a. stress
adductor
    a. canal
    a. canal syndrome
    a. hallucis
    a. hallucis tendon
    a. hiatus
    a. insertion avulsion syndrome
    a. longus
    a. magnus
    a. magnus muscle
    a. muscle strain
    a. pollicis
    a. pollicis brevis tendon
    a. sweep of thumb
    a. tubercle
adductus
    metatarsus a.
    pes a.
    true metatarsus a. (TMA)
ADEM
    acute disseminated encephalomyelitis
adenitis
    cervical lymph node tuberculous a.
    mesenteric a.
    sclerosing a.
adenoacanthoma
    endometrial a.
adenocarcinoma
    acinar a.
    acinic cell a.
    ampullary a.
    bronchiolar a.
    cervical a.
    colloid a.
    cystic a.
    distal rectal a. (DRA)
    ductal pancreatic a.
    duct cell a.
    duodenal a.
    endometrial secretory a.
    exophytic a.
    gastrointestinal tract a.
    giant cell a.

A

NOTES

13

adenocarcinoma *(continued)*
    hepatoid a.
    infiltrating a.
    intraluminal a.
    kidney a.
    lung a.
    medullary-type a.
    metastatic a.
    mucinous a.
    mucin-producing a.
    nonmucinous a.
    pancreatic ductal a.
    papillary serous a.
    poorly differentiated a. (PDA)
    renal a.
    scirrhous infiltrating a.
    secretory a.
    serous a.
    a. in situ
    small bowel a.
    stomach a.
    ulcerating a.
    urinary bladder a.
    a. of uterus
    vulvar adenoid cystic a.
adenocystic carcinoma
adenofibroma
adenofibromyoma
adenography
adenohypophysial
adenohypophysis
adenoid
    a. cystic carcinoma parotitis
    a. cystic lung carcinoma
    a. squamous cell carcinoma
    a. tonsil
    a. tumor
adenoidal-nasopharyngeal ratio (AN)
adenoleiomyofibroma
adenolipoma
adenolymphoma
adenoma
    acidophilic a.
    acinous a.
    adnexal a.
    adrenal a.
    adrenocortical a.
    apocrine a.
    autonomous thyroid a.
    basal cell a.
    basophilic brain a.
    benign oxyphilic a.
    bile duct a. (BDA)
    a. of breast
    bronchial a.
    bronchoalveolar cell a.
    bronchogenic a.
    Brunner gland a.
    carcinoma ex pleomorphic a.

carotid sheath a.
colloid a.
colonic a.
colorectal a.
cortical a.
cutaneous a.
cystic a.
ductal a.
ectopic parathyroid a.
embryonal a.
eosinophilic brain a.
fetal a.
fibroid a.
a. fibrosum
flat a.
follicular thyroid a.
Fuchs a.
functioning pituitary a.
gallbladder a.
giant villous a.
glycoprotein-secreting a.
gonadotroph cell a.
gonadotropin-secreting a.
growth hormone-producing a.
hepatic a.
hepatocellular a.
Hürthle cell a.
intraspinal a.
kidney a.
lactating a.
Leydig cell a.
liver cell a.
macrocystic a.
malignant pleomorphic a.
a. malignum
mediastinal a.
microcystic a.
mucinous a.
multifocal autonomic a.
nephrogenic bladder a.
a. of nipple
nonfunctioning pituitary a.
nonhyperfunctioning adrenal a.
oncocytic thyroid a.
oxyphilic a.
pancreatic macrocystic a.
pancreatic microcystic a.
papillary cystic a.
parathyroid a. (PA)
parotid pleomorphic a.
Pick tubular a.
pituitary a.
pleomorphic lung a.
polypoid a.
prostatic a.
proximal tubular a.
renal cortical a.
retrotracheal a.
sebaceous a.

a. sebaceum
sessile a.
small bowel a.
solitary a.
suprasellar a.
sweat duct a.
testicular tubular a.
thyroid a.
thyrotroph cell a.
toxic a.
tubulovillous colon a.
villotubular a.
villous a.
well-differentiated a.

adenoma-associated calcification
adenomatoid
a. malformation
a. odontogenic tumor
adenomatosis
adenomatous
a. goiter
a. hyperplasia
a. polyp (AP)
adenomyoma
adenomyomatosis
adenomyosarcoma
adenomyosis
diffuse a.
ureteral a.
uterine a.
adenopapillomatosis
gastric a.
adenopathy
abdominal a.
axillary a.
bilateral hilar a.
cervical a.
hemorrhagic mediastinal a.
hilar a.
mediastinal a.
mesenteric a.
metastatic a.
paratracheal a.
postinflammatory a.
pulmonary a.
reticulation with hilar a.
retrocrural a.
retroperitoneal a.
sandwich configuration a.
secondary axillary a.
thoracic a.
tuberculous mediastinal a.

widespread hyperattenuating
mediastinal a.
adenosarcoma
breast a.
Adenoscan imaging agent
adenosine
echocardiogram a.
a. echocardiography
a. stress imaging
a. stress-imaging agent
a. triphosphate
adenosis
breast a.
microglandular a.
radiation-induced sclerosing a.
sclerosing a.
adenovirus
genetically engineered oncolytic a.
Onyx-015 genetically engineered a.
a. pneumonia
adequate
a. cardiac output
a. contention
a. coronary perfusion
a. stroke volume
AD/FHD
acetabular depth-to-femoral head
diameter
adherence factor
adherent
a. pericardium
a. placenta
a. profundus tendon
a. thrombus
adhesed
adhesio interthalamica
adhesion
abdominal a.
attic a.
bandlike a.
fibrous pleural a.
inflammatory a.
intraarticular a.
pericardial diaphragmatic a.
peritendinous a.
pleuropericardial a.
pleuropulmonary a.
subacromial bursal a.
subdeltoid bursal a.
adhesive
a. arachnoiditis
a. atelectasis

NOTES

adhesive *(continued)*
   a. bursitis
   a. capsulitis
   cyanoacrylate tissue a.
   a. ileus
   a. inflammation
   Neuroacryl tissue a.
   a. periarthritis
   a. platelet
   tissue a.

ADI
   absolute dose intensity
   atlantodens interval

adiabatic
   a. demagnetization
   a. demagnetization in the rotating
    frame (ADRF)
   a. fast passage (AFP)
   a. fast scanning technique
   a. off-resonance spin locking
   a. rapid passage (ARP)
   a. slice-selective radiofrequency
    pulse

adiadochokinesia
adipiodone
adipose
   a. fold
   a. fossa
   a. ligament
   a. tissue
   a. tumor

adiposogenital dystrophy
aditus
   a. ad antrum
   a. ad pelvem
   a. orbitae
   a. pelvis
   a. vaginae

adjacent
   a. edema
   a. field x-ray dosimetry
   a. organ
   a. voxel

adjunctive
   a. mechanical thrombectomy
   a. surgical bypass
   a. therapy

adjustment
   Bonferroni a.

adjuvant
   a. analgesic drug
   a. chronotherapy
   a. irradiation
   a. radiation
   a. therapy

adjuvanticity
admaxillary gland
admedial
admedian

administration
   competitive iron a.
   contrast a.
   drug a.
   intralymphatic radioactivity a.
   intraperitoneal drug a.
   vasodilator a.

admixture lesion
adnexa
   ocular a.
   transposed a.

adnexal
   a. adenoma
   a. carcinoma
   a. condition
   a. cyst
   a. embryo
   a. metastasis
   a. torsion

adolescent
   a. hallux valgus
   a. idiopathic scoliosis (AIS)
   a. tibia vara

ADPKD
   autosomal dominant polycystic kidney
    disease

ADQ
   abductor digiti quinti

adrenal
   a. adenoma
   a. angiography
   a. artery
   bilateral large a.
   a. calcification
   a. capsule
   a. carcinoma
   a. cortex
   a. cyst
   a. cystic mass
   a. failure
   a. ganglioneuroma
   a. gland
   a. hematoma
   a. hemorrhage
   a. hyperplasia
   a. imaging
   a. incidentaloma
   a. insufficiency
   a. lesion
   a. medulla
   a. medullary disease
   a. metastasis
   a. myelolipoma
   a. neuroblastoma
   a. paraganglioma
   a. pheochromocytoma
   a. pseudocyst
   a. scan
   a. scintigraphy

a. tuberculosis
a. tumor
a. vein
a. venography
adrenal-spleen ratio (ASR)
adrenergic drug
adrenocortical
a. adenoma
a. carcinoma
a. hyperfunction
a. hyperplasia
a. macrocyst
a. neoplasm
a. secretion
a. tumor
adrenocorticosteroid
adrenocorticotropic hormone (ACTH)
adrenocorticotropin microadenoma
adrenogenital syndrome
adrenogram
adrenoleukodystrophy
adrenoleukodystrophy-
adrenomyeloneuropathy (ALD-AMN)
ADRF
adiabatic demagnetization in the rotating
frame
Adrian-Crooks cassette
ADR Ultramark 4 ultrasound
Adson maneuver
adsorption
competitive a.
adsternal
adult
a. coarctation
a. dose
a. polycystic kidney disease
a. progeria
a. respiratory distress syndrome
(ARDS)
a. rheumatoid arthritis
a. T-cell lymphoma
adult-to-adult
a.-t.-a. liver transplantation
a.-t.-a. living related liver
transplant donor
adult-type III TIE fracture
adumbration
advanced
a. breast biopsy instrumentation
(ABBI)
a. cardiac mapping
A. Cardiovascular Systems (ACS)

a. life support techniques
a. multiple-beam equalization
radiography (AMBER)
A. NMR Systems scanner
a. real-time motion analysis
(ARTMA)
a. vessel analysis (AVA)
advance directives
advancement
frontoorbital a.
vastus medialis a. (VMA)
Advantage Workstation 3.1
AdvanTeq II TENS unit
Advantx-E Legacy system
Advantx LC+ cardiovascular imaging
system
adventitia of artery
adventitial
a. fibroplasia
a. tissue
adventitious bursa
adverse effect
adynamic
a. ileus
a. intestinal obstruction
adynamic/paralytic ileus
AE
above elbow
AE amputation
Aeby
A. muscle
A. plane
AEC
Atomic Energy Commission
automatic exposure control
AEC technique
AED
automatic external defibrillator
AEG
acute erosive gastritis
Aegis sonography management system
AER
apical ectodermal ridge
aerated tissue
aeration
regional differences in a.
aerobilia
aerocele
AeroChamber
aerodigestive
a. carcinoma

NOTES

aerodigestive *(continued)*
    a. fistula
    a. tract
aerophagia
aerosol
    radioactive a.
    technetium-99m DTPA a.
    a. ventilation scan
aerosolized ^{99m}Tc DTPA imaging agent
AESOP
    automatic endoscopic system for optimal
    positioning
        AESOP Hermes-Ready system
Aestiva/5 MRI anesthesia machine
AF
    amnionic fluid
    aortic flow
    arcuate fasciculus
A-FAIR
    arrhythmia-insensitive flow-sensitive
    alternating inversion recovery
        A-FAIR imaging
        A-FAIR MRI
AFBG
    aortofemoral bypass graft
affect
    pseudobulbar a.
afferent
    a. digital nerve
    a. loop
    a. loop syndrome
    a. lymph vessel
    a. nerve lesion
    a. nipple valve
    a. view
AFI
    amnionic fluid index
AFP
    adiabatic fast passage
African
    A. Burkitt lymphoma
    A. Kaposi sarcoma
AFROC
    alternative-free response receiver
    operating characteristic
AFT
    adaptive focusing technology
afterglow
afterload
    increased ventricular a.
    left ventricular a.
afterloader
    Fletcher a.
    Henschke a.
    ^{192}I high-dose-rate remote a.
    Nucletron MicroSelectron/LDR
    remote a.
afterloading
    a. brachytherapy

high-dose-rate remote a.
    a. radiation
    a. tandem and ovoid
    a. technique
AG
    angular gyrus
aganglionic
    a. bowel
    a. megacolon
    a. segment
aganglionosis
    skip a.
Agatston
    A. calcium scoring method
    A. score
AGC
    anatomically graduated component
AGE
    angle of greatest extension
age
    anatomic a.
    biologic a.
    bone a. (BA)
    chronologic a.
    delayed bone a.
    fetal a.
    gestational a. (GA)
    indeterminate a.
    large for gestational a.
age-indeterminate infarct
agenesis
    Bayne classification of radial a.
    callosal a.
    corpus callosum a.
    gallbladder a.
    liver a.
    lumbosacral a.
    lung a.
    partial corpus callosum a.
    pulmonary artery a.
    renal a.
    sacral a.
    thymic a.
    unilateral pulmonary a.
    uterine a.
    vaginal a.
    vermian a.
agenetic
    a. fracture
    a. porencephaly
agent *(See* contrast, material, medium)
    ^{18}F estradiol imaging a.
    ^{18}F fludeoxyglucose imaging a.
    ^{18}F fluorodeoxyglucose imaging a.
    ^{18}F fluoro-DOPA imaging a.
    ^{18}F fluoroisonidazole imaging a.
    ^{18}F fluorotamoxifen imaging a.
    ^{18}F L-DOPA imaging a.
    ^{18}F *N*-methylspiperone imaging a.

^{18}F spiperone imaging a.
Acetrizoate contrast a.
AcuTect imaging a.
Adenoscan imaging a.
adenosine stress-imaging a.
aerosolized ^{99m}Tc DTPA imaging a.
air imaging a.
Altropane radioimaging a.
AMI 121, 227 contrast a.
amidotrizoic acid contrast a.
Amipaque imaging a.
Amiscan imaging a.
Angio-Conray imaging a.
Angiografin imaging a.
AngioMARK contrast a.
antifibrin antibody imaging a.
antimyosin monoclonal antibody
  imaging a.
Apomate radiopharmaceutical
  imaging a.
baby formula with ferrous sulfate
  contrast a.
Baricon imaging a.
barium sulfate imaging a.
Baro-CAT imaging a.
Barosperse imaging a.
benzamide imaging a.
Biliscopin imaging a.
Bilopaque imaging a.
Biloptin imaging a.
bioreductive a.
bis-Gd-MP imaging a.
blood oxygenation level-dependent
  contrast a.
blood pool contrast a.
bone marrow a.
bromodeoxyuridine imaging a.
bromophenol blue imaging a.
^{45}Ca imaging a.
^{11}C acetate imaging a.
calcium 45 imaging a.
calcium ipodate imaging a.
carbon imaging a.
Cardiolite imaging a.
cardioselective a.
^{11}C butanol imaging a.
^{11}C carfentanil imaging a.
CEA-Scan imaging a.
Ceretec radioisotope imaging a.
cerium silicate imaging a.
cesium chloride imaging a.
^{11}C flumazenil imaging a.

CheeTah radiopaque contrast a.
chelating a.
Cholebrine imaging a.
Choletec radionuclide imaging a.
Cholografin meglumine imaging a.
chromated Cr-51 serum albumin
  imaging a.
chromium imaging a.
^{11}C imaging a.
^{11}C-labeled cocaine imaging a.
^{11}C-labeled fatty acid imaging a.
Clariscan imaging a.
^{11}C N-methylspiperone imaging a.
^{11}C nomifensine imaging a.
Combidex MRI contrast a.
CO_2-negative imaging a.
Conray 30, 43, 400 imaging a.
contrast a.
copper imaging a.
copper-zinc superoxide dismutase
  imaging a.
^{11}C raclopride imaging a.
^{11}C thymidine imaging a.
^{64}Cu imaging a.
^{67}Cu imaging a.
^{62}Cu PTSM imaging a.
^{64}Cu-TETA-octreotide imaging a.
Cu/Zn-SOD imaging a.
cyanoacrylate imaging a.
cyanocobalamin imaging a.
Cysto-Conray contrast a.
Cysto-Conray II imaging a.
Cystografin-Dilute imaging a.
DaTSCAN imaging a.
denatured ^{99m}Tc-RBC imaging a.
depilatory a.
a. detection imaging
deuterium imaging a.
dextrose 5% in water imaging a.
diatrizoate meglumine imaging a.
diatrizoate sodium imaging a.
diethylenetriaminepentaacetic acid
  imaging a.
Digibar 190 contrast a.
dihydroxyphenylalanine imaging a.
Dionosil imaging a.
dispersing a.
dodecafluoropentane imaging a.
DOPA imaging a.
Dopascan radiopharmaceutical
  imaging a.
DTPA imaging a.

NOTES

agent *(continued)*
Dy-DTPA-BMA imaging a.
dysprosium HP-DO3A imaging a.
echo contrast a.
echo-enhancing a.
EchoGen ultrasound imaging a.
Echovist imaging a.
EDTMP imaging a.
effervescent a.
endogenous contrast a.
Eovist contrast a.
Ethiodol imaging a.
etidronate disodium imaging a.
Evans blue imaging a.
exametazime imaging a.
extracellular contrast a.
extravasated contrast a.
extravasation of contrast a.
E-Z-CAT Dry contrast a.
Feridex IV MRI contrast a.
ferucarbotran MR imaging a.
feruglose contrast a.
ferumoxide imaging a.
ferumoxsil imaging a.
ferumoxtran imaging a.
Fibrimage diagnostic imaging a.
Fluoratec imaging a.
fluorine imaging a.
fluorocarbon-based ultrasound
  contrast a.
fluorodeoxyglucose imaging a.
^{18}F sodium fluoride imaging a.
FS-069 sterile injectable sonography
  contrast a.
furosemide imaging a.
gadobenic acid imaging a.
gadobutrol imaging a.
gadodiamide imaging a.
gadolinium-based contrast a.
gadolinium oxide imaging a.
Gadolite oral suspension contrast a.
gadopentetate contrast a.
gadopentetate dimeglumine
  imaging a.
gadoteridol imaging a.
gadoversetamide contrast a.
gadoversetamide imaging a.
gallium imaging a.
Gastrografin imaging a.
GastroMARK oral imaging a.
Gastroview imaging a.
Gastrovist imaging a.
Gd-BOPTA/Dimeg imaging a.
Gd-BOPTA imaging a.
  gadobenate dimeglumine
Gd-DTPA PGTM imaging a.
Gd-DTPA with mannitol contrast a.
Gd-enhanced imaging a.
Gd-EOB-DTPA imaging a.

Gd-HP-DO3A imaging a.
Gd-153 imaging a.
glomerular filtration a.
glucagon imaging a.
glucarate imaging a.
gold Au-198 imaging a.
GSA imaging a.
hand-agitated imaging a.
hematoporphyrin derivative
  photosensitizing a. (HpD)
hepatobiliary contrast a.
Hepatolite imaging a.
Hexabrix imaging a.
high-density barium imaging a.
high-osmolar contrast a. (HOCA)
Hippuran imaging a.
Histoacryl embolic a.
D, L-HMPAO imaging a.
holmium imaging a.
human serum albumin imaging a.
HumaSPECT imaging a.
hybrid MRI imaging a.
hydrogen peroxide imaging a.
hydrophilic contrast a.
hydrosoluble contrast a.
hyoscine butylbromide imaging a.
Hypaque-Cysto imaging a.
Hypaque-76 imaging a.
Hypaque Meglumine imaging a.
Hypaque-M imaging a.
Hypaque Sodium imaging a.
hyperpolarized ^{3}He imaging a.
hyperpolarized ^{129}Xe imaging a.
Imagent GI, US imaging a.
imaging a.
imidoacetic acid imaging a.
ImmuRAID antibody imaging a.
indium imaging a.
indocyanine green imaging a.
inhaled oxygen imaging a.
intercalating a.
intratumoral a.
intravenous microbubble contrast a.
iobitridol imaging a.
iocetamic acid imaging a.
iodamine imaging a.
iodinated imaging a.
iodine-123-MIBG radioactive
  imaging a.
iodine-131-MIBG radioactive
  imaging a.
iodipamide meglumine imaging a.
iodized oil imaging a.
5-iodo-2-deoxyuridine imaging a.
Iodo-gen imaging a.
iodohippurate sodium imaging a.
Iodotope imaging a.
iohexol imaging a.
ionic paramagnetic imaging a.

iopamidol imaging a.
Iopamiron 310, 370 imaging a.
iopanoic acid imaging a.
iopentol nonionic imaging a.
iophendylate imaging a.
iopromide nonionic imaging a.
iosefamic acid imaging a.
iothalamate meglumine imaging a.
iothalamate sodium imaging a.
iotroxic acid imaging a.
ioversol imaging a.
ioxaglate meglumine imaging a.
ioxaglate sodium imaging a.
ioxilan imaging a.
ioxithalamic acid contrast a.
ipodate calcium imaging a.
ipodate sodium imaging a.
ipodic acid contrast a.
iridium imaging a.
Isovue-200, -250, -300, -370
  imaging a.
Isovue-M 200, 300 imaging a.
Isovue nonionic imaging a.
kinase C antiglioma monoclonal
  antibody imaging a.
Kinevac imaging a.
LeukoScan imaging a.
LeuTech radiolabeled imaging a.
Levovist imaging a.
ligand a.
Lipiodol myelographic imaging a.
lipophilic imaging a.
liquid embolic a.
litholytic a.
liver-specific MRI contrast a.
long-scale imaging a.
low-osmolar contrast a. (LOCA)
lymphangiographic imaging a.
Lymphazurin imaging a.
LymphoScan imaging a.
macroaggregated albumin
  imaging a.
macromolecular imaging a.
Macrotec imaging a.
magnetic resonance receptor a.
magnetite albumin imaging a.
Magnevist imaging a.
mangafodipir trisodium a.
manganese-containing contrast a.
manganese imaging a.
mannitol and saline imaging a.
MD-Gastroview imaging a.

meglumine iodipamide imaging a.
meglumine iotroxate imaging a.
methiodal sodium imaging a.
methyl methacrylate imaging a.
metrizamide imaging a.
metrizoate imaging a.
microbubble-based contrast a.
mineral oil imaging a.
monoclonal antibody imaging a.
monodisperse iodinated
  macromolecular blood pool a.
MS-325 contrast a.
MultiHance imaging a.
myelographic imaging a.
Myoscint imaging a.
Myoview imaging a.
naloxone imaging a.
nanoparticulate imaging a.
negative contrast a.
negative contrast imaging a.
NeoSpect diagnostic imaging a.
NeoTect imaging a.
Neurolite imaging a.
neurotrophic imaging a.
nicotinamide imaging a.
nimodipine imaging a.
Niopam imaging a.
NIR contrast a.
nitrogen-13 ammonia imaging a.
no-carrier-added ^{18}F imaging a.
nofetumomab diagnostic imaging a.
nonionic iodinated contrast a.
nonionic paramagnetic contrast
  imaging a.
nonnephrotoxic contrast a.
novel a.
occluding a.
OctreoScan 111 radioactive
  imaging a.
octreotide imaging a.
oil emulsion imaging a.
Omnipaque 140, 180, 240, 300,
  350 imaging a.
Omniscan imaging a.
OncoScint CR/OV breast
  imaging a.
OptiMARK contrast a.
Optiray 10, 240, 300, 320, 350
  imaging a.
Optison sterile injectable
  sonography contrast a.
Oragrafin calcium imaging a.

NOTES

agent *(continued)*
Oragrafin sodium imaging a.
oral contrast imaging a.
Oxilan imaging a.
oxygen imaging a.
palladium imaging a.
Pantopaque imaging a.
paramagnetic contrast a.
particulate embolic a.
pentagastrin imaging a.
pentavalent DMSA imaging a.
pentetic acid imaging a.
pentetreotide imaging a.
peppermint oil imaging a.
peptide imaging a.
perflubron imaging a.
perfluorocarbon imaging a.
perfusion a.
Persantine imaging a.
phenobarbital imaging a.
phosphoric acid imaging a.
phosphorus imaging a.
PMT imaging a.
polidocanol sclerosing a.
polymerizing a.
positive contrast a.
potassium imaging a.
ProHance imaging a.
propyliodone imaging a.
ProstaScint monoclonal antibody
    imaging a.
pulmonary perfusion MRI
    contrast a.
radioactive cancer-specific
    targeting a.
radioactive isotope imaging a.
radiolabeled MoAb imaging a.
radiopaque imaging a.
radiopharmaceutical a.
radioprotective a.
radiotherapeutic a.
recombinant thyrotropin contrast a.
    (rTSH)
renal cortical isotope scanning a.
Renografin-60 imaging a.
Renovist II imaging a.
Renovue-Dip imaging a.
Renovue-65 imaging a.
residual imaging a.
reticuloendothelial imaging a.
rhenium imaging a.
RIGScan CR49 imaging a.
rose bengal ^{131}I radioactive a.
rubidium chloride imaging a.
Rubratope-57 imaging a.
samarium imaging a.
satumomab pendetide imaging a.
sclerosing a.
selenium imaging a.

^{75}Se selenomethionine radioactive a.
sestamibi imaging a.
Sethotope radioactive imaging a.
SH U 508A contrast a.
sincalide imaging a.
Sinografin imaging a.
SmartPrep imaging a.
sodium and/or methylglucamine
    diatrizoate contrast a.
sodium bicarbonate imaging a.
sodium chloride imaging a.
sodium diatrizoate imaging a.
sodium iodide ring imaging a.
sodium iodohippurate imaging a.
sodium iothalamate imaging a.
sodium ipodate imaging a.
sodium meglumine ioxaglate
    contrast a.
sodium metrizoate acid contrast a.
sodium pertechnetate imaging a.
sodium tyropanoate imaging a.
solidifying a.
somatostatin imaging a.
Sonazoid contrast a.
sonicated dextrose albumin
    imaging a.
SonoRx oral ultrasound contrast a.
sorbitol 70% imaging a.
sprodiamide imaging a.
stool-tagging a.
strontium-89 imaging a.
sucrose polyester imaging a.
sulfobromophthalein imaging a.
sulfur colloid imaging a.
superparamagnetic iron oxide blood
    pool a.
superparamagnetic iron oxide
    imaging a.
tantalum imaging a.
targeted contrast a.
^{99m}Tc aggregated albumin
    imaging a.
^{99m}Tc albumin colloid imaging a.
^{99m}Tc albumin microspheres
    imaging a.
^{99m}Tc biciromab imaging a.
^{99m}Tc bicisate imaging a.
^{99m}Tc dimer captosuccinic acid
    imaging a.
^{99m}Tc disofenin imaging a.
^{99m}Tc exametazime imaging a.
^{99m}Tc furifosmin imaging a.
^{99m}Tc-galactosyl human serum
    albumin imaging a.
^{99m}Tc glucarate imaging a.
^{99m}Tc gluceptate imaging a.
^{99m}Tc GSA imaging a.
^{99m}Tc human serum albumin
    imaging a.

^{99m}Tc-labeled cerebral perfusion imaging a.
^{99m}Tc lidofenin imaging a.
^{99m}Tc mebrofenin imaging a.
^{99m}Tc medronate imaging a.
^{99m}Tc mertiatide imaging a.
^{99m}Tc microaggregated albumin imaging a.
^{99m}Tc-N-NOEt neutral myocardial perfusion imaging a.
^{99m}Tc oxidronate imaging a.
^{99m}Tc pentetate calcium trisodium imaging a.
^{99m}Tc pentetate sodium imaging a.
^{99m}Tc polyphosphate imaging a.
^{99m}Tc pyrophosphate imaging a.
^{99m}Tc sestamibi imaging a.
^{99m}Tc sodium pertechnetate imaging a.
^{99m}Tc succimer imaging a.
^{99m}Tc sulfur colloid imaging a.
^{99m}Tc teboroxime imaging a.
^{99m}Tc tetrofosmin imaging a.
teboroxime imaging a.
Techneplex imaging a.
TechneScan HDP, MAA, MAG3, PYP imaging a.
technetium imaging a.
Telepaque imaging a.
teratogenicity of contrast a.
thallium imaging a.
thallous chloride imaging a.
TheraSeed imaging a.
thorium dioxide imaging a.
Thorotrast imaging a.
tissue-specific imaging a.
Tomocat imaging a.
triiodinated imaging a.
Tyropaque imaging a.
L-tyrosine imaging a.
Ultravist 150, 240, 300, 370 contrast a.
uniphasic imaging a.
uranium imaging a.
urografin imaging a.
urokinase imaging a.
Urovist Cysto imaging a.
Urovist Meglumine Diu/CT imaging a.
Urovist Sodium 300 imaging a.
USPIO imaging a.
Varibar contrast a.

Varibar oral contrast a.
vasodilating a.
Verluma diagnostic imaging a.
Visipaque 270, 320 contrast a.
water-soluble iodinated imaging a.
water-soluble nonionic imaging a.
xenon imaging a.
xylenol orange imaging a.
age-related change
AGF
  angle of greatest flexion
Agfa
  A. ADC 70 storage phosphor system
  A. CR, PACS system
  A. LR 3300 laser imager
  A. Medical scanner
agger nasi
aggregated
  a. lymphatic follicle
  a. sludge
aggregation
  nuclear a.
aggregometer
aggregometry
aggressive
  a. angiomyxoma
  a. fibromatosis
  a. infantile fibromatosis
  a. interstitial infiltrate
  a. malignancy
  a. perivascular infiltrate
  a. tissue-protective therapy
aggressiveness
  bone tumor a.
aging gut
AGL
  anterior glenoid labrum
agnogenic
  a. myeloid metaphysis
  a. myeloid metaplasia
agnosia
  visual object a.
agonal clot
agonist
agranular leukocyte
agretope
agyria pachygria complex
ahaustral
AHI
  acetabular head index

NOTES

AHI *(continued)*
  acromiohumeral interval
  apnea-hypopnea index
Ahmed glaucoma valve
Ahn thrombectomy catheter
AHO
  acute hematogenous osteomyelitis
AHQ
  amnionic head quotient
AHR
  airway hyperreactivity
AHS
  Alpers-Huttenlocher syndrome
AI
  acceleration index
    AI 5200 diagnostic ultrasound
AICA
  anterior-inferior cerebellar artery
  anterior-inferior cerebral artery
  anterior-inferior communicating artery
Aicardi-Goutières syndrome
Aicardi syndrome
AICD
  automatic implantable cardioverter-
    defibrillator
AICS
  artery of inferior cavernous sinus
AIDS
  acquired immunodeficiency syndrome
    AIDS cholangitis
    AIDS encephalopathy
AIDS-related esophagitis
AIF
  arterial input function
AIN
  acute interstitial nephritis
AIOD
  aortoiliac occlusive disease
AIP
  acute interstitial pneumonia
AIPH
  attenuation in phantom method
    AIPH method
AIR
  automatic image registration
air
    ambient a.
    a. arthrography
    a. block
    a. bolus
    bowel loop a.
    a. bronchogram
    a. cavity
    a. cisternography
    a. collection
    colonic a.
    a. conditioner lung
    a. contrast study
    a. contrast view of the stomach

a. crescent
a. cyst
a. cystogram
a. density
a. dose
a. embolus
a. encephalography
a. enema fluoroscopic imaging
a. esophagram
a. exchange
a. expansion
extraalveolar a. (EAA)
extraluminal a.
flail a.
free intraperitoneal a.
free peritoneal a.
a. gap
a. hunger
a. imaging agent
a. inflation
a. injection
inspired a.
a. insufflation
a. interface
intracranial a.
intraluminal a.
intramural colonic a.
intraorbital a.
intraperitoneal a.
a. kerma
a. leak
a. leak complication
a. luminogram
mediastinal a.
a. monitor
a. myelography
a. plasma spray hydroxyapatite
a. plethysmography
a. pocket
a. pyelography
retrocrural a.
retroperitoneal a.
a. sac
subcutaneous a.
transradiant a.
a. trapping
a. vesicle
air/bone/tissue boundary
airborne
    a. precautions
    a. transmission
air-containing neck mass
air-contrast
    a.-c. barium enema (ACBE)
    a.-c. imaging
    a.-c. view
air-core magnet
air-crescent sign
air-driven artificial heart

air-filled
    a.-f. cyst
    a.-f. loop
    a.-f. lung
air-filtration system
airflow
    a. obstruction disease (AOD)
    unidirectional a.
air-fluid
    a.-f. level
    a.-f. line
air-gap
    a.-g. radiography
    a.-g. technique
AIRIS II MR system
air-kerma
    a.-k. rate constant
    a.-k. strength
airless
    a. lung
    a. mass
air-meniscus sign
air-soft tissue interface
airspace
    a. consolidation
    a. disease
    a. edema
    a. enlargement
    lung a.
    a. nodule
    a. opacity
    retrosternal a.
    terminal a.
    volumetry of ventilated a.
air-trapping zone
airway
    a. anatomy
    asthmatic a.
    bronchiectatic a.
    a. constriction
    dilated small a.
    a. embryology
    esophageal obturator a.
    a. fluoroscopy
    a. hyperreactivity (AHR)
    hypertonic a.
    increased a.
    large a.
    mucoid plugging of a.
    mucus-filled small a.
    a. narrowing
    a. obstruction

    oropharyngeal a.
    a. pattern
    a. pressure
    a. pressure release ventilation
    a. resistance (Raw)
    a. responsiveness
    small a.
    a. tree
    a. tuberculosis
AIS
    abbreviated injury scale
    adolescent idiopathic scoliosis
Aitken
    A. acromioclavicular injury
      classification
    A. classification of epiphysial
      fracture
    A. femoral deficiency
AIVV
    anterior internal vertebral vein
AJCC-UICC
    American Joint Committee on
      Cancer/Union International Contre le
      Cancer
      AJCC-UICC mediastinal lymph
        node classification
AKA
    above-knee amputation
Akerlund deformity
akinesis
    inferior wall a.
akinetic
    a. left ventricle
    a. segment
    a. segmental wall motion
AL
    anterolateral
ala, pl. **alae**
    collagenous perivascular a.
    a. cristae galli
    a. lobuli centralis
    sacral a.
Alagille syndrome
alanine-silicone pellet
Alanson amputation
alar
    a. bone
    a. cartilage
    a. chest
    a. dysgenesis
    a. fold
    a. ligament

NOTES

alar *(continued)*
    a. plate
    a. process
    a. spine
ALARA
    as low as reasonably achievable
    ALARA radiation dose
ALARP
    as low as readily practicable
alba
    linea a.
Albarran gland
Albers-Schönberg position
Albert position
Albini nodule
Albinus muscle
Albrecht bone
Albright
    A. hereditary osteodystrophy
    A. syndrome
Albright-McCune-Sternberg syndrome
albumin
    a. calculus
    chromium CR-51 serum a.
    Evans blue a.
    galactosyl human serum a. (GSA)
    Gd-DTPA-labeled a.
    human serum a. (HSA)
    I-labeled macroaggregated a.
    iodinated human serum a. (IHSA)
    iodinated I-131 aggregated a.
    iodinated I-125 serum a.
    iodinated I-131 serum a.
    macroaggregated a. (MAA)
    microaggregated a.
    neogalactosyl a.
    perfluorocarbon-exposed sonicated
      dextrose a. (PESDA)
    radioactive iodinated serum a.
      (RISA)
    radioiodinated serum a. (RISA)
    technetium-99m
      minimicroaggregated a.
ALCL
    anaplastic large cell lymphoma
Alcock
    A. canal
    A. test
alcohol
    polyvinyl a. (PVA)
alcoholic
    a. cirrhosis (AC)
    a. fatty liver
    a. fibrosis
    a. heart
    a. liver disease (ALD)
    a. pneumonia
ALD
    alcoholic liver disease

ALD-AMN
    adrenoleukodystrophy-
      adrenomyeloneuropathy
aldehyde
    formic a.
Alder constitutional granulation anomaly
Alder-Reilly anomaly
Alderson anthropomorphic phantom
aldolase
aldosterone-producing carcinoma
aldosterone-secreting carcinoma
Alert catheter
Alexander
    A. disease
    A. view
alexandrite laser
Alexa 1000 system
alexia
    pure word a.
AlexLAZR laser
algebraic reconstruction technique
    (ART)
algorithm
    annealing a.
    bioeffects a.
    bone a.
    bone-detail a.
    Canny edge detection a.
    Clarkson scatter-summation a.
    clustering a.
    cone-beam reconstruction a.
    contour-following a.
    Cooley-Tukey a.
    correlation a. (CR)
    decryption a.
    defuzzification a.
    3D elastic subtraction a.
    design rule check a.
    digital image processing a.
    DIP a.
    document-recognition a.
    DRC a.
    3D reconstruction a.
    3D surface detection a.
    dual-lookup table a.
    edge-enhanced error diffusion a.
    elastic subtraction a.
    encryption a.
    Feldkamp a.
    filtered back-projection a.
    fringe thinning a.
    fully automated segmentation a.
    fuzzy clustering a.
    geometric optimization a.
    high spatial frequency
      reconstruction a.
    high spatial resolution a.
    histogram equalization a.
    image reconstruction a.

image restoration a.
interpolation a.
iterative a.
K-means clustering a.
least square a.
lossy a.
mapping a.
maximum intensity projection a.
maximum likelihood a.
memory-intensive a.
mensuration a.
MIP a.
neural evaluation a.
pixel-oriented a.
Preussmann a.
quantizer-design a.
radix-2 a.
Ramesh and Pramod a.
reconstruction a.
regridding a.
restoration a.
Shinnar-LeRoux a.
SSD a.
thresholding a.
Z-interpolation a.

ALH
atypical lobular hyperplasia

aliased
a. flow
a. pixel

aliasing
a. artifact
image a.
temporal a.

Alibert-Bazin syndrome

alignment
anatomic a.
angular a.
bony a.
Cooley-Tukey a.
field a.
a. of fracture fragment
a. and registration of 3D image
rotational a.
torsion a.
transverse plane a.
vertebral body a.

alimentary
a. canal
a. tract
a. tract calcification

aliquot

alkalinity
Engel a.

Alken-Marberger nephroscope

allantoic
a. circulation
a. cyst
a. vesicle

allergic
a. bronchopulmonary aspergillosis (ABPA)
a. granulomatosis
a. pneumonia
a. reaction
a. sinusitis

allergy
iodine a.

Allis sign

Allman classification

allocation
bit-rate a.
a. of treatment

allocortex

alloesthesia

allogeneic, allogenic
a. bone marrow transplant
a. peripheral cell transplant

allograft
aortic a.
bone a.
bone-chip a.
renal a.

alloimmune disease

allowed beta transition

alloxan-Schiff staining

All-Terrain Balloon (ATB)

All-Tronics scanner

ALN
axillary lymph node

alobar holoprosencephaly

Aloka
A. color Doppler real-time 2D blood flow imaging with cine memory
A. imaging
A. linear ultrasound
A. sector ultrasound
A. SSD-1700 transducer
A. SSD ultrasound system
A. SSD ultrasound system and probe
A. ultrasound linear scanner
A. ultrasound sector scanner

NOTES

Alouette amputation
Alpers disease
Alpers-Huttenlocher syndrome (AHS)
alpha, α
    a. chamber
    a. cradle
    a. decay
    a. frequency band
    A. 21064 microprocessor
      workstation
    a. particle
    a. particle accelerator
    a. particle bombardment
    a. radiation
    a. ray
    a. sigmoid loop
    a. threshold
    a. tocopherol
alpha-M^2
    radiolabeled peptide a.-M.
alpha-particle emitter
alpine hunter's cap deformity
ALPSA
    anterior labroligamentous periosteal
    sleeve avulsion
      ALPSA lesion
alta
    patella a.
    A. reconstruction rod
    A. tibial/humeral rod
alteplase recombinant tissue plasminogen
  activator
alteration
    bilateral a.
    hemodynamic a.
    metabolic a.
altered
    a. aortic contour
    a. blood flow
    a. mediastinal contour
alternans
    pulsus a.
    strabismus convergens a.
alternated delay acquisition (ADA)
alternating
    a. calculus
    a. current
    a. hemifield stimulation
    a. sinus
alternative-free response receiver
  operating characteristic (AFROC)
alternator
    film a.
altitudinal hemianopsia
Altman classification
Altropane radioimaging agent
altus
    calcaneus a.
alumina

aluminum
    a. ion breakthrough test
    a. pneumoconiosis
ALVAD
    abdominal left ventricular assist device
alveodental ridge
alveolar
    a. atrophy
    a. basal cell carcinoma
    a. bone fracture
    a. border of mandible
    a. bronchiole
    a. canal
    a. clouding
    a. collapse
    a. consolidation
    a. consolidative process
    a. crest
    a. dead space
    a. dilatation
    a. distention
    a. duct
    a. duct emphysema
    a. echinococcosis
    a. ectasia
    a. epithelial hyperplasia
    a. foramen
    a. gland
    a. hemorrhage
    a. hydatid
    a. hypersensitivity
    a. infection
    a. infiltrate
    a. instability
    a. lung disease
    a. microlithiasis
    a. mucosal carcinoma
    a. overdistention
    a. overventilation
    a. pattern
    a. paucity
    a. pneumonia
    a. point
    a. pressure
    a. proteinosis
    a. pulmonary edema
    a. rhabdomyosarcoma
    a. ridge
    a. sac
    a. sarcoidosis
    a. septal inflammation
    a. septal necrosis
    a. septum
    a. soft-part sarcoma (ASPS)
    a. supporting bone
    a. ventilation (VA)
    a. volume
alveolar-capillary block
alveolarization

alveoli (*pl. of* alveolus)
alveolingual groove
alvcolitis
    acute extrinsic allergic a.
    chronic diffuse sclerosing a.
    chronic extrinsic allergic a.
    chronic fibrosing a.
    cryptogenic fibrosing a.
    desquamative fibrosing a.
    diffuse sclerosing a.
    extrinsic allergic a.
    fibrosing cryptogenic a.
    mural fibrosing a.
    subacute extrinsic allergic a.
alveolobuccal groove
alveolodental canal
alveologram
alveololabial groove
alveolus, pl. alveoli
    pulmonary a.
alvine calculus
alymphocytosis
alymphoplasia
Alzheimer disease (AD)
AM
    arterial malformation
Am
    americium
^{241}Am
    americium 241
amastia
AMATC
    Amplatz maceration aspiration
    thrombectomy catheter
amaurosis
    central a.
    cerebral a.
    a. fugax
    uremic a.
Amazr radiofrequency catheter ablation
AMBER
    advanced multiple-beam equalization
    radiography
ambient
    a. air
    a. segment of posterior cerebral
    artery
    a. wing of the quadrigeminal
    cistern
ambiguous genitalia
ambilevous

AMBRI
    atraumatic, multidirectional, bilateral
    radial instability
ambulatory
    a. equilibrium angiocardiography
    a. equilibrium angiography
    a. Holter echocardiography
AME
    AME bone growth stimulator
    AME PinSite shield
amebic abscess
amelanotic tumor
ameloblastic
    a. adenomatoid tumor
    a. carcinoma
    a. fibroma
    a. fibrosarcoma
    a. sarcoma
ameloblastoma of the jaw
amelogenesis imperfecta
amentia
American
    A. Academy of Orthopaedic
    Surgeons (AAOS)
    American Joint Committee on
    Cancer/Union International Contre
    le Cancer (AJCC-UICC)
    A. Board of Radiology
    A. Cancer Society (ACS)
    A. College of Radiology (ACR)
    A. Joint Committee on Cancer
    A. Medical Association
    A. Medical Association Ligament
    Injury Classification System
    A. Registry of Diagnostic Medical
    Sonographers
    A. Shared-CuraCare scanner
    A. Society of Neuroradiology
    A. Spinal Cord Injury Association
    A. Spinal Cord Injury Association
    classification
    A. Thoracic Society node station
    A. Urological Association
americium (Am)
    a. 241 (^{241}Am)
    a. radioactive source
ameroid occluder
ametriodinic acid
AMI
    acute mesenteric ischemia
    AMI 121, 227 contrast agent
amiculum, pl. amicula

NOTES

amiculum *(continued)*
    a. olivare
    a. of olive
amidotrizoic
    a. acid
    a. acid contrast agent
aminobutyrate
    gamma a.
amiodarone
    a. liver
    a. lung
Amipaque imaging agent
Amiscan imaging agent
AML
    angiomyolipoma
Ammon horn
ammonia
    anhydrous a.
ammonium excretion
amniocentesis
    therapeutic a.
amniodrainage
amniography
amnioinfusion
amnion
    a. ring
    a. rupture
    a. rupture sequence
amnionic, amniotic
    a. band
    a. band syndrome
    a. cavity
    a. duct
    a. fluid (AF)
    a. fluid embolus
    a. fluid index (AFI)
    a. fluid volume
    a. fold
    a. head quotient (AHQ)
    a. inclusion cyst
    a. membrane
    a. raphe
    a. sac
    a. sheet
amnionicity
A-mod
    amplitude modulation
A-mode
    A-m. amplitude modulation scan
    A-m. display
    A-m. echocardiography
    A-m. encephalography
amorphous
    a. fetus
    a. high signal intensity
    a. selenium
    a. selenium plate
    a. silicon

    a. silicon filmless digital x-ray detection technology
    a. silicon filmless digital x-ray detection technology device
amosite
Amoss sign
amp
    amplification
    low-pressure mercury arc amp
ampere
amphiarthrodial
amphiarthrosis
amphibole asbestos
amphoric echo
amphoteric dipolar ion
Amplatz
    A. Anchor System
    A. angiography needle
    A. Clot Buster
    A. dilator set
    A. Goose Neck snare
    A. left coronary catheter
    A. maceration aspiration thrombectomy catheter (AMATC)
    A. radiolucent handle
    A. right coronary catheter
    A. Super Stiff catheter
    A. Super Stiff guidewire
    A. technique
    A. Teflon sheath
    A. thrombectomy device
Amplatzer septal occluder device
amplification (amp)
    multiscale image detail contrast a. (Musica)
amplifier
    buffer a.
    gradient a.
    image a.
    linear a.
    log a.
    nuclear pulse a.
    pulse a.
    servo power a.
    Servox a.
    voltage a.
amplitude
    acoustic pressure a.
    a. asymmetry
    deformation a.
    gradient a.
    a. image
    a. imaging
    a. modulation (A-mod)
    output a.
    peak a.
    a. of phase encoding
    pressure a.
    septal a.

ampule
ampulla, pl. **ampullae**
    a. biliaropancreatica
    a. canaliculi lacrimalis
    a. chyli
    a. ductus deferentis
    duodenal a.
    a. duodeni
    hepatopancreatic a.
    a. hepatopancreatica
    a. membranacea anterior
    a. ossea anterior
    a. ossea lateralis
    a. ossea posterior
    phrenic a.
    rectal a.
    a. recti
    a. of semicircular canal
    a. tubae uterinae
    a. tumor
    a. of Vater
ampullar pregnancy
ampullary
    a. adenocarcinoma
    a. aneurysm
    a. carcinoma
    a. crest
    a. stenosis
amputated-foot view
amputation
    above-knee a. (AKA)
    AE a.
    Alanson a.
    Alouette a.
    Beclard a.
    below-knee a.
    Berger interscapular a.
    Bier a.
    Boyd ankle a.
    Bunge a.
    Burgess below-knee a.
    button toe a.
    Callander a.
    Carden a.
    chop a.
    Chopart hindfoot a.
    circular supracondylar a.
    closed flap a.
    congenital a.
    digital a.
    femoral head a.
    fetal a.

    fingertip a.
    fishmouth a.
    forearm a.
    Guyon a.
    Hey a.
    interscapulothoracic a.
    Jaboulay a.
    Kirk distal thigh a.
    Le Fort a.
    Lisfranc a.
    midthigh a.
    nonreplantable a.
    Pirogoff a.
    ray a.
    replantable a.
    1-stage a.
    2-stage a.
    supramalleolar open a.
    Syme ankle disarticulation a.
    Teale a.
    transcarpal a.
    transcondylar a.
    translumbar a.
    transmetatarsal a. (TMA)
    traumatic a.
    Vladimiroff-Mikulicz a.
AMRIS
    active MRI stent
AMS
    accelerator mass spectrometry
Amsterdam dwarfism
Amstutz classification
AMT-25-enhanced MR imaging
amu
    atomic mass unit
amygdala
    a. of cerebellum
    a. volume
amygdaline
amygdalofugal pathway
amygdaloid
    a. area
    a. fossa
    a. nuclear complex
    a. tubercle
amylaceum, pl. **amylacea**
    corpus a.
amyloid
    a. deposit
    a. tumor
amyloidoma

NOTES

amyloidosis
    chronic renal failure a.
    CNS a.
    GI tract a.
    heart a.
    hereditary a.
    idiopathic a.
    immunocytic a.
    kidney a.
    lung a.
    a. of multiple myeloma
    orbital a.
    primary a.
    pulmonary a.
    renal a.
    secondary a.
    senile a.
    skeletal a.
    splenic a.
    urethral a.
amyloidotic cardiomyopathy
amyotonia congenita
AN
    adenoidal-nasopharyngeal ratio
anacrotic notch
anaerobic lung abscess
anal
    a. apparatus
    a. atresia
    a. bulge
    a. canal
    a. cleft
    a. column
    a. crypt
    a. disc
    a. fascia
    a. fissure
    a. fistula
    a. intermuscular septum
    a. intersphincteric groove
    a. manometry
    a. orifice
    a. pit
    a. plate
    a. protrusion
    a. sphincter
    a. stenosis
    a. stricture
    a. vein
    a. verge
analeptic enema
analgesic nephropathy
analog, analogue
    a. computations
    dysprosium a.
    halogenated thymidine a.
    a. photo
    pyrimidine a.
    radiolabeled estrogen a.

    a. rate meter
    ^{99m}Tc-labeled phosphate a.
    technetium-99m IDA a.
analogous
analog-to-digital
    a.-t.-d. conversion quantization error
    a.-t.-d. converter
analysis, pl. **analyses**
    activation a.
    advanced real-time motion a.
     (ARTMA)
    advanced vessel a. (AVA)
    basic volume image a.
    bayesian a.
    5-bromodeoxyuridine a.
    cephalometric a.
    CEqual quantitative a.
    Cerenkov scintillation a.
    clinicopathological a.
    compartmental a.
    computer-aided image a.
    computer-assisted joint motion a.
    correlation a.
    cue-based image a.
    deconvolutional a.
    deformation-based hippocampal
     segmentation and shape a.
    diagnostic efficacy a.
    digital frequency a.
    3-dimensional a.
    direct immunofluorescence a.
    discriminant a.
    Doppler spectral a.
    Doppler waveform a.
    duplex Doppler signal a. (DDSA)
    duplex ultrasound a.
    eigenvector a.
    electrooculographic a.
    fast Fourier spectral a.
    field-fitting a.
    fission track a.
    focal and diffuse lung texture a.
    folding potential a.
    footprint a.
    Fourier a.
    fractal a.
    fractional volumetric a.
    frequency a.
    gamma spectrometric a.
    high-definition 3-dimensional a.
    image display and a. (IDA)
    intracardiac pressure waveform a.
    iodine-131 outcome a.
    isotope dilution a.
    kinetic parameter a.
    late effect a.
    least square a.
    linear regression a.
    liquid scintillation a.

multielemental neutron activation a.
multivariant regressional a.
myocardial texture a.
neutron activation a.
nuclide a.
phase a.
planar thallium with quantitative a.
pole figure texture a.
power spectral a. (PSA)
prospective a.
pulse height spectral a.
quadratic discriminant a. (QDA)
qualitative a.
quantitative a.
radiometric a.
range-gated Doppler spectral
  flow a.
rate a.
recursive partitioning a.
regression a.
residual stress a.
roentgen stereophotogrammetric a.
  (RSA)
Sassouni a.
saturation a.
sensitivity a.
signal sonographic feature a.
slope blot a.
sonographic feature a.
spectral a.
S-phase a.
stepwise regression a.
thin film a.
time-action a.
volume a.
volumetric a.
x-ray diffraction a.

analytic reconstruction
analyzer
automated biochemical a.
automated cerebral blood flow a.
ChromaVision digital a.
Dow hollow fiber a.
electronic micro a. (EMA)
Gammex RBA-5 radiation beam a.
Medigraphics a.
multichannel a. (MCA)
platelet function a. (PFA)
pulse-height a. (PHA)
single-channel a. (SCA)

anaphylactic
a. reaction
a. shock
anaphylactoid reaction
anaplasia
cancer cell a.
cerebellar a.
anaplastic
a. astrocytoma (AA)
a. cerebral glioma
a. ependymoma
a. large cell lymphoma (ALCL)
a. mixed oligoastrocytoma
a. plasmacytoma
a. thyroid carcinoma
a. tumor
anastomosis, pl. anastomoses
arterial brain a.
arteriovenous a. (AVA)
Baffe a.
bidirectional cavopulmonary a.
bile duct a.
biliary-enteric a.
Billroth I, II a.
bowel-to-bowel a.
cholecystenteric a.
cobra-head a.
coiling of a.
colocolic a.
colorectal a.
embryonic a.
end-to-side biliary-enteric a.
extradural a.
gastroenteric a.
Glenn a.
hepatic arterial a.
hepatojejunal a.
heterocladic a.
Hofmeister a.
Horsley a.
ileal pouch-anal a.
ileocolic a.
ileorectal a. (IRA)
ileotransverse colon a.
infrahepatic inferior vena cava a.
intercavernous a.
J-shaped a.
Kocher a.
Kugel a.
laser-assisted microvascular a.
left internal mammary artery a.
leptomeningeal a.

NOTES

anastomosis *(continued)*
LIMA a.
magnet compression a.
portal venous a.
portosystemic a.
splenorenal a.
stenotic esophagogastric a.
Sucquet-Hoyer a.
suprahepatic inferior vena cava a.
tracheal a.
UA to OA a.
ureteroureteral a.

anastomotic
a. aneurysm
a. arch
a. arterial circle
a. dehiscence
a. disruption
a. hemorrhage
a. leakage
a. pseudoaneurysm
a. site
a. stenosis
a. stoma
a. stricture
a. ulcer
a. vein

anastomy
donor-recipient a.

anatomic
a. age
a. alignment
a. axis
a. barrier
a. bile duct variant
a. brain classification
a. configuration
a. dead space
a. distribution
a. esophageal vestibule
a. fracture
a. genu valgus
a. image
a. landmark
a. landscape
a. localization
a. marker
a. misregistration
a. moment erratum
a. neck
a. overlay
a. plane
a. position
a. reduction
a. resolution
a. root
a. shunt flow
a. snuffbox

a. variability
a. variation
anatomically
a. dominant
a. graduated component (AGC)
anatomopathologic study
anatomy
airway a.
anomalous a.
arterial a.
basal ganglia a.
breast a.
bronchopulmonary lung segment a.
bulbourethral gland a.
carpal bone a.
chain-of-lakes a.
cochlear a.
computational a.
coronary artery a.
craniovertebral junction a.
cross-sectional lung segment a.
Daseler-Anson classification of
  plantaris muscle a.
distorted a.
endometrial a.
a. exclusion artifact
facial nerve a.
hepatic artery a.
inner ear a.
internal auditory canal a.
kidney a.
left-dominant coronary a.
lobar breast a.
Lowsley lobar a.
maxillary nerve a.
medullary venous a.
neck-space a.
normal planar MR a.
ovarian a.
pituitary gland a.
plantar compartmental a.
prostate a.
radiologic a.
renal vascular a.
right dominant coronary a.
Saltzman a.
scrotal a.
sectional segmental a.
segmental liver a.
small bowel fold a.
stapedial nerve a.
superior orbital fissure a.
teardrop pelvic a.
temporal bone a.
thoracic spine a.
trigeminal nerve a.
umbilical cord a.
uterine a.
vascular kidney a.

vascular renal a.
venous a.
zonal prostate a.
zonal uterine a.
anatomy-based extraction (ABE)
anatomy-oriented colon segmentation
  (AOCS)
anchor
  Mitek bone a.
  a. plate
  traction a.
anchoring
  a. tendon
  a. villus
anconal, anconeal
  a. fossa
anconeus muscle
anconoid
Ancure tube graft
ancyroid, ankyroid
  a. cavity
Anderson-Hutchins tibial fracture
Andren method
Andren-von Rosen line
androblastoma
androgen-independent prostate
  carcinoma
androgen-producing tumor
android pelvis
anechoic
  a. area
  a. center
  a. cyst
  a. fluid
  a. fluid collection
  a. lesion
  a. mantle
  a. mass
  a. thrombus
anembryonic pregnancy
anemic infarct
anencephaly
aneroid manometry
anesthetic drug
aneuploid cell line
AneuRx
  A. bifurcated stent-graft system
  A. endograft
  A. stent
  A. stent-graft
aneurysm
  abdominal aortic a. (AAA)

AcomA a.
acquired left ventricle a.
ampullary a.
anastomotic a.
aortic arch a.
aortic sinus a.
aortoiliac a.
arterial a.
arteriosclerotic intracranial a.
arteriosclerotic thoracoabdominal
  aortic a.
arteriovenous pulmonary a.
ascending aortic a.
aspergillotic a.
atherosclerotic aortic a.
atrial septal a.
axillary a.
bacterial a.
basilar artery a.
basilar tip a.
bifurcation a.
bland aortic a.
brachiocephalic arterial a.
brain a.
bulging a.
calcified wall of a.
cardiac ventricle a.
carotid artery a.
carotid-ophthalmic a.
cavernous sinus a.
cavity of a.
celiac artery a.
cerebral a.
circumscript a.
cirsoid a.
clinoid a.
clip ligation of a.
clipping of a.
coating of a.
coiling of a.
communicating artery a.
compound a.
congenital aortic sinus a.
congenital arteriosclerotic a.
congenital cerebral a.
congenital intracranial a.
congenital left ventricular a.
congenital pulmonary artery a.
congenital renal a.
contained leak of aortic a.
coronary artery a.
coronary vessel a.

NOTES

aneurysm *(continued)*

cranial a.
cylindroid a.
degenerative aortic a.
de novo a.
dilatation of a.
dissecting abdominal a.
dissecting aortic a.
dissecting basilar artery a.
dissecting intracranial a.
distal aortic arch a.
dome of a.
Dorendorf sign of aortic arch a.
Drummond sign of aortic a.
ductal a.
ductus arteriosus a.
ectatic a.
eggshell border of a.
embolic a.
extracerebral a.
extracranial a.
false a.
feeding artery of a.
fenestration of dissecting a.
fundus of a.
fusiform a.
Galen vein a.
giant brain a.
giant saccular a.
giant serpentine a.
hepatic artery a.
hernial a.
hunterian ligation of a.
Hunt-Kosnik classification of a.
iliac artery a.
induced thrombosis of aortic a.
infected a.
inflammatory aortic a.
infrarenal abdominal aortic a.
innominate a.
internal carotid artery a.
intracerebral a.
intracranial a. (ICA)
intracranial berry a.
intracranial saccular a.
intramural coronary artery a.
juxtarenal aortic a.
kidney a.
late false a.
lateral a.
leaking abdominal aortic a.
left ventricular a.
lower basilar a.
luetic aortic a.
malignant bone a.
miliary a.
mirror image a.
mixed a.
M1 segment a.

mural a.
mycotic aortic a.
mycotic brain a.
mycotic intracranial a.
neck of a.
neoplastic a.
nodular a.
orbital a.
oval a.
pararenal aortic a.
pelvic a.
perforating a.
popliteal artery a.
portal vein a.
posterior communicating artery a.
postinfarction ventricular a.
Pott a.
precursor sign to rupture of a.
prerenal aortic a.
prerupture of a.
P2 segment a.
pulmonary arteriovenous a.
pulmonary artery compression
  ascending aortic a.
racemose a.
Rasmussen mycotic a.
rebleeding of a.
a. remnant neck
renal artery a.
ruptured a.
sac of a.
sacciform a.
saccular cerebral a.
sacral a.
a. sac shrinkage
serpentine a.
sinus of Valsalva a.
slow-flowing giant saccular a.
spindle-shaped a.
splanchnic a.
splenic artery a.
spontaneous infantile ductal a.
spurious a.
subclavian a.
subvalvular a.
supraclinoid carotid a.
suprarenal aortic a.
suprarenal extension of a.
suprasellar a.
syphilitic aortic a.
thoracic aortic a.
thoracoabdominal aortic a.
thrombosed giant vertebral artery a.
thrombotic a.
trapping of a.
traumatic intracranial a. (TICA)
true aortic a.
true heart a.
true ventricular a.

tubular a.
uterine cirsoid a.
varicose a.
varix of a.
venous a.
ventricular septal a.
verminous a.
wide-neck carotid cavernous a.
windsock a.
a. with simple shape
worm a.

aneurysmal
a. bone cyst (ABC)
a. clip
a. coil
a. dilation
a. disease
a. dissection
a. fundus
a. hematoma
a. hemorrhage
a. neck
a. ostium
a. outpouching
a. proportion
a. rupture
a. sac
a. vein
a. wall
a. wall calcification
a. wall gas
a. widening of aorta
a. wrap
aneurysmogram
aneurysmography
AngeLase combined mapping-laser probe
Angelchik reflux prosthesis
angel-wing sign
Anger scintillation camera
angioarchitecture
angioblastic lymphadenopathy
angioblastoma
bone a.
cord a.
angiocardiogram (ACG)
angiocardiography (ACG)
ambulatory equilibrium a.
biplane a.
equilibrium radionuclide a.
exercise radionuclide a.
first-pass radionuclide exercise a.

gas a.
gated radionuclide a.
intravenous a.
radionuclide a.
rapid biplane a.
retrograde a.
right-sided a.
selective a.
transseptal a.
venous a.
Angiocath
A. Autoguard Shielded IV catheter
A. PRN catheter
angiocatheter
4F a.
angiocentric
a. immunoproliferative disorder
a. immunoproliferative lesion
a. lymphoproliferative lesion
angiocholitis
Angio-Conray imaging agent
angio-CT
superselective a.-CT
AngioDynamics
angiodynography
angiodysplasia
a. of colon
colonic a.
angioedema
angiofibroblastic
a. hyperplasia
a. proliferation
a. tendinosis
angiofibroma
juvenile nasopharyngeal a. (JNPA)
Angioflow meter system
angiofollicular
a. lymph node hyperplasia
a. and plasmacytic polyadenopathy
angiogenesis
a. gene delivery
a. tumor
angiogenic factor
Angiografin imaging agent
angiogram (*See* angiography)
balloon occlusion pulmonary a.
biplane left ventricular a.
control a.
digital subtraction a.
digital subtraction pulmonary a.
dynamic subtraction magnetic
  resonance a.

NOTES

37

angiogram *(continued)*
    fluorescein a.
    flush a.
    interventional vascular a.
    overview a.
    projection a.
    radionuclide a. (RNA)
    radionuclide cerebral a.
    spinal a.
    volume-rendered MR a.

angiographic
    a. blush
    a. catheter
    a. corkscrew artery
    a. finding
    a. guidewire
    a. muscle mass index
    a. occlusion
    a. system for unlimited rolling
    field-of-views (angioSURF)
    a. target
    a. targeting
    a. Teflon dilator

angiographically
    a. occult intracranial vascular
    malformation (AOIVM)
    a. occult vascular malformation
    (AOVM)
    a. occult vessel
    a. visualized vascular malformation
    (AVVM)

angiography *(See* angiogram)
    adrenal a.
    ambulatory equilibrium a.
    aortic arch a.
    axial a.
    basilar a.
    biliary a.
    biplane a.
    black blood magnetic resonance a.
    blood pool radionuclide a.
    blush of dye on a.
    brain capillary a.
    breath-hold contrast-enhanced three-
    dimensional MR a.
    bronchial a.
    Brown-Dodge method for a.
    cardiac-gated MR a.
    carotid a.
    catheter a.
    cavernous brain a.
    celiac a.
    cerebral a.
    CO_2 a.
    color power a.
    3-compartment wrist a.
    computed tomographic a. (CTA)
    computed tomographic pulmonary a.

computerized tomographic
    hepatic a. (CTHA)
contrast a.
contrast-enhanced magnetic
    resonance a. (CEMRA, CE-MRA)
contrast-enhanced MR a.
coronary electron beam a.
CT a.
cut-film a. (CFA)
cystic duct a.
3D contrast-enhanced MR a.
3D coronary magnetic resonance a.
3DFT magnetic resonance a.
2DFT time-of-flight MR a.
3D gadolinium-enhanced magnetic
    resonance a.
3D helical CT a.
3D inflow MR a.
directional color a. (DCA)
dobutamine thallium a.
3D phase-contrast magnetic
    resonance a.
3D rotational a.
dual-detector helical CT a.
3D volume-rendered helical CT a.
3D volume-rendering CT a.
diagnostic a.
digital celiac trunk a.
digital rotational a. (DRA)
digital subtraction a. (DSA)
digital subtraction rotational a.
3-dimensional contrast-enhanced
    MR a.
3-dimensional digital subtraction a.
    (3D-DSA)
3-dimensional magnetic
    resonance a.
2-dimensional magnetic resonance
    digital subtraction a.
dynamic tagging magnetic
    resonance a.
EBCT IV a.
ECG-synchronized digital
    subtraction a.
edge-detection a.
elastic subtraction spiral CT a.
electrocardiogram-synchronized
    digital subtraction a.
electron beam a. (EBA)
emission a.
EPISTAR subtraction a.
equilibrium radionuclide a.
extremity CT a.
femoral runoff a.
femorocerebral catheter a.
first-pass radionuclide a. (FPRNA)
fluorescein a.
FluoroPlus a.

frameless stereotactic digital
  subtraction a.
functional magnetic resonance a.
  (fMRA)
gadolinium-enhanced elliptically
  reordered three-dimensional MR a.
gadolinium-enhanced subtracted
  MR a.
gadoterate-enhanced digital
  subtraction a.
gated blood pool a.
gated equilibrium radionuclide a.
gated nuclear a.
Gd-enhanced MR a.
hand a.
helical computed tomographic a.
  (HCTA)
helical CT a.
hepatic a.
a. imaging
indocyanine green a.
innominate a.
intercostal artery a.
internal carotid a.
interventional a.
intraarterial digital subtraction a.
  (IADSA)
intraarterial stereotactic digital
  subtraction a.
intracranial MR a.
intraoperative digital subtraction a.
  (IDSA)
intravenous digital subtraction a.
  (IVDSA)
intravenous fluorescein a. (IVFA)
intravenous renal a.
intravenous stereotactic digital
  subtraction a.
left coronary a. (LCA)
left ventricular a.
low-field MR a.
magnetic resonance a. (MRA)
magnetic resonance digital
  subtraction a. (MRDSA)
magnification a.
mesenteric a.
minimum basis set magnetic
  resonance a. (MBS-MRA)
multigated a.
multiple projection biplane a.
multislab magnetic resonance a.

multislice computed tomographic a.
  (MSCTA)
noncardiac a.
nonselective a.
nontriggered phase-contrast MR a.
nuclear a.
occlusion a.
orbital a.
orthogonal view on a.
pancreatic a.
PC MR a.
peripheral MR a.
phase-contrast a.
postangioplasty a.
postembolization a.
postoperative a.
posttourniquet occlusion a.
preoperative a.
pulmonary artery wedge a.
pulmonary magnetic resonance a.
  (PMRA)
pulmonary vein wedge a.
quantitative coronary a. (QCA)
radionuclide a.
renal a.
resistive index a.
rest-and-exercise-gated nuclear a.
right coronary a. (RCA)
rotational a. (RA)
scintigraphic a.
segmented k-space time-of-flight
  MR a.
Seldinger a.
selective arterial magnetic
  resonance a.
selective presaturation MR a.
selective venous magnetic
  resonance a.
semiautomated computed
  tomography a.
single-plane a.
sitting-up view a.
spinal cord a.
stereotactic cerebral a.
subtraction a.
superselective a.
Tagarno 3SD cine projector for a.
therapeutic a.
thoracic a.
time-of-flight magnetic resonance a.
  (TOF-MRA)
transfemoral cerebral a.

NOTES

angiography *(continued)*
    transseptal a.
    transvenous digital subtraction a.
    tumor blush on a.
    ultrafast 3D MR digital
      subtraction a.
    velocity encoding on brain MR a.
    venous brain a.
    vertebral a.
    4-vessel cerebral a.
    3-vessel multiple projection
      biplane a.
    4-vessel multiple projection
      biplane a.
    visceral a.
Angioguard
AngioGuard-ex distal protection device
angioimmunoblastic
    a. lymphadenopathy
    a. lymphadenopathylike T-cell
      lymphoma
angioinfarction
angioinvasion
AngioJet
    A. thrombectomy device
    A. Xpeedior catheter
angiokeratoma
angioleiomyoma
Angiolink EVS closure device
angiolipofibroma
angiolipoma
    epidural a.
    mediastinal a.
angiolithic
    a. degeneration
    a. sarcoma
angiolymphangioma
angiolymphoid hyperplasia
angioma, pl. **angiomata**
    arterial a.
    arteriovenous interhemispheric a.
    capillary a.
    cavernous a.
    cutaneous a.
    encephalic a.
    extracerebral cavernous a.
    extraosseous a.
    intracranial cavernous a.
    intradermal a.
    a. lymphaticum
    pulmonary a.
    a. serpiginosum
    spider a.
    superficial a.
    telangiectatic a.
    a. venosum racemosum
    venous a.
AngioMARK contrast agent

Angiomat
    A. 3000, 6000 contrast delivery
      system
    A. ILLUMENA injector system
angiomatoid
    a. malignant fibrous histiocytoma
    a. tumor
angiomatosis
    cystic bone a.
    diffuse skeletal a.
    encephalotrigeminal a.
    epithelioid a.
    leptomeningeal a.
    meningofacial a.
    a. of retina
    retinal a.
    retinocerebellar a.
    visceral a.
angiomatous
    a. disease
    a. lymphoid hamartoma
    a. nasal polyp
    a. syndrome
angiomyofibroma
angiomyolipoma (AML)
    hepatic a.
    kidney a.
    renal a.
angiomyoma
angiomyosarcoma
angiomyxoma
    aggressive a.
    umbilical cord a.
angioneuromyoma
angioneurotic edema
angioosteohypertrophy syndrome
angiopathy
    cerebral amyloid a.
angioplastic meningioma
angioplasty
    excimer laser coronary a. (ELCA)
    infrainguinal percutaneous
      transluminal a.
    laser-assisted balloon a. (LABA)
    percutaneous transluminal a. (PTA)
    percutaneous transluminal
      coronary a. (PTCA)
    percutaneous transluminal renal a.
      (PTRA)
    peripheral excimer laser a. (PELA)
    peripheral laser a.
    a. sheath
    smooth excimer laser coronary a.
      (SELCA)
    transluminal balloon a.
    venous a.
    vessel reshaping by a.
angiopneumography
AngiOptic microcatheter

AngioRad radiation system
angioreticuloendothelioma of heart
angioreticuloma
    spine a.
angiosarcoma
    bone a.
    breast a.
    cavernous a.
    a. of heart
    hepatic a.
    liver a.
    parosteal soft tissue a.
    spleen a.
angioscintigraphy
angioscopic guidance
angioscopy
    virtual a. (VA)
Angio-Seal
    A.-S. carrier tube
    A.-S. closure device
    A.-S. diagnostic device
    A.-S. system
    A.-S. therapeutic device
angiosome
AngioSURF system
angiotensin-converting enzyme (ACE)
angiotherapy
    vasoocclusive a. (VAT)
angiotomomyelography
angiotropic large cell lymphoma
angitis-granulomatosis disorder
angle
    acetabular sector a. (AASA)
    acromial a.
    anorectal a. (ARA)
    antegonial a.
    anterior angulation a.
    anterior talocalcaneal a.
    a. of anteversion
    arch a.
    basal a.
    Baumann a.
    Beatson combined ankle a.
    beta a.
    bimalleolar a.
    blunting of costovertebral a.
    blurring of costophrenic a.
    board a.
    Boehler a.
    Böhler a.
    Bragg a.
    brain tumor at cerebellopontine a.

C a.
calcaneal inclination a.
calcaneal pitch a.
calcaneoplantar a.
capital epiphysis a.
capitolunate a.
cardiodiaphragmatic a.
cardiohepatic a.
cardiophrenic a.
carinal a.
carpal wrist a.
carrying a.
CCD a.
central collodiaphysial a.
cephalic a.
cephalometric a.
cerebellopontine a. (CPA)
Clarke arch a.
clivus-canal a.
Cobb scoliosis a.
Codman a.
condylar a.
congruence a.
costal a.
costolumbar a.
costophrenic a.
costosternal a.
costovertebral a. (CVA)
CP a.
craniofacial a.
craniovertebral a.
a. of declination of metatarsal
de Seze a.
distal articular set a. (DASA)
distal metatarsal articular a.
  (DMMA)
Doppler a.
dorsiflexion a. (DFA)
dorsoplantar talometatarsal a.
dorsoplantar talonavicular a.
Drennan metaphysial-epiphysial a.
duodenojejunal a.
Ebstein a.
a. electron (UE)
epigastric a.
Ernst a.
exposure a.
fan a.
femoral torsion V a.
femorotibial a. (FTA)
Ferguson a.
first-fifth intermetatarsal a.

NOTES

angle *(continued)*
    first metatarsal a.
    first-second intermetatarsal a.
    flip a.
    focal spot-to-film a.
    foot-progression a. (FPA)
    Frankfort mandibular incisor a.
    Garden a.
    gastroesophageal a.
    Gissane a.
    gonial a.
    Graf alpha a.
    Graf beta a.
    a. of greatest extension (AGE)
    a. of greatest flexion (AGF)
    hallux dorsiflexion a. (DFA)
    hallux interphalangeus a. (HIA)
    hallux valgus a. (HVA)
    hallux valgus interphalangeus a.
    hepatic a.
    hepatorenal a.
    Hibbs metatarsocalcaneal a.
    Hilgenreiner epiphysial a.
    His a.
    horizontal toit externe a.
    HTE a.
    incident a.
    a. of inclination of urethra
    a. of incongruity
    increased carrying a.
    infrasternal a.
    a. of insonation
    interbronchial a. (IA)
    intercarpal a.
    intermetatarsal a. (IMA)
    kite a.
    Konstram a.
    lateral divergence a. (LDA)
    lateral patellofemoral a.
    lateral plantar metatarsal a.
    lateral talocalcaneal a.
    lateral talometatarsal a.
    lateral tarsometatarsal a.
    Laurin a.
    a. of Lequesne and de Seze
    Lewis a.
    Lippman-Cobb a.
    Louis a.
    Ludovici a.
    Ludwig a.
    lumbar facet a.
    lumbosacral joint a.
    magnetization precession a.
    mandibular a.
    Meary metatarsotalar a.
    medial a.
    mediolateral radiocarpal a.
    Merchant a.
    metaphysial-diaphysial a.

    metaphysial-epiphysial a.
    metatarsal a.
    metatarsocalcaneal a.
    metatarsotalar a.
    metatarsus adductus a.
    metatarsus primus varus a.
     (MPVA)
    Mikulicz a.
    navicular to first metatarsal a.
    neck shaft a.
    nidus a.
    nutation a.
    obliterated costophrenic a.
    occipitocervical a.
    a. of orientation
    patellofemoral a.
    Pauwel a.
    pelvic femoral a.
    phase a.
    phrenopericardial a.
    Pirogoff a.
    plantar metatarsal a.
    pontine a.
    posterior urethrovesical a. (PUVA)
    precession a.
    proximal articular set a.
    psoas shadow a.
    pulse flip a.
    Q a.
    QRST a.
    radiocarpal a.
    Ranke a.
    resting forefoot supination a.
    a. of rib
    Rolando a.
    rotation a.
    sacrohorizontal a.
    sacrovertebral a.
    scapular a.
    set a.
    Sharp a.
    slip a.
    sphenoid a.
    spinographic a.
    splenic a.
    splenorenal a.
    sternal a.
    sternoclavicular a.
    subcarinal a. (SA)
    substernal a.
    subtalar a.
    sulcus a.
    surgical a.
    talar tilt a.
    talocalcaneal a.
    talocrural a.
    talohorizontal a.
    talometatarsal a.
    talonavicular a.

tarsometatarsal a.
thigh-foot a. (TFA)
tibiocalcaneal a.
tibiofemoral a. (TFA)
tibiotalar a.
tip a.
tracheal bifurcation a.
tracheobronchial a.
transmalleolar axis-thigh a.
transmetatarsal-thigh a.
urethral a.
urethrovesical a. (UVA)
valgus carrying a.
a. variation resolution
varus metatarsophalangeal a.
venous brain a.
venous neck a.
vertebrophrenic a.
vertical-center-anterior a.
vesicourethral a.
wedge isodose a.
Welcher basal a.
Welcker a.
Wiberg a.
Wiltze a.
xiphoid a.

angled
a. craniocaudal view
a. Glidewire
a. pleural tube
a. slice

angled-tip catheter
Angle-Iron skull immobilizer
angles of trigone
Angström
A. law
A. unit

angular
a. alignment
a. artery
a. bolster
a. curvature
a. deformity
a. deviation
a. frequency
a. gyrus (AG)
a. momentum
a. notch
a. process of orbit
a. sampling
a. vein
a. velocity

angularis
a. body
incisura a.
a. sulcus

angulated
a. catheter
a. fracture
a. lesion
a. segment

angulation
anterior a.
bowel loop a.
caudal-cranial a.
cephalic a.
coronal a.
cranial a.
craniocaudal needle a.
forefoot a.
gantry a.
kyphotic a.
palmar a.
posttraumatic a.
spinal a.
a. of spine
valgus a.
varus a.
volar a.

angulator
angulus of stomach
anhaustral colonic gas pattern
anhydrous ammonia
ani
aniline carcinoma
anisotrophy
anisotropic
a. 3D imaging
a. resolution
a. rotation
a. tissue
a. volume study

anisotropically
a. rotational diffusion (ARD)
a. rotational diffusion imaging

anisotropy
brain diffusion a.
curvature a.
decreased diffusion a.
diffusional a.
a. factor
fractional a. (FA)
functional diffusion a.

NOTES

anisotropy *(continued)*
 magnetic a.
 a. map
anisura
ankle
 athlete's a.
 a. bone
 disc of a.
 eccentric axis of rotation of a.
 eversion of a.
 fused a.
 a. fusion
 a. immobilizer
 a. instability
 inversion injury of a.
 a. inversion injury
 a. joint
 a. joint complex
 laciniate ligament of a.
 a. mortise
 a. mortise axis
 a. mortise fracture
 a. mortise widening
 neuropathic a.
 a. swelling
 synthetic graft bypass to a.
 a. systolic pressure
 tailor's a.
 transmalleolar a.
 twisted a.
ankle-arm
 a.-a. index (AAI)
 a.-a. pressure
ankle-brachial (AB)
 a.-b. index (ABI)
 a.-b. pressure measurement
 a.-b. pressure ratio
ankle immobilizer
ankylosing
 a. hyperostosis
 a. spondylitis
ankylosis
 bony a.
 extracapsular a.
 false a.
 fibrous a.
 intracapsular a.
 joint a.
 ligamentous a.
 shoulder a.
 spurious a.
 vertebral a.
ankyroid *(var. of* ancyroid)
anlage, pl. **anlagen**
 cartilaginous a.
 pancreatic dorsal a.
 ventral pancreatic a.
ANMR Insta-scan MR scanner
Ann Arbor classification

annealing
 a. algorithm
 simulated a.
annihilation
 a. coincidence detection (ACD)
 a. photon
 a. radiation
 a. reaction
annotated imaging
annotation
annular *(var. of* anular)
annulus *(var. of* anulus)
ano
 fissure in a.
 fistula in a.
anococcygeal
 a. body
 a. ligament
 a. raphe
anodal block
anode
 molybdenum a.
 a. ray
 rhodium a.
 rotating a.
 stationary a.
 a. tube
 a. tube reloading
 tungsten a.
anode-cathode axis
anodontia
anogenital
 a. band
 a. raphe
anomalad
 Robin a.
anomalous
 a. anatomy
 a. branching
 a. bronchus
 a. craniovertebral junction
 a. development
 a. distribution
 a. insertion
 a. left coronary artery
 a. left pulmonary artery
 a. muscle
 a. origin
 a. origin of artery
 a. pathway
 a. pulmonary venous connection
 a. pulmonary venous return
 a. right coronary artery
 a. right subclavian artery
 a. vessel
anomaly, pl. **anomalies**
 Alder constitutional granulation a.
 Alder-Reilly a.
 anorectal a.

aortic arch a.
associated a.
atlas a.
atrioventricular junction a.
axis a.
back-angle a.
bell-clapper a. (BCA)
cardiac a.
cardiovascular a.
cervical rib a.
cloacal a.
conjoined nerve root a.
conotruncal congenital a.
cranial a.
craniofacial a.
craniovertebral a.
Cruveilhier-Baumgarten a.
cutaneous vascular a.
double-inlet ventricle a.
duplication a.
Ebstein a.
extracardiac a.
fast-flow vascular a.
fetal cardiac a.
fetal chest a.
fetal CNS a.
fetal gastrointestinal a.
fetal heart a.
fetal neck a.
fetal urinary tract a.
Freund a.
gastrointestinal fetal a.
genitourinary a.
heart a.
intracranial leptomeningeal
  vascular a.
jugular bulb a.
kidney a.
limb reduction a.
May-Hegglin a.
Michel a.
migrational a.
Mondini a.
müllerian duct a.
multiple congenital anomalies
  (MCA)
numerary renal a.
occipitoatlantoaxial a.
presacral a.
radial ray a.
renal a.
rotation a.

segmentation a.
Shone a.
slow-flow vascular a.
spinal a.
structural a.
Taussig-Bing a.
tricuspid valve a.
Uhl a.
Undritz a.
urachal a.
urinary tract a.
uterine duplication a.
in utero detection of cardiac a.
vascular a.
vena cava a.
venous a.
vertebral segmentation a.
Zahn a.
anonymous vein
anophthalmia
anorectal
  a. angle (ARA)
  a. anomaly
  a. atresia
  a. dysgenesis
  a. fistula
  a. junction (ARJ)
  a. line
  a. lymph node
  a. malformation
  a. manometry
  a. ring
  a. tuberculosis
anorectum
anovaginal fistula
anovular ovarian follicle
anoxia
  brain a.
  cerebral a.
  perinatal a.
anoxic
  a. encephalopathy
  a. ischemia
Anrep effect
ansa, pl. **ansae**
  a. of Vieussens
anserine
  a. bursa
  a. bursitis
anserinus
  pes a.
antacid

NOTES

antagonist
anteater nose
antebrachial
    a. fascia
    a. vein
antebrachium
antecedent sign
antecolic
antecubital
    a. fossa
    a. space
    a. vein
anteflexed uterus
anteflexion
antegonial
    a. angle
    a. notch
antegrade
    a. aortography
    a. bile flow
    a. blood flow
    a. cystography
    a. diastolic flow
    a. fast pathway
    a. femoral artery catheterization
    a. filling of vessel
    a. perfusion
    a. perfusion pressure measurement
    (APPM)
    a. pressure study
    a. puncture
    a. pyelography
    a. pyelography imaging
    a. refractory period
    a. transluminal balloon dilatation
    a. ureteral stenting
    a. urography
    a. venography
antepartum hemorrhage
anteprostatic gland
anterior
    a. abdominal wall
    ampulla membranacea a.
    ampulla ossea a.
    a. angulation
    a. angulation angle
    a. aspect
    a. atlas arch
    a. atrial myocardial bundle
    a. axillary line (AAL)
    a. band
    a. band of colon
    a. basal bronchus
    a. border
    a. border of heart
    a. bowing of sternum
    a. bowing tibia
    a. capsular distance (ACD)
    a. capsular shift

a. cardiac vein
a. central beaking
a. central indentation
a. cerebral artery (ACA)
a. cerebral artery crawling under skull
a. cervical fusion (ACF)
a. choroidal artery
a. clear space
a. colliculus
a. column fracture
a. column of spine
a. commissure (AC)
a. commissure-posterior commissure (AC-PC)
a. communicating artery (ACoA, AcomA)
a. communicating artery complex
a. communicating artery distribution infarct
a. compartment syndrome
a. condylar canal
a. condyloid foramen
a. cord syndrome
a. coronary plexus
a. corpus
a. corticospinal tract
a. cranial base lesion
a. cruciate deficit of knee
a. cruciate ligament (ACL)
a. cruciate ligament injury
a. current (AC) generator
a. curvature
a. cusp
a. cutaneous branch
a. descending artery
a. dislocation
a. drawer sign
a. epidural fat
a. exenteration
a. fascicular block
a. feet view
a. fibular ligament
a. fontanelle
a. fornix of vagina
a. glenoid labrum (AGL)
a. gray column
a. gray column of cord
a. horn
a. horn cell disease
a. horn of spinal cord
a. humeral line
a. hypothalamus
a. iliac crest
a. impingement syndrome
a. inferior tibiofibular ligament
a. intercostal artery
a. interhemispheric cistern
a. interhemispheric fissure

a. internal vertebral vein (AIVV)
a. internodal pathway
a. internodal tract of Bachmann
a. interventricular groove
a. intervertebral disc
a. joint capsule thickening
a. jugular vein
a. junction line
a. labral avulsion
a. labral disruption
a. labroligamentous periosteal sleeve avulsion (ALPSA)
a. labroligamentous periosteal sleeve avulsion lesion
a. leaflet prolapse
a. maxillary spine
a. median fissure
a. mediastinal compartment
a. mediastinal mass
a. mediastinum
a. meningeal artery
a. metatarsal arch
a. midbody of corpus callosum
a. motion of posterior mitral valve leaflet
a. myocardial infarct
a. oblique position
a. osteophyte
a. palatine foramen
a. palatine suture
a. papillary muscle (APM)
a. pararenal space (APS)
a. parietal lesion
a. pillar of fauces
a. precordium
a. predominance
a. projection
a. pulmonary plexus
a. recess of ischiorectal fossa
a. rectus fascia
a. rectus sheath
a. sacral foramen
a. sacral meningocele
a. sagittal diameter (ASD)
scalenus a.
a. scalloping of vertebra
a. semicircular canal
a. semilunar valve
a. septal myocardial infarct
serratus a. (SA)
a. spinal artery
a. spinal artery stroke

a. spinal artery syndrome
a. spinal ligament calcification
a. spine fusion (ASF)
a. spinocerebellar tract
a. spinothalamic tract
a. spur
a. surface of pancreas
a. synchondrosis intraoccipital
a. talar dome
a. talocalcaneal angle
a. talofibular ligament (ATF)
a. tarsal tunnel syndrome
a. temporal branch of posterior cerebral artery
a. terminal vein (ATV)
a. thalamotomy
a. thoracic meningocele
a. tibial artery
a. tibial bowing
a. tibial compartment
tibialis a.
a. tibial subluxation
a. tibial tendon
a. tibiofibular ligament
a. tibiotalar ligament
a. tip of temporal lobe
a. tracheal displacement
a. tracking
a. tricuspid valve leaflet
a. urethra
a. urethral injury
a. vertebral body margin
a. wall antral ulcer
a. wall motion
a. wall myocardial infarct
a. wedging
anterior-inferior
a.-i. cerebellar artery (AICA)
a.-i. cerebral artery (AICA)
a.-i. communicating artery (AICA)
a.-i. iliac spine
anterior-posterior
a.-p. flow direction
a.-p., posterior-anterior view
anterior-superior iliac spine (ASIS)
anterior-to-posterior sagittal canal diameter
anteroapical
a. defect
a. trabecular septum
anterobasal segment
anterochiasmatic lesion

NOTES

anterofundal placenta
anterograde
  a. block
  a. peristalsis
anteroinferior
  a. corner fracture
  a. dislocation
  a. myocardial infarct
  a. triangular fragment
anterolateral (AL)
  a. abdominal wall
  a. aspect
  a. compression fracture
  a. fontanelle
  a. groove
  a. gutter
  a. impingement
  a. impingement syndrome
  a. myocardial infarct
  a. rotary knee instability
  a. segment
  a. surface
  a. system
  a. white matter of cord
anterolisthesis
anteromedial
  a. superior humeral head impaction
  a. surface
anteromedian groove
anteroposterior (AP)
  a. aspect
  a. axis
  a. diameter
  a. dimension
  a. film
  a. iliac spine
  a. lordotic projection
  a. position
  a. talocalcaneal (APTC)
  a. tube
  a. view
anteroposterior-posteroanterior (AP-PA)
anteroseptal
  a. commissure
  a. myocardial infarct
antetorsion
  femoral a.
anteversion
  acetabular a. (AA)
  angle of a.
  femoral a.
  Magilligan technique for measuring
    neutral a.
anteverted uterus
anthracosilicosis
anthracosis
anthracotic material
anthracycline-induced myocardial
  damage

anthrax
  a. exposure
  inhalation a.
  a. pneumonia
anthrocotic tuberculosis
Anthron heparinized catheter
anthropoid pelvis
anthropologic baseline
anthropometric imaging
anthropometry
  3D surface a.
anthropomorphic baseline
antiadrenergic drug
antiaggregation
antialiasing technique
antibody
  a. half-life
  a. labeling
  radiolabeled a.
  ^{99m}Tc-labeled antigranulocyte a.
antibody-conjugated paramagnetic
  liposome (ACPL)
antibody-labeled circulating granulocyte
anti-CEA
  radiolabeled a.-C.
anticoagulant bleed
anticoagulant-related bleed
anticoagulation
anticoincidence circuit
anticonvulsant drug
antidepressant drug
antidysrhythmic
antiemetic
antiestrogen radiologic therapy
antiferromagnetism
antifibrin
  a. antibody imaging
  a. antibody imaging agent
  a. scintigraphy
antigen
  a. expression
  HLA-A3 histocompatibility a.
  HLA-B7 histocompatibility a.
  HLA-B14 histocompatibility a.
  human leukocyte a. (HLA)
antigen-modulated mini-stem-cell
  transplant
antigravity muscle
antihyperlipidemic
antiidiotypic affinity chromatography
antimesenteric
  a. border
  a. border of distal ileum
  a. fat pad
antimesocolic side of cecum
antimuscarinic drug
antimyosin monoclonal antibody imaging
  agent
antineutrino

antiparticle
antiproton
antipsychotic drug
antipyretic
antiradial technique
antiscatter grid
antisense oligonucleotide
antisiphon device
antitragohelicine fissure
antitubercular therapy
Antopol-Goldman lesion
antra (*pl. of* antrum)
antral
- a. beaking
- a. edema
- a. gastritis
- a. G-cell hyperplasia
- a. mucosal diaphragm
- a. mucosal thickening
- a. padding
- a. polyp
- a. pouch
- a. sphincter
- a. stasis
- a. stenosis
- a. stomach narrowing
- a. stricture
- a. ulcer
- a. web

antrochoanal polyp
antroduodenal motility
antropyloric
- a. canal
- a. muscle thickness (APT)

antrum, pl. **antra**
- aditus ad a.
- cardiac a.
- gastric a.
- Highmore a.
- a. of Highmore
- Malacarne a.
- mastoid a.
- maxillary a.
- prepyloric a.
- pyloric a.
- retained gastric a.
- a. of stomach
- Willis a.

anular, annular
- a. abscess
- a. appearance
- a. array

- a. array transducer
- a. calcification
- a. constricting lesion
- a. detector
- a. dilatation
- a. disc bulge
- a. disruption
- a. epiphysis
- a. esophageal stricture
- a. fiber
- a. fibrosis
- a. foreshortening
- a. fracture
- a. hypoplasia
- a. lamellae
- a. ligament
- a. ligament of trachea
- a. pancreas
- a. phased-array hyperthermia
- a. placement
- a. placenta
- a. rim of cartilage
- a. tear
- a. tear classification
- a. tear extent
- a. tear pattern

anuloaortic ectasia
anulospiral organ
anulus, annulus
- aortic valve a.
- atrioventricular a.
- bulging a.
- calcified a.
- a. fibrosus
- fissure of a.
- friable a.
- mitral valve of a.
- a. ovalis
- periphery of a.
- posterior a.
- pulmonary valve a.
- redundant scallop of posterior a.
- septal tricuspid a.
- tricuspid valve a.
- a. umbilicalis
- valve a.
- Vieussens a.
- Zinn a.

anus
- ectopic a.
- imperforate a.
- levator a.'s

NOTES

anvil bone
AO
 aorta
 aortic opening
 Arbeitsgemeinschaft für
  Osteosynthesefragen
  AO ankle fracture classification
  AO classification of ankle fracture
  AO tension band
AO/AC
 aortic valve opening to aortic valve
  closing ratio
AOCS
 anatomy-oriented colon segmentation
AOD
 airflow obstruction disease
AO-Danis-Weber ankle fracture
 classification
AOIVM
 angiographically occult intracranial
  vascular malformation
aorta, pl. **aortae (AO)**
 abdominal a.
 aneurysmal widening of a.
 ascending a. (AA)
 ascending hypoplasia of a.
 bifurcation of a.
 biventricular origin of a.
 biventricular transposed a.
 brachiocephalic trunk of a.
 calcified a.
 central a.
 cervical a.
 coarctation of a.
 descending thoracic a.
 dextropositioned a.
 dilated descending a.
 distal a.
 D-malposition of a.
 double arch a.
 double-barrel a.
 draped a.
 dynamic a.
 ectasia of a.
 elongated a.
 feminine a.
 Hodgson aneurysmal dilatation
  of a.
 infantile coarctation of a.
 infrarenal abdominal a.
 intramural hematoma of a.
 juxtaductal coarctation of a.
 kinked a.
 L-malposition of a.
 native a.
 occlusion a.
 overriding a.
 pericardial a.
 porcelain a.

postductal coarctation of a.
proximal a.
pseudocoarctation of a.
recoarctation of a.
reconstruction of a.
retroesophageal a.
reversed coarctation of a.
small feminine a.
stenosis of a.
supraceliac a.
supradiaphragmatic a.
symptomatic coarctation of a.
terminal a.
thoracic a.
thoracoabdominal a.
tortuous a.
transposed a.
tulip bulb a.
uncoiling ascending a.
uncoiling descending a.
unwinding of a.
ventral a.
widening of a.
wide tortuous a.
aorta-left ventricular fistula
aorta-right ventricular fistula
aortic
 a. allograft
 a. anulus abscess
 a. aperture
 a. arch
 a. arch aneurysm
 a. arch angiography
 a. arch anomaly
 a. arch atresia
 a. arch calcification
 a. arch interruption
 a. arch lesion
 a. arch malformation
 a. arch obstruction
 a. atherosclerosis
 a. attenuation
 a. bifurcation
 a. body tumor
 a. bulb
 a. button
 a. cannulation
 a. cartilage
 a. closure (AC)
 a. coarctation
 a. cuff
 a. cusp
 a. cusp separation
 a. deviation
 a. diameter (AD)
 a. dilation
 a. dissection
 a. distensibility
 a. elongation

a. flow (AF)
a. flow volume
a. foramen
a. gland
a. graft infection
a. hiatus
a. idiopathic necrosis
a. impedance
a. incisura
a. inflammation
a. inflow
a. insult
a. intimal dehiscence
a. intramural hematoma
a. isthmus
a. kinking
a. knob
a. knuckle
a. lumen
a. lymph node
a. motion artifact
a. nipple
a. nipple sign
a. node metastasis
a. notch
a. opening (AO)
a. opening of heart
a. orifice
a. ostium
a. outflow gradient
a. outflow obstruction
a. override
a. oxygen saturation
a. paravalvular leak
a. penetrating ulcer
a. plexus
a. prominence
a. pseudoaneurysm
a. pullback
a. reconstruction
a. regurgitation (AR)
a. root
a. root cineangiography
a. root diameter
a. root dilatation
a. root dimension
a. root echocardiography
a. root homograft
a. root pressure
a. root ratio
a. root replacement
a. runoff

a. rupture
a. sac
a. sclerosis
a. segment
a. septal defect
a. septum
a. shag
a. sinotubular junction
a. sinus aneurysm
a. sinus to right ventricle fistula
a. spindle
a. stenosis (AS)
a. stiffness
a. stump blowout
a. thromboembolism
a. thrombosis
a. tract complex hypoplasia
a. transsection
a. tube graft
a. valve (AoV)
a. valve anulus
a. valve area (AVA)
a. valve atresia
a. valve calcification
a. valve calcium quantification with MSCT
a. valve calcium score
a. valve deformity
a. valve echocardiography
a. valve endocarditis
a. valve gradient (AVG)
a. valve lesion
a. valve nodule
a. valve obstruction
a. valve opening
a. valve opening to aortic valve closing ratio (AO/AC)
a. valve peak instantaneous gradient
a. valve pressure gradient
a. valve replacement (AVR)
a. valve sinus
a. valve thickening
a. valvular disease (AVD)
a. valvular incompetence
a. valvular insufficiency
a. vasa vasorum
a. vent suction line
a. vestibule of ventricle
a. wall thickening
a. window

NOTES

aortic *(continued)*
    a. window node
    a. wrap
aortic-brachiocephalic (ABC)
    a.-b. injury
aortic-enteric fistula
aortic-left ventricular tunnel
aorticopulmonary *(var. of*
    aortopulmonary)
aorticorenal
    a. ganglion
    a. graft
aortitis
    infectious a.
    luetic a.
    a. syndrome
    Takayasu a.
aortobifemoral reconstruction
aortobiliac bypass
aortocaval fistula
aortocoronary valve
aortoduodenal fistula
aortoenteric fistula
aortoesophageal fistula
aortofemoral
    a. arteriography
    a. bypass graft (AFBG)
    a. runoff
aortogastric
aortogram
    arch a.
    transbrachial arch a.
aortography
    abdominal a.
    antegrade a.
    arch a.
    ascending a.
    balloon occlusive a.
    biplanar a.
    catheter a.
    contrast a.
    countercurrent a.
    digital subtraction a.
    flush a.
    a. imaging
    intravenous a.
    lumbar a.
    postangioplasty a.
    preembolization a.
    renal a.
    retrograde femoral a.
    retrograde transaxillary a.
    retrograde transfemoral a.
    retrograde translumbar a.
    selective visceral a.
    supravalvular a.
    thoracic arch a.
    translumbar a. (TLA)
    ultrasonic a.

    venous a.
    visceral a.
aortoiliac
    a. aneurysm
    a. bypass graft
    a. inflow assessment
    a. inflow system
    a. obstruction
    a. occlusive disease (AIOD)
    a. stenosis
    a. thrombosis
aortoiliofemoral artery
aortojejunal fistula
aortomegaly
    diffuse a.
aortoplasty
    balloon a.
    patch-graft a.
    posterior patch a.
    subclavian flap a.
    a. with patch graft
aortopulmonary, aorticopulmonary
    a. fenestration
    a. fistula
    a. mediastinal stripe
    a. septal defect
    a. septum
    a. trunk
    a. window
    a. window mass
aortosclerosis
aortoseptal continuity
aortosigmoid fistula
aortovelography
    transcutaneous a. (TAV)
aortoventriculoplasty
AoV
    aortic valve
AOVM
    angiographically occult vascular
    malformation
AP
    adenomatous polyp
    anteroposterior
        AP inversion stress vagina view
        AP malleolar bisection
        AP projection
        AP supine portable view
apallic syndrome
APC-3, APC-4 collimator
ape hand of syringomyelia
apelike hand
aperiodic
    a. complex
    a. functional MR imaging
    a. wave
aperistalsis
    esophageal a.

aperistaltic
   a. distal ureteral segment
   a. esophagus
aperta
   spina bifida a.
apertura, pl. **aperturae**
   a. externa aqueductus vestibuli
   a. externa canaliculi cochleae
   a. lateralis ventriculi quarti
   a. mediana ventriculi quarti
   a. pelvis inferior
   a. pelvis superior
   a. piriformis
   a. sinus frontalis
   a. sinus sphenoidalis
   a. thoracis inferior
   a. thoracis superior
   a. tympanica canaliculi chordae
     tympani
aperture
   aortic a.
   coded-image a.
   a. diaphragm
   superior thoracic a.
apex, pl. **apices**
   a. beat
   a. of bladder
   A. 409, 415 camera
   cardiac a.
   a. cordis
   displaced left ventricular a.
   duodenal bulb a. (DBA)
   external ring a.
   a. of femur
   a. of fibula
   F point of cardiac a.
   a. of head of patella
   a. of heart
   Koch triangle a.
   left ventricular a.
   lung a.
   orbital a.
   petrous a.
   a. of petrous portion of temporal
     bone
   A. Plus excimer laser
   a. of prostate
   right ventricular a. (RVA)
   sternal a.
   systolic retraction of a.
   true a. (TA)

   uptilted cardiac a.
   ventricular a.
apexcardiogram, apex cardiogram (ACG)
   derived value on a. (dD/dt)
aphalangia
apheresis catheter
aphtha, pl. **aphthae**
aphthoid ulcer
aphthous stomach ulcer
apical
   a. aspect
   a. atelectasis
   a. bronchus
   a. canaliculus
   a. cap
   a. capping
   a. cap sign
   a. 2-chamber view
     echocardiography
   a. 5-chamber view
     echocardiography
   a. complex
   a. corn
   a. defect
   a. dip
   a. duodenal ulcer
   a. ectodermal ridge (AER)
   a. fenestration
   a. foramen
   a. gland
   a. granuloma
   a. hypokinesis
   a. hypoperfusion
   a. impulse
   a. infiltrate
   a. lesion
   a. ligament
   a. lordotic projection
   a. lordotic view
   a. lymph node
   a. myocardial infarct
   a. notch
   a. petrositis
   a. pleural thickening
   a. pneumonia
   a. posterior artery
   a. process
   a. pulse
   a. scarring
   a. segment
   a. short-axis slice
   a. and subcostal 4-chambered view

NOTES

apical *(continued)*
    a. surface of heart
    a. suture
    a. thinning
    a. tissue
    a. wall
    a. wall motion
    a. window
apical-lateral wall myocardial infarct
apically directed chest tube
apical pulse
apices *(pl. of* apex)
apicoposterior
    a. bronchus
    a. segment
apiculate waveform
aplasia
    bilateral semicircular canal a.
    cerebellar a.
    cochlea a.
    a. of deep vein
    deep venous a.
    lung a.
    Michel a.
    pulmonary a.
    radial a.
aplastic uterus
APLD
    automated percutaneous lumbar
      discectomy
APM
    anterior papillary muscle
apnea-bradycardia ratio
apnea-hypopnea index (AHI)
apocrine
    a. adenoma
    a. carcinoma
    a. cyst
    a. metaplasia
    a. sweat gland
Apogee
    A. CX100, CX200
      echocardiography system
    A. RX400 diagnostic ultrasound
      system
Apollo DXA bone densitometry system
Apomate radiopharmaceutical imaging
    agent
aponeurosis, pl. **aponeuroses**
    bicipital a.
    digital a.
    epicranial a.
    external oblique a.
    flexor carpi ulnaris a.
    internal oblique a.
    palmar a.
    plantar a.
    tendon a.

aponeurotic
    a. band
    a. fibroma
    a. portion of diaphragm
    a. tendon
    a. triangle
    a. troika
apophysial, apophyseal
    a. fracture
    a. injury
    a. joint
    a. lesion
    a. point
    a. pouch
apophysis, pl. **apophyses**
    bone lesion a.
    calcaneal a.
    fragmentation of a.
    a. of Rau
    rim a.
    ring a.
apophysitis
    calcaneal a.
    iliac a.
apoplexy
    cerebellar a.
    delayed pineal a.
    mesenteric a.
    pineal a.
    pituitary a.
    postpartum pituitary a.
    pulmonary artery a.
    pulmonary vein a.
apoptic
    a. body
    a. nuclear fragment
aporic gland
apotentiality
    cerebral a.
APP
    average pixel projection
AP-PA
    anteroposterior-posteroanterior
    AP-PA skull block
    AP-PA skull immobilizer
apparatus
    Acuson 128 a.
    anal a.
    electrooculogram a.
    extensor a.
    Hilal embolization a.
    Jaquet a.
    juxtaglomerular a. (JGA)
    mitral a.
    oculomotor a.
    stereotactic a.
    valvular a.
    vestibular a.
    zero time of the x-ray a.

apparent
a. diffusion coefficient (ADC)
a. paramagnetism
a. volume of distribution (Vd)

appearance
anular a.
apple-core a.
apple-peel a.
applesauce a.
asymmetric target a.
ball-in-hand a.
ball-on-spoon a.
banding a.
batwing a.
beaded necklace a.
beaked a.
beaten brass a.
beaten silver a.
beaver-tail a.
bilaminar a.
birdlike a.
blade-of-grass a.
blown-out a.
bone-within-bone a.
bubblelike a.
bull-neck a.
bull's eye a.
bunch of-grapes a.
butterfly a.
candle dripping a.
catheter tip hockey-stick a.
cauliflower a.
chisellike truncated a.
Christmas tree a.
cobblestone a.
cobra-head a.
cobweb a.
cockscomb a.
coffee-bean a.
coiled spring a.
collar-button a.
colonic lead-pipe a.
constant level a. (CLEAR)
corkscrew a.
cottage loaf a.
cotton ball a.
cotton-wool a.
crabmeatlike a.
crazy-paving a.
cystic a.
double-bubble a.
double-bulb a.

double-halo a.
drooping lily a.
drumstick a.
dumbbell a.
duodenal teardrop a.
echogenic a.
Erlenmeyer flask a.
feathery a.
featureless a.
figure-8 a.
fine-speckled a.
fish flesh a.
fishnet a.
flame a.
frayed-string a.
froglike a.
frondlike a.
ground-glass a.
hair-on-end a.
hammered-brass a.
hammered-silver a.
heterogeneous a.
hole-within-hole a.
holly leaf a.
homogeneous a.
Honda sign a.
honeycomb a.
horseshoe a.
hot-cross bun a.
ill-defined a.
inverse comma a.
inverted-T a.
irregular tapered a.
isodense a.
jail-bar a.
jelly-belly a.
kernel-of-corn a.
lacelike a.
leafless tree a.
light bulb a.
lobulated saccular a.
lollipop tree a.
Mickey Mouse a.
mixed-echo a.
molar tooth a.
moth-eaten a.
mottled a.
"mouse-ear" a.
multiseptate a.
mushroom a.
Neptune trident a.
nodular a.

NOTES

appearance *(continued)*
    nodule-in-a-nodule a.
    onion peel a.
    onionskin a.
    owl's eye a.
    pancake a.
    panda a.
    partial tubular a.
    pencil-in-cup a.
    picket fence a.
    picture frame a.
    pistol-grip a.
    pluglike a.
    polka-dot a.
    popcornlike a.
    pruned tree a.
    pruned-tree a.
    pseudopost Billroth I a.
    pseudotumor a.
    punched-out a.
    radial scarlike mammographic a.
    railroad track a.
    reticulogranular a.
    ringlike a.
    rounded a.
    rugger jersey a.
    saber-shin a.
    sandwich a.
    sausage-shaped a.
    sawtooth a.
    scalloped a.
    scottie dog a.
    septate a.
    serpentine a.
    serrated a.
    shading a.
    shell-of-bone a.
    smooth tapered a.
    snake's head a.
    soap-bubble a.
    spadelike a.
    spiderweb a.
    spiral a.
    spongy a.
    stacked-coin a.
    stained-glass a.
    stepladder a.
    stippled a.
    string-of-beads a.
    string-of-pearls a.
    stumped off a.
    sunburst a.
    sun-ray a.
    Swiss Alps a.
    Swiss cheese a.
    tam-o-shanter a.
    target a.
    teardrop a.
    thumbprint a.

    tram-track a.
    tree-in-winter bile duct a.
    trefoil a.
    trilaminar a.
    trilayer a.
    twisted small bowel ribbon a.
    ventricle batwing a.
    violin-string a.
    waferlike a.
    walking-stick a.
    waterfall a.
    weblike a.
    well-defined a.
    whirlpool a.
    whorled a.
    windsock a.
    wine glass a.
    wormy a.
    yin-yang a.
    zebra stripe a.

appendage
    atrial a.
    cecal a.
    coccygeal a.
    epiploic a.
    inverted left atrial a.
    left atrial a. (LAA)
    left auricular a. (LAA)
    right atrial a. (RAA)
    testicular torsion a.
    truncated atrial a.
    vermicular a.
    wide-based, blunt-ended, right-sided,
      atrial a.

appendiceal
    a. abscess
    a. carcinoma
    a. intussusception
    a. lesion
    a. mass
    a. stump

appendicolith *(var. of* appendolith*)*
appendicolithiasis *(var. of*
  appendolithiasis*)*
appendicular
    a. bone mass measurement
    a. lymph node
    a. skeleton
    a. vein
appendiculare
    skeleton a.
appendix, pl. **appendices**
    cecal a.
    double a.
    ensiform a.
    a. of epididymis
    epiploic a.
    a. epiploica
    filiform a.

Morgagni a.
a. mucocele
paracecal a.
perforated gangrenous a.
retrocecal a.
retroileal a.
a. rupture
subcecal a.
a. testis
a. of ventricle of larynx
vermicular a.
vermiform a.
vesiculosa a.
xiphoid a.
appendolith, appendicolith
appendolithiasis, appendicolithiasis
apperceptive mass
apple-core
a.-c. appearance
a.-c. carcinoma
a.-c. lesion
a.-c. tumor
apple-peel
a.-p. appearance
a.-p. appearance of GI tract
a.-p. bowel
a.-p. syndrome
applesauce appearance
application
infradiaphragmatic a.
interstitial radioelement a.
intracavitary radioelement a.
ribbon a.
surface radioelement a.
application-specific integrated circuit
(ASIC)
applicator
beam-therapy a.
beta-ray a.
Burnett a.
colpostat a.
Henschke seed a.
intracavitary afterloading a.
LITT a.
Mick seed a.
Nucletron a.
perfused needle a.
RFA with perfused needle a.
small LITT a.
^{90}Sr-loaded eye a.
standard LITT a.

Syed-Puthawala-Hedger
esophageal a.
tandem a.
Wang a.
APPM
antegrade perfusion pressure
measurement
apposing articular surface
apposition
bone-to-bone a.
bony a.
close a.
fracture in close a.
a. of leaflet
margin of a.
Appraise monitor
approach
axillofemoral a.
bipediculate a.
brachial artery a.
catheter-directed a.
direct transtorcular a.
endovascular embolization
femoral a.
femoral artery a.
femoral venous a.
flow-directed a.
hybrid a.
interscalene a.
mask-based a.
organ-sparing treatment a.
palpation-guided a.
particle a.
pencil-beam a.
posterior retrocrural a.
posterior transcaval a.
pterional transsylvian a.
retrograde femoral arterial a.
skull-base a.
tourniquet-directed a.
unipediculate a.
approximation
Born a.
apron
abdominal a.
lead-rubber a.
quadriceps a.
a. shield
APS
anterior pararenal space
APT
antropyloric muscle thickness

NOTES

APT *(continued)*
    attached proton test
    automatic peak tracking
APTC
    anteroposterior talocalcaneal
AQP4 expression
aquagenic
AquariusBLUE 3D imaging
AquariusNET 2D/3D medical imaging server
AquaSens FMS 1000 fluid monitoring system
aqueduct
    cerebral a.
    cochlear a.
    a. compression
    forking of sylvian a.
    gliosis of sylvian a.
    mesencephalon a.
    midbrain a.
    Monro a.
    a. stenosis
    sylvian a.
    a. of Sylvius
    ventricular a.
    vestibular a.
aqueductal
    a. CSF stroke volume
    a. forking
    a. jet
    a. obstruction
    a. occlusion
    a. stenosis
aqueous
    a. solution
    a. vein
Aquilion
    A. combined CT-fluoroscopy scanner
    A. plus V-detector CT scanner
AR
    aortic regurgitation
    atrial rate
ARA
    American Rheumatism Association
    anorectal angle
arabinsylguanosine triphosphate
arachnodactilia
arachnodactyly CHD
arachnoid
    a. brain cyst
    a. canal
    a. diverticulum
    a. fibrosis
    a. granulation
    a. granulation calcification
    a. loculation of the spine
    pia a.
    a. retrocerebellar pouch

    a. space
    a. spine cyst
    a. of uncus
    a. villi obstruction
    a. villus
arachnoidal
    a. foramen
    a. gliomatosis
arachnoidea mater encephali
arachnoiditis
    adhesive a.
    cystic a.
    fibrosing a.
Arantius
    A. canal
    A. ligament
    A. nodule
    nodulus A.
    A. ventricle
Arbeitsgemeinschaft für Osteosynthesefragen (AO)
arborescens
    lipoma a.
arborescent
arborization
    a. block
    cervical mucus a.
    a. of duct
    a. pattern
    pulmonary a.
arborize
arboroid
arc
    bregmatolambdoid a.
    nasobregmatic a.
    nasooccipital a.
    pulmonary a.
    a. radiotherapy
    reflex a.
    a. ring
    a. therapy
    a. welder's lung
arcade
    collateral a.
    a. of Frohse
    Frohse ligamentous a.
    gastroepiploic a.
    mitral a.
    septal a.
    Struthers a.
    subpleural pulmonary a.
    superficialis a.
Arcelin view
arch
    anastomotic a.
    a. angle
    anterior atlas a.
    anterior metatarsal a.
    a. of aorta abnormality

aortic a.
a. aortogram
a. aortography
articular a.
atlas a.
azygous a.
a. bar
a. of bone
carpal a.
cervical aortic a.
chimney-shaped high aortic a.
circumflex retroesophageal a.
congenital interruption of aortic a.
coracoacromial a.
cortical kidney a.
deep a.
distal aortic a.
double aortic a.
ductal a.
embryonic aortic a.
embryonic branchial a.
a. of fauces
first branchial a.
flattened a.
a. of foot
fourth branchial a.
a. fracture
Hapad metatarsal a.
hemal a.
high a.
Hillock a.
hyoid a.
hypochordal a.
hypoplastic aortic a.
keystone of calcar a.
a. length index
longitudinal a.
lung a.
medial a.
midaortic a.
mural a.
neural vertebral a.
osseocartilaginous a.
osseoligamentous a.
palmar arterial a.
plantar arterial a.
posterior metatarsal a.
posterior neural a.
posterior turn of the aortic a.
pubic a.
retroesophageal a.
right aortic a.

right-sided a.
Riolan a.
a. rupture
second branchial a.
subpubic a.
superciliary a.
superficial palmar arterial a.
target a.
tarsal a.
third branchial a.
tortuous aortic a.
transverse aortic a.
vertebral a.
Zimmerman a.
zygomatic a.
arched crest
archenteric canal
archicortex
arching of mitral valve leaflet
arch-isthmic junction
architectural
> a. alterations of bone
> a. distortion
> a. disturbance
> a. effacement
> a. pattern
> a. symmetry
architecture
> bony a.
> brain a.
> disorganized a.
> ductal a.
> foot a.
> hepatic a.
> internal a.
> intestinal villous a.
> intranodal a.
> lobular a.
> lung a.
> microstructural a.
> mural a.
> trabecular a.
archival system
arciform vein
Arco classification
arcuate
> a. artery
> a. complex
> a. crest
> a. eminence
> a. fasciculus (AF)
> a. fiber involvement

NOTES

arcuate *(continued)*
    a. ligament
    a. movement
    a. nucleus
    a. uterus
    a. vein
    a. vessel
arcuatus
    pes a.
    talipes a.
    uterus a.
ARD
    anisotropically rotational diffusion
ARDS
    acute respiratory distress syndrome
    adult respiratory distress syndrome
area
    a. of abnormal density
    amygdaloid a.
    anechoic a.
    aortic valve a. (AVA)
    arrhythmogenic a.
    Bamberger a.
    bare a.
    body surface a. (BSA)
    Broca a.
    Brodmann a.
    callosal a.
    cardiac frontal a.
    cluster of radiolucent a. (CORLA)
    cortical motor a.
    cross-sectional a. (CSA)
    cystic-malacic a.
    denervated a.
    a. of denudation
    echo-free a.
    echo-poor a.
    effective balloon-dilated a. (EBDA)
    fat-density a.
    fractional a.
    a. gastrica
    gastrohepatic bare a.
    Gorlin formula for aortic valve a.
    Gorlin formula for mitral valve a.
    Hatle method to calculate mitral
      valve a.
    hilar a.
    hot a.
    hyperechoic a.
    hypodense a.
    hypoechoic a.
    hypometabolic a.
    a. of increased radiolabeling
    infraclavicular a.
    infrahilar a.
    ischemic a.
    lenticular a.
    a. of lucency
    luminal a.

    lytic a.
    metabolically inert a.
    midsternal a.
    mitral regurgitant signal a.
    mitral valve a. (MVA)
    motor a.
    olfactory a.
    parietal association a.
    parietooccipital a.
    parietotemporal a.
    peak a.
    periaortic a.
    perihilar a.
    periportal a.
    pharyngeal a.
    photon-deficient a.
    photopenic a.
    postcricoid a.
    premotor a.
    proliferation a.
    a. prostrema
    proximal isovelocity surface a.
      (PISA)
    puboischial a.
    pulmonary valve a.
    pulmonic a.
    punched-out a.
    radiodensity a.
    radiolucent a.
    rarefied a.
    regurgitant orifice a. (ROA)
    retrocardiac a.
    retroperitoneal a.
    retrosternal a.
    Rolando a.
    sclerotic a.
    scrotal a.
    septal a.
    skip a.
    sonolucent a.
    speech a.
    stenosis a.
    subglottic a.
    subhepatic a.
    suprapubic a.
    transverse cranial a.
    tricuspid valve a.
    a. under the curve (AUC)
    valve a.
    visual word form a. (VWFA)
    water density a.
    watershed a.
    Wernicke a.
    xiphopubic a.
    zygomaticomalar a.
area/hemidiameter variation
area-length method for ejection fraction
Arelin method
areola of bone

areolar
a. connective tissue
a. plane
ARF
acute renal failure
acute respiratory failure
ArF excimer laser
argentaffinoma
argon
a. beam coagulator (ABC)
a. laser
a. laser trabeculectomy (ATL)
argon/krypton laser
argon-pumped dye laser
Argus camera
arhinencephaly
ARJ
anorectal junction
arm
Leyla a.
linebacker's a.
outrigger a.
PinPoint stereotactic a.
scanning a.
Armanni-Ebstein lesion
arm-down image
arm-lung time
armored heart
arms-up positioning
arm-up image
Arnold
A. canal
A. convolution
Arnold-Chiari
A.-C. deformity
A.-C. malformation
A.-C. syndrome
aromatic solvent-induced shift (ASIS)
ARP
adiabatic rapid passage
ARPKD
autosomal recessive polycystic kidney disease
arrangement
string-of-pearls nuclear a.
array
Acuson 5-MHz linear a.
anular a.
coil a.
convex linear a.
detector a.
electrode a.

gate a.
high-density linear a.
linear electrode a.
linear phased a.
9- to 5-MHz convex a.
multiple coil a.
NMR quadrature detection a.
parallel a.
a. processor
satellite-borne phased a. (SBPA)
silicon diode a.
a. spatial sensitivity encoding technique (ASSET)
symmetric phased a.
thin-film transistor a.
virtual a.
voxel a.
arrays
multiple-coil a.
arrest
circulatory a.
electrical circulatory a.
epiphysial a.
flow a.
growth plate a.
intermittent sinus a.
a. reaction
sinus a.
transient sinus a.
arrested circulation
arrhenoblastoma
arrhinencephaly
arrhythmia
a. circuit
a. mapping system
a. mapping system catheter
venography-related a.
arrhythmia-insensitive
a.-i. flow-sensitive alternating inversion recovery (A-FAIR)
a.-i. flow-sensitive alternating IR
arrhythmic myocardial infarct
arrhythmogenic
a. area
a. border zone
a. myocardial tissue ablation catheter
a. right ventricular cardiomyopathy
a. right ventricular dysplasia (ARVD)
arrow
A. catheter

NOTES

arrow *(continued)*
    A. Fischell EVAN Needle
    A. PICC line
    A. Twin Cath
ArrowFlex sheath
ARROWgard
    A. Blue Line catheter
    A. Blue Plus multilumen central
    venous catheter kit
arrowhead sign
Arrow-Howes multilumen catheter
Arrow-Trerotola
    A.-T. percutaneous thrombectomy
    device
    A.-T. percutaneous thrombolytic
    device
ARS
    acute radiation syndrome
ART
    algebraic reconstruction technique
    ART transducer
artefact *(var. of* artifact)
arteria, pl. **arteriae**
    a. lusoria
    a. radicularis anterior magna
    a. radicularis magna of
    Adamkiewicz
arterial
    a. access
    a. anatomy
    a. aneurysm
    a. angioma
    a. avulsion
    a. blockage
    a. brachiocephalic trunk
    a. brain anastomosis
    a. brain displacement
    a. branch
    a. bulb
    a. bypass graft
    a. calcification
    a. canal
    a. cannulation
    a. capillary
    a. circle
    a. circle of Willis
    a. collateral
    a. cone
    a. cutoff
    a. deficiency pattern
    a. degenerative disease
    a. dilatation
    a. dilatation and rupture
    a. dimension
    a. duct
    a. embolus
    a. endothelium
    a. fenestration
    a. flow-phase image

    a. gland
    a. groove
    a. hemorrhage
    a. hyperemia
    a. hypertension
    a. hypotension
    a. infusion
    a. input function (AIF)
    a. insufficiency
    a. intima
    a. invasion
    a. kinking
    a. ligament
    a. linear density
    a. lumen
    a. malformation (AM)
    a. narrowing
    a. nephrosclerosis
    a. obstruction
    a. occlusion
    a. opacification
    a. oxygen saturation
    a. patency
    a. peak systolic pressure
    a. phase
    a. plaque
    a. port catheter system
    a. portography
    a. pseudoaneurysm
    a. pulsatility
    a. pulsation artifact
    a. puncture site closure device
    a. return
    a. runoff
    a. sclerosis
    a. scrotum supply
    a. segment
    a. sheath
    a. spasm
    a. steal
    a. stenosis
    a. sump effect
    a. thrombosis
    a. tonus
    a. topography
    a. tree
    a. varix
    a. vein
    a. wall
    a. wall dissection
    a. wall thickness
    a. waveform
arterial-arterial fistula
arterialization
    hypervascular a.
    a. of venous blood
arterial-portal fistula
arteriobiliary fistula
arteriocapillary sclerosis

arteriococcygeal gland
arteriogenic impotence
arteriogram
arteriography
    abdominal visceral a.
    aortofemoral a.
    axillary a.
    balloon occlusion a.
    bilateral carotid a.
    biplane pelvic a.
    biplane quantitative coronary a.
    brachial a.
    brachiocephalic a.
    bronchial a.
    carotid cerebral a.
    catheter a.
    celiac a.
    cerebral a.
    cine coronary a.
    completion a.
    contrast a.
    coronary a.
    cortical kidney a.
    CT a.
    delayed phase of a.
    3D hepatic a.
    digital subtraction a. (DSA)
    documentary a.
    femoral runoff a.
    hepatic a.
    infrahepatic a.
    intraoperative a.
    ipsilateral antegrade a.
    Judkins coronary a.
    longitudinal a.
    lumbar a.
    mesenteric a.
    operative a.
    pancreatic a.
    pelvic a.
    percutaneous femoral a.
    peripheral a.
    postdilatation a.
    proximity a.
    pulmonary a.
    quantitative coronary a. (QCA)
    renal a.
    retrograde a.
    ring blush on cerebral a.
    runoff a.
    selective cerebral a.
    selective coronary a.
    selective visceral a.
    Sones selective coronary a.
    spinal a.
    spiral computed tomography a.
    (SCTA)
    splenic a.
    subclavian a.
    superior mesenteric a.
    transfemoral a.
    vertebral a.
    4-vessel a.
    visceral a.
    wedge a.
    x-ray a. (XRA)
arteriohepatic dysplasia
arteriolar
    a. ischemic ulcer
    a. narrowing
    a. necrosis
    a. resistance
    a. sclerosis
arteriole
    reactive a.
arteriole-capillary-venous bed
arteriolovenular bridge
arteriomyomatosis
arteriopathy
    plexogenic pulmonary a.
arterioportobiliary fistula
arterioportography
    computed tomography with a.
    (CTAP)
arteriorenal
arteriosclerosis
    calcific a.
    cerebral a.
    coronary a.
    generalized a.
    hyaline a.
    hypertensive a.
    idiopathic pulmonary a. (IPA)
    infantile a.
    intimal a.
    kidney a.
    medial a.
    Mönckeberg a.
    a. obliterans (ASO)
    obliterative a.
    obscuration a.
    obstructing embolus a.
    peripheral a.
    presenile a.

NOTES

arteriosclerosis *(continued)*
    pulmonary a.
    renal a.
    senile a.
arteriosclerotic
    a. cardiovascular disease (ASCVD)
    a. deposit
    a. heart disease (ASHD)
    a. intracranial aneurysm
    a. kidney
    a. occlusive disease
    a. peripheral vascular disease
    a. plaque
    a. thoracoabdominal aortic
      aneurysm
arteriosinusoidal penile fistula
arteriostenosis
arteriosum
    cor a.
    ligamentum a.
arteriosus
    calcified ductus a.
    ductus a.
    embryonic truncus a.
    patent ductus a. (PDA)
    persistent ductus a.
    persistent truncus a. (PTA)
    premature closure of ductus a.
    pseudotruncus a.
    railroad track ductus a.
    reversed ductus a.
    silent patent ductus a.
    truncus a.
arteriovascular calcification
arteriovenous (AV)
    a. anastomosis (AVA)
    a. brain malformation
    a. colon malformation
    a. cord malformation
    a. fistula (AVF)
    a. fistula transplant
    a. hemangioma
    a. interhemispheric angioma
    a. kidney malformation
    a. malformation (AVM)
    a. malformation nidus
    a. pressure gradient
    a. pulmonary aneurysm
    a. shunt imaging
    a. varix
arteritis, pl. **arteritides**
    carotid artery a.
    cranial granulomatous a.
    luetic a.
    Takayasu a.
    temporal granulomatous a.
artery
    A1-A5 segment of anterior
      cerebral a.

Abbott a.
abdominal aortic a.
aberrant a.
aberrant right subclavian a.
accessory middle cerebral a.
accessory right renal a.
accessory right uterine a.
Adamkiewicz a.
adrenal a.
adventitia of a.
ambient segment of posterior
  cerebral a.
angiographic corkscrew a.
angular a.
anomalous left coronary a.
anomalous left pulmonary a.
anomalous origin of a.
anomalous right coronary a.
anomalous right subclavian a.
anterior cerebral a. (ACA)
anterior choroidal a.
anterior communicating a. (ACoA,
  AcomA)
anterior descending a.
anterior-inferior cerebellar a.
  (AICA)
anterior-inferior cerebral a. (AICA)
anterior-inferior communicating a.
  (AICA)
anterior intercostal a.
anterior meningeal a.
anterior spinal a.
anterior temporal branch of
  posterior cerebral a.
anterior tibial a.
aortoiliofemoral a.
apical posterior a.
arcuate a.
ascending frontoparietal a.
ascending pharyngeal a.
atrial circumflex a.
atrioventricular node a. (AVNA)
auricular a.
axillary a.
azygos anterior cerebral a.
basal cerebral a.
basal perforating a.
basilar a.
beading of a.
bifurcation of anterior
  communicating a.
bifurcation of internal carotid a.
blocked a.
brachial a.
brachiocephalic a.
branch of a.
bronchial a.
a. bronchus ratio (ABR)
buckled innominate a.

bulbourethral a.
calcarine a.
calcific a.
callosomarginal a.
candelabra a.
cannulated a.
caroticotympanic a.
carotid a.
cavernous segment of internal
  carotid a.
C1-C5 segment of internal
  carotid a.
celiac branch a.
central a.
cerebellar a.
cerebellolabyrinthine a.
cerebral a.
cervical segment of internal
  carotid a.
CF a.
choroidal pericallosal a.
circumflex coronary a.
circumflex groove a.
colic a.
collateral circulation in compression
  of a.
common carotid a. (CCA)
common femoral a.
common hepatic a.
common iliac a.
common peroneal a.
communicating a.
complete transposition of great a.
congenital absence of pulmonary a.
congenital aneurysm of
  pulmonary a.
congenitally corrected transposition
  of great a.
contralateral a.
conus a.
a. of conus medullaris
corduroy a.
corkscrew appearance of hepatic a.
coronary a.
corrected transposition of great a.
cortical a.
costocervical a.
course of a.
cremasteric a.
CX a.
cystic a.
deep a.

deferential a.
deltoid branch of posterior tibial a.
descending septal a.
dextrotransposition of great a.
diagonal branch of a.
a. diameter
dilated pulmonary a.
diminutive interlobar right
  pulmonary a.
dissection of a.
distal circumflex marginal a.
dominant left coronary a.
dominant right coronary a.
dorsal a.
Drummond marginal a.
ductus deferens a.
duodenal a.
duplex ultrasound carotid a.
dural a.
dynamic entrapment of vertebral a.
eccentric coronary a.
ectatic carotid a.
elastic recoil of a.
en passage feeder a.
a. entrapment
epicardial coronary a.
ethmoidal a.
external carotid a. (ECA)
external iliac a.
extracranial vertebral a.
extradural a.
facial a.
falx a.
familial fibromuscular dysplasia
  of a.
feeder a.
feeding branch of a.
femoral a.
femoropopliteal a.
fenestration of basilar a.
first diagonal branch a.
first obtuse marginal a.
FP a.
friable a.
frontal a.
frontopolar a.
fusiform narrowing of a.
gastric a.
gastroduodenal a.
gastroepiploic a.
gonadal a.
helicine a.

NOTES

artery *(continued)*

hepatic a.
Heubner a.
high left main diagonal a.
hilar a.
horizontal segment of middle
  cerebral a.
hyaloid a.
hypogastric a.
idiopathic dilated pulmonary a.
ileocolic a.
iliac a.
iliofemoral a.
a. of inferior cavernous sinus
  (AICS)
inferior epigastric a.
inferior mesenteric a. (IMA)
infragastric infragenicular
  popliteal a.
infrageniculate popliteal a.
innominate a.
insular segment of middle
  cerebral a.
intercostal a.
interlobar a.
intermediate coronary a.
internal aberrant carotid a.
internal carotid a. (ICA)
internal iliac a.
internal mammary a. (IMA)
internal pudendal a.
internal thoracic a. (ITA)
intraacinar pulmonary a.
intracavernous internal carotid a.
intracerebral a.
intracranial vertebral a.
invisible main pulmonary a.
ipsilateral downstream a.
Kugel a.
a. of labyrinth
labyrinthine a.
lacrimal a.
left anterior descending a.
left atrioventricular groove a.
left circumflex coronary a.
left common carotid a.
left common femoral a.
left coronary a. (LCA)
left descending a. (LDA)
left gastric a.
left internal carotid a. (LICA)
left internal mammary a. (LIMA)
left main coronary a. (LMCA)
left pulmonary a. (LPA)
lenticulostriate a.
leptomeningeal a.
lingual a.
lumbar a.
main pulmonary a. (MPA)

mainstem coronary a.
major aorticopulmonary collateral a.
mammary a.
marginal branch of left circumflex
  coronary a.
marginal branch of right
  coronary a.
marginal circumflex a.
maxillary a.
medial plantar a.
median sacral a.
medullary a.
meningeal a.
meningohypophysial a.
mesencephalic a.
mesenteric a.
middle cerebral a. (MCA)
middle meningeal a.
M1-M5 segment of middle
  cerebral a.
multiple aortopulmonary
  collateral a. (MAPCA)
musculophrenic a.
narrowing of a.
native coronary a.
nodular induration of temporal a.
obtuse marginal coronary a.
occipital a.
occlusion of a.
OM a.
omphalomesenteric a.
opercular segment of middle
  cerebral a.
operculofrontal a.
ophthalmic a.
origin of a.
a. ostium
ovarian a. (OA)
overriding great a.
pancreaticoduodenal a.
paracentral a.
paramalleolar a.
paramedian thalamic a.
paramedian thalamopeduncular a.
parietal middle cerebral a.
parietooccipital branch of posterior
  cerebellar a.
partial transposition of great a.
patency of a.
peduncular segment of superior
  cerebellar a.
pelvic a.
penile a.
a. of Percheron
perforating a.
pericallosal a.
perimedial renal fibroplasia a.
periosteal a.
peripancreatic a.

peroneal a.
persistent primitive trigeminal a.
persistent sciatic a
petrous segment of internal
  carotid a.
pharyngeal a.
phrenic a.
pipestem a.
plantar metatarsal a.
plaque-containing a.
pontine a.
popliteal a.
posterior aorta transposition of
  great a.
posterior cerebral a. (PCA)
posterior choroidal a.
posterior circumflex humeral a.
posterior communicating a. (PCA,
  PCoA)
posterior descending a. (PDA)
posterior inferior cerebellar a.
  (PICA)
posterior intercostal a.
posterior parietal a.
posterior spinal a.
posterior temporal a.
posterior tibial a.
posterolateral spinal a.
posttemporal middle cerebral a.
P1-P4 segment of posterior
  cerebral a.
precentral a.
precommunicating segment of
  anterior cerebral a.
precommunicating segment of
  posterior cerebral a.
prefrontal a.
premammillary a.
primitive acoustic a.
primitive hypoglossal a.
primitive trigeminal a. (PTA)
profunda femoris a.
proper hepatic a. (PHA)
proximal anterior descending a.
proximal anterior tibial a.
proximal circumflex a.
proximal digital a.
proximal left anterior descending a.
proximal popliteal a.
pterygoid a.
pulmonary a. (PA)

quadrigeminal segment of posterior
  cerebral a.
radial digital a.
radicular a.
radiculomedullary a.
radiculospinal a.
radiomedullary a.
ramus intermedius a.
ramus medialis a.
recanalized a.
a. reconstitution
reconstitution of blood flow in a.
reconstitution via profunda a.
redundant carotid a.
renal a.
reperfused a.
resilient a.
retinal a.
retroesophageal right subclavian a.
right coronary a. (RCA)
right descending pulmonary a.
  (RDPA)
right femoral a.
right ileocolic a.
right inferior epigastric a.
right internal iliac a.
right internal jugular a.
right ovarian a.
right pulmonary a. (RPA)
right ventricular branch of right
  coronary a.
Riolan a.
rolandic a.
round ligament a.
scalp branch of external carotid a.
sclerotic coronary a.
segmental branch of a.
septal perforator a.
shared coronary a.
side-by-side transposition of
  great a.
single umbilical a.
sinuatrial node a.
sinus nodal a.
a. spectrum
spermatic a.
spinal a.
splenial branch of posterior
  cerebral a.
splenic a. (SA)
stapedial a.
stenotic coronary a.

NOTES

artery (*continued*)
  subclavian a.
  subcostal a.
  subscapular a.
  sudden blockage of coronary a.
  sulcocommissural a.
  superdominant left anterior
    descending a.
  superficial external pudendal a.
  superficial femoral a. (SFA)
  superficial temporal a.
  superior bronchial a.
  superior cerebellar a. (SCA)
  superior epigastric a.
  superior genicular a.
  superior intercostal a.
  superior mesenteric a. (SMA)
  superior pulmonary a.
  superior thyroid a.
  supernormal a.
  supraclinoid segment of internal
    carotid a.
  supraorbital a.
  supratrochlear a.
  surgically corrected transposition of
    the great a.
  takeoff of a.
  telencephalic ventriculofugal a.
  temporal a.
  temporooccipital a.
  terminal segment of posterior
    cerebral a.
  testicular a.
  thalamocaudate a.
  thalamogeniculate a.
  thalamoperforating a.
  thoracoacromial a.
  thoracodorsal a.
  thrombosed intraaortic a.
  thrombotic pulmonary a. (TPA)
  thyrocervical trunk of subclavian a.
  thyroid a.
  tibial a.
  translocation of coronary a.
  transposition of great a. (TGA)
  trifurcation of a.
  truncal a.
  twig of a.
  ulnar digital a.
  umbilical a. (UA)
  uterine a. (UA)
  ventriculofugal a.
  vertebral a. (VA)
  vertebrobasilar a.
  vidian a.
  visceral a.
  weakened a.
  a. of Willis
artery-aortic velocity ratio

arterylike pattern of enhancement
artery-vein-nerve bundle
arthrempyesis
arthritic talonavicular change
arthritis, pl. **arthritides**
  adult rheumatoid a.
  a. arthrogram
  Bekhterev a.
  Cedell-Magnusson classification
    of a.
  cystic rheumatoid a.
  degenerative a.
  destructive brucellar a.
  facet joint a.
  gouty a.
  hand/wrist a.
  infectious a.
  inflammatory bowel disease a.
  Jaccoud a.
  juvenile rheumatoid a. (JRA)
  Kellgren a.
  lunohamate a.
  metatarsophalangeal joint a.
  mixed rheumatoid and
    degenerative a.
  a. mutilans
  pancarpal destructive a.
  posttraumatic a.
  reactive a.
  Reiter syndrome a.
  rheumatoid a.
  septic a.
  seronegative rheumatoid a.
  a. syphilitica deformans (ASD)
  systemic juvenile rheumatoid a.
  traumatic a.
  tuberculous a.
ArthroCare Coblation-based cosmetic
  surgery system
arthrodesed digit
arthrodial cartilage
arthrogram
  arthritis a.
arthrography
  air a.
  3-compartment a.
  coronal computed tomographic a.
    (CCTA)
  CT a.
  double-contrast a.
  Gordon-Brostrom single-contrast a.
  a. imaging
  indirect MR a.
  joint a.
  magnetic resonance a.
  MR a.
  opaque a.
  saline-enhanced MR a.
  single-contrast a.

temporomandibular joint a.
vacuum a.
arthrogryposis multiplex congenita
arthroosteitis
pustulotic a.
arthropathy
Charcot a.
crystal deposition a.
dialysis a.
facet a.
gouty a.
Jaccoud a.
neuropathic a.
pyrophosphate a.
rotator cuff a.
urate a.
arthrophyte
arthroplasty
total knee a. (TKA)
arthropneumoradiography
ArthroProbe laser system
arthropyosis
arthroscintigraphy
arthroscope
Citscope disposable a.
arthroscopic decompression
arthroscopy
second-look a.
arthrosis
crystal-induced a.
a. deformans
degenerative a.
spiral a.
arthrotomography
contrast computed a.
a. of shoulder
articular
a. arch
a. calculus
a. capsule
a. cartilage
a. cartilage attenuation
a. cartilage degeneration
a. cartilage violation
a. cartilage volume
a. cortex
a. crest
a. derangement
a. disc
a. eminence
a. erosion
a. facet

a. fluid
a. fossa
a. fragment
a. gout
a. hand disorder
a. instability
intercarpal a.
a. labrum
a. lamella
a. lamella of bone
a. mass separation fracture
a. meniscus
a. metaplasia
a. network
a. pillar fracture
a. pit
a. process
a. process of vertebra
a. rheumatism
a. surface
a. tubercle
a. tubercle of temporal bone
a. vascular circle
a. wrist disorder
articularis
meniscus a.
articulated skeleton
articulating surface
articulation
acromioclavicular a.
atlantoaxial a.
calcaneocuboid a.
carpometacarpal a.
carporadial a.
condylar a.
congruent a.
costovertebral a.
DIP a.
disturbance of a.
femoral a.
fixation a.
humeroradial a.
humeroulnar a.
intercarpal a.
intermetacarpal a.
interphalangeal a.
interval a.
joint a.
metacarpophalangeal a.
occipitocervical a.
patellofemoral a.
PIP a.

NOTES

articulation (*continued*)
    pisotriquetral a.
    posterior membrane a.
    proximal interphalangeal joint a.
    radiocapitellar a.
    radiocarpal a.
    radiohumeral a.
    radiolunate a.
    radioscaphoid a.
    radioulnar a.
    sacroiliac a.
    scapuloclavicular a.
    subluxation a.
    subtalar a.
    talocalcaneal a.
    talocalcaneonavicular a.
    talonavicular a.
    tarsometatarsal a.
    thorax a.
    tibiofibular a.
    triquetropisiform a.
    zygapophysial a.
articulography
    electromagnetic a. (EMA)
artifact, artefact
    acoustic a.
    aliasing a.
    anatomy exclusion a.
    aortic motion a.
    arterial pulsation a.
    asymmetric a.
    attenuation a.
    barium a.
    baseline a.
    beam-hardening a.
    beamlike a.
    black boundary a.
    black comet a.
    blooming a.
    blur a.
    bone-hardening a.
    bounce-point a.
    bowel gas a.
    brace a.
    breast a.
    breathing a.
    broadband noise detection error a.
    bulk susceptibility a.
    calibration failure a.
    catheter impact a.
    catheter tip motion a.
    catheter tip position a.
    catheter whip a.
    center line a.
    central point a.
    chastity ring a.
    chemical shift a.
    clothing a.
    coin a.

    color Doppler twinkling a.
    comet-tail a.
    computer-generated a.
    construction a.
    corduroy a.
    crescent a.
    crinkle a.
    cross-talk effect a.
    crush a.
    CSF pulsation a.
    data-clipping detection error a.
    data spike detection error a.
    DC offset a.
    developer a.
    direct current offset a.
    dirty film a.
    double-exposure drift a.
    eddy current a.
    eddy ringing a.
    edge-boundary a.
    edge misalignment a.
    edge ringing a.
    a. effect
    effusion a.
    end-pressure a.
    entry slice phenomenon a.
    equipment a.
    external a.
    eyebrow ring a.
    faulty radiofrequency shielding a.
    ferromagnetic a.
    fingerprint mark a.
    flow effect a.
    flow-induced a.
    flow-related a.
    fluid-flow a.
    fog a.
    foldover a.
    foreign material a.
    gaseous oxygen a.
    geophagia a.
    ghosting a.
    glass eye a.
    glove phenomenon a.
    hair a.
    half-moon a.
    hardening a.
    hot-spot a.
    a. image
    image postprocessing error a.
    imaging timing a.
    imbalance of gain a.
    imbalance of phase a.
    india ink a.
    intensifying screen a.
    intravascular stent a.
    iron overload a.
    kink a.
    kissing a.

large clothing a.
large susceptibility a.
lettering a.
linear a.
lipid a.
lip ring a.
low attenuation pulsation a.
low signal intensity a.
magic angle effect a.
magnetic susceptibility a.
main magnetic field
 inhomogeneity a.
mercury a.
metallic a.
micrometallic a.
minus-density a.
mirror-image a.
misregistration a.
mitral regurgitation a.
moiré fringes a.
mosaic a.
motion a.
movement a.
muscle a.
navel ring a.
nipple ring a.
noise spike a.
nose ring a.
orbit a.
out-of-slice a.
overlying attenuation a.
pacemaker a.
pacing a.
paramagnetic a.
partial volume effect a.
patient motion a.
pellet a.
phase discontinuity a.
phase-encoding motion a.
phase-shift a.
pica a.
pick-off a.
plus-density a.
popliteal artery pulsation a.
posterior ghosting a.
processor-related a.
a. pronunciation
propagation speed a.
pseudofracture a.
pulsation a.
quadrature phase detector a.
radiofrequency overflow a.

radiofrequency spatial distribution
 problem reconstruction a.
range ambiguity a.
reconstruction a.
respiratory motion a.
reticulation a.
reverberation a.
ring-down a.
roller mark a.
scintigraphy a.
screen craze a.
side lobe a.
signal drop-out a.
skin crease a.
skin fold a.
skin lesion a.
slice overlap a.
slice profile a.
spatial misregistration a.
spatial offset image a.
split image a.
stairstep a.
star a.
stent-related a.
stimulated echo a.
streak a.
streaklike a.
subcutaneous injection of
 contrast a.
summation shadow a.
superimposition a.
suppression of heart pulsation a.
surgical a.
susceptibility a.
swallowing a.
swamp-static a.
T a.
T1-contamination a.
temporal instability a.
tongue stud a.
tree a.
truncation band a.
twinkling a.
velocity a.
venetian blind a.
view insufficiency a.
voluming a.
wheelchair a.
white noise a.
wraparound ghosting a.
wrapped a.
wrinkle a.

NOTES

artifact *(continued)*
    zebra stripe a.
    zero-fill a.
    zipper a.
artifactitious
artifactual
    a. gap
    a. lucency
artificial
    a. active acquired immunity
    a. cardiac valve
    a. fracture
    a. heart
    a. lumen narrowing
    a. lung
    a. neural network
    a. passive acquired immunity
    a. pleural effusion procedure
    a. pneumothorax
    a. radioactivity
ARTMA
    advanced real-time motion analysis
    ARTMA virtual patient technology
Artoscan
    A. MRI imaging
    A. MRI scanner
    A. MRI system
ARVD
    arrhythmogenic right ventricular
    dysplasia
Arvidsson dimension-length method for ventricular volume
aryepiglottic
    a. cyst
    a. fold
    a. fold carcinoma
    a. fold neurofibroma
    a. fold width
arytenoid
    a. cartilage
    a. sparing
arytenoidal articular surface
AS
    aortic stenosis
as
    as low as readily practicable (ALARP)
    as low as reasonably achievable (ALARA)
asbestos
    amphibole a.
    blue a.
    a. body
    brown a.
    chrysotile a.
    crocidolite a.
    a. exposure
    a. fiber
    a. pleural plaque
    serpentine a.
    white a.
asbestos-induced pleural fibrosis
asbestosis
    pulmonary a.
asbestos-related
    a.-r. lung carcinoma
    a.-r. mesothelioma
    a.-r. pleural disease
    a.-r. pleural effusion
    a.-r. pleural thickening
A-scan
    A-s. imaging
    A-s. ultrasound
ascendant follicle
ascending
    a. aorta (AA)
    a. aorta dilatation
    a. aorta hypoplasia
    a. aortic aneurysm
    a. aortography
    a. cholangitis
    a. colon
    a. contrast MR phlebogram
    a. contrast phlebography
    a. contrast phlebography imaging
    a. contrast venography
    a. frontal convolution
    a. frontoparietal (ASFP)
    a. frontoparietal artery
    a. hypoplasia of aorta
    a. lumbar vein
    a. medullary vein thrombosis
    a. parietal convolution
    a. parietal gyrus
    a. pharyngeal artery
    a. process
    a. pyelography
    a. ramus of ischium
    a. tract
    a. urography
Ascent guiding catheter
Aschoff
    A. node
    A. nodule
Aschoff-Tawara node
ascites
    chylous a.
    a. due to bile leak
    fetal a.
    gelatinous a.
    massive a.
    neonatal a.
    pancreatic a.
    urine a.
ascitic fluid
ASCVD
    arteriosclerotic cardiovascular disease
    atherosclerotic cardiovascular disease

ASD
    anterior sagittal diameter
    arthritis syphilitica deformans
    atrial septal defect
Aselli pancreas
asepsis
        medical a.
        surgical a.
aseptic necrosis
ASF
    anterior spine fusion
ASFP
    ascending frontoparietal
ASH
    asymmetric septal hypertrophy
ASHD
    arteriosclerotic heart disease
Asherson syndrome
Ashhurst-Bromer classification of ankle fracture
Ashhurst fracture classification system
ash leaf patch
Ashman
        A. index
        A. phenomenon
ASHN
    acute sclerosing hyaline necrosis
ASIC
    application-specific integrated circuit
        ASIC circuit
ASIS
    anterior-superior iliac spine
    aromatic solvent-induced shift
Askin thoracopulmonary neuroepithelial tumor
A·S·KMerit safety access kit
Ask-Upmark kidney
ASO
    arteriosclerosis obliterans
    atherosclerosis obliterans
asoma
aspect
        anterior a.
        anterolateral a.
        anteroposterior a.
        apical a.
        axial a.
        dorsal a.
        dorsolateral a.
        dorsoplantar a.
        inferior a.
        infrapatellar a.

        lateral a.
        lordotic a.
        medial a.
        mediolateral a.
        mesial a.
        plantar a.
        posterior a.
        posterolateral a.
        proximal a.
        superior a.
        superolateral a.
        ventral a.
Aspen
        A. digital ultrasound system
        A. sonography unit
        A. ultrasound system
aspergilloma
aspergillosis
        allergic bronchopulmonary a. (ABPA)
        bronchopulmonary a.
        chronic necrotizing a.
        invasive pulmonary a. (IPA)
        necrotizing a.
        noninvasive a.
        primary a.
        pulmonary a.
        saprophytic a.
        semiinvasive a.
aspergillotic
        a. aneurysm
        a. granuloma
***Aspergillus* cerebral abscess**
asphyxia
        fetal a.
        perinatal a.
asphyxial renal trauma
asphyxia-related renal necrosis
asphyxiating
        a. thoracic dysplasia
        a. thoracic dystrophy
aspiration
        barium a.
        a. biopsy
        a. biopsy needle
        breast cyst a.
        CT-guided needle a.
        endoscopic ultrasound-guided fine needle a. (EUS-FNA)
        fine-needle a.
        meconium a.
        a. of ova

NOTES

aspiration *(continued)*
    pleural fluid a.
    a. pneumonia
    a. pneumonitis
    pulmonary a.
    tracheal a.
    transbronchial needle a. (TBNA)
    transtracheal a.
    ultrasonic a.
    ultrasound-guided cyst a.
    ultrasound-guided transthoracic
      needle a.
aspirator
    Cavitron Ultrasonic Surgical A.
      (CUSA)
    Sonocut ultrasonic a.
Aspire continuous imaging system
aSpire covered stent
asplenia syndrome R
asplenic
ASPS
    alveolar soft-part sarcoma
ASPVD
    atherosclerotic peripheral vascular disease
ASR
    adrenal-spleen ratio
assay
    Accuclot D-dimer a.
    Clauss a.
    erythropoietin a.
    immunofluorimetric a.
    radiometric a.
    renal vein renin a.
assembly
    linear array-hydrophone a.
assessment
    activity a.
    aortoiliac inflow a.
    BFM arm impairment a.,
      Brunnstrom-Fugl-Meyer arm
      impairment a.
    diagnostic and therapeutic
      technology a.
    Doppler a.
    hemodynamic a.
    indicator dilution method of
      perfusion a.
    invasive a.
    in vivo stereologic a.
    lumen a.
    myocardial function a.
    noninvasive a.
    qualitative a.
    quantitative Doppler a.
    real-time a.
    regional wall motion a.
    sonographic a.
    transmetallation a.

    ultrasonic a.
    vascular a.
ASSET
    array spatial sensitivity encoding
      technique
assimilation
    atlantooccipital a.
    a. pelvis
assist
    intraaortic balloon a.
assistance
    fluoroscopic a.
Assmann
    A. focus
    A. tuberculous infiltrate
associated
    a. anomaly
    a. imaging characteristic
    a. sequestrum
association
    a. cortex of parietal lobe
    a. fiber
    VATER a.
Assurant balloon-expanded stent
AST
    above-selected threshold
astatine (At)
asterixis
asteroid body
asthmatic
    a. airway
    a. bronchitis
    a. pneumonia
astragalar bone
astragalocalcanean bone
astragalocrural bone
astragaloscaphoid bone
astragalotibial bone
astragalus
    aviator's a.
    a. bone
    fracture of a.
astroblastoma
astrocytic
    a. gliosis
    a. hamartoma
    a. proliferation
    a. tumor
astrocytoma
    anaplastic a. (AA)
    calcified a.
    cerebellar a.
    cerebral a.
    chiasmatic-hypothalamic pilocytic a.
    CNS juvenile pilocytic a.
    a. cord
    cystic pilocytic a.
    desmoplastic infantile a.
    gemistocytic a.

giant cell a.
high-grade infiltrative a.
infiltrative a.
juvenile orbital pilocytic a.
juvenile pilocytic a. (JPA)
low-grade a.
macrocystic pilocytic cerebellar a.
microcystic pilocytic cerebellar a.
multifocal anaplastic a.
orbital juvenile pilocytic a.
pilocytic a.
piloid a.
protoplasmic a.
radiation-treated a.
retinal a.
solid pilocytic a.
subependymal giant cell a.
supratentorial a.
temporoinsular a.
well-differentiated a.

astroglial tumor
asymmetric
a. appearance time
a. artifact
a. bile duct
a. breast density
a. closure of cusp
a. data sampling
a. echo
a. intrauterine growth retardation
a. IUGR
a. limb uptake
a. "look-up" table
a. lung opacity
a. negative T-wave
a. pulmonary congestion
a. septal hypertrophy (ASH)
a. signal change
a. target appearance
a. thorax

asymmetry
amplitude a.
congestive a.
facial a.
focal a.
frontal horn a.
hypertrophic a.
interhemispheric a.
left-right a.
limb-length a.
narrowing a.
septal a.

skull a.
thoracic a.
asymptomatic
a. coarctation
a. gallstone
a. hydrocephalus
a. hypertrophy
asynchronous transfer mode (ATM)
asynergic myocardium
asynergy
infarct-localized a.
left ventricular a.
regional a.
segmental a.
asystolic pause
AT
acceleration time
At
astatine
ATAI
acute traumatic aortic injury
atavistic epiphysis
ataxia
Friedreich a.
a. telangiectasia
ATB
All-Terrain Balloon
ATB PTA ablation catheter
atelectasis
absorption a.
acquired a.
acute a.
adhesive a.
apical a.
band of a.
basilar a.
bibasilar discoid a.
bronchopulmonary a.
chronic a.
cicatricial a.
compressive a.
confluent areas of a.
congenital a.
congestive a.
dependent a.
disclike a.
discoid a.
initial a.
lobar resorption a.
lobular a.
lower pulmonary lobe a.
middle pulmonary lobe a.

NOTES

atelectasis *(continued)*
    nonobstructive a.
    obstructive a.
    passive a.
    patchy a.
    peripheral parenchymal a.
    platelike a.
    postobstructive a.
    postoperative resorption a.
    primary a.
    reabsorption a.
    relaxation a.
    resorption a.
    resorptive a.
    rounded a.
    secondary a.
    segmental resorption a.
    slowly developing a.
    streak of a.
    subsegmental bibasilar a.
    subsegmental lower lobe a.
    upper pulmonary lobe a.
atelectatic
    a. asbestos pseudotumor
    a. lung
atelosteogenesis
atenna
    loopless a.
ATF
   anterior talofibular ligament
atherectomy
    directional coronary a. (DCA)
    extraction catheter a.
    percutaneous a.
    percutaneous coronary rotational a. (PCRA)
    peripheral directional a.
    retrograde a.
    rotational a. (RA)
    rotational coronary a. (RCA)
    Simpson a.
    transcutaneous extraction catheter a.
    transluminal a.
AtheroCath
    A. Bantam coronary atherectomy catheter
    DVI Simpson A.
atheroembolic renal disease
atheroembolism
atherogenesis
atherolysis
    ultrasonic a.
atherolytic
atheroma
    carotid bifurcation a.
    coral reef a.
    a. molding
    protruding a.
    resection of mobile aortic arch a.

atheromatosis
atheromatous
    a. abscess
    a. debris
    a. degeneration
    a. embolus
    a. lesion
    a. material
    a. plaque
    a. stenosis
    a. ulcer
atherosclerosis
    accelerated a.
    aortic a.
    carotid a.
    coronary a.
    extracranial carotid artery a.
    fatty streak a.
    fibrous plaque a.
    intimal a.
    intracranial carotid artery a.
    juxtarenal aortic a.
    native a.
    a. obliterans (ASO)
    pararenal aortic a.
    premature a.
    Strokes Outcome and Neuroimaging of Intracranial A. (SONIA)
    virulent a.
atherosclerotic
    a. aortic aneurysm
    a. aortic ulcer
    a. calcification
    a. cardiovascular disease (ASCVD)
    a. carotid artery disease (ACAD)
    a. change
    a. debris
    a. fatty streak
    a. lesion
    a. narrowing
    a. occlusive syndrome
    a. peripheral vascular disease (ASPVD)
    a. stenosis
atherostenosis
atherothrombotic brain infarct
AtheroTrack catheter
Athlete GT coronary guidewire
athlete's
    a. ankle
    a. heart
    a. pseudonephritis
Atkin epiphysial fracture
ATL
   argon laser trabeculectomy
    ATL HDI 5000 color Doppler
    ATL HDI 3000, 3500, 4000, 5000 ultrasound system

ATL Mark 600 real-time sector scanner
ATL Neurosector real-time scanner
ATL Ultramark 8, 9
ATL ultrasound system
atlantal ligament
Atlantis SR IVUS catheter
atlantoaxial
   a. articulation
   a. instability
   a. interval
   a. joint
   a. relationship
   a. rotary displacement
   a. rotary fixation
   a. separation
   a. subluxation
atlantodens interval (ADI)
atlantodental
atlantomastoid
atlantooccipital
   a. assimilation
   a. dislocation
   a. fusion
   a. joint
   a. junction
   a. membrane
   a. separation
atlantoodontoid
atlas
   a. anomaly
   a. arch
   bifid a.
   A. 2.0 diagnostic ultrasound system
   a. facet
   a. fracture
   Greulich and Pyle a.
   a. matching
   a. occipitalization
   a. odontoid distance
   rachischisis of a.
   split a.
   standard a.
   transverse ligament of a.
ATM
   asynchronous transfer mode
   ATM mode
atmospheric pressure
ATN
   acute tubular necrosis
   autonomous thyroid nodule

atom
   activated a.
   Bohr a.
   excited a.
   ionized a.
   labeled a.
   nuclear a.
   radioactive a.
   recoil a.
   stripped a.
   tagged a.
atomic
   a. absorption spectrophotometry
   a. absorption spectroscopy
   a. energy
   A. Energy Commission (AEC)
   a. mass unit (amu)
   a. volume
atomization
atonic
   a. esophagus
   a. ureter
   a. urinary bladder
atony, atonia
   chronic gastric a.
   collecting system a.
   gastric a.
   intestinal a.
   renal collecting system a.
   sphincter a.
   stomach a.
   urinary bladder a.
atopic
atopy
atraumatic
   a., multidirectional, bilateral radial instability (AMBRI)
   a. occlusion of vessel
atresia
   anal a.
   anorectal a.
   aortic arch a.
   aortic valve a.
   bile duct a.
   biliary a.
   bowel a.
   bronchial a.
   choanal a.
   colonic a.
   congenital biliary a.
   congenital intestinal a.
   congenital laryngeal a.

NOTES

atresia *(continued)*
    diffuse aortic a.
    duodenal a.
    esophageal a.
    external auditory canal a.
    extrahepatic biliary a. (EBA)
    familial a.
    ileal a.
    infundibular a.
    inner ear a.
    intestinal congenital a.
    intrahepatic a. (IHA)
    intrahepatic biliary a.
    laryngeal a.
    mitral valve a.
    nasopharyngeal a.
    phenobarbital biliary a.
    prepyloric a.
    pulmonary artery a.
    pulmonary valve a.
    pulmonary vein a.
    pulmonic a.
    small bowel a.
    tricuspid valve a.
    urethral a.
    valvular a.
    ventricular a.
atresic
atretic
    a. aortic segment
    a. cephalocele
    a. ovarian follicle
    a. segment
    a. tube
atria *(pl. of* atrium)
atrial
    a. activation time
    a. appendage
    a. appendage juxtaposition
    a. bigeminal rhythm
    a. canal
    a. cannulation
    a. circumflex artery
    a. complex
    a. cuff
    a. disc
    a. diverticulum of brain
    a. dome
    a. echo
    a. ectopic automatic tachycardia
    a. electrogram
    a. emptying volume
    a. fetal flutter
    a. fibrillation
    a. focus
    a. infarct
    a. inhibited (AAI)
    a. irritability

    a. isomerism
    a. kick
    a. mesenchymoma
    a. myxoma
    a. ostium primum defect
    a. partition
    a. pressure
    a. rate (AR)
    a. septal aneurysm
    a. septal defect (ASD)
    a. septal defect occlusion
    a. septal resection
    a. septostomy
    a. septum
    a. situs
    a. situs solitus
    a. standstill
    a. systole
    a. thrombosis
    a. transposition
atrialized ventricle
atrial-phase volumetric function
atriocaval junction
atriofascicular tract
atriography
    contrast left a.
    negative contrast left a.
atrio-His
    a.-H. bypass tract
    a.-H. fiber
    a.-H. pathway
atriohisian
atrioventricular (AV)
    a. anulus
    a. band
    a. block
    a. bundle
    a. canal
    a. canal defect
    a. connection
    a. gradient
    a. groove
    a. groove branch
    a. junction
    a. junction anomaly
    a. nodal bypass tract
    a. nodal node mesothelioma
    a. nodal orifice
    a. nodal ostium
    a. nodal reentry tachycardia
    a. nodal rhythm
    a. nodal septal defect
    a. nodal septum
    a. nodal valve
    a. node
    a. node artery (AVNA)
    a. septal defect (AVSD)
    a. sulcus

a. time
a. trunk
atrium, pl. **atria**
    accessory a.
    common a.
    a. dextrum cordis
    giant left a.
    high right a. (HRA)
    left a. (LA)
    low right a. (LRA)
    low septal right a.
    maximal volume of left a.
    nontrabeculated a.
    oblique vein of left a.
    a. pulmonale
    pulmonary a.
    respiratory a.
    right a. (RA)
    shunt with normal left a.
    single a.
    a. sinistrum
    a. sinistrum cordis
    stenosing ring of left a.
    thin-walled a.
    trabeculated a.
    ventricular a.
atrophic
    a. brain lesion
    a. breast
    a. cirrhosis
    a. degeneration
    a. emphysema
    a. fracture
    a. gastritis
    a. inflammation
    a. kidney
    a. nonunion
    a. pyelonephritis
    a. thrombosis
    a. villus
atrophie
    a. blanch
    a. noire
atrophied ovary
atrophy
    alveolar a.
    back pressure a.
    bone a.
    brachial a.
    brain a.
    brown a.
    cerebellar a.

cerebral surface a.
compensatory a.
compression a.
cord a.
cortical a.
degenerative a.
denervation a.
dentatorubral a.
divopontocerebellar a.
dorsum sellae a.
eccentric a.
focal a.
frontotemporal a.
gastric a.
hemisphere a.
hippocampal a.
Hoffmann a.
interstitial a.
kidney a.
lesser a.
lobar lung a.
multiple system a. (MSA)
olivopontocerebellar a.
optic nerve a.
pallidoluysian a.
pancreatic a.
parenchymatous a.
physiologic a.
postinflammatory renal a.
postischemic a.
postmenopausal uterine a.
postobstructive renal a.
primary optic a.
progressive encephalopathy with
    edema, hypsarrhythmia, and
    optic a. (PEHO)
radiation-induced cerebral a.
reflux a.
renal reflux a.
seminal vesicle a.
small bowel fold a.
spinal cord a.
spinal muscular a. (SMA)
subacute denervation a.
subcortical Sudeck osteoporotic a.
Sudeck a.
sulcal a.
temporal horn a.
vascular villous a.
villous a.
attached proton test (APT)

NOTES

attachment
   abnormal umbilical cord a.
   biopsy-guided a.
   capsular a.
   central rhomboid a.
   cerebellar a.
   commissural a.
   dural a.
   epicardial a.
   fibroosseous a.
   fibrous a.
   Hudson a.
   intimate a.
   lateral pterygoid tendinous a.
   ligamentous a.
   meniscocapsular a.
   meniscofemoral a.
   meniscotibial a.
   mesenteric a.
   Pearson a.
   peritoneal a.
   tendinous a.
   tendon-to-bone a.
   tentorium cerebelli a. (TCA)
   vascular pterygoid a.
attack
   transient ischemic a. (TIA)
attenuate
attenuated
   a. cortical surface
   a. dura
   a. image
   a. intercarpal articular cartilage
   a. ligament
   a. lumen
attenuating
attenuation
   aortic a.
   articular cartilage a.
   a. artifact
   beam a.
   breast a.
   a. coefficient
   a. compensation
   a. correction
   CT correction a.
   decreased a.
   diaphragmatic a.
   diffuse low a.
   digital beam a.
   a. effect
   expiratory a.
   focal a.
   gamma ray a.
   ground-glass a.
   hemidiaphragm a.
   a. imaging
   increased a.
   inhomogeneous a.

   a. level
   linear a.
   low a.
   a. measurement
   near-water a.
   nonuniform a.
   a. in phantom method (AIPH)
   photon a.
   a. scan
   signal a.
   tendon a.
   theophylline a.
   a. threshold
   ultrasonic a.
   a. value
   valve a.
   x-ray a.
attenuation-based on-line modulation of the tube current
attenuation-corrected image
attenuation-correction coefficient
attenuator
attic
   a. adhesion
   a. cholesteatoma
   a. recess
   a. temporal bone
attitude
   fetal a.
attritional
   a. pattern change
   a. tear
attrition rupture of tendon
ATV
   anterior terminal vein
atypical
   a. aortic valve stenosis
   a. benign fibrous histiocytoma
   a. brain teratoma
   a. bronchial pneumonia
   a. carcinoid
   a. chondrocyte
   a. ductal hyperplasia
   a. epithelium
   a. finding
   a. interstitial pneumonia
   a. lobular breast hyperplasia
   a. lobular hyperplasia (ALH)
   a. measles pneumonia
   a. medullary carcinoma
   a. meningioma
   a. primary pneumonia
   a. regenerative hyperplasia
   a. renal cyst
   a. subisthmic coarctation
   a. tuberculosis
   a. verrucous endocarditis
   a. vessel colposcopic pattern

AUC
    area under the curve
^{198}**Au colloid**
auditory
    a. canal
    a. capsule
    a. cartilage
    a. cortex
    a. ganglion
    a. pit
    a. plate
    a. process
    a. tube
    a. vein
    a. vesicle
Auerbach
    myenteric plexus of A.
Auer body
Auger
    A. effect
    A. electron
Auger-electron emitter
augmentation
    bladder a.
    a. mammoplasty
    mechanical a.
    thiol a.
augmented
    a. breast
    a. cardiac output
    a. filling
    a. filling of right ventricle
    a. pressure colostogram
    a. stroke volume
Aunt Minnie sign
aura
    A. desktop laser
    A. Laser helical scanner
    uncinate a.
aural thermometer
auricle
    left a.
    right a.
auricular
    a. artery
    a. canaliculus
    a. cartilage
    a. complex
    a. fissure
    a. ganglion
    a. ligament
    a. line

    a. lymph node
    a. muscle
    a. notch
    a. point
    a. surface
    a. triangle
    a. tubercle
    a. vein
auriculoventricular groove
Aurora
    A. dedicated breast MRI system
    A. diode-based dental laser system
    A. diode soft-tissue laser
    A. MR breast imaging system scanner
auscultatory finding
Aussies-Isseis unstable scoliosis
Austin Flint phenomenon
Auth Rotablator atherectomy catheter
autoattenuation correction method
autocalibration k-space profile
autocancellation
AutoCAT intraaortic balloon pump
autocorrelation function
Autocorrelator
autoerythrocyte sensitization syndrome
autofluorescence
autofluoroscope
    digital a.
autofusion
autogenous
    a. bone
    a. hemodialysis fistula
    a. vein
    a. vein bypass graft
autograft
    bridge a.
    double a.
autohistoradiograph
autoimmune
    a. phenomenon
    a. response
    a. sialadenitis
autologous
    a. blood clot
    a. bone marrow rescue
    a. bone marrow transplant
    a. labeled leukocyte
    a. patch graft
    a. pericardium
    a. stem-cell transplantation

NOTES

autologous (*continued*)
   a. vein graft
   a. white cell localization
automated
   a. airway tree segmentation method
   a. angle-encoder system
   a. biochemical analyzer
   a. biopsy gun
   a. biopsy system
   a. border detection by
   echocardiography
   a. cardiac flow measurement
   (ACM)
   a. cardiac flow measurement
   ultrasound
   a. cellular imaging system (ACIS)
   a. cerebral blood flow analyzer
   a. computed axial tomography
   (ACAT)
   a. gamma counter
   a. gun-needle device
   a. Hough transform
   a. infusion system
   a. large-core breast biopsy
   2.1-mm a. biopsy needle
   a. percutaneous lumbar discectomy
   (APLD)
   a. polyp detection
   a. quantification
automatic
   a. bladder
   a. collimator
   a. endoscopic system for optimal
   positioning (AESOP)
   a. exposure control (AEC)
   a. external defibrillator (AED)
   a. extraction
   a. image registration (AIR)
   a. implantable cardioverter-
   defibrillator (AICD)
   a. lumen edge segmentation
   a. lung nodule segmentation
   a. motion correction
   a. peak tracking (APT)
   a. spring-loaded biopsy device
   a. vessel tracking technique
automaticity
   sinus node a.
automotility factor
autonephrectomy
autonomic
   a. denervation
   a. insufficiency
   a. nerve block
   a. nervous system
   a. plexus
autonomous
   a. thyroid adenoma
   a. thyroid nodule (ATN)

**AutoPAP 300 QC automatic Pap
screener**
autoparenchymatous metaphysis
autoprescanning
autopsy
   digital a.
autoradiogram
autoradiograph
autoradiographic
   a. localization
   a. technique
autoradiography
   quantitative track etch a.
autoregressive moving average
autoregulation of cerebral blood flow
autosomal
   a. dominant benign form of
   osteopetrosis
   a. dominant polycystic kidney
   disease (ADPKD)
   a. recessive polycystic kidney
   disease (ARPKD)
AutoSPECT
autosplenectomy
autostereoscopic
autotomogram
autotomographic
autotomography
autotopagnosia
autotransformer formula
autotriggering software
auxiliary
   a. CT tabletop
   a. ventricle
AV
   arteriovenous
   atrioventricular
   AV node
   AV Wenckebach heart block
AVA
   advanced vessel analysis
   aortic valve area
   arteriovenous anastomosis
availability
   PET measurement of dopamine
   receptor a.
Avantx LC angiography suite
avascular
   a. bone necrosis
   a. brain mass
   a. cortical infarction necrosis
   a. femoral head necrosis
   a. fibrocartilage
   a. kidney mass
   a. necrosis (AVN)
   a. necrosis lunate
   a. renal mass
   a. tarsal scaphoid necrosis
   a. vertebral body necrosis

avascularity
AVD
    aortic valvular disease
AVE
    AVE Bridge Flexible balloon-expanded stent
    AVE Bridge SE self-expanding stent
    AVE bridge stainless steel balloon-expandable stent
    AVE stent
Avellis syndrome
Avera breast imaging system
average
    autoregressive moving a.
    a. diffusivity histogram
    a. gradient number
    number of signal a. (NSA)
    a. pixel projection (APP)
    a. positron energy
    a. radiation dose
    signal a.
    spatial average-pulse a. (SAPA)
    spatial average-temporal a. (SATA)
    spatial peak-temporal a. (SPTA)
    time-weighted a.
averaged
    number of signals a. (NSA)
averaging
    motion a.
    multiple a.
    partial volume a.
    spike a.
    volume a.
AVF
    arteriovenous fistula
    spinal dural AVF
AVG
    aortic valve gradient
aviator's astragalus
axis
    calcar a.
Aviva mammography system
AVM
    arteriovenous malformation
    intradural spinal AVM
    pial AVM
    AVM radiotherapy
AVN
    avascular necrosis
AVNA
    atrioventricular node artery

Avogadro
    A. constant
    A. law
    A. number (Λ)
    A. postulate
Avotec
    A. MR-compatible headphones
    A. MR-compatible liquid crystal display goggles
AVR
    aortic valve replacement
AVSD
    atrioventricular septal defect
avulse
avulsed
    a. fracture fragment
    a. ligament
    a. retinaculum
avulsion
    anterior labral a.
    anterior labroligamentous periosteal sleeve a. (ALPSA)
    arterial a.
    bony humeral a.
    a. chip fracture
    coracoid tip a.
    epiphysis a.
    iatrogenic a.
    lumbar root a.
    nail plate a.
    peroneus longus muscle a.
    posterior labroscapular periosteal a. (POLPSA)
    spinal nerve root a.
    spinous process a.
    a. stress fracture
    testicular artery a.
    traumatic a.
    venous a.
avulsive cortical irregularity
AVVM
    angiographically visualized vascular malformation
A-wave pressure
awl
    Mark II Kodros radiolucent a.
axes (*pl. of* axis)
axial
    a. acetabular index (AAI)
    a. angiography
    a. aspect

NOTES

axial *(continued)*
   a. BMD center with agreed joint protocol
   a. breath-hold gradient-echo cine magnetic resonance imaging
   a. carpal dislocation
   a. celloidin section
   a. cineangiography
   a. compression fracture
   a. compression injury
   a. dimension
   a. echo planar diffusion weighted imaging
   a. fat-suppressed T2-weighted image
   a. grade echo imaging
   a. gradient echo image
   a. hiatal hernia
   horizontal long a.
   a. joint dissection
   a. left anterior oblique ventriculogram
   a. loading injury
   a. load 3-part, 2-plane fracture
   a. load teardrop fracture
   a. localizer
   a. manual traction test
   multiecho a.
   a. multiplanar reformation technique
   a. musculature
   a. neuritis
   a. orientation
   a. osteomalacia
   a. plane
   a. plane imaging
   a. plate
   a. projection
   a. proton-density-weighted image
   a. radiograph
   a. resolution
   a. rotation
   a. scan
   a. sesamoid view
   a. single shot fast spin-echo
   a. skeleton
   a. slice
   a. spin density
   a. surface
   a. transabdominal image
   a. transverse tomography
   a. T1-SE protocol
   a. 0.2T T1-weighted spin-echo imaging
   a. unenhanced CT scan
   a. wall
   a. weight loading
axiale
   skeleton a.
axilla, pl. **axillae**

axillary
   a. adenopathy
   a. aneurysm
   a. arteriography
   a. artery
   a. cavity
   a. fascia
   a. fossa
   a. hematoma
   a. irradiation
   a. line
   a. lymphadenopathy
   a. lymph node (ALN)
   a. muscle
   a. node involvement
   a. node metastasis
   a. plexus
   a. pouch
   a. projection
   a. sheath
   a. space
   a. sweat gland
   a. tail of Spence
   a. tail view
   a. triangle
   a. tumor downstaging
   a. ultrasonography
   a. vein
   a. vein traumatic thrombosis
   a. vessel
axillary-axillary bypass graft
axillary-brachial bypass graft
axillary-femoral bypass graft
axillary-femorofemoral bypass graft
axillobifemoral bypass graft
axillofemoral approach
axillosubclavian vein thrombosis
axiolabiolingual plane
axiomesiodistal plane
axipetal
axis, pl. **axes**
   anatomic a.
   ankle mortise a.
   anode-cathode a.
   a. anomaly
   anteroposterior a.
   basibregmatic a.
   basicranial a.
   bimalleolar foot a.
   a. body
   bowel a.
   carpal axes
   celiac a.
   condylar a.
   coordinate a.
   cortical hinge a.
   craniocaudal a.
   craniospinal a.
   distal reference a. (DRA)

enteroinsular a.
femoral shaft a.
a. fracture
a. of heart
horizontal long a.
HPA a.
hypothalamic-pituitary a.
hypothalamic-pituitary-adrenal a.
hypothalamic-pituitary-gonadal a.
hypothalamoneurohypophysial a.
leg a.
a. ligament
long a.
longitudinal a.
mechanical a.
metatarsal a.
midpapillary short a.
normal a.
pendulous reference a. (PRA)
renal a.
single a.
spinal a.
subtalar a.
T a.
transcondylar a. (TCA)
transporionic a.
vertical a.
vertical-long a.
weightbearing a.
X a.
Y a.
Z a.
3-axis gradient coil

axon
    obliquely oriented a.
axonal
    a. cylinder
    a. shearing
    a. transport impairment
axonopathic neurogenic thoracic outlet syndrome
Ayerza syndrome
azotemic osteodystrophy
azygoesophageal
    a. line
    a. recess
azygogram
azygography
azygos
    a. anterior cerebral artery
    a. artery of vagina
    a. blood flow
    a. continuation
    a. continuation of inferior vena cava
    a. fissure
    a. hematoma cap
    a. lobe of lung
    a. lymph node
    nodus arcus venae a.
    a. vein
    a. vein distention
    a. vein enlargement
azygous arch
Azzopardi tumor

NOTES

B

B level of esophagus
B ring of esophagus
B scan
B-19036 chelate
B6 bronchus sign
BA
bone age
Ba
point Ba
BabyFace
B. 3D surface rendering accessory
B. 3D surface rendering accessory device
baby formula with ferrous sulfate contrast agent
babyPAC ventilator
Baccelli sign of pleural effusion
Bachmann
anterior internodal tract of B.
B. bundle
bacillary embolus
back
b. crease
b. pressure atrophy
b. projection
b. stroke volume
back-angle anomaly
backbleeding
backfire fracture
backflow
b. of blood
pyelolymphatic b.
pyelorenal b.
pyelotubular b.
pyelovenous b.
venous b.
backflux
background (BKG)
b. activity
b. count
b. density
b. erase
b. radiation
b. slowing
b. subtraction
b. subtraction technique
back-knee deformity
backlit digitizer
backrush of blood into left ventricle
backscatter
b. of blood
b. electron
b. factor (BSF)
b. peak

backscattered
b. power
b. radiation
back-to-back configuration
backup of blood
backward
b. curvature
b. flow
b. heart failure
backwash ileitis
bacterial
b. aneurysm
b. cholangitis
b. endocarditis
b. ependymitis
b. epiglottitis
b. nephritis
b. osteomyelitis
b. pneumonitis
b. sinusitis
b. toxin
badge
film b.
ring b.
BAE
bronchial artery embolization
Baehr-Lohlein lesion
Baer plane
Baerveldt glaucoma drainage implant
Baeyer-Villiger oxidation
Baffe anastomosis
baffled tunnel
baffle leak
BaFT
barium meal and follow-through
Bäfverstedt syndrome
bag
b. of bagassosis
balloon b.
bile b.
Tedlar b.
bagasse
bagassosis
bag of b.
BAI
basion axial interval
Baillinger
inner stripe of B.
bail-lock knee joint
baja
patella b.
baker's leg
BAK interbody fusion system
balance
mass b.

balanced
- b. circulation
- b. fast-field-echo pulse
- b. gradient
- b. hemivertebra
- b. ischemia
- b. pneumoperitoneum

balanced-gradient technique
balancing subdural hematoma
bald gastric fundus
Balint syndrome
Balkan
- B. fracture frame
- B. nephritis
- B. nephropathy

ball
- b. catcher view
- b. of foot
- fungus b.
- keratin urinary tract b.
- kidney fungus b.
- lung fungus b.
- B. method
- mobile fat b.
- myelin b.
- renal fungus b.
- sludge b.

ball-and-socket
- b.-a.-s. ankle mortise
- b.-a.-s. epiphysis
- b.-a.-s. joint

ball-catcher projection
ballerina-foot pattern
8-ball hemorrhage
ball-in-hand appearance
ballistic
- b. injury
- b. material

ballistocardiography
ball-occluder valve
ball-on-spoon appearance
balloon
- All-Terrain B. (ATB)
- b. aortoplasty
- b. atrial septostomy
- b. bag
- Bardex b.
- barium enema retention b.
- b. biliary catheter
- Blue Max high-pressure b.
- b. bronchoplasty
- b. catheter fenestration
- b. catheterization
- b. cholangiogram
- b. counterpulsation
- cryoplasty b.
- cutting b.
- b. dilatation
- b. dilator

- b. dissector
- Duralyn b.
- b. embolectomy catheter
- b. epiphysis
- b. expulsion imaging
- b. fenestration
- GuardWire distal b.
- high-pressure Blue Max b.
- b. inflation
- kissing b.
- low-compliance, fixed diameter b.
- b. mitral valvoplasty
- 7 × 40-mm percutaneous
  transluminal angioplasty b.
- nondetachable b.
- b. occlusion
- b. occlusion arteriography
- b. occlusion pulmonary angiogram
- b. occlusion tolerance test
- b. occlusive aortography
- OPTA 5 angioplasty b.
- Optiplast Centurion b.
- Penta b.
- percutaneous intraaortic b.
- PET b.
- pressure-detachable silicone b.
- b. proctogram
- b. PTA catheter
- b. pump
- radiofrequency b.
- rectal b.
- b. remodeling
- scintigraphic b.
- self-sealing latex b.
- b. tamponade
- b. test occlusion
- b. test occlusion imaging
- b. topography
- b. tuboplasty
- Ultrathin Diamond b.
- USCI PET b.
- b. valvotomy
- waist in b.
- windowed b.

ballooned
- b. floor of ventricle
- b. sella

balloon-expandable stent
ballooning
- b. degeneration
- disc b.
- b. mitral cusp
- b. of vertebral interspace

balloon-occluded
- b.-o. arterial infusion
- b.-o. transvenous obliteration

balloon-related trauma
balloon-retriever technique
balloon-shaped heart

B

2-balloon technique
balloon-tipped angiographic catheter
ball-tip microcatheter
ball-type valve
ball-valve
    b.-v. obstruction
    b.-v. thrombus
    b.-v. tumor
Baló concentric sclerosis
BALT
    bronchus-associated lymphoid tissue
Bamberger area
Bamberger-Marie disease
bamboo spine
banana
    b. fracture
    b. sign
banana-shaped uterine cavity
Bancaud phenomenon
band
    aberrant b.
    alpha frequency b.
    amnionic b.
    anogenital b.
    anterior b.
    AO tension b.
    aponeurotic b.
    b. of atelectasis
    atrioventricular b.
    b. of Broca
    Broca diagonal b.
    calf b.
    Clado b.
    conduction b.
    constriction b.
    dark Mach b.
    dense metaphysial b.
    b. of density
    b. of deossification
    echogenic b.
    external b.
    fascial b.
    fibroelastic b.
    fibromuscular b.
    fibrous b.
    free band of colon b.
    Gennari b.
    H b.
    Harris b.
    b. heterotopia
    His b.
    Hunter-Schreger b.

    hypoechoic b.
    iliotibial b.
    intercaval b.
    internal b.
    intratesticular b.
    IT b.
    Ladd b.
    Lane b.
    lateral b.
    longitudinal b.
    low signal intensity fibrous b.
    low signal intensity peripheral b.
    lucent b.
    Mach b.
    Maissiat b.
    Marlex b.
    Meckel b.
    mesocolic b.
    metaphysial lucent b.
    moderator b.
    myocardial b. (MB)
    negative Mach b.
    omental b.
    parenchymal fibrous b.
    parenchymal lung b.
    Parham-Martin b.
    parietal b.
    peritoneal b.
    posterior tracheal b.
    pretendinous b.
    radiofrequency saturation b.
    Reil b.
    saturation b.
    scar b.
    septal b.
    septomarginal b.
    septum b.
    serpiginous b.
    silicone elastomer b.
    Simonart b.
    spatial presaturation b.
    tendinous b.
    b. tenodesis
    tracheal b.
    transverse b.
    valence b.
    vascular b.
    walking saturation b.
    Z b.
bandage
    Esmarch b.
bandaletta

NOTES

bandbox resonance
bandelette
banding
    b. appearance
    halftone b.
bandlike
    b. adhesion
    b. margin
    b. shadow
bandpass filter
Bankart
    B. dislocation
    B. fracture
    B. lesion
Bannayan-Riley-Ruvalcaba syndrome
Banti syndrome
Banyan emergency kit
BAP
    brightness area product
bar
    arch b.
    Bill b.
    bony b.
    cartilaginous b.
    cecal b.
    congenital b.
    coracoclavicular b.
    cricopharyngeal b.
    b. defect
    fibrous b.
    hyoid b.
    median b.
    parallel-line-equal-space b.
    Passavant b.
    physial b.
    PLES b.
    unsegmented vertebral b.
barber-chair position
Bard
    B. CPS system
    B. Monoply reusable core biopsy
        instrument
    B. percutaneous cardiopulmonary
        support system
    B. rotary atherectomy device
    B. Safety Excalibur catheter
    B. Saxx Stent
Bardex
    B. balloon
    B. Lubricath catheter
Bardinet ligament
BardPort
    B. low-profile port
    B. MRI full size port
bare area
Baricon imaging agent
baritosis
barium
    b. artifact

    b. aspiration
    b. bolus
    double tracking of b.
    b. enema (BE)
    b. enema imaging
    b. enema retention balloon
    b. enema through colostomy
    b. enema with air contrast
    b. esophagram
    flocculation of b.
    b. fluoride
    b. fluorochloride
    b. follow-through examination
    fragmentation of b.
    high-density b.
    holdup in flow of b.
    hydrophilic nonflocculating b.
    b. injection
    b. injection through colostomy
    b. lead sulfate
    b. meal
    b. meal and follow-through (BaFT)
    b. meal study
    b. mixture
    b. pill
    b. platinocyanoide
    b. pneumoconiosis
    pocketing of b.
    b. powder
    b. radiography
    reflux of b.
    residual b.
    retained b.
    retention of b.
    b. segmentation
    sterile b.
    b. strontium sulfate
    b. sulfate ($BaSO_4$)
    b. sulfate contrast medium
    b. sulfate imaging agent
    b. suspension
    b. swallow
    b. swallow imaging
    b. titanate
    b. vaginography
barium-based fecal tagging
barium-filled colon
barium-impregnated poppet
barium-sulfate impregnated shunt
barium-water esophagram
barked injury
Barkow ligament
Barlow
    B. hip instability test
    B. syndrome
Baro-CAT imaging agent
baroreceptor
    b. bulb
    carotid bulb b.

B

Barosperse imaging agent
barotrauma
    intrapulmonary b.
    pulmonary b.
barrel chest
Barré-Lieou syndrome
barreling distortion
barrel-shaped
    b.-s. lesion
    b.-s. stone
Barrett
    B. epithelium
    B. esophagus
    B. ulcer
barrier
    anatomic b.
    b. beam
    blood-brain b. (BBB)
    blood-spinal cord b. (BSCB)
    blood-thymus b.
    contrast absorption b.
    incompetent blood-brain b.
    radiation b.
Bart abdominoperipheral angiography unit
Barth hernia
Bartholin
    B. duct
    B. gland
Barton fracture
Barton-Smith fracture
Bartter syndrome
basal
    b. angle
    b. arachnoid cistern
    b. bone
    b. cell adenoma
    b. cell carcinoma
    b. cell nevus syndrome
    b. cell papilloma
    b. cerebral artery
    b. chorda
    b. descent
    b. extension
    b. ganglia anatomy
    b. ganglia calcification
    b. ganglia of cerebellum
    b. ganglia echogenic focus
    b. ganglia hematoma
    b. ganglia infarct
    b. ganglion
    b. ganglionic change

    b. hypodense ganglia lesion
    b. joint
    b. joint of thumb
    b. lamella
    b. layer
    b. neck fracture
    b. nucleus
    b. perforating artery
    b. placenta vein
    b. plate
    b. ridge
    b. segmental bronchus
    b. short-axis slice
    b. short-axis view
    b. skull fracture
    b. sphincter
    b. surface
    b. tuberculosis
    b. vein of Rosenthal (BVR)
    b. zone
bascule
    cecal b.
base
    b. of bladder
    b. of brain
    cranial b.
    b. deficit
    b. density
    Dycal b.
    b. of finger
    b. fog
    b. of heart
    invagination skull b.
    lung b.
    b. of metacarpal
    orbital b.
    b. of phalanx
    b. projection
    respiratory disturbance of acid b.
    b. of skull (BOS)
    b. of skull foramen
    b. of thumb
    b. of toe
    ulcer b.
    b. view
baseball
    b. bat shape
    b. finger
    b. finger fracture
    b. pitcher's elbow
    b. shoulder
Basedow goiter

NOTES

91

baseline
    anthropologic b.
    anthropomorphic b.
    b. artifact
    b. of bulb
    b. chest x-ray
    b. correction
    b. mammography
    radiographic b.
    Reid b. (RBL)
    reproducible b.
    return to b.
    b. tenting
    b. view
bases (*pl. of* basis)
basial
basialis
basibregmatic axis
basic
    b. cycle length (BCL)
    b. drive cycle length (BDCL)
    b. life support (BLS)
    b. volume image analysis
basicervical fracture
basicranial axis
basicranium
basilar
    b. angiography
    b. artery
    b. artery aneurysm
    b. artery bifurcation
    b. artery ectasia
    b. artery insufficiency
    b. artery syndrome
    b. atelectasis
    b. block skull positioner
    b. cartilage
    b. cistern
    b. crest
    b. femoral neck fracture
    b. fibrosis
    b. groove
    b. impression
    b. intracerebral hemorrhage
    b. invagination
    b. line
    b. occlusion
    b. part of occipital bone
    b. pleural scarring
    b. plexus
    b. pneumonitis
    b. pneumothorax
    b. pons
    b. predominance
    b. process
    b. projection
    b. reticular opacity
    b. sinus
    b. skull fracture

    b. spine
    b. sulcus
    b. suture
    b. tip aneurysm
    b. vertebra
    b. zone infiltrate
basilar pons
basilic vein
basin
    positive node b.
basioccipital bone
basiocciput
    b. hypoplasia
    b. tumor
basion
    b. axial interval (BAI)
    b. dens interval (BDI)
basipharyngeal canal
basis, pl. **bases**
    b. imaging with selective inversion-
      prepared
    b. pontis
basisphenoid bone
basivertebral
    b. vein
    b. venous complex
basket
    b. cell
    double b.
    b. guidewire
    Highflex large stone retrieval b.
basket-like calcification
basket-weave pattern
BaSO$_4$
    barium sulfate
basophilic, basophil
    b. brain adenoma
    b. leukocyte
    b. series
basovertical projection
BAT
    B-mode acquisition and targeting
    bolus arrival time
    BAT system
Bateman classification of full-thickness
    tears
batimastat
Batson
    B. plexus
    B. vertebral brain system
battledore placenta
Battle sign
batwing
    b. appearance
    b. configuration
    b. configuration of ventricle
    b. distribution
    b. edema
    b. formation

b. lung consolidation
b. shadow
Baudelocque diameter
Bauer-Temno biopsy needle
Bauhin valve
Baumann angle
Baumgarten recess
bauxite
b. fibrosis of lung
b. pneumoconiosis
Baxter PMT device
bayesian
b. analysis
b. calculation
b. formula
b. image estimation (BIE)
b. technique
Bayes theorem
Bayle granulation
Bayler-Pinneau method
Bayliss effect
Baylor total artificial heart
Bayne
B. classification
B. classification of radial agenesis
bayonet
b. deformity
b. dislocation
b. fracture
b. fracture position
b. leg
bayoneting of fracture fragment
Bazex syndrome
BBB
blood-brain barrier
BBB breakdown
BBBB
bilateral bundle-branch block
BBC
biceps, brachialis, coracobrachialis
BBC muscles
BBD
benign breast disease
BBO
benign biliary obstruction
BBR
bundle-branch reentry
BCA
bell-clapper anomaly
B-cell
B.-c. monocytoid lymphoma
B.-c. tumor

BCI
bicaudate index
BCL
basic cycle length
BD
below diaphragm
BD Insyte Autoguard shielded
intravenous catheter
B-D
Becton-Dickinson
B-D bone marrow biopsy needle
B-D FAC scan
BDA
bile duct adenoma
BDCL
basic drive cycle length
BDI
basion dens interval
BDM
border detection method
BE
barium enema
beach-chair position
bead
b. block
immunomagnetic b.
methyl methacrylate b.
packed b.
Sephadex b.
targeting b.
bead-chain
b.-c. cystogram
b.-c. cystography
beaded
b. bile duct
b. bronchus
b. ductal dilatation
b. hepatic duct
b. necklace appearance
b. pancreatic duct
b. rib
b. septal thickening
b. septum sign
b. ureter
beading
b. of artery
rosary b.
b. of vessel
beak
dorsal talar b.
b. fracture

NOTES

beak (*continued*)
    b. ligament
    b. sign
beaked
    b. appearance
    b. cervicomedullary junction
    b. pelvis
    b. vertebra
beaking
    anterior central b.
    antral b.
    central b.
    b. of head of talus
    inferior b.
    talar b.
    talonavicular b.
    tectal b.
beaklike
    b. configuration
    b. narrowing
    b. osteophyte formation
beak-shaped nose
Beall valve
BEAM
    brain electrical activity mapping
beam
    b. attenuation
    barrier b.
    blended b.
    broad b.
    cobalt-60 b.
    cone b.
    coplanar b.
    CT scanner b.
    b. current
    b. diffraction
    electron b.
    b. energy
    b. eye view (BEV)
    fan b.
    b. filtration
    flattening filter b.
    gaussian mode profile laser b.
    b. geometry
    b. hardening
    helium ion b.
    b. intensity
    intensity-modulated photon b.
    laser b.
    lateral opposed b.
    b. limitation
    Lucite b.
    megavoltage treatment b.
    b. monitor
    monochromatic x-ray b.
    multifield b.
    narrow b.
    noncoplanar therapy b.

    open b.
    parallel-opposed b.'s
    b. pattern
    pencil electron b.
    pion b.
    b. pitch
    primary b.
    proton b.
    b. quality comparison
    radiation b.
    b. restrictor
    b. shaper
    sound b.
    b. splitter
    b. steering
    b. therapy
    useful b.
    wedged-pair b.
    x-ray b.
beam-bending magnet
beam-hardening
    b.-h. artifact
    b.-h. effect
beamlike artifact
beam-modifying device
beam's
    b. eye view (BEV)
    b. eye view dosimetry
beam-splitter
beam-splitting mirror
beam-therapy applicator
bear's
    b. claw ulcer
    b. paw hand
beat
    apex b.
    ectopic b.
    escape b.
    inferolateral displacement of
      apical b.
    ventricular capture b. (VCB)
    ventricular ectopic b. (VEB)
    ventricular premature b. (VPB)
    ventricular pseudoperfusion b.
beaten
    b. brass appearance
    b. brass skull
    b. silver appearance
    b. silver appearance of skull
Beath view
beat-knee syndrome
Beatson
    B. combined ankle angle
    B. combined ankle length
beat-to-beat variability
beaver-tail appearance
Bechthold
Beck triad
Beckwith-Wiedemann syndrome

Beclard
>B. amputation
>B. hernia

Beclere position

becquerel (Bq)

Becton-Dickinson
>B.-Dickinson (B-D)
>B.-Dickinson FAC scan

BED
>bioeffect dose
>biologically equivalent dose

bed
>arteriole-capillary-venous b.
>bladder b.
>distal tissue b.
>draining lymphatic b.
>gallbladder b.
>hepatic b.
>ipsilateral jugular lymphatic b.
>liver b.
>lumpectomy b.
>peritubular vascular b.
>portal vascular b.
>primary tumor b.
>prostatic b.
>pulmonary vascular b.
>b. of rib
>skeletal b.
>stomach b.
>tumor b.
>vascular b.

Bednar tumor

bedroom fracture

bedside radiography

beer
>b. heart
>B. law

Beevor sign

Behnken unit

Behr syndrome

BEI
>butanol-extractable iodine

Bekhterev
>B. arthritis
>B. layer

Bell
>B. brachydactyly
>B. phenomenon

bell-and-clapper deformity

bell-clapper anomaly (BCA)

2-bellied muscle

Bellini
>duct of B.
>B. ligament
>papillary duct of B.

bellomedullary

bell-shaped thorax

belly
>bubble of the b.
>b. of muscle

below diaphragm (BD)

below-knee amputation

Benassi
>B. method
>B. position

bend
>dorsal b.
>hand-shaped b.
>kneelike b.

bending fracture

Bends asbestos pleurisy

benediction posture

Benedict-Talbot body surface area method

beneficial atrial septal defect

bengal
>I-labeled rose b.

benign
>b. adrenal mass
>b. asbestos-related pleural disease
>b. biliary obstruction (BBO)
>b. biliary stricture
>b. breast calcification
>b. breast disease (BBD)
>b. cerebellar ectopia
>b. chondroblastoma
>b. conal cyst
>b. congenital Wilms tumor
>b. cortical defect
>b. duct ectasia
>b. duodenal tumor
>b. fetal hamartoma
>b. fibrous bone lesion
>b. fibrous bone tumor
>b. fibrous histiocytoma
>b. gastric ulcer
>b. infiltrate
>b. intracranial hypertension
>b. intraductal papilloma
>b. lung tumor
>b. lymphadenopathy
>b. lymphoepithelial lesion
>b. lymphoepithelial parotid tumor

NOTES

benign *(continued)*
- b. lymphoma of rectum
- b. lymphoproliferative lesion
- b. meningeal fibrosis
- b. mesenchymoma
- b. mesothelioma
- b. metastasizing leiomyoma
- b. mixed tumor parotitis
- b. neoplasm
- b. nephrosclerosis
- b. node
- b. osteoblastoma
- b. osteochondroma
- b. ovarian tumor
- b. oxyphilic adenoma
- b. papillary stenosis
- b. peptic stricture
- b. pleural fibroma
- b. prostatic hyperplasia (BPH)
- b. prostatic hypertrophy (BPH)
- b. sclerosing ductal proliferation
- b. small bowel tumor
- b. subdural effusion
- b. teratoid mediastinum tumor
- b. teratoma
- b. thymoma
- b. tracheobronchial stenosis
- b. urethral tumor
- b. vascular lesion

benign-appearing pattern
Benink tarsal index
Benjamin
- B. binocular slimline laryngoscope
- B. pediatric laryngoscope

Bennett
- B. comminuted fracture
- B. dislocation
- B. lesion

Benoist penetrometer
bent-knee pelvic tilt
benzamide imaging agent
benzocaine
benzoic
- b. acid
- b. acid contrast medium

bEPI
  blipped echo planar imaging
Berdon syndrome
Berenstein catheter
Berger interscapular amputation
Bergman
- B. fiber
- B. sign

Bergonie-Tribondeau law
beriberi heart
berkelium
Berman angiographic catheter
Bernard canal
Bernard-Horner syndrome

Bernard-Soulier syndrome
Berndt-Hardy talar dome classification
Bernoulli
- B. effect
- B. equation

Bernstein catheter
Berry
- B. aneurysm rupture
- B. ligament

Bertel
- B. method
- B. position

Bertillon cephalometer
Bertin
  column of B.
- B. ligament
  septum of B.

Bertolotti syndrome
berylliosis
  acute b.
  chronic b.
beryllium
- b. granuloma
- b. mammography x-ray tube window

best-guess technique
beta, β
- b. amyloid senile plaque
- b. angle
- b. decay
- b. detection
- b. emission
- b. emitter
- b. particle
- b. radiation
- b. ray
- b. transition

Beta-Cath
- B.-C. system
- B.-C. system catheter

beta-emitting isotope
beta-minus decay
beta-plus decay
beta-ray
- b.-r. applicator
- b.-r. ophthalmic plaque therapy
- b.-r. spectrometer

betatron
Bethesda unit
Beuren syndrome
BEV
  beam's eye view
  billion electron volt
beveled
- b. electron beam cone
- b. margin
- b. needle

bezoar

BFI
  bifrontal index
B$_O$ field variation
BFM
  Brunnstrom-Fugl-Meyer
    BFM arm impairment assessment
BGO
  $Bi_4Ge_3O_{12}$
  bismuth-germanate detector
    BGO crystal
BH4 precursor
Biad
    B. camera
    B. SPECT imaging system
Biafine RF
Bianchi nodule
bias
    lead-time b.
    length-time b.
    minimizing b.
    overdiagnostic b.
    selection b.
    self-selection b.
    time-to-treatment b.
biatrial
    b. hypertrophy
    b. myxoma
biaxial
BIB
  biliointestinal bypass
bibasally
bibasilar
    b. bronchopneumonia
    b. discoid atelectasis
Bible printer's lung
bicameral uterus
bicanalicular sphincter
BICAP
  bipolar circumactive probe
    BICAP unit
bicaudate
    b. index (BCI)
    b. ratio
bicaval cannulation
biceps
    b., brachialis, coracobrachialis (BBC)
    b., brachialis, coracobrachialis muscles
    b. brachialis tendon
    b. brachii tendon
    b. femoris muscle

    b. femoris tendon
    short head of b.
biceps-labral complex
bicerebral infarct
Bichat
    B. canal
    B. foramen
    B. ligament
    B. membrane
bicipital
    b. aponeurosis
    b. bursitis
    b. fascia
    b. groove
    b. groove view
    b. rib
    b. synovial sheath
    b. tendon
    b. tendon sheath
    b. tuberosity
bicisate
bicollis
    bicornis b.
    bicornuate b.
bicommissural aortic valve
biconcave
    b. deformity
    b. depression
    b. disc
biconcavity
bicondylar
    b. T-shaped fracture
    b. Y-shaped fracture
biconvex
bicornis
    b. bicollis
    b. uterus
bicornuate
    b. bicollis
    b. uterus
bicoronal synostosis
bicortical
    b. iliac bone
    b. screw
Bicor Top
bicristal diameter
bicuspid
    b. aortic valve
    b. atrioventricular valve
    b. valvular aortic stenosis
bicycle
    b. ergometer

NOTES

B

bicycle *(continued)*
>   b. exercise radionuclide
>   ventriculogram
>   b. exercise stress test
>   b. spoke fracture

Bid-Gd mesoporphyrine
bidirectional
>   b. cavopulmonary anastomosis
>   b. interface
>   b. shunt

BIE
>   bayesian image estimation

Biello criterion
Bielschowsky stain
Bier amputation
Bierman needle
biexponential fitting of left ventricular curve
bifascicular bundle branch block
bifemoral graft
bifid
>   b. aortic branch
>   b. atlas
>   b. biceps tendon
>   b. pelvis
>   b. pons
>   b. precordial impulse
>   b. rib
>   b. thumb deformity
>   b. ureter

bifida
>   spina b.

bifidum
>   cranium b.

bifocal manipulation with distraction
biforate uterus
bifrontal
>   b. index (BFI)
>   b. oligodendroglioma

bifurcate
bifurcated ligament
bifurcating branch
bifurcatio, pl. **bifurcationes**
>   b. aortae
>   b. aortica
>   b. carotidis
>   b. tracheae
>   b. trunci pulmonalis

bifurcation
>   b. aneurysm
>   b. of anterior communicating artery
>   b. of aorta
>   aortic b.
>   basilar artery b.
>   carotid artery b.
>   common bile duct b.
>   common carotid artery b.
>   b. graft
>   hepatic duct b.

>   iliac b.
>   b. of internal carotid artery
>   b. lesion
>   b. lymph node
>   middle cerebral artery b.
>   patent b.
>   pulmonary artery b.
>   pulmonary trunk b.
>   tracheal b.
>   b. of trunk
>   ureteral bud b.

Bigelow ligament
bigeminal
>   b. pattern
>   b. pregnancy

Bi$_4$Ge$_3$O$_{12}$ (BGO)
Bigliani
>   B. classification
>   B. and Morrison method

big rib sign
bihemispheral insult
biischial diameter
bilaminar
>   b. appearance
>   b. zone

bilateral
>   b. alteration
>   b. anterior chest bulge
>   b. arachnoid cyst
>   b. breast coil
>   b. bronchogram
>   b. bundle-branch block (BBBB)
>   b. carotid arteriography
>   b. carotid stenosis
>   b. choroid plexus cyst
>   b. consolidation
>   b. cortical necrosis
>   b. diaphragmatic elevation
>   b. diffuse increased uptake
>   b. ductal ectasia
>   b. dysplasia epiphysialis hemimelica
>   b. elevation of diaphragm
>   b. fetal chest mass
>   b. hallux valgus
>   b. hilar adenopathy
>   b. hydrocephalus
>   b. hyperlucent lung
>   b. iliac crest
>   b. iliopsoas abscess
>   b. incomplete ureteral injury
>   b. infarct
>   b. interstitial pulmonary infiltrate
>   b. intrafacetal dislocation
>   b. invasive lobular carcinoma
>   b. juxtafoveal telangiectasis
>   b. large adrenal
>   b. large kidney
>   b. left-sidedness
>   b. lesion

B

b. locked facets
b. lower lobe pneumonia
b. myocutaneous graft
b. narrowing of urinary bladder
b. obstruction
b. occlusion
b. orbital frontal cortex
b. pleural tube
b. reduction of tracer uptake
b. renal mass
b. right-sidedness
b. semicircular canal aplasia
b. small kidney
b. striopallidodentate calcinosis
b. superior parietal hypometabolism
b. superior vena cava
b. symmetry
b. upper lobe cavitary infiltrate
b. vagotomy effect
bilaterality
bilaterally symmetric
bile
b. bag
b. capillary
concentrated b.
b. concretion
b. duct
b. duct adenoma (BDA)
b. duct anastomosis
b. duct atresia
b. duct carcinoma
b. duct cystadenoma
b. duct dilatation
b. duct dyskinesia
b. duct filling defect
b. duct gas
b. duct imaging
b. duct infundibulum
b. duct lumen
b. duct multiple hamartoma
b. duct narrowing
b. duct pressure
b. duct proliferation
b. duct scan
b. duct stone
b. duct stricture
b. encrustation
b. extravasation
b. flow
b. flow obstruction
gastric reflux of b.
b. lake

b. leakage
lithogenic b.
b. papilla
b. peritonitis
b. plug
b. pulmonary embolus
b. reflux
b. reflux gastritis
b. stasis
b. tree
bileaflet valve
bile-tagged 3D magnetic resonance colonography
bilharzial
b. carcinoma
b. granuloma
bilharziasis
cardiopulmonary b.
protopulmonary b.
biliary
b. angiography
b. atresia
b. calculus
b. canal
b. cirrhosis
b. cirrhotic liver
b. colic
b. cystadenoma
b. decompression
b. dilatation
b. drainage
b. drainage catheter
b. duct
b. dyskinesia
b. dyssynergia
b. endoprosthesis
b. excretion bowel activity
b. fistula
b. hypoplasia
b. lithotripsy
b. manometry
b. microhamartoma
b. mud
b. obstruction syndrome
b. passage
b. piecemeal necrosis
b. plexus
b. saturation index
b. sludge
b. stent
b. stricture
b. structure

NOTES

biliary *(continued)*
- b. system
- b. tract
- b. tract carcinoma
- b. tract CT scan imaging
- b. tract disease
- b. tract obstruction
- b. tract stone
- b. tree
- b. tree compression
- b. tree gas
- b. tree obstruction

biliary-cutaneous fistula
biliary-duodenal
- b.-d. fistula
- b.-d. pressure gradient

biliary-enteric
- b.-e. anastomosis
- b.-e. fistula

biliary-to-bowel transit
BiliBed phototherapy system
Biligram
bilinear rotation decoupling (BIRD)
bilioenteric fistula
biliointestinal bypass (BIB)
biliopancreatic
- b. bypass
- b. diversion
- b. shunt

bilious bronchial pneumonia
bilirubinate stone
Biliscopin imaging agent
Bilivistan
Bill bar
billion electron volt (BEV)
billowing
- b. mitral valve
- b. mitral valve prolapse

Billroth
- B. I, II anastomosis
- B. I, II gastroduodenostomy
- B. I, II gastrojejunostomy

bilobate placenta
bilobed
- b. configuration
- b. gallbladder
- b. mass
- b. polypoid lesion

bilobulation
bilocular
- b. disc
- b. stomach
- b. uterus

biloculare
- cor b.

biloma
- b. in gallbladder fossa
- intrahepatic b.
- subphrenic b.

Bilopaque imaging agent
Biloptin imaging agent
bimalleolar
- b. angle
- b. ankle fracture
- b. foot axis

bimastoid line
BimOdal Slice Select (BOSS)
bimolecular
binarized image
binary
- b. digit
- b. image
- b. imaging
- b. opacity table
- b. similarity coefficient

bind
- ^{99m}Tc Ceretec b.

binding
- b. energy
- ionic b.
- receptor b.
- b. site

Bing-Horton syndrome
binned
binning
- projection b.

binocular stereoscope
Binswanger
- B. disease
- B. encephalopathy

bioabsorbable
- b. Dexon suture
- b. sheath-delivered vascular device

bioassay
- erythropoietin b.

biocavity laser
biodegradable
- b. collagen plug
- b. implant
- b. magnetic microcluster
- b. stent

BiodivYsio stent
bioeffect
- b. dose (BED)
- thermal b.

bioeffects algorithm
biograph molecular imaging system
bio-heat equation
bioimpedance
- needle-tip b.

biologic
- b. age
- b. half-life
- b. osteosynthesis
- b. variation
- b. window

B

biological
    b. half-life
    b. tissue valve
biologically equivalent dose (BED)
biology
    radiation b.
biomagnetometer
    Magnes b.
biomarker
biomechanical
    b. imbalance
    b. stress
biomechanically normal spine
biomechanics of limb-length discrepancy
biomedical radiography
biometry
    fetal b.
    longitudinal ultrasonic b.
biomicroscopy
    slit-lamp b.
    ultrasound b. (UBM)
biomodulator
biomolecular reaction
bionucleonic
biophysical
    b. limitation
    b. profile score (BPS)
BioPince needle
biopotential
    induced b.
bioprosthesis
    ProCol vascular b.
biopsy
    aspiration b.
    automated large-core breast b.
    blind b.
    bone marrow b.
    breast b.
    computerized tomography-guided
      needle b.
    core needle b.
    CT-directed b.
    CT-guided needle b.
    CT-guided percutaneous b.
    CT-guided transsternal core b.
    curved needle b.
    excisional b.
    fetal liver b.
    fetal skin b.
    fine-needle aspiration b.
    guided b.
    interactive MR-guided b.

    intramedullary tumor b.
    large-core ultrasound-guided b.
    Monopty core b.
    MRI-guided breast b.
    needle b.
    b. needle
    needle-guided excisional b.
    needle-localized breast b. (NLBB)
    percutaneous transhepatic
      endoluminal biliary b.
    percutaneous transhepatic liver b.
    percutaneous transthoracic needle b.
      (PTNB)
    placenta b.
    point-in-space stereotactic b.
    sentinel node localization and b.
    skeletal b.
    StereoGuide stereotactic needle
      core b.
    stereotactic breast b.
    stereotactic core needle b. (SCNB)
    stereotactic percutaneous needle b.
    stereotactic vacuum-assisted b.
    stereotactic vacuum-assisted
      breast b. (SVABB)
    stereotaxic core needle b.
    systematic ultrasound-guided b.
    transbronchial lung b.
    b. transducer
    transjugular liver b. (TJLB, TLB)
    transthoracic needle aspiration b.
      (TTNAB)
    ultrasound-guided anterior subcostal
      liver b.
    ultrasound-guided core b.
    ultrasound-guided large core-
      needle b.
    ultrasound-guided stereotactic b.
    ultrasound-guided vacuum-assisted b.
    vacuum-assisted b.
    vacuum-assisted core b.
    vacuum-assisted imaging-guided b.
    ventricular endomyocardial b.
    virtual bone b.
biopsy-guided attachment
Biopsys mammotome
bioptome
Biopty
    B. biopsy gun
    B. cut needle
bioreductive agent
Biosense-guided LMR

NOTES

Biosound AU3, AU4, AU5 system
BioSpec
> B. MR imaging system
> B. MR imaging system scanner

BioSphere Medical
bioterrorism exposure
Biotrack coagulation monitor
biotransformation
BioZ system
biparietal
> b. bossing
> b. diameter (BPD)
> b. lesion
> b. plane
> b. suture

biparietotemporal hypometabolism
bipartite
> b. fracture
> b. patella
> b. sesamoid bone
> b. uterus

bipartition
> facial b.

bipedal lymphangiography
bipediculate approach
bipennate muscle
bipenniform muscles of hand
biperforate
biphasic
> b. acquisition
> b. breast tumor
> b. contrast-enhanced helical CT
> b. CT
> b. curve
> b. helical CT scan
> b. injection protocol
> b. magnetic resonance

biplanar
> b. aortography
> b. MR imaging guidance
> b. transducer

biplane
> b. angiocardiography
> b. angiography
> b. axial film
> b. cineangiography
> b. cinefluorography
> b. DSA unit
> b. fluoroscopy
> b. image intensifier system
> b. left ventricular angiogram
> b. orthogonal view
> b. pelvic arteriography
> b. pelvic oblique study
> b. projection
> b. quantitative coronary
>   arteriography
> b. radiograph
> b. screening

> b. sector probe
> b. sector scanner
> b. system
> b. transesophageal echocardiography
> b. ventriculogram

bipolar
> b. circumactive probe (BICAP)
> b. gradient
> b. hip replacement
> b. lead
> b. pacemaker

BI-RADS
> Breast Imaging Reporting and Data
>   System

biramous
BIRD
> bilinear rotation decoupling

bird
> b. breeder's lung
> b. fancier's lung
> b. handler's lung

bird-beak
> b.-b. configuration or narrowing
> b.-b. esophagus
> b.-b. taper at esophagogastric
>   junction

bird-cage
> b.-c. coil designed for wrist
>   imaging
> b.-c. head coil
> b.-c. resonator
> b.-c. splint

bird-headed dwarfism
birdlike appearance
bird's
> b. eye view
> b. nest filter
> b. nest lesion

birefringent
birhinal phantosmia
birth canal
BIS
> Bispectral Index Sensor

bisacodyl tannex
bisacromial diameter
bisagittal ridge
bisection
> AP malleolar b.

biseptate
bisferious pulse rhythm
bis-gadolinium-mesoporphyrine (bis-Gd-MP)
bis-Gd-MP
> bis-gadolinium-mesoporphyrine
>   bis-Gd-MP imaging agent

bismethylamide
> gadolinium diethylenetriamine
>   pentaacetic acid b. (Gd-DTPA-BMA)

bis(methylamide)
dysprosium
diethylenetriaminepentaacetic acid-
b. (Dy-DTPA-BMA)
dysprosium DTPA-b. (Dy-DTPA-
BMA)
bismuth
b. contrast medium
b. germanate-68
b. germinate
b. injection
bismuth-germanate detector (BGO)
Bispectral Index Sensor (BIS)
1,4-bis(5-phenyloxazol-2-yl)benzene
bispinous diameter
bistephanic
bistratal
bit CT
bite
b. jumping
b. plane
biteblock
Oxyguard endoscopy b.
bitemporal diameter
bitewing (BW)
b. film
b. radiograph
bit-rate allocation
bituberous diameter
bivalve
biventricular
b. assist device (BVAD)
b. configuration
b. enlargement
b. hypertrophy
b. origin of aorta
b. support (BVS)
b. transposed aorta
bizarre
b. parosteal osteochondromatous
proliferation
b. subparosteal osteochondromatous
proliferation
Björk-Shiley heart valve
BKG
background
black
b. blood cardiac image
b. blood magnetic resonance
angiography
b. blood method
b. blood sequence

b. blood technique
b. blood T2-weighted inversion-
recovery MR imaging
b. boundary artifact
b. comet artifact
b. echo writing
b. epidermoid
b. faceted stone
b. hole
b. lung
b. lung disease
b. star breast lesion
b. and white (BW)
black-dot heel
Blackett-Healy method
Blackfan-Diamond syndrome
bladder
apex of b.
atonic urinary b.
b. augmentation
automatic b.
base of b.
b. bed
bilateral narrowing of urinary b.
b. capacity
b. carcinoma
centrally uninhibited b.
contracted b.
b. contractility study
b. contusion trauma
b. distention
b. diverticulitis
b. diverticulum
b. dome
b. dysfunction
b. endometriosis
b. exstrophy
b. flap hematoma
flat-top b.
b. floor
b. fundus
b. hemorrhage
hourglass b.
hypertrophic b.
b. hypertrophy
hypotonic b.
b. incontinence
intraperitoneal rupture of b.
kidneys, ureters, b. (KUB)
b. laceration
b. map
neck of b.

NOTES

103

bladder *(continued)*
    b. neck contracture
    b. neck position
    b. outlet obstruction
    papilloma of b.
    pear-shaped urinary b.
    b. perforation
    b. pheochromocytoma
    refluxing spastic neurogenic b.
    b. rupture
    sensory paralytic b.
    shrunken b.
    smooth-walled b.
    b. stasis
    b. stone
    teardrop b.
    thickened b.
    transurethral resection of b.
    trigone of b.
    b. tumor
    uninhibited b.
    urinary blunt trauma b.
    uvula of b.
    b. volume
    b. wall
    b. wall calcification
    b. wall thickness
BladderManager ultrasound device
bladder-prostate rhabdomyosarcoma
BladderScan ultrasound
blade
    b. bone
    b. of grass sign
    b. plate
blade-of-grass
    b.-o.-g. appearance
    b.-o.-g. osteolysis
Blake pouch
Blalock shunt
Blalock-Taussig shunt
blanch
    atrophie b.
Blancophor, blankophor
    B. FFG, SV solution
bland
    b. aortic aneurysm
    b. embolus
    b. infarct
Bland-Garland-White syndrome
blank scan
blank-to-trues ratio
BLAST
    broad-use linear acquisition speed-up
     technique
     k-t BLAST
blast chest
blastic
    b. lesion
    b. metastasis

    b. metastatic prostate carcinoma
    b. phase
    b. transformation
    b. variant
blastocytoma
blastoma
    parenchymal b.
    pleuropulmonary b.
bleb
    emphysematous b.
    oval aneurysm with b.
    ruptured emphysematous b.
    subpleural b.
Bleck metatarsus adductus classification
bleed
    anticoagulant b.
    anticoagulant-related b.
    gel b.
    herald b.
    intraparenchymal b.
    subcapsular b.
    technetium-99m pertechnetate GI b.
    technetium-99m sulfur colloid
     GI b.
    tumor-related spontaneous b.
bleeding
    first-trimester b.
    gastrointestinal b.
    hepatic b.
    b. into brain parenchyma
    intracystic b.
    intrapericardial b.
    b. lesion
    perirenal b.
    b. point
    b. polyp
    renal anticoagulant-related b.
    b. scintigraphy
    b. site
    splenic b.
    b. ulcer
    b. uterus
blended
    b. beam
    b. beam technique
blennorrhagic swelling
blepharoncus
Blesovsky syndrome
Blessig cyst
blind
    b. biopsy
    b. dimple
    b. enema
    b. foramen
    b. gut
    b. intestine
    b. loop syndrome
    b. percutaneous puncture of
     subclavian vein

b. pouch syndrome
b. segment
b. upper esophageal pouch
blink mode
blipped echo planar imaging (bEPI)
blister
    bone b.
    fracture b.
blistering lesion
Bloch
    B. equation
    B. scale
block
    air b.
    alveolar-capillary b.
    anodal b.
    anterior fascicular b.
    anterograde b.
    AP-PA skull b.
    arborization b.
    atrioventricular b.
    autonomic nerve b.
    AV Wenckebach heart b.
    bead b.
    bifascicular bundle branch b.
    bilateral bundle-branch b. (BBBB)
    bone b.
    brachial plexus b.
    bundle-branch heart b.
    celiac ganglion b.
    celiac plexus b.
    Cerrobend b.
    cervical, skull, and shoulder b.
    complete atrioventricular b. (CAVB)
    complete congenital heart b.
    complete fetal heart b.
    complete heart b. (CHB)
    conduction b.
    congenital heart b.
    congenital symptomatic AV b.
    continuous psoas compartment b.
    (CPCB)
    CT-guided superior hypogastric
      plexus b.
    custom shielding b.
    deceleration-dependent b.
    b. detector
    divisional b.
    donor heart-lung b.
    dual lateral skull b.
    entrance b.
    exit b.

false bundle-branch b.
fascicular b.
filler b.
first-degree AV b.
first-degree heart b.
fixed third-degree AV b.
ganglion impar b.
heart b.
high-grade AV b.
incomplete atrioventricular b.
  (IAVB)
incomplete heart b.
incomplete left bundle-branch b.
  (ILBBB)
incomplete right bundle-branch b.
  (IRBBB)
inflammatory heart b.
infra-His b.
intercostal nerve b.
intermittent third-degree AV b.
interventricular b.
intraatrial b.
intra-His b.
intranodal b.
intravenous b.
intraventricular b. (IVB)
intraventricular conduction b.
intraventricular heart b.
inverted-Y b.
ipsilateral bundle-branch b.
irregular b.
left anterior fascicular b. (LAFB)
left anterior hemiblock b.
left bundle-branch b. (LBBB)
lumbar sympathetic b.
mantle b.
midline mucosa-sparing b.
b. motor task
mucosa-sparing b.
multiple b.'s
b. paradigm
paroxysmal AV b.
partial heart b.
periinfarction b.
pixel b.
8×8-pixel b.
posterior fascicular b.
pseudo-AV b.
retrograde b.
right bundle-branch b. (RBBB)
second-degree AV b.
second-degree heart b.

B

NOTES

block (*continued*)
 simple b.
 sinuatrial b. (SAB)
 sinuatrial exit b.
 sinus node exit b.
 stellate ganglion b.
 subarachnoid nerve b.
 subarachnoid phenol b.
 superior hypogastric plexus b.
 suprahisian b.
 sympathetic b.
 third-degree AV b.
 third-degree heart b.
 transient AV b.
 transmission b.
 trifascicular b.
 unidirectional b.
 unifascicular b.
 ventricular b.
 ventriculoatrial b.
 b. vertebra
 vesicular b.
 Wenckebach AV b.
 Wilson b.
blockade
 celiac plexus b.
 neural b.
 sympathetic b.
blockage
 arterial b.
 bronchus b.
 pulmonary artery b.
 ventricular catheter b.
blocked
 b. artery
 b. bronchus
 b. pleurisy
 b. shunt tube
 b. vertex field
blocker
 calcium channel b.
blocker's exostosis
blocking factor
Blom-Singer tracheoesophageal fistula
blood
 arterialization of venous b.
 backflow of b.
 backscatter of b.
 backup of b.
 b. channel
 b. clearance half-time
 b. clot
 deoxygenated b.
 egress of b.
 epidural b.
 extravasated b.
 b. flow
 b. flow extraction fraction
 b. flow imaging

b. flow measurement
b. flowmetry
b. flow pattern
b. flow redistribution
b. flow reserve
b. flow response
b. flow study
b. flow velocity
hydrostatic pressure of b.
hyperattenuated b.
b. inflow
intracerebral b.
intraparenchymal b.
intraventricular b.
b. leak
left-to-right shunting of b.
marked shunting of b.
mixed venous b.
occult b.
b. oxygenation level-dependent
 (BOLD)
b. oxygenation level-dependent
 contrast agent
b. oxygenation level-dependent
 effect
b. oxygenation level-dependent-
 functional magnetic resonance
 imaging (BOLD-fMRI)
b. oxygenation level-dependent
 response
b. oxygen level-dependent contrast
 imaging
b. oxygen level-dependent fMRI
 method
parenchymal b.
b. patch
b. perfusion
b. perfusion monitor (BPM)
peripheral b.
periportal tracking of b.
b. plate thrombus
b. pool
b. pool activity
b. pool contrast agent
b. pool imaging
b. pool phase
b. pool radionuclide angiography
b. pool radionuclide
 cardioangiography
b. pool radionuclide
 echocardiography
b. pool radionuclide scan
b. pool scintigraphy
b. pressure
b. pressure response
right-to-left shunting of b.
shunted b.
b. sludge
splanchnic b.

subdural b.
upstream b.
vascular b.
venous b.
b. vessel
b. vessel invasion
b. vessel kinking
b. vessel thermography
b. vessel tumor
b. viscosity reduction
b. volume
b. volume per minute
blood-brain
b.-b. barrier (BBB)
b.-b. barrier disruption
blood-clotting mechanism
blood-containment needle
blood-filled bone sponge
bloodless
b. fluid
b. zone of necrosis
blood-spinal cord barrier (BSCB)
blood-thymus barrier
blood-to-fat contrast ratio
blood-to-myocardium
b.-t.-m. contrast ratio
b.-t.-m. contrast of TrueFISP
blood-tumor-barrier leakage
blooming
b. artifact
b. focal spot
signal b.
Blount
B. disease
B. tibia vara
blow-in fracture
blowing pneumothorax
blown-out appearance
blow-on-blow
blowout
aortic stump b.
bone lesion b.
b. bone lesion
b. fracture
b. lesion of posterior vertebral element
b. view projection
BLS
basic life support
BLS techniques
blue
b. asbestos

B. Max high-pressure balloon
B. Max high-pressure reinforced polyethylene balloon catheter
b. rubber-bleb nevus syndrome
blueberry muffin syndrome
blue-digit syndrome
blue-toe syndrome
Blumberg sign
Blumenbach
B. clivus
B. plane
Blumensaat line
Blumenthal lesion
Blumer rectal shelf
blunt
b. border of lung
b. chest trauma
b. gastrointestinal trauma
b. injury
b. pancreatic trauma
b. trauma gallbladder
b. trauma kidney
blunted
b. ejection fraction
b. mucosal fold
b. posterior sulcus
blunt-end sialogram needle
blunting
calyceal b.
costophrenic angle b.
b. of costovertebral angle
haustral b.
b. of valve
blur
b. artifact
focal spot b.
geometric b.
motion b.
object-plane b.
blurred-image tomogram
blurring
b. of aortic knob
b. of costophrenic angle
b. of disc margin
radial b.
radiographic b.
blurting
blush
angiographic b.
choroid plexus b.
cortical b.
b. of dye on angiography

NOTES

B

blush *(continued)*
    kidney papillary b.
    marrow b.
    myocardial b.
    b. on imaging
    periventricular b.
    physiologic uterine b.
    pregnancy-induced uterine b.
    renal parenchymal b.
    tumor b.
    vascular b.
BMC
    bone mineral content
BMD
    bone mineral density
BMIPP SPECT scan imaging
B-mode
    B-m. acquisition and targeting
      (BAT)
    B-m. brightness modulation scan
    B-m. display
    B-m. echocardiography
    B-m. echography
    B-m. imaging
    longitudinal B-m.
    pseudocolor B-m.
    B-m. ultrascan
    B-m. ultrasound
BMP
    bone marrow pressure
BMS
    bulk magnetic susceptibility
Bo
    Bolton point (craniometric)
    Bo field mapping
board
    b. angle
    immobilizer b.
    right-angled isosceles triangle b.
boat-shaped heart
Bochdalek
    B. foramen
    B. gap
    B. hernia
    B. muscle
body
    angularis b.
    anococcygeal b.
    apoptic b.
    asbestos b.
    asteroid b.
    b. atomic number
    Auer b.
    axis b.
    b. background activity
    b. box plethysmography
    b. burden
    calcific round b.
    calcified pineal b.

cancer b.
carotid b.
caudate b.
b. cavity
coccygeal b.
b. coil
b. coil imaging
b. composition measurement
compressed b.
b. contour orbit
dense b.
diffuse low signal replacement of
    vertebral b.
elementary b.
embryoid b.
enlargement of vertebral b.
b. of epididymis
esophageal b.
b. of femur
ferruginous b.
flat vertebral b.
foreign b. (FB)
free b.
b. of gallbladder
geniculate b.
glenoid labral ovoid b.
b. glomus
b. habitus
H-shaped vertebral b.
b. interface
intraarticular loose b.
intraluminal foreign b.
intraocular foreign b.
intravascular foreign b.
juxtarestiform b.
ketone b.
lamellar b.
lateral geniculate b.
loose intraarticular b.
Luys b.
malpighian b.
mamillary b.
b. mass index
Masson b.
b. mechanics
medial geniculate b.
metallic foreign b. (MFB)
Michaelis-Gutmann b.
Mott b.
multilaminar b.
b. of nail
navicular b.
nonradiopaque foreign b.
no-threshold b.
opaque foreign b.
ossified b.
osteochondral loose b.
osteochondrotic loose b.
pacchionian b.

b. of the pancreas
pearly b.
pharmacoradiologic disimpaction of
  esophageal foreign b.
Pick b.
picture frame pattern of
  vertebral b.
pineal b.
psammoma b.
radiopaque foreign b.
restiform b.
retained foreign b.
rhinencephalic mamillary b.
rice joint b.
Russell b.
scalloping of margin of
  vertebral b.
b. scanning
b. of scapula
scapular b.
Schaumann b.
Schiller-Duval b.
b. section radiography
b. section radiography imaging
Seidelin b.
small vertebral b.
squared vertebral b.
b. stalk
b. of the stomach
b. surface area (BSA)
b. surface area calculation
b. surface laplacian mapping
  (BSLM)
b. surface potential mapping
Symington b.
threshold b.
thyroid psammoma b.
tracheobronchial foreign b.
trapezoid b.
uterine b.
b. of uterus
Verocay b.
b. of vertebra
vesalianum of vertebral b.
b. wall
Weibel-Palade b.
b. weight
Zuckerkandl b.
body-coil-based contrast-enchanced MRA
body-coil MRI
Boehler angle
Boerhaave syndrome

boggy
  b. synovitis
  b. synovium
Bogros space
Böhler angle
Bohr
  B. atom
  B. effect
  B. equation
  B. magneton
  B. radius
  B. theory
BOLD
  blood oxygenation level-dependent
    BOLD contrast functional MRI
    BOLD contrast imaging
    BOLD effect
    BOLD response
    BOLD signal
    BOLD time course change
BOLD-fMRI
  blood oxygenation level-dependent-
    functional magnetic resonance imaging
bolster
  angular b.
  breast b.
  b. finger
  knee arthrography b.
Bolton
  B. plane
  B. point (craniometric) (Bo)
  B. triangle
Bolton-nasion
  B.-n. line
  B.-n. plane
Boltzmann
  B. distribution
  B. equation
bolus
  air b.
  b. arrival time (BAT)
  barium b.
  CARE b.
  b. challenge imaging
  b. challenge test
  b. chase
  b. chase image
  b. chase imaging technique
  b. chase technique
  contrast b.
  b. contrast enhancement
  b. dose

NOTES

bolus *(continued)*
dynamic b.
electron b.
intravenous b.
b. intravenous injection
marshmallow b.
b. passage perfusion measurement
radioactive b.
simple b.
special b.
b. tagging
test b.
b. timing
tracer b.
b. tracking
b. transit
water b.
bolus-chase stepping-table 3D MRA
bombard
bombardment
alpha particle b.
end of saturated b. (EOSB)
neutron b.
bond
valence b.
wedge b.
bone (os)
b. abscess
accessory multangular b.
accessory navicular b.
accessory sesamoid b.
acetabular b.
acromial b.
adamantinoma of long b.
b. age (BA)
b. age imaging
b. age ratio
alar b.
Albrecht b.
b. algorithm
b. allograft
alveolar supporting b.
b. angioblastoma
b. angiosarcoma
ankle b.
anvil b.
apex of petrous portion of
  temporal b.
arch of b.
architectural alterations of b.
areola of b.
articular lamella of b.
articular tubercle of temporal b.
astragalar b.
astragalocalcanean b.
astragalocrural b.
astragaloscaphoid b.
astragalotibial b.
astragalus b.

b. atrophy
attic temporal b.
autogenous b.
basal b.
basilar part of occipital b.
basioccipital b.
basisphenoid b.
bicortical iliac b.
bipartite sesamoid b.
blade b.
b. blister
b. block
bowed long b.
breast b.
bregmatic b.
brittle b.
bundle b.
calcaneal b.
calvarial b.
b. canaliculus
cancellated b.
candle-wax appearance of b.
cannon b.
b. capillary hemangioma
capitate b.
b. carcinoma
carpal navicular b.
cartilage b.
cavalry b.
b. cement
b. center
central b.
chalky b.
cheek b.
chevron b.
b. chip
b. chloroma
b. coccidioidomycosis
coccygeal b.
coccyx b.
coffin b.
compact b.
b. computed tomography
condylar part of occipital b.
continuity of b.
b. contusion
convoluted b.
b. core
b. cortex
cortical b.
corticocancellous b.
costal b.
coxal b.
cranial b.
cribriform b.
b. crisis
cubital b.
cuboid b.
cuneiform b.

dancer's b.
dead b.
b. debris
b. demineralization
dense structure of b.
b. densitometer
b. densitometry
b. density imaging
b. density measurement
b. density study
depression of nasal b.
dermal b.
detecting Down syndrome by
  ultrasound of the nose b.
devitalized allogeneic b.
devitalized portion of b.
diastasis of cranial b.
dimple of b.
displaced fragment of b.
dorsal talonavicular b.
b. dysplasia
b. dystrophy
eburnated b.
b. echinococcosis
b. end
endochondral b.
entrapped plantar sesamoid b.
epactal b.
epihyal b.
epihyoid b.
epiphysis b.
epipteric b.
episternal b.
erosion of epiphysial b.
ethmoid b.
exoccipital b.
exoccipital part of occipital b.
b. expansion
facial b.
femoral b.
fencer's b.
b. fibrosarcoma
fibular sesamoid b.
first cuneiform b.
b. fixation device
b. fixation plate
flank b.
b. flap
flat b.
b. formation
b. formation cloaca
fourth turbinated b.

b. fracture
fracture running length of b.
b. fragment
frontal b.
Goethe b.
gracile b.
b. graft
greater multangular b.
great toe sesamoid b.
growth center of b.
b. growth stimulator
hallux sesamoid b.
hamate b.
b. hardening
heel b.
heterotopic b.
hip b.
b. histology
b. histomorphometry
hollow b.
hooked b.
humeral b.
hyoid b.
hyperplastic b.
b. hypertrophy
iliac cancellous b.
immature b.
b. implant
b. implantation cyst
incisive b.
incomplete fracture of b.
incus b.
b. infarct
infected b.
inferior turbinated b.
inflammation of b.
b. ingrowth
b. injury radiation
inner table of frontal b.
innominate b.
intermaxillary b.
intermediate cuneiform b.
interparietal b.
b. interstice
intracartilaginous b.
intrachondral b.
intramembranous b.
irregular b.
ischial b.
b. island
jaw b.
knuckle b.

NOTES

bone *(continued)*
  lacrimal b.
  b. lacuna
  lamellar b.
  lateral part of occipital b.
  lateral sesamoid b.
  b. length imaging
  b. length study
  lenticular b.
  lentiform b.
  b. lesion apophysis
  b. lesion blowout
  b. lesion epiphysis
  b. lesion of rib
  b. and limb growth velocity ratio
  lingual b.
  b. lipoma
  long b.
  long axis of b.
  lunate b.
  lunocapitate b.
  luxated b.
  b. lymphoma
  malar b.
  malignant fibrous histiocytoma
    of b. (MFH-B)
  malleolus b.
  marble b.
  b. marrow
  b. marrow agent
  b. marrow biopsy
  b. marrow boundary
  b. marrow depression
  b. marrow dose
  b. marrow edema
  b. marrow edema pattern on MR
    imaging
  b. marrow edema syndrome
  b. marrow embolus
  b. marrow fibrosis
  b. marrow hypoplasia
  b. marrow infiltrate
  b. marrow lesion
  b. marrow lymphoid hyperplasia
  b. marrow microenvironment
  b. marrow myeloid precursor
  b. marrow pressure (BMP)
  b. marrow purging
  b. marrow relapse
  b. marrow rescue
  b. marrow scan
  b. marrow scintigraphy
  b. marrow stroma
  b. marrow toxicity
  b. marrow transplant
  b. mastocytosis
  mastoid b.
  b. maturation
  mature b.

  maxillary b.
  medial cuneiform b.
  medial sesamoid b.
  medullary b.
  membrane of b.
  mesocuneiform b.
  metacarpal b.
  b. metastasis
  metatarsal b.
  b. microarchitecture
  middle cuneiform b.
  middle turbinate b.
  b. mineral content (BMC)
  b. mineral content imaging
  b. mineral content study
  b. mineral density (BMD)
  b. mineral immobilization
  b. mineralization
  morcellized b.
  b. morphogenetic activity
  mortise of b.
  multangular b.
  nasal b.
  navicular b.
  b. neck
  necrotic b.
  b. neoplasm
  Nicoll b.
  occipital b.
  odontoid b.
  omovertebral b.
  orbicular b.
  orbital b.
  orbitosphenoidal b.
  os calcis b.
  osteonal b.
  osteopenic b.
  osteoporosis of b.
  osteoporotic b.
  b. overdevelopment
  b. oxalosis
  Paget disease of b.
  pagetoid b.
  palatine b.
  parietal b.
  b. particle
  pedal b.
  pelvic b.
  perichondral b.
  periosteal b.
  periotic b.
  peroneal b.
  petrosal b.
  petrous temporal b.
  phalangeal b.
  phantom b.
  b. phase image
  b. phase imaging
  b. pinhole

B

Pirie b.
pisiform b.
b. plug
pneumatic b.
pole of scaphoid b.
porous b.
postsphenoid b.
posttraumatic atrophy of b.
postulnar b.
b. powder
preinterparietal b.
premaxillary b.
presphenoid b.
primitive b.
proliferation of b.
prominence of b.
pterygoid b.
pubic b.
b. pulley
pyramidal b.
quadrilateral b.
b. quantitative CT (BQCT)
radial b.
b. radiation absorption
Recklinghausen disease of b.
refractured b.
b. remodeling
replacement b.
b. resorption
reticulated b.
rider's b.
ring-of-b.
rudimentary b.
sacral b.
b. sarcoidosis
scaphoid b.
scapular b.
b. scintiscan imaging
sclerosed temporal b.
b. screw
scroll b.
second cuneiform b.
b. seeker
semilunar b.
septal b.
sesamoid b.
b. shaft
shank b.
shin b.
short b.
sieve b.
b. sliver

solid b.
sphenoid b.
sphenoidal turbinated b.
splintered b.
spoke b.
spongy b.
b. spur
squamous part of frontal b.
squamous part of occipital b.
squamous part of temporal b.
stirrup b.
b. strut
subchondral b.
subperiosteal new b.
b. substance
b. substitute
superior turbinated b.
supernumerary sesamoid b.
supracollicular spike of cortical b.
suprainterparietal b.
supraoccipital b.
suprapharyngeal b.
suprasternal b.
supreme turbinate b.
b. surface
b. survey
sutural b.
b. syphilis
tail b.
talus b.
target b.
tarsal b.
temporal b.
thick b.
thigh b.
thoracic b.
tibia b.
tibial sesamoid b.
trabecular b.
trabeculated b.
trapezium b.
trapezoid b.
triangular b.
triquetral b.
b. tuberculosis
tuberculous b.
tubular b.
b. tumor
b. tumor aggressiveness
tumor-bearing b.
b. tumor matrix
b. tumor scalloping

NOTES

bone *(continued)*
    turbinate b.
    b. turnover
    tympanic b.
    ulnar b.
    ulnar sesamoid b.
    unciform b.
    b. unloading
    upper jaw b.
    vascular b.
    vesalian b.
    vomer b.
    weightbearing b.
    b. window
    wing of sphenoid b.
    wormian b.
    woven b.
    wrist triquetrum b.
    b. xanthogranuloma
    xiphoid b.
    zygomatic b.
bone-air interface
bone-chip allograft
bone-detail algorithm
bone-forming
    b.-f. bone tumor
    b.-f. sarcoma
bone-hardening artifact
bone-implant interface
bonelet
bone-on-bone contact
bone-tendon-bone graft
bone-tendon exposure
bone-to-bone apposition
bone-within-bone
    b.-w.-b. appearance
    b.-w.-b. vertebra
Bonferroni adjustment
bonnet
    gluteal b.
Bonopty needle system
bony
    b. abnormality
    b. alignment
    b. ankylosis
    b. apposition
    b. architecture
    b. bar
    b. bridge
    b. callus
    b. callus formation
    b. change
    b. coalition
    b. contusion
    b. cortex interruption
    b. decompression
    b. defect
    b. deformity

    b. degeneration
    b. deposit
    b. destruction
    b. disruption
    b. eburnation
    b. encroachment
    b. enlargement
    b. erosion
    b. excrescence
    b. exostosis
    b. fossa
    b. fusion
    b. glenoid marrow fat
    b. glenoid rim
    b. healing
    b. heart
    b. humeral avulsion
    b. hyperostosis
    b. island
    b. labyrinth
    b. lysis
    b. necrosis
    b. nonunion
    b. orbit
    b. osteophyte
    b. overgrowth
    b. pelvis
    b. plate
    b. process
    b. projection from vertebra
    b. proliferation
    b. prominence
    b. protuberance
    b. rarefaction
    b. reabsorption
    b. remodeling
    b. ridge
    b. sclerosis
    b. semicircular canal
    b. sequestrum
    b. shadow
    b. skeleton
    b. skull landmark
    b. spicule
    b. spurring
    b. stability
    b. structure
    b. suture
    b. thoracic cage
    b. thorax
    b. tissue
    b. trabecula
    b. trabecular injury
    b. trabecular pattern
    b. tuft of finger
    b. union
    b. vertebra projection
boomerang tendon

BOOP
bronchiolitis obliterans with organizing
pneumonia
**Boorman classification of gastric
carcinoma**
boost
brachytherapy b.
b. dose
electron-beam b.
GK-SRS b.
interstitial b.
b. therapy
booster heart
boot-shaped heart
boot-top fracture
border
anterior b.
antimesenteric b.
cardiac b.
ciliated b.
corticated b.
crescentic b.
b. detection method (BDM)
diaphragmatic b.
echocardiographic automated b.
gradually tapering b.
heart b.
inferior b.
interosseous b.
irregular b.
lateral b.
left sternal b. (LSB)
lobulated b.
lower sternal b. (LSB)
medial b.
mediastinal b.
mesenteric b.
midleft sternal b.
overhanging b.
peripheral b.
posterior b.
rounded convex b.
scalloped b.
scapulovertebral b.
sclerotic b.
serpiginous low signal intensity b.
shagging of cardiac b.
shaggy heart b.
smooth b.
spiculated b.
sternal b.
sternocleidomastoid muscle b.

straight anterior vertebral b.
superior b.
tapering b.
thin b.
upper sternal b.
well-defined b.
b. zone
borderline
b. cardiomegaly
b. heart size
b. malignancy
b. normal
Borell and Fernström method
Borg scale of treadmill exertion
Born
B. approximation
B. method
boron
b. counter
b. neutron capture
BOS
base of skull
Bosniak classification
BOSS
BimOdal Slice Select
boss
carpal b.
parietal b.
bossa
bosselated
b. stone
b. surface
bosselation
bossing
biparietal b.
frontal b.
occipital b.
Bosworth
B. bone peg insertion
B. fracture
Botallo
B. duct
B. foramen
B. ligament
pervious duct of B.
both-bone fracture
both-column fracture
botryoid
b. rhabdomyosarcoma
b. sarcoma
Böttcher canal

NOTES

B

115

Bouchard
    B. disease
    B. node
bougienage technique
Bouillaud disease
bounce-point artifact
bouncing
    ligamentous b.
bound
    Cramer-Rao minimum variance b.
      (CR-MVB)
    b. electron
boundary
    air/bone/tissue b.
    bone marrow b.
    b. edge
    horizontal b.
    b. layer
    tumor b.
bouquet
    fixed shaped coplanar or nonplanar
      radiation beam b.
Bourgery ligament
Bourneville disease
Bourneville-Pringle disease
Boutin thoracoscope
boutonnière
    b. deformity
    b. dislocation
Bouveret syndrome
Bovero muscle
bovine heart xenograft
Bowditch effect
bowed
    b. legs
    b. long bone
    b. micromelia
bowel
    aganglionic b.
    apple-peel b.
    b. atresia
    b. axis
    b. and bladder dysfunction
    b. caliber
    b. carcinoma
    b. content
    b. continuity
    corkscrew appearance of small b.
    dead b.
    dilated dry small b.
    dilated fetal b.
    dilated loops of b.
    dilated wet small b.
    distal small b.
    b. distention
    echogenic fetal b.
    fixed segment of b.
    fluid-filled loop of b.
    free-floating loop of b.

    functional immaturity of b.
    b. gangrene
    b. gas
    b. gas artifact
    b. gas pattern
    herniated b.
    hoop-shaped loops of b.
    b. incontinence
    b. infarct
    b. intussusception
    ischemic b.
    kinked b.
    large b.
    b. loop
    b. loop air
    b. loop angulation
    b. loop dilatation
    b. loop fixation
    b. lumen
    b. migration
    b. motion
    b. movement
    b. mucosa
    multiple loops of small b.
    multiple stenotic lesions of
      small b.
    b. necrosis
    normal caliber b.
    b. obstruction
    b. perforation
    b. peristalsis
    pleating of small b.
    b. preparation
    proximal small b.
    b. pseudoobstruction
    ribbon b.
    b. secretion
    b. serosal endometrial implant
    shaggy contour to b.
    b. shock
    small b.
    b. sound
    b. spasm
    b. stenosis
    b. stoma
    strangulated b.
    b. wall
    b. wall hematoma
    b. wall penetration
bowel-to-bowel anastomosis
bowing
    anterior tibial b.
    b. deformity
    b. fracture
    b. of mitral valve leaflet
    b. of tendon
bowleg
bowler hat sign
bowler's thumb

Bowman
>B. capsule
>B. disc
>B. muscle
>B. probe
>B. space

bowstring
>b. sign
>b. tear

bowstringing
bow-tie sign
box
>carpal b.
>ligamentous b.
>mammographic view b.
>shadow b.
>view b.

box-and-whisker plot
boxer knuckle
boxer's
>b. elbow
>b. fracture

boxlike cardiomegaly
Boyd
>B. ankle amputation
>B. formula
>B. perforating vein
>B. type II fracture

Boyden
>B. sphincter
>B. test meal

Boyd-Griffin trochanteric fracture classification
Bozzolo sign
BP
>bronchopleural
>bronchopulmonary
>bypass
>>BP fistula
>>Imagent BP
>>BP MR

BPD
>biparietal diameter
>bronchopulmonary dysplasia

BPFM
>bronchopulmonary foregut malformation

BPH
>benign prostatic hyperplasia
>benign prostatic hypertrophy

BPM
>blood perfusion monitor

BPS
>biophysical profile score
>>fetal BPS

Bq
>becquerel

BQCT
>bone quantitative CT

Bracco A-C-D solution
brace artifact
bracelet
>^{89}Sr b.

brachia (*pl. of* brachium)
brachial
>b. arteriography
>b. artery
>b. artery approach
>b. artery compression
>b. artery cuff pressure
>b. artery end-diastolic pressure
>b. artery peak systolic pressure
>b. artery pulse pressure
>b. atrophy
>b. fascia
>b. lymph node
>b. plexus
>b. plexus birth injury
>b. plexus block
>b. plexus compression
>b. plexus infiltrate
>b. plexus neuritis
>b. plexus tendon
>b. pulse
>b. vein

brachial-basilar insufficiency
brachialis tendon
brachicephaly
brachii
>triceps b.

brachiocephalic
>b. arterial aneurysm
>b. arteriography
>b. artery
>b. artery stenting
>b. artery thrombolysis
>b. branch
>b. ischemia
>b. lymph node
>b. stent
>b. trunk
>b. trunk of aorta
>b. vein
>b. vessel

NOTES

brachiocubital
brachioradialis
    b. muscle
    b. tendon
brachium, pl. **brachia**
    b. of colliculus
    b. conjunctivum
    b. pontis
Bracht-Wachter lesion
brachycephalic head shape
brachycephaly
brachydactyly
    Bell b.
    Christian b.
    Mohn-Wriedt b.
brachymetatarsia
brachypellic pelvis
BrachySeed
    B. implant
    B. PD-103 implant
brachytelephalangic type of cystic fibrosis
brachytherapy
    afterloading b.
    b. boost
    endovascular b.
    episcleral plaque b.
    b. implant removal
    interstitial b.
    intracavitary application b.
    intraluminal b.
    IOHDR b.
    permanent b.
    remote afterloading b. (RAB)
    Ultraseed b.
    vascular b.
bracing
    fracture b.
bradyphemic
bradyphrenia
Bragard sign
Bragg
    B. angle
    B. curve
    B. equation
    B. ionization peak
    B. law
    B. peak radiosurgery
    B. spectrometer
Bragg-Gray cavity
braided diagnostic catheter
brain
    b. abscess
    b. activation study
    b. activity
    b. anatomy classification
    b. aneurysm
    b. anoxia
    b. architecture

    atrial diverticulum of b.
    b. atrophy
    base of b.
    b. bridging vein
    Broca motor speech area of b.
    buckling cortical b.
    b. calcification hemangioma
    b. candle dripping
    b. capillary angiography
    b. carcinoma
    b. cavernoma
    b. concussion
    b. contusion
    b. cyst
    b. death
    b. degeneration
    b. diffusion anisotropy
    dura mater of b.
    b. dysfunction
    b. dysgerminoma
    b. edema
    edematous b.
    b. electrical activity mapping (BEAM)
    eloquent area of b.
    b. empyema
    b. ependymoma
    b. fiber tracking
    b. fissure
    b. function
    b. geography
    b. Glx/Cr ratio
    b. hamartoma
    b. hematoma
    b. homeostasis
    horseshoe configuration of b.
    b. imaging radiopharmaceutical
    b. incidentaloma
    b. infarct
    inflammation of b.
    insular region of b.
    b. ischemia
    b. laceration
    left b.
    b. lesion
    b. lipoma
    b. lymphoma
    b. mantle
    b. mass
    b. mass in jugular foramen
    meninx of b.
    b. metastasis
    b. paragonimiasis
    b. parenchyma
    b. perfusion
    b. perfusion reserve
    b. perfusion scintigraphy
    b. perfusion SPECT
    b. plasticity

b. proton magnetic resonance spectroscopy
b. region vesicle
right b.
sagging b.
b. scan
b. scan imaging
b. shrinkage
silent area of b.
smooth b.
softening of b.
split b.
b. stem
b. stenosis hemorrhage
b. structure
b. substance
b. surface matching technique
b. swelling
b. tissue herniation
b. tuber
b. tuberculoma
b. tumor
b. tumor at cerebellopontine angle
b. tumor classification
unicameral b.
Virchow-Robin space of b.
b. volume
b. water content
water on b.
watershed zone in b.
wet b.
b. window
brain-core gradient
BrainLAB VectorVision neuronavigation system
brainstem
b. compression
b. demyelination
b. displacement
b. edema
b. encephalitis
b. ependymoma
b. glioma
b. hemorrhage
b. infarct
b. ischemia
b. lesion
b. pyramidal tract
reticular formation of b.
b. reticular formation
tegmentum of b.
brain-to-background ratio

BrainVoyager interactive software
braking radiation
branch
acute marginal b.
anterior cutaneous b.
arterial b.
b. of artery
atrioventricular groove b.
bifid aortic b.
bifurcating b.
brachiocephalic b.
bronchial b.
bronchus b.
cardiac b.
caudal b.
circumflex b.
collateral b.
cortical b.
cutaneous lateral b.
b. decay
diagonal b.
digital b.
distal b.
dorsal b.
b. duct
feeding b.
first major diagonal b.
first septal perforator b.
geniculate b.
inferior cardiac b.
inferior wall b.
intrahepatic portal vein b.
large obtuse marginal b.
left bundle b.
marginal b.
midmarginal b.
motor b.
muscular b.
musculophrenic b.
nonlingular b.
obtuse marginal b. (OMB)
paired parietal b.
paired visceral b.
pancreatic duct b.
perforating b.
phalangeal b.
b. point
posterior descending b.
posterior intercostal b.
posterior ventricular b.
premammillary b.
proper digital nerve b.

NOTES

branch *(continued)*
  pruning of pancreatic duct b.
  pudendal b.
  b. pulmonary artery stenosis
  ramus intermedius artery b.
  ramus medialis artery b.
  right bundle b.
  second diagonal b.
  segmental renal artery b.
  septal perforating b.
  side b.
  sinuatrial b.
  subcostal b.
  subsegmental renal artery b.
  sulcocommissural b.
  superior phrenic b.
  thalamoperforating b.
  unpaired parietal b.
  unpaired visceral b.
  ventral b.
  ventricular b.
branched
  b. calculus
  b. chain
branches of vein
branchial
  b. cartilage
  b. cleft cyst
  b. cleft development
  b. duct
  b. efferent column
  b. fistula
  b. pouch
  b. sinus
branching
  anomalous b.
  b. calcification
  b. centrilobar opacity
  b. decay
  b. fraction
  b. line
  b. linear structure
  mirror-image brachiocephalic b.
  b. pattern
  b. ratio
  right aortic arch with mirror
    image b.
  b. tubular structure
Brasdor method
Brasfield scoring system
Braun
  B. canal
  B. tumor
Braune muscle
Braunwald-Cutter valve
Braunwald sign
BRCA2 genes

bread-and-butter
  b.-a.-b. heart
  b.-a.-b. pericarditis
bread loaf technique
breadth
  photopeak b.
breakdown
  BBB b.
breakthrough
  normal perfusion pressure b.
  b. vasodilation
  b. visualization
breast
  b. abscess
  accessory b.
  adenoma of b.
  b. adenosarcoma
  b. adenosis
  b. anatomy
  b. angiosarcoma
  b. artifact
  atrophic b.
  b. attenuation
  augmented b.
  b. biopsy
  b. bolster
  b. bone
  b. cancer risk factor
  b. cancer screening
  B. cancer system 2100
  b. carcinoma
  central solitary papilloma b.
  b. coil
  compression of b.
  b. cyst
  b. cyst aspiration
  cystic disease of b.
  b. degeneration
  b. edema
  b. embryology
  fascia of b.
  b. fat necrosis
  b. fibroadenolipoma
  b. fibroadenoma
  b. fibroadenomatosis
  fibrocystic b.
  b. fibrosis
  b. hamartoma
  b. hematoma
  b. hyperplasia
  B. Imaging Reporting and Data
    System (BI-RADS)
  b. irradiation
  b. lesion
  b. lipofibroadenoma
  b. lipoma
  lobule b.
  b. localizer
  b. lymphoma

b. mammographic technique
b. metastasis
b. microcalcification
Miraluma nuclear scan of b.
b. mucocele
b. neoplasm
b. papilloma
b. parenchyma
b. phyllode tumor
b. pneumocystography
b. popcorn calcification
prepubertal female b.
b. prosthesis rupture
b. pseudolymphoma
radiographic-dense b.
round cancer of b.
b. sarcoma
b. shadow
shoemaker's b.
b. skin thickening
b. sonography
stromal pattern of b.
tail of b.
b. thrombophlebitis
b. tissue
b. tissue displacement
b. traction
b. trigger point
b. ultrasound
variocele tumor of b.
breastbone
BreastScan IR system
breaststroker's knee
breath-hold
b.-h. cine-MR
b.-h. contrast-enhanced MRI
b.-h. contrast-enhanced three-
dimensional MR angiography
b.-h. cycle
b.-h. fast-recovery fast SE pulse
sequence
b.-h. fast spin-echo image
b.-h. gradient-recalled echo
sequence
b.-h. imaging
b.-h. MR cholangiography
b.-h. MRCP
b.-h. scanning
b.-h. segmented k-space gradient-
echo imaging
b.-h. technique
b.-h. turbo spin-echo

b.-h. T1-weighted gradient echo
imaging
b.-h. T1-weighted MP-GRE MR
imaging
b.-h. ungated imaging
b.-h. velocity-encoded cine MR
imaging
breathing
b. artifact
b. feedback
free b.
breath pentane measurement
breech presentation
breeder reactor
bregma
bregmatic
b. bone
b. fontanelle
bregmatolambdoid arc
bregmatomastoid suture
Bremer
B. AirFlo Vest
B. Halo Crown system
bremsstrahlung
b. process
b. radiation
b. scan
Brenner tumor
Breschet canal
Brescia-Cimino
B.-C. fistula
B. C. graft
Breslow classification
Brett sun
Breuerton view of hand
breve
vinculum b.
Brevi-Kath epidural catheter
brevis
abductor pollicis b. (APB)
coxa b.
extensor carpi radialis b. (ECRB)
extensor digitorum b. (EDB)
extensor pollicis b. (EPB)
flexor digiti minimi b.
flexor digiti quinti b. (FDQB)
flexor digitorum b.
flexor hallucis b.
flexor pollicis b.
palmaris b.
split peroneus b.
b. tendon

NOTES

bridge
    arteriolovenular b.
    b. autograft
    bony b.
    b. circuit
    interthalamic b.
    intraductal b.
    loop ostomy b.
    mucosal b.
    muscular b.
    myocardial b.
    nasal b.
    osseous b.
    osteophytic b.
    portal-to-portal b.
    skin b.
    transphysial bone b.
    ventral b.
    Wheatstone b.
bridged loop-gap resonator
bridging
    b. callus
    b. defect
    b. necrosis
    b. osteophyte
    physial bony b.
bright
    b. contrast enhancement
    b. cystic focus
    b. echo
    b. fatty marrow
    b. layer
    b. pixel value
    b. signal
    b. signal intensity
bright-field imaging
brightly
    b. echogenic focus
    b. increased renal parenchymal
      echogenicity
brightness
    b. area product (BAP)
    b. gain
    b. mode
    b. modulation
    b. modulation scan
brightness-time curve
bright-signal-intensity tumor
Brilliance 109 MP PC monitor
brim
    pelvic b.
    b. of pelvis
    quadrilateral b.
    b. sign
brimstone liver
brisement therapy
brisk wall motion
Brissaud syndrome

Brite
    80-cm 8F B. Tip guide catheter
    B. Tip 5F–10F guiding catheter
BriteSmile laser
British thermal unit
brittle
    b. bone
    b. bone disease
broad
    b. beam
    b. fascia
    b. ligament
    b. ligament hernia
    b. ligament pregnancy
    b. maxillary ridge
broadband
    b. noise detection error artifact
    b. transducer
broad-based
    b.-b. disc protrusion
    b.-b. polyp
broad-beam
    b.-b. absorption
    b.-b. scattering
Broadbent-Bolton plane
broadening
    dipolar b.
    quadripolar signal b.
    spectral b.
broad-use linear acquisition speed-up technique (BLAST)
Broca
    B. area
    band of B.
    B. convolution
    B. diagonal band
    B. gyrus
    B. index
    B. motor speech area of brain
    B. pudendal pouch
    B. region
Brockenbrough needle
Brödel bloodless line of incision
Broden
    B. position
    B. view
Broders tumor index classification
Brodie
    B. bursa
    B. disease
    B. knee
    B. ligament
    B. metaphysial abscess
Brodmann
    B. area
    B. cytoarchitectonic field
broken bough pattern
bromide
    perfluorooctyl b. (PFOB)

B

brominated oil
bromine-76 bromospirone
brominized oil contrast medium
bromodeoxyuridine
    b. imaging agent
    b. labeling index
5-bromodeoxyuridine analysis
bromophenol blue imaging agent
bromospirone
    bromine-76 b.
bronchi (*pl. of* bronchus)
bronchial
    b. adenoma
    b. angiography
    b. anular cartilage
    b. arteriography
    b. artery
    b. artery embolization (BAE)
    b. atresia
    b. branch
    b. bud
    b. calculus
    b. caliber
    b. carcinoid tumor
    b. carcinoma
    b. cleft cyst
    b. collateral circulation
    b. cuff sign
    b. dehiscence
    b. diameter
    b. dilatation
    b. distortion
    b. erosion
    b. fracture
    b. groove
    b. inflammation
    b. kinking
    b. lumen
    b. mucocele
    b. mucosa
    b. obstruction
    b. polyp
    b. provocation imaging
    b. provocation testing
    b. reactivity
    b. rupture
    b. septum
    b. sinus
    b. smooth muscle spasm
    b. spur
    b. stenosis
    b. stenting

    b. stricture
    b. tract
    b. tree
    b. tube
    b. vein
    b. vessel
    b. wall thickening
bronchiectasis
    acquired b.
    capillary b.
    central b.
    congenital b.
    cylindrical b.
    cystic b.
    distal b.
    dry b.
    follicular b.
    fusiform b.
    Polynesian b.
    postinfectious b.
    recurrent b.
    reversible b.
    saccular b.
    b. traction
    tuberculous b.
    tubular b.
    varicose b.
bronchiectasis-ethmoid sinusitis
bronchiectatic
    b. airway
    b. cyst
    b. pattern
bronchiolar
    b. adenocarcinoma
    b. carcinoma
    b. dilatation
    b. edema
    b. emphysema
    b. narrowing
    b. obstruction
bronchiole
    alveolar b.
    conducting b.
    irreversible narrowing of b.
    lobular b.
    membranous b.
    respiratory b.
    terminal b.
    tree-in-bud b.
bronchiolectasis
    traction b.
bronchioli (*pl. of* bronchiolus)

NOTES

bronchiolitis
    cellular b.
    constrictive b.
    diffuse aspiration b.
    exudative b.
    b. fibrosa obliterans
    follicular b.
    b. obliterans with organizing
      pneumonia (BOOP)
    obliterative b.
    pediatric b.
    proliferative b.
    respiratory b.
    smoker's b.
    vesicular b.
bronchioloalveolar
    b. carcinoma
    b. cell carcinoma
bronchiolocentric
bronchiolus, pl. **bronchioli**
bronchitis
    asthmatic b.
    follicular b.
    irritant b.
Bronchitrac L catheter
bronchoadenitis
bronchoalveolar
    b. carcinoma
    b. cell adenoma
bronchoarterial bundle
bronchobiliary fistula
bronchocavernous
bronchocavitary fistula
bronchocele
bronchocentric
    b. granulomatosis
    b. inflammatory infiltrate
bronchoconstriction
    exercise-induced b.
    isocapnic hyperventilation-induced b.
bronchoconstrictor
bronchocutaneous fistula
bronchodilation, bronchodilatation
bronchodilator effect
bronchoesophageal fistula
bronchogenic
    b. adenoma
    b. carcinoma
    b. duplication cyst
bronchogram
    air b.
    bilateral b.
    Cope method b.
    fiberoptic b.
    fluid-filled b.
    b. imaging
    mucinous b.
    mucous b.
    scattered air b.

    Swiss cheese air b.
    tantalum b.
    unilateral b.
bronchography
    Cope-method b.
    percutaneous transtracheal b.
broncholith
broncholithiasis
bronchomalacia
bronchomediastinal lymph trunk
bronchomotor effect
bronchoplasty
    balloon b.
bronchoplegia
bronchopleural (BP)
    b. fistula
bronchopleuropneumonia
bronchopneumonia
    bibasilar b.
    hemorrhagic b.
    hypostatic b.
    inhalation b.
    b. pattern
    subacute b.
    tuberculous b.
bronchopneumonitis
bronchopulmonary (BP)
    b. aspergillosis
    b. atelectasis
    b. dysplasia (BPD)
    b. fistula
    b. foregut
    b. foregut malformation (BPFM)
    b. lung segment anatomy
    b. lymph node
    b. marking
    b. neoplasm
    b. segment
    b. sequestration
bronchoradiography
bronchorrhea
bronchoscope
    Storz infant b.
bronchoscopy
    fiberoptic b. (FOB)
    virtual b. (VB)
bronchosinusitis
bronchospasm
    paradoxic b.
bronchospastic effect
bronchostaxis
bronchostenosis
bronchotracheal
bronchovascular
    b. anatomy cross-section
    b. bundle
    b. marking
    b. pattern

bronchovesicular marking
bronchus, pl. **bronchi**
  anomalous b.
  anterior basal b.
  apical b.
  apicoposterior b.
  basal segmental b.
  beaded b.
  b. blockage
  blocked b.
  b. branch
  cardiac segmental b.
  contracted b.
  depression of left mainstem b.
  dilated b.
  distended central bronchi
  ectatic b.
  edematous b.
  epiarterial b.
  extrapulmonary b.
  fractured b.
  granulomatous inflammation of b.
  hyparterial b.
  inferior lobe b.
  inflamed b.
  intermediate b.
  b. intermedius
  intrapulmonary b.
  inverted-T-appearance mainstem b.
  lateral basal segmental b.
  left main stem b.
  left primary b.
  lingular b.
  lobar b.
  mainstem b.
  major b.
  medial basal segmental b.
  medium-sized b.
  middle lobe b.
  mucoid impaction of b.
  nonlingular branch of upper
    lobe b.
  normal-appearing b.
  posterior basal segmental b.
  primary left b.
  primary right b.
  principal b.
  right lobe b.
  right mainstem b.
  right primary b.
  secondary b.
  secretion-filled b.

  segmental b.
  b. sign
  b. stem
  subapical b.
  subsegmental b.
  superior lobe b.
  superior segmental b.
  tracheal b.
bronchus-associated lymphoid tissue
  (BALT)
bronchus-to-pulmonary artery ratio
bronzed sclerosing encephalitis
bronze liver
Brooker periarticular heterotopic
  ossification classification
Brooke tumor
Broselow-Luten Pediatric System
Broviac long-term catheter
brow-down
  b.-d. position
  b.-d. projection
  b.-d. skull view
brown
  b. asbestos
  b. atrophy
  b. cell cyst
  b. edema
  b. fat origin
  b. induration of lung
  b. tumor
  b. tumor of hyperparathyroidism
Brown-Dodge method for angiography
brownian water motion
Brown-Roberts-Wells (BRW)
  B.-R.-W. CT stereotactic guide
  B.-R.-W. frame
  B.-R.-W. stereotactic system
  B.-R.-W. technique
Brown-Séquard
  B.-S. lesion
  B.-S. syndrome
brow presentation
brow-up
  b.-u. position
  b.-u. projection
  b.-u. skull view
brucellar
  b. myositis
  b. osteomyelitis
  b. synovitis
Bruch gland
Bruch disease

NOTES

Brücke muscle
Brudzinski sign
Bruel-Kjaer
    B.-K. transvaginal ultrasound probe
    B.-K. ultrasound
    B.-K. ultrasound scanner
Brugada syndrome
Bruker
    B. AMX 300 NMR spectrometer
    B. console
    B. CSI Omega MR system
    B. minispec measuring device
    B. PC-10 relaxometer
    B. scanner
    B. TC-10 relaxometer
Brunner
    B. gland
    B. gland adenoma
    B. gland hyperplasia
    B. gland hypertrophy
Brunnstrom-Fugl-Meyer (BFM)
    B.-F.-M. arm impairment
      assessment
brush
    Castaneda thrombolytic b.
    Cragg-Castaneda thrombolytic b.
    Cragg thrombolytic b.
BRW
    Brown-Roberts-Wells
    BRW CT stereotaxic guide
    BRW stereotactic system
Bryant
    B. sign
    B. triangle
BSA
    body surface area
B-scan imaging
BSCB
    blood-spinal cord barrier
BSF
    backscatter factor
BSLM
    body surface laplacian mapping
bubble
    b. of the belly
    encapsulated gas b.
    free gas b.
    Garren-Edwards gastric b.
    gas b.
    gastric air b.
    GEG b.
    intragastric b.
    microscopic air b.
    b. oxygenator
    b. sign
    stomach b.
    b. ventriculography
bubblebreaker
bubblelike appearance

bubbling lesion
bubbly
    b. bone lesion
    b. bulb
    b. lung
    b. opacity
    b. pattern
bubonulus
bucca, pl. **buccae**
buccal
    b. cavity
    b. groove
    b. mucosa
    b. mucosal carcinoma
    b. shelf
    b. space
    b. space infection
    b. surface
buccinator
    b. crest
    b. lymph node
buccogingival ridge
buccolingual plane
bucconeural duct
buccopharyngeal fascia
Buck
    B. extension
    B. fascia
bucket-handle
    b.-h. meniscus tear
    b.-h. pattern of fracture
    b.-h. pelvic fracture
Buckland-Wright macroradiography
buckle
    b. fracture
    wire-fixation b.
buckled innominate artery
buckling
    b. cortical brain
    innominate artery b.
bucky
    chest b.
    B. diaphragm
    B. digital x-ray device
    B. film
    B. grid
    oscillating B.
    B. ray
    B. tomogram
    B. view
bud
    accessory ureteral b.
    bronchial b.
    capillary b.
    dorsal pancreatic b.
    end b.
    limb b.
    ureteral b.

vascular b.
ventral pancreatic b.
Budd
    B. cirrhosis
    B. syndrome
Budd-Chiari syndrome
Budge
    ciliospinal center of B.
budgerigar fancier's lung
Budin-Chandler anteversion
  determination
Budin joint
buffalo
    b. hump
    B. malleolar rule
buffer amplifier
Buford complex
Buhl desquamative pneumonia
bulb
    aortic b.
    arterial b.
    baroreceptor b.
    baseline of b.
    bubbly b.
    carotid b.
    dehiscent jugular b.
    dental b.
    duodenal b.
    end b.
    heart b.
    high jugular b. (HJB)
    inferior jugular vein b.
    internal jugular b.
    b. of occipital horn of lateral
      ventricle
    olfactory b.
    b. of penis
    b. of posterior horn of lateral
      ventricle
    sinovaginal b.
    superior jugular vein b.
    b. ureterography
    b. of vein
bulbar
    b. abnormality
    b. intracerebral hemorrhage
    b. peptic ulcer
    b. ridge
    b. septum
    b. swelling
    b. tract

bulbi
    b. muscle
    phthisis b.
bulbocavernosus muscle
bulbocavernous gland
bulbomembranous urethral rupture
bulbosity
bulbospongiosus muscle of penis
bulbourethral
    b. artery
    b. gland
    b. gland anatomy
    b. gland lesion
bulbous
    b. configuration
    b. costochondral junction
    b. enlargement
    b. stump
    b. urethra
bulbous-tip stiff malleable cannula
bulbus cordis
bulge
    anal b.
    anular disc b.
    bilateral anterior chest b.
    disc b.
    epiphrenic b.
    inguinal b.
    late systolic b.
    palpable presystolic b.
    parasternal b.
    precordial b.
    suprasternal b.
bulging
    b. aneurysm
    b. anulus
    b. dura
    b. fontanelle
    b. lung fissure
    b. precordium
bulk
    b. laxative
    b. magnetic susceptibility (BMS)
    b. magnetization vector
    mediastinal b.
    muscle b.
    b. susceptibility artifact
bulky tumor
bulla, pl. **bullae**
    emphysematous b.
    ethmoidal b.
    b. formation

NOTES

Bullard laryngoscope
bullet
    hollow-point b.
    b. kit culture medium
    metallic track of b.
    stabilizing b.
    tripoint b.
bullet-shaped vertebra
Bull method
bull-neck appearance
bullosa
    concha b.
    junctional epidermolysis b.
bullous
    b. disorder
    b. edema
    b. edema of bladder wall
    b. emphysema
    b. emphysema of intestine
    b. lung disease
bull's
    b. eye appearance
    b. eye configuration
    b. eye deformity
    b. eye image
    b. eye imaging
    b. eye lesion
    b. eye polar map
    b. eye technique
    b. eye view
bump
    hip b.
    inion b.
    runner's b.
    splenic b.
bumper fracture
bunamiodyl
bunch-of-grapes appearance
bundle
    aberrant b.
    anterior atrial myocardial b.
    artery-vein-nerve b.
    atrioventricular b.
    Bachmann b.
    b. bone
    bronchoarterial b.
    bronchovascular b.
    central bronchovascular b.
    common b.
    fascicular b.
    fiberoptic b.
    Flechsig b.
    b. function
    Gierke respiratory b.
    Gowers b.
    His b.
    intercostal neuromuscular b.
    James b.
    Keith sinuatrial b.

    b. of Kent
    Kent-His b.
    Mahaim b.
    main b.
    middle perforating collagen b.
    neurovascular b.
    Pick b.
    Probst callosal b.
    Schultze b.
    sinuatrial b.
    Thorel b.
    vascular b.
    b. of Vicq d'Azyr
bundle-branch
    b.-b. heart block
    b.-b. reentry (BBR)
Bunge amputation
bunion formation
bunk-bed fracture
Bunsen-type valve
Burdach
    column of B.
burden
    body b.
    maximum permissible body b.
    tumor b.
Burger scalene triangle
Burgess below-knee amputation
buried tonsil
Burke-type metaphysial dysplasia
Burkhalter-Reyes method of phalangeal
    fracture
Burkitt-like lymphoma
Burkitt lymphoma
burn
    b. boutonnière deformity
    radiation b.
    x-ray b.
burned-out
    b.-o. colon
    b.-o. mucosa
    b.-o. tabes
    b.-o. tumor
    b.-o. tumor of testis
Burnett
    B. applicator
    B. BiDirectional TMJ device
    B. cylinder
burning
    selective hole b.
burnout
    detail b.
Burns ligament
Burrow vein
bursa, pl. **bursae**
    Achilles b.
    adventitious b.
    anserine b.
    Brodie b.

calcaneal b.
coracoid b.
deltoid b.
b. exostotica
b. of Fabricius
Fleischmann b.
flexor b.
gastrocnemius b.
gastrocnemius-semimembranosus b.
iliopsoas b.
infrapatellar b.
interligamentous b.
intermediate b.
intermetatarsophalangeal b.
intraligamentous b.
intratendinous b.
ischiogluteal b.
lateral epicondylar b.
Luschka b.
MCL b.
medial epicondylar b.
Monro b.
olecranon b.
omental b.
patellar b.
pes anserine b.
plantar b.
popliteus b.
premalleolar b.
prepatellar b.
radial b.
retrocalcaneal b.
semimembranosus b.
semimembranosus-tibial collateral
    ligament b.
subacromial b.
subacromial-subdeltoid b.
subdeltoid b.
subgluteus maximus b.
subgluteus medius b.
submetatarsal b.
subscapular b.
subtendinous b.
superficial tendo-Achilles b.
suprapatellar b.
synovial b.
tendo-Achilles b.
tibial collateral ligament b.
trochanteric b.
ulnar b.
bursal
b. calcification

b. flap
b. fluid
b. inflammation
b. osteochondromatosis
b. sac
bursitis
adhesive b.
anserine b.
bicipital b.
calcaneal b.
calcific b.
chronic retrocalcaneal b.
cubital b.
distended scapulothoracic b.
iliopsoas b.
infracalcaneal b.
intermetatarsal b.
intermetatarsophalangeal b.
intertubercular b.
ischial b.
ischiogluteal b.
olecranon b.
patellar b.
pes anserinus b.
posterior calcaneal b.
prepatellar b.
pseudotrochanteric b.
radiohumeral b.
retrocalcaneal b.
SA-SD b.
septic b.
subacromial b.
subacromial-subdeltoid septic b.
subcoracoid b.
subdeltoid b.
Tornwaldt b.
trochanteric b.
bursography
bursolith
burst
b. fracture
b. injury
respiratory b.
burst-forming unit
bursting
b. dislocation
b. fracture
b. pressure
Buschke-Löwenstein tumor
buster
Amplatz Clot B.
butanol-extractable iodine (BEI)

NOTES

Butcher staging classification
butterfly
  b. appearance
  b. breast shadow
  b. coil
  b. configuration
  b. distribution
  b. effect
  b. fracture
  b. fracture fragment
  b. glioblastoma
  b. glioma
  b. lesion
  b. lymphoma
  b. pattern
  b. pattern of infiltrate
  b. vertebra
butterfly-wing vertebra
Butterworth
  B. filter
  10-pole B. filter
button
  aortic b.
  duodenal b.
  full-thickness Carrel b.
  Kistner tracheal b.
  patellar b.
  b. procedure
  b. sequestrum eosinophilic
    granuloma
  b. sequestrum skull
  subdural b.
  b. toe amputation
  tracheal B b.
buttoned device
buttonhole
  b. deformity
  b. fracture

  b. mitral stenosis
  b. opening
  radiopaque wire of
    counteroccluder b.
  b. rupture
  b. tear
buttressing
  medial femoral b.
buttress plate
butyral
  polyvinyl b. (PVB)
BV2 needle
BVAD
  biventricular assist device
BVR
  basal vein of Rosenthal
BVS
  biventricular support
BW
  bitewing
  black and white
Bx Velocity stent
bypass (BP)
  adjunctive surgical b.
  aortobiliac b.
  biliointestinal b. (BIB)
  biliopancreatic b.
  b. circuit
  extracranial-intracranial b.
  b. failure
  b. graft
  iliofemoral crossover b.
  jejunoileal b. (JIB)
byproduct material
byssinosis
bystander effect
byte mode
B-zone small lymphocytic lymphoma

C
- carbon
- coulomb
  - C angle
  - C loop
  - C loop of duodenum
  - C scan
  - C sign
  - C sign sensitivity

^{11}C
- carbon 11
  - ^{11}C acetate imaging agent
  - ^{11}C butanol imaging agent
  - ^{11}C carbon monoxide
  - ^{11}C carfentanil imaging agent
  - ^{11}C deoxyglucose
  - ^{11}C flumazenil imaging agent
  - ^{11}C imaging agent
  - ^{11}C L-159
  - ^{11}C L-methylmethionine
  - ^{11}C lumazenil
  - ^{11}C methionine
  - ^{11}C methoxystaurosporine
  - ^{11}C N-methylspiperone imaging agent
  - ^{11}C N-methylspiroperidol
  - ^{11}C nomifensine imaging agent
  - ^{11}C palmitate
  - ^{11}C palmitic acid radioactive
  - ^{11}C raclopride imaging agent
  - ^{11}C thymidine imaging agent

^{12}C
- carbon 12

^{13}C
- carbon 13

^{14}C
- carbon 14
  - ^{14}C lactose breath test

C-150 LXP EBT scanner
C1-C5 segment of internal carotid artery
C-60 teletherapy
Ca
- calcium

^{47}Ca, Ca-47
- calcium 47

^{45}Ca, Ca-45
- calcium 45
  - ^{45}Ca imaging agent

CA15-3 RIA
CAAS
- cardiovascular angiography analysis system
  - CAAS QCA system

CABBS
- computer-assisted blood background subtraction

CABG
- coronary artery bypass graft

cable
- FlexStrand c.

Cabrol composite graft procedure
CABS
- coronary artery bypass surgery

CAC
- coronary artery calcification

CACG
- cineangiocardiogram

CACS
- coronary artery calcium score
  - CACS threshold

CAD
- computer-aided detection
- computer-aided diagnosis
  - RapidScreen RS-2000 CAD

cadaveric renal transplant
CAD-evaluated mammogram
cadmium (Cd)
- c. iodide detector

CADstream
CADx SecondLook system
caesium iodide scintillator
Caffey
- C. hyperostosis
- C. syndrome

Caffey-Kempe syndrome
cage
- bony thoracic c.
- Faraday c.
- Harms c.
- metallic c.
- osseocartilaginous thoracic c.
- threaded fusion c. (TFC)

CAH
- congenital adrenal hyperplasia

caisson disease
Cajal
- nucleus of C.

cake
- c. kidney
- omental c.

cake-glaze consistency
calcaneal
- c. apophysis
- c. apophysitis
- c. articular surface
- c. avulsion fracture
- c. bone
- c. bursa

calcaneal *(continued)*
  c. bursa inflammation
  c. bursitis
  c. displaced fracture
  c. inclination angle
  c. pitch
  c. pitch angle
  c. process
  c. spur
  c. stress fracture
  c. tendon
  c. tubercle
  c. tuberosity
calcanei (*pl. of* calcaneus)
calcaneocavus
  c. foot
  pes c.
  talipes calcaneus c.
  talipes cavus c.
calcaneoclavicular ligament
calcaneocuboid
  c. articulation
  c. joint
  c. ligament
calcaneofibular ligament (CFL)
calcaneonavicular
  c. coalition
  c. ligament
calcaneoplantar angle
calcaneotibial
  c. fusion
  c. ligament
calcaneovalgocavus
calcaneovalgus
  c. flatfoot
  pes c.
calcaneovarus deformity
calcaneus, pl. **calcanei**
  c. altus
  c. deformity
  pes c.
  sulcus calcanei
  talipes c.
  tendo c.
  thalamic fracture of c.
calcar
  c. avis
  c. femorale
  c. pedis
  pivot of c.
calcareous
  c. degeneration
  c. deposit
  c. infiltrate
  c. metastasis
  c. renal calculus
calcarine
  c. artery
  c. cortex

  c. fissure
  c. sulcus
calciferous canal
calcific
  c. arteriosclerosis
  c. artery
  c. bicuspid valvular stenosis
  c. bursitis
  c. cochleitis
  c. density
  c. discitis
  c. matrix
  c. myonecrosis
  c. round body
  c. senile aortic valvular stenosis
  c. shadow
  c. spur
  c. tendinitis
  c. tendinosis
calcificans
  chondrodysplasia c.
  chondroplasia c.
  liponecrosis macrocystica c.
  liponecrosis microcystica c.
calcification
  abdominal wall c.
  adenoma-associated c.
  adrenal c.
  alimentary tract c.
  aneurysmal wall c.
  anterior spinal ligament c.
  anular c.
  aortic arch c.
  aortic valve c.
  arachnoid granulation c.
  arterial c.
  arteriovascular c.
  atherosclerotic c.
  basal ganglia c.
  c. of basal ganglion
  basket-like c.
  benign breast c.
  bladder wall c.
  branching c.
  breast popcorn c.
  bursal c.
  calcium c.
  calcium phosphate c.
  cardiac c.
  carotid artery c.
  cartilage c.
  casting breast c.
  cerebral c.
  chicken-wire c.
  choroid plexus c.
  clustered c.
  coarse c.
  conglomerate c.
  coronary artery c. (CAC)

costal cartilage c.
curvilinear c.
defined and homogeneous c.
dentate nuclei c.
dermal breast c.
diffuse abdominal c.
diffuse stippled c.
disc c.
dural c.
dystrophic soft tissue c.
eggshell c.
eggshell breast c.
eggshell nodal c.
falx c.
female genital tract c.
fetal intraabdominal c.
fine c.
fingertip c.
flaky c.
flocculent focus of c.
fluffy and amorphous c.
focal alimentary tract c.
focus of c.
free body c.
genital tract c.
glial tumor c.
granular c.
gyriform c.
habenular commissure c.
heart valve c.
hepatic c.
idiopathic pleural c.
inadequate calvarial c.
inadequate cranial c.
intervertebral cartilage c.
intervertebral disc c.
intraabdominal c.
intraabdominal fetal c.
intracardiac c.
intracranial physiologic c.
intraductal c.
intraocular c.
intratumoral c.
involutional breast c.
inwardly displaced c.
irregular c.
isolated clustered c.'s
kidney c.
laminated c.
layering c.
ligamentous c.
c. line

linear c.
liver c.
lobular breast c.
lucent-centered c.
lung popcorn c.
lymph node eggshell c.
male genital tract c.
malignant breast c.
medial collateral ligament c.
medullary c.
meniscus-shaped c.
mesenteric c.
metastatic soft tissue c.
milk-of-calcium c.
mitral ring c.
mitral valve c.
Mönckeberg c.
mottled c.
mulberry-type c.
multiple pulmonary c.
myocardial c.
c. of myocardium
needle-shaped breast c.
neoplastic c.
node c.
normal c.
oyster-pearl breast c.
pancreatic c.
paraarticular c.
paraspinal c.
parentheseslike c.
parietal pericardial c.
pathologic intracranial c.
pearllike breast c.
Pellegrini-Stieda c.
periarticular c.
pericardial c.
periductal c.
peritendinous c.
periventricular c.
phlebolithlike c.
pineal gland c.
plaquing c.
pleomorphic c.
pleural c.
popcorn c.
popcornlike c.
poppy seedlike c.
postbiopsy eggshell c.
postradiation c.
premature c.
psammomatous c.

NOTES

calcification *(continued)*
    pulmonary c.
    punctate c.
    railroad track c.
    renal c.
    retroperitoneal c.
    ricelike muscle c.
    ring-and-arc c.
    ring apophysis c.
    rod-shaped c.
    scrotal c.
    sebaceous gland c.
    secondary c.
    secretory c.
    sella turcica c.
    semilunar c.
    skin c.
    snowflakelike c.
    splenic c.
    stippled c.
    subanular c.
    suprasellar mass c.
    sutural c.
    suture c.
    target c.
    teacup breast c.
    teacup-shaped c.
    thrombus c.
    thyroid adenoma c.
    tramline cortical c.
    tram-track ductus arteriosus c.
    tram-track gyral c.
    tram-track renal cortical necrosis c.
    tumoral c.
    urinary bladder wall c.
    valvular leaflet c.
    vascular abdominal c.
    venous c.
    visceral pericardial c.
    wall c.

calcified
    c. amorphous tumor
    c. anulus
    c. aorta
    c. aortic valve
    c. astrocytoma
    c. brain mass
    c. cartilage
    c. cysticercus granuloma
    c. density structure
    c. ductus arteriosus
    c. fetus
    c. fibroadenoma
    c. fibroid
    c. fibroma
    c. free fragment
    c. granuloma
    c. intracranial mass
    c. kidney mass

    c. lesion
    c. lung nodule
    c. lymph node
    c. medullary defect
    c. myocardial tuberculoma
    c. nodularity
    c. ovarian metastases
    c. pericardial cyst
    c. pericardium
    c. pineal body
    c. pineal gland
    c. plaque
    c. renal mass
    c. sclerosis
    c. sequestra of low signal intensity
    c. thrombus
    c. wall of aneurysm

calciform lobe

calcifying
    c. Malherbe epithelioma
    c. metastasis

calcinosis
    bilateral striopallidodentate c.
    c. circumscripta
    cutis c.
    generalized c.
    interstitial c.
    tumoral c.
    c. universalis

calcis
    os c.
    trigonum c.

calcium (Ca)
    c. 45 (^{45}Ca, Ca-45)
    c. 47 (^{47}Ca, Ca-47)
    c. bile soap
    c. calcification
    c. channel blocker
    c. debris
    c. hydroxyapatite
    c. hydroxyapatite deposition disease
    c. 45 imaging agent
    c. infiltrate
    intracardiac c.
    c. ion
    c. ipodate imaging agent
    c. layering
    liquid c.
    c. metabolism
    milk of c.
    c. phosphate calcification
    c. pyrophosphate deposition disease (CPPD)
    c. pyrophosphate dihydrate crystal deposition
    c. pyrophosphate dihydrate deposition disease
    c. pyrophosphate dihydrate hand
    c. salt deposit

c. scoring
c. scoring software
sedimented c.
c. sign
c. tungstate
calcium/oxyanion-containing particle
calculated
    c. clearance time
    c. image
    c. resistance
calculation
    bayesian c.
    body surface area c.
    Cerenkov c.
    contrast-to-noise c.
    gap c.
    magnitude c.
    Monte Carlo c.
    multiplane dosage c.
    radiation dosimetry c.
    signal-to-noise c.
    spectrophotometric c.
    velocity c.
    volume implant c.
calculi (*pl. of* calculus)
calculogram
calculography
calculous
    c. cholecystitis
    c. cirrhosis
calculus, pl. **calculi**
    albumin c.
    alternating c.
    alvine c.
    articular c.
    biliary c.
    branched c.
    bronchial c.
    calcareous renal c.
    cat's eye c.
    colloid c.
    coral c.
    cystic c.
    cystine c.
    decubitus c.
    dendritic c.
    echogenic c.
    encysted c.
    fibrinous c.
    gallbladder c.
    gastric hemic c.
    gonecystic c.

hemic c.
hemp seed c.
hepatic c.
impacted c.
indigo c.
intestinal c.
intrahepatic biliary c.
joint c.
kidney c.
lacteal c.
lucent c.
lung c.
mammary c.
matrix c.
metabolic c.
mulberry c.
nephritic c.
noncalcareous renal c.
nonopaque c.
obstructive c.
opaque c.
pancreatic c.
pocketed c.
primary vesical c.
prostatic c.
radiopaque vesical c.
renal c.
salivary c.
spermatic c.
staghorn c.
Steinstrasse c.
stomach c.
stonelike c.
struvite c.
submandibular duct c.
urate c.
ureteral c.
urethral c.
uric acid c.
urinary bladder c.
urinary tract c.
urostealith c.
vesicle c.
xanthic c.
Caldani ligament
Caldwell
    C. method
    C. occipitofrontal view
    C. position
    C. projection
    C. view

NOTES

Caldwell-Moloy classification
calf, pl. **calves**
    c. band
    c. vein thrombosis
calf-foot station
caliber
    bowel c.
    bronchial c.
    internal c.
    luminal c.
    medium c.
    modest c.
    narrow c.
    normal bladder c.
    spinal cord c.
    tracheal c.
    vessel c.
    wide c.
calibrate
calibrated
    c. leak
    c. tris-acryl gelatin microsphere
calibration
    absolute-peak efficiency c.
    catheter c.
    cross c.
    E-dial c.
    c. factor
    c. failure artifact
    film density c.
    c. method
calibrator
    accuracy c.
    digital isotope c.
    dose c.
    isotope c.
    radioisotope c.
caliceal (*var. of* calyceal)
caliectasis
    focal c.
    localized c.
californium (Cf)
californium 252 (^{252}Cf)
caliper
    restraint c.
calix (*var. of* calyx)
Callander amputation
callosal
    c. agenesis
    c. area
    c. dysgenesis
    c. formation
    c. gyrus
    c. lesion
    c. sulcus
callosomarginal
    c. artery
    c. fissure

callosum
    anterior midbody of corpus c.
    corpus c.
    genu of corpus c.
    isthmus of corpus c.
    posterior midbody of corpus c.
    rostral body of corpus c.
    rostrum of corpus c.
    splenium of corpus c.
callous
callus
    bony c.
    bridging c.
    central c.
    definitive c.
    c. deposit
    endosteal c.
    ensheathing c.
    external c.
    exuberant c.
    florid c.
    c. formation
    fracture c.
    intermediate c.
    permanent c.
    provisional c.
    tumoral c.
    c. weld
Calot triangle
calvaneovalgus
    pes c.
calvaria, pl. **calvariae**
    external table of c.
    internal table of c.
calvarial
    c. bone
    c. echogenicity
    c. fracture
Calvé
    septal cusp of C.
    C. vertebra plane
Calvé-Legg-Perthes disease
Calvé-Perthes disease
calves (*pl. of* calf)
calyceal, caliceal
    c. abnormality
    c. blunting
    c. clubbing
    c. dilatation
    c. diverticulum
    c. nephrostolithotomy
    c. system
Calypso Rely catheter
calyx, calix, pl. **calyces**
    cupping of c.
    major c.
    minor c.
    renal c.

spiderlike c.
c. tube
CAM
complementary and alternative medicine
computer-assisted myelography
camera
ADAC MCD Vertex Plus MCD
gamma c.
Anger scintillation c.
Apex 409, 415 c.
Argus c.
Biad c.
CerASPECT c.
CFA digital c.
charge-coupled device TV c.
CID c.
Cidtech c.
cine c.
Circon video c.
coincidence gamma c.
coincident gamma c.
crystal gamma c.
data c.
Digirad gamma c.
DSI c.
dual-head coincidence c.
dual single-crystal gamma c.
electron diffraction c.
Elscint APEX 409-AG ECT c.
Elscint APEX 009 Precursor c.
Elscint dual-detector cardiac c.
Elscint Dual-Head Helix c.
gamma c.
gantry-free gamma c.
GE 400AC/T; STAR II c.
GE gamma c.
Genesys c.
GE Neurocam c.
GE single-detector SPECT-
capable c.
GE Starcam single-crystal
tomographic scintillation c.
Haifa c.
4-head c.
Helix c.
Hitachi SPECT 2000H-40 c.
hybrid PET/SPECT c.
infrared c.
integral uniformity scintillation c.
isocon c.
Israel c.
large field of view gamma c.

MedX c.
multicrystal gamma c.
multiformat c.
multiple-headed gamma c.
nuclear medicine c.
Orthicon c.
Picker c.
pinhole c.
Pixsys FlashPoint c.
positron scintillation c.
PULSEcdc compact gamma c.
PULSEcdc gamma c.
radioisotope c.
radionuclide c.
R&F c.
rotating gamma c.
Scanditronix 1024-7B c.
Scinticore multicrystal
scintillation c.
scintillation c.
Shimadzu HeadTome Set-031 c.
Siemens gamma c.
Siemens Orbiter large-field-of-
view c.
single-head rotating gamma c.
SKYLight gantry-free nuclear
medicine gamma c.
slip-ring c.
Sopha DSX1 c.
Sophy c.
SP6 c.
Starcam c.
Strichman SME-810 c.
Technicare c.
Toshiba GGA 9300 c.
Trionix c.
Trionix-Triad c.
triple-head gamma c.
variable-angle gamma c.
Vertex c.
video display c.
video pill c.
Vision c.
cameral fistula
Cameron method
Camino
C. intracranial catheter
C. microventricular bolt catheter
Campbell ligament
Camper
C. chiasm
C. fascia

NOTES

C

Camper *(continued)*
    C. ligament
    C. line
Camp grid cassette
camptocormia
camptodactyly
camptomelic dysplasia
Camurati-Engelmann disease
CAMV
    congenital anomaly of mitral valve
canal
    abdominal c.
    accessory c.
    acoustic c.
    adductor c.
    Alcock c.
    alimentary c.
    alveolar c.
    alveolodental c.
    ampulla of semicircular c.
    anal c.
    anterior condylar c.
    anterior semicircular c.
    antropyloric c.
    arachnoid c.
    Arantius c.
    archenteric c.
    Arnold c.
    arterial c.
    atrial c.
    atrioventricular c.
    auditory c.
    basipharyngeal c.
    Bernard c.
    Bichat c.
    biliary c.
    birth c.
    bony semicircular c.
    Böttcher c.
    Braun c.
    Breschet c.
    calciferous c.
    caroticotympanic c.
    carotid c.
    carpal c.
    caudal c.
    central spinal c.
    cerebrospinal c.
    cervical c.
    cervicoaxillary c.
    ciliary c.
    Civinini c.
    Cloquet c.
    cochlear c.
    common atrioventricular c.
    complex atrioventricular c.
    condylar c.
    condyloid c.
    connecting c.

Corti c.
Cotunnius c.
craniopharyngeal c.
crural c.
Cuvier c.
c. decompression
deferent c.
diploic c.
Dorello c.
Dupuytren c.
endocervical c.
endometrial fluid in c.
ethmoid c.
eustachian c.
facial nerve c.
fallopian c.
femoral medullary c.
Ferrein c.
flexor c.
Fontana c.
galactophorous c.
ganglionic c.
Gartner c.
gastric c.
genital c.
gray horns in spinal c.
greater palatine c.
gubernacular c.
Guyon c.
gynecophoric c.
Hannover c.
haversian c.
hemal c.
Henle c.
Hensen c.
Hering c.
hernia c.
Hirschfeld c.
His c.
Huguier c.
Hunter c.
Huschke c.
hyaloid c.
hydrops c.
hypoglossal c.
iliac c.
incisive c.
inferior dental c.
infraorbital c.
inguinal c.
interfacial c.
internal auditory c.
intersacral c.
intestinal c.
intramedullary c.
Jacobson c.
Kovalevsky c.
lacrimal c.
Lambert c.

lateral semicircular c.
Löwenberg c.
lumbar spinal c.
lumbosacral c.
lymphatic c.
mandibular c.
marrow c.
mastoid c.
maxillary c.
medullary c.
mental c.
Müller c.
musculotubal c.
narrowing of spinal c.
nasal c.
nasolacrimal c.
nasopalatine c.
neural c.
neurenteric c.
notochordal c.
Nuck c.
olfactory c.
optic c.
orbital c.
palatine c.
palatomaxillary c.
palatovaginal c.
paraurethral c.
parturient c.
pelvic c.
pericardioperitoneal c.
persistent common
  atrioventricular c.
petrous carotid c.
pharyngeal c.
pleural c.
pleuropericardial c.
pleuroperitoneal c.
pneumoenteric c.
portal c.
posterior semicircular c.
principal artery of pterygoid c.
pterygoid c.
pterygopalatine c.
pudendal c.
pulmoaortic c.
pulp c.
pyloric c.
recurrent c.
Reichert c.
Rivinus c.
Rosenthal c.

sacculocochlear c.
sacculoutricular c.
sacral c.
Santorini c.
c. of Scarpa
Schlemm c.
scleral c.
semicircular c.
c. septum
sheathing c.
small internal auditory c.
sphenopalatine c.
sphenopharyngeal c.
spinal cord c.
c. stenosis
Stensen c.
Stilling c.
c. of stomach
subsartorial c.
Sucquet-Hoyer c.
supraorbital c.
target c.
tarsal c.
temporal c.
Theile c.
tibial medullary c.
tight spinal c.
tubal c.
tubotympanic c.
umbilical c.
uniting c.
urogenital c.
uterine c.
uterocervical c.
uterovaginal c.
utriculosaccular c.
vaginal c.
ventricular c.
Verneuil c.
vertebral c.
vesicourethral c.
vestibular c.
vidian c.
Volkmann c.
vomerine c.
vomerorostral c.
vomerovaginal c.
vulvouterine c.
widened optic c.
zygomaticofacial c.
zygomaticotemporal c.

NOTES

Canale-Kelly talar neck fracture classification
canalicular
    c. duct
    c. sphincter
canaliculus, pl. **canaliculi**
    apical c.
    auricular c.
    bone c.
    cochlear c.
    haversian c.
    innominate c.
canalization
Canavan disease
Canavan-van Bogaert-Bertrand disease
cancellated bone
cancellation
    fat-water signal c.
    phase c.
cancellous
    c. bone chip
    c. hematopoietic marrow
    c. osteoid osteoma
    c. screw
    c. tissue
cancer (*See* carcinoma)
    American Joint Committee on
      Cancer/Union International Contre
      le C. (AJCC-UICC)
    c. body
    c. cell anaplasia
    c. embolus
    hereditary nonpolyposis colorectal c.
      (HNPCC)
    radiation-induced c.
    c. of unknown primary (CUP)
cancerization
    field c.
cancriform
cancroid
candela
    c. lithotripsy
    C. 405-nm pulsed dye laser
candelabra
    c. artery
    sylvian c.
candida
    c. enteritis
    c. esophagitis
candidate lesion
candle
    c. drip disc
    c. dripping appearance
    c. wax dripping
candle-flame osteolysis
candle-guttering
candle-wax appearance of bone

candy-wrapper
    c.-w. effect
    c.-w. stenosis
caniocervical junction
cannon
    c. bone
    C. point
Cannon-Boehm point
cannula
    bulbous-tip stiff malleable c.
    Fluoro Tip c.
    indwelling c.
    metallic tip c.
    ultrasonic lithotripter c.
cannulated
    c. artery
    c. central vein
    percutaneously c.
cannulation
    aortic c.
    arterial c.
    atrial c.
    bicaval c.
    direct caval c.
    endoscopic retrograde pancreatic
      duct c.
    left atrial c.
    ostial c.
    retrograde c.
    selective c.
    single-cannula atrial c.
    2-stage venous c.
    subselective c.
    venoarterial c.
    venous c.
    venovenous c.
Canny edge detection algorithm
Canon scanner
Cantelli sign
canthomeatal line
canthus, pl. **canthi**
    outer c.
Cantlie line
Cantor tube
Cantrell pentalogy
caoutchouc
    silicone c.
cap
    apical c.
    azygos hematoma c.
    cartilaginous c.
    duodenal c.
    fibrous c.
    hilar c.
    left pleural apical hematoma c.
    phrygian c.
    c. plate
    pleural apical hematoma c.

pyloric c.
thin fibrous c.
capacious vein
capacitative calcium entry
capacitator
MOS c.
capacitive
c. interaction
c. reactance
capacity
bladder c.
closing c.
cranial c.
decreased vital c.
diffusing c.
dye-binding c. (DBC)
functional bladder c.
functional residual c.
gastric c.
limited oxidative c.
lung c.
residual volume/total lung c.
(RV/TLC)
respiratory c.
secretory c.
total lung c.
urinary bladder c.
vasodilatory c.
vital c. (VC)
Capener
triangle of C.
capillaritis
capillary, pl. **capillaries**
c. angioma
arterial c.
bile c.
c. blockade perfusion C-mode scan
c. blood flow
c. blood volume
c. bronchiectasis
c. bud
c. congestion
continuous c.
c. density
c. embolus
c. endothelium
c. filling
c. filling time
c. hemangioblastoma
c. hemangioendothelioma
c. hemangioma

c. hemorrhage
c. hydrostatic pressure
c. lake
c. leak
c. leak syndrome
c. loop
lymph c.
c. lymphangioma
c. lymphatic space invasion
c. malformation
Meigs c.
c. perfusion
c. permeability
c. pneumonia
c. pulsation
c. refill
ruptured c.
sinusoidal c.
c. telangiectasia
telangiectasia brain c.
c. tube
c. valve
c. vein
venous c.
c. vessel
c. wall
c. wedge pressure
capillary-lymphatic malformation (CLM)
capita (*pl. of* caput)
capital
c. epiphysis (CE)
c. epiphysis angle
c. extension
c. femoral epiphysis
c. flexor
c. fragment
capitate
c. bone
c. facet
c. fracture
c. hamate joint
c. soft spot
capitella
capitellar fracture
capitellum
humeral c.
capitis
fovea c.
capitolunate
c. angle
c. joint

NOTES

capitular
    c. epiphysis
    c. process
capitulum, pl. **capitula**
    c. costae
    c. fibulae
    c. humeri
    c. mandibula
    c. radiale humeri fracture
    c. radii
    c. ulnae
Caplan
    C. nodule
    C. syndrome
capping
    apical c.
    c. cyst
capsular
    c. attachment
    c. contracture
    c. drop lesion
    c. imbrication
    c. infarct
    c. insertion
    c. ligament
    c. plane
    c. reefing
    c. space
    c. thickening
    c. thrombosis
capsule
    adrenal c.
    articular c.
    auditory c.
    Bowman c.
    cartilage c.
    cricoarytenoid articular c.
    cricothyroid articular c.
    dorsal c.
    external c.
    facet joint c.
    fatty renal c.
    fibrous renal c.
    Gerota c.
    Given imaging capsule/M2A c.
    glenoid labrum c.
    Glisson c.
    hepatic c.
    hour-glass constriction of hip c.
    hypointense fibrous c.
    internal c.
    joint c.
    limb of anterior c.
    liver c.
    M2A c.
    M2A Swallowable Imaging C.
    medial carpal c.
    metatarsophalangeal c.
    organ c.

    otic c.
    plantar c.
    posterolateral c.
    prostate c.
    redundant c.
    renal c.
    rim of c.
    Sitzmarks c.
    splenic c.
    suprasellar c.
    talonavicular c.
    thyroid c.
    tissue c.
    tumor c.
    volar c.
    wrist c.
capsulitis
    adhesive c.
capsulocaudate infarct
capsulolabral complex
capsuloma
capsuloperiosteal envelope
capsuloputaminal infarct
capsuloputaminocaudate infarct
capsulorrhaphy
captopril-enhanced renal scintigraphy
captopril renogram
captopril-stimulated renal imaging
capture
    boron neutron c.
    cross-section c.
    electron c.
    gamma ray c.
    K c.
    resonance c.
caput, pl. **capita**
    c. cecum
    c. medusae
carbogen radiosensitizer
Carbomedics valve
carbon (C)
    c. 11 (^{11}C)
    c. 12 (^{12}C)
    c. 13 (^{13}C)
    c. 14 (^{14}C)
    c. dioxide (CO_2)
    c. dioxide generator
    c. dioxide laser
    double-bonded c.
    c. fiber-reinforced plastic
    c. imaging agent
    c. metabolism
    c. monoxide
    c. 13 spectroscopy
carbuncle
    renal c.
Carcassonne ligament
carcinogenesis
    radiation c.

carcinoid
  atypical c.
  colorectal c.
  c. GI tract
  c. syndrome
  thymic c.
  c. tumor
carcinoma, pl. **carcinomata, carcinomas**
  acinar pancreatic cell c.
  acinic cell c.
  adenocystic c.
  adenoid cystic lung c.
  adenoid squamous cell c.
  adnexal c.
  adrenal c.
  adrenocortical c.
  aerodigestive c.
  aldosterone-producing c.
  aldosterone-secreting c.
  alveolar basal cell c.
  alveolar mucosal c.
  ameloblastic c.
  ampullary c.
  anaplastic thyroid c.
  androgen-independent prostate c.
  aniline c.
  apocrine c.
  appendiceal c.
  apple-core c.
  aryepiglottic fold c.
  asbestos-related lung c.
  atypical medullary c.
  basal cell c.
  bilateral invasive lobular c.
  bile duct c.
  bilharzial c.
  biliary tract c.
  bladder c.
  blastic metastatic prostate c.
  bone c.
  Boorman classification of gastric c.
  bowel c.
  brain c.
  breast c.
  bronchial c.
  bronchiolar c.
  bronchioloalveolar c.
  bronchioloalveolar cell c.
  bronchoalveolar c.
  bronchogenic c.
  buccal mucosal c.
  cavitary squamous cell c.

  cavitating c.
  cecal c.
  cerebriform c.
  cholangiocellular c.
  chorionic c.
  choroid plexus c.
  clay pipe c.
  colloid c.
  colon c.
  colorectal c.
  comedo–basal cell c.
  conjugal c.
  contact c.
  corpus c.
  cortisol-producing c.
  cribriform c.
  cylindrical c.
  cylindromatous c.
  cystic renal cell c.
  dendritic c.
  differentiated c. (DC)
  distal bile duct c. (DBDC)
  ductal papillary c.
  ductal in situ breast c.
  duct cell c.
  embryonal cell c.
  encephaloid c.
  c. en cuirasse
  endobronchial c.
  endometrial c.
  endometrioid ovarian c.
  epidermal c.
  epidermoid lung c.
  epiglottic c.
  epithelial-myoepithelial c.
  epithelial ovarian c.
  esophageal c.
  ethmoid sinus c.
  exophytic c.
  c. ex pleomorphic adenoma
  extensive intraductal c. (EIC)
  extrahepatic bile duct c.
  extrapulmonary small cell c.
  fallopian tube c.
  false cord c.
  fibrolamellar hepatocellular c.
  FIGO stage c.
  flat colorectal c.
  focal lobular c.
  follicular thyroid c.
  gallbladder c.
  gastric remnant c.

C

NOTES

143

carcinoma *(continued)*
    gastric stump c.
    gastroesophageal junction c.
    gastrointestinal c.
    gelatinous c.
    genital c.
    genitourinary c.
    giant cell lung c.
    gingival c.
    glandular c.
    glans c.
    glottic c.
    granulosa cell c.
    hard palate c.
    head and neck c.
    hepatic c.
    hepatobiliary c.
    hepatocellular c. (HCC)
    hereditary nonpolyposis colorectal c.
      (HNPCC)
    hormone-receptor negative c.
    hormone-resistant prostate c.
    hyopharyngeal c.
    hypernephroid c.
    hypervascular hepatocellular c.
    hypopharyngeal c.
    infantile embryonal c.
    infiltrating ductal c.
    infiltrating esophageal c.
    infiltrating lobular c.
    inflammatory breast c. (IBC)
    intracystic breast c.
    intraductal c. (IDC)
    intraductal papillary c.
    intrahepatic biliary c.
    invasive breast c.
    invasive lobular c.
    jugular node metastatic c.
    juvenile embryonal c.
    known primary c.
    Kulchitsky cell c. (KCC)
    large cell neuroendocrine c.
      (LCNEC)
    large cell undifferentiated c.
    laryngeal c.
    lenticular c.
    leptomeningeal c.
    linitis plastica c.
    lobular c.
    locoregional breast c.
    lung c.
    mammographically occult c.
    maxillary sinus c.
    medullary breast c.
    medullary thyroid c.
    meibomian gland c.
    melanotic c.
    Merkel cell c.
    mesometanephric c.

metachronous transitional cell c.
metaplastic c.
metastatic urothelial c.
micropapillary c.
missed bronchogenic c.
mucin-hypersecreting c.
mucinous c.
mucinous breast c.
mucin-producing c.
mucoepidermoid c.
mucous c.
multicentric basal cell c.
multicentric invasive lobular c.
multifocal breast c.
multifocal invasive lobular c.
nasopharyngeal c. (NPC)
nasopharyngeal squamous cell c.
necrotic renal cell c.
neuroendocrine small-cell c.
nevoid basal cell c.
node-negative c.
node-positive c.
noncalcified c.
non-small cell lung c. (NSCLC)
oat cell c.
occult papillary c.
occult thyroid c.
osteoid c.
ovarian c.
Paget c.
palpatory T-stage prostate c.
pancreatic c.
papillary breast c.
papillary renal cell c.
papillary serous c.
papillary thyroid c.
paranasal sinus c.
parathyroid c.
perforating colorectal c.
periampullary c.
peripheral bronchogenic c.
pharyngeal wall c.
pigmented basal cell c.
piriform sinus c.
platinum-resistant ovarian c.
polypoid c.
postcricoid c.
posterior pharyngeal wall c.
preinvasive c.
prickle cell c.
primary hepatocellular c.
primary intraosseous c.
primary neuroendocrine small-cell c.
prostate c.
prostatic c.
pulmonary squamous cell c.
radiation-induced c.
rectal c.
rectosigmoid c.

renal c.
resectable colorectal c.
retinoblastoma hereditary human c.
retromolar trigone c.
salivary gland c.
scar c.
schistosomal bladder c.
schneiderian c.
scirrhous breast c.
sclerosing basal cell c.
sclerosing hepatic c. (SHC)
sebaceous c.
secretory c.
serous c.
sessile nodular c.
sigmoid c.
signet ring cell c.
c. simplex
sinonasal c.
c. in situ
skin c.
small bowel c.
small-cell cribriform c.
small-cell lung c. (SCLC)
small-cell undifferentiated c.
small intestine c.
small round cell c.
soft palate c.
solid circumscribed breast c.
solid and papillary pancreatic c.
spiculated c.
splenic flexure c.
sporadic colorectal c.
string cell c.
stump c.
subareolar c.
subglottic c.
superficial basal cell c.
superficial depressed c.
superficial spreading esophageal c.
superficial spreading stomach c.
supraglottic c.
suture line c.
sweat gland c.
synchronous transitional cell c.
telangiectatic c.
terminal c.
testicular c.
testis c.
thymic c.
thyroid c.
tongue c.

tonsil c.
tonsillar c.
trabecular c.
transitional cell c. (TCC)
transitional kidney cell c.
transitional urinary bladder cell c.
transition ureteral cell c.
transverse colon c.
tripartite duodenal c.
tubular breast c.
typical medullary c.
ulcerative esophageal c.
undifferentiated nasopharyngeal c.
unresectable colorectal c.
urachal c.
ureteral c.
urothelial c.
uterine cervix c.
uterine corpus c.
uterine papillary serous c. (UPSC)
vaginal c.
varicoid esophageal c.
verrucous c.
villous c.
vocal cord c.
vulvar c.
vulvovaginal c.
Walker c.
wolffian duct c.
carcinomatosa
carcinomatosis
lymphangitic c.
lymphatic c.
peritoneal c.
c. peritonei
carcinomatosum
carcinomatous
c. cavitary metastasis
c. implant
c. myelopathy
c. myopathy
c. neuromyopathy
c. subacute cerebellar degeneration
carcinosarcoma
embryonal c.
esophageal c.
renal c.
Walker c.
carcinosis
abdominal c.
carcinostatic
Carden amputation

NOTES

cardia
- crescent of c.
- gastric c.
- patulous c.

cardiac
- c. anomaly
- c. antrum
- c. apex
- C. Assist intraaortic balloon catheter
- c. atrial shunt
- c. blood pool imaging
- c. border
- c. branch
- c. calcification
- c. catheterization
- c. catheterization imaging
- c. chamber
- c. cirrhosis
- c. compression
- c. congestion
- c. contractility
- c. creep
- c. decompensation
- c. decompression
- c. decortication
- c. denervation
- c. diameter
- c. dilatation
- c. disturbance syndrome
- c. effusion
- c. failure
- c. fibroma
- c. fibrosarcoma
- c. filling pressure
- c. fossa
- c. frontal area
- c. ganglion
- c. gating
- c. gating compensation
- c. glycoside
- c. hamartoma
- c. hemangioma
- c. hydatidosis
- c. hypertrophy
- c. hypokinesis
- c. impression
- c. impression on liver
- c. incisura
- c. index (CI)
- c. infarct
- c. insufficiency
- c. inversion
- c. irradiation
- c. irritability
- c. ischemia
- c. laminography
- c. lipoma
- c. long axis view
- c. lymphangioma
- c. mapping
- c. margin
- c. mogul
- c. monitor
- c. MRI
- c. muscle
- c. muscle fiber
- c. muscle inflammation
- c. myocyte
- c. myxoma
- c. node
- c. notch
- c. oblique reformatting
- c. obstruction
- c. orifice
- c. osteosarcoma
- c. output (CO, Q)
- c. output echocardiography
- c. output measurement
- c. output video densitometry
- c. overload
- c. perforation
- c. PET
- c. phase
- c. plexus
- c. polyp
- c. position
- c. positron emission tomography imaging
- C. Protect
- c. pulmonary edema
- c. pulse duplicator
- c. pumping ability
- c. radiography
- c. radiography imaging
- c. recovery
- c. reserve
- c. rhabdomyoma
- c. rhabdomyosarcoma
- c. rupture
- c. sarcoidosis
- c. sarcoma
- c. scan
- c. scintigraphy
- c. scintigraphy ejection fraction
- c. segment
- c. segmental bronchus
- c. series
- c. shadow
- c. shape
- c. shock
- c. shock wave therapy (CSWT)
- c. short axis view
- c. shunt detection
- c. silhouette
- c. silhouette enlargement
- c. situs invertus
- c. situs solitus

c. skeleton
c. sling
c. standstill
C. STATus
c. steady state
c. stomach
c. tamponade
c. teratoma
c. thrombosis
c. tumor
c. valve
c. valve mucoid degeneration
c. valvular lesion
c. vasculature
c. vein
c. ventricle aneurysm
c. ventriculography
C. View probe
c. volume
c. waist
c. wall motion
c. wall motion imaging

cardiac-gated
    c.-g. MR angiography
    c.-g. PGSE sequence
    c.-g. quantitative computed
      tomography
    c.-g. respiration
    c.-g. study

Cardima Pathfinder microcatheter
cardinal
    c. event
    c. finding
    c. ligament
    c. point
    c. sign
    c. vein

cardioangiography
    blood pool radionuclide c.
    retrograde c.

CardioBeeper CB-12L cardiac monitor
CardioCard
cardiochalasia
CardioCoil coronary stent
cardiocutaneous syndrome
Cardio Data MK3 Holter scanner
cardiodiaphragmatic angle
cardioesophageal (CE)
    c. junction

CardioGen-82
cardiogenesis

cardiogenic
    c. embolic stroke
    c. embolus
    c. plate
    c. pulmonary edema
    c. shock
    c. shock heart

cardiogram
    ultrasonic c. (UCG)

cardiographic
cardiography
    M-mode c.
    radionuclide c.
    ultrasonic c.

cardiohepatic
    c. angle
    c. triangle

cardiohepatomegaly
cardioinhibitory response
cardiokymography (CKG)
Cardiolite
    C. imaging agent
    C. scan imaging
    technetium-tagged C.
    C. Tl-201

Cardiomed
    C. Bodysoft epidural catheter
    C. endotracheal ventilation catheter

cardiomediastinal shadow
cardiomegaly
    borderline c.
    boxlike c.
    funnellike c.
    globular c.
    iatrogenic c.

cardiomotility
cardiomyopathic degeneration
cardiomyopathy
    amyloidotic c.
    arrhythmogenic right ventricular c.
    concentric hypertrophic c.
    congenital dilated c.
    congestive c.
    constrictive c.
    degenerative c.
    diabetic c.
    diffuse symmetric hypertrophied c.
    dilated c. (DCM)
    dystrophinopathic c.
    end-stage c.
    familial hypertrophic c. (FHC)
    Friedreich ataxic c.

NOTES

cardiomyopathy *(continued)*
    hypertrophic c. (HCM)
    hypertrophic obstructive c. (HOC, HOCM)
    idiopathic dilated c. (IDC)
    idiopathic restrictive c.
    infantile c.
    infectious c.
    infiltrative c.
    ischemic congestive c.
    left ventricular c.
    metabolic c.
    nonischemic congestive c.
    nonobstructive c.
    obliterative c.
    obstructive hypertrophic c.
    peripartum dilated c.
    postmyocarditis dilated c.
    postpartum c.
    restrictive c.
    right-sided c.
    right ventricular c.
    tachycardia-induced c.
    toxic c.
cardionecrosis
cardiophrenic
    c. angle
    c. junction
    c. right-angle mass
cardiopneumatic
cardioptosis
    Wenckebach c.
cardiopulmonary
    c. abnormality
    c. bilharziasis
    c. disease
    c. edema
    c. insufficiency
    c. support system
cardiopyloric
cardiorenal disease
cardiorespiratory sign
cardiorrhexis
cardioscan
Cardioscint
cardiosclerosis
CardioSEAL occluder
cardioselective agent
cardiospasm
cardiosplenic syndrome
cardiosynchronous stimulation
CardioTec scan
cardiothoracic
    c. index
    c. ratio (CT, CTR)
    c. trauma
cardiothymic
    c. shadow
    c. silhouette

cardiothyrotoxicosis
cardiotocogram
cardiotocography imaging
cardiotopometry
cardiovalvular
cardiovascular
    c. accident (CVA)
    c. angiography analysis system (CAAS)
    c. anomaly
    c. computed tomographic scanner (CVCT)
    c. disease (CD, CVD)
    c. imaging technique
    c. malformation
    c. pressure
    c. radioisotope scan and function imaging
    c. radiology
    c. renal disease
    c. shadow
    c. shunt
    c. silhouette
    c. system
cardioverter-defibrillator
    automatic implantable c.-d. (AICD)
cardiovolume
    multislice c. (MSCV)
carditis
    acute lethal c.
    Lyme c.
care
    home infusion c.
CARE bolus
CareGraph skin dose mapping software
Carey-Coons soft stent biliary endoprosthesis
carina, pl. **carinae**
    mainstem c.
    sharp c.
    c. of trachea
carinal
    c. angle
    c. angle narrowing
    c. lesion
Carleton spot
C-arm
    C-a. DSA system
    C-a. fluoroscopic control
    C-a. fluoroscopy
    Mini 6000 C-a.
    C-a. portable x-ray unit
    Siremobile Iso-C3d isocentric C-a.
Carman sign
Carnesale-Stewart-Barnes hip dislocation classification
Carnett sign

Carney
  C. syndrome
  C. triad
Carnoy solution
Caroli disease
caroticocavernous fistula
caroticoclinoid ligament
caroticojugular spine
caroticotympanic
  c. artery
  c. canal
carotid
  c. angiography
  c. artery
  c. artery aneurysm
  c. artery arteritis
  c. artery bifurcation
  c. artery calcification
  c. artery disease
  c. artery dissection trauma
  c. artery ischemia
  c. artery kinking
  c. artery occlusion
  c. artery plaque
  c. artery stenosis
  c. artery stenting
  c. atherosclerosis
  c. atherosclerotic disease
  c. bifurcation atheroma
  c. blowout syndrome
  c. body
  c. body tumor
  c. bulb
  c. bulb baroreceptor
  c. canal
  c. cerebral arteriography
  c. circulation
  c. cistern
  c. compression tonography
  c. disobliteration
  c. distribution TIA
  c. duct
  c. duplex imaging
  c. duplex study
  c. duplex ultrasound
  c. ejection time
  c. endarterectomy (CEA)
  external c.
  c. foramen
  c. ganglion
  c. gland
  c. groove

  c. hemorrhage
  internal c.
  c. lumen
  c. occlusive disease
  c. phonoangiography
  c. plaque hematoma
  c. plexus
  c. pulse
  c. pulse peak
  c. pulse tracing
  c. pulse upstroke
  c. revascularization endarterectomy
    stent trial
  c. sheath
  c. sheath adenoma
  c. shudder
  c. sinus
  c. sinus hypersensitivity
  c. sinus imaging
  c. sinus syndrome (CSS)
  c. siphon
  c. sonography
  c. space
  c. space mass
  c. string sign
  c. sulcus
  c. triangle
  c. tubercle
  c. vein
  c. velocity
  c. and vertebral artery transluminal
    (CAVATAS)
  c. wall
carotid-carotid venous bypass graft
carotid-cavernous
  c.-c. fistula (CCF)
  c.-c. fistula occlusion
  c.-c. sinus fistula
carotid-dural fistula
carotidis
  bifurcatio c.
carotid-jugular fistula
carotid-ophthalmic aneurysm
carotid pulse
carotid-subclavian transposition
Carotid-Wallstent Monorail
carpal
  c. arch
  c. articular surface
  c. axes
  c. bone anatomy
  c. bone stress fracture

NOTES

149

carpal *(continued)*
   c. boss
   c. box
   c. canal
   c. coalition
   c. content ratio
   c. deviation
   c. groove
   c. height index
   c. height ratio
   c. navicular
   c. navicular bone
   c. navicular fracture
   c. row
   c. scaphoid bone fracture
   c. tunnel
   c. tunnel projection
   c. tunnel syndrome
   c. tunnel view
   c. wrist angle
Carpentier-Edwards ring
Carpentier ring
carpet
   c. lesion
   c. lesion of colon
   c. polyp
carpometacarpal
   c. articulation
   c. fusion
   c. joint (CMC)
   c. joint fracture
   c. ligament
carpophalangeal joint
carporadial articulation
carpotarsal osteolysis
carpus, pl. **carpi**
   adaptive c.
   cuneiform bone of c.
   ulnar translocation of c.
carrier
   c. added radionuclide
   c. free radionuclide
   ^{67}Ga GABA uptake c.
   c. protein
   radionuclide c.
   c. tube
carrier-free
   c.-f. isotope
   c.-f. radioisotope
   c.-f. separation
   c.-f. separation process
carrier-mediated transport system
Carrington disease
carrot-shaped trachea
Carr-Purcell (CP)
   C.-P. sequence
Carr-Purcell-Meiboom-Gill (CPMG)
   C.-P.-M.-G. sequence
carrying angle

Carson procedure
Carter equation
Carter-Rowe view
cartesian reference coordinate system
cartilage
   absent bronchial c.
   accessory nasal c.
   alar c.
   anular rim of c.
   aortic c.
   arthrodial c.
   articular c.
   arytenoid c.
   attenuated intercarpal articular c.
   auditory c.
   auricular c.
   basilar c.
   c. bone
   branchial c.
   bronchial anular c.
   c. calcification
   calcified c.
   c. capsule
   ciliary c.
   circumferential c.
   conchal c.
   connecting c.
   corniculate c.
   costal intraarticular c.
   cricoid c.
   cricothyroid c.
   cuneiform c.
   delayed gadolinium-enhanced
     magnetic resonance imaging of c.
     (dGEMRIC)
   delayed gadolinium-enhanced MRI
     of c.
   elastic c.
   c. endplate
   ensiform c.
   epiglottic c.
   epiphysial c.
   facet c.
   falciform c.
   fibroelastic c.
   fibrous c.
   flaking of c.
   floating c.
   free flap of c.
   c. hair hypoplasia
   hyaline articular c.
   interarticular c.
   c. island
   c. joint space
   c. lacuna
   laryngeal c.
   liplike projection of c.
   loss of elasticity of c.
   c. matrix

ossified c.
osteoarthritic c.
patellofemoral articular c.
physial c.
pitted c.
pulmonary c.
quadrangle c.
rim of c.
roughened c.
scored c.
semilunar c.
shelling off of c.
softening of c.
sternal c.
c. stroma
swelling of c.
tag of c.
talar dome articular c.
thinned c.
thyroid c.
tracheal c.
triradiate c.
unossified c.
xiphoid c.
Y c.
yellow c.
cartilage-capped exostosis
cartilage-containing giant cell tumor
cartilage-forming bone tumor
cartilaginous
c. acetabulum
c. anlage
c. bar
c. cap
c. cap of phalangeal head
c. degeneration
c. disc
c. endplate
c. epiphysis
c. growth plate
c. growth plate disorder
c. hamartoma
c. joint surface
c. lesion
c. metaplasia
c. node
c. nodule
c. ring
c. septum
c. soft-tissue tumor
c. synchondrosis

c. tissue
c. viscerocranium
CARTO EP navigation system
cartographic projection
cartwheel fracture
Carvallo sign
Cary-Coon biliary stent
CAS
coronary artery scan
coronary artery spasm
CAS imaging
cascade
diagnostic c.
gamma c.
c. stomach
c. system
time-dependent metabolic c.
caseating granuloma
caseous
c. necrosis
c. pneumonia
Casser
C. ligament
C. muscle
casserian
c. ligament
c. muscle
cassette
Adrian-Crooks c.
Camp grid c.
Curix film screen c.
film screen c.
CAST
computer automated scan technology
Castaneda thrombolytic brush
casting breast calcification
Castleman
C. disease
C. lymphoma
cast-off x-ray (COX)
CAT
computerized axial tomography
catamenial pneumothorax
catapophysis
cataract
radiation c.
catarrhal pneumonia
catastrophe
vascular c.
catecholamine-producing tumor
catechol-*O*-methyltransferase

NOTES

category
    iliac PTA c. 1–4
    Rutherford-Becker claudication c.
      1–5
catenary system
cath
    catheter
    Arrow Twin Cath
cathartic colon
catheter (cath)
    abscess drainage c.
    Abscession drainage c.
    Accu-Vu sizing c.
    Achiever balloon dilatation c.
    Ackrad balloon-bearing c.
    ACS balloon c.
    ACS Concorde c.
    ACS Endura coronary dilation c.
    ACS OTW Photon coronary
      dilatation c.
    ACS RX Comet coronary
      dilatation c.
    ACS Tourguide II guiding c.
    AcuNav ultrasound c.
    Ahn thrombectomy c.
    Alert c.
    Amplatz left coronary c.
    Amplatz maceration aspiration
      thrombectomy c. (AMATC)
    Amplatz right coronary c.
    Amplatz Super Stiff c.
    Angiocath Autoguard Shielded
      IV c.
    Angiocath PRN c.
    angiographic c.
    c. angiography
    AngioJet Xpeedior c.
    angled-tip c.
    angulated c.
    Anthron heparinized c.
    c. aortography
    apheresis c.
    arrhythmia mapping system c.
    arrhythmogenic myocardial tissue
      ablation c.
    Arrow c.
    ARROWgard Blue Line c.
    Arrow-Howes multilumen c.
    c. arteriography
    Ascent guiding c.
    ATB PTA ablation c.
    AtheroCath Bantam coronary
      atherectomy c.
    AtheroTrack c.
    Atlantis SR IVUS c.
    Auth Rotablator atherectomy c.
    balloon biliary c.
    balloon embolectomy c.
    balloon PTA c.

    balloon-tipped angiographic c.
    Bardex Lubricath c.
    Bard Safety Excalibur c.
    BD Insyte Autoguard shielded
      intravenous c.
    Berenstein c.
    Berman angiographic c.
    Bernstein c.
    Beta-Cath system c.
    biliary drainage c.
    Blue Max high-pressure reinforced
      polyethylene balloon c.
    braided diagnostic c.
    Brevi-Kath epidural c.
    Brite Tip 5F–10F guiding c.
    Bronchitrac L c.
    Broviac long-term c.
    c. bursting pressure
    c. calibration
    Calypso Rely c.
    Camino intracranial c.
    Camino microventricular bolt c.
    Cardiac Assist intraaortic balloon c.
    Cardiomed Bodysoft epidural c.
    Cardiomed endotracheal
      ventilation c.
    Caud-A-Kath c.
    central venous c. (CVC)
    Centurion PTA balloon dilatation c.
    Cheetah angioplasty c.
    Chemo-Port c.
    c. cholangiogram
    cholangiography c.
    CliniCath peripherally inserted c.
    80-cm 8F Brite Tip guide c.
    coaxillary directed c.
    Cobra 1 c.
    Cobra 2 c.
    Cobra diagnostic c.
    cobra-shaped c.
    c. coiling sign
    Comfort Cath I c.
    Comfort Cath II c.
    condom c.
    conductance c.
    Conquest balloon dilatation c.
    Conquest PTA balloon dilatation c.
    contrast-filled c.
    Cook-Cope type loop c.
    Cope locking-loop c.
    Cope loop c.
    Cordis Brite Tip 5F–10F
      guiding c.
    Cordis Predator PTCA balloon c.
    coudé c.
    Cragg-McNamara multiple side-hole
      infusion c.
    cutting balloon c.
    Datascope c.

Dawson-Mueller drainage c.
decompression c.
Derek Harwood-Nash c.
directional atherectomy c.
double-J indwelling c.
double-J ureteral c.
double lumen central venous c.
drainage c.
dual-lumen silicone
  hemodialysis/apheresis c.
Du Pen long-term epidural c.
EchoMark c.
electrothermal c.
Endosound endoscopic ultrasound c.
Envoy 6F guiding c.
Epimed spring guide c.
EPT-Dx steerable diagnostic c.
Equinox occlusion balloon c.
ERCP c.
c. exit site
Explorer 360-degree rotational
  diagnostic c.
Explorer ST fixed curve
  diagnostic c.
Export c.
Express PTCA c.
external biliary drainage c.
Fast-Cath introducer c.
FasTracker c.
c. fixation
Flexima biliary drainage c.
Flexi-Tip ureteral c.
fluid-filled c.
Fogarty Adherent Clot c.
Fogarty balloon embolectomy c.
Fogarty Thru-Lumen c.
8-French guiding c.
9-French guiding c.
French tip c.
gastrojejunostomy c.
gastrostomy c.
Glide Cobra c.
Greenfield c.
Grollman pigtail c.
Groshong distal-valve c.
Grüntzig balloon dilatation c.
H1 c.
Headhunter c.
helium-filled balloon c.
hemodialysis c.
Hickman long-term c.
Hickman tunneled indwelling c.

hockey-stick c.
Hopkins hook-guiding c.
H/S Elliptosphere balloon c.
HSG c.
Hydrolyser hydrodynamic
  thrombectomy c.
hydrophilic-coated guiding c.
hysterosalpingography c.
ILUS c.
Imager II c.
c. impact artifact
impeller basket c.
implantable access c.
indwelling Foley c.
Infuse-a-Port c.
infusion c.
c. insertion
Insyte Autoguard Shielded IV c.
internal/external c.
intraarterial chemotherapy c.
IntraCardiac Echocardiography
  IVUS c.
Intracath c.
intraluminal ultrasound c.
intravascular ultrasound c.
IVUS c.
JB1 c.
jejunostomy c.
Jography angiographic c.
Judkins 4 diagnostic c.
Judkins left coronary c.
Judkins right coronary c.
jugular c.
c. kinking
Kumpe c.
large-bore c.
LifeJet c.
8-lumen manometric c.
Maglinte c.
Malecot nephrostomy c.
MammoSite radiation therapy
  system c. (MammoSite RTS
  catheter)
MammoSite RTS c.
  MammoSite radiation therapy
  system catheter
c. mapping
MediPort c.
Medi-tech c.
Medtronic c.
Mercator atrial high-density
  array c.

NOTES

153

catheter *(continued)*
Mewissen infusion c.
micromanometer-tipped c.
MicroMewi multiple sidehole
  infusion c.
c. migration
Motarjeme c.
MR-trackable intramyocardial
  injection c.
multiaccess c.
multielectrode c.
multiple-side-hole infusion c.
multipurpose c.
multi-sideport infusion c.
multislit c.
Navarre c.
Navarre drainage c.
Navi-Star ablation c.
Nd:YAG laser c.
NephroMax balloon c.
nephrostomy c.
nondetachable balloon c.
nontunneled c.
nylon c.
Oasis triple-lumen c.
c. obstruction
Omni Flush 3F, 4F, 5F c.
Omni Selective 0-3 c.
OneStep paracentesis drainage c.
Opticath c.
Opti-Flow dialysis c.
Opti-Plast balloon dilatation c.
OptiQue c.
Oracle MegaSonics c.
Oracle Micro Plus c.
Oracle PTCA c.
PASV c.
PE c.
percutaneous cavity drainage c.
percutaneous cholecystotomy c.
peripherally inserted central c.
  (PICC)
peritoneal dialysis c.
pigtail c.
c. placement
Polaris-Dx steerable diagnostic c.
Polaris X steerable diagnostic c.
polyethylene c.
polypropylene c.
Possis AngioJet Xpeedior c.
Proforma c.
PU c.
Pulse-Spray/PRO infusion c.
PVC c.
quantum Monorail balloon c.
RadPICC c.
Ranfac cholangiographic c.
Rapid Transit c.

Reddick cystic duct
  cholangiogram c.
Resolution ultrasonic c.
Resolve non-locking draining c.
Ring biliary drainage c.
Rosch hepatic c.
rotatable pigtail c.
Royal Flush 4F pigtail c.
Rusch c.
Saf-T-Intima integrated IV c.
Schneider Guider c.
SCOOP model polyurethane
  intratracheal c.
self-retaining Cope loop pigtail c.
c. sheath
Sidewinder c.
Sidewinder diagnostic c.
Silverhawk c.
Simmons c.
Simpson directional atherectomy c.
single-curved Cobra c.
Softouch c.
Soft-Tip c.
Soft Torque uterine c.
Soft-Vu angiographic c.
solid-state manometry c.
Sonicath Ultra imaging c.
Spyglass angiography c.
Steerocath-Dx octapolar and valve
  mapping c.
Stimucath continuous nerve
  block c.
straight end-hole c.
straight side-hole c.
sump drainage c.
Swan-Ganz balloon c.
Tamp c.
Teflon c.
temporary pacing c.
Temp Tip drainage c.
Tenckhoff c.
thermodilution c.
thin-walled c.
c. tip
c. tip hockey-stick appearance
c. tip motion
c. tip motion artifact
c. tip position
c. tip position artifact
Torcon blue c.
Tracker 10 c.
Tracker Excel c.
transducer-tipped c.
transhepatic c.
TRAX c.
tunneled c.
UltraICE c.
Ultra ICE 9F/9 MHz c.
Uni-Fuse infusion c.

Van Aman pulmonary pigtail c.
Van Sonnenberg sump c.
Vaxcel peripherally inserted c.
ventriculography c.
visceral c.
water-infusion c.
c. whip artifact
c. with preformed curves
Z-MED balloon c.

catheter-based
c.-b. inducible enhancers of gene expression
c.-b. interventional MRI
c.-b. intervention technique

catheter-borne sector transducer
catheter-delivered platinum coil
catheter-directed
c.-d. approach
c.-d. extremity thrombolysis
c.-d. fenestration
c.-d. interventional procedure
c.-d. thrombolytic therapy
c.-d. urokinase

catheter-induced
c.-i. coronary artery spasm
c.-i. embolus
c.-i. pulmonary artery hemorrhage
c.-i. subclavian vein thrombosis
c.-i. thromboembolization
c.-i. vasospasm

catheterization
antegrade femoral artery c.
balloon c.
cardiac c.
high brachial artery c.
interventional c.
left axillary artery c.
left heart c.
retrograde femoral artery c.
right heart c.
Seldinger c.
superior petrosal sinus c.
superselective mesenteric artery c.
therapeutic cardiac c.

catheter-securing technique
catheter-skin interface
catheter-tissue contact
Cathflo Activase
cathode
c. glow
c. ray
c. ray tube (CRT)

CathScanner ultrasound imaging system
CathTrack catheter locator system
cation
paramagnetic c.
CAT-MIBI image fusion
cat phantom
cat's
c. cry syndrome
c. eye calculus
c. eye reflex
c. tail configuration

cauda, pl. **caudae**
c. equina
c. equina compression
c. equina syndrome (CES)

caudad projection
Caud-A-Kath catheter
caudal
c. branch
c. canal
c. direction
c. flexure
c. ligament
c. pharyngeal complex
c. pons
c. projection
c. regression
c. regression syndrome
c. sheath
c. tilt
c. vertebra
c. view

caudal-cranial angulation
caudalward
caudate
c. body
c. lobe
c. lobe of liver
c. nucleus
c. process
c. vein
c. volume

caudocranial
c. projection
c. tangential view

caudothalamic groove
cauliflower appearance
cauliflower-shaped filling defect
caustic esophagitis
cava
azygos continuation of inferior vena c.

C

NOTES

cava *(continued)*
    bilateral superior vena c.
    collapsed inferior vena c.
    duplicated inferior vena c.
    inferior vena c. (IVC)
    infrahepatic vena c.
    juxtarenal c.
    membranous obstruction of inferior
      vena c.
    paired inferior vena c.
    persistent left inferior vena c.
    persistent left superior vena c.
    redirection of inferior vena c.
    retrohepatic vena c.
    sinus of vena c.
    superior bilateral vena c.
    superior vena c. (SVC)
    suprahepatic vena c.
    thrombosed filter-bearing inferior
      vena c.
    transposition of inferior vena c.
    vena c.
cavagram
    inferior vena c.
caval
    c. filter
    c. fold
    c. lymph node
    c. opening
    c. tourniquet
    c. valve
cavalry bone
CAVATAS
    carotid and vertebral artery transluminal
    CAVATAS trial
CAVB
    complete atrioventricular block
cavernoma
    brain c.
    portal vein c.
cavernosa
cavernosogram
cavernosography
    corpora c.
cavernosometry
cavernous
    c. angioma
    c. angiosarcoma
    c. brain angiography
    c. brain hemangioma
    c. groove
    c. lymphangioma
    c. malformation
    c. plexus
    c. portal vein transformation
    c. portion
    c. segment of internal carotid
      artery
    c. sinus

    c. sinus aneurysm
    c. sinus fistula
    c. sinus lesion
    c. sinus meningioma
    c. sinus syndrome
    c. tissue
    c. transfer of portal vein
    c. transformation of portal vein
    c. tumor
    c. urethra
caviar lesion
cavitary
    c. consolidation
    c. dilatation
    c. fluid
    c. infiltrate
    c. lung lesion
    c. mass
    c. metastasis
    c. prostatitis
    c. pulmonary lesion
    c. small bowel lesion
    c. space
    c. squamous cell carcinoma
    c. tuberculosis
cavitate
cavitating
    c. carcinoma
    c. lung metastasis
    c. lung nodule
    c. neoplasm
    c. pattern
    c. pneumonia
cavitation
    collapse c.
    crescent of c.
    lobar c.
    pulmonary c.
    stable c.
    transient c.
Cavitron Ultrasonic Surgical Aspirator
    (CUSA)
cavity
    abdominal c.
    abdominopelvic c.
    absorption c.
    acetabular c.
    air c.
    amnionic c.
    ancyroid c.
    c. of aneurysm
    axillary c.
    banana-shaped uterine c.
    body c.
    Bragg-Gray c.
    buccal c.
    chest c.
    cleavage c.
    coexistent c.

cotyloid c.
cranial c.
crown c.
dome-shaped roof of pleural c.
embryonic abdominal c.
endometrial c.
epidural c.
funnel-shaped c.
glenoid c.
grape-skin lung c.
greater sac of peritoneal c.
intraperitoneal c.
joint c.
c. lavage
lesser sac of peritoneal c.
lung c.
marrow c.
Meckel c.
medullary c.
midcarpal joint c.
miniature uterine c.
multiple thin-walled lung c.
nasal c.
orbital c.
pericardial c.
peritoneal c.
pleural c.
popliteal c.
pulmonary c.
resection c.
retroperitoneal c.
saclike c.
septum pellucidum c.
sigmoid c.
sinonasal c.
sinus c.
Stafne idiopathic bone c.
subarachnoid c.
subchondral cystic c.
subdural c.
surgically created resection c.
synovial c.
syringohydromyelic c.
syrinx c.
thin-walled lung c.
thoracic c.
trigeminal c.
tubular c.
tympanic c.
uterine c.
ventricular c.

c. volume
c. wall
cavoatrial junction
cavogram
cavography
cavopulmonary connection
cavovalgus
    pes c.
    talipes c.
cavovarus
    c. deformity
    pes c.
cavum
    c. septum pellucidum
    c. veli interpositi
cavus
    c. deformity
    global c.
    local c.
    pes c.
    posttraumatic c.
    talipes c.
Cayler syndrome
CBCL
    cutaneous B-cell lymphoma
CBD
    common bile duct
CBDE
    common bile duct exploration
CBF
    cerebral blood flow
        CBF index
CBFV
    coronary blood flow velocity
CBI
    convergent beam irradiation
CBT
    corticobulbar tract
CBV
    cerebral blood volume
CBV-CBF
    cerebral blood volume to cerebral blood
        flow ratio
C-C
    convexoconcave
        C-C heart valve
cc
    cubic centimeter
CCA
    common carotid artery

NOTES

C

CCAM
congenital cystic adenomatoid
malformation
CCD
central collodiaphysial
charge-coupled device
CCD angle
CCD detector
CCD photodetector
CCDS
color-coded duplex sonography
CCF
carotid-cavernous fistula
CCRT
computer-controlled conformal radiation
therapy
CCT
cranial computed tomography
CCTA
coronal computed tomographic
arthrography
CD
cardiovascular disease
cluster of differentiation
coincidence detection
color Doppler
Crohn disease
Cd
cadmium
CDFI
color-coded Doppler flow imaging
CDH
congenital dislocation of hip
CDI
color Doppler imaging
CDR
computed dental radiography
CDRPan digital x-ray system
CDS
color Doppler sonography
CDUS
color Doppler ultrasound
microbubble-enhanced CDUS
CE
capital epiphysis
cardioesophageal
CE angle of Wiberg
CE junction
CEA
carotid endarterectomy
CEA-Scan
CEA-S. diagnostic imaging
CEA-S. imaging agent
cebocephaly
ceca (*pl. of* cecum)
cecal
c. appendage
c. appendix
c. bar

c. bascule
c. carcinoma
c. deformity
c. filling defect
c. fold
c. foramen
c. hernia
c. ileus
c. recess
c. serosa
c. sphincter
c. thickening
c. volvulus
cecocutaneous fistula
cecostomy
percutaneous c.
CECT
contrast enhanced computed tomography
cecum, pl. **ceca**
antimesocolic side of c.
caput c.
coned c.
conic c.
conical c.
c. diameter
kidney-shaped distended c.
c. mobile
subhepatic c.
Cedell
C. fracture
C. fracture of talus
Cedell-Magnusson
C.-M. arthritis classification
C.-M. classification of arthritis
Ceelen-Gellerstedt syndrome
CE-FAST
contrast-enhanced Fourier-acquired
steady state
CE-FAST scan
Celestin tube
celiac
c. angiography
c. arteriography
c. artery aneurysm
c. artery compression syndrome
c. artery dissection
c. axis
c. axis occlusion
c. axis syndrome
c. branch artery
c. disease
c. ganglion
c. ganglion block
c. lymph node
c. lymph node metastasis
c. plexus
c. plexus block
c. plexus blockade

c. plexus neurolysis, endoscopic
ultrasound-guided
c. trunk
celiacography
celiectasia
celioma
celiomesenteric trunk
celioscopy
celiotomy
cell
basket c.
cerebellar granule c.
chromium-heated red blood c.
encroaching endothelial c.
epithelial c.
ethmoid air c.
glomerular mesangial c.
homophilic Purkinje c.
human aortic smooth muscle c.
^{111}In-labeled white blood c.
Kulchitsky c.
morulalike epithelial c.
Onodi c.
pluripotential bronchial epithelial
stem c.
c. polarization
polygonal elongate c.
c. preparation bone marrow uptake
protein-nucleic acid synthesis in
tumor c.
Rael c.
red blood c. (RBC)
Rieder c.
Schwann c.
tagged red c.
tanned red c. (TRC)
technetium-99m red blood c.
(^{99m}Tc-RBC)
technetium-tagged red blood c.
totipotential stem c.
c. tumor
white blood c. (WBC)
Zimmerman c.
cella medix index
cell-dose threshold
celloidin section
CellSeek technology
cellular
c. binding site
c. bronchiolitis
c. embolus

c. fibroadenoma
c. tumor
cellule formation
cellulitis
iodine 131–induced c.
orbital c.
celomic
c. metaphysis
c. pouch
CEM
central extensor mechanism
Cemax/Icon PACS system
cement
bone c.
c. line
c. mantle
radiopaque bone c.
residual c.
cemental
c. dysplasia
c. fracture
cementation
cementifying fibroma
cementinoma
cementoblastoma
cementoma
gigantiform c.
cementoosseous dysplasia
cementoossifying fibroma
cementoplasty
percutaneous c.
cementosis
cementum
CE-MRA
contrast-enhanced magnetic resonance
angiography
CEMRA
contrast-enhanced magnetic resonance
angiography
3D CEMRA
Cencit surface scanner
Centauri Er:YAG dental laser system
center
accessory ossification c.
anechoic c.
bone c.
cortical c.
diaphysial c.
elbow bone c.
emetic c.
enlargement with low-density lymph
node c.

NOTES

center (*continued*)
  epileptogenic c.
  epiphysial fetal bone c.
  epiphysial ossification c.
  femoral ossification c.
  fetal epiphysial bone c.
  c. of gravity
  c. line artifact
  lucent c.
  C. of Metabolic and Experimental
    Imaging
  ossification c.
  ovoid ossification c.
  swallowing c.
  tibial tubercle ossification c.
  vertebral body ossification c.
  window c.
center-edge
  c.-e. angle of Lequesne
  c.-e. angle of Wiberg
center-to-center distance
centigray (cGy)
centimeter (cm)
  cubic c. (cc)
central
  c. airway disease
  c. amaurosis
  c. aorta
  c. aortic pressure
  c. artery
  c. axis depth dose
  c. beaking
  c. blood volume
  c. bone
  c. bronchiectasis
  c. bronchovascular bundle
  c. caged ball occluder valve
  c. caged disc occluder valve
  c. callus
  c. canal stenosis
  c. cavity of cerebrum
  c. cementifying fibroma
  c. cerebellar fissure
  c. cervical cord syndrome
  c. channel
  c. chondrosarcoma
  c. collodiaphysial (CCD)
  c. collodiaphysial angle
  c. dislocation
  c. extensor mechanism (CEM)
  c. fat signal intensity
  c. fatty hilum
  c. fibrosarcoma
  c. fracture
  c. groove
  c. gyrus
  c. hemorrhagic component
  c. herniation
  c. high-signal intensity stripe

  c. hilar structure
  c. horn
  c. indentation
  c. intraluminal saturation stripe
  c. intrasubstance signal intensity
  c. lung distance (CLD)
  c. lymph node
  c. medullary bone lesion
  c. necrosis
  c. nervous system (CNS)
  c. nervous system tumor
  c. neurocytoma
  c. neurofibromatosis
  c. nidus of high-intensity marrow
  c. ossifying fibroma
  c. osteosarcoma
  c. pancreatic lesion scar
  c. perineal tendon
  c. pit
  c. placenta previa
  c. pneumonia
  c. point artifact
  c. pontine
  c. pontine myelinolysis
  c. ray (CR)
  c. rhomboid attachment
  c. sacral line (CSL)
  c. sinus lipomatosis
  c. solitary papilloma breast
  c. spinal canal
  c. spinal cord syrinx
  c. spinal stenosis
  c. splanchnic venous thrombosis
    (CSVT)
  c. sulcus
  c. tegmental tract (CTT)
  c. tendon diaphragm
  c. vein
  c. venous access
  c. venous catheter (CVC)
  c. venous drainage
  c. venous line position
  c. venous obstruction
  c. venous pressure (CVP)
  c. venous pressure line
  c. vertebral osteomyelitis
centralis
  fovea c.
centrally
  c. ordered phase encoding
  c. uninhibited bladder
centriacinar emphysema
centriciput
centrifugation
  discontinuous density gradient c.
centrilobar opacity
centrilobular
  c. congestion
  c. distribution

c. emphysema
c. lesion
c. micronodule
c. necrosis
c. nodule
c. region of liver
c. shadow
centroblast
centroblastic lymphoma
centrocytelike type
centrocytic lymphoma
centrocytoid
centroid
endocardial c.
epicardial c.
floating endocardial c.
floating epicardial c.
myocardial c.
centroid-based maximum intensity projection
centromere
centrum
c. commune
c. ovale
c. semiovale
c. semiovale pattern
Centurion PTA balloon dilatation catheter
cephalad-caudad direction
cephalad direction
cephalhematoma (*var. of* cephalohematoma)
cephalic
c. angle
c. angulation
c. arch stenosis
c. flexure
c. index
c. pole
c. presentation
c. presentation of fetus
c. tilt view
c. triangle
c. vein
c. ventricle
cephalization of blood flow
cephalized vessel
cephalocaudad
cephalocele
atretic c.
occipital c.
oral c.
sincipital c.
cephalofacial proportionality
cephalogram imaging
cephalohematocele
cephalohematoma, cephalhematoma
parietal c.
cephalomedullary nail fracture
cephalometer
Bertillon c.
cephalometric
c. analysis
c. angle
c. radiograph
cephalometry
radiographic c.
ultrasonic c.
cephalopelvic
c. disproportion (CPD)
c. disproportion index
cephalopelvimetry
cephalosporin
cephalostat
cephalosyndactyly
Vogt c.
CEqual quantitative analysis
CerASPECT
C. camera
C. system
ceratocricoid ligament
cerebella (*pl. of* cerebellum)
cerebellar
c. anaplasia
c. aplasia
c. apoplexy
c. artery
c. astrocytoma
c. atrophy
c. attachment
c. cortex
c. cystic mass
c. degeneration
c. diaschisis
c. ectopia
c. epidermoid
c. fiber
c. folia
c. gliosarcoma
c. granule cell
c. hemisphere
c. hemorrhage
c. heterotopia

NOTES

C

cerebellar *(continued)*
  c. hypoperfusion
  c. hypoplasia
  c. infarct
  c. notch
  c. pathway
  c. peduncle
  c. peg
  c. sarcoma
  c. syndrome
  c. tonsil
  c. tract
  c. uvula
  c. vermis
  c. vermis hypoplasia, oligophrenia,
    congenital ataxia, ocular
    coloboma, hepatic fibrosis
    (COACH)
  c. view
  c. volume
cerebelli
  falx c.
  gyrus c.
  mediastinum c.
  tentorium c.
  vallecula c.
cerebellitis
cerebellolabyrinthine artery
cerebellomedullary cistern
cerebelloolivary degeneration
cerebellopontine
  c. angle (CPA)
  c. angle meningioma
  c. angle tumor
  c. cistern
  c. cisternography
  c. recess
cerebelloretinal
  c. hemangioblastoma
  c. hemangioblastomatosis
cerebellum, pl. **cerebella**
  amygdala of c.
  basal ganglia of c.
  dentate nucleus of c.
  fetal c.
  flocculonodular lobe of c.
  Gowers bundle in c.
  inverse c.
  midline c.
  petrosal c.
  towering c.
cerebra (*pl. of* cerebrum)
cerebral
  c. abscess
  c. amaurosis
  c. amyloid angiopathy
  c. aneurysm
  c. angiography
  c. anoxia

  c. apotentiality
  c. aqueduct
  c. arterial circle
  c. arteriography
  c. arteriosclerosis
  c. arteriovenous fistula
  c. arteriovenous malformation
  c. artery
  c. artery infarct
  c. artery stenosis
  c. astrocytoma
  c. blood flow (CBF)
  c. blood flow study
  c. blood vessel
  c. blood volume (CBV)
  c. blood volume to cerebral blood
    flow ratio (CBV-CBF)
  c. blood volume map
  c. calcification
  c. circulation
  c. circulation time
  c. commissure
  c. congestion
  c. contrast medium
  c. contusion
  c. convexity
  c. convolution
  c. cortex
  c. cortical gyral pattern
  c. CT venography
  c. cyst
  c. death
  c. dominance
  c. dysfunction
  c. edema
  c. embolism
  c. fat embolus
  c. fissure
  c. flexure
  c. flow image technique
  c. gammography
  c. gigantism
  c. glioma
  c. gyri interdigitation
  c. hemiatrophy
  c. hemidecortication
  c. hemisphere
  c. hemorrhage
  c. herniation
  c. hypoperfusion
  c. hypotension
  c. inflammatory disease
  c. infundibulum
  c. ischemia
  c. ischemic event
  c. lesion
  c. lymphoma
  c. malformation classification
  c. mantle

c. metabolic oxygen consumption
c. metabolic rate of oxygen (CMRO$_2$)
c. metabolism
c. metastasis
c. microarteriovenous malformation (micro-AVM)
c. microembolism
c. neuroblastoma
c. nodule
c. operculum
c. palsy pathological fracture
c. parenchyma
c. peduncle
c. perfusion pressure (CPP)
c. perfusion SPECT imaging
c. perfusion SPECT scan
c. perfusion study
c. pneumoencephalography
c. pneumography
c. pneumonia
c. porosis
c. radionecrosis
c. revascularization
c. ridge
c. salt wasting
c. scintigraphy
c. shunt
c. sinovenous occlusion
c. sinusography
c. SPECT
c. steal syndrome
c. sulcus
c. surface
c. surface atrophy
c. thrombophlebitis
c. toxoplasmosis
c. vascular microlattice
c. vasculature
c. vasoreactivity
c. vasospasm
c. vein
c. venous sinus
c. venous sinus thrombosis (CVST)
c. venous thrombosis
c. ventricle
c. ventricular shunt connector
c. ventriculography
c. vesicle
c. Whipple disease
c. white matter hypoplasia

c. xenon-enhanced blood flow (X-CDF)
cerebri
choana c.
commotio c.
contusio c.
falx c.
fornix c.
gliomatosis c.
gyri c.
hypophysis c.
mediastinum c.
pseudotumor c. (PTC)
cerebriform carcinoma
cerebritis
sinusitis c.
cerebrohepatorenal syndrome (CHRS)
cerebromacular degeneration (CMD)
cerebromeningeal intracerebral hemorrhage
cerebropontocerebellar pathway
cerebroside lipidosis
cerebrospinal
c. canal
c. fluid (CSF)
c. fluid circulation
c. fluid-containing lesion
c. fluid diversion
c. fluid fistula
c. fluid flow measurement
c. fluid flow waveform
c. fluid leak
c. fluid obstruction
c. fluid pathway
c. fluid shunt function
c. fluid volume
cerebrotendinous xanthomatosis
cerebrovascular
c. accident (CVA)
c. aneurysmal clip
c. insufficiency
c. insult
c. malformation
c. occlusive disease
c. stroke
cerebrum, pl. cerebra
central cavity of c.
cistern of lateral fossa of c.
cortex of c.
degenerative disease in c.
c. demyelination
first ventricle of c.

C

NOTES

cerebrum *(continued)*
    great vein of c.
    lateral ventricle of c.
    second ventricle of c.
    third ventricle of c.
Cerenkov
    C. calculation
    C. count
    C. counter
    C. measurement
    C. radiation
    C. radiation production
    C. scintillation analysis
Ceretec
    C. brain imaging
    C. radioisotope imaging agent
    ^{99m}Tc C.
cerium-doped lutetium oxyorthosilicate (LSO)
cerium silicate imaging agent
ceroid gallbladder granuloma
Cerrobend block
cervical
    c. adenocarcinoma
    c. adenopathy
    c. aorta
    c. aortic arch
    c. canal
    c. cord
    c. cord lesion
    c. CSF systole
    c. CT
    c. disc
    c. disc disease
    c. disc herniation
    c. disc syndrome
    c. dysplasia
    c. enlargement
    c. esophagostomy
    c. esophagus
    c. eversion
    c. facet dislocation
    c. fascia
    c. flexure
    c. flush
    c. fusion of spine
    c. ganglion
    c. heart
    c. interbody fusion
    c. intraepithelial neoplasm
    c. length
    c. loop
    c. lordosis
    c. lordotic curvature
    c. lymph node tuberculous adenitis
    c. magnetic resonance phlebography (CMRP)
    c. meningocele
    c. mover ligament

    c. mucus arborization
    c. muscle
    c. musculature
    c. myelography
    c. nerve root
    c. neural foramen
    c. osteophyte
    c. outlet
    c. pain syndrome
    c. paratracheal lymph node
    c. pleura
    c. plexus
    c. polyp
    c. pregnancy
    c. rest
    c. rib
    c. rib anomaly
    c. rib syndrome
    c. sarcoma
    c. segment of internal carotid artery
    c. sinus
    c. skull pillow
    c., skull, and shoulder block
    c. spine curve
    c. spine dens view
    c. spine fracture
    c. spine fusion
    c. spine injury
    c. spine spondylosis
    c. spondylotic myelopathy (CSM)
    c. spondylotic radiculopathy
    c. stenosis
    c. stroma
    c. structure
    c. synostosis
    c. synspondylism
    c. syringomyelia
    c. thymic cyst
    c. triangle
    c. tumor
    c. vein
    c. vertebra
    c. vesicle
cervices (*pl. of* cervix)
cervicitis
cervicoaxillary canal
cervicocerebral
cervicocranium
cervicography
cervicomedullary
    c. junction
    c. kink
cervicooccipital fusion
cervicothoracic
    c. ganglion
    c. junction
    c. sagittal scout image
cervicothoracolumbar

cervicotrochanteric fracture
cervigram
cervix, pl. **cervices**
> cockscomb appearance of c.
> double c.
> incompetent c.
> c. uteri
> uterine c.

CES
> cauda equina syndrome

cesium
> c. 137 (^{137}Cs, Cs 137)
> c. 139 (^{139}Cs)
> c. chloride imaging agent
> c. implant
> c. iodide input phosphor
> c. iodide scintillator
> c. needle
> c. with barium 137m

Cestan-Chenais syndrome
cestodic tuberculosis
CF
> common femoral
> CF artery

Cf
> californium

^{252}Cf
> californium 252

CF-200Z Olympus colonoscope
CFA
> cut-film angiography
> CFA digital camera

CFD
> color-flow Doppler

CFI
> color-flow imaging

CFL
> calcaneofibular ligament

C-flex stent
CFR
> coronary flow reserve

CF-UM3 echocolonoscope
CGI
> common gateway interface

CGR biplane angiographic system
cGy
> centigray

CH20 Kernal and slim 2 profile
Chaddock sign
chain
> branched c.
> c. cystogram

c. cystourethrography
heavy c.
image c.
internal mammary lymphatic c.
J c.
jugulodigastric c.
c. of lakes deformity
Markov c.
obturator nodal c.
sympathetic c.

chain-of-lakes anatomy
chalasia
chalky bone
challenge
> solid bolus c.

chamber
> abnormal dimensions of cardiac c.
> alpha c.
> cardiac c.
> cloud c.
> c. compression
> defective communication between
>   cardiac c.'s
> c. dilatation
> c. enlargement
> false aneurysmal c.
> c. of heart
> hydraulic c.
> infundibular c.
> ion c.
> ionization c.
> irradiation c.
> left atrial c.
> left ventricular c.
> multiwire proportional c.
> personal ionization c.
> pocket c.
> reduced compliance of c.
> reentrant well c.
> right atrial c.
> right ventricular c.
> rudimentary outlet c.
> rudimentary ventricular c.
> spark c.
> c. volume
> well-type ionization c.
> Wilson cloud c.

4-chamber
> 4-c. apical view
> 4-c. echocardiography
> 4-c. hypertrophy
> 4-c. plane

NOTES

2-chamber echocardiography
3-chambered heart
Chamberlain
    C. line
    C. procedure
Chamberlain-Towne view
champagne
    c. glass iliac wing
    c. glass pelvis
    c. glass ureter
champagne-bottle legs
chance
    c. equivalent
    C. spinal fracture
change
    age-related c.
    arthritic talonavicular c.
    asymmetric signal c.
    atherosclerotic c.
    attritional pattern c.
    basal ganglionic c.
    BOLD time course c.
    bony c.
    consolidative c.
    cystic c.
    deep gray matter nucleus c.
    degenerative osseous c.
    drug-induced brain c.
    dynamic cervical c.
    dystrophic c.
    E-A c.
    epithelial degenerative c.
    fibrocystic c.
    fibrotic c.
    fMRI signal c.
    focal degenerative c.
    high-signal-intensity ischemic c.
    hydropic c.
    interstitial c.
    interval c.
    ischemic c.
    lytic c.
    marrow signal c.
    mural c.
    myxoid degenerative c.
    nonspecific c.
    osteoarthritic c.
    papillary apocrine c.
    parenchymal c.
    paroxysmal c.
    pathophysiologic c.
    pelvicalyceal c.
    pleural c.
    polyneuropathy, organomegaly, endocrinopathy, monoclonal gammopathy, skin c.'s (POEMS)
    postbiopsy c.
    postsurgical c.
    posttherapy c.
    postthoracotomy c.
    precancerous c.
    prediverticular c.
    preslip c.
    proliferative c.
    pulmonary parenchymal c.
    radiation-induced c.
    radiation-related ischemic c.
    reciprocal c.
    residual interstitial c.
    residual limb-shaped c.
    roentgenographic c.
    senescent c.
    senile c.
    serial c.
    signal c.
    spinal endplate c.
    spondylitic c.
    spongiform c.
    stenotic c.
    vasomotor c.
change-of-angle view
changer
    Elema roll-film c.
    film c.
    Franklin c.
    Puck film c.
    rapid film c.
    Sanchez-Perez cassette c.
    Schonander film c.
    serial film c.
channel
    aberrant vascular c.
    blood c.
    central c.
    collateral venous c.
    deep venous c.
    dentate output c.
    engorged collateral venous c.
    enlarged vascular c.
    false c.
    gastric c.
    haversian c.
    Lambert c.
    lymphatic c.
    pancreaticobiliary common c.
    pyloric c.
    c. pyloric ulcer
    thread-and-streaks vascular c.
    true c.
    vascular c.
2-channel phased-array RF receiver coil system
chaotic heart
Chaoul
    C. therapy
    C. voltage x-ray tube

Chaput
    C. fracture
    C. tubercle
characteristic
    alternative-free response receiver
        operating c. (AFROC)
    associated imaging c.
    contrast transfer c.
    c. curve
    echo c.
    c. emission
    excitatory pulse c.
    c. finding
    generator c.
    pathognomonic imaging c.
    c. radiation
    receiver operating c. (ROC)
    signal c.
    suspension c.
    tip dispersion c.
    c. x-ray
characterization
    tissue c.
charcoal
    dextran-coated c.
Charcot
    C. arthropathy
    C. chondroma
    C. cirrhosis
    C. deformity
    C. foot
    C. fracture
    C. joint
    C. spine
    C. triad
Charcot-Bouchard intracerebral microaneurysm
Charcot-Marie-Tooth (CMT)
    C.-M.-T. disease
charge
    homogeneous positive c.
charge-coupled
    c.-c. device (CCD)
    c.-c. device scanner
    c.-c. device TV camera
charged-particle radiosurgery
charge injection device (CID)
charge-injection device
CHARM
    chunk acquisition and reconstruction
        method

chart
    Segre c.
    x-ray tube rating c.
chase bolus imaging technique
chaser
    saline c.
Chassaignac muscle
Chassard-Lapiné
    C.-L. position
    C.-L. projection
    C.-L. view
chastity ring artifact
Chauffard point
chauffeur's fracture
Chausse
    C. III projection
    third projection of C.
    C. view
Chaussier
    C. line
    C. projection
    C. view
CHB
    complete heart block
CHD
    common hepatic duct
    congenital heart defect
    congenital heart disease
        arachnodactyly CHD
        oligemia-related cyanotic CHD
        plethora-related cyanotic CHD
check
    design rule c. (DRC)
Check-Flo sheath
Checkmate system
checkrein
    c. deformity
    c. ligament
check-valve
    c.-v. mechanism
    c.-v. sheath
Chédiak-Steinbrinck-Higashi syndrome
cheek bone
cheese
    c. handler's lung
    c. washer's lung
cheese-wiring
cheesy pneumonia
Cheetah angioplasty catheter
CheeTah radiopaque contrast agent
cheirolumbar
cheiromegaly

NOTES

167

cheirospasm
chelate
    B-19036 c.
    Cr-HIDA c.
    gadolinium c.
    Gd-HIDA c.
chelating agent
chelonian pneumonia
chemical
    c. dosimeter
    c. peritonitis
    c. pleurodesis
    c. pneumonia
    c. pneumonitis
    c. potential energy
    c. pulmonary edema
    c. ray
    c. shift
    c. shift artifact
    c. shift imaging (CSI)
    c. shift imaging technique
    c. shift ratio
    c. shift reference
    c. shift selective suppression
      technique
    c. shift spatial offset
chemically-induced
    c.-i. dynamic nuclear depolarization
      (CIDNP)
    c.-i. dynamic nuclear polarization
chemical-selective
    c.-s. fat-saturation imaging
    c.-s. fat-saturation MR
chemiluminescence
chemisorb
chemisorption
chemistry
    nuclear c.
    radiation c.
    radiopharmaceutical c.
chemodectoma
    chest c.
chemoembolization
    HCC c.
    hepatic c.
    segmental transcatheter arterial c.
    c. solution
    therapeutic c.
    transarterial c. (TACE)
    transcatheter arterial c. (TACE)
    transcatheter hepatic arterial c.
    transcatheter oily c.
chemohyperthermia
    intraperitoneal c.
Chemo-Port
    C.-P. catheter
    C.-P. vascular access system
chemotherapy
    CT-guided intraarterial c.

    intraarterial c.
    intralesional c.
chemotoxic reaction
chemsat fat suppression
chenodeoxycholic acid
Chen-Smith image coder
Cherenkov effect
cherubism
CHESS
    Cornell high energy synchrotron source
      CHESS method
chest
    alar c.
    barrel c.
    blast c.
    c. bucky
    c. cavity
    c. chemodectoma
    cobbler's c.
    cylindrical c.
    dirty c.
    c. empyema
    expiratory c.
    c. film
    flail c.
    c. fluke lung
    c. fluoroscopy
    foveated c.
    funnel c.
    globular c.
    hollow c.
    hourglass c.
    jail-bar c.
    keeled c.
    c. lead
    narrow c.
    paralytic c.
    c. phantom
    phthinoid c.
    pigeon c.
    pneumonectomy c.
    pterygoid c.
    c. radiology
    symmetric c.
    tetrahedron c.
    c. tube
    c. view
    c. wall
    c. wall hamartoma
    c. wall lateral xeromammogram
    c. wall lesion
    c. wall mesenchymoma
    c. wall neuroblastoma
    c. wall paradoxic motion
    c. wall retraction
    c. wall rhabdomyosarcoma
    c. wall trauma
    c. x-ray (CXR)

chevron
  c. bone
  c. fracture
  c. fusion
CHF
  congenital hepatic fibrosis
  congestive heart failure
CHI
  closed head injury
Chiari
  C. formation
  C. I–II malformation
  C. I–IV lesion
Chiari-associated syringomyelia
chiasm, chiasma
  Camper c.
  c. of digit of hand
  optic c.
chiasmal
  c. compression
  c. lesion
chiasmata, pl. **chiasma**
chiasmatic
  c. cistern
  c. defect
  c. groove
chiasmatic-hypothalamic pilocytic astrocytoma
chiasmaticus
  sulcus c.
Chiba
  C. needle
  C. percutaneous cholangiogram
chicken-wire calcification
Chilaiditi
  C. sign
  C. syndrome
CHILD
  congenital hemidysplasia with
  ichthyosiform erythroderma and limb
  defects
  CHILD syndrome
childhood
  c. discitis
  c. fracture
  c. osteomyelitis
  c. rhabdomyosarcoma
Child-Pugh
  C.-P. classification
  C.-P. liver function classification
  A, B, C

chimera
  radiation c.
chimney-shaped high aortic arch
Chinese fluke liver
chin-occiput piece
chip
  bone c.
  cancellous bone c.
  corticocancellous bone c.
  c. fracture
chisel fracture
chisellike truncated appearance
chloride
  ^{111}In c.
  magnesium c.
  manganese c.
  polyvinyl c. (PVC)
  stannous c.
  strontium-89 c.
  thallium-201 c.
  Tl-201 c.
  triphenyltetrazolium c. (TTC)
  xenon c. (XeCl)
chloriodized oil
chlormerodrin accumulation test
chlormerodrin-cysteine complex
chloroma
  bone c.
  gastric c.
  c. granulocytic sarcoma
  kidney c.
choana cerebri
choanal
  c. atresia
  c. polyp
chocolate
  c. cyst
  c. joint effusion
cholangiectasis
  extrahepatic c.
cholangiocarcinoma
  extrahepatic c.
  hilar c.
  intrahepatic c.
  peripheral c. (PCC)
Cholangiocath
cholangiocatheter
cholangiocellular carcinoma
cholangiodrainage
cholangiodysplastic pseudocirrhosis
cholangiofibromatosis

NOTES

cholangiogram
    balloon c.
    catheter c.
    Chiba percutaneous c.
    common duct c.
    contrast selective c.
    cystic duct c.
    drip infusion c. (DIC)
    endoscopic retrograde c. (ERC)
    fine-needle transhepatic c. (FNTC)
    intraoperative c.
    intravenous c. (IVC)
    magnetic resonance c. (MRC)
    operative c.
    percutaneous transhepatic c. (PTC, PTCA, PTHC)
    retrograde c.
    serial c.
    single-shot MR c.
    transhepatic c. (THC)
    transjugular c.
    T-tube c. (TTC)
cholangiography
    breath-hold MR c.
    c. catheter
    computed tomographic c.
    cystic duct c.
    delayed operative c.
    direct percutaneous transhepatic c.
    drip infusion c. (DIC)
    endoscopic c. (ERC)
    c. imaging
    intraoperative c.
    intravenous c.
    percutaneous hepatobiliary c.
    percutaneous transhepatic c. (PTHC)
    postoperative c.
    transabdominal c.
    T-tube c.
cholangiohepatitis
    Oriental c.
cholangiolithiasis
cholangiopancreatography
    endoscopic percutaneous c.
    endoscopic retrograde c. (ERCP)
    kinematic MR c.
    magnetic resonance c. (MRCP)
cholangioscopy
    contrast-enhanced virtual MR c.
cholangiotomogram
cholangiovenous communication
cholangitic biliary cirrhosis
cholangitis
    acute nonsuppurative ascending c.
    acute obstructive c.
    acute suppurative ascending c.
    AIDS c.
    ascending c.
    bacterial c.

    chronic nonsuppurative destructive c.
    fibrous obliterative c.
    intrahepatic sclerosing c.
    nonsuppurative ascending c.
    nonsuppurative destructive c.
    primary sclerosing c.
    progressive suppurative c.
    pyogenic c.
    recurrent pyogenic c.
    sclerosing c.
    secondary sclerosing c.
    septic c.
    suppurative ascending c.
Cholebrine imaging agent
cholecystectomy
    endoscopic laser c.
cholecystenteric
    c. anastomosis
    c. fistula
cholecystitis
    acalculous c.
    acute c.
    calculous c.
    chronic c.
    emphysematous c.
    gangrenous c.
    gaseous c.
    c. glandularis proliferans
    lipid c.
    perforated c.
    c. with cholelithiasis
    xanthogranulomatous c.
cholecystocholangiography
cholecystocholangitis
cholecystocholedochal fistula
cholecystocholedochostomy
    percutaneous c.
cholecystocolic fistula
cholecystocutaneous fistula
cholecystoduodenal
    c. fistula
    c. ligament
cholecystoduodenocolic
    c. fistula
    c. fold
cholecystogram
    Graham-Cole c.
    oral c. (OCG)
cholecystography
    intravenous c.
    oral c.
    post fatty meal c.
cholecystokinetic food
cholecystokinin cholescintigraphy
cholecystolithiasis
cholecystomegaly
cholecystopaque
cholecystopathy

cholecystoptosis
cholecystosis
    hyperplastic c.
cholecystosonography
cholecystostomy
    percutaneous transhepatic c.
    ultrasound-guided percutaneous c.
choledochal
    c. cyst
    c. sphincter
choledochal-colonic fistula
choledochocele
choledochocholedochostomy
choledochoduodenal
    c. fistula
    c. junctional stenosis
choledochofiberscope
    Olympus CHF-BP30
      transduodenal c.
choledochogram
choledochograph
choledochography
choledochojejunostomy stricture
choledocholithiasis
choledochopancreatic ductal junction
choledochoscope
choledochoscopy
    percutaneous c.
choledochostomy
choledochous duct
cholegraphy
cholelith, chololith
cholelithiasis
    cholecystitis with c.
cholelithoptysis
cholescintigraphy
    cholecystokinin c.
    radionuclide c.
    sincalide c.
cholescintography
cholestasis, cholestasia
    intrahepatic c.
cholestatic liver disease
cholesteatoma
    attic c.
    congenital c.
    ear c.
    GU tract c.
    inflammatory c.
    pars flaccida c.
    pars tensa c.
    primary acquired c.

    primary CNS c.
    primary temporal bone c.
    secondary acquired c.
cholesterinosis, cholesterolosis,
  cholesterosis
cholesterol
    c. debris
    c. ear cyst
    c. ear granuloma
    c. embolus
    c. gallbladder polyp
    c. gallstone
    I-labeled c.
cholesterol-based scintigraphy
cholesterol-containing brain lesion
Choletec radionuclide imaging agent
Cholografin
    C. meglumine
    C. meglumine imaging agent
chololith (*var. of* cholelith)
chondral
    c. defect
    c. fracture
    c. fragment
chondrification
chondritis
chondroblastic osteosarcoma
chondroblastoma
    benign c.
    c. straddling
chondrocalcinosis
    familial c.
chondrocyte
    atypical c.
    c. degeneration
    epiphysial c.
    regenerative c.
chondrodiastasis
chondrodysplasia
    c. calcificans
    Jansen-type metaphysial c.
    McKusick-type metaphysial c.
    metaphysial c.
    c. punctata
    Schmid-like metaphysial c.
chondrodystrophia
    c. calcificans congenita
    c. fetalis
chondrodystrophy
chondroectodermal dysplasia
chondrofibroma
chondrogenic tumor

NOTES

chondrogladiolar
chondroid
    c. matrix
    c. syringoma
    c. tissue
chondroid-origin tumor
chondroitin sulfate iron colloid-enhanced MRI
chondrolipoma
chondrolysis
    posttraumatic c.
chondroma
    Charcot c.
    extraskeletal c.
    joint c.
    juxtacortical c.
    soft tissue c.
chondromalacia
    c. patella
    patellar c.
    ulnar c.
    c. with fibrillation
    c. with surface fraying
chondromanubrial
chondromatosis
    Henderson-Jones c.
    secondary c.
    synovial c.
chondromatous hamartoma
chondromyofibroma
chondromyxoid fibroma (CMF)
chondromyxoma
chondromyxosarcoma
chondronecrosis
chondroosteodystrophy
chondrophyte
chondroplasia calcificans
chondroporosis
chondrosarcoma
    central c.
    endosteal c.
    exostotic c.
    extraskeletal mesenchymal c.
    juxtacortical c.
    malignant c.
    mesenchymal c.
    myxoid extraskeletal c.
    parosteal c.
    peripheral c.
chondrosarcomatosis
chondrosteoma
chondrosternal junction
chondroxiphoid ligament
chop amputation
Chopart
    C. fracture
    C. fracture-dislocation
    C. hindfoot amputation
    C. joint

chopper
    McIlwain tissue c.
Chopper-Dixon fat suppression imaging
Choquet fuzzy integral
choracobrachialis
chord
    contiguous parallel c.
    multiple c.'s
chorda, pl. **chordae**
    basal c.
    cleft c.
    commissural c.
    first-order c.
    c. magna
    second-order c.
    strut c.
    third-order c.
    c. tympani
chordal rupture
chordate
chordocarcinoma
chordoepithelioma
chordoma
    clivus c.
    sacral c.
    sacrococcygeal c.
    sphenooccipital c.
    spinal c.
    vertebral c.
chordosarcoma
chorioallantoic placenta
chorioamnionic
    c. elevation
    c. separation
chorioangioma
choriocarcinoma
    esophageal c.
    gestational c.
    ovarian c.
    primary ovarian c.
    testicular c.
choriodecidua
choriodecidual reaction
chorionic
    c. carcinoma
    c. disc
    c. gonadotropin
    c. sac
    c. tissue
chorionicity
choristoma
    middle ear c.
    renal c.
choroid
    c. glomera
    c. plexus
    c. plexus blush
    c. plexus calcification
    c. plexus carcinoma

c. plexus cyst
c. plexus hemorrhage
c. plexus neoplasm
c. plexus papilloma
c. point
c. vein

choroidal
c. fissure
c. hemangioma
lateral posterior c. (LPCh)
medial posterior c. (MPCh)
c. neovascularization (CNV)
c. osteoma
c. pericallosal artery

choroidal-hippocampal fissure complex
choroidea
tela c.
choroideum
glomus c.
Christian brachydactyly
Christmas tree appearance
chromaffin
c. paraganglioma
c. tumor
chromated Cr-51 serum albumin imaging agent
chromatic spectrum
chromatid-type aberration
chromatogram
chromatographic-fluorometric technique
chromatographic separation
chromatography
antiidiotypic affinity c.
DEAE-Sephadex A-25 c.
gas-liquid phase c. (GLPC)
high-performance liquid c.
high-performance size-exclusion c.
high-pressure liquid c.
ion-exchange c.
ChromaVision digital analyzer
chromic phosphate suspension
chromium (Cr)
c. CR-51 serum albumin
c. imaging agent
c. phosphate
chromium-heated red blood cell
chromium:yttrium-aluminum-garnet
erbium c.-a.-g. (ErCr:YAG)
chromophobe
kidney carcinoma c.
pituitary adenoma c.
chromoscopy time

chronic
c. abdominal inflammation
c. airway obstruction
c. alveolar infiltrate
c. atelectasis
c. atrophic duodenitis
c. atrophic pyelonephritis
c. berylliosis
c. beryllium disease
c. breast abscess
c. calcifying pancreatitis
c. cerebral ischemia
c. cholecystitis
c. communicating hydrocephalus
c. constrictive state
c. diffuse confluent lung opacity
c. diffuse reticulation
c. diffuse sclerosing alveolitis
c. diverticulitis
c. duodenal ileus
c. edema
c. esophagitis
c. extrinsic allergic alveolitis
c. fibrosing alveolitis
c. fibrosing mesenteritis
c. fissure
c. friction and impingement
c. functional instability
c. gastric atony
c. gastritis
c. glomerulonephritis
c. heart failure
c. hemodynamic overload
c. hepatitis
c. hereditary nephritis
c. hydronephrosis
c. hypertrophic emphysema
c. idiopathic intestinal pseudoobstruction (CIIP)
c. ileus duodenum
c. infantile hyperostosis
c. insufficiency of vein
c. interstitial pneumonia
c. interstitial salpingitis
c. interstitial simulating airspace lung disease
c. irritation
c. ischemic brain infarct
c. ligament complex laxity
c. ligamentous injury
c. lung thromboembolism
c. lymphedematous limb

NOTES

173

chronic *(continued)*
    c. lymphocytic leukemia
    c. lymphocytic thyroiditis
    c. mesenteric ischemia (CMI)
    c. multifocal ill-defined lung
      opacity
    c. myeloid leukemia
    c. necrotizing aspergillosis
    c. nonsuppurative destructive
      cholangitis
    c. obstructive emphysema
    c. obstructive lung disease (COLD)
    c. obstructive pancreatitis
    c. obstructive pulmonary disease
      (COPD)
    c. obstructive uropathy
    c. outward force
    c. overuse syndrome
    c. parenchymal hemorrhage
    c. partial epilepsy
    c. passive congestion
    c. peptic ulcer
    c. periaortitis
    c. peripheral arterial disease
      (CPAD)
    c. phase
    c. pleurisy
    c. pneumonitis
    c. posttraumatic aortic
      pseudoaneurysm
    c. pulmonary emphysema (CPE)
    c. recurrent dislocation
    c. recurrent multifocal osteomyelitis
    c. recurrent sialadenitis
    c. renal failure (CRF)
    c. renal failure amyloidosis
    c. renal infarct
    c. renal vein thrombosis
    c. reserve flow
    c. respiratory decompensation
    c. retrocalcaneal bursitis
    c. sclerosing osteomyelitis
    c. simple silicosis
    c. sinusitis
    c. sprain
    c. subdural hematoma (CSDH)
    c. subperitoneal sclerosis
    c. tamponade
    c. testicular torsion
    c. tuberculous emphysema
    c. ulcerative colitis (CUC)
    c. venous insufficiency
    c. venous stasis
chronologic age
chronology
    imaging c.
chronotherapy
    adjuvant c.
chronotropic incompetence

chronotropy
CHRS
    cerebrohepatorenal syndrome
CHRYS CO_2 laser
chrysotile asbestos
**chunk acquisition and reconstruction
    method (CHARM)**
Churg-Strauss syndrome
chyle
    c. cistern
    effused c.
    c. fistula
    c. leak
    c. vessel
chyli
    ampulla c.
    cisterna c.
chyliferous vessel
chylocele
    nonfilarial c.
chyloma
chylomediastinum
chylopericardium
chylothorax
    postoperative c.
chylous
    c. ascites
    c. effusion
    c. fistula
    c. leakage
CI
    cardiac index
    confidence interval
    continuous imaging
Ci
    curie
cicatricial
    c. atelectasis
    c. kidney
    c. stricture
CID
    charge injection device
    CID camera
CIDNP
    chemically-induced dynamic nuclear
      depolarization
Cidtech camera
cigarroa formula
CIIP
    chronic idiopathic intestinal
      pseudoobstruction
ciliaris
    zonula c.
ciliary
    c. canal
    c. cartilage
    c. ganglionic plexus
    c. ligament

c. ring
c. vein
ciliated border
ciliospinal center of Budge
Cimino
C. AV shunt
C. dialysis shunt
cine
c. acquisition
c. camera
c. coronary arteriography
c. CT
c. CT imaging
c. CT scan
c. CT scanner
c. film
c. fistulogram
c. gradient-echo MR imaging
c. gradient-echo sequence
c. gradient magnetic resonance imaging
c. left ventriculogram
c. loop
c. magnetic resonance function image
c. magnetic resonance tagging
C. Memory with color flow Doppler imaging
c. mode
c. MRI
parallel c.
c. phase contrast imaging
c. projector
c. raw data
segmented c.
c. study
velocity-encoded c. (VEC)
c. view
c. view imaging
c. view in MUGA scan
cineangiocardiogram (CACG)
cineangiocardiography
cineangiogram
ventricular c.
cineangiography
aortic root c.
axial c.
biplane c.
coronary c.
radionuclide c.
selective coronary c.

cinearteriography
Judkins selective left coronary c.
cine-based viewing
cinebronchogram
cinecardioangiography
cinedefecogram
cinedensigraphy
cine-encoded image
cineesophagogram
cine-FFE breath-hold sequence
cinefluorography
biplane c.
cinefluoroscopy
valve c.
cine-gated imaging
cine-loop
cinematography
cinematoradiography
cinemicrography
cine-mode display
cine-MR
breath-hold c.-MR
cinepharyngoesophagogram
cinephlebography
cineportography
cineradiographic view
cineradiography imaging
cinereum
tuber c.
cineroentgenofluorography
cineroentgenography
cineurography
cineventriculogram
cineventriculography
cingulate
c. gyrus
c. herniation
c. sulcus
cingulum, pl. **cingula**
cipher
transposition c.
circadian
c. continuous infusion
c. pattern
c. periodicity
c. variation
circle
anastomotic arterial c.
arterial c.
articular vascular c.
cerebral arterial c.
c. of confusion

NOTES

C

circle *(continued)*
    c. loop biliary drainage
    c. of Vieussens
    c. of Willis
    c. wire nephrostomy
Circon video camera
circuit
    anticoincidence c.
    application-specific integrated c.
      (ASIC)
    arrhythmia c.
    ASIC c.
    bridge c.
    bypass c.
    coincidence c.
    doubly broadband triple-resonance
      NMR probe c.
    macroreentrant c.
    magnetic c.
    magnetoresistive sensor c.
    microreentrant c.
    phototube output c.
    quad resonance NMR probe c.
    reentry c.
    shunting c.
    triple-resonance NMR probe c.
circular
    c. dichroism spectroscopy
    c. fold
    c. lesion
    c. muscle
    c. plane
    c. polarization wave
    c. polarized volume head coil
    c. sinus
    c. supracondylar amputation
    c. syncytium
    c. tomosynthesis
circularly polarized coil
circulating blood volume
circulation
    allantoic c.
    arrested c.
    balanced c.
    bronchial collateral c.
    carotid c.
    cerebral c.
    cerebrospinal fluid c.
    codominant c.
    c. collapse
    collateral mesenteric c.
    compensatory c.
    cutaneous collateral c.
    derivative c.
    devoid of c.
    c. disturbance
    extracardiac collateral c.
    extracorporeal c.
    extracranial carotid c.

    extracranial cerebral c.
    c. failure
    fetal c.
    greater c.
    high-impedance c.
    intervillous c.
    intraaneurysmal flow c.
    intracranial c.
    Korotkoff test for collateral c.
    microvascular c.
    peripheral c.
    persistent fetal c.
    placental c.
    portosystemic collateral c.
    posterior fossa c.
    pulmonary arterial c.
    reduced c.
    c. shock
    spiderweb c.
    c. stasis
    systemic arterial c.
    thebesian c.
    thoracoabdominal venous
      collateral c.
    c. time (CT)
    uteroplacental c.
    venous c.
    vertebrobasilar c.
    c. volume
circulator
    sequential c.
circulatory
    c. arrest
    c. compromise
    c. embarrassment
    c. impairment
circumaortic left renal vein
circumaxillary
circumcaval ureter
circumduction
circumduction-adduction shoulder
    maneuver
circumference
    abdominal c. (AC)
    femur length to abdominal c.
    fetal abdominal c.
    c. of fetal head
    fetal head c.
    fetal thoracic c.
    head c. (HC)
    head circumference-to-abdominal c.
      (HC-AC)
    thoracic c. (TC)
circumferential
    c. cartilage
    c. echo-dense layer
    c. extremity coil
    c. fibrocartilage
    c. fracture

c. lamella
c. narrowing
c. shortening
c. thickening
c. venous stenosis

circumflex (CX)
c. branch
c. coronary artery
c. groove artery
humeral c.
left c. (LCF, LCX)
c. retroesophageal arch
c. system
c. vein
c. vessel

circummarginate placenta
circummesencephalic cistern
circumscribed
c. edema
c. infiltrate
c. lesion
c. margin
c. mass
c. nodule
c. pleurisy

circumscripta
calcinosis c.
myositis ossificans c.
osteoporosis c.

circumscript aneurysm
circumvallate papilla
circumventricular organ
cirrhosis
acholangic biliary c.
acute juvenile c.
alcoholic c. (AC)
atrophic c.
biliary c.
Budd c.
calculous c.
cardiac c.
Charcot c.
cholangitic biliary c.
congestive c.
Cruveilhier-Baumgarten c.
cryptogenic c.
decompensated alcoholic c.
diffuse c.
end-stage c.
fatty c.
focal biliary c.
frank c.

glabrous c.
Hanot c.
hepatic c.
hypertrophic c.
Indian childhood c.
juvenile c.
liver c.
macrolobular c.
medionodular c.
metabolic c.
microlobular c.
micronodular c.
multilobular c.
nutritional c.
obstructive biliary c.
periportal c.
pipestem c.
porta c.
posthepatic c.
postnecrotic c.
primary biliary c.
progressive familial c.
pulmonary c.
secondary biliary c.
septal c.
stasis c.
Todd c.
toxic c.
unilobular c.
vascular c.

cirrhosis-related fibrosis
cirrhotic
c. gastritis
c. inflammation
c. liver
c. nodule

cirsoid
c. aneurysm
c. placenta

cis-11beta-methoxy-17alpha-iodovinyl-estradiol (Z-MIVE)
cistern
ambient wing of the
quadrigeminal c.
anterior interhemispheric c.
basal arachnoid c.
basilar c.
carotid c.
cerebellomedullary c.
cerebellopontine c.
c. of chiasma
chiasmatic c.

NOTES

cistern *(continued)*
    chyle c.
    circummesencephalic c.
    crural c.
    c. effacement
    great c.
    increased basilar c.
    c. indium
    interpeduncular c. (IPC)
    c. isotope
    c. of lamina terminalis
    c. of lateral fossa of cerebrum
    mesencephalic c.
    opticochiasmatic c.
    c. oxygen
    parasellar c.
    c. of Pecquet
    perimesencephalic c.
    pontine c.
    posterior c.
    prepontine c.
    quadrigeminal plate c.
    c. radioisotope
    subarachnoid c.
    suprasellar subarachnoid c.
    sylvian c.
    c. of Sylvius
    terminal c.
    trigeminal c.
cisterna
    c. chyli
    c. magna
    c. magna effacement
cisternal
    c. herniation
    c. puncture
    c. space
cisternogram
    CT c.
    metrizamide CT c.
cisternography
    air c.
    cerebellopontine c.
    computed tomography c.
    CT c.
    gas CT c.
    c. imaging
    isotopic c.
    Katzman infusion of
     radionuclide c.
    metrizamide computed
     tomography c. (MCTC)
    oxygen c.
    Pantopaque c.
    radioisotope c.
    radionuclide c.
cisternomyelography
citrate
    clomiphene c.

fentanyl c.
ferrous c.
gallium-67 c.
manganese c.
Citscope disposable arthroscope
CIVI
    continuous intravenous infusion
Civinini
    C. canal
    C. ligament
CJD
    Creutzfeldt-Jakob disease
CKG
    cardiokymography
    CKG imaging
C-labeled
^{11}C-labeled
    ^{11}C-l. cocaine
    ^{11}C-l. cocaine imaging agent
    ^{11}C-l. fatty acid imaging agent
Clado
    C. band
    C. ligament
    C. point
clamshell double umbrella occluder
Clariscan imaging agent
Clarke
    C. arch angle
    C. column
Clarke-Hadefield syndrome
Clark malignant melanoma classification
Clarkson scatter-summation algorithm
Clarus spinescope
classical
    c. nephroblastoma
    c. osteosarcoma
    c. scattering
classic carpal tunnel view
classification
    AAOS acetabular abnormalities c.
    acromioclavicular injury c.
    Aitken acromioclavicular injury c.
    AJCC-UICC mediastinal lymph
     node c.
    Allman c.
    Altman c.
    American Spinal Cord Injury
     Association c.
    Amstutz c.
    anatomic brain c.
    Ann Arbor c.
    anular tear c.
    AO ankle fracture c.
    AO-Danis-Weber ankle fracture c.
    Arco c.
    Bayne c.
    Berndt-Hardy talar dome c.
    Bigliani c.
    Bleck metatarsus adductus c.

Bosniak c.
Boyd-Griffin trochanteric fracture c.
brain anatomy c.
brain tumor c.
Breslow c.
Broders tumor index c.
Brooker periarticular heterotopic ossification c.
Butcher staging c.
Caldwell-Moloy c.
Canale-Kelly talar neck fracture c.
Carnesale-Stewart-Barnes hip dislocation c.
Cedell-Magnusson arthritis c.
cerebral malformation c.
Child-Pugh c.
Child-Pugh liver function c. A, B, C
Clark malignant melanoma c.
CNS anomaly c.
CNS tumor c.
Colonna hip fracture c.
congenital heart disease c.
Copeland-Kavat metatarsophalangeal dislocation c.
Couinaud c.
Danis-Weber ankle fracture c.
D'Antonio acetabular c.
DeBakey aortic c.
Delbet hip fracture c.
Denis c.
Dickhaut-DeLee discoid meniscus c.
distance-based block c.
Essex-Lopresti calcaneal fracture c.
Evans intertrochanteric fracture c.
Fielding-Magliato subtrochanteric fracture c.
fracture c.
Fränkel spinal cord injury c.
Freeman calcaneal fracture c.
Fries score for rheumatoid arthritis c.
Frykman distal radius fracture c.
Galassi arachnoidal cyst c.
Garden femoral neck fracture c.
Gertzbein seatbelt injury c.
Glasscock-Jackson c.
Goldsmith and Woodburne c.
Graf hip dysplasia c.
Grantham femur fracture c.
Gumley seatbelt injury c.

Gustilo-Anderson tibial plafond fracture c.
Hahn-Steinthal capitellum fracture c.
Hansen fracture c.
Hardy-Clapham sesamoid c.
Hawkins talar neck fracture c.
Herbert-Fisher fracture c.
Hinchey c.
Hohl tibial condylar fracture c.
Holdsworth spinal fracture c.
Hughston Clinic injury c.
Hunt-Kosnik c.
Hyams grading of esthesioneuroblastoma c.
Jahss dislocation c.
Jones c.
Judet epiphysial fracture c.
Kalamchi-Dawe congenital tibial deficiency c.
Kazangia and Converse facial fracture c.
Kernohan brain tumor c.
Key-Conwell pelvic fracture c.
Kiel non-Hodgkin lymphoma c.
Kilfoyle condylar fracture c.
Kimura c.
King-Moe c.
Kistler subarachnoid hemorrhage c.
Klatskin tumor c.
Kocher-Lorenz capitellum fracture c.
Kostuik-Errico spinal stability c.
Kyle fracture c.
Lauge-Hansen ankle fracture c.
Lie c.
Mason radial fracture c.
Mazur ankle evaluation c.
McCabe-Fletcher c.
McLain-Weinstein spinal tumor c.
Melone distal radius fracture c.
Merland perimedullary arteriovenous fistula c.
Meyer-McKeever tibial fracture c.
Michels c.
Milch elbow fracture c.
Mink-Deutsch c.
Mitchell c.
Modic disc abnormality c.
mulberry-type c.
Müller humerus fracture c.
multiaxial c.

NOTES

179

classification *(continued)*
Neer-Horowitz humerus fracture c.
Neviaser frozen shoulder c.
Newman radial fracture c.
Nurick spondylosis c.
NYHA congestive heart failure c.
O'Brien radial fracture c.
Ogden epiphysial fracture c.
Olerud and Molander fracture c.
osteoarthritis grading c.
Ovadia-Beals tibial plafond
    fracture c.
Papile c.
Pauwel femoral neck fracture c.
percentage c.
pineal gland tumor c.
Pipkin femoral fracture c.
pneumoconiosis c.
Poland epiphysial fracture c.
Potter c.
primary CNS tumor c.
Rappaport c.
Ratliff avascular necrosis c.
REAL c.
rickets c.
Riemann c.
Riordan club hand c.
Riseborough-Radin intercondylar
    fracture c.
Robson staging c.
Rockwood acromioclavicular
    injury c.
Rowe calcaneal fracture c.
Rowe-Lowell fracture-dislocation c.
Ruedi-Allgower tibial plafond
    fracture c.
Runyon c.
Russell-Rubinstein cerebrovascular
    malformation c.
Salter-Harris growth plate injury c.
Salter-Harris-Rang epiphysial
    fracture c.
Schatzker fracture c.
Severin c.
Shelton femur fracture c.
Smith sesamoid position c.
Snyder c.
soft tissue lesion c.
Sorbie calcaneal fracture c.
Stanford aortic dissection c.
Steinberg c.
Steinbrocker rheumatoid arthritis c.
Steinert epiphysial fracture c.
Steward-Milford fracture c.
talocalcaneal index c.
Thompson-Epstein femoral
    fracture c.
Todani c.
Tronzo intertrochanteric fracture c.

Trunkey fracture c.
Vostal radial fracture c.
Watanabe discoid meniscus c.
Watson-Jones tibial tubercle
    avulsion fracture c.
Werner c.
WHO c.
Wiberg patellar types c.
Wilkins radial fracture c.
Winquist-Hansen femoral fracture c.
Wiseman c.
Wolfe breast carcinoma c.
Working Formulation c.
World Health Organization c.

clasticus
conus c.

Claude syndrome

claudication
c. of jaw
lifestyle-limiting c.

Clauss
C. assay
C. method

claustrum, pl. **claustra**

clavicle
absence of outer end of c.
penciling of the distal c.

clavicular
c. birth fracture
c. facet
c. head of sternocleidomastoid
c. notch
c. osteitis condensans

clavipectoral
c. fascia
c. triangle

clavus
interdigital c.

clawfoot deformity

clawhand deformity

clawtoe deformity

clay
c. pipe carcinoma
c. shoveler's fracture

Claybrook sign

CLD
central lung distance

clean shadow

cleansing enema

CLEAR
constant level appearance
CLEAR technique

clear
c. cell neoplasm of ovary
c. cell sarcoma
c. endpoint
enemas until c.
c. zone

clearance
> c. curve
> c. half-time
> isotope c.
> multicompartment c.
> multiple-sample c.
> c. phase ventilation scan
> radioactive xenon c.
> radioaerosol c.
> renal c.
> single-sample c.

Clearview CO$_2$ laser
cleavage
> c. cavity
> c. fracture
> plane of c.
> c. tear

cleaved cell lymphoma
Cleaves
> C. method
> C. position

cleaving
> plaque c.

cleft
> anal c.
> c. chorda
> coronal c.
> c. face syndrome
> facial c.
> first visceral c.
> full-thickness c.
> gill c.
> Hahn c.
> intergluteal c.
> interinnominoabdominal c.
> intranuclear c.
> intravertebral body vacuum c.
> lateral facial c.
> median facial c.
> median lip c.
> meniscal c.
> midline longitudinal pontine c.
> c. mitral valve
> neural arch c.
> pudendal c.
> radiolucent c.
> retrosomatic c.
> spinal cord c.
> c. spine
> splenic c.
> synaptic c.
> vacuum c.

> ventricular c.
> c. vertebra

cleidocranial
> c. dysostosis
> c. dysplasia

Cleland ligament
Clements-Nakayama position
clenched fist view
Cleopatra view
Clerc-Levy-Cristico syndrome
climbing fiber
clinical
> c. complete response
> c. correlation
> c. feature
> c. parameter
> c. partial response
> c. target volume (CTV)

clinically isolated syndrome
CliniCath peripherally inserted catheter
clinicopathological analysis
clinodactyly
> factitious c.
> traumatic c.

clinoid
> c. aneurysm
> c. ligament
> c. process

clinoparietal line
clip
> aneurysmal c.
> cerebrovascular aneurysmal c.
> c. ligation of aneurysm
> sternal c.

clip-editing plane
clipping
> c. of aneurysm
> ureteric c.

clival meningioma
clivus, pl. **clivi**
> Blumenbach c.
> c. chordoma
> c. meningioma tumor
> c. metastasis

clivus-canal angle
CLM
> capillary-lymphatic malformation

cloaca, pl. **cloacae**
> bone formation c.

cloacal
> c. anomaly
> c. exstrophy

NOTES

cloacal *(continued)*
    c. formation
    c. malformation
    c. plate
cloaking
    periosteal c.
    perivascular c.
clock cycle
clockwise whirlpool sign
clomiphene citrate
cloning
    subtraction c.
clonogen number
Cloquet
    C. canal
    C. fascia
    hyaloid canal of C.
    C. inguinal lymph node
    C. ligament
close apposition
closed
    c. conducting loop
    c. core transformer
    c. dislocation
    c. exstrophy
    c. flap amputation
    c. fontanelle
    c. fracture
    c. head injury (CHI)
    c. pneumothorax
    c. reduction
    c. spinal dysraphism
closed-break fracture
closed-fist configuration
closed-loop intestinal obstruction
closed-mouth view
closer
    Perclose 6F C.
    C. percutaneous suture-mediated
        closure device
close-space thin-section scanning
close-up view
closing
    c. capacity
    c. slope
    c. velocity
    c. volume
closure
    abrupt vessel c.
    aortic c. (AC)
    c. device
    growth center c.
    incomplete c.
    native aortic valve c.
    physial c.
    premature valve c.
    sandwich patch c.
    Stanford type B dissection c.
    threatened vessel c.

    tricuspid valve c.
    valve c.
    VasoSeal elite vascular c.
    velopharyngeal c.
Clo-Sur PAD closure device
clot
    agonal c.
    autologous blood c.
    blood c.
    internal c.
    intramural c.
    isoechoic c.
    c. lysis
    c. maceration
    marantic c.
    mural c.
    passive c.
    plastic c.
    preformed c.
    c. removal by laser thrombolysis
    c. retraction
    saddle c.
    subarachnoid c.
    subdural c.
clot-filled lumen
clothesline injury
clothing artifact
cloud
    c. chamber
    electron c.
clouding
    alveolar c.
cloudy
    c. sinus
    c. swelling of heart
cloverleaf
    c. deformity
    c. plate
    c. skull
cloverleaf-shaped lumen
Cloward bone graft
clubbed
    c. finger
    c. penis
clubbing
    calyceal c.
clubfoot deformity
clubhand deformity
club-shaped conus
cluneal nerve
cluster
    activated voxel c.
    c. of differentiation (CD)
    grapelike c.
    c. of grapes lung
    K-means c.
    microcalcification c.
    c. of radiolucent area (CORLA)

clustered
    c. calcification
    c. data
clustering algorithm
Clutton painful joint
clysis
Clysodrast
CM
    contrast medium
        iodinated intravascular CM
cm
    centimeter
CMC
    carpometacarpal joint
CMD
    cerebromacular degeneration
    corticomedullary differentiation
^{11}C-methionine
    ^{11}C-m. PET scan
    ^{11}C-m. positron emission
        tomography (MET-PET)
CMF
    chondromyxoid fibroma
CMI
    chronic mesenteric ischemia
CMJ
    corticomedullary junction
        CMJ imaging
CMOS
    complementary metal oxide
        semiconductor
CMR
    congenital mitral regurgitation
CMRO$_2$
    cerebral metabolic rate of oxygen
CMRP
    cervical magnetic resonance
        phlebography
CMS
    compliance matching stent
CMT
    Charcot-Marie-Tooth
CMV
    cytomegalovirus
        CMV encephalitis
CNR, C/N
    contrast-to-noise ratio
CNS
    central nervous system
        CNS amyloidosis
        CNS anomaly classification
        CNS cortical hamartoma

        CNS empyema
        CNS fibromuscular dysplasia
        CNS ghost tumor
        CNS juvenile pilocytic astrocytoma
        CNS multifocal tumor
        CNS teratoma
        CNS toxoplasmosis
        CNS tumor classification
CNV
    choroidal neovascularization
CO
    cardiac output
CO$_2$
    carbon dioxide
        CO_2 angiography
        CO_2 cylinder
        CO_2 generator
        CO_2 insufflation
        CO_2 laser
        CO_2 retention
Co
    cobalt
^{57}Co
    cobalt 57
^{58}Co
    cobalt 58
^{60}Co
    cobalt 60
COACH
    cerebellar vermis hypoplasia,
        oligophrenia, congenital ataxia, ocular
        coloboma, hepatic fibrosis
        COACH syndrome
coadaptation
coagulation
    disseminated intravascular c. (DIC)
    laser c.
    microwave tumor c.
    c. necrosis
coagulator
    argon beam c. (ABC)
coagulography
coagulopathy
    intravascular consumption c.
coal
    c. macule
    c. miner's lung
    c. tar
    c. worker's lung
    c. worker's pneumoconiosis (CWP)
coalesce
coalescence

NOTES

coalescent granuloma
coalition
> bony c.
> calcaneonavicular c.
> carpal c.
> fibrous c.
> intercarpal c.
> lunate-triquetral c.
> Minaar classification of c.
> osseous c.
> talocalcaneal c.
> talonavicular c.
> target c.
> tarsal c.
> c. view

coanalgesic
coaptation point
coapted leaflet
coarctation
> abdominal aortic c.
> adult c.
> c. of aorta
> aortic c.
> asymptomatic c.
> atypical subisthmic c.
> congenital isthmic c.
> infantile c.
> isthmic c.
> juxtaductal aortic c.
> localized c.
> postductal aortic c.
> preductal aortic c.
> reversed c.
> c. syndrome
> thoracic aortic c.

coarcted segment
coarse
> c. bronchovascular marking
> c. calcification
> c. injection
> c. linear opacity
> c. lung reticulation
> c. microcalcification
> c. nodularity
> c. pattern
> c. reticular opacity

coarsening
coated
> enteric c.

coat hanger osteochondroma
coating
> c. of aneurysm
> Hydro-Sil c.

Coats disease
coaxial
> 17-gauge c. Temno needle
> c. micropuncture needle set
> c. sheath cut-biopsy needle

> c. sheath technique
> c. steering

coaxially
> pass c.

coaxillary directed catheter
cobalt (Co)
> c. 57 (^{57}Co)
> c. 58 (^{58}Co)
> c. 60 (^{60}Co)
> c. alloy stent
> c. 60 beam therapy unit
> c. megavoltage machine
> c. pneumopathy
> radioactive c.
> c. radioactive source

cobalt-60
> c.-60 beam
> c.-60 gamma knife radiosurgical
> treatment

cobalt-chromium-molybdenum alloy metal implant
cobalt-chromium-tungsten-nickel alloy metal implant
Cobatope-57
Cobb
> C. measurement
> C. measurement of scoliosis
> C. method
> C. method of measuring kyphosis
> C. scoliosis angle
> C. syndrome

cobbler's chest
cobblestone
> c. appearance
> c. appearance of bile duct
> c. appearance of the colon
> c. appearance duodenum
> c. appearance eosinophilic
> gastroenteritis
> c. appearance esophagus
> c. appearance lymphoma
> c. appearance stomach
> c. degeneration
> c. ileum
> c. lissencephaly
> c. mucosa
> c. pattern
> c. sign

cobblestoning
Coblation
Cobra
> C. 1 catheter
> C. 2 catheter
> C. diagnostic catheter

cobra-eye sign
cobra-head
> c.-h. anastomosis
> c.-h. appearance

c.-h. effect
c.-h. ureter
cobra-shaped catheter
cobweb
    c. appearance
    c. pattern
cocaine
    ^{11}C-labeled c.
coccidioidoma
coccidioidomycosis
    bone c.
    disseminated c.
    latent c.
    lung c.
    Posadas-Wernicke c.
    primary c.
    progressive c.
    secondary c.
coccygeal
    c. appendage
    c. body
    c. bone
    c. ganglion
    c. gland
    c. ligament
    c. plexus
    c. sinus
    c. spine
    c. vertebra
    c. vestige
    c. whorl
coccygeopubic diameter
coccygeus
    vortex c.
coccyx, pl. **coccyges**
    c. bone
    c. fracture
cochlea, pl. **cochleae**
    c. aplasia
    single-cavity c.
cochleae
    apertura externa canaliculi c.
cochlear
    c. anatomy
    c. aqueduct
    c. canal
    c. canaliculus
    c. duct
    c. implant
    c. labyrinth
    c. lesion
    c. nerve

    c. otosclerosis
    c. recess
    c. root
cochleariform process
cochlearis
    stria vascularis ductus c.
cochleate uterus
cochleitis
    calcific c.
    ossifying c.
Cockayne syndrome
cocking injury
cock-robin position
cockscomb
    c. appearance
    c. appearance of cervix
    c. papilloma
cocktail
    renal c.
cock-up deformity
Co-Cr-Mo alloy metal implant
Co-Cr-W-Ni alloy implant metal
cocurrent flow-related enhancement
COD
    computerized optical densitometry
CoDe
    coincidence detection
Code and Carlson radiograph
coded-aperture imaging
coded-image aperture
coder
    Chen-Smith image c.
    ICS c.
    improved c. (ICS)
codfish
    c. deformity
    c. vertebra
Codivilla extension
Codman
    C. angle
    C. Cranioplastic Type 1 Slow Set
    C. Medos programmable valve
    C. sign
    C. triangle
    C. tumor
codominant
    c. circulation
    c. vessel
coefficient
    absorption c.
    apparent diffusion c. (ADC)
    attenuation c.

C

NOTES

coefficient *(continued)*
> attenuation-correction c.
> binary similarity c.
> c. conversion
> correlation c.
> curve fit c.
> diffusion c.
> effective mass attenuation c.
> Fourier c.
> linear absorption c.
> linear attenuation c.
> mass absorption c.
> mass attenuation c.
> Ostwald solubility c. (Λ)
> partition c.
> Pearson correlation c.
> reflection c.
> Spearman correlation c.
> stiffness c.
> uniform attenuation c.
> c. of variation (c.v.)
> viscosity c.

coeur en sabot
coexistent
> c. cavity
> c. intravoxel fat and water

coffee
> c. grounds material
> c. worker's lung

coffee-bean appearance
coffin bone
Cogan lid twitch sign
cognitive
> c. fMRI
> c. functional MR imaging

cogwheel sign
coherence
> multiple quantum c.
> phase c.

coherent
> C. CO_2 surgical laser
> c. scattering
> steady-state c.
> C. UltraPulse 5000C laser
> C. VersaPulse device

coil
> aneurysmal c.
> c. array
> 3-axis gradient c.
> bilateral breast c.
> bird-cage head c.
> body c.
> breast c.
> butterfly c.
> catheter-delivered platinum c.
> circularly polarized c.
> circular polarized volume head c.
> circumferential extremity c.

> c. closure of coronary artery fistula
> collagen-filled interlocking detachable c.
> conventional head c.
> coupled array c.
> crossed c.
> custom-curved c.
> DCS-10, DCS-18 mechanically detachable platinum c.
> dedicated phased-array c.
> dedicated shoulder c.
> c. delivery
> c. deposition
> detachable platinum c.
> detector c.
> double breast c.
> electrically detachable c.
> 2-element phased array c.
> 4-element phased array c.
> embedding of stent c.
> c. embolization
> endoanal c.
> endoesophageal MRI c.
> endorectal c.
> endoscopic quadrature radiofrequency c.
> endovaginal c.
> endovascular c.
> extremity c.
> fat-suppressed body c.
> field-profiling c.
> flexible radiofrequency c.
> flexible surface c.
> free fibered c.
> GDC-10 soft c.
> c. geometry
> Gianturco occlusion c.
> Gianturco-Wallace-Anderson c.
> Gianturco-Wallace-Chuang c.
> Gianturco wool-tufted wire c.
> Golay c.
> gonion gradient c.
> Gore 1.5T torso array MRI surface c.
> gradient sheet c.
> Guglielmi detachable c. (GDC)
> head c.
> Helmholtz c.
> high-speed gradient c.
> Hipper twist release c.
> immediately detachable c.
> Intercept Vascular 0.030^2 internal MR c.
> interlocking detachable c. (IDC)
> c.'s of intestine
> intrarectal c.
> intravascular c.
> in vitro evaluation of c.

Jackson c.
linearly polarized c.
liver c.
c. loading
local c.
local gradient c.
Maxwell c.
MDS c.
mechanically detachable platinum c.
Medrad MRInnervu endorectal
  colon probe c.
micronester platinum
  embolization c.
c. migration
2-mm/3-cm c.
2-mm/6-cm c.
3 mm x 6 cm interlocking
  detachable c.
4 mm x 8 cm interlocking
  detachable c.
modified bird-cage c.
MRCP using HASTE with a
  phased array c.
multiply tuned c.
neck c.
nester c.
opposed loop-pair quadrature
  NMR c.
orthogonal radiofrequency c.
parallel data acquisition c.
pelvic phased-array c.
phased array c.
phased-array surface c.
phased-array torso c.
planar circular c.
platinum c.
posterior neck surface c.
c. protrusion
proximal c.
pushable c.
quadrature body c.
quadrature cervical spine c.
quadrature head c.
quadrature radiofrequency
  receiver c.
quadrature terminal latency
  surface c.
quadrature transmit/receive head c.
radiofrequency c.
radiofrequency transmitter-receiver c.
receive-only circular surface c.
receiver c.

RF c.
right ventricular c.
saddle c.
c. selection
send-receive phased-array
  extremity c.
sensing c.
c. sensitive encoding
shielded gradient c.
shim c.
shoulder surface c.
solenoid surface c.
stainless steel c.
steel c.
Stylet esophageal MRI c.
surface c.
Surgi-Vision MRI c.
switchable c.
thrombogenic c.
Tornado c.
torso phased-array c. (TPAC)
transmit-receive c.
transmitter c.
TriSpan detachable c.
twist-release c.
c. vascular stent
volume c.
VortXX c.
whole-volume c.
wool c.
wrist quadrature phased-array
  surface c.
2 (x) 3, 4, 5, 6 fibered Guglielmi
  detachable c.

coiled
  c. spring appearance
  c. spring pattern
  c. spring sign
coiling
  c. of anastomosis
  c. of aneurysm
coil-to-vessel diameter
coin
  c. artifact
  fracture en c.
  c. lesion
  c. lesion of lung
  c. test
coincidence
  c. circuit
  counting c.
  c. detection (CD, CoDe)

NOTES

coincidence *(continued)*
  c. detection mode
  c. detection positron emission
    tomography
  c. detection scan
  c. event
  c. gamma camera
  c. imaging
  c. imaging scanner
  loss c.
  sum peak c.
coincidence-resolving window
coincidence-summing correction
coincident gamma camera
coin-on-edge vertebra
Coiter muscle
Colapinto
  C. needle
  C. sheath
Colbert method
COLD
  chronic obstructive lung disease
cold
  c. breast abscess
  c. defect
  c. defect renal scintigraphy
  c. lesion
  c. nodule thyroid
  c. quartz lamp germicidal lamp
  c. spine abscess
  c. spot
  c. spot myocardial imaging
  c. thyroid nodule
colectasia
coli
  elastin deposition in taeniae c.
  familial polyposis c.
  haustra c.
  melanosis c.
  pneumatosis c.
colic
  c. artery
  biliary c.
  c. impression
  c. omentum
  c. plexus
  renal c.
  c. sphincter
  c. surface
  c. vein
colitis
  chronic ulcerative c. (CUC)
  Crohn c.
  c. cystica profunda
  focal c.
  fulminant c.
  fulminating ulcerative c.
  granulomatous transmural c.
  ischemic c.

myxomembranous c.
  c. polyposa
  pseudomembranous c.
  radiation-induced c.
  regional c.
  single-stripe c. (SSC)
  transmural c.
  ulcerative c. (UC)
  c. ulcerosa gravis
collagen
  c. defect type I, II
  c. fiber separation
  c. fibril
  c. fragmentation
  c. mediated closure device
  microfibrillar c.
  c. plug
  c. plug device
  c. tissue proliferation
**collagen-filled interlocking detachable
  coil**
collagenosis
  mediastinal c.
collagenous
  c. perivascular ala
  c. structure
  c. tissue
collapse
  acinar c.
  acute vertebral c.
  alveolar c.
  c. cavitation
  circulation c.
  jugular venous pressure c.
  scapholunate advanced c. (SLAC)
  scapholunate arthritic c.
  subchondral c.
  vertebral body c.
collapsed
  c. distal ileum
  c. inferior vena cava
  c. lobe
  c. lung
  c. lung field
  c. subpectoral implant
collapsing cord sign
collar
  Cowboy C.
  implant c.
  periosteal bone c.
  periportal c.
  c. sign
  tension c.
collarbone
collar-button
  c.-b. abscess
  c.-b. appearance
  c.-b. chest lesion
  c.-b. ulcer

collateral
c. arcade
arterial c.
c. blood flow
c. blood supply
c. branch
c. circulation in compression of
    artery
cross-scrotal c.
developed c.
c. edema
c. eminence
c. fissure
gastroesophageal c.
c. hyperemia
c. ligament
c. ligament of knee
c. mesenteric circulation
parasitized c.
portosystemic c.
c. sulcus
c. system
tributary c.
c. trigone
venous c.
c. venous channel
c. vessel
collateralization
collecting
c. system
c. system atony
c. system filling defect
c. system opacification
c. tube
c. tubule
c. venous pouch
c. vessel
collection
abdominal air c.
air c.
anechoic fluid c.
complex abdominal fluid c.
complex fluid c.
c. of contrast material
crescentic c.
EAA c.
extraalveolar air c.
extraaxial fluid c.
extracerebral fluid c.
fluid c.
gas c.
hypoechoic fluid c.

intratendinous fluid c.
list mode data c.
mottled gas c.
pancreatic fluid c.
periarticular fluid c.
pericholecystic fluid c.
perifascial fluidlike c.
perinephric fluid c.
peripancreatic fluid c.
periprosthetic fluid c.
pleural fluid c.
posttraumatic subcapsular hepatic
    fluid c.
retrocerebellar CSF c.
retromammary fluid c.
saccular c.
collective paramagnetism
Colles
C. fascia
C. fracture
C. ligament
Collet-Sicard syndrome
colli
fibromatosis c.
pterygium c.
vertebrae c.
collicular fracture
colliculus, pl. **colliculi**
anterior c.
brachium of c.
facial c.
fused colliculi
inferior c.
plicae colliculi
posterior c.
seminal c.
superior c.
Collier sign
collimated slice width
collimating system
collimation
c. CT
detector c.
dynamic multileaf c.
electronic c.
c. imaging
lead c.
narrow c.
c. scanning
c. scintillation detector
secondary c.
submillimeter c.

NOTES

189

collimation *(continued)*
    tertiary c.
    c. width
collimator
    APC-3, APC-4 c.
    automatic c.
    converging c.
    converging-hole c.
    diverging c.
    dual-shaped c.
    Eureka c.
    c. exchange effect
    fan-beam c.
    focusing c.
    heart-shaped c.
    c. helmet
    high-resolution c.
    high-resolution, fan-beam c.
    high-resolution multileaf c.
    LEAP c.
    LEUHR fan beam c.
    LEUHR parallel-hole c.
    Leur-par c.
    long-bore c.
    low-energy c.
    medium-energy c.
    Micro-Cast c.
    multihole c.
    multileaf c. (MLC)
    multirod c.
    parallel-hole medium sensitivity c.
    pinhole c.
    c. plugging pattern
    c. scattering
    single-hole c.
    slant hole c.
    slat c.
    slit c.
    thick-septa c.
    thin-septa c.
    triple-leaf c.
    ultra-high-resolution, parallel-hole c.
colliquative necrosis
collision
    c. detecting
    elastic c.
    c. tumor
collodiaphysial
    central c. (CCD)
colloid
    c. adenocarcinoma
    c. adenoma
    [198]Au c.
    c. calculus
    c. carcinoma
    c. cyst
    c. cystadenoma
    c. cystic tumor
    c. cyst of third ventricle

    c. degeneration
    c. goiter
    minimicroaggregated albumin c.
    c. oncotic pressure (COP)
    radioactive c.
    radiogold c.
    c. shift
    c. shift on scan
    sulfur c.
    [99mTc] sulfur c.
    TechneScan Sulfur C.
    technetium-99m antimony
      trisulfide c.
    technetium-99m minimicroaggregated
      albumin c.
    technetium-sulfur c.
colloidal
    c. brain cyst
    c. chromic phosphorus
    c. sulfur
    c. suspension
colobomatous cyst
colocolic
    c. anastomosis
    c. fistula
    c. intussusception
colocutaneous fistula
colography
    CT c.
Colombo count
colon
    accessory sign c.
    angiodysplasia of c.
    anterior band of c.
    ascending c.
    barium-filled c.
    burned-out c.
    c. carcinoma
    carpet lesion of c.
    cathartic c.
    cobblestone appearance of the c.
    coned-down appearance of c.
    Crohn disease of c.
    c. cutoff sign
    c. cyst duplication
    descending c.
    distal c.
    double-tracking c.
    c. duplication
    epithelial c.
    fecal-filled c.
    free band of c.
    giant c.
    hepatodiaphragmatic interposition
      of c. (HDIC)
    hypoganglionosis of c.
    iliac c.
    inflammation of c.
    intramural air in c.

irritable c.
jejunization of c.
c. kinking
knuckle of c.
lateral reflection of c.
left c.
c. margin
mesosigmoid c.
midsigmoid c.
pelvic c.
perisigmoid c.
proximal c.
c. pseudostricture
right c.
sigmoid c.
spastic c.
c. stenting
thumbprinting appearance of the c.
transverse c.

colonic
  c. activity
  c. adenoma
  c. adenomatous polyp
  c. air
  c. angiodysplasia
  c. apple-core lesion
  c. atresia
  c. carpet lesion
  c. dilatation
  c. distention
  c. diverticular hemorrhage
  c. diverticulitis
  c. diverticulosis
  c. diverticulum
  c. duplication cyst
  c. evacuation
  c. filling defect
  c. fistula
  c. flexure
  c. gas composition
  c. hamartomatous polyp
  c. haustra
  c. ileus
  c. interposition
  c. involvement of endometriosis
  c. lead-pipe appearance
  c. loop
  c. motility
  c. mucosal excretion
  c. myenteric plexus
  c. narrowing
  c. necrosis

c. neoplasm
c. obstruction
c. perforation
c. pit
c. pseudoobstruction
c. saddle lesion
c. spasm
c. stricture
c. transit time
c. ulcer
c. urticaria pattern
c. varix
c. volvulus

colonization
  saprophytic c.
Colonna hip fracture classification
colonography
  bile-tagged 3D magnetic
    resonance c.
  computed tomographic c. (CTC)
  computed tomography c. (CTC)
  CT c.
  MR c.
  Virtual CT c.
  volume-rendered CT c.
colonoscope
  CF-200Z Olympus c.
  Olympus CF-1T100L c.
  Olympus CF-200Z c.
colonoscopy
  virtual c.
ColonoSight system
colony-forming unit
coloproctitis
coloptosis
color
  c. amplitude imaging
  c. Doppler (CD)
  c. Doppler imaging (CDI)
  c. Doppler recording
  c. Doppler signal
  c. Doppler sonography (CDS)
  c. Doppler twinkling artifact
  c. Doppler ultrasound (CDUS)
  c. duplex interrogation
  c. duplex ultrasound
  c. encoded brain MR imaging
  c. gain
  c. kinesis
  c. power angiography
  c. power transcranial Doppler
    sonography

NOTES

C

color *(continued)*
    c. power transcranial Doppler ultrasound
    c. space conversion
    c. space interpolation
    c. space interpolator
    c. spectrum
    c. velocity imaging
    c. void
color-coded
    c.-c. Doppler flow imaging (CDFI)
    c.-c. duplex sonography (CCDS)
    c.-c. duplex ultrasound
    c.-c. guidewire
    c.-c. pulmonary blood flow imaging
    c.-c. real-time sonography
    c.-c. real-time ultrasound
colorectal (CR)
    c. adenoma
    c. anastomosis
    c. cancer endoscopy
    c. carcinoid
    c. carcinoma
    c. duplication
    c. hemorrhage
    c. lymphoma
    c. mucosa
    c. polyp
colorectal/ovarian (CR/OV)
color-flame scale
color-flow
    c.-f. Doppler (CFD)
    c.-f. Doppler imaging
    c.-f. Doppler real-time 2D blood flow imaging
    c.-f. Doppler sonography
    c.-f. duplex imaging
    c.-f. duplex scan
    c.-f. imaging (CFI)
    c.-f. imaging Doppler echocardiography
    c.-f. mapping
colorimetric
    c. color reproduction
    c. test
color-scale image
coloscopy
    endocervical canal c.
colosigmoid resection
colostogram
    augmented pressure c.
colostomy
    barium enema through c.
    barium injection through c.
    fecal diversion c.
colovaginal fistula
colovesical fistula
colpocele

colpocephaly
colpoptosis
colposcopy
colpostat applicator
column
    anal c.
    anterior gray c.
    c. of Bertin
    branchial efferent c.
    c. of Burdach
    Clarke c.
    contrast medium c.
    corrugated air c.
    dye c.
    extraction c.
    c. extraction method
    Gowers c.
    head of barium c.
    intermediolateral gray c.
    Lissauer c.
    c. mode sinogram image
    c. of Morgagni
    Quick Spin Sephadex G-50 c.
    renal c.
    thoracolumbar spine c.
    variceal c.
    vertebral c.
    weighted spin-echo c.
columnar-lined esophagus
columnar metaphysis
2-column injury
3-column injury
columnization of contrast material
column-mode sinogram imaging
Colyte bowel preparation
COMBI
    continuous moving bed (MR) imaging
Combidex MRI contrast agent
combination
    c. flow and pressure load
    molybdenum-molybdenum target filter c. (Mo-Mo)
    molybdenum-rhodium target filter c. (Mo-Rh)
    rhodium-rhodium target filter c. (Rh-Rh)
    target-filter c.
combined
    c. anatomic registration
    c. CT-fluoroscopy scanner
    c. CT-PET
    c. dynamic 2D and bolus-chase 3D acquisitions
    c. flexion-distraction injury and burst fracture
    c. leukocyte-marrow imaging
    c. multisection diffuse-weighted and hemodynamically weighted echo-planar MR

c. Myoscint/thallium imaging
c. pregnancy
c. radial-ulnar-humeral fracture
c. ^{99m}Tc-DMSA and ^{99m}Tc-DTPA scanning
c. thallium-Tc-HMPAO imaging
c. transmission-emission scintiphoto
c. ventilation-perfusion scintigraphy

comb sign
comedo
    c. necrosis
    c. pattern
comedo–basal cell carcinoma
comedomastitis
comedo-type DCIS
comet-tail
    c.-t. artifact
    c.-t. artifact gallbladder
    c.-t. sign
comfort
    C. Cath I catheter
    C. Cath II catheter
comitans
    vena c.
comma-shaped
    c.-s. crus
    c.-s. duodenum
commemorative sign
commencement of vessel
comminuted
    c. bursting fracture
    c. intraarticular fracture
    c. teardrop fracture
commission
    (U.S.) Nuclear Regulatory C. (NRC)
commissural
    c. attachment
    c. chorda
    c. function
    c. leaflet
    c. point
commissure
    anterior c. (AC)
    anterior commissure-posterior c. (AC-PC)
    anteroseptal c.
    cerebral c.
    fused c.
    gray c.
    mitral valve c.
    posterior c. (PC)

scalloped c.
tectum c.
temporal limb of the anterior c.
valve c.
vestigial c.
white matter c.

common
    c. atrioventricular canal
    c. atrium
    c. basal vein
    c. bile duct (CBD)
    c. bile duct bifurcation
    c. bile duct diverticulum
    c. bile duct exploration (CBDE)
    c. bile duct obstruction
    c. bile duct spontaneous perforation
    c. bile duct stone
    c. bile duct stricture
    c. bundle
    c. cardinal vein
    c. carotid artery (CCA)
    c. carotid artery bifurcation
    c. carotid plexus
    c. cavity phenomenon
    c. duct cholangiogram
    c. duct dilatation
    c. dural sac
    c. extensor tendinosis
    c. facial vein
    c. femoral (CF)
    c. femoral artery
    c. femoral vein
    c. gall duct
    c. gateway interface (CGI)
    c. hepatic artery
    c. hepatic duct (CHD)
    c. iliac artery
    c. iliac lymph node
    c. peroneal artery
    c. pulmonary vein stenosis
    c. synovial flexor sheath
    c. tendinous ring
    c. tendon
commotio cerebri
commune
    centrum c.
    crus c.
    mesenterium c.
    persistent ostium atrioventriculare c.
communicating
    c. artery
    c. artery aneurysm

NOTES

communicating *(continued)*
  c. cavernous ectasia
  c. cyst
  c. fistula
  c. hydrocephalus
  c. syringomyelia
  c. vein
  c. vein incompetence
communication
  cholangiovenous c.
  fistulous gas c.
  interatrial c.
  macrofistulous arteriovenous c.
  Medical Ultrasound Three-
    Dimensional Portable
    Advanced C.'s (MUSTPAC)
  peritoneopleural c.
  pleuroperitoneal c.
communis
  extensor digitorum c. (EDC)
community-acquired pneumonia
Comolli sign
compact
  c. bone
  c. fibrillar echotexture
  c. island
  c. osteoma
companion
  c. lymph node
  c. shadow
  c. vein
comparative value
comparator
  public sector c. (PSC)
comparison
  beam quality c.
  c. film
  histopathologic c.
  c. view
  yield c.
compartment
  anterior mediastinal c.
  anterior tibial c.
  deep posterior c.
  distal radioulnar joint c.
  extensor c.
  extracellular c.
  extradural c.
  extravascular c.
  fifth c.
  fourth c.
  iliopsoas c.
  infracolic c.
  infratentorial c.
  lateral c.
  medial c.
  midcarpal c.
  patellofemoral c.
  peribronchovascular interstitial c.

  perirenal c.
  plantar c.
  posterior c.
  posterolateral c.
  posteromedial c.
  radiocarpal c.
  sixth c.
  superficial posterior c.
  supracolic c.
  supramesocolic c.
  c. syndrome
  vascular c.
  wrist extensor c.
3-compartment
  3-c. arthrography
  3-c. system
  3-c. wrist angiography
compartmental
  c. analysis
  c. modeling
  c. radioimmunoglobulin therapy
compartmentalization
2-compartment system
COMPASS stereotactic system
compensated
  c. composite spin-lock pulse
  c. congestive heart failure
  c. hydrocephalus
compensating filter
compensation
  attenuation c.
  cardiac gating c.
  depth c.
  flow c. (FC)
  gradient c.
  respiratory c.
  scatter c.
  second-order c.
  section-select flow c.
  supratentorial flow c.
  time gain c. (TGC)
  velocity c.
compensator
  multivane intensity modulation c.
    (MIMIC)
  scattering foil c.
  tissue deficit c.
compensatory
  c. atrophy
  c. capillary filling
  c. circulation
  c. cortical activation
  c. deformity
  c. emphysema
  c. enlargement
  c. enlargement of ventricle
  c. hyperplasia
  c. lobe hyperexpansion
  c. mechanism

c. nodular kidney hypertrophy
c. pause
competence of ureterovesical junction
competent ileocecal valve
competitive
   c. adsorption
   c. inhibition
   c. iron administration
complementary
   c. and alternative medicine (CAM)
   c. hypertrophy
   c. metal oxide semiconductor
     (CMOS)
   c. spatial modulation of
     magnetization (CSPAMM)
complete
   c. anatomic cure
   c. atrioventricular block (CAVB)
   c. atrioventricular dissociation
   c. bladder emptying
   c. bowel obstruction
   c. congenital heart block
   c. dislocation
   c. duplication
   c. fetal heart block
   c. fracture
   c. heart block (CHB)
   c. myelography
   c. nerve lesion
   c. occlusion
   c. placenta previa
   c. situs inversus
   c. small bowel malrotation
   c. stent expansion
   c. stress/rest study
   c. tear
   c. transposition of great artery
   c. vascular stasis
completed stroke
completion arteriography
complex, pl. **complexes**
   c. abdominal fluid collection
   agyria pachygria c.
   amygdaloid nuclear c.
   c. anatomic relationship
   ankle joint c.
   c. anorectal fistula
   anterior communicating artery c.
   aperiodic c.
   apical c.
   arcuate c.
   atrial c.

c. atrioventricular canal
auricular c.
basivertebral venous c.
biceps-labral c.
c. breast cyst
Buford c.
capsulolabral c.
caudal pharyngeal c.
chlormerodrin-cysteine c.
choroidal-hippocampal fissure c.
complex blocking c.
compound dislocation c.
c. conjugate
Dandy-Walker c.
discoligamentous c.
eighth cranial nerve c.
Eisenmenger c.
epispadia exstrophy c.
c. extraperitoneal rupture
fabellofibular c.
fibrocartilage c.
c. fluid collection
foot-ankle c.
frontonasal dysplasia
  malformation c.
gadolinium c.
gallium-transferrin c.
gastrocnemius-soleus c.
gastroduodenal artery c.
Ghon c.
Ghon-Sachs c.
growth plate c.
hallux sesamoid c.
hallux valgus-metatarsus primus
  varus c.
hindfoot joint c.
hippocampal-amygdaloid c.
hypoperfusion c.
hypovolemic c.
inferior glenohumeral ligament
  labral c. (IGLLC)
inverted-Y c.
Kirklin meniscal c.
labral capsular c.
labral-ligamentous c.
labrum-ligament c.
lateral collateral ligament c.
ligamentous c.
limb-body wall c.
Lutembacher c.
mantle c.
mastoid c.

C

NOTES

complex *(continued)*
medial collateral ligament c. (MCLC)
mesenteric adenitis-ileitis c.
metal chelate c.
Michaelis c.
multiform ventricular c.
c. myxoma
nipple-areolar c.
ostiomeatal c.
outer anular/posterior longitudinal ligament c.
oxidized c.
pelvic mass c.
c. periosteal reaction
c. platinum microcoil
preintegration c.
primary c.
pulmonary sling c.
Ranke c.
renal sinus c.
respiratory chain c. I–VI
c. sclerosing lesion (CSL)
sesamoid c.
shoulder labral capsular c.
c. simple fracture
sling ring c.
c. solid and cystic mass
subluxation c.
c. subtraction
superior olivary c.
syndesmotic ligament c.
tibiocalcaneal joint c.
transluminal coronary artery angioplasty c.
transposition c.
triangular fibrocartilaginous c. (TFCC)
VATER c.
ventricular premature c. (VPC)
vertebrobasilar c.
c. of vessel
VIII nerve c.
von Meyenburg c.
zygomatic c. (ZMC)
zygomaticomaxillary c. (ZMC)
zygomaxillary c. (ZMC)

compliance
craniospinal c.
lung c.
c. matching stent (CMS)
reduced pulmonary c.

complicated
c. dislocation
c. fracture
c. myoma
c. pneumoconiosis
c. renal cyst

c. scleroderma
c. silicosis

complication
air leak c.
graft-related c.
ischemic c.
nonfetal c.
pleuropulmonary c.

component
anatomically graduated c. (AGC)
central hemorrhagic c.
cystic c.
dispersive c.
extensive intraductal c. (EIC)
extracellular matrix c.
frequency c.
irregularly layered astrocytic c.
irregularly layered neuronal c.
markedly accentuated pulmonic c.
mitral c.
obstructive c.
secretory c.
solid c.

composite
c. aortic valve
c. fracture
c. pulse
c. signal

composition
colonic gas c.
hydropic c.
renal stone mineral c.

compound
c. aneurysm
c. comminuted fracture
c. complex fracture
c. dislocation
c. dislocation complex
lipophilic c.
PET c.
c. pregnancy
c. presentation
radiolabeled c.
reference c.
c. skull fracture
thorium c.
titanium c.
unsaturated c.

compressed body
compressibility and phasicity study
compression
aqueduct c.
c. atrophy
biliary tree c.
brachial artery c.
brachial plexus c.
brainstem c.
c. of breast
cardiac c.

cauda equina c.
chamber c.
chiasmal c.
coned-down spot c.
contrecoup c.
cord c.
c. device
double-spot c.
external pneumatic calf c.
extrinsic bladder c.
fenestrated alphanumeric c.
fingerprint image c.
c. flexion injury
c. fracture
image c.
interfragmental c.
intrinsic c.
irreversible c.
lossless image data c.
lossy image data c.
magnification and spot c.
manual c.
multiplanar c.
nerve root c.
c. neuropathy
neurovascular c.
optic nerve c.
orbital mass c.
c. paddle
pancake c.
plaque c.
c. plate
c. plate and screw
radicular c.
c. ratio
real-time c.
root c.
c. sonography
spinal cord c.
spot c.
subchondral trabecular c.
symptomatic metastatic spinal
  cord c.
c. syndrome
thermal c.
c. ultrasonography
ultrasound-guided c.
ultrasound-guided
  pseudoaneurysm c.
vascular esophageal c.
vascular tracheal c.
wavelet c.

compressive
　　c. atelectasis
　　c. edema
　　c. hyperextension injury
compromise
　　circulatory c.
　　respiratory c.
　　vascular c.
compromised
　　c. flow
　　c. pregnancy
　　c. ventricular function
Compton
　　C. coherent scattering densitometry
　　C. edge
　　C. effect
　　C. electron
　　C. interaction
　　C. scattering
　　C. scattering cross-section
　　C. scattering photon
　　C. suppression spectrometer
　　C. suppression system
　　C. wavelength
Compuscan
　　C. Hittman computerized
　　　electrocardioscanner
　　C. Hittman computerized imaging
computation
　　analog c.
computational anatomy
computed
　　c. dental radiography (CDR)
　　c. ejection fraction
　　c. myelography
　　c. radiography (CR)
　　c. radiology (CR)
　　c. tomographic angiography (CTA)
　　c. tomographic cholangiography
　　c. tomographic colonography (CTC)
　　c. tomographic cystography
　　c. tomographic dacryocystography
　　c. tomographic enteroclysis
　　c. tomographic lymphography (CT-LG)
　　c. tomographic pulmonary angiography
　　c. tomography (CT)
　　c. tomography cisternography
　　c. tomography colonography (CTC)
　　c. tomography dose index (CTDI)

NOTES

computed *(continued)*
- c. tomography during arterial portography (CTAP)
- c. tomography fluoroscopy (CTF)
- c. tomography-guided percutaneous radiofrequency denervation of the sacroiliac joint
- c. tomography laser mammography (CTLM)
- c. tomography lymphography (CT-LG)
- c. tomography scan
- c. tomography with arterioportography (CTAP)
- c. transmission tomography
- c. transmission tomography imaging

computer
- c. automated scan technology (CAST)
- c. fusion imaging
- image reconstruction c.
- c. information system
- c. method
- c. strain-gauge plethysmography (CSGP)
- c. subtraction technique

computer-aided
- c.-a. detection (CAD)
- c.-a. diagnosis (CAD)
- c.-a. diagnosis scheme
- c.-a. image analysis
- c.-a. polyp detection

computer-assisted
- c.-a. blood background subtraction (CABBS)
- c.-a. intracranial navigation
- c.-a. joint motion analysis
- c.-a. myelography (CAM)
- c.-a. resection of cerebral arteriovenous malformation
- c.-a. stereotactic resection
- c.-a. volumetric stereotaxis

computer-controlled conformal radiation therapy (CCRT)

computer-generated
- c.-g. artifact
- c.-g. image

computerized
- c. axial tomography (CAT)
- c. cranial tomography
- c. fluoroscopy
- c. optical densitometry (COD)
- c. radiography
- c. radiotherapy
- c. texture analysis of lung nodules and lung parenchyma
- C. Thermal Imaging system
- c. tomographic hepatic angiography (CTHA)

- c. tomographic holography (CTH)
- c. tomography guidance
- c. tomography-guided needle biopsy
- c. tomography/magnetic resonance (CT/MR)
- c. transverse axial image
- c. transverse axial tomography (CTAT)

conal
- c. cyst
- c. papillary muscle
- c. septum
- c. ventricular septal defect

concatenation of shadows

Concato disease

concave skull disc

concavity
- posterior c.

concavoconvex

concealed
- c. hemorrhage
- c. penis

concentrated bile

concentration
- deoxyhemoglobin c.
- directional gradient c. (DGC)
- hypertensive contrast c.
- maximum permissible c.
- methylene diphosphonate (MDP) c.
- NAWM metabolite c.
- organ-specific c.
- Poisson distributed activity c.
- c. of radionuclide
- synaptic dopamine c.
- time-dependent xenon c.
- c. times time ($C \times T$)

concentration-time curve

concentric
- c. anular tear
- c. atherosclerotic plaque
- c. circle technique
- c. contraction
- c. fibroma
- c. heart hypertrophy
- c. hernia
- c. herniation
- c. hourglass stenosis
- c. hypertrophic cardiomyopathy
- c. lamella
- c. lesion
- c. narrowing
- c. pantomography
- c. reduction

concentrica
- encephalitis periaxialis c.

concept
- gooseneck c.
- line integral c.

no-threshold c.
ring-of-bone c.

concertina pattern
concha, pl. **conchae**
    c. bullosa
    nasal c.
conchal
    c. cartilage
    c. crest
concomitant
    c. boost radiation therapy
    c. defect
    c. finding
    c. infarct
    c. pneumonia
    c. tracheal injury
concordance
    c. of MR finding
    radiologic-pathologic c.
    situs c.
concordant result
concretion
    bile c.
    fecal c.
concussion
    brain c.
    spinal c.
condensans
    clavicular osteitis c.
condition
    adnexal c.
    grade 0, 2 insonation c.
    insonation c.
    nonfetal uterine c.
    nonthromboembolic c.
conditioned reflex (CR)
condom catheter
conductance catheter
conducting bronchiole
conduction
    c. band
    c. block
    interval intraatrial c.
    nodal c.
    c. ratio
    reciprocating c.
    retrograde ventriculoatrial c.
    ventriculoatrial c.
    zone of slow c.
conductive
    c. development
    c. loop

conductivity
    thermal c.
    tissue c.
    vascular hydraulic c.
conductor
    fiberoptic c.
    c. resistivity
conduit
    detour c.
    ileal c.
    intestinal c.
    nonvalved c.
    right ventricle-pulmonary artery c.
    urinary c.
    c. valve
    ventriculoarterial c.
condylar
    c. angle
    c. articulation
    c. axis
    c. canal
    c. emissary vein
    c. flare
    c. fossa
    c. part of occipital bone
    c. plate
    c. skull hypoplasia
    c. split fracture
    c. translation
condyle
    c. cord
    external c.
    femoral c.
    lateral c.
    mandibular c.
    medial c.
    occipital c.
    tibial c.
condyloid
    c. canal
    c. joint
    c. process
condyloma, pl. **condylomata**
    c. urethra acuminata
condylomatous atypia lesion
condylus tertius
cone
    arterial c.
    c. beam
    beveled electron beam c.
    c. disc
    c. epiphysis

NOTES

cone (*continued*)
    c. of extraocular muscle
    medullary c.
    parenchymal c.
    c. spot compression view
    transvaginal c.
cone-beam
    c.-b. image
    c.-b. reconstruction algorithm
coned
    c. cecum
    c. down
    c. panoramic tomogram
coned-down
    c.-d. appearance of colon
    c.-d. compression view
    c.-d. radiograph
    c.-d. spot compression
    c.-d. view
CO_2-negative imaging agent
confidence interval (CI)
configuration
    adaptic detector c.
    anatomic c.
    back-to-back c.
    batwing c.
    beaklike c.
    bilobed c.
    biventricular c.
    bulbous c.
    bull's eye c.
    butterfly c.
    cat's tail c.
    closed-fist c.
    Cupid's bow c.
    cylindrical c.
    discoid c.
    dome-and-dart c.
    double-halo c.
    expansile c.
    fishmouth mitral valve c.
    geriatric c.
    globular c.
    Helmholtz c.
    hexagonal c.
    horizontal dipole c.
    horseshoe c.
    hourglass c.
    hybrid detector c.
    inverted-Y c.
    isosceles triangular c.
    left ventricular c.
    lock-washer c.
    masslike c.
    molar tooth c.
    mosaic detector c.
    multilobular c.
    octagonal c.
    reverse 3 c.

    ringlike c.
    rosary bead c.
    sandwich c.
    sawtooth c.
    scalloped luminal c.
    shepherd's crook c.
    sigmoid-shaped c.
    snowman c.
    stellate c.
    streaklike c.
    surface c.
    swallowtail c.
    T c.
    tentorium keyhole c.
    thoracic cage c.
    tombstone pelvis c.
    triangle c.
    triple-peak cerebellum c.
    unidirectional lead c.
    water-bottle c.
    winged c.
    wooden shoe c.
    Y c.
configurational formula
confinement
    regional tumor c.
confluence
    pulmonary c.
    stellate c.
    c. of vascular marking
confluens sinuum
confluent
    c. areas of atelectasis
    c. consolidation
    c. fibrosis
    c. infiltrate
confocal image
conformal
    c. neutron and photon radiation
        therapy
    c. radiation therapy (CRT)
Conformexx biliary stent
confusion
    circle of c.
congenita
    amyotonia c.
    arthrogryposis multiplex c.
    chondrodystrophia calcificans c.
congenital
    c. abnormality
    c. absence of kidney
    c. absence of pulmonary artery
    c. absence of pulmonary valve
    c. absence of thymus
    c. adrenal hyperplasia (CAH)
    c. adrenocortical hyperplasia
    c. adrenogenital syndrome
    c. amputation
    c. aneurysm of pulmonary artery

c. anomaly of mitral valve (CAMV)
c. aortic regurgitation
c. aortic sinus aneurysm
c. arteriosclerotic aneurysm
c. atelectasis
c. bar
c. biliary atresia
c. bipartite scaphoid
c. bronchiectasis
c. bronchogenic cyst
c. cardiac tumor
c. cerebral aneurysm
c. cholesteatoma
c. cystic adenomatoid malformation (CCAM)
c. cystic dilatation
c. cystic neck lesion
c. deformity
c. diaphragmatic hernia
c. diffuse fibromatosis
c. dilated cardiomyopathy
c. dislocation of hip (CDH)
c. disorder
c. duodenal obstruction
c. dysplasia of hip
c. Finnish nephrosis
c. fracture
c. generalized fibromatosis
c. goiter
c. heart block
c. heart defect (CHD)
c. heart disease (CHD)
c. heart disease classification
c. heart malformation
c. hemidysplasia with ichthyosiform erythroderma and limb defects (CHILD)
c. hemiplegia
c. hepatic cyst
c. hepatic fibrosis (CHF)
c. hip dislocation
c. hip dysplasia
c. hippocampal sclerosis
c. hydrocele
c. hydrocephalus
c. hydronephrosis
c. infiltrating lipomatosis of the face
c. interruption of aortic arch
c. intestinal atresia
c. intracranial aneurysm

c. isthmic coarctation
c. kidney fibrosarcoma
c. laryngeal atresia
c. laxity of ligament
c. left-sided outflow obstruction
c. left ventricular aneurysm
c. leukodystrophy
c. liver fibrosis
c. lobar emphysema
c. lobar hyperinflation
c. lymphangiectasia of intestine
c. lymphangiectasis
c. mediastinal arterial variant
c. megacalyx
c. megacolon
c. mesoblastic nephroma
c. mitral regurgitation (CMR)
c. muscular dystrophy
c. nasal mass
c. pelviureteric junction obstruction
c. pericardial absence
c. pneumothorax
c. polyvalvular dysplasia
c. pulmonary arteriovenous fistula
c. pulmonary artery aneurysm
c. pulmonary valve insufficiency
c. pulmonary venolobar syndrome
c. radioulnar synostosis
c. renal aneurysm
c. renal hypoplasia
c. renal osteodystrophy
c. ring
c. scoliosis
c. splenomegaly
c. stenosis of pulmonary vein
c. stippled epiphysis
c. subpulmonic obstruction
c. symptomatic AV block
c. tibia vara
c. tracheobiliary fistula
c. tracheobronchomegaly
c. tracheomalacia
c. ureteric obstruction
c. urethral diverticulum
c. urethral stricture
c. vascular-bone syndrome (CVBS)
c. vascular malformation (CVM)
c. vertical talus
c. vesicoureteral reflux

congenitally
c. absent pericardium
c. corrected transposition

NOTES

congenitally (*continued*)
    c. corrected transposition of great artery
    c. short esophagus
congested
    c. kidney
    c. pleura
congestion
    active c.
    asymmetric pulmonary c.
    capillary c.
    cardiac c.
    centrilobular c.
    cerebral c.
    chronic passive c.
    hepatic c.
    hypostatic c.
    c. index
    intravascular c.
    passive hepatic c.
    passive vascular c.
    pulmonary vascular c.
    pulmonary venous c. (PVC)
    splenic c.
    symmetric pulmonary c.
    vascular c.
    venous heart c.
congestive
    c. asymmetry
    c. atelectasis
    c. brain swelling
    c. cardiomyopathy
    c. cirrhosis
    c. heart failure (CHF)
    c. splenomegaly
conglomerate
    c. calcification
    c. mass
    nonspecific c.
    c. opacity
    c. pulmonary nodule
conglutinating complement absorption test
congruence
    c. angle
    patellofemoral c.
congruent
    c. articulation
    c. point
    c. reduction
    c. signal intensity abnormality
conical
    c. cecum
    c. heart
    c. mass
conic cecum
conjoined
    c. cusp
    c. nerve root anomaly

    c. root sleeve
    c. tendon
    c. twin
conjugal carcinoma
conjugate
    complex c.
    c. diameter
    c. foramen
    c. gradient
    c. ligament
conjunctival vein
conjunctivum
    brachium c.
connate teeth
connectedness
    theory of fuzzy c.
connecting
    c. canal
    c. cartilage
    c. plate
    c. tubule
connection
    anomalous pulmonary venous c.
    atrioventricular c.
    cavopulmonary c.
    corticocerebellar c.
    partial anomalous pulmonary venous c.
    partial pulmonary venous c.
    rostral c.
    slip-in c.
    total anomalous pulmonary venous c.
    ventriculoarterial c.
    wispy c.
connective
    c. tissue
    c. tissue disease
    c. tissue fibrous tumor
    c. tissue neoplasm
    c. tissue proliferation
    c. tissue septum
connector
    cerebral ventricular shunt c.
Conn syndrome
conoid
    c. ligament
    c. process
    c. tubercle
conotruncal congenital anomaly
conoventricular defect
Conquest
    C. balloon dilatation catheter
    C. PTA balloon dilatation catheter
Conrad-Bugg trapping of soft tissue in ankle fracture
Conrad-Crosby bone marrow biopsy needle
Conradi-Hünermann syndrome

Conradi line
Conray 30, 43, 400 imaging agent
conscious sedation
consecutive dislocation
consistency
    cake-glaze c.
    glaze c.
console
    Bruker c.
    direct display c. (DDC)
    Siemens Satellite CT evaluation c.
consolidated
    c. infiltrate
    c. lung
consolidation
    airspace c.
    alveolar c.
    batwing lung c.
    bilateral c.
    cavitary c.
    confluent c.
    dense c.
    discrete area of c.
    exudative c.
    fracture line of c.
    hemorrhage c.
    ill-defined c.
    lobar c.
    lung parenchyma c.
    nonhomogeneous c.
    parenchymal c.
    patchy area of c.
    peripheral c.
    pulmonary c.
    segmental bronchus c.
    solid c.
    symmetric c.
    unilateral c.
consolidative
    c. change
    c. pneumonia
    c. process
conspicuity
    lesion c.
constant
    air-kerma rate c.
    Avogadro c.
    coupling c.
    decay c.
    disintegration c.
    equilibrium dissociation c.
    equilibrium dose c.

    c. infusion excretory urogram
    c. level appearance (CLEAR)
    maximum amplitude c.
    c. permeability
    permeability c.
    Planck c.
    radioactive c. (Λ)
    c. tilt wave
    time c.
    transformation c.
    T2 time c.
constant-load treadmill testing
constellation
    c. of findings
    c. of symptoms
constituent
    plaque c.
constitutional
    c. osteosclerosis
    c. symptom
constrained Wallgraft endoprosthesis
constricting esophageal lesion
constriction
    airway c.
    c. band
    c. band syndrome
    ductal c.
    hourglass c.
    occult pericardial c.
    postglomerular arteriolar c.
    c. ring
    supraanular c.
    tangential c.
    waistlike c.
constrictive
    c. bronchiolitis
    c. cardiomyopathy
    c. pericarditis
construction artifact
consultation
    curbstone c.
consumption
    cerebral metabolic oxygen c.
    myocardial oxygen c.
    oxygen c. (QO_2)
contact
    bone-on-bone c.
    c. B-scan ultrasound
    c. carcinoma
    catheter-tissue c.
    c. effect
    c. image

NOTES

contact (*continued*)
    c. lateral view
    poor screen/film c.
    c. precautions
    c. radiation therapy
    c. radiograph
    c. radiotherapy
    screen-film c.
    stent-vessel wall c.
    c. transscleral laser
      cytophotocoagulation (CTLC)
contained
    c. aneurysmal rupture
    c. aortic rupture
    c. disc
    c. leak
    c. leak of aortic aneurysm
contamination
    radionuclide c.
    venous c.
content
    abdominal c.
    bone mineral c. (BMC)
    bowel c.
    brain water c.
    digestive tract c.
    disc water c.
    fat-suppressing c.
    femoral triangular c.
    gastric c.
    herniated abdominal c.
    homogenous echogenic uterine c.
    intestinal c.
    intravascular c.
    macromolecular c.
    overlying bowel c.
    retrograde flow of gastric c.
    small bowel c.
    tissue water c.
    venous oxygen c.
contention
    adequate c.
contiguous
    c. articular surface
    c. image
    c. interleaved axial section
    c. loop
    c. organ involvement
    c. parallel chord
    c. scan
    c. segment
    c. slice
    c. slice MEMP
    c. slice multiecho multiplane
      (CSMEMP)
    c. supramarginal gyrus
    c. ventricular septal defect

continent
    c. diversion
    c. urinary diversion
continent urinary diversion
continuation
    azygos c.
continuity
    aortoseptal c.
    c. of bone
    bowel c.
    c. equation
    pancreatic-enteric c.
continuous
    c. arterial spin-labeling perfusion
      MR
    c. capillary
    c. diaphragm sign
    c. hyperfractionated accelerated
      radiation therapy
    c. hyperfractionated accelerated
      radiotherapy
    c. hyperthermic peritoneal perfusion
    c. imaging (CI)
    c. intravenous infusion (CIVI)
    c. mode
    c. moving bed (MR) imaging
      (COMBI)
    c. psoas compartment block
      (CPCB)
    c. scanning
    c. scan thermograph
    c. suture graft inclusion technique
      (CSGIT)
    c. volumetric acquisition
    c. wave (CW)
    c. x-ray spectrum
continuous-loop exercise
  echocardiography
continuous-wave
    c.-w. Doppler echocardiography
    c.-w. Doppler imaging
    c.-w. Doppler recording
    c.-w. Doppler ultrasound system
    c.-w. laser system
    c.-w. NMR
continuum
    Dandy-Walker c.
contour
    altered aortic c.
    altered mediastinal c.
    convex outward c.
    Cupid's bow c.
    diaphragmatic c.
    double diaphragm c.
    c. extraction
    irregular hazy luminal c.
    isodose c.
    lobulated c.
    local bulge of kidney c.

local bulge renal c.
c. mapping
patellar c.
reniform c.
S c.
sawtooth irregularity of bowel c.
scalloping c.
C. SE microsphere
smooth c.
undulating c.
vascular c.

contoured tilting compression mammography

contour-following algorithm

contracted
c. bladder
c. bronchus
c. gallbladder
c. kidney
c. pelvis

contractile
c. function
c. pattern
c. reserve
c. ring dysphagia
c. stricture
c. work index

contractility
cardiac c.
c. index
myocardial c.

contraction
c. band necrosis
concentric c.
esophageal c.
focal myometrial c.
kissing c.
myometrial c.
nodal premature c.
peristaltic c.
phasic c.
premature nodal c. (PNC)
premature ventricular c. (PVC)
ringlike c.
c. stress test (CST)
uterine c.
ventricular premature c. (VPC)
ventricular segmental c.

contracture
bladder neck c.
capsular c.
c. deformity

Dupuytren c.
elbow c.
fixed flexion c.
flexion c.
flexion-adduction c.
gastrocnemius-soleus c.
hip flexion c.
ischemic c.
joint c.
knee flexion c.
muscle c.
myocardial c.
myostatic c.
scar c.
secondary c.
soft tissue c.
Volkmann ischemic c.
web c.

contralateral
c. artery
c. hypertrophy
c. kidney
c. lung
c. sign
c. subtraction technique
c. vessel

contrast (*See* agent, material, medium)
c. absorption barrier
c. administration
c. agent
c. angiography
c. aortography
c. arteriography
barium enema with air c.
c. bolus
c. computed arthrotomography
CT scan with c.
c. data
c. ductography
dynamic susceptibility c. (DSC)
echo c.
c. echocardiography
c. enema
c. enhanced computed tomography (CECT)
c. enhancement
c. enhancement of computed tomographic imaging
c. enhancement pattern
c. esophagram
c. extravasation
image c.

NOTES

contrast *(continued)*
  c. inhomogeneity
  c. injection
  intraarticular c.
  c. laryngography
  c. left atriography
  c. loading
  long-scale c.
  c. lymphangiography
  magnetization transfer c. (MTC)
  c. material
  c. material-enhanced scanning
  c. material instillation
  c. media adverse effect
  c. media excretion
  c. media–induced nephropathy
  c. media leakage
  c. media nephrotoxicity
  c. medium (CM)
  c. medium column
  c. medium–induced pulmonary
    vascular hyperpermeability
  c. medium washout
  near-resonance spin-lock c.
  c. opacification
  phase c. (PC)
  c. precipitation
  puddling of c.
  radiographic c.
  c. radiography
  c. resolution
  c. selective cholangiogram
  c. sensitivity
  short scale c.
  small particle iron oxide c.
  soft tissue c.
  spontaneous echo c.
  subject c.
  c. subtraction mammography
  time-to-peak c. (TPC)
  tissue c.
  c. transesophageal
    echocardiography:yttrium-aluminum-
    garnet (CTE:YAG)
  c. transfer characteristic
  unsharp mask-type c.
  c. uptake
  c. venography
  c. ventriculogram
  c. window level
  c. window width
contrast-enhanced
  c.-e. color Doppler
  c.-e. computed tomography
  c.-e. CT
  c.-e. CT with saline flush
    technique
  3-dimensional c.-e. (3DCE)
  c.-e. dynamic snapshot

  c.-e. echocardiography
  c.-e. FAST
  c.-e. Fourier-acquired steady state
    (CE-FAST)
  c.-e. fundamental imaging
  c.-e. magnetic resonance
    angiography (CEMRA, CE-MRA)
  c.-e. magnetic resonance imaging
  c.-e. MR
  c.-e. MRA
  c.-e. MR angiography
  c.-e. MR image
  c.-e. near-infrared laser
    mammography
  c.-e. power Doppler
  c.-e. radiographic examination
  c.-e. T1-GRE imaging
  c.-e. transrectal sonography
  c.-e. T1-weighted fat-suppressed
    image
  c.-e. T1-weighted spin-echo high-
    field-strength MR imaging
  c.-e. ultrasound
  c.-e. virtual MR cholangioscopy
contrast-enhancing parametric imaging
contrast-filled
  c.-f. catheter
  c.-f. stomach
contrast-improvement factor
contrast-induced renal failure
contrast-to-noise
  c.-t.-n. calculation
  c.-t.-n. ratio (CNR, C/N)
contrecoup
  c. compression
  c. fracture
  c. injury
  c. mechanism
control
  c. angiogram
  automatic exposure c. (AEC)
  C-arm fluoroscopic c.
  dynamic range c. (DRC)
  fluoroscopic c.
  image c.
  intravenous accurate c. (IVAC)
  locoregional c.
  radiofrequency radiographic c.
  radiographic c.
  radiopharmaceutical quality c.
  roentgenographic c.
  scintigraphy quality c.
  SPECT quality c.
  Spli-Prest negative c.
  Spli-Prest positive c.
  time-varied gain c.
controlled ventricular response
controller
  IMED Gemini PC-2 volumetric c.

contusio cerebri
contusion
>bone c.
>bony c.
>brain c.
>cerebral c.
>frontal lobe c.
>lung c.
>myocardial c.
>osseous bone c.
>c. pneumonia
>pontine c.
>pulmonary c.
>rib c.
>soft tissue c.
>urinary bladder c.

conus
>c. arteriosus medullaris
>c. artery
>c. branch ostia
>c. clasticus
>club-shaped c.
>c. elasticus
>c. eye
>c. hypoplasia
>c. ligament
>c. medullaris lesion
>c. medullaris position
>c. septum
>c. tip

conventional
>c. head coil
>c. hysterography
>c. osteosarcoma
>c. planar imaging (CPI)
>c. processor
>c. pulse sequence
>c. radiograph
>c. spin-echo imaging
>c. study
>c. tomography
>c. transverse cross-sectional image
>c. ultrashort echo time (CUTE)
>c. venography

conventionally fractionated stereotactic radiation therapy
convergence zone
convergent
>c. beam irradiation (CBI)
>C. color Doppler
>c. color Doppler imaging

converging collimator

converging-hole collimator
conversion
>coefficient c.
>color space c.
>c. defect
>c. efficiency
>c. electron
>internal c.
>c. ratio
>spontaneous c.
>thoracofemoral c.

converter
>analog-to-digital c.
>digital-to-analog c. (DAC)
>image c.
>motion-compensating format c.
>multiplying digital-to-analog c. (MDAC)
>real-time format c.
>scan c.

convex
>c. border of stomach
>c. linear array
>9- to 5-MHz c. array
>c. outward contour
>c. posterior margin

convexity
>cerebral c.
>frontocentral c.
>c. lesion
>c. of lung
>c. meningioma
>paratracheal c.
>parietal c.
>soft tissue c.

convexobasia
convexoconcave (C-C)
>c. heart valve

convoluted
>c. bone
>c. T-cell lymphoma
>c. tubule

convolution
>Arnold c.
>ascending frontal c.
>ascending parietal c.
>Broca c.
>cerebral c.
>Gratiolet c.
>Heschl c.
>c. mask

NOTES

convolution *(continued)*
    occipitotemporal c.
    Zuckerkandl c.
convolutional
    c. differencing
    c. impression
    c. marking
    c. pattern
Cook-Cope type loop catheter
Cook enforcer
cookie
    c. bite lesion
    c. cutter lesion
coolant
Cooley-Tukey
    C.-T. algorithm
    C.-T. alignment
CoolGlide laser
Coolidge
    C. transformer
    C. x-ray tube
cooling
    tissue c.
Coopernail sign
Cooper suspensory ligament
coordinate
    c. axis
    Talairach c.
    c.'s for target lesion
coordination
    meniscocondylar c.
COP
    colloid oncotic pressure
COPD
    chronic obstructive pulmonary disease
    emphysematous COPD
Cope
    C. biopsy needle
    C. locking-loop catheter
    C. loop
    C. loop catheter
    C. loop nephrostomy
    C. mandril guidewire
    C. method bronchogram
    C. point
**Copeland-Kavat metatarsophalangeal
dislocation classification**
Cope-method bronchography
coplanar
    c. beam
    c. contour point
copper (Cu)
    c. 64 (^{64}Cu)
    c. 67 (^{67}Cu)
    c. filtration
    c. imaging agent
    c. 7, T intrauterine device
    c. wire effect
copper-vapor pulsed laser

copper-zinc
    c.-z. superoxide dismutase (Cu/Zn-SOD)
    c.-z. superoxide dismutase imaging agent
coprecipitation
coprolith
coprostasis
copy
    magnification hard c.
coracoacromial
    c. arch
    c. ligament
    c. process
coracobrachialis
coracoclavicular
    c. bar
    c. joint
    c. ligament
    c. space
coracohumeral ligament
coracoid
    c. bursa
    c. fracture
    c. notch
    c. process
    c. tip avulsion
    c. tuberosity
coral
    c. calculus
    c. reef atheroma
    c. thrombus
cord
    c. angioblastoma
    anterior gray column of c.
    anterior horn of spinal c.
    anterolateral white matter of c.
    astrocytoma c.
    c. atrophy
    cervical c.
    c. compression
    condyle c.
    c. deformation
    dura mater of spinal c.
    c. edema
    c. embarrassment
    ependymoma c.
    c. epidural extramedullary lesion
    false vocal c.
    fibrous c.
    hepatic c.
    c. intradural extramedullary mass
    c. intramedullary lesion
    medullary c.
    meninx of spinal c.
    mucoid degeneration of
      umbilical c.
    multiple focal lesions of spinal c.
    noncoiled umbilical c.

nuchal c.
posterior gray column of c.
c. presentation
pretendinous c.
c. prolapse
prolapse of umbilical c.
reactive cyst c.
c. remodeling
ropelike c.
rostral spinal c.
c. sign
size of spinal c.
spermatic c.
spinal c.
split spinal c.
straight c.
c. structure
c. subarachnoid space ratio
tethered spinal c.
thoracic spinal c.
transsection of spinal c.
true vocal c.
umbilical c.
velamentous insertion of c.
2-vessel umbilical c.
3-vessel umbilical c.
vocal c.
Weitbrecht c.
white commissure of spinal c.
cordate pelvis
cordiform pelvis
cordis
apex c.
atrium dextrum c.
atrium sinistrum c.
C. Brite Tip 5F–10F guiding catheter
bulbus c.
chordae tendineae c.
crux c.
ectopia c.
C. endovascular system
fetal ectopia c.
fossa ovalis c.
C. injector
C. multipurpose access port
C. Palmaz Corinthian stent
C. Palmaz Schatz long medium stent
C. Predator PTCA balloon catheter
C. sheath

C. Smart Nitinol stent
ventriculus c.
vortex c.
cordlike
c. mass
c. trunk
cordocentesis
therapeutic c.
Cordonnier ureteroileal loop
corduroy
c. artery
c. artifact
c. cloth pattern
core
c. biopsy needle
bone c.
C. bone biopsy needle
fibrovascular c.
ischemic c.
c. needle biopsy
nitinol wire c.
coregistered
c. MRI
c. scan
coregistration
image c.
morphologic and physiologic image c.
c. paradigm
CORI computerized endoscopic report generator
Corinthian stainless steel balloon-expandable stent
corkscrew
c. appearance
c. appearance of esophagus
c. appearance of hepatic artery
c. appearance of small bowel
c. pattern
c. ureter
c. vessel
CORLA
cluster of radiolucent area
corn
apical c.
corneae
vertex c.
corneal
c. facet
c. tube

NOTES

Cornell
    C. high energy synchrotron source (CHESS)
    C. protocol
corner
    c. film
    c. fracture
    c. of knee
cornflake esophageal motility study
corniculate
    c. cartilage
    c. tubercle
corniculopharyngeal ligament
cornu, pl. **cornua**
    c. of sacrum
    c. of uterus
cornual
    c. ectopic pregnancy
    c. implantation
corona, pl. **coronae, coronas**
coronal
    c. angulation
    c. bending view
    c. cleft
    c. cleft vertebra
    c. computed tomographic arthrography (CCTA)
    c. ECD brain SPECT image
    c. FLAIR MRI
    c. GRE MR image
    c. maximum-intensity projection
    c. oblique technique
    c. orientation
    c. planar image
    c. plane
    c. proton-density-weighted fast spin-echo image
    c. reconstruction
    c. reconstruction view
    c. reformation
    c. scan
    c. section
    c. slab
    c. slice
    c. SPIR image
    c. suture
    c. suture synostosis
    c. T1-weighted image
corona radiata
coronary
    c. arteriography
    c. arteriosclerosis
    c. arteriosystemic fistula
    c. arteriovenous fistula
    c. artery
    c. artery anatomy
    c. artery aneurysm
    c. artery bypass graft (CABG)
    c. artery bypass graft patency

    c. artery bypass surgery (CABS)
    c. artery calcification (CAC)
    c. artery calcium score (CACS)
    c. artery cameral fistula
    c. artery disease
    c. artery dominance
    c. artery ectasia
    c. artery embolus
    c. artery of heart
    c. artery lesion
    c. artery malformation
    c. artery ostium
    c. artery-pulmonary artery fistula
    c. artery to right ventricular fistula
    c. artery scan (CAS)
    c. artery scan imaging
    c. artery spasm (CAS)
    c. artery steal syndrome
    c. artery stenosis
    c. artery of stomach
    c. artery tree
    c. atherosclerosis
    c. blood flow
    c. blood flow velocity (CBFV)
    c. cineangiography
    c. cusp
    c. electron beam angiography
    c. embolism
    c. flow reserve (CFR)
    c. groove
    c. insufficiency
    c. ischemia
    c. ligament
    c. luminal stenosis
    c. node
    c. occlusion
    c. orifice
    c. ostial revascularization
    c. ostial stenosis
    c. perfusion gradient
    c. perfusion pressure
    c. plexus
    proximal c. (PCS)
    c. radiation therapy (CRT)
    c. remodeling
    c. reserve flow (CRF)
    c. sclerosis
    c. sinus (CS)
    c. sinus CT
    c. sinus electrogram
    c. sinus os
    c. sinus ostium
    c. sinus retroperfusion
    c. sinus root
    c. sinus of Valsalva
    c. sinus valve
    c. stenosis index (CSI)
    c. sulcus
    c. tendon

c. thrombosis
c. vascular resistance
c. vascular resistance index (CVRI)
c. vein
c. vessel aneurysm
c. vessel geometry
c. wedge pressure
coronary-subclavian steal syndrome
coronas (*pl. of* corona)
coronoid
c. fossa
c. of mandibula
c. process
c. process fracture
c. of ulna
Coroskop Plus cardiac angiography system
corpora (*pl. of* corpus)
corpulence
corpulent
corpus, pl. **corpora**
c. albicans cyst
c. amylaceum
anterior c.
c. callosum
c. callosum agenesis
c. callosum dysgenesis
c. callosum hypoplasia, retardation, adducted thumbs, spastic paraparesis, and hydrocephalus (CRASH)
c. callosum lipoma
c. callosum ring-enhancing lesion
c. carcinoma
corpora cavernosa penis
corpora cavernosography
c. cavernosonography imaging
corpora fornicis
c. hemorrhagicum
c. luteal cyst
c. luteum cyst
c. luteum hematoma
c. medullare
corpora restiformia
c. spongiosum
c. spongiosum penis
c. sterni
c. striatum
c. uteri
corpuscular radiation
corrected
c. gradient echo phase imaging

c. sinus node recovery time
c. thrombosis in myocardial infarction frame count (CTFC)
c. transposition of great artery
correction
accidental c.
adaptive c.
attenuation c.
automatic motion c.
baseline c.
coincidence-summing c.
degree of c.
3D motion c.
echo phase c. (EPC)
fuzzy logic contrast c.
inhomogeneity c.
multiilluminant color c.
navigator-guided motion c.
on-the-fly random c.
phase c.
Picker SPECT attenuation c.
prospective acquisition c. (PACE)
scatter c.
second-order c.
section timing c.
summing c.
surface variable-attenuation c.
correlation (CR)
c. algorithm (CR)
c. analysis
clinical c.
c. coefficient
false-negative c.
functional c.
histologic c.
histopathologic CT c.
imaging-anatomic c.
imaging-pathologic c.
mammographic-histopathologic c.
morphologic c.
pathologic c.
radiologic-anatomic c.
radiologic-pathologic c.
c. time
in vivo c.
correlative
c. diagnostic imaging
c. Doppler study
c. pertechnetate thyroid imaging
Correra line
corresponding ray
Corrigan sign

NOTES

corrosive
  c. esophagitis
  c. gastritis
corrugated
  c. air column
  c. fat pad surface
Cortenema retention enema
cortex, pl. **cortices**
  adrenal c.
  articular c.
  auditory c.
  bilateral orbital frontal c.
  bone c.
  calcarine c.
  cerebellar c.
  cerebral c.
  c. of cerebrum
  eloquent c.
  entorhinal c.
  femoral c.
  frontal c.
  frontoparietal parasagittal c.
  increased renal echogenicity c.
  inner adrenal c.
  lymphatic c.
  mesial-frontal c.
  motor c.
  nonolfactory c.
  opercular c.
  orbitofrontal c.
  ovarian c.
  parastriate c.
  parietal c.
  patchy atrophy of renal c.
  perirolandic parietal c.
  peristriate c.
  perisylvian c.
  postrolandic parietal c.
  premotor c.
  primary auditory c.
  primary motor c. (PMC)
  primary visual c.
  pyramidal layer of cerebral c.
  rarefaction of c.
  renal c.
  renin-angiotensin-dependent outer c.
  rolandic c.
  sensorimotor c.
  somatosensory c.
  striate c.
  ventral occipitotemporal (visual) c.
    (VOTC)
  visual c.
Corti
  C. canal
  C. organ
cortical
  c. abrasion
  c. activity

  c. adenoma
  c. artery
  c. atrophy
  c. blush
  c. bone
  c. bone infarct
  c. bone lesion
  c. bone resorption
  c. branch
  c. center
  c. cerebellar degeneration
  c. defect
  c. deficit
  c. desmoid
  c. destruction
  c. diffusion restriction
  c. dysfunction
  c. dysplasia
  c. flattening
  c. fracture
  c. fragment
  c. gray matter
  c. hamartoma
  c. hinge axis
  c. hyperintensity
  c. hyperostosis
  c. hypointensity
  c. intracerebral hemorrhage
  c. ischemia
  c. kidney arch
  c. kidney arteriography
  c. kidney necrosis
  c. liquoral space
  c. mapping
  c. margin
  c. motor area
  c. nephrocalcinosis
  c. nodular hyperplasia
  c. nodule
  c. notching
  c. osteoid osteoma
  c. plate
  c. renal cyst
  c. rim nephrogram
  c. rim sign
  c. scalloping
  c. scarring of kidney
  c. scintigraphy
  c. signet ring shadow
  c. sulcus
  c. thinning
  c. thumb
  c. tissue
  c. transgression
  c. tuber
  c. vein
  c. vein sign
  c. vein thrombosis
  c. venous reflux

c. white matter
c. window
corticale
    cryptostroma c.
corticated border
cortices (*pl. of* cortex)
corticobasal ganglionic degeneration
corticobulbar tract (CBT)
corticocallosal dysgenesis
corticocancellous
    c. bone
    c. bone chip
    c. strut
corticocerebellar connection
corticogram
corticography
corticomedullary
    c. differentiation (CMD)
    c. junction (CMJ)
    c. phase
corticopontine tract
corticorubral tract
corticospinal
    c. motor pathway
    c. pathway lesion
    c. tract (CST)
corticosteroid-induced osteoporosis
corticostriatospinal degeneration
cortisol-producing carcinoma
corundum smelter's lung
Corvita endoluminal graft
cosine
    c. curve
    c. transform
cosmic radiation
costa
    c. fluctuans decima
    c. retraction
costal
    c. angle
    c. bone
    c. cartilage calcification
    c. facet
    c. groove
    c. intraarticular cartilage
    c. margin
    c. notch
    c. osteoma
    c. part of diaphragm
    c. pit
    c. pleura
    c. pleurisy

c. process
c. sulcus
c. surface
c. tubercle
c. tuberosity
costimulatory molecule
costoaxillary vein
costocervical
    c. artery
    c. trunk
costochondral
    c. joint
    c. junction
    c. junction separation
costochondritis
costoclavicular
    c. ligament
    c. line
    c. maneuver
    c. syndrome
    c. test
costocolic
    c. fold
    c. ligament
costodiaphragmatic
    c. margin
    c. recess
    c. recess of pleura
costolateral
costolumbar angle
costomediastinal
    c. recess
    c. sinus
costophrenic (CP)
    c. angle
    c. angle blunting
    c. recess
    c. septal line
    c. sinus
    c. sulcus
costopleural
costosternal angle
costotransverse
    c. foramen
    c. joint
    c. ligament
costovertebral
    c. angle (CVA)
    c. articulation
    c. joint
costoxiphoid ligament
COSY H-1 MR spectroscopy

NOTES

Cotrel-Dubousset system
cottage loaf appearance
cotton
  C. ankle fracture
  c. ball appearance
  c. fiber embolus
cotton-wool
  c.-w. appearance
  c.-w. spot
Cotunnius canal
cotyloid
  c. cavity
  c. ligament
couch view
coudé catheter
cough
  c. fracture of rib
  c. resonance
Couinaud
  C. classification
  C. liver segment 1–8
coulomb (C)
  c. force
  C. law
Coulter counter
coumarin pulsed dye laser
count
  absolute granulocyte c.
  background c.
  Cerenkov c.
  Colombo c.
  corrected thrombosis in myocardial
    infarction frame c. (CTFC)
  c. density
  direct liquid scintillation c.
  filament-nonfilament c.
  noise effective c. (NEC)
  out-of-field c.
  c. per plane
  random c.
  c. rate
  scattered c.
count-density threshold
counter
  automated gamma c.
  boron c.
  Cerenkov c.
  Coulter c.
  event c.
  gamma ray c.
  gamma well c.
  Geiger c.
  Geiger-Müller c.
  ionization c.
  proportional c.
  radiation c.
  scaler c.
  scintillation c.

  well c.
  whole-body c.
countercurrent
  c. aortography
  c. flow-related enhancement
counteroccluder
counterpulsation
  balloon c.
  diastolic c.
  intraaortic balloon c.
  mechanical c.
counterstimulation
counting
  c. coincidence
  double-label c.
  c. rate meter
  whole-body c.
coupled array coil
couplet
  ventricular premature contraction c.
coupling
  c. constant
  dipole c.
  dipole-dipole c.
  dynamic c.
  electric quadrupole c.
  c. exchange
  c. gel
  hyperfine c.
  magnetic dipole-dipole c.
  scalar c.
  spin c.
  spin-spin c.
  static c.
Cournand arteriography needle
Cournand-Grino angiography needle
course
  c. of artery
  extracranial c.
  midlateral c.
  relapsing c.
  remitting c.
  signal time c.
  undulating c.
coursing
  c. of gas
  c. vessel
Courvoisier
  C. gallbladder
  C. law
  C. sign
Courvoisier-Terrier syndrome
Couvelaire uterus
coverage
  interleaved k-space c.
  spiral k-space c.
covered stent
Cowboy Collar

Cowden
    C. disease
    C. syndrome
cow horn deformity
Cowper
    C. gland lesion
    C. ligament
COX
    cast-off x-ray
    cyclooxygenase
    cytochrome c oxidase
    COX deficiency
coxa, pl. **coxae**
    c. adducta
    c. brevis
    c. flexa
    c. magna
    os coxae
    c. plana
    c. saltans
    c. senilis
    c. valga
    c. valga deformity
    c. vara
    c. vara deformity
coxal bone
coxarthrosis
    Postel destructive c.
coxitis fugax
Cox sterilizer and incinerator unit
CP
    Carr-Purcell
    costophrenic
    cross-polarization
    CP angle
    CP sequence
CPA
    cerebellopontine angle
CPAD
    chronic peripheral arterial disease
CPCB
    continuous psoas compartment block
CPD
    cephalopelvic disproportion
CPE
    chronic pulmonary emphysema
C-PET scanner
CPI
    conventional planar imaging
cpm
    cycle per minute

CPMG
    Carr-Purcell-Meiboom-Gill
    CPMG sequence
CPP
    cerebral perfusion pressure
CPPD
    calcium pyrophosphate deposition disease
    CPPD arthritis of hand
CPR
    curved multiplanar reformation
cps
    cycle per second
CR
    central ray
    colorectal
    computed radiography
    computed radiology
    conditioned reflex
    correlation
    correlation algorithm
    crown-rump length
CR103
    OncoScint CR103
Cr
    chromium
CR-39 nuclear tract detector
crabmeatlike appearance
crack
    c. fracture
    hairline c.
cracked-pot resonance
cradle
    alpha c.
    CT scan c.
    Spectrum DG-P pediatric c.
Cragg
    C. EndoPro stent-graft
    C. Endopro system I covered stent
    C. FX-wire
    C. stent
    C. thrombolytic brush
Cragg-Castaneda thrombolytic brush
Cragg-McNamara multiple side-hole
    infusion catheter
Cramer-Rao minimum variance bound
    (CR-MVB)
Crampton
    C. line
    C. muscle
crania (*pl. of* cranium)
cranial
    c. aneurysm

C

NOTES

cranial (*continued*)
  c. angled view
  c. angulation
  c. anomaly
  c. base
  c. bone
  c. capacity
  c. cavity
  c. computed tomography (CCT)
  c. diameter
  c. fixation plate
  c. flexure
  c. fontanelle
  c. foramen
  c. fossa
  c. granulomatous arteritis
  c. irradiation
  c. meningocele
  c. nerve
  c. nerve involvement
  c. nerve neoplasm
  c. nerve sheath tumor
  c. nerve sign
  c. nucleus
  c. osteopetrosis
  c. ridge
  c. root
  c. sinus
  c. suture
  c. synostosis
  c. ultrasound
  c. vault
  c. vertebra
  c. vessel
cranii
  pneumatocele c.
  synchondroses c.
  vertex c.
craniocaudal, craniocaudad
  c. axis
  c. needle angulation
  c. projection
  c. view
craniocervical junction
craniofacial
  c. angle
  c. anomaly
  c. dysjunction
  c. dysjunction fracture
  c. dysostosis
  c. notch
  c. pain syndrome
  c. plexiform neurofibroma
  c. remodeling
  c. synostosis
craniography
craniolacunia
craniomandibular syndrome

craniometric
  c. diameter
  c. point
cranioorbital deformity
craniopagus twin
craniopharyngeal
  c. canal
  c. duct
craniopharyngioma
  adamantinomatous c.
  ectopic c.
  nasopharyngeal c.
cranioschisis
craniosclerosis
cranioskeletal dysplasia
craniospinal
  c. axis
  c. axis radiation therapy
  c. compliance
  c. hemangioblastoma
craniostenosis, pl. **craniostenoses**
craniosynostosis, pl. **craniosynostoses**
  c. syndrome
craniotabes
craniotelencephalic dysplasia
craniotomy defect
craniotrypesis
craniovertebral
  c. angle
  c. anomaly
  c. junction
  c. junction anatomy
cranium, pl. **crania**
  c. bifidum
  c. bifidum occultum
  fetal c.
  split c.
  vertex of bony c.
crankshaft phenomenon
CRASH
  corpus callosum hypoplasia, retardation, adducted thumbs, spastic paraparesis, and hydrocephalus
  CRASH syndrome
crater
  ulcer c.
craterlike ulcer
crazy-paving
  c.-p. appearance
  c.-p. pattern
Cr-chromate-labeled red cell technique
CRE
  cumulative radiation effect
C-reactive protein level
crease
  back c.
  infragluteal c.
  inframammary c.

inguinal c.
stellate c.
creation
percutaneous peritoneovenous
shunt c.
Cree leukoencephalopathy
creep
cardiac c.
diaphragmatic c.
periosteal c.
creeping epithelialization
cremaster
cremasteric
c. artery
c. fascia
crescendo TIA
crescent
air c.
c. artifact
c. of cardia
c. of cavitation
c. of gas
c. hip line
c. sign
crescentic
c. border
c. collection
c. lumen
c. submucosal fold
crescent-in-doughnut sign
crescent-shaped
c.-s. fibrocartilaginous disc
c.-s. glomerulonephritis
cross-correlation technique
crest
acoustic c.
acousticofacial c.
alveolar c.
ampullary c.
anterior iliac c.
arched c.
arcuate c.
articular c.
basilar c.
bilateral iliac c.
buccinator c.
conchal c.
deltoid c.
dental c.
ethmoidal c.
falciform c.
frontal c.

ganglionic c.
gingival c.
gyral c.
iliac c.
infundibuloventricular c.
intertrochanteric c.
posterior iliac c.
pubic c.
sacral c.
supraventricular c. (SVC)
terminal c.
tibial c.
urethral c.
CREST syndrome
Creutzfeldt-Jakob disease (CJD)
crevice
nonpolar c.
CRF
chronic renal failure
coronary reserve flow
Cr-HIDA chelate
cribrate
cribration
cribriform
c. bone
c. carcinoma
c. DCIS
c. fascia
c. pattern
c. plate
c. process
cricket bat shape
cricoarytenoid articular capsule
cricoesophageal tendon
cricoid cartilage
cricopharyngeal
c. achalasia
c. bar
c. diameter
c. diverticulum
c. ligament
c. sphincter
cricopharyngeus muscle
cricothyreotomy
cricothyroid
c. articular capsule
c. cartilage
c. ligament
c. membrane
cricotracheal ligament
cri-du-chat syndrome
crimp stop

NOTES

crinkle artifact
crinkling
    mucosal c.
    patch c.
crisis, pl. crises
    bone c.
crisscross heart
crista
    c. galli
    c. pulmonis
    c. supraventricularis
    c. terminalis
criteria
    goodness-of-match c.
    Rose c.
criterion, pl. criteria
    Biello c.
    error-sum c.
    interpretive c.
    Jones c.
    morphologic c.
    Nyquist c.
    PIOPED criteria
    radiographic c.
    Schumacher c.
    Schwartz c.
    c. standard
critical
    c. coronary stenosis
    c. dose table
    c. lesion
    c. mass
    c. organ
    c. valvular stenosis
CRL
    crown-rump length
Cr-labeled red blood cell technique
CR-MVB
    Cramer-Rao minimum variance bound
crocidolite asbestos
Crohn
    C. colitis
    C. disease (CD)
    C. disease of colon
    C. duodenitis
    C. granulomatous enteritis
    C. ileitis
    C. ileocolitis
    C. jejunitis
    C. regional enteritis
Crohn-like lymphoid reaction
Crone-Renkin index of permeability
Cronkhite-Canada syndrome
Cronqvist cranial index
Crookes
    C. space
    C. tube
cross
    c. calibration

    c. ligament
    c. section
    c. slice
cross-aortic
crossbar symptom of Fränkel
cross-collateralization
cross-correlation technique
cross-ectopic kidney
crossed
    c. cerebellar diaschisis
    c. coil
    c. embolus
    c. upstream and downstream
crossed-coil design
crossed-fused renal ectopia
cross-filling
cross-fire
    c.-f. radiation therapy
    c.-f. treatment
cross-fogging
cross-hatch grid
cross-linked silicone gel
cross-organ and self-absorbed dose
cross-over
    c.-o. of activity
    femorofemoral c.-o.
cross-pelvic collateral vessel
cross-polarization (CP)
cross-scrotal collateral
cross-section
    bronchovascular anatomy c.-s.
    c.-s. capture
    Compton scattering c.-s.
    elastic c.-s.
    normalized c.-s.
    pharynx c.-s.
    thigh muscle c.-s.
    vertebral c.-s.
cross-sectional
    c.-s. area (CSA)
    c.-s. area stenosis
    c.-s. 2-dimensional echocardiography
    c.-s. imaging
    c.-s. lung segment anatomy
    c.-s. modality
    c.-s. pattern
    c.-s. plane
    c.-s. transverse projection
    c.-s. ultrasonographic image
    c.-s. zone
cross-table
    c.-t. lateral film
    c.-t. lateral position
    c.-t. lateral projection
    c.-t. lateral view (CTLV)
    c.-t. leg immobilizer
cross-talk effect artifact
cross-trigonal tunnel
cross-union

Crouzon syndrome
CR/OV
    colorectal/ovarian
crowded dentition
crowding of bronchovascular marking
Crowe pilot point
Crow-Fukase syndrome
crown
    c. cavity
    halo c.
    c. indemnity
    c. tubercle
crown-heel length
crown-rump length (CR, CRL)
CRT
    cathode ray tube
    conformal radiation therapy
    coronary radiation therapy
    3D CRT
CrTmEr
crucial angle of Gissane
cruciate
    c. eminence
    c. ligament
    c. orientation
cruciatum cruris ligament
cruciform
    c. eminence
    c. ligament
crunch
    mediastinal c.
crural
    c. canal
    c. cistern
    c. cistern widening
    c. fascia
    c. fossa
    c. septum
    c. sheath
    c. triangle
crus, pl. **crura**
    comma-shaped c.
    c. commune
    c. cupula
    c. of the diaphragm
    diaphragmatic c.
    displaced c.
    c. dome
    c. hiatus
    lateral c.
    left c.
    medial c.

    muscular c.
    c. of penis
    c. pericardium
    c. pleura
    right c.
crush
    c. artifact
    c. fracture
    c. injury
    c. kidney
    c. preparation
    c. syndrome
    thoracic c.
crushed
    c. eggshell fracture
    c. tissue
Cruveilhier
    C. fascia
    C. joint
    C. ligament
    C. nodule
    C. ulcer
Cruveilhier-Baumgarten
    C.-B. anomaly
    C.-B. cirrhosis
crux cordis
cryogen
CRYOguide ultrasound guidance system
CryoHit tumor ablation system
cryomagnet
cryoplasty balloon
cryoprobe
cryosection
cryostable magnet
cryotherapy
crypt
    c. abscess
    anal c.
    enamel c.
    epithelium c.
    ileal c.
    Lieberkühn c.
    Luschka c.
    Morgagni c.
cryptic vascular malformation (CVM)
cryptococcal
    c. meningitis
    c. spondylitis
cryptococcoma
    focal parenchymal c.
cryptococcosis
    intracranial c.

NOTES

cryptogenic
- c. cirrhosis
- c. fibrosing alveolitis
- c. organizing pneumonia

cryptorchidism

cryptostroma corticale

crystal
- BGO c.
- c. deposition arthropathy
- c. deposition disease
- c. field theory
- c. gamma camera
- pyrophosphate c.
- scintillation c.

CrystalEyes endoscopic video system

crystal-induced arthrosis

crystalline phosphor detector

crystallogram

crystallography
- x-ray c.

CS
- coronary sinus

^{139}Cs
- cesium 139

^{137}Cs, Cs 137
- cesium 137
  - ^{137}Cs point source

CSA
- cross-sectional area

CSDH
- chronic subdural hematoma

CSF
- cerebrospinal fluid
  - CSF 14-3-3 isoform
  - CSF oscillatory motion
  - CSF 14-3-3 protein
  - CSF pulsation artifact
  - CSF systole length
  - CSF ventricular systole

CSF-suppressed T2-weighted 3D MP-RAGE MR imaging

CSGIT
- continuous suture graft inclusion technique

CSGP
- computer strain-gauge plethysmography

CSI
- chemical shift imaging
- coronary stenosis index
- craniospinal irradiation
  - risk-adapted CSI
  - CSI spectroscopy

CSL
- central sacral line
- complex sclerosing lesion

CSM
- cervical spondylotic myelopathy

CSMEMP
- contiguous slice multiecho multiplane

CSPAMM
- complementary spatial modulation of magnetization

C-spine pseudosubluxation

CSS
- carotid sinus syndrome

CST
- contraction stress test
- corticospinal tract

CSVT
- central splanchnic venous thrombosis

CSWT
- cardiac shock wave therapy

CT
- cardiothoracic ratio
- circulation time
- computed tomography
  - CT angiography
  - CT arteriography
  - CT arthrography
  - CT attenuation value
  - biphasic CT
  - biphasic contrast-enhanced helical CT
  - bit CT
  - CT body scanner
  - bone quantitative CT (BQCT)
  - CT bone window
  - CT bone window photography
  - cervical CT
  - cine CT
  - CT cisternogram
  - CT cisternography
  - collimation CT
  - CT colography
  - CT colonography
  - contrast-enhanced CT
  - coronary sinus CT
  - CT correction attenuation
  - 3D drip infusion cholangiography CT
  - CT densitometer
  - CT densitometry
  - 3D portography using multislice helical CT
  - 3D processed ultrafast CT
  - dual-energy CT
  - dual-isotope single-photon emission CT
  - dual-phase CT
  - dynamic contrast-enhanced CT
  - electrocardiogram-gated multislice spiral CT
  - enhanced CT
  - expiratory CT
  - fast dynamic volumetric x-ray CT
  - gestalt impression on CT
  - HeartView CT

helical biphasic contrast-enhanced
  CT (HBCT)
helical thin-section CT
high spatial resolution cine CT
CT imaging error
indirect CT
intravascular contrast-enhanced CT
Marconi/Elscint MxTwin CT
CT Max 640 scanner
multidetector CT (MDCT)
multidetector helical CT
multidetector-row CT (MDCT)
multiphasic helical CT
multislice CT
multislice spiral CT (MSCT)
CT myelography
noncontrast head CT (NCCT)
non-ECG-assisted multidetector row
  CT
nonenhanced CT
CT number
perfusion CT
CT Perfusion 2 software
2-phase helical CT
postmyelography CT
Proceed vascular interventional CT
CT pulmonary venography (CTPV)
quantitative spirometrically
  controlled CT
CT ratio
CT reconstruction image
renal helical CT
CT scan
CT scan cradle
CT scan gantry
CT scanner beam
CT scan with contrast
CT scan with renal stone protocol
CT sialography
single-detector helical CT
single-photon emission CT
single-slice helical CT
slip-ring CT
SOMATOM Plus 4 CT
spiral multidetector CT
spiral volumetric CT
stable Xenon CT
CT stereotactic guide
surgical simulation CT
thallium-201 single-photon emission
  CT
thin-section CT

thin-slice CT
CT tracheobronchography
triphasic spiral CT
twin-beam CT
ultrafast CT
CT unit
W3000 helical CT
xenon-enhanced CT
Z-dependent CT

C × T
  concentration times time

CT9000, 9800 scanner

CTA
  computed tomographic angiography
    helical CTA
    CTA image
    multidetector CTA
    single-detector CTA
    single-slice CTA

CT-aided volumetry

CTAP
  computed tomography during arterial
    portography
  computed tomography with
    arterioportography

CTAT
  computerized transverse axial
    tomography
    CTAT imaging

CT-based virual tracheobronchoscopy

CTC
  computed tomographic colonography
  computed tomography colonography

CTDI
  computed tomography dose index

CT-directed
    CT-d. biopsy
    CT-d. hook-wire localization
    CT-d. puncture

C-telopeptide
    type II collagen C-t.

CT-enteroclysis
    helical CT-e. (HCTE)

**CT-estimated superimposed hydrostatic
pressure**

CTE:YAG
  contrast transesophageal
    echocardiography:yttrium-aluminum-
    garnet
    CTE:YAG laser

CTF
  computed tomography fluoroscopy

NOTES

CTFC
    corrected thrombosis in myocardial
      infarction frame count
CT-guided
    CT-g. intraarterial chemotherapy
    CT-g. needle aspiration
    CT-g. needle biopsy
    CT-g. percutaneous biopsy
    CT-g. percutaneous endoscopic
      gastrostomy
    CT-g. percutaneous excision
    CT-g. stereotactic surgery
    CT-g. superior hypogastric plexus
      block
    CT-g. transsternal core biopsy
    CT-g. ultrasound
CTH
    computerized tomographic holography
CTHA
    computerized tomographic hepatic
      angiography
CTI
    C. 933/04 ECAT scanner
    C. 931 PET scanner
CTLC
    contact transscleral laser
      cytophotocoagulation
      Nd:YAG CTLC
CT-LG
    computed tomographic lymphography
    computed tomography lymphography
CTLM
    computed tomography laser
      mammography
CTLV
    cross-table lateral view
CTMM
    metrizamide-assisted computed
      tomography
CT/MR
    computerized tomography/magnetic
      resonance
**CT/MRI-compatible stereotactic head
frame**
CT/MRI-defined
    CT/MRI-d. tumor slice image
    CT/MRI-d. tumor volume image
CT, MR peritoneography
CT-PET
    combined C.-P.
CTPV
    CT pulmonary venography
CTR
    cardiothoracic ratio
C-Trak hand-held gamma detector
CT/SPECT fusion imaging
CTT
    central tegmental tract

CTV
    clinical target volume
CU
Cu
    copper
⁶⁴Cu
    copper 64
      ^{64}Cu imaging agent
⁶⁷Cu
    copper 67
      ^{67}Cu imaging agent
cube vertex
cubic
    c. centimeter (cc)
    c. convolution interpolation
    c. voxel
cubital
    c. bone
    c. bursitis
    c. fossa
    c. lymph node
    c. tunnel
    c. tunnel retinaculum
    c. tunnel syndrome
cubitocarpal
cubitoradial
cubitus
    c. valgus
    c. valgus deformity
    c. varus
    c. varus deformity
cuboid
    c. bone
    c. fracture
cuboidal articular surface
cuboideonavicular ligament
cubonavicular joint
CUC
    chronic ulcerative colitis
cue-based image analysis
cuff
    c. abscess
    aortic c.
    atrial c.
    inflow c.
    musculotendinous c.
    pressure c.
    rectal muscle c.
    right atrial c.
    rotator c.
    suprahepatic caval c.
    vaginal c.
cuffed endotracheal tube
cuffing
    peribronchial c.
    perivascular c.
CUG
    cystourethrogram

cuirasse
    carcinoma en c.
    cor en c.
cul-de-sac
    Douglas c.-d.-s.
    dural c.-d.-s.
Culiner theory
Cullen sign
culpocephaly
culprit
    c. lesion
    c. stenosis
    c. vessel
cumulative
    c. dose
    c. radiation effect (CRE)
cumulus oophorus
cuneatus
    funiculus c.
cuneiform
    c. bone
    c. bone of carpus
    c. cartilage
    c. fracture
    c. fracture-dislocation
    c. joint
    c. lobe
    c. mortise
    c. tubercle
cuneocerebellar tract
cuneocuboid ligament
cuneonavicular ligament
CUP
    cancer of unknown primary
cup
    acetabular c.
    Diogenes c.
    migration of acetabular c.
    prosthetic c.
    retroversion of acetabular c.
cup-and-spill stomach
cupboard
    RF-shielded c.
Cupid's
    C. bow configuration
    C. bow contour
cupola sign
cupping
    c. of acromion
    c. of calyx
^{62}Cu PTSM imaging agent
cupula, pl. **cupulae**

crus c.
diaphragmatic c.
gas c.
pleural c.
curative irradiation
curbstone consultation
cure
    complete anatomic c.
Curie
    C. effect
    C. law
curie (Ci)
curie-hour
curietherapy
curium
Curix
    C. Capacity Plus film processing
      system
    C. film screen cassette
    C. Ultra UV-L film
curlicue ureter
curling
    c. esophagus
    C. ulcer
curly toe deformity
Currarino triad
current
    alternating c.
    attenuation-based on-line modulation
      of the tube c.
    beam c.
    direct c. (DC)
    eddy c.
    gradient drive c.
    ionization c.
    c. leak
    c. line distortion
    3-phase c.
    pulsating c.
    pulsing c.
    saturation c.
    single-phase c.
    tube c.
    unidirectional c.
    unmodulated radiofrequency c.
    variable tube c.
Curry intravascular retriever set
curtain
    subaortic c.
curvature
    angular c.
    c. anisotropy

C

NOTES

curvature *(continued)*
    anterior c.
    backward c.
    cervical lordotic c.
    dorsal kyphotic c.
    fibroid c.
    flattening of normal lordotic c.
    gingival c.
    kyphotic c.
    lumbar c.
    radius of c.
    stomach c.

curve
    area under the c. (AUC)
    biexponential fitting of left
      ventricular c.
    biphasic c.
    Bragg c.
    brightness-time c.
    catheter with preformed c.'s
    cervical spine c.
    characteristic c.
    clearance c.
    concentration-time c.
    cosine c.
    depth-dose c.
    c. of duodenum
    dye dilution c.
    elimination c.
    c. fit coefficient
    flattening of normal lumbar c.
    flow-time c.
    fractionated dose-survival c.
    Frank-Starling c.
    free induction delay c.
    full-width at half-maximum of
      lorentzian c.
    gaussian c.
    glow c.
    Harrison c.
    H and D c.
    Hurter and Driffield c.
    indicator dilution c.
    indocyanine dilution c.
    isoclosed c.
    isodose c.
    kinetic c.
    lordotic c.
    lorentzian c.
    loss of sigmoid c.
    lumbar lordotic c.
    lung count c.
    normal lordotic c.
    pulmonary time activity c.
    renal flow c.
    renogram c.
    ROC c.
    sensitometric c.
    sigmoid density c.
    signal intensity time c.
    spline c.
    Starling c.
    stress-strain c.
    superincumbent spinal c.
    thoracic spine c.
    time-activity c.
    time-attenuation c.
    time-density c.
    time intensity c. (TIC)
    ventricular function c.
    videodensity c.
    washout c.

curved
    c. multiplanar reformation (CPR)
    c. needle biopsy
    c. planar reformation
    c. radiolucent line
    c. reconstruction
    c. vessel

curve-fit

curvilinear
    c. calcification
    c. defect
    c. density
    c. reconstruction
    c. subpleural line
    c. threshold shoulder

CUSA
    Cavitron Ultrasonic Surgical Aspirator

Cushing
    C. disease
    C. phenomenon
    C. syndrome
    C. triad
    C. ulcer

Cushing-Rokitansky ulcer

cushion
    c. defect
    endocardial c.
    foam c.

cusp
    accessory c.
    anterior c.
    aortic c.
    asymmetric closure of c.
    ballooning mitral c.
    conjoined c.
    coronary c.
    c. degeneration
    dysplastic c.
    c. fenestration
    fibrocalcific c.
    fishmouth c.
    fusion of c.
    intact valve c.
    left coronary c.
    left pulmonary c.
    mitral valve c.

c. motion
noncoronary c.
perforated aortic c.
posterior c.
prolapse of right aortic valve c.
pulmonary valve c.
right coronary c.
ruptured aortic c.
semilunar valve c.
septal c.
c. shot
tricuspid valve c.
valve c.
custom-curved coil
custom-fabricated graft
custom shielding block
cut
c. and cine film
high-resolution coronal c.
off-center c.
scalpel c.
tangential c.
tomographic c.
cutaneous
c. adenoma
c. angioma
c. B-cell lymphoma (CBCL)
c. collateral circulation
c. fissure
c. lateral branch
c. lymphoscintigraphy
c. necrotizing venulitis
c. nodule
c. pit
c. pneumocystosis
c. ridge
c. T-cell lymphoma
c. twig
c. vascular anomaly
c. vein
CUTE
conventional ultrashort echo time
^{64}Cu-TETA-octreotide imaging agent
cut-film
c.-f. angiography (CFA)
c.-f. technique
cuticular overgrowth
cutis
atrophia c.
c. calcinosis
osteoma c.
tuberculosis verrucosa c.

cutoff
arterial c.
c. sign
cutting
c. balloon
c. balloon catheter
Cuvier
C. canal
C. duct
Cu/Zn-SOD
copper-zinc superoxide dismutase
Cu/Zn-SOD imaging agent
c.v.
coefficient of variation
CVA
cardiovascular accident
cerebrovascular accident
costovertebral angle
CVBS
congenital vascular-bone syndrome
CVC
central venous catheter
CVCT
cardiovascular computed tomographic scanner
CVD
cardiovascular disease
CVIS information system
CVM
congenital vascular malformation
cryptic vascular malformation
CVP
central venous pressure
CVRI
coronary vascular resistance index
CVST
cerebral venous sinus thrombosis
CW
continuous wave
C-wave pressure
CWP
coal worker's pneumoconiosis
CX
circumflex
CX artery
CXR
chest x-ray
cyanoacrylate
N-butyl c. (NBCA)
c. imaging agent
c. tissue adhesive
cyanoacrylate imaging agent

NOTES

cyanocobalamin
  c. Co (cobalt)
  c. imaging agent
  radioactive c.
cyanocobalamin Co 57, 58, 60
cyanotic
  c. congenital heart disease
  c. kidney
Cyber 170/720
CyberKnife
  C. Express device
  C. stereotactic radiosurgery system
Cyberware 3D scanning system
Cybex ergometer
cycle
  breath-hold c.
  clock c.
  Krebs c.
  pentose c.
  c. per minute (cpm)
  c. per second (cps)
  c. time
  tricarboxylic acid c.
cycle-length window
cyclic
  c. adenosine monophosphate
  c. guanosine monophosphate
  c. guanosine triphosphate
  c. idiopathic edema
cycling
  phase c.
cyclooxygenase (COX)
  c. deficiency
cyclopia
cyclops lesion
cyclosporin nephrotoxicity
cyclotron
  medical c.
  multiparticle c.
  negative-ion c.
  positive-ion c.
  c. radiation
CY color space
cylinder
  abdominal compression c.
  axonal c.
  Burnett c.
  CO_2 c.
  dome c.
  Fletcher-Delclos dome c.
  sum of c. (SOC)
  vaginal c.
cylindrical
  c. bronchiectasis
  c. carcinoma
  c. chest
  c. configuration
  c. format
  c. map projection

  c. projection map
  c. thorax
cylindrical-ablation scheme
cylindroid aneurysm
cylindroma
  lung c.
  c. parotitis
cylindromatous carcinoma
cylindrosarcoma
cyllosis
Cyma line
Cypher stent
Cyriax syndrome
cyst
  acoustic c.
  acquired hepatic c.
  adnexal c.
  adrenal c.
  air c.
  air-filled c.
  allantoic c.
  amnionic inclusion c.
  anechoic c.
  aneurysmal bone c. (ABC)
  apocrine c.
  arachnoid brain c.
  arachnoid spine c.
  aryepiglottic c.
  atypical renal c.
  benign conal c.
  bilateral arachnoid c.
  bilateral choroid plexus c.
  Blessig c.
  bone implantation c.
  brain c.
  branchial cleft c.
  breast c.
  bronchial cleft c.
  bronchiectatic c.
  bronchogenic duplication c.
  brown cell c.
  calcified pericardial c.
  capping c.
  cerebral c.
  cervical thymic c.
  chocolate c.
  choledochal c.
  cholesterol ear c.
  choroid plexus c.
  colloid c.
  colloidal brain c.
  colobomatous c.
  colonic duplication c.
  communicating c.
  complex breast c.
  complicated renal c.
  conal c.
  congenital bronchogenic c.
  congenital hepatic c.

corpus albicans c.
corpus luteal c.
corpus luteum c.
cortical renal c.
cysticercus c.
Dandy-Walker c.
daughter c.
decidual c.
dental c.
dentigerous c.
dermoid c.
dermoid ovarian c.
dorsal enterogenous c.
duplication c.
echinococcal c.
endodermal c.
endometrial c.
endometriotic c.
enteric duplication c.
enterogenous c.
entrapped ovarian c.
ependymal c.
epidermal inclusion c.
epididymal c.
epidural arachnoid c.
epithelial inclusion c.
esophageal duplication c.
expansile aneurysmal bone c.
extradural arachnoid c.
extraparenchymal c.
false splenic c.
first branchial cleft c.
fluid-filled c.
follicular ovarian c.
foregut c.
functional ovarian c.
ganglion c.
Gartner duct c.
gastric duplication c.
gastrointestinal c.
gurgling c.
hemorrhagic corpus luteum c.
hemorrhagic ovarian c.
hepatic c.
honeycomb c.
hydatid heart c.
hydatid lung c.
hydatid mediastinum c.
implantation c.
inclusion c.
interhemispheric c.
interosseous c.

intracranial dermoid c.
intraduodenal choledochal c.
intradural arachnoid c.
intramedullary epidermoid c.
intrameniscal c.
intraneural ganglion c.
intraosseous keratin c.
intraparenchymal c.
intrapulmonary bronchogenic c.
intrasellar Rathke cleft c.
intraspinal dermoid c.
intraspinal enteric c.
intraspinal epidermoid c.
intraspinal neurenteric c.
intratesticular c.
intrathoracic c.
intratumoral c.
intraventricular cryptococcal c.
joint c.
keratin testicular c.
kidney c.
Kimura-type choledochal c.
leptomeningeal arachnoid c.
lipid c.
liver c.
lumbar synovial c.
lung c.
luteal c.
mammary c.
mediastinal bronchogenic c.
mediastinal dorsal enteric c.
mediastinal duplication c.
meibomian c.
mesenteric c.
mesothelial c.
midline of brain c.
milk of calcium urinary tract c.
morgagnian c.
mucinous c.
mucous retention c.
müllerian duct c.
multilocular renal c.
multiple pulmonary c.'s
multiple thyroid c.'s
myxoid c.
nabothian c.
nasolabial c.
nasopharyngeal mucous retention c.
neoplastic c.
neuroenteric c.
noncommunicating c.
nonneoplastic c.

NOTES

cyst *(continued)*
    nuchal c.
    odontogenic c.
    oil c.
    omental c.
    omphalomesenteric duct c.
    orbital blood c.
    orbital chocolate c.
    orbital dermoid c.
    ovarian dermoid c.
    ovarian follicular c.
    ovarian image signature c.
    ovarian retention c.
    pancreatic c.
    paraglenoid c.
    paralabral c.
    parameniscal c.
    paramesonephric duct c.
    paraovarian c.
    parapelvic c.
    parapharyngeal space c.
    parathyroid c.
    paratubal serous c.
    paraurethral c.
    parovarian c.
    pelvic chocolate c.
    peribiliary c.
    pericaliceal c.
    pericardial duplication c.
    perineural arachnoid c.
    perineural sacral c.
    peripelvic c.
    peritoneal inclusion c.
    peritumoral c.
    physiologic ovarian c.
    pilonidal c.
    pineal c.
    pituitary c.
    placental septal c.
    pleural c.
    pleuropericardial c.
    c. or polyp
    pontine hydatid c.
    popliteal c.
    porencephalic c.
    posterior fossa c.
    postmenopausal adnexal c.
    posttraumatic oil c.
    posttraumatic spinal cord c.
    primordial tooth c.
    prostatic c.
    pulmonary c.
    pyelogenic c.
    racemose c.
    radicular c.
    Rathke cleft c.
    reactive spinal c.
    rectal duplication c.
    regressed c.
    renal sinus c.
    retention c.
    retrocerebellar arachnoid c.
    retroperitoneal c.
    sacral c.
    c. sclerosis
    sebaceous c.
    secondary archnoid c.
    second branchial cleft c.
    seminal vesicle c.
    septal placenta c.
    serous intraparenchymatous c.
    simple bone c.
    simple breast c.
    simple cortical renal c.
    small bowel duplication c.
    solitary bone c.
    spinal hydatid c.
    splenic epidermoid c.
    subarachnoid c.
    subarticular c.
    subchondral c.
    subcortical c.
    subependymal c.
    subpleural air c.
    syndrome with multiple cortical
      renal c.
    synovial c.
    synovium-filled degenerative c.
    tailgut c.
    talar dome c.
    Tarlov c.
    tarsal c.
    tectal c.
    tension c.
    testicular c.
    theca-lutein ovarian c.
    thick-walled c.
    thin-walled c.
    thoracic duct c.
    thymic c.
    thyroglossal duct c.
    thyroid c.
    Todani type c.
    Tornwaldt c.
    traumatic bone c.
    traumatic lipid c.
    traumatic lung c.
    tunica albuginea c.
    umbilical cord c.
    unicameral bone c.
    unilocular c.
    urachal c.
    wolffian c.

cystadenocarcinoma
    mucinous ovarian c.
    ovarian serous c.
    pancreatic c.

pseudomucinous c.
serous c.
cystadenofibroma
ovarian c.
cystadenoma
bile duct c.
biliary c.
colloid c.
endometrioid c.
glycogen-rich pancreatic c.
c. lymphomatosum
macrocystic c.
mucinous c.
ovarian c.
pancreas c.
papillary epididymal c.
serous c.
thyroid c.
cystic
c. adenocarcinoma
c. adenoma
c. adenomatoid malformation
c. airspace HRCT
c. appearance
c. arachnoiditis
c. area thyroid
c. artery
c. bone angiomatosis
c. breast disease
c. breast mass
c. bronchiectasis
c. calculus
c. change
c. component
c. degeneration
c. dilatation
c. disease of breast
c. duct angiography
c. duct cholangiogram
c. duct cholangiography
c. duct lumen
c. duct obstruction
c. duct remnant
c. duct remnant stone
c. duct stump
c. endometrial hyperplasia
c. epididymis lesion
c. fibrosis
c. fibrous dysplasia
c. fistula
c. fluid
c. gall duct

c. ganglioglioma
c. glandular hyperplasia
c. glioma
c. goiter
c. hemangioblastoma
c. hyperplasia photomicrograph
c. intracranial fetal lesion
c. intraparenchymal meningioma
c. kidney
c. kidney disease
c. liver lesion
c. lymph node
c. lysis
c. mastoplasia
c. medial necrosis
c. medionecrosis
c. mesothelioma
c. metastasis
c. myelomalacia
c. myelopathy
c. neck hygroma
c. nephroma
c. orbital hygroma
c. osteofibromatosis
c. ovarian disease
c. ovary
c. partially differentiated
nephroblastoma
c. pattern
c. pilocytic astrocytoma
c. plexus
c. pneumatosis
c. polyp
c. process
c. pulmonary emphysema
c. renal cell carcinoma
c. rheumatoid arthritis
c. sac
c. splenic lesion
c. splenic neoplasm
c. structure
c. teratoma
c. teratomatous mass
c. tuberculosis
c. tuberculous osteomyelitis
c. tumor
c. vein
c. wall
cystica
cystitis c.
mastitis fibrosa c.
osteitis fibrosa c.

NOTES

cystica *(continued)*
>> pyelitis c.
>> pyeloureteritis c.
>> ureteritis c.

cystic-choledochal junction
cysticercus
>> c. cyst
>> c. granuloma

cystic-malacic area
cysticohepatic triangle
cystine
>> c. calculus
>> c. stone

cystinosis
>> nephropathic c.

cystitis
>> c. cystica
>> emphysematous c.
>> interstitial c.
>> radiation c.
>> tuberculous c.

cystoatrial shunt
cystocarcinoma
cystocele
>> protrusion of c.

cystocolpoproctography
Cysto-Conray
>> C.-C. contrast agent
>> C.-C. II imaging agent

cystoduodenal ligament
cystofiberscope
cystofibroma
Cystografin
Cystografin-Dilute imaging agent
cystogram
>> air c.
>> bead-chain c.
>> chain c.
>> delayed c.
>> double voiding c.
>> excretory c.
>> postdrainage c.
>> radioisotope voiding c.
>> radionuclide c.
>> radiopharmaceutical voiding c.
>> retrograde c. (RC)
>> stress c.
>> triple-voiding c.
>> voiding c.

cystography
>> antegrade c.
>> bead-chain c.
>> computed tomographic c.
>> c. imaging
>> radionuclide c.
>> retrograde c.
>> triple-voiding c.

cystoid

cystoma
cystomatous
cystometrography
cystomorphous
cystoplasty
>> ileocecal c.

cystopyelography
cystoradiogram
cystoradiography
cystosarcoma phyllodes
cystoscope
cystoscopic urography
cystoscopy
>> virtual c.
>> virtual reality flexible c.

cystosonography
>> echo-enhanced c.

cystostomy
cystoureterogram
cystoureterography
cystourethrogram (CUG)
>> lateral c.
>> micturating c. (MCU)
>> voiding c. (VCU, VCUG)

cystourethrography
>> chain c.
>> expression c.
>> isotope voiding c. (IVCU)
>> micturating c.
>> micturition c.
>> radionuclide voiding c.
>> retrograde c.
>> video c.
>> voiding c. (VCU, VCUG)

cystourethroscopy imaging
cytochrome c oxidase (COX)
cytomegalovirus (CMV)
>> c. encephalitis
>> c. esophagitis

Cytomel suppression
cytometer
>> FACScan flow c.

cytometry
>> DNA flow c.
>> flow c.
>> image c.
>> laser scanning c. (LSC)
>> multicolor flow c.

cytophotocoagulation
>> contact transscleral laser c. (CTLC)

cytophotometry
>> DNA c.

cytoskeletal
>> c. misalignment
>> c. perturbation

cytotoxic
>> c. edema
>> c. edema of gray matter

D

3D (continued)

3D postprocessing technique
3D pre-filtering
3D processed ultrafast computerized imaging
3D processed ultrafast CT
3D projection reconstruction imaging
3D proton MR spectroscopy
3D pulse design
3D radiation treatment planning
3D reconstructed target
3D reconstruction
3D reconstruction algorithm
3D reformatting
3D RODEO
3D rotating delivery of excitation off-resonance
3D rotational angiography
3D RTP
3D shape of neuroanatomic structure
3D spatial encoding
3D spoiled gradient-recalled echo sequence
3D stereotactic surface projection
3D superficial liposculpture
3D surface anthropometry
3D surface detection algorithm
3D surface digitizer
3D surface digitizer scanner
3D surface rendering
3D technique
3D time-of-flight magnetic resonance angiographic sequence
3D transesophageal echocardiographic sequence
3D transesophageal echocardiography
3D turbo fluid-attentuated inversion recovery
3D turbo SE imaging
3D T1-weighted gradient-echo imaging
3D ultrasound reconstruction imaging
3D ultrasound volumetry
3D VIEWNIX software system
3D volume
3D volume-rendered helical CT angiography
3D volume-rendering CT angiography
3D volume-rendering reconstruction image
3D volume-rendering technique
3D volume technique

4D

4-dimensional
    4D US imagine

D$_{max}$

maximum density

Da

dalton

DAC

digital-to-analog converter

Dacron-coated microcoil
Dacron-covered stent graft
Dacron stent
dacryoadenitis
dacryocystitis
dacryocystocele
dacryocystogram
dacryocystography

computed tomographic d.
d. imaging
magnetic resonance d.
radiopharmaceutical d.

dacryocystorhinostomy

endoscopic laser d.

dacryoscintigraphy
dactylitis

tuberculous d.

dagger sign
Dagradi classification of esophageal varix
DAI

diffuse axonal injury
    DAI in vivo

Dalen-Fuchs nodule
DALM

dysplasia with associated lesion or mass

dalton (D, Da)
damage

anthracycline-induced myocardial d.
diffuse alveolar d.
drug-induced pulmonary d.
endothelial d.
fatigue d.
focal d.
hemisphere d.
hypoxic brain d.
ischemic brain d.
physial d.
projection fiber d.
renal vascular d.
seminiferous tubular d.
U-fiber d.
valvular d.
vascular cord d.

dammed-up cerebrospinal fluid
dampened

d. obstructive pulse
d. pulsatile flow
d. waveform

dampening
    Doppler waveform d.
damping of catheter tip pressure
Damus-Kaye-Stansel (DKS)
dancer's
    d. bone
    d. foot malformation
    d. fracture
Dance sign
Dandy-Walker
    D.-W. complex
    D.-W. continuum
    D.-W. cyst
    D.-W. deformity
    D.-W. malformation
    D.-W. spectrum
    D.-W. syndrome
    D.-W. variant
dangling choroid plexus
Danis-Weber
    D.-W. ankle fracture classification
    D.-W. fracture
DANTE
    delay alternating with nutation for
    tailored excitation
    DANTE sequence
DANTE-selective pulse
D'Antonio acetabular classification
DAP
    dose area product
dark
    d. lung
    d. Mach band
    d. pixel value
    d. region
    d. signal intensity
    d. signal intensity rim
darkfield
    d. imaging
    d. microscopy
darkroom error
Darkschewitsch
    nucleus of D.
Darrach-Hughston-Milch fracture
dartoic tissue
dartos muscle
darwinian tubercle
DAS
    data-acquisition system
DASA
    distal articular set angle

Daseler-Anson classification of plantaris muscle anatomy
dashboard fracture
DAT
    digital axial tomography
    symmetric loss of DAT
data, sing. **datum**
    d. acquisition
    d. acquisition time
    d. camera
    cine raw d.
    d. clipping detection error
    clustered d.
    d. collection system
    contrast d.
    emission and transmission d.
    ferrokinetic d.
    functional d.
    mask d.
    d. pitch
    radiology outcomes d.
    relaxivity d.
    rotating raw cine d.
    d. set
    d. spike detection error
    d. spike detection error artifact
    stereotactic d.
    transmission d.
    volume rendering of helical CT d.
    volumetric image d.
data-acquisition system (DAS)
data-clipping detection error artifact
Datascope catheter
dataset
    isotropic d.
dating
    second-trimester gestational d.
    third-trimester gestational d.
DaTSCAN
    D. imager
    D. imaging agent
datum (*sing. of* data)
Daubenton
    D. line
    D. plane
daughter
    d. abscess
    d. cyst
    d. element
    d. isotope
    d. nuclide

D

NOTES

DAVF
  dural arteriovenous fistula
David Letterman sign
Davidson shunt
Davies
    D. endocardial fibrosis
    D. endomyocardial fibrosis
Davies-Colley syndrome
da Vinci surgical system
Davis intubated pyelotomy
Dawbarn sign
Dawson finger
Dawson-Mueller drainage catheter
daylight processor
d'Azyr
    bundle of Vicq d.
DBA
  duodenal bulb apex
DBC
  dye-binding capacity
DBDC
  distal bile duct carcinoma
DBM
  demineralized bone matrix
DC
  differentiated carcinoma
  direct current
    DC offset artifact
DCA
  directional color angiography
  directional coronary atherectomy
DCBE
  double-contrast barium enema
DCCF
  dural carotid cavernous fistula
3DCE
  3-dimensional contrast-enhanced
DCE-MRI
  dynamic contrast-enhanced magnetic
    resonance imaging
3DCE-T1-MRA
DCIS
  ductal carcinoma in situ
    comedo-type DCIS
    cribriform DCIS
    micropapillary DCIS
    papillary DCIS
    solid DCIS
    Van Nuys Prognostic Index for
      DCIS
DCM
  dilated cardiomyopathy
DCO
  distal clavicle osteolysis
    nontraumatic DCO
DCS
  distal coronary sinus
**DCS-10, DCS-18 mechanically
  detachable platinum coil**

1D-CSI
  1-dimensional chemical-shift imaging
DCT
  discrete cosine transform
  dynamic computed tomography
DDC
  direct display console
DDD
  double-dose delay
  dual-mode, dual-pacing, dual-sensing
dD/dt
  derived value on apexcardiogram
DDFP
  dodecafluoropentane
DDH
  developmental dysplasia of hip
DDREF
  dose/dose-rate effective factor
DDSA
  duplex Doppler signal analysis
    Integris V-3000 DDSA
3D-DSA
  3-dimensional digital subtraction
    angiography
    3D-DSA image
DE
  dose equivalent
de
    de Broglie wavelength
    de Lange syndrome
    de Morsier syndrome
    de Musset sign
    de novo aneurysm
    de novo lesion
    de Quervain disease
    de Quervain fracture
    de Quervain thyroiditis
    de Seze angle
deactivation
dead
    d. bone
    d. bowel
    d. space
    d. time
    d. time loss
    d. tissue
DEAE-Sephadex A-25 chromatography
death
    brain d.
    cerebral d.
    early fetal d.
    fetal d.
    imminent d.
    intermediate fetal d.
    late fetal d.
    quadrant of d.
    sudden cardiac d.
DeBakey aortic classification
deblurring technique

debris
> atheromatous d.
> atherosclerotic d.
> bone d.
> calcium d.
> cholesterol d.
> echogenic d.
> embolic d.
> extraarticular d.
> foreign d.
> gelatinous d.
> grumous d.
> intimal d.
> intraarticular d.
> intraluminal d.
> joint d.
> layering d.
> metallic d.
> necrotic d.
> particulate d.
> thallium d.

debris-fluid level
DEC
> direction-encoded color mapping

decade scaler
decalcification
decalcified dorsum sella
decannulation
decay
> alpha d.
> beta d.
> beta-minus d.
> beta-plus d.
> branch d.
> branching d.
> d. constant
> energy d.
> d. equation
> exponential d.
> free-induction d. (FID)
> isomeric d.
> isotope d.
> d. mode
> nuclear d.
> positron d.
> d. product
> radioactive d.
> repeated free-induction d.
> d. scheme
> d. series
> d. time

decay-activating factor

deceleration-dependent block
deceleration time
decelerative injury
dechondrification
decidua
decidual
> d. cyst
> d. fissure
> d. sac

decidualized endometrium
deciduate placenta
deciduous
decima
> costa fluctuans d.

decimalized variance map
decision matrix
decline
> ADC d.

declotting
decoding
> document image d. (DID)
> Viterbi d.

decompensated
> d. alcoholic cirrhosis
> d. congestive heart failure

decompensation
> cardiac d.
> chronic respiratory d.
> end-stage adult cardiac d.
> end-stage fetal cardiac d.
> hemodynamic d.
> ischemic d.
> respiratory d.
> singular valve d. (SVD)
> ventricular d.

decomposition
> 3-level Haar wavelet d.
> linear prediction with singular
>   value d.

decompression
> arthroscopic d.
> biliary d.
> bony d.
> canal d.
> cardiac d.
> d. catheter
> endoscopic d.
> foramen magnum d.
> d. of fracture
> gastric d.
> hydrostatic d.
> intestinal d.

D

NOTES

decompression *(continued)*
    microvascular d.
    percutaneous transhepatic d.
    peripheral nerve d.
    portal d.
    d. sickness
    spinal cord d.
    surgical d.
    transduodenal endoscopic d.
    transpedicular d.
    tube d.
    d. tube
    variceal d.
    venous d.
deconditioned exercise response
deconditioning
deconvolution
    d. method
    d. technique
deconvolutional analysis
decortication
    cardiac d.
    heart d.
    lung d.
decoupling
    bilinear rotation d. (BIRD)
decrease
    intraluminal attenuation d.
    split renal function d.
decreased
    d. activity
    d. attenuation
    d. cerebral blood flow
    d. closing velocity
    d. diffusion anisotropy
    d. distal perfusion
    d. E-to-F slope
    d. intensity
    d. peripheral vascular resistance
    d. peristalsis
    d. placenta size
    d. pulmonary vascularity
    d. stroke volume
    d. systemic resistance
    d. thyroid radiotracer uptake
    d. tidal volume
    d. uptake of radiotracer
    d. vital capacity
decrement
    scan d.
decryption algorithm
DecThreads software
decubitus
    d. calculus
    d. film
    d. pad
    d. position

    d. radiograph
    d. ulcer
    d. view
decussate
decussation
dedicated
    d. head scanner
    d. linear accelerator
    d. mammography system
    d. PET scanner
    d. phased-array coil
    d. shoulder coil
    d. viewer
dedifferentiated
    d. liposarcoma
    d. parosteal osteosarcoma
dedifferentiation
deep
    d. arch
    d. artery
    d. cardiac plexus
    d. collateral ligament
    d. Doppler velocity interrogation
    d. fascia
    d. fascia of penis
    d. gray matter nucleus change
    d. interloop abscess
    d. lymphatic vessel
    d. muscle
    d. myometrial invasion
    d. to the nipple
    d. pelvic abscess
    d. perineal pouch
    d. posterior compartment
    d. roentgen ray therapy
    d. sedation
    d. sulcus sign
    d. tumor
    d. vein
    d. vein system of leg
    d. venous aplasia
    d. venous channel
    d. venous incompetence
    d. venous insufficiency (DVI)
    d. venous occlusion
    d. venous thromboembolization
    d. venous thrombosis (DVT)
    d. white ischemia matter
    d. white matter track
deep-seated
    d.-s. lesion
    d.-s. tumor
deep-shelled acetabulum
deexcitation
default display protocol
defecating proctogram
defecogram

defecography

dynamic open magnetic
   resonance d.
open magnetic resonance d.

defect

abdominal wall d.
anteroapical d.
aortic septal d.
aortopulmonary septal d.
apical d.
atrial ostium primum d.
atrial septal d. (ASD)
atrioventricular canal d.
atrioventricular nodal septal d.
atrioventricular septal d. (AVSD)
bar d.
beneficial atrial septal d.
benign cortical d.
bile duct filling d.
bony d.
bridging d.
calcified medullary d.
cauliflower-shaped filling d.
cecal filling d.
chiasmatic d.
chondral d.
cold d.
collecting system filling d.
colonic filling d.
conal ventricular septal d.
concomitant d.
congenital heart d. (CHD)
congenital hemidysplasia with
   ichthyosiform erythroderma and
   limb d.'s (CHILD)
conoventricular d.
contiguous ventricular septal d.
conversion d.
cortical d.
craniotomy d.
curvilinear d.
cushion d.
developmental d.
discoid filling d.
duodenal filling d.
Eisenmenger d.
endocardial cushion d. (ECD)
endocardial cushion ventricular
   septal d.
esophageal filling d.
extradural d.
extrinsic filling d.

extrinsic ureteral d.
fetal abdominal wall d.
fibrous cortical d.
fibrous medullary d.
fibrous metaphysial-diaphysial d.
field d.
filling d.
fixed intracavitary filling d.
fixed perfusion d.
flap valve ventricular septal d.
focal liver scintigraphic d.
focal plaquelike d.
frondlike filling d.
frontal d.
fusiform d.
fusion d.
gallbladder filling d.
gastric remnant filling d.
global cortical d.
gouge d.
hatchet d.
hernia d.
high d.
Hill-Sachs d. (HSD)
hot d.
incisura d.
inferoapical d.
infracristal ventricular septal d.
infundibular ventricular septal d.
interatrial septal d.
intercalary d.
interventricular septal d. (IVSD)
intraarterial filling d.
intraatrial filling d.
intracavitary filling d.
intraductal breast filling d.
intraluminal filling d.
intramural filling d.
intravascular filling d.
intrinsic filling d.
inverted umbrella d.
ischemic d.
joint capsule d.
junctional cortical d.
junctional parenchymal kidney d.
juxtaarterial ventricular septal d.
juxtatricuspid ventricular septal d.
linear d.
lingular mandibular bony d.
   (LMBD)
lobulated filling d.
lucent d.

D

NOTES

defect *(continued)*
luminal d.
lung perfusion d.
luteal phase d.
malaligned atrioventricular septal d.
mapping of d.
mass d.
membranous ventricular septal d.
metaphysial fibrous d.
monoradicular filling d.
multiple colon filling d.'s
multiple small bowel filling d.'s
mural d.
muscular ventricular septal d.
neural tube d. (NTD)
nonexpansile well-demarcated
  multilocular bone d.
nonexpansile well-demarcated
  unilocular bone d.
nonsubperiosteal cortical d.
nonuniform rotational d. (NURD)
obstructive ventilatory d.
open neural tube d.
organification d.
osseous d.
osteocartilaginous d.
osteochondral d. (OCD)
osteophytic d.
ostium primum atrial septal d.
ostium secundum atrial septal d.
pars interarticularis d.
partial atrioventricular canal d.
pear-shaped d.
pericardial d.
perimembranous ventricular
  septal d.
photopenic d.
plaquelike linear d.
plication d.
pneumoenteric d.
polypoid filling d.
porta hepatis d.
postcricoid d.
posteroapical d.
postinfarction ventriculoseptal d.
postoperative skull d.
punched-out bony d.
radial ray d.
radiolucent linear filling d.
resolving ischemic neurologic d.
restrictive ventilatory d.
reversible ischemic d.
right ventricular conduction d.
Roger ventricular septal d.
scan d.
scintigraphic perfusion d.
secundum atrial septal d.
segmental bone d.
segmental bronchus d.

septal d. (SD)
septation septal d.
septum transversum d.
serpiginous luminal filling d.
sessile filling d.
single colonic filling d.
sinus venosus atrial septal d.
small bowel filling d.
soft tissue d.
solitary small bowel filling d.
spontaneous closure of d.
stellate d.
stomach filling d.
subcortical d.
subperiosteal cortical d.
subsegmental perfusion d.
superior caval d.
superior marginal d.
supracristal ventricular septal d.
Swiss cheese ventricular septal d.
thyroid organification d.
thyroid trapping d.
transient perfusion d.
trapping thyroid d.
triangular d.
trochlear d.
tumor d.
type I (supracristal) ventricular
  septal d.
type II (infracristal) ventricular
  septal d.
type IV (muscular) ventricular
  septal d.
ureteral filling d.
valvular cardiac d.
venous d.
ventilation d.
ventilation-perfusion d.
ventral hernia d.
ventricular septal d. (VSD)
wedge-shaped d.
wire-related d.

defective
d. communication between cardiac
  chambers
d. volume regulation delay

deferens, pl. **deferentia**
ductus d.
vas d.

deferent
d. canal
d. duct

deferential
d. artery
d. plexus

defibrillation
rectilinear biphasic waveform for
  external d.

defibrillator
    automatic external d. (AED)
defibrination syndrome
deficiency
    acyl CoA oxidase d.
    Aitken femoral d.
    COX d.
    cyclooxygenase d.
    photon d.
    proximal focal femoral d. (PFFD)
    RDS-like d.
    sphingomyelinase d.
    surfactant d.
deficit
    base d.
    cortical d.
    focal d.
    hand motor d.
    lateralization d.
    posterior column d.
    reversible ischemic neurologic d.
    significant residual d.
    space d.
defined and homogeneous calcification
definition
    ground-glass d.
    loss of d.
    pseudopolyp d.
definitive
    d. abnormality
    d. callus
Definity
    D. injectable suspension
    D. suspension for IV injection
deflation
deflection
    fracture simple and depressed full-scale d. (FSD)
    intrinsic d.
deflector
    tip d.
defluorescence
defluxion
deformability
deformable
    d. manipulation
    d. template
deformans
    arthritis syphilitica d. (ASD)
    arthrosis d.
    osteitis d.
    osteochondrodystrophia d.

    ostitis d.
    Paget osteitis d.
    spondylitis d.
    spondylosis d.
deformation
    d. amplitude
    cord d.
    d. posterior plagiocephaly
    shear-strain d.
deformation-based
    d.-b. hippocampal segmentation and shape analysis
    d.-b. surface-rendered image
deformity
    Åkerlund d.
    alpine hunter's cap d.
    angular d.
    aortic valve d.
    Arnold-Chiari d.
    back-knee d.
    bayonet d.
    bell-and-clapper d.
    biconcave d.
    bifid thumb d.
    bony d.
    boutonnière d.
    bowing d.
    bull's eye d.
    burn boutonnière d.
    buttonhole d.
    calcaneovarus d.
    calcaneus d.
    cavovarus d.
    cavus d.
    cecal d.
    chain of lakes d.
    Charcot d.
    checkrein d.
    clawfoot d.
    clawhand d.
    clawtoe d.
    cloverleaf d.
    clubfoot d.
    clubhand d.
    cock-up d.
    codfish d.
    compensatory d.
    congenital d.
    contracture d.
    cow horn d.
    coxa valga d.
    coxa vara d.

NOTES

D

deformity (*continued*)

cranioorbital d.
cubitus valgus d.
cubitus varus d.
curly toe d.
Dandy-Walker d.
digital d.
digitus flexus d.
dinner-fork d.
duodenal bulb d.
endometrial surface d.
equinovalgus d.
equinovarus hindfoot d.
equinus d.
Erlenmeyer-flask-like d.
eversion-external rotation d.
femoral head d.
flatfoot d.
flexible spastic equinovarus d.
flexion d.
foot d.
forefoot abduction d.
fracture d.
funnel chest d.
garden spade d.
gastric wall d.
genu valgum d.
genu varum d.
gibbous d.
gooseneck outflow tract d.
gunstock d.
Haglund d.
hallux flexus d.
hallux malleus d.
hallux rigidus d.
hallux valgus d.
hallux varus d.
hammertoe d.
hatchet-head d.
Hill-Sachs d.
hindbrain d.
hindfoot d.
hockey-stick tricuspid valve d.
hourglass d.
humpback d.
Ilfeld-Holder d.
internal rotation d.
intrinsic minus d.
intrinsic plus d.
J-hook d.
joint d.
J-sella d.
keyhole d.
Kirner d.
kleeblatschädel d.
Klippel-Feil d.
knock-knee d.
lanceolate d.
lobster-claw d.

Madelung d.
mallet-finger d.
mermaid d.
metatarsus adductocavus d.
metatarsus adductovarus d.
metatarsus adductus d.
metatarsus atavicus d.
metatarsus latus d.
metatarsus primus varus d.
metatarsus varus d.
Michel d.
mitral valve d.
nasal tip d.
neuropathic midfoot d.
pannus d.
parachute mitral valve d.
pectus carinatum d.
pectus excavatum d.
pencil-in-cup d.
penciling d.
pencillike d.
pencil-point metatarsal d.
perigastric d.
pes arcuatus clawfoot d.
pes cavus clawfoot d.
pes planovalgus d.
pes planus d.
phrygian cap d.
pigeon-breast d.
ping-pong ball d.
pistol-grip femur d.
planovalgus foot d.
plantar flexion-inversion d.
postoperative thoracic d.
procurvature d.
pseudo-Hurler d.
pulmonary valve d.
recurvatum d.
reduction d.
rocker d.
rocker-bottom foot d.
rolled edge d.
rotational d.
rotoscoliotic d.
roundback d.
round shoulder d.
saber-shin d.
sandal-gap d.
scimitar d.
seal-fin d.
shepherd's crook d.
snowman d.
spastic equinovarus d.
spastic hindfoot valgus d.
splayfoot d.
split foot d.
spondylitic d.
Sprengel d.
static foot d.

subtrochanteric varus d.
supination d.
supratip nasal tip d.
swan-neck finger d.
talus foot d.
thoracic d.
thumb-in-palm d.
torsion d.
trefoil d.
tricuspid valve d.
trigger finger d.
triphalangeal thumb d.
turned-up pulp d.
ulnar drift d.
valgus heel d.
varus d.
Velpeau d.
vertical talus foot d.
VISI d.
Volkmann d.
wasp-tail d.
wedging d.
whistling d.
Whitehead d.
windblown d.
windswept d.
defuzzification algorithm
degenerated
    d. fibroadenoma
    d. tissue
    d. uterine leiomyoma
degeneration
    acquired hepatocerebral d.
    angiolithic d.
    articular cartilage d.
    atheromatous d.
    atrophic d.
    ballooning d.
    bony d.
    brain d.
    breast d.
    calcareous d.
    carcinomatous subacute cerebellar d.
    cardiac valve mucoid d.
    cardiomyopathic d.
    cartilaginous d.
    cerebellar d.
    cerebelloolivary d.
    cerebromacular d. (CMD)
    chondrocyte d.
    cobblestone d.
    colloid d.

cortical cerebellar d.
corticobasal ganglionic d.
corticostriatospinal d.
cusp d.
cystic d.
disc d.
Doyne honeycomb d.
dystrophic d.
esophageal d.
facet d.
fatty d.
fibrinous d.
fibroid d.
gliosis-induced microcystic d.
granulovacuolar d.
gray matter d.
heart d.
hepatic d.
hepatocerebral d.
hepatolenticular d.
Holmes cortical cerebellar d.
honeycomb d.
hyaline d.
hydropic d.
hypertensive vascular d.
hypertrophic olivary d.
internal d.
intimal d.
intrameniscal mucoid d.
liquefaction d.
malignant d.
Menzel olivopontocerebellar d.
microcystic d.
mitral valve myxomatous d.
Mönckeberg d.
mucinous d.
mucoid umbilical cord d.
mucous d.
mural d.
muscular d.
myocardial cellular d.
myocardial fibrous d.
myxomatous d.
olivary d.
olivopontocerebellar d. (OPCD)
d. of pancreas
pancreatic d.
paraneoplastic cerebellar d.
parenchymatous cerebellar d.
paving-stone d.
primary progressive cerebellar d.
progressive d.

D

NOTES

degeneration *(continued)*
    Regnauld-type great toe d.
    renal tubular d.
    retinal d.
    retrograde d.
    rim d.
    sclerotic d.
    secondary d.
    senile d.
    spinal d.
    spinocerebellar d.
    spongiform d.
    spongy white matter d.
    striatonigral d.
    subacute combined spinal cord d.
    testicular d.
    thyroid d.
    trabecular d.
    traumatic d.
    wallerian d.
    wear-and-tear d.
    Zenker d.
degenerative
    d. aortic aneurysm
    d. arthritis
    d. arthrosis
    d. atrioventricular node disease
    d. atrophy
    d. brain disease
    d. cardiomyopathy
    d. dementia
    d. disc
    d. disc disease
    d. disease in cerebrum
    d. horizontal cleavage tear
    d. joint disease (DJD)
    d. liver
    d. microcystic formation
    d. narrowing
    d. nuclear pattern
    d. osseous change
    d. osteoarthritis
    d. spinal instability
    d. spondylolisthesis
    d. spondylosis
    d. spur
    d. spurring
deglutition
    d. disorder
    d. mechanism
    muscle of d.
    d. pneumonia
Degos syndrome
degradable starch microsphere
degradation
    fibrinogen d.
    d. of image
    image quality d.
    motion d.

degraded
    d. liver
    d. photon
degranulation
degree
    d. of correction
    d. of head rotation
    d. of inspiration
    d. of neck obliquity
    noncircularity d.
80-degree linear interpolation
45-degree spinal wedge
55-degree tomography wedge
dehalogenation
dehiscence
    anastomotic d.
    aortic intimal d.
    bronchial d.
    Killian's d.
    valve d.
    wound d.
dehiscent jugular bulb
dehydration-induced renal dysfunction
dehydrogenase
    succinate d. (SDH)
DEI
    diffraction-enhanced imaging
Dejerine-Roussy
    thalamic syndrome of D.-R.
Dejerine sign
Delarnette scanner
delay
    d. alternating with nutation for
      tailored excitation (DANTE)
    defective volume regulation d.
    double-dose d. (DDD)
    interscan d. (ID)
    intraventricular conduction d.
    phase d.
    postinjection scan d.
    readout d.
    regrowth d.
    regular wedge d.
    regurgitant flow d.
    regurgitant lesion d.
    temporal phase d.
    d. time selection
    transition d. (TD)
    trigger d. (TD)
    upfront d.
delayed
    d. bone age
    d. bone imaging
    d. closure of suture
    d. cystogram
    d. development
    d. eclampsia
    d. excretion of contrast medium
    d. film

d. fracture union
d. gadolinium-enhanced magnetic resonance imaging of cartilage (dGEMRIC)
d. gadolinium-enhanced MRI of cartilage
d. gastric emptying
d. hydrocephalus
d. myelination
d. operative cholangiography
d. phase
d. phase of arteriography
d. phase image
d. phase scanning
d. pineal apoplexy
d. posttraumatic myelopathy
d. resolution of pneumonia
d. rupture spleen
d. small bowel transit
d. splenic rupture
d. transit time
d. transport of tracer
d. traumatic intracerebral hematoma (DTICH)
d. traumatic intracerebral hemorrhage
d. unilateral nephrogram
d. visualization
d. washout

Delbet
D. hip fracture classification
D. sign
deleterious effect
delimitation
delineation
lumen d.
delivered
d. by balloon inflation
d. total dose (DTD)
delivery
angiogenesis gene d.
coil d.
intracavitary d.
intravascular angiogenesis gene d.
percutaneous endometrial drug d.
timed bolus d.
transcutaneous angiogenesis gene d.
viral vector d.
Delmege sign of tuberculosis
delphian lymph node
delta, δ
D. 32 digital stereotactic system

d. pressure/delta time (dP/dt)
d. ray
d. sign
D. 32 TACT 3-dimensional breast imaging system
DELTAmanager MedImage system
deltoid
d. branch of posterior tibial artery
d. bursa
d. crest
d. eminence
d. fascia
d. ligament
d. tuberosity
deltoideopectoral
d. triangle
d. trigone
deltopectoral
d. groove
d. lymph node
demagnetization
adiabatic d.
d. field effect
demarcate
demarcation
d. line
nidus d.
shelllike d.
dementia
degenerative d.
multiinfarct d.
subcortical ischemic vascular d.
Demianoff sign
demifacet
demineralization
bone d.
demineralized
d. bone matrix (DBM)
d. bony structure
demise
embryo d.
d. of fetus
imminent d.
intrauterine d.
demodulator
Demons-Meigs syndrome
demyelinating disease
demyelination
brainstem d.
cerebrum d.
intramedullary d.
large-fiber d.

NOTES

D

demyelination *(continued)*
  leopard skin d.
  posterior column d.
  postinfectious d.
  segmental d.
  tigroid d.
  white matter d.
demyelinative disorder
DeMyer system of cerebral malformation
denatured
  d. ^{99m}Tc-RBC
  d. ^{99m}Tc-RBC imaging agent
dendritic
  d. calculus
  d. carcinoma
  d. gynecomastia
  d. lesion
  d. spine
  d. vegetation
dendrocytoma
denervated area
denervation
  d. atrophy
  autonomic d.
  cardiac d.
  sympathetic d.
Denis
  D. classification
  D. classification of spinal fracture
Dennis tube
Denonvilliers
  D. fascia
  D. ligament
dens
  d. in dente
  d. fracture
  hypoplasia of d.
  d. view
  d. view of cervical spine
dense
  d. abdominal veins
  d. body
  d. brain mass
  d. cerebral mass
  d. connective tissue
  d. consolidation
  d. echo
  d. enhancing brain lesion
  d. lung lesion
  d. MCA sign
  d. metaphysial band
  d. rib
  d. scar
  d. structure of bone
densitometer
  accuDEXA bone d.
  Achilles d.
  bone d.

CT d.
DEXA dual-energy x-ray absorptiometry d.
DEXAscan bone d.
DPX-IQ d.
dual-photon d.
dynamic spiral CT lung d.
Expert-XL d.
Hologic 2000 d.
Lunar DPX d.
Lunar Expert d.
Norland XR26 bone d.
OsteoView digital bone d.
pDEXA x-ray peripheral bone d.
Prodigy bone d.
QDR-1500 bone d.
QDR-2000 bone d.
Sahara portable bone d.
single-photon d.
video d.
densitometric measurement
densitometry
  bone d.
  cardiac output video d.
  Compton coherent scattering d.
  computerized optical d. (COD)
  CT d.
  dual-photon d.
  dynamic spiral CT lung d.
  Norland bone d.
  photon d.
  QCT 3000 system for bone d.
  quantitative CT d.
  spirometrically controlled CT lung d.
  d. z score
density
  air d.
  area of abnormal d.
  arterial linear d.
  asymmetric breast d.
  axial spin d.
  background d.
  band of d.
  base d.
  bone mineral d. (BMD)
  calcific d.
  capillary d.
  count d.
  curvilinear d.
  diffuse increase in breast d.
  diffuse reticular d.
  diffuse reticulogranular lung d.
  discrete perihilar d.
  d. discrimination
  double d.
  echo d.
  echo-spin d.
  endoluminal d.

energy flux d.
d. equalization filter
falx increased d.
fat d.
fibroglandular d.
fluid d.
focal asymmetric d.
ground-glass d.
hazy d.
homogeneous soft tissue d.
hydrogen spin d.
ill-defined breast d.
ill-defined multifocal lung d.
increased bone d.
increased splenic d.
inherent d.
integrated optical d. (IOD)
ionization d.
lamellar body d. (LBD)
linear d.
low d.
lung d.
magnetic flux d.
d. matrix theory
maximum d. (D_{max})
metallic d.
minimum pixel d.
mixed fat-water breast lesion d.
mottled d.
multiple pleural d.'s
near-water d.
nodular d.
optic d. (OD)
patchy area of d.
peak count d.
perihilar d.
photon d.
pleural d.
proton-d.
pulmonary d.
radiographic d.
radiolucent d.
radiopaque d.
reticulogranular pulmonary d.
retroareolar d.
retrocardiac d.
segmental lung d.
soft tissue d.
spicular d.
spin d.
spleen d.
strands of increased d.

streak of increased d.
subareolar breast d.
tissue d.
T-score measurement of bone
   mineral d.
tubular lung d.
urographic d.
variation in d.
water d.
wedge-shaped d.

densography
dental
   d. bulb
   d. contrast material
   d. crest
   d. cyst
   d. granuloma
   d. groove
   d. neck
   d. polyp
   d. radiography
   d. radiology
   d. ridge
   d. root
   d. sac
   d. scan
   d. shelf
   d. tubercle
Dentalaser
   Multi-Operatory D. (MOD)
DentaScan
   D. imaging
   D. multiplanar reformation
dentata
   vertebra d.
dentate
   d. fascia
   d. fissure
   d. fracture
   d. gyrus
   d. ligament
   d. line
   d. nuclei
   d. nuclei calcification
   d. nucleus of cerebellum
   d. output channel
   d. suture
   d. suture of skull
dentatoolivary pathway
dentatorubral atrophy
dentatothalamic tract
DentCAM

NOTES

D

dente
>dens in d.

denticulate
>d. ligament
>d. suture

dentiform
dentigerous cyst
dentin
dentinal
>d. sheath
>d. tubule

dentinogenesis imperfecta
dentition
>crowded d.

dentoskeletal relationship
denture-supporting structure
Dent-X intraoral x-ray unit
denudation
>area of d.

denutrition
Denver shunt
Denys-Drash tumor
Denys syndrome
deossification
>band of d.

6-deoxy-1-galactose
deoxygenated blood
deoxyglucose
>^{11}C d.

2-deoxyglucose
>2-fluoro 2-d. (FDG)

deoxyhemoglobin concentration
deoxyribonucleic acid (DNA)
dependence
>quadratic d.
>relaxation rate frequency d.
>solvent water TI frequency d.

dependency reaction
dependent
>d. atelectasis
>d. edema fluid resorption
>d. extracellular fluid accumulation
>d. lung
>d. opacity
>d. pouch of Douglas

dephase-rephase magnitude subtraction technique
dephasing
>d. gradient
>intraluminal d.
>intravoxel d.
>odd-echo d.
>rapid d.
>signal d.
>spin d.

depicted Hounsfield unit
depiction
>magnetic resonance d.
>d. of vasculature

depilatory agent
depletion
>intravascular volume d.

deployed stent
deployment
>stent d.

depolarization
>chemically-induced dynamic nuclear d. (CIDNP)
>ventricular premature d. (VPD)

deposit
>amyloid d.
>arteriosclerotic d.
>bony d.
>calcareous d.
>calcium salt d.
>callus d.
>endochondral bone d.
>intramuscular hemosiderin d.
>pericardium calcareous d.

deposition
>calcium pyrophosphate dihydrate crystal d.
>coil d.
>radiotracer d.
>d. of tracer

depreotide
>^{99m}Tc d.
>technetium-99m d.

depressed
>d. diaphragm
>d. ejection fraction
>d. right ventricular contractile function
>d. skull fracture

depression
>biconcave d.
>bone marrow d.
>fragment d.
>hemidiaphragm d.
>iodinated CM-induced cardiac d.
>iodinated contrast material-induced cardiac d.
>d. of left mainstem bronchus
>marginal kidney d.
>myocardial d.
>d. of nasal bone
>pacchionian d.
>parasagittal d.
>reciprocal d.
>d. of renal margin
>sinus node d.
>spinal cord d.
>tibial plateau d.
>translucent d.
>ventricular d.

depression-type intraarticular fracture
deprivation dwarfism

depth
>acetabular d.
>d. compensation
>d. dose
>d. dose distribution
>lumbosacral spine d.
>midplane d.
>photon interaction d.
>d. pulse
>d. resolution
>scatterer d.
>signal d.
>skin d.
>target d.
>d. of tumor invasion assessed by EUS

depth-dose curve
depth-pulse technique
depth-resolved surface spectroscopy (DRESS)
DER
>dual-energy radiograph

deranged tissue development
derangement
>articular d.
>disc d.
>internal d.
>longitudinal transarticular d.
>painful disc d.
>soft tissue d.

derby hat fracture
Derek Harwood-Nash catheter
Derenzo equation
derivative
>d. circulation
>pyridone d.

derived value on apexcardiogram (dD/dt)
Derma
>D. K laser
>D. 20 laser

dermal
>d. bone
>d. breast calcification
>d. duct tumor
>d. sinus tract

DermaLase laser
dermal-subcutaneous fat interface
dermatoarthritis
>lipoid d.

dermatofibrosarcoma protuberans

dermoid
>d. cyst
>mediastinum d.
>monodermal d.
>ovarian d.
>d. ovarian cyst
>d. plug
>spinal d.
>d. tumor

derotate
derotation
DES
>diffuse esophageal spasm
>DES exposure

Desault
>D. dislocation
>D. fracture

descending
>d. aorta dissection
>d. colon
>d. duodenum
>left anterior d. (LAD)
>d. septal artery
>d. thoracic aorta
>d. tract
>d. urography
>d. venography

descent
>basal d.
>epididymal d.
>perineal d.

desert rheumatism
desiccated
desiccation
>disc d.

design
>crossed-coil d.
>3D pulse d.
>factorial d.
>Hanafy piano-concave transducer d.
>over-the-wire d.
>PORT radiofrequency electrode d.
>pulse d.
>d. rule check (DRC)
>d. rule check algorithm

Desilets-Hoffman introducer
desmectasis
desmocytoma
desmofibromatosis
desmoid
>cortical d.
>extraabdominal d.

D

NOTES

desmoid *(continued)*
    d. lesion
    periosteal d.
    subperiosteal d.
    d. tumor
desmoma
desmoplasia
desmoplastic
    d. fibroma
    d. infantile astrocytoma
    d. reaction
    d. response
    d. small round-cell tumor (DSRCT)
desmosis
desmosome
d'Espine sign
desquamated epithelial breast hyperplasia
desquamative
    d. fibrosing alveolitis
    d. interstitial pneumonia (DIP)
destroy and replace method
destruction
    bony d.
    cortical d.
    geographic bone d.
    moth-eaten bone d.
    mucosal d.
    pattern of d.
    permeative bone d.
    sellar d.
    temporomandibular joint d.
    d. of tissue
    trabecular d.
destructive
    d. bone lesion
    d. brucellar arthritis
    d. discovertebral lesion
    d. interference technique
    d. process
    d. spondyloarthropathy
    d. tumor
detachable
    d. balloon-modified reducing stent
    d. platinum coil
detail
    d. burnout
    exquisite d.
    fetal d.
    fine d.
    intraluminal d.
    rib d.
    suboptimal d.
    trabecular bone d.
detectability
    lesion d.
detecting
    collision d.

    d. Down syndrome by ultrasound of the nose bone
    d. module
detection
    annihilation coincidence d. (ACD)
    automated polyp d.
    beta d.
    cardiac shunt d.
    coincidence d. (CD, CoDe)
    computer-aided d. (CAD)
    computer-aided polyp d.
    d. echocardiography
    edge d. (ED)
    focus d.
    ICP-AES d.
    magnetic resonance d.
    molecular coincidence d. (MCD)
    occult d.
    photooptical d.
    quadrature d.
    radioactivity d.
    radwaste radioactivity d.
    sonographic d.
    d. threshold
    turbidimetric d.
    d. zone
detective quantum efficiency (DQE)
detector
    Add-On Bucky direct x-ray d.
    anular d.
    d. array
    bismuth-germanate d. (BGO)
    block d.
    cadmium iodide d.
    CCD d.
    d. coil
    d. collimation
    collimation scintillation d.
    CR-39 nuclear tract d.
    crystalline phosphor d.
    C-Trak hand-held gamma d.
    dielectric track d.
    digital amorphous silicon flat-panel d.
    digital x-ray d.
    diode d.
    Doppler ultrasonic blood flow d.
    Doppler ultrasonic velocity d.
    element-specific d.
    flame ionization d.
    flat-plate d.
    gamma probe radiation d.
    gas-filled d.
    GE d.
    Geiger-Müller d.
    glass tract d.
    HPGe d.
    ionization d.
    kinestatic charge d. (KCD)

NaI d.
Neoprobe 1000, 1500 portable
   radioisotope d.
Neoprobe radioactivity d.
passive track d.
Pediatric Ingesta Scan metal d.
phase-sensitive d.
planar d.
quadrature phase d. (QPD)
radiation d.
rature d.
ring d.
scintillation d.
semiconductor d.
Si (Li) d.
slot-scanning d.
sodium iodide d.
solid-state nuclear track d.
d. system
thallium-activated sodium iodine d.
Thoravision selenium x-ray d.
tissue-equivalent d.
Wang-Binford edge d.
x-ray d.
16-detector PET system
determinant
   sequential d.
determination
   Budin-Chandler anteversion d.
   d. of lung volume
   particle size d.
   void d.
deterministic effect
detorsion
   spontaneous d.
detour conduit
detritus
detrusor
   d. hyperreflexia
   d. instability
   d. muscle
Detsky modified cardiac risk index
detunable elliptic transmission line
   resonator
deuterium imaging agent
deuterium-tritium generator
deuteron, deuton
Deutschländer disease
devascularization
   paraesophagogastric d.
developed collateral
developer artifact

development
   anomalous d.
   branchial cleft d.
   conductive d.
   delayed d.
   deranged tissue d.
   distal bone marrow d.
   endocardial cushion d.
   interval d.
   lymphatic d.
   metacarpophalangeal bone
      marrow d.
   metatarsophalangeal bone marrow d.
   tibia bone marrow d.
developmental
   d. defect
   d. dysplasia of hip (DDH)
   d. groove
Deventer
   D. diameter
   D. pelvis
deviated mediastinum
deviation
   angular d.
   aortic d.
   carpal d.
   fracture d.
   left axis d. (LAD)
   mean d.
   mediastinal d.
   needle d.
   radial d.
   right axis d. (RAD)
   rotary d.
   septal d.
   significant axis d.
   standard d.
   tracheal d.
   ulnar d.
   ureter d.
   valgus d.
   varus d.
device (*See also* machine, scanner,
   system, unit)
   abdominal left ventricular assist d.
   (ALVAD)
   Accunet distal protection d.
   amorphous silicon filmless digital
      x-ray detection technology d.
   Amplatzer septal occluder d.
   Amplatz thrombectomy d.
   AngioGuard-ex distal protection d.

D

NOTES

device *(continued)*
AngioJet thrombectomy d.
Angiolink EVS closure d.
Angio-Seal closure d.
Angio-Seal diagnostic d.
Angio-Seal therapeutic d.
antisiphon d.
Arrow-Trerotola percutaneous
   thrombectomy d.
Arrow-Trerotola percutaneous
   thrombolytic d.
arterial puncture site closure d.
automated gun-needle d.
automatic spring-loaded biopsy d.
BabyFace 3D surface rendering
   accessory d.
Bard rotary atherectomy d.
Baxter PMT d.
beam-modifying d.
bioabsorbable sheath-delivered
   vascular d.
biventricular assist d. (BVAD)
BladderManager ultrasound d.
bone fixation d.
Bruker minispec measuring d.
Bucky digital x-ray d.
Burnett BiDirectional TMJ d.
buttoned d.
CardioBeeper CB-12L cardiac d.
charge-coupled d. (CCD)
charge-injection d.
charge injection d. (CID)
Closer percutaneous suture-mediated
   closure d.
closure d.
Clo-Sur PAD closure d.
Coherent VersaPulse d.
collagen mediated closure d.
collagen plug d.
compression d.
copper 7, T intrauterine d.
CyberKnife Express d.
directional atherectomy d.
DirectRay direct-to-digital image
   capture d.
Duett arterial puncture site
   closure d.
Duett closure d.
Duett diagnostic d.
Duett therapeutic d.
DynaWell medical compression d.
Electro-Acuscope d.
electrooptical d.
Endostaple d.
EVS mechanical closure d.
external fixation d.
FemoStop compression d.
Filter Wire distal protection d.
FloWire ultrasound d.

Gelbfish-Endovasc d.
Glucoband electronic scanning d.
halo d.
hemostatic puncture closure d.
HiSonic ultrasonic bone conduction
   hearing d.
H2 Score office-based diagnostic d.
Hysterocath
   hysterosalpingography d.
Ilizarov d.
implantable vascular access d.
internal fixation d.
intramedullary fixation d.
intraoperative d.
Kendall sequential compression d.
kinematic wrist d.
Laser Lancet laser d.
left ventricular assist d. (LVAD)
lost intrauterine d.
magnetic induction d.
MammoReader mammogram d.
Mobin-Uddin umbrella
   endoluminal d.
Molteno double plate drainage d.
Molteno single plate drainage d.
MultiDop P, T, X transcranial
   Doppler d.
nail-plate d.
NB200 vascular access d.
Neuroshield distal protection d.
nonferromagnetic positioning d.
Nuclear Magnetic Device Lypoo
   Profile d.
Oasis thrombectomy d.
Omnisense multisite QUS d.
Optical Path Difference-Scan
   optical d.
OsteoAnalyzer bone densitometry d.
Palpagraph breast mapping d.
Perclose arterial closure d.
Perclose diagnostic d.
Perclose therapeutic d.
Percusurg distal protection d.
percutaneous arterial closure d.
percutaneous suture-mediated
   arteriotomy closure d.
percutaneous suture-mediated
   closure d.
percutaneous vascular surgical d.
Pigg-O-Stat pediatric positioning d.
Prostar-Techstar suture-mediated
   closure d.
Prostar XL 8, 10 suture mediated
   closure d.
RadStat hemostasis d.
Rashkind double umbrella d.
rheolytic mechanical
   thrombectomy d.
right ventricular assist d. (RVAD)

scaling d.
ScopeGuide magnetic resonance
  imaging d.
ScopeGuide MRI d.
Second Look breast imaging d.
Sideris buttoned double-disc d.
Siemens Magnetom Vision whole-
  body MR d.
Sonoline Sierra ultrasound
  imaging d.
SonoSite 180 hand-carried
  ultrasound d.
Sonotron electronic therapeutic d.
spinal fixation d.
spot film d.
stereotactic d.
superconducting quantum
  interference d. (SQUID)
SuperStitch closure d.
synchronization d.
Syvek Patch closure d.
Telos radiographic stress d.
T-fastener d.
The Closer arterial puncture site
  closure d.
thrombectomy d.
Trak Back pullback d.
Trerotola thrombectomy d.
TriSpan aneurysm neck-bride d.
tube d.
vascular access d.
vascular hemostatic d. (VHD)
VasoSeal closure d.
VasoSeal diagnostic d.
VasoSeal ES, VHD arterial
  puncture site closure d.
VasoSeal therapeutic d.
venous access d.
ventricular assist d.
VHD closure d.
woggle d.
X-Press suture-mediated closure d.
device-independent (DVI)
devitalized
  d. allogeneic bone
  d. portion of bone
  d. tissue
devoid of circulation
DEXA
  dual-energy x-ray absorptiometry
  DEXA bone density scan imaging

DEXA dual-energy x-ray
  absorptiometry densitometer
  DEXA scan
dexamethasone suppression test imaging
DEXAscan bone densitometer
dexter
  cor triatriatum d.
**Dexter-Grossman classification of mitral
  regurgitation**
dextrad
dextral
dextran
  Gd-DTPA-labeled d.
  iron d.
  technetium-99m d.
dextran-coated charcoal
dextrocardia
dextroconcave
dextrogastria
dextro loop (D-loop)
dextroposition
dextropositioned aorta
dextrorotary scoliosis
dextrorotoscoliosis
dextroscoliosis
dextrose 5% in water imaging agent
dextrosinistral
dextrotransposition of great artery
dextrotropic
dextroversion of heart
dextrum
  cor d.
DFA
  dorsiflexion angle
  hallux dorsiflexion angle
DFI
  dye fluorescence index
DFP
  diastolic filling pressure
DFS
  distraction-flexion staging
DFT
  discrete Fourier transform
2DFT
  2-dimensional Fourier transform
    2DFT method
    2DFT time-of-flight MR
      angiography
3DFT
  3-dimensional Fourier transform
    3DFT gradient-echo MR imaging

D

NOTES

3DFT *(continued)*
3DFT magnetic resonance
angiography
3DFT volume imaging
DGC
directional gradient concentration
dGEMRIC
delayed gadolinium-enhanced magnetic
resonance imaging of cartilage
DGHAL
Doppler-guided hemorrhoid artery
ligation
DGR
duodenogastric reflux
DHCT
dual-phase helical computed tomography
DHS screw
DI
diagnostic imaging
Di
D. Guglielmo disease
D. Guglielmo syndrome
diabetes
gestational d.
d. mellitus, type 1
d. mellitus, type 2
diabetic
d. cardiomyopathy
d. gastroparesis
d. ketoacidosis
d. mastopathy
d. nephropathy
diacondylar fracture
diagniol
DIAGNOdent laser
diagnosis, pl. **diagnoses**
computer-aided d. (CAD)
prenatal d.
prospective investigation of
pulmonary embolus d. (PIOPED)
radiologic d.
roentgenographic d.
sonographic d.
ultrasound d.
Diagnost 120
diagnostic
d. angiography
d. cascade
d. efficacy analysis
d. imaging (DI)
d. mammography
d. modality
d. pneumoperitoneum
d. pneumothorax
d. procedure
d. puncture
d. radiation
d. radioiodine scanning (DxRaI)
d. radiology

d. radiopharmaceutical
d. range ultrasound
d. skull series
d. teleradiology
d. and therapeutic technology
assessment
d. x-ray camera and imaging
source
d. yield
diagonal
d. branch
d. branch of artery
d. conjugate diameter
diagram
energy level d. (ELD)
Ladder d.
marker-channel d.
Zurich growth centile d.
diagrammatic radiography
dialysis
d. arthropathy
d. fistula
d. shunt
d. tube
diamagnetic
d. shift
d. substance
d. susceptibility
diamagnetism
Landau d.
diametaphysial
diametaphysis
diameter
acetabular depth-to-femoral head d.
(AD/FHD)
anterior sagittal d. (ASD)
anterior-to-posterior sagittal canal d.
anteroposterior d.
aortic d. (AD)
aortic root d.
artery d.
Baudelocque d.
bicristal d.
biischial d.
biparietal d. (BPD)
bisacromial d.
bispinous d.
bitemporal d.
bituberous d.
bronchial d.
cardiac d.
cecum d.
coccygeopubic d.
coil-to-vessel d.
conjugate d.
cranial d.
craniometric d.
cricopharyngeal d.
Deventer d.

diagonal conjugate d.
film d.
frontomental d.
frontooccipital d.
gestational sac d.
GS d.
increased anteroposterior d.
increment in luminal d.
inferior longitudinal d.
intercristal d.
internal d. (ID)
internal conjugate d.
intertubercular d.
left anterior internal d. (LAID)
left ventricular internal d. (LVID)
Löhlein d., Loehlein d.
lumen d.
maximum anteroposterior d.
maximum short-axis d. (MSAD)
mean sac d. (MSD)
mentooccipital d.
mentoparietal d.
midsagittal d. (MSD)
minimal luminal d. (MLD)
minimal port d. (MPD)
narrow anteroposterior d.
d. obliqua pelvis
oblique d.
occipitofrontal d. (OFD)
occipitomental d.
orthonormal d.
parietal d.
pelvic d.
posterotransverse d.
pyloric d.
right ventricular internal d. (RVID)
sacropubic d.
sagittal canal d. (SCD)
spinal cord d.
spleen d.
stenosis d.
suboccipitobregmatic d.
temporal d.
d. transversa pelvis
transverse cerebellar d. (TCD)
transverse pelvic d.
ureter d.
valve d.
vertebromammary d.
vertical d.
vessel d.
yolk sac d.

diametric pelvic fracture
diamniotic pregnancy
Diamond-Blackfan syndrome
diapedesis
diaphanography
diaphanoscope
diaphragm
    above d. (AD)
    accessory d.
    antral mucosal d.
    aperture d.
    aponeurotic portion of d.
    below d. (BD)
    bilateral elevation of d.
    Bucky d.
    central tendon d.
    costal part of d.
    crus of the d.
    depressed d.
    dome of d.
    duodenal d.
    d. duplication
    elevated d.
    d. embryology
    eventration of d.
    excursion of d.
    flattening of d.
    free air under d.
    gastric d.
    inferior vena cava d.
    leaf of d.
    lumbar part of d.
    median arcuate ligament of d.
    muscular crus of d.
    paralysis of d.
    pelvic d.
    polyarcuate d.
    Potter-Bucky d.
    respiratory d.
    sella turcica d.
    sternal part of d.
    sternocostal part of d.
    tenting of d.
    thoracoabdominal d.
    traumatic rupture of d. (TRD)
    urogenital d.
    vertebral part of d.
diaphragma sella
diaphragmatic
    d. attenuation
    d. border
    d. contour

D

NOTES

diaphragmatic *(continued)*
   d. creep
   d. crus
   d. cupula
   d. dome
   d. echo
   d. elevation
   d. esophageal hiatus
   d. eventration
   d. fascia
   d. hernia
   d. hump
   d. ligament
   d. lymph node
   d. myocardial infarct (DMI)
   d. paralysis
   d. pericardium
   d. pleura
   d. pleurisy
   d. rupture
   d. sarcoma
   d. segment
   d. slip
   d. surface
   d. surface of heart
   d. surface of liver
diaphysial, diaphyseal
   d. aclasis
   d. bone length ratio
   d. center
   d. cortical mortise
   d. dysplasia
   d. fracture
   d. lesion
   d. ossification
   d. sclerosis
diaphysial-epiphysial fusion
diaphysis, pl. **diaphyses**
diaphysitis
   luetic d.
diaplasis
diapositive
diarthrodial intervertebral joint
diarthrosis
diaschisis
   cerebellar d.
   crossed cerebellar d.
   ipsilateral cortical d.
diascope
diascopy
Diasonics
   D. ultrasound
   D. ultrasound scanner
diastasis
   d. of cranial bone
   fracture d.
   d. heart period
   d. of suture

   syndesmotic d.
   tibiofibular d.
diastatic
   d. fracture
   d. lambdoid suture
diastematomyelia
   spinal d.
diastolic
   d. atrial volume
   d. counterpulsation
   d. depolarization phase
   d. depolarization pulse
   d. doming
   d. filling period
   d. filling pressure (DFP)
   d. gating
   d. gradient
   d. heart failure
   d. left ventricular index
   d. notch impedance
   d. overload
   d. perfusion pressure
   d. perfusion time
   d. pressure-time index (DPTI)
   d. pseudogating
   d. regurgitant velocity
   d. reserve
   d. velocity ratio
   d. zero flow
diastrophic
   d. dwarfism
   d. dysplasia
diathermic
   d. loop
   d. vascular occlusion
diathermy ultrasound
diathesis, pl. **diatheses**
   hypertensive d.
diatrizoate
   meglumine d.
   d. meglumine imaging agent
   methylglucamine d.
   d. sodium imaging agent
diatrizoic acid contrast medium
DIC
   disseminated intravascular coagulation
   drip infusion cholangiogram
   drip infusion cholangiography
dicephalus
dichorionic, dichorial
   d. diamniotic twin pregnancy
dichorionic-diamniotic twin
dichromate
   d. dosimeter
   d. dosimetry
Dickhaut-DeLee discoid meniscus classification
Dickinson
   Becton D. (B-D)

DICOM
  Digital Imaging and Communications in
    Medicine
  DICOM format
DICOM-3 compatible digital computer
format
dicondylar fracture
Dicopac test
dicrotic notch
DID
  document image decoding
DIDA
  dimethyl iminodiacetic acid
didactylism
didelphia
  uterine d.
didelphic uterus
didelphys
  uterine d.
dielectric track detector
diencephalic herniation
diencephalon, pl. **diencephala**
die-punch fracture
DIET
  DIET fast SE imaging
  DIET method of fat suppression
diet cola and metoclopramide syrup
diethylenetriaminepentaacetic
  d. acid (DTPA)
  d. acid imaging agent
Dieulafoy
  D. disease
  D. lesion
  D. vascular malformation
DiFerrante syndrome
difference
  field-echo d.
  hemispheric regional
    lateralization d.
  potential d.
  rib-vertebral angle d.
  transient hepatic attenuation d.
    (THAD)
differencing
  convolutional d.
  d. fiber
  d. filter
differential
  d. diagnosis bone lesion
  d. diagnostic lung mass feature
  d. interference contrast microscopy
  renal function d.

scintillation camera linearity d.
scintillation camera uniformity d.
d. signal
d. uniformity
d. uptake ratio
d. washout
differentiated carcinoma (DC)
differentiation
  cluster of d. (CD)
  corticomedullary d. (CMD)
  gray matter–white matter d.
  gray-white d.
  liposarcomatous d.
  nuclear anular d.
difficult-to-treat vascular lesion
diffracting Doppler transducer
diffraction
  beam d.
  high-resolution d.
  high-temperature d.
  low-temperature d.
  d. pattern
  d. peak
  x-ray d.
diffraction-enhanced imaging (DEI)
diffuse
  d. abdominal calcification
  d. adenomyosis
  d. aggressive lymphoma
  d. aggressive polymorphous
    infiltrate
  d. airspace disease
  d. airspace opacity
  d. alveolar damage
  d. alveolar interstitial infiltrate
  d. aortic atresia
  d. aortic dilatation
  d. aortomegaly
  d. arterial ectasia
  d. arteriolar spasm
  d. aspiration bronchiolitis
  d. axonal injury (DAI)
  d. bacterial nephritis
  d. bilateral alveolar infiltrate
  d. cerebral histiocytosis
  d. cirrhosis
  d. CNS sclerosis
  d. contrast agent distribution
    pattern
  d. dilation of esophagus
  d. edema
  d. emphysema

D

NOTES

diffuse *(continued)*
- d. enlargement of the thymus
- d. esophageal spasm (DES)
- d. fatty liver infiltrate
- d. fibrosis type
- d. fine lung reticulation
- d. gallbladder wall thickening
- d. ganglion
- d. haziness
- d. hepatic enlargement
- d. hyperemia
- d. idiopathic skeletal hyperostosis (DISH)
- d. increase in breast density
- d. infection
- d. inflammation
- d. intermediate lymphocytic lymphoma
- d. interstitial pulmonary fibrosis (DIPF)
- d. intimal thickening
- d. irregularity
- d. large-cell lymphoma (DLCL)
- d. leiomyomatosis
- d. liver enlargement
- d. low attenuation
- d. low signal replacement of vertebral body
- d. lung uptake
- d. lymphangioma
- d. malformation
- d. malignant peritoneal mesothelioma
- d. mixed small- and large-cell lymphoma
- d. mottling
- d. mucosal polyposis
- d. multinodular infarction
- d. myelinoclastic sclerosis
- d. narrowing
- d. necrosis
- d. necrotizing leukoencephalopathy
- d. osteosclerosis
- d. panbronchiolitis
- d. pancreatitis
- d. parenchymal lung disease
- d. periapical sclerosing osteitis
- d. pericarditis
- d. perivascular infiltrate
- d. pleural thickening
- d. pleurisy
- d. pneumonia
- d. pneumonitis
- d. pulmonary alveolar hemorrhage
- d. pulmonary neuroendocrine cell hyperplasia
- d. reflector
- d. reticular density
- d. reticulogranular lung density
- d. reticulonodular infiltrate
- d. sarcomatosis
- d. scleroderma
- d. sclerosing alveolitis
- d. signal hyperintensity
- d. skeletal angiomatosis
- d. skeletal metastasis
- d. small-cell lymphocytic lymphoma
- d. spasm of esophagus
- d. spatial distribution
- d. spondylosis
- d. stenosis
- d. stippled calcification
- d. subarachnoid hemorrhage
- d. symmetric hypertrophied cardiomyopathy
- d. synovial lipoma
- d. thymic enlargement
- d. toxic goiter
- d. ulcerative lesion
- d. uterine enlargement
- d. ventricular hypokinesis
- d. white matter injury

diffusible tracer
diffusing capacity
diffusion
- anisotropically rotational d. (ARD)
- d. anisotropy thresholding
- d. characteristics of water
- d. coefficient
- directional d.
- d. encoding strength
- d. factor
- Fick first law of d.
- d. gradient
- d. magnetic resonance imaging
- molecular d.
- d. MRI
- d. pulse sequence
- restricted d.
- restricted water d.
- d. scan
- spectral d.
- d. spectroscopy
- spin d.
- d. tension (DT)
- d. tension imaging (DTI)
- d. tensor (DT)
- d. tensor imaging (DTI)
- d. tensor MR imaging
- thermal d.
- d. time
- translational d.

diffusional anisotropy
diffusion-perfusion mismatch
diffusion/perfusion snapshot FLASH (DPSF)
diffusion-sensitive sequence
diffusion-sensitizing gradient

diffusion-weighted
> d.-w. echo planar imaging
> d.-w. image
> d.-w. imaging (DWI)
> d.-w. magnetic resonance imaging
> d.-w. MR imaging
> d.-w. pulse sequence
> d.-w. scanning

diffusivity
> mean d.
> white matter d.

diffusum
> papilloma d.

digastric
> d. fossa
> d. groove
> d. impression
> d. line
> d. muscle
> d. notch
> d. triangle

DiGeorge syndrome

digestive
> d. system
> d. tract
> d. tract content
> d. tube

digestive-respiratory fistula

DIGGEST
> direct imaging of local gradients by
> group echo selection tomography

Digibar 190 contrast agent

Digirad
> D. gamma camera
> D. 2020 TC imager
> D. 2020tc imager

Digiscope
> Direx D.

digit
> accessory d.
> arthrodesed d.
> binary d.
> fibroosseous pseudotumor of d.
> flail d.
> photoplethysmographic d.
> replanted d.
> sausage d.
> supernumerary d.
> syndactylization of d.

digital
> d. abdominal radiograph

> d. Add-On Bucky image
> acquisition imaging system
> D. Add-On Bucky radiographic
> detector image acquisition system
> d. amorphous silicon flat-panel
> detector
> d. amputation
> d. aponeurosis
> d. artery of foot
> d. artery of hand
> d. autofluoroscope
> d. autopsy
> d. axial tomography (DAT)
> d. beam attenuation
> d. branch
> d. celiac trunk angiography
> d. chest imaging
> d. chest imaging system
> d. chest radiograph
> d. deformity
> d. ejection fraction
> D. Equipment system
> d. extensor tendon
> d. flat-panel amorphous silicon
> detector-radiography system
> d. flexor tendon
> d. fluorography
> d. fluoroscopy
> d. fossa
> d. free hepatic venography
> d. frequency analysis
> d. fundus imager
> d. gray scale
> d. high-speed endoscopy
> d. holography system
> d. image processing algorithm
> D. Imaging and Communications in
> Medicine (DICOM)
> d. imaging processing (DIP)
> d. isotope calibrator
> d. livedo reticularis infarct
> d. mammographic system
> d. mammography
> d. marking
> D. Medical system
> d. neuroma
> D. OsteoView 2000
> d. parabola
> d. plethysmography
> d. process of fat
> d. pulsed fluoroscopy (DPF)
> d. radiography (DR)

D

NOTES

digital *(continued)*
 d. radiography imaging
 d. ray
 d. rectal evacuation
 d. reformatting knee MRI
 d. road mapping
 d. rotational angiography (DRA)
 d. runoff
 d. sampling rate
 d. selenium-based chest imaging
  system
 d. storage
 d. subtraction
 d. subtraction angiogram
 d. subtraction angiography (DSA)
 d. subtraction aortography
 d. subtraction arteriography (DSA)
 d. subtraction film
 d. subtraction mammography
  (DSM)
 d. subtraction pulmonary angiogram
 d. subtraction rotational angiography
 d. subtraction technique
 d. subtraction ventriculogram
 d. tomosynthesis
 D. Traumex system
 d. unraveling
 d. vascular imaging (DVI, DVI
  mode)
 d. vein
 d. videoangiography
 d. video gastrointestinal radiography
 d. x-ray detector
digitalization noise
digitally
 d. fused CT and radiolabeled
  imaging
 d. fused CT and radiolabeled
  monoclonal antibody SPECT
  image
 d. reconstructed radiograph (DRR)
digital-to-analog converter (DAC)
digitate ectasia
digiti (*pl. of* digitus)
digitization
digitized
 d. contact mammogram
 d. CT slice
 d. film image
 d. spinography
digitizer
 backlit d.
 3D surface d.
 laser d.
 multiple jointed d.
 multisensor structured light
  range d.
 Polhemus 3D d.

digitorum
 extensor d.
Digitron
 D. digital subtraction imaging
  system
 D. Koordinat angiography
  equipment
dihydropyrimidine dehydrogenase
 activity
dihydroxyphenylalanine (DOPA)
 d. imaging agent
diiodotyrosine
dilacerated tooth root
dilatation, dilation
 alveolar d.
 d. of aneurysm
 antegrade transluminal balloon d.
 anular d.
 aortic root d.
 arterial d.
 ascending aorta d.
 balloon d.
 beaded ductal d.
 bile duct d.
 biliary d.
 bowel loop d.
 bronchial d.
 bronchiolar d.
 calyceal d.
 cardiac d.
 cavitary d.
 chamber d.
 colonic d.
 common duct d.
 congenital cystic d.
 cystic d.
 diffuse aortic d.
 distal ureteral d.
 ductal d.
 Eder-Puestow d.
 esophageal d.
 extrahepatic biliary cystic d.
 fusiform d.
 gaseous d.
 gastric d.
 hepatic web d.
 d. and hypertrophy
 idiopathic pulmonary artery d.
 idiopathic right atrial d.
 intestinal d.
 intrahepatic biliary cystic d.
 intrahepatic biliary ductal d.
 intrahepatic biliary tract d.
 intraluminal d.
 junctional d.
 left ventricular d.
 megacolon d.
 multiple mural d.'s
 mural d.

myocardial d.
pancreatic duct d.
paradoxic colon d.
pelvicalyceal d.
percutaneous transluminal balloon d.
periportal sinusoidal d.
pharmacologic d.
poststenotic d.
prestenotic d.
probe d.
prognathic d.
proximal esophagitis d.
pulmonary artery d.
pulmonary trunk idiopathic d.
pulmonary valve stenosis d.
rectal d.
respiratory bronchiolar d.
right ventricular d.
saccular d.
stress-induced left ventricular d.
sulcal d.
sulcus d.
d. of sulcus
thickened irregular small bowel
  fold d.
thickened smooth small bowel
  fold d.
tortuous vein d.
track d.
transient left ventricular d.
transluminal d.
tubular d.
d. of ureter
ureteral d.
vein d.
d. of ventricle
ventricular wall d.
Virchow-Robin space d.
Wirsung d.

dilated

d. aortic root
d. bile duct
d. bowel loop
d. bronchus
d. cardiomyopathy (DCM)
d. collateral vein
d. descending aorta
d. dry small bowel
d. duodenum
d. esophagus
d. fetal bowel
d. gallbladder

d. intercavernous sinus
d. intrahepatic duct
d. loops of bowel
d. lymphatic
d. mammary duct
d. myocardium
d. pulmonary artery
d. pulmonary trunk
d. rete testis
d. small airway
d. subareolar duct
d. ureter
d. ventricle
d. wet small bowel

dilation

aneurysmal d.
aortic d.
proximal d.

dilator

angiographic Teflon d.
balloon d.
Teflon d.
Teflon fascial d.
telescopic aerial d.

dilution

isotopic d.
ultrasound d.

DIMAQ integrated ultrasound
workstation

dimeglumine

gadopentetate d. (Gd-DTPA)
gadopentetate d. (Gd-DTPA)
Magnevist gadopentate d.

dimension

abnormal heart chamber d.
absolute artery d.
anteroposterior d.
aortic root d.
arterial d.
axial d.
fractal d. (FD)
intraluminal d.
intrathoracic d.
left ventricular diastolic d. (LVdd)
left ventricular end-diastolic d.
  (LVEDD)
left ventricular end-systolic d.
  (LVESD)
left ventricular internal diastolic d.
  (LVIDd, LVIDD)
lumbar spine d.
luminal d.

NOTES

D

dimension *(continued)*
    right ventricular d. (RVD)
    spleen d.
1-dimensional
    1-d. chemical-shift imaging (1D-CSI)
    1-d. phase encoding
2-dimensional (2D) *(See* 2D*)*
    2-d. cross-sectional echocardiography
    2-d. echocardiography (TDE)
    2-d. Fourier transform (2DFT)
    2-d. magnetic resonance digital subtraction angiography
    2-d. time-of-flight (2D TOF)
3-dimensional (3D) *(See* 3D*)*
    3-d. analysis
    3-d. conformal radiotherapy
    3-d. contrast-enhanced (3DCE)
    3-d. contrast-enhanced MR angiography
    3-d. digital subtraction angiography (3D-DSA)
    3-d. Fourier transform (3DFT)
    3-d. Fourier transform volume image
    3-d. magnetic resonance angiography
    3-D. Perfusion/Motion Map software
    3-d. trabecular bone microstructure
4-dimensional (4D) *(See* 4D*)*
    4-d. image
    4-d. imaging
dimer
    d. captosuccinic acid (DMSA)
    ethyl cysteinate d. (ECD)
    ionic hexaiodinated d.
    ^{99m}Tc ethyl cysteinate d. (EDC)
    ^{99m}technetium L-ethyl cysteinate d.
    technetium-99m ethyl cysteinate d. (^{99m}Tc-ECD)
    D. x
dimerization
3,4-dimethoxyphenyl-ethylamine (DMPE)
dimethyl iminodiacetic acid (DIDA)
dimethylsuccinic acid
diminished
    d. airway perfusion
    d. lung volume
    d. marrow signal intensity
    d. systemic perfusion
diminutive
    d. interlobar right pulmonary artery
    d. vessel
dimple
    blind d.
    d. of bone
    pretibial d.

dinner-fork deformity
diode
    d. detector
    infrared light-emitting d.
    d. laser
    d. measurement
    Palomar SLP1000 d.
    PIN d.
    positive-intrinsic-negative d.
    Zener d.
diodone
Diodrast
Diogenes cup
Diomed
    D. EVLT laser
    D. 630 PDT laser model T2USA
Dionosil imaging agent
dioxide
    carbon d. (CO_2)
    radiopaque medium thorium d.
    titanium d.
DIP
    desquamative interstitial pneumonia
    digital imaging processing
    distal interphalangeal
    DIP algorithm
    DIP articulation
    DIP joint
dip
    apical d.
    d. phenomenon
    septal d.
DIPF
    diffuse interstitial pulmonary fibrosis
diphosphate
    dipyridoxal d.
    manganese dipyridoxyl d.
diphosphine
    lipophilic cationic d.
diphosphonate
    methylene d. (MDP)
diplegia spinalis brachialis traumatica
diploë
diplogram
diploic
    d. canal
    d. vein
diplomyelia
dipolar
    d. broadening
    d. interaction
dipole
    d. coupling
    electric d.
    d. field
    magnetic d.
dipole-dipole
    d.-d. coupling
    d.-d. interaction

proton electron d.-d.
d.-d. relaxation rate
diprosopus
DIPS
 direct intrahepatic portacaval shunt
dipygus
dipyridamole
 d. echocardiography
 d. echocardiography imaging
 d. handgrip imaging
 d. handgrip test
 d. infusion imaging
 d. technetium-99m-2-methoxy
   isobutyl
 d. technetium-99m-2-methoxy
   isobutyl isonitrile
 d. thallium-201 imaging
 d. thallium-201 scintigraphy
 d. thallium stress imaging
 d. thallium ventriculogram
dipyridoxal diphosphate
direct
 d. caval cannulation
 d. current (DC)
 d. current generator
 d. current offset artifact
 d. digital radiography
 d. display console (DDC)
 d. embolus
 d. Fourier transformation imaging
 d. fracture
 d. imaging of local gradients by
   group echo selection tomography
   (DIGGEST)
 d. immunofluorescence analysis
 d. inguinal hernia
 d. intrahepatic portacaval shunt
   (DIPS)
 d. liquid scintillation count
 d. needle puncture
 d. percutaneous transhepatic
   cholangiography
 d. puncture MR phlebogram
 d. puncture phlebography
 d. radiation
 d. radioiodination
 d. ray
 d. slice
 d. spiral computed tomography
   venography
 d. splenoportography
 d. transtorcular approach

 d. venography
 d. vision spectroscope
 d. visualization
direct-contact transmission
direction
 aboral d.
 anterior-posterior flow d.
 caudal d.
 cephalad d.
 cephalad-caudad d.
 mediolateral flow d.
 noncollinear d.
 phase-encoding d.
 superior-inferior flow d.
 white matter tract d.
directional
 d. atherectomy catheter
 d. atherectomy device
 d. color angiography (DCA)
 d. coronary atherectomy (DCA)
 d. diffusion
 d. gradient concentration (DGC)
direction-encoded color mapping (DEC)
directives
 advance d.
director
 grooved d.
DirectRay direct-to-digital image capture device
DirectView CR 900 imaging system
Direx
 D. Digiscope
 D. Thermex
 D. Tripter
dirty
 d. acoustic shadowing
 d. chest
 d. fat
 d. film artifact
 d. mass
 d. necrosis
disappearance
 d. frequency
 d. slope
disappearing
 d. bone disease
 d. fetus
disarray
 myocardial d.
disarticulation
 hip d.

D

NOTES

disc, disk

acromioclavicular joint d.
anal d.
d. of ankle
anterior intervertebral d.
articular d.
atrial d.
d. ballooning
biconcave d.
bilocular d.
Bowman d.
d. bulge
d. calcification
candle drip d.
cartilaginous d.
cervical d.
chorionic d.
concave skull d.
cone d.
contained d.
crescent-shaped fibrocartilaginous d.
d. degeneration
degenerative d.
d. derangement
d. desiccation
d. disease
d. displacement
distal radioulnar d.
embryonic d.
d. of endocardium
Engelmann d.
epiphysial d.
extruded d.
d. extrusion
fibrocartilaginous d.
fibrous ring of d.
fixation d.
d. fragment
frayed d.
growth d.
H d.
herniated intervertebral d. (HID)
d. herniation
hydrodynamic potential of d.
interarticular d.
d. interspace
intervertebral d.
isotropic d.
kidney d.
d. lesion
locking d.
lumbar d.
lumbosacral d.
magnetic d.
mandibular d.
d. margin
massive herniated d.
d. maturation
midline herniation of d.

Molnar d.
d. morphology
occult residual herniated d.
d. ossification
d. oxygenator
placental d.
d. plication
d. poppet
protruded d.
d. protrusion
rectangular d.
ruptured d.
sequestered d.
d. sequestration
d. space
d. space height
d. space infection
d. space narrowing
spheric d.
sternoclavicular joint d.
tactile d.
temporomandibular joint d.
thoracic d.
thoracolumbar vertebral d.
d. tissue
triangular d.
unilocular d.
vertebral d.
d. water content
Winchester d.

discectomy, diskectomy

automated percutaneous lumbar d.
(APLD)
percutaneous automated d.
same-day microsurgical arthroscopic
lateral-approach laser-assisted
fluoroscopic d.
stereotactic percutaneous lumbar d.

discernible venous motion

discharge

periodic synchronous d. (PSD)
sympathetic d.
d. tube

discharging tubule

disci (*pl. of* discus)

discitis, diskitis

calcific d.
childhood d.
juvenile calcific d.
septic d.

disclike atelectasis

discogenic

d. disease
d. osteophyte

discogram, diskogram

intervertebral d.
intranuclear d.

discographer, diskographer

discographic technique

discography, diskography
discoid
    d. atelectasis
    d. chest mass
    d. configuration
    d. filling defect
    d. kidney
    d. lateral meniscus
    d. shadow
discoligamentous complex
disconnected
    d. duct syndrome
    d. pancreatic duct syndrome
discontinuous
    d. density gradient
    d. density gradient centrifugation
    d. imaging
    d. scanning
discordance
    radiologic-pathologic d.
discordant
    d. finding
    d. nodule thyroid
    d. thyroid nodule
    d. twin
discovertebral
    d. infection
    d. osteomyelitis
    d. spondylitis
Discovery
    D. LS imaging system
    D. LS, ST^4 PET/CT scanner
discrepancy
    biomechanics of limb-length d.
    leg-length d. (LLD)
    limb-length d. (LLD)
discrete
    d. area of consolidation
    d. area of effusion
    d. bleeding source
    d. cosine transform (DCT)
    d. focal stenosis
    d. Fourier transform (DFT)
    d. hyperintense focus
    d. hyperintense signal intensity
    d. lesion
    d. mass
    d. narrowing
    d. perihilar density
    d. plaque
    d. pulmonary nodule
    d. segment of normal esophagus

    d. subaortic stenosis
    d. subvalvular aortic stenosis
    (DSAS)
    d. tumor
discriminant analysis
discriminate
discrimination
    density d.
discriminator setting
disc-shaped bone graft
disc-thecal sac interface
disc-to-magnetic
    d.-t.-m. field
    d.-t.-m. field orientation
disc-type valve
discus, pl. **disci**
DISE
    driven inversion spin echo
disease
    acquired cystic kidney d.
    acquired occupational lung d.
    acquired renal cystic d.
    active parenchymal d.
    acyanotic congenital heart d.
    Addison d.
    adrenal medullary d.
    adult polycystic kidney d.
    airflow obstruction d. (AOD)
    airspace d.
    alcoholic liver d. (ALD)
    Alexander d.
    alloimmune d.
    Alpers d.
    alveolar lung d.
    Alzheimer d. (AD)
    aneurysmal d.
    angiomatous d.
    anterior horn cell d.
    aortic valvular d. (AVD)
    aortoiliac occlusive d. (AIOD)
    arterial degenerative d.
    arteriosclerotic cardiovascular d.
    (ASCVD)
    arteriosclerotic heart d. (ASHD)
    arteriosclerotic occlusive d.
    arteriosclerotic peripheral
    vascular d.
    asbestos-related pleural d.
    atheroembolic renal d.
    atherosclerotic cardiovascular d.
    (ASCVD)

D

NOTES

disease *(continued)*
  atherosclerotic carotid artery d.
   (ACAD)
  atherosclerotic peripheral vascular d.
   (ASPVD)
  autosomal dominant polycystic
   kidney d. (ADPKD)
  autosomal recessive polycystic
   kidney d. (ARPKD)
  Bamberger-Marie d.
  benign asbestos-related pleural d.
  benign breast d. (BBD)
  biliary tract d.
  Binswanger d.
  black lung d.
  Blount d.
  Bouchard d.
  Bouillaud d.
  Bourneville d.
  Bourneville-Pringle d.
  brittle bone d.
  Brodie d.
  Bruck d.
  bullous lung d.
  caisson d.
  calcium hydroxyapatite
   deposition d.
  calcium pyrophosphate deposition d.
   (CPPD)
  calcium pyrophosphate dihydrate
   deposition d.
  Calvé-Legg-Perthes d.
  Calvé-Perthes d.
  Camurati-Engelmann d.
  Canavan d.
  Canavan-van Bogaert-Bertrand d.
  cardiopulmonary d.
  cardiorenal d.
  cardiovascular d. (CD, CVD)
  cardiovascular renal d.
  Caroli d.
  carotid artery d.
  carotid atherosclerotic d.
  carotid occlusive d.
  Carrington d.
  Castleman d.
  celiac d.
  central airway d.
  cerebral inflammatory d.
  cerebral Whipple d.
  cerebrovascular occlusive d.
  cervical disc d.
  Charcot-Marie-Tooth d.
  cholestatic liver d.
  chronic beryllium d.
  chronic interstitial simulating
   airspace lung d.
  chronic obstructive lung d. (COLD)

  chronic obstructive pulmonary d.
   (COPD)
  chronic peripheral arterial d.
   (CPAD)
  Coats d.
  Concato d.
  congenital heart d. (CHD)
  connective tissue d.
  coronary artery d.
  Cowden d.
  Creutzfeldt-Jakob d. (CJD)
  Crohn d. (CD)
  crystal deposition d.
  Cushing d.
  cyanotic congenital heart d.
  cystic breast d.
  cystic kidney d.
  cystic ovarian d.
  degenerative atrioventricular node d.
  degenerative brain d.
  degenerative disc d.
  degenerative joint d. (DJD)
  demyelinating d.
  de Quervain d.
  Deutschländer d.
  Dieulafoy d.
  diffuse airspace d.
  diffuse parenchymal lung d.
  Di Guglielmo d.
  disappearing bone d.
  disc d.
  discogenic d.
  disseminated d.
  diverticular colon d.
  Duroziez mitral stenosis d.
  Ekman-Lobstein d.
  end-stage lung d.
  end-stage renal d.
  Engelmann d.
  eosinophilic lung d.
  Erb d.
  Erdheim-Chester d.
  extracolonic d.
  extracranial carotid artery
   occlusive d.
  extramammary Paget d.
  extrathoracic d.
  Fahr d.
  Fairbank d.
  Favre d.
  fibrocystic breast d.
  fibrocystic lung d.
  first trimester gestational
   trophoblastic d.
  Flatau-Schilder d.
  flax-dresser d.
  focal lung d.
  focal small-bowel d.
  Fong d.

Forestier d.
Freiberg d.
Friedreich d.
Fukuyama congenital muscular d.
 (FCMD)
Gandy-Nanta d.
Garré d.
gastroesophageal reflux d. (GERD)
Gaucher d.
Gee-Herter d.
Gee-Thaysen d.
Gerstmann-Sträussler-Scheinker d.
gestational trophoblastic d. (GTD)
Gilchrist d.
Glénard d.
Gorham d.
Graves d.
heart d. (HD)
heavy-chain d.
Heberden d.
hepatic vein d.
hepatic venoocclusive d.
hepatobiliary d.
hepatocerebral d.
Hirschsprung d. (HD)
Hodgkin d. (HD)
Hodgson d.
Hoffa d.
Horton d.
Hunter d.
Huppert d.
hyaline membrane d. (HMD)
hydroxyapatite deposition d.
 (HADD)
hypertensive cardiovascular d.
hypertensive renal d.
hypertensive vascular d.
idiopathic mural endomyocardial d.
ileocolic d.
iliocaval d.
immunoproliferative small
 intestine d. (IPSID)
infantile polycystic kidney d.
infectious heart d.
inflammatory bowel d.
interfollicular Hodgkin d.
interstitial fibrotic lung d.
intracranial stenoocclusive d.
intrasynovial d.
ischemic bowel d.
Jaffe-Lichtenstein d.
Jansen d.

Jansky-Bielschowsky d.
juvenile autosomal recessive
 polycystic d.
juvenile Paget d.
Kahler d.
Kawasaki d.
Keinböck d.
Keshan d.
Kikuchi d.
Kikuchi-Fujimoto d.
Kinnier-Wilson d.
Köhler d.
Krabbe d.
Kugelberg-Welander d.
Kussmaul-Maier d.
kyphoscoliotic heart d.
Legg-Calvé-Perthes d. (LCP)
Leigh d.
leptomeningeal d.
Libman-Sacks endocarditis d.
Lichtenstein-Jaffe d.
light chain deposition d. (LCDD)
liver hydatid d.
local nodal d.
locoregional d.
maple bark d.
maple syrup urine d.
marble bone d.
Marchiafava-Bignami d.
Marie-Bamberger d.
Marie-Strümpell d.
Martin d.
medullary cystic d.
Ménétrier d.
Ménière d.
mesenteric Weber-Christian d.
metabolic bone d.
metastatic d.
microvascular d.
Mikulicz d.
miliary lung d.
miliary parenchymal d.
Milroy d.
mixed connective-tissue d. (MCTD)
Mondor d.
monostotic Paget d.
moyamoya d.
multicentric Castleman d. (MCD)
multiple gland d.
multisegment d.
muscle-eye-brain d.
mushroom picker's d.

D

NOTES

disease *(continued)*

neonatal wet lung d.
neurodegenerative d.
Niemann-Pick d.
Nievergelt d.
nodal d.
nodular lung d.
nodular sclerosis Hodgkin d.
nodular thyroid d.
no evidence of d. (NED)
no evidence of recurrent d. (NERD)
nonatherosclerotic d.
Norrie d.
obstructive airway d.
obstructive lung d.
obstructive pulmonary d. (OPD)
occlusive cerebrovascular d.
occupational lung d.
Ollier d.
optic chiasm d.
Ormond d.
Osgood-Schlatter d.
Osler d.
osseous metastatic d.
Otto d.
Paas d.
Paget jaw d.
pancreatic d.
pancreaticobiliary d.
Panner d.
Parenti-Fraccaro d.
Pelizaeus-Merzbacher d.
Pellegrini-Stieda d.
pelvic inflammatory d.
peptic ulcer d. (PUD)
pericardial d.
perihilar lung d.
periodontal d.
peripheral airspace d.
peripheral arterial d.
peripheral arterial occlusive d. (PAOD)
peripheral lung d.
peripheral vascular d. (PVD)
peripheral vascular occlusive d.
Perthes d.
Peyronie d.
Pfaundler-Hurler d.
Pfeiffer d.
Pick d.
pleural d.
Plummer d.
polycystic kidney d.
polycystic liver d.
polycystic ovarian d. (PCOD)
Pompe d.
popliteal artery occlusive d.
posttransplant coronary artery d.

Pott d.
prediverticular d.
Preiser d.
primary pigmented nodular adrenocortical d.
pseudo-Whipple d.
pulmonary embolic septic d.
pulmonary interstitial d.
pulmonary thromboembolic d.
Pyle d.
radiation-induced liver d. (RILD)
ragpicker's d.
reactive airway d. (RAD)
renal cystic d.
renal parenchymal d.
renovascular d.
respiratory bronchiolitis-associated interstitial lung d. (RB-ILD)
restrictive lung d.
restrictive myocardial d.
reticulonodular lung d.
reversible airway d.
rheumatic heart d.
rheumatic valvular d.
rheumatoid lung d.
Ribbing d.
Roger d.
Rosai-Dorfman d.
Rutherford clinical stage (peripheral vascular d.)
Ruysch d.
sacroiliac d.
Salla d.
Santavuori-Haltia d.
Scheuermann d.
Schilder d.
Schmid d.
Schmorl d.
Sever d.
Shaver d.
silo-filler's d.
Simmond d.
Sinding-Larsen-Johansson d. (SLJD)
single-vessel d.
small bowel d.
Spielmeyer-Vogt d.
Still d.
subarachnoid metastatic d.
subarachnoid space d.
synchronous d.
systemic granulomatous d.
Takayasu d.
thromboembolic d. (TED)
thromboembolic lung d.
thyrocardiac d.
thyroid d.
tibial artery d.
tibioperoneal occlusive d.
toxic lung d.

Trevor d.
Uhl d.
ulcer d.
"undercalling" d.
upper lung d.
upper respiratory tract d.
valvular d. (VD)
valvular heart d.
van Buchem d.
vanishing bone d.
Vaquez d.
variant Creutzfeldt-Jacob d. (vCJD)
vascular occlusive d.
venous occlusive d.
venous thromboembolic d. (VTED)
venous thrombotic d.
vertebrobasilar d.
3-vessel coronary d.
von Recklinghausen d.
von Willebrand d.
Voorhoeve d.
Vrolik d.
Warburg d.
Warfarin-Aspirin Symptomatic
  Intracranial D. (WASID)
Werdnig-Hoffmann d.
Werner classification (thyroid
  eye d.)
Westphal-Strümpell d.
Whipple d.
white matter d.
Wilson d.
Winiwarter-Buerger d.
Zuska d.
disease-free vessel
DISH
  diffuse idiopathic skeletal hyperostosis
dishpan fracture
DISI
  dorsal intercalated segmental instability
disintegration
  d. constant
  myofibrillar d.
  nuclear d.
  radioactive d.
  d. rate
  spontaneous d.
disintegrator
  electrohydraulic d.
disjointing
disk (*var. of* disc)
Disk-Criminator

diskectomy (*var. of* discectomy)
diskitis (*var. of* discitis)
diskogram (*var. of* discogram)
diskographer (*var. of* discographer)
diskography (*var. of* discography)
dislocated
  d. hip
  d. knee
dislocation
  anterior d.
  anteroinferior d.
  atlantooccipital d.
  axial carpal d.
  Bankart d.
  bayonet d.
  Bennett d.
  bilateral intrafacetal d.
  boutonnière d.
  bursting d.
  central d.
  cervical facet d.
  chronic recurrent d.
  closed d.
  complete d.
  complicated d.
  compound d.
  congenital hip d.
  consecutive d.
  Desault d.
  divergent d.
  dysplasia d.
  facet d.
  fracture d.
  frank d.
  glenohumeral d.
  Hill-Sachs d.
  hip d.
  hyperextension d.
  incomplete d.
  interfacetal d.
  interphalangeal d.
  irreducible dorsal d.
  isolated d.
  joint d.
  Kienböck d.
  Lisfranc d.
  lunate d.
  midcarpal d.
  milkmaid's elbow d.
  Monteggia d.
  Nélaton d.
  open d.

D

NOTES

dislocation *(continued)*
    partial d.
    d. of patella
    patellar d.
    pathologic d.
    perilunar d.
    perilunate d.
    primitive d.
    radiocarpal d.
    recent d.
    recurrent d.
    rotational d.
    scapholunate d.
    shoulder d.
    simple d.
    Smith d.
    sternoclavicular d.
    subastragalar d.
    subspinous d.
    tibiofemoral joint d.
    tibiotarsal d.
    transradial styloid perilunate d.
    transscaphoid perilunate d.
    traumatic d.
    triquetrolunate d.
    unilateral facet d.
    unilateral interfacetal d.
    unilateral intrafacetal d.
    upward and backward d.
    upward lens d.
    volar d.
    wrist d.
dislodgement
    partial d.
dismutase
    copper-zinc superoxide d. (Cu/Zn-SOD)
    superoxide d.
disobliteration
    carotid d.
disodium
    pamidronate d.
disofenin
    technetium-99m d.
disorder
    angiocentric immunoproliferative d.
    angitis-granulomatosis d.
    articular hand d.
    articular wrist d.
    bullous d.
    cartilaginous growth plate d.
    congenital d.
    deglutition d.
    demyelinative d.
    drug-induced bullous d.
    esophageal functional d.
    esophageal morphologic d.
    esophageal motility d.
    evacuation d.

    functional d.
    gastric motor d.
    infectious pulmonary d.
    intractable bleeding d.
    lymphoproliferative d.
    metabolic bone d.
    migration d.
    motility d.
    myeloproliferative d.
    neurogenic d.
    nonspecific esophageal motility d. (NEMD)
    patellofemoral d.
    posttransplant lymphoproliferative d.
    pulmonary lymphoid d.
    surfactant deficiency d. (SDD)
    systemic d.
    underlying d.
disorganized
    d. architecture
    d. folia
dispenser
    film d.
dispersing agent
dispersion
    gradient-induced phase d.
    intravoxel phase d.
    d. mode
dispersive component
disphenoid extraction
displaced
    d. crus
    d. fracture
    d. fracture fragment
    d. fragment of bone
    d. gallbladder
    d. left paraspinal line
    d. left ventricular apex
    d. osteochondral fragment
    d. vertebra
displacement
    anterior tracheal d.
    arterial brain d.
    atlantoaxial rotary d.
    d. of bowel gas
    brainstem d.
    d. of brain vessel
    breast tissue d.
    disc d.
    Ellis Jones peroneal d.
    esophageal d.
    d. field-fitting MR imaging
    hilar d.
    inferior d.
    d. of interhemispheric fissure
    left apexcardiogram, calibrated d. (LACD)
    mediastinum d.
    palmar d.

d. placentogram (DPG)
radial epiphysial d.
retroperitoneal fat stripe d.
rotational d.
superolateral d.
tracheal d.

display
A-mode d.
B-mode d.
cine-mode d.
d. coordinate system
dynamic volume-rendered d.
image d.
M-mode d.
multiparametric color composite d.
multiplanar d. (MPD)
real-time d.
segmentation method for real-
time d.
shaded surface d.
stack mode d.
static image d.
surface shaded d. (SSD)
d. system
tile mode d.

disposable thermometer
disproportion
cephalopelvic d. (CPD)
fetal-pelvic d.
fetal ventricular heart d.
fiber-type d.
ventricular d.

disproportionate upper septal thickening
disrupted plaque
disruption
anastomotic d.
anterior labral d.
anular d.
blood-brain barrier d.
bony d.
d. of cartilaginous synchondrosis
d. of duct
epiglottic d.
facet capsule d.
glenoid articular rim d. (GARD)
glenolabral articular cartilage d.
(GLAD)
ligamentous d.
lymphatic needle d.
myofascial d.
retinacular d.
skeletal d.

superior peroneal retinaculum d.
supraspinous ligament d.
trabecular d.
traumatic aortic d.
volar radiocarpal ligament d.

dissecans
osteochondritis d.
osteochondrosis d.

dissecting
d. abdominal aneurysm
d. aortic aneurysm
d. aortic hematoma
d. basilar artery aneurysm
d. intracranial aneurysm
d. intramural hematoma

dissection
aneurysmal d.
aortic d.
arterial wall d.
d. of artery
axial joint d.
celiac artery d.
descending aorta d.
esophageal d.
extensive d.
extracapsular d.
extrapericardial d.
familial aortic d.
groin d.
intimal-medial d.
medial d.
renal artery d.
sentinel node d.
sharp d.
spiral d.
spontaneous carotid d.
spontaneous coronary artery d.
(SCAD)
Stanford type B aortic d.
subintimal d.
thoracic aortic d.
d. tubercle
type-B aortic d.
vertebral arterial d.

dissector
balloon d.

disseminated
d. CNS histoplasmosis
d. coccidioidomycosis
d. disease
d. inflammation
d. intravascular coagulation (DIC)

D

NOTES

disseminated *(continued)*
    d. intravascular coagulation
      syndrome
    d. lipogranulomatosis
    d. necrotizing leukoencephalopathy
    d. sclerosis
    d. tuberculosis
dissemination
    hematogenous d.
    lymphogenous d.
    d. pattern
Disse space
dissociation
    complete atrioventricular d.
    electromechanical d. (EMD)
    interference d.
    scapholunate d.
dissociative instability
dissolution of gallstone
distal
    d. acinar emphysema
    d. aorta
    d. aortic arch
    d. aortic arch aneurysm
    d. articular set angle (DASA)
    d. bile duct
    d. bile duct carcinoma (DBDC)
    d. blind stomach
    d. bone marrow development
    d. branch
    d. bronchiectasis
    d. bulbar septum
    d. carpal row
    d. circumflex marginal artery
    d. clavicle osteolysis (DCO)
    d. colon
    d. common bile duct obstruction
    d. convoluted tubule
    d. coronary perfusion pressure
    d. coronary sinus (DCS)
    d. duodenum
    d. embolization
    d. esophageal ring
    d. femoral epiphysial fracture
    d. femur
    d. humoral fracture
    d. ileitis
    d. interphalangeal (DIP)
    d. interphalangeal joint
    d. intestinal obstruction syndrome
    d. leak type I
    d. leg cross section
    d. line of reference (DLR)
    d. lobular emphysema
    d. metatarsal articular angle
      (DMMA)
    d. occlusal distention
    d. radial fracture
    d. radioulnar disc

    d. radioulnar joint (DRUJ)
    d. radioulnar joint compartment
    d. radioulnar subluxation
    d. rectal adenocarcinoma (DRA)
    d. reference axis (DRA)
    d. runoff
    d. runoff vessel
    d. segment
    d. shift
    d. small bowel
    d. splenorenal shunt
    d. surface
    d. tibial physis
    d. tibiofibular syndesmosis
    d. tissue bed
    d. ureteral dilatation
distalward
distance
    acromiohumeral d.
    anterior capsular d. (ACD)
    atlas odontoid d.
    center-to-center d.
    central lung d. (CLD)
    Doppler-derived stroke d.
    fanning of the interspinous d.
    film-focus d.
    film tube d.
    flexion interspinous d. (FID)
    focal film d. (FFD)
    focal spot-to-object d.
    focus object d. (FOD)
    focus-skin d. (FSD)
    interarch d.
    intercaudate d.
    interlaminar d.
    internuclear d.
    interopercular d.
    interorbital d.
    interpedicular d.
    interridge d.
    interslice d.
    interspinous d. (ISD)
    interuncal d. (IUD)
    object-film d. (OFD)
    pisoscaphoid d.
    posterior capsular d. (PCD)
    probe-surface d.
    source-film d. (SFD)
    source-skin d. (SSD)
    source-surface d. (SSD)
    source-to-image receptor d. (SID)
    source-tray d. (STD)
    surface d.
    target-film d. (TFD)
    target-skin d. (TSD)
    teardrop d. (TDD)
    ulnotriquetral d.
    widened teardrop d.
distance-based block classification

distant
    d. metastasis
    d. spread
distended
    d. abdomen
    d. central bronchi
    d. gallbladder
    d. kidney
    d. scapulothoracic bursitis
    d. stomach
    d. vein
distensibility
    aortic d.
distensible
distention, distension
    abdominal d.
    alveolar d.
    azygos vein d.
    bladder d.
    bowel d.
    colonic d.
    distal occlusal d.
    d. of esophagogastric region
    gaseous d.
    gastric d.
    hydraulic d.
    intestinal d.
    jugular venous d.
    luminal d.
    maximal radiographic d.
    passive venous d.
    pelvicalyceal d.
    postvagotomy small-bowel d.
    radiographic d.
    d. ratio
    rectal d.
    ureteral d.
    venous d.
    vesical d.
distinction
    loss of d.
distorted
    d. anatomy
    d. mucosal fold
distortion
    architectural d.
    barreling d.
    bronchial d.
    current line d.
    focal d.
    geometric d.
    image d.

    pincushion d.
    radiographic pincushion d.
    S d.
    spiculated d.
    Y-shaped d.
distraction
    bifocal manipulation with d.
    d. of fracture
    d. gap
    d. hyperflexion injury
    joint d.
    d. osteogenesis
    physial d.
    segment d.
    small-step d.
    soft tissue d.
distraction-flexion staging (DFS)
distractor
    intramedullary skeletal kinetic d.
        (ISKD)
distribution
    anatomic d.
    anomalous d.
    apparent volume of d. (Vd)
    batwing d.
    Boltzmann d.
    butterfly d.
    centrilobular d.
    depth dose d.
    diffuse spatial d.
    dose d.
    gaussian d.
    geometric d.
    harness-shaped d.
    homogeneous susceptibility d.
    homogeneous thallium d.
    inhomogeneous tracer d.
    interstitial lung disease d.
    loop d.
    lung infiltrate d.
    maxwellian d.
    mottled d.
    normal variant fluorodeoxyglucose
        uptake d.
    normal whole body
        fluorodeoxyglucose d.
    peribronchial d.
    perivascular d.
    Poisson d.
    radioactivity d.
    rapid d.
    regional myocardial mass d.

D

NOTES

distribution *(continued)*
 reverse d.
 rimlike calcium d.
 spatial d.
 spatial dose d.
 spectral noise d.
 symmetric d.
 thallium-201 uptake and d.
 trace element d.
 d. transformer
 uniform d.
 unusual marrow d.
distributive shock
disturbance
 architectural d.
 d. of articulation
 circulation d.
disturbed orientation
disuse osteoporosis
diuresis
 d. renogram
 d. urogram
diuretic
 d. radionuclide urography
 d. renal imaging
 d. renal scan
 d. renography
Diva laparoscopic morcellator
divergent
 d. dislocation
 d. ray projection
 d. spiculated pattern
diverging
 d. collimator
 d. meniscus
diversion
 biliopancreatic d.
 cerebrospinal fluid d.
 continent d.
 continent urinary d.
 urinary d.
 ventriculoperitoneal d.
diversity segment
diverticular
 d. abscess
 d. colon disease
 d. prostatitis
diverticulitis
 acute d.
 bladder d.
 chronic d.
 colonic d.
 Meckel d.
 sigmoid d.
diverticulogram
diverticulosis
 colonic d.
 intramural esophageal d.

jejunal d.
 tracheal d.
diverticulum
 acquired urethral d.
 arachnoid d.
 bladder d.
 calyceal d.
 colonic d.
 common bile duct d.
 congenital urethral d.
 cricopharyngeal d.
 divisional block d.
 dorsal d.
 ductus d.
 duodenal intraluminal d.
 esophageal d.
 fallopian tube d.
 false d.
 fourth ventricle d.
 functional d.
 gallbladder d.
 Ganser d.
 gastric d.
 giant sigmoid d.
 Graser d.
 hepatic d.
 Hutch d.
 hypopharyngeal d.
 interaorticobronchial d.
 interbronchial d.
 intestinal d.
 intraluminal duodenal d. (IDD)
 intramural d.
 inverted Meckel d.
 jejunal d.
 jejunoileal d.
 juxtapapillary d.
 Kirchner d.
 Kommerell d.
 Kumeral d.
 Meckel d.
 metanephric d.
 midesophageal d.
 Nuck d.
 paraureteral d.
 perforated d.
 periampullary d.
 pharyngoesophageal d.
 pulsion d.
 pyelocalyceal d.
 Rokitansky d.
 roofless fourth ventricle d.
 sigmoid d.
 small bowel d.
 stomach d.
 thoracic pulsion d.
 thoracic root sleeve d.
 traction d.
 urachal d.

urethral d.
urinary bladder d.
Vater d.
vesical d.
windsock d.
Zenker d.
diverting stoma
divided dose
diving goiter
division
mandibular d.
maxillary d.
ureteral d.
divisional
d. block
d. block diverticulum
divisionary line
divisum
pancreas d.
pancreatic d.
divopontocerebellar atrophy
Dixon
D. fat-fraction measurement
D. method of phase unwrapping
D. quantitative chemical shift
image
dizygotic twin
DJD
degenerative joint disease
DJF
duodenojejunal flexure
DJJ
duodenojejunal junction
DKS
Damus-Kaye-Stansel
DKS procedure
DLCL
diffuse large-cell lymphoma
limited-stage DLCL
D, L-HMPAO imaging agent
D-loop
dextro loop
ventricular D-l.
D-l. ventricular situs
DLP
dose-length product
DLR
distal line of reference
D-malposition of aorta
DMI
diaphragmatic myocardial infarct

DMMA
distal metatarsal articular angle
DMPE
3,4-dimethoxyphenyl-ethylamine
DMSA
dimer captosuccinic acid
(V)-dimer captosuccinic acid
^{99m}Tc (V) DMSA
DNA
deoxyribonucleic acid
DNA cytophotometry
DNA flow cytometry
DNA microinjection technique
DNET
dysembryoplastic neuroepithelial tumor
DNP
dynamic nuclear polarization
DNR
dose nonuniformity ratio
DOBI
dynamic optical breast imaging system
DOBI system
dobutamine
low-dose d. (LDD)
d. stress echocardiography (DSE)
d. thallium angiography
DOBV
double-outlet both ventricles
doctrine
Monroe-Kellie d.
documentary arteriography
document image decoding (DID)
document-recognition algorithm
Dodd perforating vein group
dodecafluoropentane (DDFP)
d. imaging agent
Dodge
D. area-length method for
ventricular volume
D. method for ejection fraction
D. principle
Dodick Laser Photolysis System
Doerner-Hoskins distribution law
dolens
phlegmasia cerulea d.
dolichocephalic
dolichocephaly
dolichocolon
dolichoectasia
vertebrobasilar d.
dolichoesophagus
dolichopellic pelvis

D

NOTES

dolichosigmoid
dolichostenomelia
DoLi S extracorporeal shock wave lithotripter
DOLV
    double-outlet left ventricle
domain
        dose rate d.
        extracellular d.
        Fourier d.
        frequency d.
        magnetic d.
        scene d.
        spatial frequency d.
        time d.
dome
        d. of aneurysm
        anterior talar d.
        atrial d.
        bladder d.
        crus d.
        d. cylinder
        d. of diaphragm
        diaphragmatic d.
        d. fracture
        lateral talar d.
        liver d.
        shoulder d.
        talar d.
        weightbearing acetabular d.
dome-and-dart configuration
dome-shaped
        d.-s. heart
        d.-s. roof of pleural cavity
dome-to-neck ratio
dominance
        cerebral d.
        coronary artery d.
        orbitofrontal d.
dominant
        anatomically d.
        d. follicle
        d. hemisphere
        d. hemisphere infarct
        d. hemisphere lesion
        hepatic arterial d.
        d. left coronary artery
        portal venous d.
        d. right coronary artery
        d. vessel
doming
        diastolic d.
        d. of leaflet
        d. of valve
donor
        adult-to-adult living related liver
          transplant d.
        d. graft
        d. heart

        d. heart-lung block
        d. site
        d. twin
donor-recipient anastomy
"don't touch" lesion
DOPA
        dihydroxyphenylalanine
        DOPA imaging agent
dopaminergic dysfunction
dopamine transporter
Dopascan radiopharmaceutical imaging agent
doped water
Doppler
        D. angle
        D. ankle systolic pressure
        D. assessment
        ATL HDI 5000 color D.
        D. blood flow monitor
        D. blood flow velocity signal
        D. blood pressure
        color D. (CD)
        color-flow D. (CFD)
        D. color-flow imaging
        D. color-flow mapping
        D. continuous-wave
          echocardiography
        contrast-enhanced color D.
        contrast-enhanced power D.
        Convergent color D.
        duplex B-mode D.
        D. effect
        D. equation
        D. flow echocardiographic probe
        D. flow index
        D. flowmeter
        D. flowmetry
        D. flow probe study
        D. flow signal enhancement
        D. frequency shift
        D. frequency spectrum
        D. gain
        gray-scale D.
        high-frequency D. (HFD)
        high pulse repetition frequency D.
        D. insonation
        D. interrogation
        intraoperative D.
        multigate D.
        D. ovary signal
        periorbital bidirectional D.
        pocket D.
        power D.
        D. pulse
        pulsed-wave D.
        D. pulsed-wave echocardiography
        range-gated pulsed D.
        real-time D.
        renal D.

D. Resistive Index (DRI)
D. shift frequency
D. shift principle
D. signal enhancement
D. sonography
D. sonography of the SMA
SonoSite pulsed wave D.
spectral D.
D. spectral analysis
D. spectral waveform
D. study of blood flow
D. System 97
D. tissue imaging (DTI)
transcranial D. (TCD)
transcranial color-coded D.
D. tricuspid regurgitation
D. ultrasonic blood flow detector
D. ultrasonic fetal heart monitor
D. ultrasonic velocity detector
D. ultrasonic velocity detector
  segmental plethysmography
D. ultrasonography imaging
D. ultrasound
D. ultrasound segmental blood
  pressure testing
D. venous examination
D. venous imaging
D. VWF
D. waveform analysis
D. waveform dampening
Doppler-derived stroke distance
Doppler-guided hemorrhoid artery
  ligation (DGHAL)
Dorello canal
Dorendorf
D. sign
D. sign of aortic arch aneurysm
dormancy
tumor d.
Dornier
D. compact lithotripter
D. HM3, HM4 lithotripter
D. scanner
Dor reconstruction
dorsad
dorsal
d. abdominal wall
d. artery
d. artery of penis
d. aspect
d. bend

d. branch
d. capsule
d. decubitus position
d. dermal sinus
d. diverticulum
d. enteric fistula
d. enteric sinus
d. enterogenous cyst
d. induction
d. induction error
d. intercalated segmental instability
  (DISI)
d. interossei
d. kyphotic curvature
d. meningocele
d. metacarpal ligament
d. muscle
d. nerve of penis
d. pancreas
d. pancreatic bud
d. penile vein
d. plate
d. point
d. primary ramus
d. ramus of spinal nerve
d. recumbent position
d. ridge
d. rim
d. rim distal radial fracture
d. root entry zone (DREZ)
d. root entry zone lesion
d. root ganglion (DRG)
d. scapular
d. spinal cord horn
d. spine
d. spinocerebellar tract
d. subaponeurotic space
d. subcutaneous space
d. talar beak
d. talonavicular bone
d. tubercle
d. vertebra
d. view
d. wing fracture
d. wrist ligament
dorsalis
funiculus d.
d. pedis
d. pedis pulse
tabes d.
dorsalward

NOTES

275

dorsiflexion
    d. angle (DFA)
    d. view
dorsiflexor
dorsispinal vein
dorsoanterior
dorsocephalad
dorsolateral
    d. aspect
    d. tract
dorsomedial
    d. nucleus
    d. thalamotomy
dorsoplantar
    d. aspect
    d. projection
    d. talometatarsal angle
    d. talonavicular angle
    d. view
dorsoposterior
dorsoradial
dorsorostral
dorsosacral position
dorsum
    d. pedis
    d. of penis
    d. sella
    d. sellae atrophy
DORV
    double-outlet right ventricle
dose
    absorbed d. (AD)
    adult d.
    air d.
    d. area product (DAP)
    bioeffect d. (BED)
    biologically equivalent d. (BED)
    bolus d.
    boost d.
    d. calibrator
    central axis depth d.
    cross-organ and self-absorbed d.
    cumulative d.
    delivered total d. (DTD)
    depth d.
    d. distribution
    divided d.
    doubling d.
    epilation d.
    d. equivalent (DE)
    d. equivalent radiation
    exit d.
    exposure d.
    ^{67}Ga higher d.
    genetically significant d.
    glandular d.
    gonadal d.
    Haut-Einheits-Dosis unit skin d.
    incremental d.

    d. infiltration
    integral d.
    iodine d.
    isoeffect d.
    d. kernel
    lethal d.
    matched peripheral d. (MPD)
    mean central d. (MCD)
    mean gonad d.
    median lethal d.
    d. nonuniformity ratio (DNR)
    peak skin d. (PSD)
    percentage depth d. (PDD)
    radiation adsorbed d. (rad)
    d. rate domain
    reference d.
    scatter d.
    skin d.
    tapering d.
    threshold d.
    threshold erythema d.
    tissue tolerance d. (TTD)
    tracer d.
dose-area product meter
dose/dose-rate effective factor (DDREF)
dose-length product (DLP)
dose-limiting toxicity
dose-surface histogram
dose-time relationship
dose-volume
    d.-v. histogram (DVH)
    d.-v. relationship
dosimeter
    chemical d.
    dichromate d.
    electronic d.
    Gardray d.
    high-dose film d.
    LiF thermoluminescence d.
    pencil d.
    pocket d.
    silicon diode d.
    sucrose d.
    thermoluminescent d. (TLD)
    ultraviolet fluorescent d.
    Victoreen d.
dosimetric penumbra
dosimetrist
dosimetry
    adjacent field x-ray d.
    beam's eye view d.
    dichromate d.
    electron d.
    4-field x-ray d.
    free-radical d.
    Fricke d.
    high-dose film d.
    large-field x-ray d.
    LiF thermoluminescence d.

marrow d.
medical internal radiation d.
  (MIRD)
phantom d.
pion d.
polymer d.
radiation d.
radiopharmaceutical d.
single x-ray d.
thermoluminescence d.
transmission d.
x-ray d.

Dos Santos aortography needle
dot

d. scan
subpleural d.

DOTA
tetraazacyclododecanetetraacetic acid
dot-and-dash pattern
Dotter

D. effect
D. tube

dottering effect
double

d. aortic arch
d. aortic arch of Edwards
d. appendix
d. arch aorta
d. autograft
d. basket
d. breast coil
d. camelback sign of knee
d. cervix
d. coronary orifice
d. decidual sac
d. decidual sac sign
d. density
d. density heart
d. density sign
d. diaphragm contour
d. diaphragm sign
d. duct sign
d. emission
d. fracture
d. gallbladder
d. helical CT scan
d. injection
d. inversion recovery sequence
d. kidney
d. label
d. lesion sign
d. line sign

d. lumen
d. lumen central venous catheter
d. outflow
d. outline
d. penis
d. pleurisy
d. pneumonia
d. pulse interlaced echo imaging
d. reverse alpha sigmoid loop
d. systolic apical impulse
d. tracking of barium
d. track sign
d. uterus
d. vagina
d. voiding cystogram
d. wall sign

double-arc gallbladder shadow
double-barrel

d.-b. aorta
d.-b. esophagus
d.-b. lumen

double-bleb sign
double-bonded carbon
double-bubble

d.-b. appearance
d.-b. shadow
d.-b. sign

double-bulb appearance
double-channel endoscope
double-contrast

d.-c. arthrography
d.-c. arthrotomography of shoulder
d.-c. barium enema (DCBE)
d.-c. barium meal
d.-c. barium study
d.-c. esophagography
d.-c. eversion examination
d.-c. laryngography
d.-c. radiograph
d.-c. radiography
d.-c. roentgenography
d.-c. technique
d.-c. visualization

double-dose

d.-d. delay (DDD)
d.-d. delayed-contrast MRI
d.-d. gadolinium imaging

double-echo

d.-e. Broglie Wavelength
d.-e. method

double-exposed rib
double-exposure drift artifact

D

NOTES

double-freeze technique
double-halo
    d.-h. appearance
    d.-h. configuration
    d.-h. sign
double-helical CT imaging
double-helix
    d.-h. acquisition
    d.-h. prostatic stent
double-inlet
    d.-i. left ventricle
    d.-i. single ventricle
    d.-i. ventricle anomaly
double-J
    d.-J indwelling catheter
    d.-J stent placement
    d.-J ureteral catheter
    d.-J ureteral stent
double-label counting
double-lumen
    d.-l. breast implant
    d.-l. endoprosthesis
double-mode steady state
double-mouthed uterus
double-outlet
    d.-o. both ventricles (DOBV)
    d.-o. left ventricle (DOLV)
    d.-o. right ventricle (DORV)
double-phase technetium-99m sestamibi imaging
double-pigtail endoprosthesis
double-populated detector ring
double-power injector
double-probe pH study
double-ring
    d.-r. esophageal sign
    d.-r. esophagus
double-spin echo proton spectroscopy
double-spiral CT arterial portography
double-spot compression
double-stem silicone lesser MP implant
double-strand scission
double-throw
    single-pole d.-t. (SPDT)
double-tracking colon
double-umbrella technique
double-wire atherectomy technique
doubling dose
doubly broadband triple-resonance NMR probe circuit
doughnut
    GE Signa 0.5T double d.
    d. kidney
    d. lesion
    d. magnet
    d. sign
    d. transformer
doughy mass

Douglas
    D. cul-de-sac
    dependent pouch of D.
    D. fold
    D. ligament
    D. rectouterine pouch
Dow
    D. hollow fiber analyzer
    D. method for measuring cardiac output
dowager's hump
dowel
    iliac d.
dowel-shaped bone graft
down
    coned d.
    ramp d.
    D. syndrome
downhill varix
downscatter
downsloping
downstaging
    axillary tumor d.
downstream
    crossed upstream and d.
    d. sampling method
downward
    d. displacement of apical impulse
    d. slope
    d. vergence
Dox-Spheres
Doyne honeycomb degeneration
DPA
    dual-photon absorptiometry
dP/dt
    delta pressure/delta time
    peak dP/dt
DPF
    digital pulsed fluoroscopy
DPG
    displacement placentogram
DPR
    dynamic planar reconstructor
DPSF
    diffusion/perfusion snapshot FLASH
DPTA
    DPTA CSF flow study
    ^{99m}Tc-DPTA
DPTI
    diastolic pressure-time index
DPX-IQ densitometer
DQE
    detective quantum efficiency
DR
    digital radiography
DRA
    digital rotational angiography
    distal rectal adenocarcinoma
    distal reference axis

dragon pyelogram
drain
external ventricular d. (EVD)
occlusive d.
radiopaque d.
retroperitoneal d.
rubber d.
sump d.
drainage
aberrant venous d.
biliary d.
d. catheter
central venous d.
circle loop biliary d.
enteric exocrine d.
external-internal d.
extrapleural d.
gaseous d.
guided d.
imaging guided catheter d.
infradiaphragmatic totally anomalous
pulmonary venous d.
internal biliary d.
intrathoracic catheter d.
pancreatic pseudocyst d.
percutaneous d.
percutaneous abscess d.
percutaneous antegrade biliary d.
percutaneous biliary d. (PBD)
percutaneous catheter d. (PCD)
percutaneous transhepatic d. (pTL)
percutaneous transhepatic biliary d.
(PTBD)
percutaneous transhepatic
cholangial d. (PTCD)
pulmonary venous d.
spondylodiskitis d.
spontaneous d.
total anomalous pulmonary
venous d. (TAPVD)
transhepatic d.
transvaginal ultrasound-guided d.
tube d.
venous d.
ventricular d.
water-sealed d.
draining
d. lymphatic bed
d. sinus
d. with venous pressure
drain-out film
draped aorta

Drash syndrome
DRC
design rule check
dynamic range control
DRC algorithm
Drennan metaphysial-epiphysial angle
DRESS
depth-resolved surface spectroscopy
dressing
pressure applied d. (PAD)
Dressler syndrome
DREZ
dorsal root entry zone
DREZ lesion
DRG
dorsal root ganglion
DRI
Doppler Resistive Index
Driffield
Hurter and D. (H and D)
drift
field d.
radial d.
drifting wedge pressure
drill
lithoclast miniature pneumatic d.
magnetic resonance
imaging–compatible piezoelectric
power d.
drink
drip
d. infusion cholangiogram (DIC)
d. infusion cholangiography (DIC)
d. infusion pyelography
d. infusion technique
d. infusion urography
dripping
brain candle d.
candle wax d.
driven
d. equilibrium Fourier transform
d. equilibrium Fourier transform
technique
d. inversion spin echo (DISE)
dromedary hump
drooping
d. lily appearance
d. lily sign
d. shoulder
drop
d. finger
d. foot

NOTES

drop *(continued)*
    d. heart
    d. metastasis
    d. shoulder
    d. test for pneumoperitoneum
drop-lock ring
dropped stone
drowned lung
DRR
    digitally reconstructed radiograph
drug
    adjuvant analgesic d.
    d. administration
    adrenergic d.
    anesthetic d.
    antiadrenergic d.
    anticonvulsant d.
    antidepressant d.
    antimuscarinic d.
    antipsychotic d.
    d. efflux
    d. fraction
    macromolecular d.
    psychotherapeutic d.
    slow-channel blocking d.
    d. tolerance
drug-induced
    d.-i. bone marrow suppression
    d.-i. brain abnormality
    d.-i. brain change
    d.-i. bullous disorder
    d.-i. drug resistance
    d.-i. erythematous lupus
    d.-i. esophagitis
    d.-i. nephrotoxicity
    d.-i. pneumonitis
    d.-i. pulmonary damage
drug-resistant
    d.-r. extratemporal epilepsy
    d.-r. tumor
DRUJ
    distal radioulnar joint
Drummond
    D. marginal artery
    D. sign
    D. sign of aortic aneurysm
drum spur
drumstick
    d. appearance
    d. phalanx
drusen
    optic nerve d.
dry
    d. bowel preparation
    d. bronchiectasis
    d. heat sterilizer and incinerator unit
    d. laser imaging
    d. pleurisy
    d. swallow
dryer system
Drystar dry imager
DryView laser imaging system
DS
    duplex sonography
DSA
    digital subtraction angiography
    digital subtraction arteriography
    DSA image
    infrainguinal DSA
DSAS
    discrete subvalvular aortic stenosis
DSC
    dynamic susceptibility contrast
    DSC MR imaging
3-Dscope laparoscope
DSE
    dobutamine stress echocardiography
D-shaped vessel lumen
DSI camera
DSM
    digital subtraction mammography
DSR
    dynamic spatial reconstructor
    DSR scanner
DSRCT
    desmoplastic small round-cell tumor
DT
    diffusion tension
    diffusion tensor
    DT MR imaging
DTD
    delivered total dose
DTI
    diffusion tension imaging
    diffusion tensor imaging
    Doppler tissue imaging
DTICH
    delayed traumatic intracerebral hematoma
D-to-E slope
DTPA
    diethylenetriaminepentaacetic acid
    DTPA imaging agent
    ^{111}In DTPA
    DTPA renography
    technetium-99m DMSA, DTPA
    ytterbium-169 DTPA
DTU-215 cardiac digital stimulator
DTU-one UltraSure imaging system
DU
    duplex ultrasound
dual
    d. atrioventricular node pathway
    d. blood supply
    d. gradient-recalled echo pulse sequence
    d. intracoronary scintigraphy

d. isotope imaging
d. isotope scanning
d. lateral hand positioner
d. lateral skull block
d. leg immobilizer
d. lookup table
d. oblique hand positioner
d. photon
d. plate
d. popliteal vein
d. single-crystal gamma camera
d. transverse linear-array sonogram
d. ventricle
dual-balloon method
dual-coil imaging
dual-contrast study
dual-demand pacing mode
dual-detector helical CT angiography
dual-echo
d.-e. chemical shift gradient-echo MRI
d.-e. DIET fast spin-echo imaging
d.-e. and DT MR imaging
d.-e. interleaved spiral out-in imaging
d.-e. sequence
d.-e. turbo spin-echo
dual-emulsion mammography film
dual-energy
d.-e. CT
d.-e. imaging
d.-e. linear accelerator
d.-e. mammography
d.-e. radiograph (DER)
d.-e. subtraction
d.-e. x-ray absorptiometry (DEXA, DXA)
d.-e. x-ray absorptiometry densitometer
dual-head
d.-h. coincidence camera
d.-h. coincidence detection system
d.-h. SPECT
dual-isotope
d.-i. single-photon emission CT
d.-i. SPECT
d.-i. subtraction technique
d.-i. TI 201
dual-lookup table algorithm

dual-lumen silicone hemodialysis/apheresis catheter
dual-mode, dual-pacing, dual-sensing (DDD)
dual-phase
d.-p. CT
d.-p. helical computed tomography (DHCT)
d.-p. scan
d.-p. ^{99m}Tc-sestamibi imaging
dual-photon
d.-p. absorptiometry (DPA)
d.-p. densitometer
d.-p. densitometry
dual-probe rectilinear scanner
dual-sensing
dual-mode, dual-pacing, d.-s. (DDD)
dual-shaped collimator
dual-tracer imaging
Dubin-Johnson syndrome
Duchenne
D. muscular dystrophy
D. sign
duct
aberrant intrahepatic bile d.
accessory hepatic d.
accessory pancreatic d.
alveolar d.
amnionic d.
arborization of d.
arterial d.
asymmetric bile d.
Bartholin d.
beaded bile d.
beaded hepatic d.
beaded pancreatic d.
d. of Bellini
bile d.
biliary d.
Botallo d.
branch d.
branchial d.
bucconeural d.
canalicular d.
carotid d.
d. cell adenocarcinoma
d. cell carcinoma
choledochous d.
cobblestone appearance of bile d.
cochlear d.
common bile d. (CBD)

NOTES

duct *(continued)*
    common gall d.
    common hepatic d. (CHD)
    craniopharyngeal d.
    Cuvier d.
    cystic gall d.
    deferent d.
    dilated bile d.
    dilated intrahepatic d.
    dilated mammary d.
    dilated subareolar d.
    disruption of d.
    distal bile d.
    duodenal end of dorsal d.
    duodenal end of main d.
    efferent d.
    ejaculatory d.
    endolymphatic d.
    excretory d.
    extrahepatic bile d.
    extralobular terminal d.
    focally dilated d.
    frontonasal d.
    fusiform widening of d.
    galactophorous d.
    gall d.
    Gartner d.
    genital d.
    hepatic d.
    hypophysial Rathke d.
    infundibulum of bile d.
    interlobular bile d.
    intrahepatic bile d.
    intralobular terminal d.
    involution of d.
    lacrimal d.
    lactiferous d.
    d. lumen
    lymph d.
    lymphatic d.
    main pancreatic d. (MPD)
    main papillary d. (MPD)
    mammary d.
    middle extrahepatic bile d.
    müllerian d.
    nasofrontal d.
    nasolacrimal d.
    nipplelike common bile d.
    normal caliber d.
    d. obstruction
    omphalomesenteric d.
    pancreatic d.
    paramesonephric d.
    paraurethral d.
    parotid d.
    percutaneous dilatation of biliary d.
    perilobular d.
    preampullary portion of bile d.
    prepapillary bile d.

    prostatic d.
    proximal part of dorsal d.
    pruned-tree-appearance bile d.
    pseudocalculus bile d.
    Rathke d.
    rat-tail common bile d.
    right hepatic d.
    Rivinus d.
    ruptured thoracic d.
    Santorini d.
    solitary dilated d.
    sphincter of bile d.
    spontaneous perforation of common
      bile d.
    Stensen d.
    subareolar d.
    submandibular d.
    subvesical d.
    terminal bile d.
    thoracic d.
    thyroglossal d.
    transabdominal catheterization of
      thoracic d.
    Vater d.
    vitelline d.
    Wharton d.
    Wirsung d.
    wolffian d.

ductal
    d. adenoma
    d. aneurysm
    d. arch
    d. architecture
    d. breast microcalcification
    d. carcinoma in situ (DCIS)
    d. constriction
    d. dilatation
    d. ectasia
    d. epithelial hyperplasia
    d. epithelium
    d. pancreatic adenocarcinoma
    d. papillary carcinoma
    d. papilloma
    d. pattern
    d. remnant
    d. in situ breast carcinoma
ductectatic
    d. mucinous cystic neoplasm
    d. mucinous tumor
ductogram
    mammary d.
ductography
    contrast d.
    peroral retrograde
      pancreaticobiliary d.
duct-penetrating sign
ductular
ductule
ductus, pl. **ductus**

d. aneriosus
d. arteriosus
d. arteriosus aneurysm
d. arteriosus occlusion
d. arteriosus patency
d. deferens
d. deferens artery
d. diverticulum
d. infundibulum
d. of Kommerell
recanalized d.
d. venosus
d. venosus patency
window d.

Duett
D. arterial puncture site closure device
D. closure device
D. diagnostic device
D. therapeutic device

Dulcolax bowel preparation
dullness
left border of cardiac d. (LBCD)
triangular area of d.

dumbbell
d. appearance
d. brain mass
d. lesion
d. loculation
d. needle
d. neurofibroma
d. shape
d. tumor

dumbbell-shaped shadow
dumbbell-type neuroblastoma
dummy source
dumping
d. stomach
d. syndrome

Duncan placenta
Dunlop-Shands view
duodenal
d. adenocarcinoma
d. ampulla
d. artery
d. atresia
d. bulb
d. bulb apex (DBA)
d. bulb deformity
d. button
d. cap
d. C loop

d. diaphragm
d. duplication
d. end of dorsal duct
d. end of main duct
d. erosion
d. filling defect
d. fossa
d. gastrinoma
d. hernia
d. hourglass stenosis
d. impression
d. intraluminal diverticulum
d. leiomyosarcoma
d. ligament
d. loop
d. lumen
d. narrowing
d. papilla
d. polyp
d. segment
d. sphincter
d. stricture
d. stump
d. sweep
d. teardrop appearance
d. terminus
d. ulcer
d. ulcer perforation
d. varix
d. vein
d. villus
d. wall hamartoma
d. web

duodenal-gastric outlet obstruction
duodeni
ampulla d.
duodenitis
chronic atrophic d.
Crohn d.
erosive d.
hemorrhagic d.
duodenobiliary
d. pressure gradient
d. reflux
duodenocolic fistula
duodenogastric reflux (DGR)
duodenogastroesophageal reflux
duodenogastroscopy
duodenogram
duodenography
hypotonic d.
d. imaging

D

NOTES

duodenojejunal
> d. angle
> d. flexure (DJF)
> d. fold
> d. fossa
> d. junction (DJJ)
> d. recess
> d. sphincter

duodenojejunitis

duodenomesocolic fold

duodenopancreatic
> d. fistula
> d. reflux

duodenorenal ligament

duodenoscope
> Olympus JF1T10 d.
> Olympus JF1T10 fiberoptic d.

duodenum
> chronic ileus d.
> C loop of d.
> cobblestone appearance d.
> comma-shaped d.
> curve of d.
> descending d.
> dilated d.
> distal d.
> d. extrinsic pressure effect
> first portion of d.
> d. inversum
> d. malignant tumor
> d. megabulbus
> mobile d.
> onion-shaped dilatation of d.
> postbulbar d.
> scarified d.
> scarred d.
> second portion of d.
> supravaterian d.
> suspensory muscle of d.
> third portion of d.
> d. water trap
> widened sweep d.
> windsock appearance of d.

duografin

Du Pen long-term epidural catheter

duplex
> d. B-mode Doppler
> d. B-mode ultrasound
> d. carotid imaging
> d. carotid ultrasound
> d. Doppler imaging
> d. Doppler signal analysis (DDSA)
> d. Doppler ultrasound
> d. echocardiography
> d. scanner
> d. screening test
> d. sonography (DS)
> d. ultrasound (DU)
> d. ultrasound analysis
> d. ultrasound carotid artery
> d. ultrasound error
> d. uterus

duplex-pulsed
> d.-p. Doppler sonography
> d.-p. Doppler ultrasound

duplicated
> d. inferior vena cava
> d. renal collecting system

duplication
> d. anomaly
> colon d.
> colon cyst d.
> colorectal d.
> complete d.
> d. cyst
> diaphragm d.
> duodenal d.
> esophageal d.
> foregut d.
> gallbladder d.
> hindgut d.
> incomplete ureteral d.
> inferior vena cava d.
> intestinal d.
> d. of left kidney
> partial ureter d.
> renal d.
> d. of right kidney
> thoracoabdominal d.
> ureteral d.

duplicator
> cardiac pulse d.

DuPont
> D. Cronex x-ray film
> D. scanner

Dupré muscle

Dupuytren
> D. canal
> D. contracture
> D. fracture
> D. sign

dura
> attenuated d.
> bulging d.
> effacement of d.
> lamina d.
> d. mater
> d. mater of brain
> d. mater of spinal cord
> d. mater venous sinus

dural
> d. arachnoid lymphoma
> d. arteriovenous fistula (DAVF)
> d. arteriovenous malformation
> d. artery
> d. attachment
> d. calcification
> d. carotid cavernous fistula (DCCF)

d. cul-de-sac
d. ectasia
d. fold
d. hematoma
d. impingement
d. ossification
d. root pouch
d. sac
d. sac effacement
d. sheath
d. sinus occlusion
d. sinus thrombosis infarct
d. tail
d. tear
d. venous sinus
d. venous sinus thrombosis
Duralyn balloon
Duran ring
Dürck node
Duret
D. hemorrhage
D. lesion
Durham flatfoot
durocutaneous fistula
duroliopaque
Duroziez
D. mitral stenosis disease
D. sign
durum
heloma d.
osteoma d.
papilloma d.
DUS
dynamic ultrasound of shoulder
Duverney
D. foramen
D. fracture
D. gland
D. muscle
DVH
dose-volume histogram
DVI
deep venous insufficiency
device-independent
digital vascular imaging
DVI mode
DVI Simpson AtheroCath
3D-VIEWNIX software system
DVT
deep venous thrombosis
dwarfism
achondroplastic d.

acromelic d.
Amsterdam d.
bird-headed d.
deprivation d.
diastrophic d.
late-onset d.
lethal d.
Lorain-Lévi d.
mesomelic d.
metatrophic d.
micromelic d.
nonlethal d.
pituitary d.
renal d.
Russell-Silver d.
thanatophoric d.
Walt Disney d.
dwarf pelvis
dwell position
DWI
diffusion-weighted imaging
Dwyer correction of scoliosis
DXA
dual-energy x-ray absorptiometry
DxRaI
diagnostic radioiodine scanning
Dy
dysprosium
Dycal base
dyclonine
Dy-DTPA-BMA
dysprosium diethylenetriaminepentaacetic
acid-bis(methylamide)
dysprosium DTPA-bis(methylamide)
Dy-DTPA-BMA imaging agent
dye
d. column
d. dilution curve
d. extravasation
fill-and-spill of d.
d. fluorescence index (DFI)
halogenated phenolphthalein d.
indentation of myelography d.
indocyanine green d.
d. injection technique
d. laser
d. laser system
lipophilic d.
d. punch fracture
d. reduction spot test

NOTES

D

dye *(continued)*
    rose bengal d.
    d. uptake
dye-binding capacity (DBC)
2-dye method
¹⁶⁶Dy generator
Dyggve-Melchior-Clausen dysplasia
Dyke-Davidoff-Masson syndrome
Dynabead
Dynalink
    D. 0.018 self-expanding stent
    D. 0.035 self-expanding stent
dynamic
    d. acquisition
    d. antral scintigraphy
    d. aorta
    d. axial fixator
    d. beat filtration
    d. bolus
    d. bolus tracking technique
    d. cervical change
    d. computed tomography (DCT)
    d. computed tomography
      mammography
    d. computerized tomography
    d. conformal therapy
    d. contrast-enhanced CT
    d. contrast-enhanced magnetic
      resonance imaging (DCE-MRI)
    d. contrast-enhanced MRI
    d. contrast-enhanced subtraction MR
      imaging
    d. contrast-enhanced subtraction
      study
    d. coupling
    d. CT scan
    d. emission scan
    d. enhancement
    d. entrapment of vertebral artery
    d. filtering
    d. focusing
    d. ileus
    d. image
    d. lineshape effect
    d. liver imaging
    d. lung
    d. magnetic resonance imaging
    d. multileaf collimation
    d. nuclear polarization (DNP)
    d. open magnetic resonance
      defecography
    d. optical breast imaging system
      (DOBI)
    d. pedobarography
    d. planar reconstructor (DPR)
    d. pulmonary hyperinflation
    d. radiation therapy
    d. radionuclide renal scintigraphy
    d. radiotherapy

    d. range
    d. range control (DRC)
    d. renal imaging
    d. scintigraphy imaging
    d. series
    d. snapshot
    d. sonography
    d. spatial reconstructor (DSR)
    d. spiral CT lung densitometer
    d. spiral CT lung densitometry
    d. stabilizer
    d. stereotactic radiosurgery
    d. subaortic stenosis
    d. subtraction magnetic resonance
      angiogram
    d. supine study
    d. susceptibility contrast (DSC)
    d. susceptibility contrast magnetic
      resonance imaging
    d. tagging magnetic resonance
      angiography
    d. ultrasound of shoulder (DUS)
    d. ventilation He-MRI
    d. volume imaging
    d. volume-rendered display
    d. volumetric SPECT
    d. wedge
    d. weightbearing cervical magnetic
      resonance imaging
dynamic-condenser electrometer
dynamic-contrast MRI
dynamite heart
Dynapix
DynaRad portable x-ray system
DynaWell medical compression device
dyne
dynode
dynography
dysarthria clumsy hand syndrome
dysautonomia
    familial d.
dyschezia
dyschondroplasia
dyschondrosteosis
dyschromia
dyscollagenosis
dyscrasic fracture
dysembryoplastic neuroepithelial tumor
    (DNET)
dysfunction
    bladder d.
    bowel and bladder d.
    brain d.
    cerebral d.
    cortical d.
    dehydration-induced renal d.
    dopaminergic d.
    frontal lobe d.
    hepatocellular d.

left ventricular d. (LVD)
lower esophageal sphincter d.
oropharyngeal d.
positional d.
regional myocardial d.
renal d.
reversible temporary myocardial d.
right ventricular d. (RVD)
salivary gland d.
sinuatrial node d.
sinus node d.
small airway d.
sphincter d.
swallowing d.
testis d.
valvular d.
ventilatory d.
ventricular d.

dysfunctional
d. autogenous hemodialysis fistula
d. kidney

dysgenesis
alar d.
anorectal d.
callosal d.
corpus callosum d.
corticocallosal d.
epiphysial d.
gonadal d.
hindbrain d.
mixed gonadal d.
ovarian d.
renal tubular d.
sacral d.
sacrolumbar d.
segmental spinal d. (SSD)
thyroid d.
tubular d.

dysgenetic kidney

dysgerminoma
brain d.
mediastinum d.
ovarian d.
pineal d.

dysjunction
craniofacial d.

dyskeratosis, pl. **dyskeratoses**
kidney d.

dyskinesia, dyskinesis
bile duct d.
biliary d.

regional d.
tardive d.

dyskinetic
d. cerebral palsy
d. segmental wall motion
d. segmental wall motion
  abnormality
d. septum

dysmaturity
pulmonary d.

dysmorphism
lobar d.

dysmotile esophagus

dysmotility
esophageal d.

dysmyelination

dysosteogenesis

dysostosis, pl. **dysostoses**
cleidocranial d.
craniofacial d.
epiphysial d.
mandibulofacial d.
metaphysial d.
d. multiplex
mutational d.

dysphagia
contractile ring d.
esophageal d.
d. inflammatoria
liquid food d.
d. lusoria
oropharyngeal d.
d. paralytica
postvagotomy d.
preesophageal d.
progressive d.
sideropenic d.
soft food d.
solid food d.
d. spastica
vallecular d.
d. valsalviana

dysplasia
acetabular residual d.
acromelic d.
acromesomelic d.
acropectorovertebral d.
arrhythmogenic right ventricular d.
  (ARVD)
arteriohepatic d.
asphyxiating thoracic d.
bone d.

D

NOTES

dysplasia *(continued)*
    bronchopulmonary d. (BPD)
    Burke-type metaphysial d.
    camptomelic d.
    cemental d.
    cementoosseous d.
    cervical d.
    chondroectodermal d.
    cleidocranial d.
    CNS fibromuscular d.
    congenital hip d.
    congenital polyvalvular d.
    cortical d.
    cranioskeletal d.
    craniotelencephalic d.
    cystic fibrous d.
    diaphysial d.
    diastrophic d.
    d. dislocation
    Dyggve-Melchior-Clausen d.
    endocardial d.
    epiarticular osteochondromatous d.
    epiphysial d.
    d. epiphysialis hemimelica
    d. epiphysialis multiplex
    d. epiphysialis punctata
    external auditory canal d.
    familial arterial fibromuscular d.
    fetal musculoskeletal d.
    fibromuscular d.
    fibrous temporal bone d.
    focal cerebellar d.
    focal cortical d.
    foot d.
    frontonasal d.
    hip d.
    idiopathic diffuse cerebellar d.
    isolated focal cerebellar cortical d.
    Jansen metaphysial d.
    Joubert focal cerebellar d.
    Kniest d.
    lethal bone d.
    lethal musculoskeletal d.
    mammary d.
    McKusick-type metaphysial d.
    mesodermal d.
    mesomelic d.
    metaphysial d.
    metatrophic d.
    Meyer d.
    micromelic d.
    microscopic cortical d.
    Mondini d.
    monostotic fibrous d.
    multicystic d.
    multiple epiphysial d.
    Namaqualand hip d.
    neuroectodermal d.

    nonlethal d.
    nonsyndromic focal cerebellar d.
    obstructive renal d.
    odontoid d.
    osseous d.
    osteofibrous d.
    periapical cemental d.
    perimedial d.
    periosteal d.
    polyostotic fibrous d.
    polypoid d.
    Potter d.
    progressive diaphysial d. (PDD)
    pulmonary valve d.
    Pyle d.
    renal artery fibromuscular d.
    retinal d.
    retroareolar d.
    rhizomelic d.
    right ventricular d.
    Scheibe d.
    Schmid-type metaphysial d.
    septooptic d.
    sheetlike d.
    short limb d.
    skeletal d.
    sphenoid d.
    spondylocostal d.
    spondyloepiphysial d.
    spondylothoracic d.
    Streeter d.
    tapetoretinal d.
    Taylor type d.
    testis d.
    thanatophoric d.
    thoracic d.
    thymic d.
    transmantle d.
    tricuspid valve d.
    variable cerebral d.
    ventricular d.
    ventriculoradial d.
    d. with associated lesion or mass
        (DALM)
dysplasia-associated lesion
dysplasia-carcinoma sequence
dysplastic
    d. cerebellar gangliocytoma
    d. cusp
    d. kidney
    d. liver nodule
    d. meniscus
    d. pulmonary valve
dysprosium (Dy)
    d. analog
    d. diethylenetriaminepentaacetic
        acid-bis(methylamide) (Dy-DTPA-
        BMA)

d. DTPA-bis(methylamide) (Dy-DTPA-BMA)

d. HP-DO3A imaging agent

dysprosium-DTPA

dysprosium-holmium (166Dy-166Ho) in vivo generator

dysraphia

    tectocerebellar d.

dysraphic spine

dysraphism

    closed spinal d.

    occult spinal d.

dysregulation

    vertigo/orthostatic d.

dysrhythmia of fetal heart

dyssynergia, dyssynergy

    biliary d.

    Ramsay Hunt cerebellar myoclonic d.

    regional d.

    segmental d.

dystocia

    fetal d.

    labor d.

    shoulder d.

dystonia

dystonic reaction

dystopia

dystrophic

    d. change

    d. degeneration

    d. soft tissue calcification

dystrophinopathic cardiomyopathy

dystrophy

    adiposogenital d.

    asphyxiating thoracic d.

    bone d.

    congenital muscular d.

    Duchenne muscular d.

    Fukuyama congenital muscular d. (FCMD)

    infantile thoracic d.

    limb-girdle muscular d.

    merosin-deficient congenital muscular d.

    muscular d.

    neuraxonal d.

    oculopharyngeal d.

    reflex sympathetic d.

    Sudeck d.

    sympathetic d.

NOTES

D

E

E plane
E point of cardiac apex pulse
E point on echocardiography
E point to septal separation
(EPSS)
E sign on x-ray

E₁

prostaglandin E_1

E-A

E-A change
E-A wave ratio

EAA

extraalveolar air
EAA collection

Eagle-Barrett syndrome
ealamus scriptorius
ear

e. cholesteatoma
frontal horn Mickey Mouse e.
inner e.
middle e.

early

e. bone scintigraphy
e. echo
e. endovascular treatment
e. fetal death
e. opening of valve
e. osteoarthritis
e. osteomyelitis
e. pneumonitis
c. repolarization pattern
e. segmental opacification
e. stromal invasion
e. systolic peak (ESP)
e. venous filling

early-phase termination
Eastman Kodak scanner
Easy Wallstent stent
Eaton agent pneumonia
EBA

electron beam angiography
extrahepatic biliary atresia

EBCT

electron-beam computed tomography
EBCT IV angiography
volume-mode EBCT

EBDA

effective balloon-dilated area

EBER

electron beam electroreflectance

EBIORT

electron-beam intraoperative radiotherapy

EBRT

external beam radiation therapy

Ebstein

E. angle
E. anomaly
E. lesion
E. malformation
E. sign

EBT

electron-beam tomography
EBT scanner

eburnated bone
eburnation

bony e.
trapezium-metacarpal e. (TME)

eburneum

osteoma e.

ECA

external carotid artery

E-CABG

endoscopic coronary artery bypass graft

E.CAM dual-head emission imaging
system
ECAT

emission computerized axial tomography
ECAT Reveal PET/CT imaging
system

eccentric

e. atherosclerotic plaque
e. atrophy
e. axis of rotation of ankle
e. coronary artery
e. enhancing nodule
e. epicenter
e. ledge
e. left ventricular hypertrophy
e. medullary bone lesion
e. monocuspid disc valve
e. narrowing
e. pantomography
e. restenosis lesion
e. stenosis
e. vessel

eccentrically placed lumen
eccentricity index
ecchondroma
Eccocee CS ultrasound system
eccrine angiomatous hamartoma
ECD

endocardial cushion defect
ethyl cysteinate dimer
^{99m}Tc ECD

ECE

extracapsular extension

ECG, EKG

echocardiogram
echocardiography

ECG *(continued)*
electrocardiogram
electrocardiography
    ECG trigger
ECG-gated
    ECG-g. multislice
    ECG-g. multislice MR imaging
    ECG-g. spin echo
    ECG-g. spin-echo MR imaging
ECG-synchronized digital subtraction angiography
ECG-triggered
    ECG-t., flow-compensated gradient echo image
    ECG-t. image
    ECG-t. phase contrast cine-gradient-echo sequence
echinococcal
    e. abscess
    e. cyst
echinococcosis
    alveolar e.
    bone e.
    liver e.
    lung e.
echo, pl. **echoes**
    amphoric e.
    asymmetric e.
    atrial e.
    bright e.
    e. characteristic
    e. contrast
    e. contrast agent
    e. delay time (TE)
    dense e.
    e. density
    3D gradient e.
    diaphragmatic e.
    3D magnetization-prepared rapid gradient e.
    driven inversion spin e. (DISE)
    early e.
    ECG-gated spin e.
    endometrial e.
    enhanced fast gradient e. (efgre)
    e. enhancement
    even distribution of echoes
    fast-field e. (FFE)
    fast spoiled gradient-recalled e. (FSPGR)
    fat-suppressed spin e.
    FID-acquired e. (FAcE)
    field e. (FE)
    field e. acquisition with short repetition time and echo reduction (FASTER)
    e. FLASH MR
    fuzzy e.

generalized interferography using spin echoes and stimulated echoes (GINSEST)
generation e.
gradient-recalled e.
gradient-refocused e. (GRE)
gradient-spin e.
hepatic pattern e.
high-amplitude e.
highly mobile e.
highly reflective e.
homogeneous e.
e. image
e. imaging
inhomogeneous e.
internal e.
linear e.
low-amplitude internal e.
low-level e.
magnetization-prepared rapid acquisition gradient e. (MP-RAGE)
median level e.
metallic e.
mirrorlike e.
multiplanar gradient-recalled e.
multiple spin e.
navigator e.
offset radiofrequency spin e.
out-of-phase gradient e.
partial saturation spin e.
particulate e.
e. pattern
pencil-beam navigator e.
e. phase correction (EPC)
e. planar readout
e. plane imaging
pulsed-gradient spin e. (PGSE)
e. ranging
rapid acquisition spin e. (RASE)
rapid gradient e. (RAGE)
e. reflectivity
renal sinus e.
e. rephasing
reverberation e.
RF spin e.
ring-down e.
salvo of echoes
SENSE with half-Fourier single-shot turbo spin e. (SShTSE)
shower of echoes
e. signature
simulated e.
single-shot fast spin e. (SSFSE)
sludgelike intraluminal e.
smokelike e.
solid e.
sonographic e.
e. space

specular e.
spin e.
spin-echo using repeated gradient
  echoes
spoiled gradient e. (SGE)
standard single e.
stimulated e. (STE)
supraventricular venous e.
swirling smokelike echoes
symmetric e.
e. texture
thick e.
e. time (TE)
e. time chemical shift imaging
time of formation of RF spin-echo
  when adjusted to be different
  from gradient spin-e. (TER)
E. Tip trocar needle
e. train
e. train echo time (T_E)
turbo gradient-refocused e.
  (turboGRE)
T1-weighted spin e.
ultrasonographic e.
ventricular e.
echoaortography
echocardiogram (ECG, EKG)
  e. adenosine
  e. planar imaging
echocardiographic
  e. automated border
  e. gating
echocardiography (ECG, EKG)
  adenosine e.
  ambulatory Holter e.
  A-mode e.
  aortic root e.
  aortic valve e.
  apical 2-chamber view e.
  apical 5-chamber view e.
  automated border detection by e.
  biplane transesophageal e.
  blood pool radionuclide e.
  B-mode e.
  cardiac output e.
  2-chamber e.
  4-chamber e.
  color-flow imaging Doppler e.
  continuous-loop exercise e.
  continuous-wave Doppler e.
  contrast e.
  contrast-enhanced e.

cross-sectional 2-dimensional e.
detection e.
2-dimensional e. (TDE)
2-dimensional cross sectional e.
dipyridamole e.
dobutamine stress e. (DSE)
Doppler continuous-wave e.
Doppler pulsed-wave e.
3D transesophageal e.
duplex e.
epicardial Doppler e.
E point on e.
exercise e.
Feigenbaum e.
fetal e.
high-pulse repetition frequency
  Doppler e.
H-mode e.
hypokinesis on e.
e. imaging
intracardiac e. (ICE)
intracoronary contrast e.
intraoperative cardioplegic
  contrast e.
Levovist myocardial contrast e.
Meridian e.
mitral valve e.
M-mode e.
multiplanar transesophageal e.
myocardial contrast e. (MCE)
myocardial perfusion e.
parasternal long-axis view e.
parasternal short-axis view e.
pharmacologic stress e.
postcontrast e.
postexercise e.
postinjection e.
postmyocardial infarction e.
precontrast e.
preinjection e.
premyocardial infarction e.
pulsed Doppler transesophageal e.
pulsed-wave Doppler e.
quantitative Levovist myocardial
  contrast e.
real-time e.
resting e.
resting myocardial e.
short axis view e.
stress e.
subcostal short-axis view e.
supine bicycle stress e.

E

NOTES

echocardiography *(continued)*
    THI e.
    transesophageal e. (TEE)
    transthoracic 3-dimensional e.
    ultrasound e.
    ventricular wall motion e.
Echo-Coat ultrasound biopsy needle
echocolonoscope
    CF-UM3 e.
echo-dense
    e.-d. layer
    e.-d. pattern
    e.-d. valve
echoencephalogram
echoencephalograph
    midline e.
echoencephalography
echoendoscope
    FG-36UX scanning e.
    linear array e.
    Olympus GF-UM2, GF-UM3 e.
    Olympus GIF-1T10 e.
    Olympus JF-UM20 e.
    Olympus VU-M2 e.
    Olympus XIF-UM3 e.
echo-enhanced cystosonography
echo-enhancer
    pulmonary stable e.-e.
echo-enhancing agent
EchoEye
    E. 3-D ultrasound imaging system
    E. ultrasound imaging system
echo-free
    e.-f. area
    e.-f. central zone
    e.-f. layer
    e.-f. space
echogastroscope
EchoGen-enhanced ultrasound
echogenic
    e. appearance
    e. band
    e. calculus
    e. debris
    e. fetal bowel
    e. focus
    e. intraluminal thrombus
    e. liver
    e. liver metastasis
    e. mass
    e. nodule
    e. noise
    e. periphery
    e. plaque
    e. plug
    e. ring
    e. solid lesion
    e. star burst sign
    e. tumor

echogenicity
    brightly increased renal
      parenchymal e.
    calvarial e.
    focally increased renal e.
    generalized increased liver e.
    increased e.
    internal e.
    normal e.
    parenchymal e.
    periventricular e. (PVE)
    e. scatterer
    ultrasound e.
EchoGen ultrasound imaging agent
echogram
    mitral valve e.
echographer
echographia
echography
    B-mode e.
    ophthalmic biometry by
      ultrasound e.
    transrectal e.
    transvaginal e.
echoic
echoicity
echoing
echolaminography
echolocation
echolucent
    e. pattern
    e. plaque
EchoMark catheter
echonography
echophonocardiography
    M-mode e.
echo-planar
    e.-p. diffusion-weighted imaging
    e.-p. FLAIR imaging
    e.-p. GRE T2*-weighted imaging
    e.-p. image
    e.-p. imaging (EPI)
    e.-p. imaging method
    e.-p. pulse sequence
echo-poor
    e.-p. area
    e.-p. areas of environment
    e.-p. testis
echo-ranging
Echospeed
    E. Signa LX 1.5 T scanner
    E. 1.5T MR machine
echo-speed gradient
echo-spin density
echo-tagging technique
echotexture
    compact fibrillar e.
    internal e.
    mottled e.

echo-train
  e.-t. length (ETL)
  e.-t. value
Echovist imaging agent
ECI
  ensemble contrast imaging
Eck fistula
eclampsia
  delayed e.
eclipse
  e. effect lung
  E. MR System
  E. TENS unit
  E. TMR laser
ECRB
  extensor carpi radialis brevis
  ECRB muscle
ECRL
  extensor carpi radialis longus
  ECRL muscle
ECS
  electrocerebral silence
ECT
  emission computed tomography
ectasia
  alveolar e.
  anuloaortic e.
  e. of aorta
  basilar artery e.
  benign duct e.
  bilateral ductal e.
  communicating cavernous e.
  coronary artery e.
  diffuse arterial e.
  digitate e.
  ductal e.
  dural e.
  gonadal venous e.
  mammary duct e.
  moniliform e.
  renal tubular e.
  saccular e.
  seminiferous tubular e.
  tubular e.
  vascular colon e.
ectatic
  e. aneurysm
  e. aortic valve
  e. bronchus
  e. carotid artery
  e. emphysema

ectocardia
ectodermal groove
ectomesenchyme
ectopia
  benign cerebellar e.
  cerebellar e.
  e. cordis
  crossed-fused renal e.
  longitudinal renal e.
  posterior pituitary gland e.
  testicular e.
  tonsillar e.
  transverse testicular e.
ectopic
  e. ACTH syndrome
  e. anus
  e. beat
  e. bone growth
  e. craniopharyngioma
  e. endometrial tissue
  e. firing nociceptor
  e. focus
  e. gallbladder
  e. gland
  e. impulse
  e. intracavernous pituitary
    microadenoma
  e. intraluminal gallstone
  e. kidney
  e. meningioma
  e. ossification
  e. pancreas
  e. parathyroid
  e. parathyroid adenoma
  e. pinealoma
  e. pregnancy (EP)
  e. spleen
  e. testis
  e. thymus
  e. thyroid tissue
  e. ureter
  e. ureterocele
  e. varices
  e. varix
ectopy
EC-TRICKS
  Elliptical Centric-Time Resolved Imaging
  of Contrast Kinetics
ectrodactyly-ectodermal
  e.-e. dysplasia-clefting
  e.-e. dysplasia-clefting syndrome

E

NOTES

ECU
    extensor carpi ulnaris
        ECU muscle
ED
    edge detection
    effective dose
EDAMS
    encephaloduroarteriomyosynangiosis
EDAS
    encephaloduroarteriosynangiosis
EDB
    extensor digitorum brevis
        EDB muscle
EDC
    extensor digitorum communis
    ^{99m}Tc ethyl cysteinate dimer
        EDC muscle
eddy
    e. current
    e. current artifact
    e. current mapping
    e. formation
    e. ringing artifact
edema
    acute interstitial lung e.
    acute pulmonary e.
    adjacent e.
    airspace e.
    alveolar pulmonary e.
    angioneurotic e.
    antral e.
    batwing e.
    bone marrow e.
    brain e.
    brainstem e.
    breast e.
    bronchiolar e.
    brown e.
    bullous e.
    cardiac pulmonary e.
    cardiogenic pulmonary e.
    cardiopulmonary e.
    cerebral e.
    chemical pulmonary e.
    chronic e.
    circumscribed e.
    collateral e.
    compressive e.
    cord e.
    cyclic idiopathic e.
    cytotoxic e.
    diffuse e.
    e. of epididymis
    fetal scalp e.
    fingerprint e.
    e. fluid
    focal e.
    frank pulmonary e.
    fulminant pulmonary e.

generalized pulmonary e.
gravitational e.
gut e.
hemorrhagic pulmonary e.
high-altitude pulmonary e. (HAPE)
hypervolemic pulmonary e.
idiopathic e.
ileocecal e.
inflammatory e.
intercellular e.
interstitial pulmonary e.
intracompartmental e.
intraosseous e.
laryngeal e.
leg e.
liver e.
local e.
localized e.
lung e.
lymphatic e.
lymphaticovenous secondary e.
malignant brain e.
massive ovarian e.
massive pulmonary hemorrhagic e.
mediastinal fat e.
mild e.
negative image pulmonary e.
e. neonatorum
nephrotic e.
nerve root e.
neurogenic pulmonary e.
neuronal cytotoxic e.
noncardiac pulmonary e.
noncardiogenic pulmonary e.
orbital e.
osmotic e.
ovarian e.
paroxysmal pulmonary e.
passive e.
patchy e.
e. pattern
pericholecystic e.
pericystic e.
perifocal e.
perihilar e.
perineoplastic e.
periorbital e.
peripheral vasogenic e.
peritumoral e.
perivascular e.
permeability pulmonary e.
placental e.
preosteonecrosis marrow e.
pulmonary e. (PE)
reactive marrow e.
reexpansion pulmonary e.
renal e.
reperfusion lung e.
reversible vasogenic e.

solid e.
stasis e.
stomal e.
subchondral marrow e.
subcutaneous e.
subglottic e.
supraglottic e.
terminal e.
testicular posttraumatic e.
thalamic e.
trace e.
transient bone marrow e.
umbilical cord e.
unilateral pulmonary e.
vasogenic e.
venous e.
vernal e.
visceral e.
white matter e.

edematous
e. brain
e. bronchus
e. gallbladder
e. kidney
e. pancreatitis
e. pleura
e. tissue

Eder-Puestow dilatation

edge
boundary e.
Compton e.
e. detection (ED)
e. effect
e. enhancement
leading e.
ligament reflecting e.
ligament shelving e.
liver e.
e. misalignment artifact
e. packing
patellar e.
e. response function (ERF)
e. ringing
e. ringing artifact
sawtooth e.
e. shadow
shelving e. of Poupart ligament
e. stenosis
sternal e.
tentorial e.
ulcer with heaped-up e.'s

edge-boundary artifact

edge-detection
e.-d. angiography
e.-d. procedure

edge-enhanced error diffusion algorithm

edge-region pixel

EDH
epidural hematoma

E-dial calibration

Edison
E. effect
E. fluoroscope

editing
spectral e.

EDL
extensor digiti longus
EDL muscle

EDQ
extensor digiti quinti
EDQ muscle

EDR
exposure data recognizer

EDSS
expanded-disability status scale

EDTMP
ethylenediaminetetramethylene
phosphonic acid
EDTMP imaging agent

education
Projects in Medical E. (PRIME)

Edwards
double aortic arch of E.
E. Fogarty
E. syndrome
E. Thrombex PMT system

EDXRF
energy-dispersive x-ray fluorescence
EDXRF spectrometer

EEG
electroencephalography

EF
ejection fraction

efaproxiral

EFF
electromagnetic focusing field

effaced mucosal fold

effacement
architectural e.
cistern e.
cisterna magna e.
e. of dura
dural sac e.
mesencephalic cistern e.

NOTES

effacement *(continued)*
    nerve root sheath e.
    pelvocalyceal e.
    sulcus e.
    ventricle e.

effect
    abscopal e.
    adverse e.
    Anrep e.
    arterial sump e.
    artifact e.
    attenuation e.
    Auger e.
    Bayliss e.
    beam-hardening e.
    Bernoulli e.
    bilateral vagotomy e.
    blood oxygenation level-dependent e.
    Bohr e.
    BOLD e.
    Bowditch e.
    bronchodilator e.
    bronchomotor e.
    bronchospastic e.
    butterfly e.
    bystander e.
    candy-wrapper e.
    Cherenkov e.
    cobra-head e.
    collimator exchange e.
    Compton e.
    contact e.
    contrast media adverse e.
    copper wire e.
    cumulative radiation e. (CRE)
    Curie e.
    deleterious e.
    demagnetization field e.
    deterministic e.
    Doppler e.
    Dotter e.
    dottering e.
    duodenum extrinsic pressure e.
    dynamic lineshape e.
    edge e.
    Edison e.
    first-pass e.
    flow-related enhancement e.
    flow void e.
    gastrointestinal adverse e.
    genitourinary adverse e.
    halo e.
    heel e.
    hematocrit e.
    hemispheral mass e.
    hemodynamic e.
    isotope e.
    lag e.
    Laplace e.
    localized mass e.
    Mach band e.
    Macklin e.
    macromolecular hydration e.
    magic angle e.
    magnetization transfer e.
    magnetohydrodynamic e.
    masquerading e.
    mass e.
    methemoglobin e.
    missile e.
    multilog e.
    neurotoxic e.
    nozzle e.
    nuclear Overhauser e.
    osmotic e.
    outflow e.
    Overhauser e.
    oxygen e.
    pacemaker e.
    pad e.
    paramagnetic e.
    passive loss of correlation e.
    phase e.
    phase-shift e.
    photoechoic e.
    photoelectric e.
    photographic e. (PE)
    photonuclear e.
    piezoelectric e.
    pinchcock e.
    postvagotomy e.
    priming e.
    purse-stringing e.
    radiation e.
    radiographic e.
    reservoir e.
    Russell e.
    sausage segment e.
    scalar e.
    side e.
    silver wire e.
    sink e.
    skin e.
    skin-sparing e.
    snowplow e.
    sonic e.
    star e.
    steal e.
    stochastic e.
    susceptibility e.
    systematic relaxation e.
    T2 dephasing e.
    teratogenic e.
    thermal e.
    time-of-flight e.
    tracheal mass e.
    vagatomy e.

vasodilatory e.
Venturi e.
Volta e.
Warburg e.
washboard e.
wash-in e.
washout e.
Wolff-Chaikoff e.
effective
e. atomic number
e. balloon-dilated area (EBDA)
e. focal spot size
e. half-life
e. mass attenuation coefficient
e. path length (EPL)
e. pulmonary blood flow (EPBF)
e. pulmonic index
e. refractory period (ERP)
e. renal plasma flow (ERFP, ERPF)
e. section thickness
e. transverse relation time
effectiveness
relative biologic e. (RBE)
effector/target cell interaction
efferent
e. arteriolar resistance
e. digital nerve
e. duct
e. ductule of testis
e. loop
e. loop obstruction
e. lymph vessel
e. nipple valve
e. view
effervescent agent
efficacy study
efficiency
absolute e.
conversion e.
detective quantum e. (DQE)
full-energy peak e.
geometric e.
geometrical e.
intrinsic e.
kidney extraction e.
quantum detection e. (QDE)
valvular e.
window e.
efficient relaxation time
effluents
radioactive e.

efflux
drug e.
e. inhibitor
e. pump
effort
inspiratory e.
respiratory e.
shallow inspiratory e.
suboptimal e.
e. thrombosis
ventilatory e.
voluntary e. (VE)
effort-dependent
effused chyle
effusion
e. artifact
asbestos-related pleural e.
Baccelli sign of pleural e.
benign subdural e.
cardiac e.
chocolate joint e.
chylous e.
discrete area of e.
epidural e.
exudative pleural e.
fetal pleural e.
free pleural e.
hemorrhagic pleural e.
inflammatory joint e.
ipsilateral pleural e.
joint e.
Karplus sign of pleural e.
Kellock sign of pleural e.
knee joint e.
large volume joint e.
layering e.
left-sided pleural e.
liquid pleural e.
loculated pleural e.
malignant pleural e.
massive pleural e.
milky e.
moderate-sized volume joint e.
noninflammatory joint e.
parapneumonic e.
pericardial e. (PE)
peritoneal e.
pleural e.
pleuropericardial e.
pseudochylous e.
serofibrinous pericardial e.
serous e.

E

NOTES

effusion *(continued)*
    e. shadow
    subdeltoid bursal e.
    subdural e.
    subpleural e.
    subpulmonic e.
    taut pericardial e.
    transient pleural e.
    transudative pleural e.
    tuberculous e.
    unilateral pleural e.
EFG
    electric field gradient
efgre
    enhanced fast gradient echo
    fast acquisition with multiphase
      efgre (FAME)
EFOV
    extended-field-of view technique
EFW
    estimated fetal weight
EG
    esophagogastric
Egan mammography
EGD
    esophagogastroduodenoscopy
egg-on-its-side heart
egg-shaped orbit
eggshell
    e. border of aneurysm
    e. breast calcification
    e. calcification
    e. calcification of lymph node
    e. nodal calcification
egress of blood
Egyptian splenomegaly
EHL
    electrohydraulic lithotripsy
    extensor hallucis longus
Ehlers-Danlos syndrome
EHM
    extrahepatic metastasis
EHT
    electrohydrothermal electrode
EIC
    extensive intraductal carcinoma
    extensive intraductal component
eigenvector
    e. analysis
    principal e.
eighth
    e. cranial nerve complex
    e. nerve tumor
Eindhoven magnet
einsteinium (Es)
einsteinium 255 (^{255}Es)
Einthoven triangle

EIP
    extensor indicis proprius
    EIP muscle
EIS
    electrical impedance scanning
    EIS spot
    targeted EIS
Eisenmenger
    E. complex
    E. defect
    E. group
    E. reaction
    E. syndrome
EIT
    electrical impedance tomography
ejaculatory duct
ejection
    e. fraction (EF)
    e. fraction by first-pass technique
    e. phase index
    e. time (ET)
EJV
    external jugular vein
EKG *(var. of* ECG)
    echocardiogram
    echocardiography
    electrocardiogram
Eklund
    E. technique
    E. view
Ekman-Lobstein disease
EKY
    electrokymogram
EL2-LS2 flexible video laparoscope
EL2-TF410 laparoscope
El-Ahwany classification of humeral supracondylar fracture
elastance
    maximum ventricular e.
elastic
    e. cartilage
    e. collision
    e. cross-section
    e. imaging
    e. recoil of artery
    e. scattering spectroscopy
    e. stable intramedullary nailing (ESIN)
    e. subtraction algorithm
    e. subtraction spiral CT angiography
elasticity
elasticum
    pseudoxanthoma e.
elasticus
    conus e.
elastin deposition in taeniae coli
elastofibroma

elastography
    magnetic resonance e. (MRE)
elastomyofibrosis
elastosis
elbow
    above e. (AE)
    baseball pitcher's e.
    e. bone center
    boxer's e.
    e. contracture
    e. coronal scan
    e. extensor tendon
    floating e.
    e. fracture
    golfer's e.
    javelin thrower's e.
    e. joint
    milkmaid's e.
    nursemaid's e.
    reverse tennis e.
    tennis e.
    thrower's e.
    wrestler's e.
ELCA
    excimer laser coronary angioplasty
    ELCA laser
ELD
    energy level diagram
elective TIPS
electric
    e. dipole
    e. field gradient (EFG)
    e. generator
    e. induction
    e. interaction
    e. joint fluoroscopy
    e. joint fluoroscopy imaging
    e. quadrupole coupling
    e. stimulation
    e. syringe
electrical
    e. activity
    e. circulatory arrest
    e. grounding pad
    e. impedance scanning (EIS)
    e. impedance tomography (EIT)
    e. potential energy
electrically
    e. activated implant
    e. detachable coil
Electro-Acuscope device
electrocardiogram (ECG, EKG)

    resting e.
    signal-averaged e. (SAECG, SaECG)
    e. tracing
    e. trigger
electrocardiogram-gated
    e.-g. high-speed X-ray computed tomography
    e.-g. MRI
    e.-g. MRI imaging
    e.-g. multislice spiral CT
    e.-g. multislice spiral CT of heart
    e.-g. SPECT
    e.-g. tomography
electrocardiogram-synchronized digital subtraction angiography
electrocardiographic
    e. gating
    e. trigger method
    e. variant
electrocardiograph triggering
electrocardiography (ECG, EKG)
electrocardiography-gated echo-planar imaging
electrocardiophonogram
electrocardioscanner
    Compuscan Hittman computerized e.
electrocautery
    endoluminal radiofrequency e.
    monopolar radiofrequency e.
electrocerebral silence (ECS)
electrocoagulation
    intraluminal e.
electrode
    e. array
    electrohydrothermal e. (EHT)
    esophageal pill e.
    Medelec DMG 50 Teflon-coated monopolar e.
    e. monitoring
    monopolar e.
    MRI-compatible e.
    patch e.
    polarographic needle e.
    subcutaneous array e.
electrodesiccation
electrodiagnosis
electrodiagnostic imaging

NOTES

electroencephalogram
    flat e.
    isoelectric e.
electroencephalography (EEG)
    intracranial e.
    quantitative e. (QEEG)
electrogastrogram
electrogastrograph
electrogram
    atrial e.
    coronary sinus e.
    esophageal e.
    high right atrial e. (HRA)
    His bundle e. (HBE)
    intraatrial e.
    intracardiac e.
    right ventricular e.
    right ventricular apical e.
    RVA e.
    sinus node e.
electrography
electrohydraulic
    e. disintegrator
    e. fragmentation
    e. lithotripsy (EHL)
    e. probe
    e. shockwave lithotripsy
electrohydrothermal electrode (EHT)
electrohysterogram
electrohysterography
electrokymogram (EKY)
electrokymograph
electroluminescent sensitometer
electrolytic reduction
electromagnet
    structured coil e.
electromagnetic (EM)
    e. absorption
    e. articulography (EMA)
    e. blood flow imaging
    e. blood flow study
    e. energy
    e. field
    e. flow probe
    e. focusing field (EFF)
    e. induction
    e. interference (EMI)
    e. interference scan
    e. modeling
    e. radiation
    e. radiation exposure
    e. spectrum
    e. unit (emu)
    e. wave
electromagnetism
electromechanical dissociation (EMD)

electrometer
    dynamic-condenser e.
    vibrating-reed e.
electromotive force (emf)
electromyogram (EMG)
electromyography (EMG)
electron
    angle e. (UE)
    e. arc therapy
    Auger e.
    backscatter e.
    e. beam
    e. beam angiography (EBA)
    e. beam CT scanner
    e. beam electroreflectance (EBER)
    e. beam therapy
    e. beam tomography
    e. bolus
    bound e.
    e. capture
    e. cloud
    Compton e.
    conversion e.
    e. diffraction camera
    e. dosimetry
    emission e.
    e. equilibrium loss
    excited e.
    e. flow
    e. flux
    free e.
    e. gun
    internal conversion e.
    K e.
    L e.
    e. linear accelerator
    e. microscopy
    e. multiplier tube
    e. neutrino
    e. orbit
    orbital e.
    oscillating e.
    e. paramagnetic resonance (EPR)
    e. paramagnetic resonance spatial
      imaging
    positive e.
    e. radiography
    e. radiography imaging
    recoil e.
    secondary e.
    e. spin
    e. spin resonance (ESR)
    e. stream
    e. theory
    transition e.
    e. valence
    e. volt (eV, ev)
electron-beam
    e.-b. boost

e.-b. computed tomography (EBCT)
e.-b. CT-derived CAC score
e.-b. intraoperative radiotherapy (EBIORT)
e.-b. tomography (EBT)
electron-capture decay mode
electron-dense
electroneuromyography
electronic
e. atlas of hippocampus
e. collimation
e. dosimeter
e. focusing field
e. independent beam steering
e. linear array transducer
e. magnification
e. micro analyzer (EMA)
e. picture acquisition
e. portal imaging
e. stabilization
e. thermometer
electronic thermometer
electron-photon field matching
electron-positron pair
electrooculogram apparatus
electrooculographic analysis
electrooptical device
electropherogram
electrophilic radioiodination
electrophysiologic mapping
electrophysiology (EP)
electropolished stent
electroradiology
electroradiometer
electroreflectance
electron beam e. (EBER)
electroretinogram (ERG)
flicker e.
electroscope
electrospray ionization mass spectroscopy
electrostatic
e. generator
e. imaging
e. imaging system
e. potential
electrothermal catheter
electrovectorcardiogram
electrovectorcardiography
Elema roll-film changer

element
blowout lesion of posterior vertebral e.
daughter e.
estrogen-response e. (ERE)
fibroglandular e.
infiltrative hemorrhagic e.
inflammatory e.
neoplastic destruction of spinal e.
parent e.
picture e.
radioactive e.
resolution e.
e. subluxation
volume e.
voxel e.
elementary
e. body
e. fracture
8000-element linear array CCD scanner
2-element phased array coil
4-element phased array coil
element-specific detector
elephant
e. ears pelvis
e. trunk graft
e. trunk technique
elephantiasis neuromatosa
elevated
e. diaphragm
e. gradient
e. leg support
e. lower esophageal sphincter resting pressure
e. retinal hamartoma
elevation
bilateral diaphragmatic e.
chorioamnionic e.
diaphragmatic e.
periosteal e.
unilateral diaphragmatic e.
elevatus
hallux e.
ELF
extremely low frequency
elimination
e. curve
e. half-life
e. kinetics
pyelography by e.
Elite
VasoSeal E.

NOTES

Ellestad protocol
ellipsoid
    e. joint
    e. lesion
    e. method
elliptic, elliptical
    e. centric acquisition
    e. lumen
ellipticity index
Ellis
    E. Jones peroneal displacement
    E. line
    E. technique for Barton fracture
Ellis-Garland line
Ellis-van Creveld syndrome
Eloesser procedure
elongated
    e. aorta
    e. heart
    e. mass
    e. structure
elongation
    aortic e.
    e. and tortuosity
    e. of ventricle
eloquent
    e. area of brain
    e. cortex
ELPS
    excessive lateral pressure syndrome
Elscint
    E. APEX 409-AG ECT camera
    E. APEX 009 Precursor camera
    E. dual-detector cardiac camera
    E. Dual-Head Helix camera
    E. Excel 905 scanner
    E. MR scanner
    E. Prestige MRI system
    E. Twin CT scanner
elution
elutriation
ELVT
    endolaser venous therapy
EM
    electromagnetic
EMA
    electromagnetic articulography
    electronic micro analyzer
emanation
    actinium e.
    radium e.
    thorium e.
emanatorium
emanon
emanotherapy
embarrassment
    circulatory e.
    cord e.

    nerve root e.
    respiratory e.
Embden-Meyerhof glycolytic pathway
embedding of stent coil
EmboGold microsphere
embolectomy
    percutaneous e.
emboli (*pl. of* embolus)
embolic
    e. aneurysm
    e. cerebral infarct
    e. debris
    e. event
    e. material
    e. necrosis
    e. obstruction
    e. occlusion
    e. phenomenon
    e. pneumonia
    e. shower
    e. stroke
embolism
    cerebral e.
    coronary e.
    venography-related air e.
    venous e.
embolization
    bronchial artery e. (BAE)
    N-butyl-2-cyanoacrylate e.
    coil e.
    distal e.
    fibroid e.
    Guglielmi detachable coil e.
    Lipiodol e.
    nontarget e.
    ovarian vein e.
    paradoxic e.
    particulate arterial e.
    platinum coil e.
    polyvinyl alcohol particle e.
    pulmonary artery e.
    SAP-MS transarterial e.
    spontaneous hemodialysis catheter
      fracture and e.
    testicular vein e.
    transcatheter arterial e. (TAE)
    e. transcatheter therapy
    transhepatic variceal e.
    uterine artery e. (UAE)
    uterine fibroid e. (UFE)
embolotherapy
    percutaneous e.
embolus, pl. **emboli**
    air e.
    amnionic fluid e.
    arterial e.
    atheromatous e.
    bacillary e.
    bile pulmonary e.

bland e.
bone marrow e.
cancer e.
capillary e.
cardiogenic e.
catheter-induced e.
cellular e.
cerebral fat e.
cholesterol e.
coronary artery e.
cotton fiber e.
crossed e.
direct e.
fat e.
fibrin platelet e.
foam e.
foreign body e.
hematogenous e.
infective e.
intracranial e.
intraluminal e.
lymphogenous e.
massive e.
e. migration
miliary e.
multiple emboli
obturating e.
occluding spring e.
oil e.
pantaloon e.
paradoxic cerebral e.
peripheral e.
plasmodium e.
platelet-fibrin e.
polyurethane foam e.
prosthetic valve e.
pulmonary e. (PE)
pulmonary venous-systemic air e.
pyemic e.
recurrent e.
renal cholesterol e.
retinal e.
retrograde e.
riding e.
saddle e.
septic pulmonary e.
silent cerebral e.
straddling e.
submassive pulmonary e.
therapeutic e.
thrombus e.
trichinous e.

tumor e.
venous thrombosis e.
visceral e.
Embosphere
E. microsphere
embosphere particle
embryo
adnexal e.
e. demise
e. size
embryogenesis
embryoid body
embryology
airway e.
breast e.
diaphragm e.
genital tract e.
reproductive tract e.
urogenital e.
embryonal
e. adenoma
e. carcinosarcoma
e. cell carcinoma
e. liver sarcoma
e. ovary teratoma
e. rhabdomyosarcoma
e. tumor
e. vein
embryonic
e. abdominal cavity
e. anastomosis
e. aortic arch
e. branchial arch
e. disc
e. organizer
e. ovary
e. period
e. sac
e. truncus arteriosus
e. tumor
e. umbilical vein
embryopathy
warfarin e.
embryotoxon
posterior e.
EMD
electromechanical dissociation
EMED scanner
emetic center
EMF
endomyocardial fibrosis

NOTES

E

emf
electromotive force
EMG
electromyogram
electromyography
Neuropack 4, 8 EMG
EMI
electromagnetic interference
EMI brain scanner
EMI CT 500 scanner
EMI 7070 scanner
EMI unit
eminence
arcuate e.
articular e.
collateral e.
cruciate e.
cruciform e.
deltoid e.
facial e.
frontal e.
genital e.
hypothenar e.
iliopectineal e.
iliopubic e.
intercondylar e.
malar e.
medial e.
occipital e.
parietal e.
pyramidal e.
thenar e.
thyroid e.
tibial intercondylar e.
emissary
e. sphenoidal foramen
e. vein
emission
e. angiography
beta e.
characteristic e.
e. computed tomography (ECT)
e. computer-assisted tomography
e. computerized axial tomography (ECAT)
double e.
e. electron
filament e.
gamma e.
e. hepatogram
induced acoustic e.
negatron e.
photoelectric e.
e. probability
radioactive e.
e. range
e. renography
source of e.
spectral e.

stimulated acoustic e. (SAE)
thermonic e.
e. tomography
e. and transmission data
emitter
alpha-particle e.
Auger-electron e.
beta e.
gamma e.
EMP
extramedullary plasmacytoma
emphysema
alveolar duct e.
atrophic e.
bronchiolar e.
bullous e.
centriacinar e.
centrilobular e.
chronic hypertrophic e.
chronic obstructive e.
chronic pulmonary e. (CPE)
chronic tuberculous e.
compensatory e.
congenital lobar e.
cystic pulmonary e.
diffuse e.
distal acinar e.
distal lobular e.
ectatic e.
false e.
focal-dust e.
gangrenous e.
gastric e.
generalized e.
giant bullous e.
glass blower's e.
hypoplastic e.
idiopathic unilobar e.
increased marking of e.
infantile lobar e.
interlobular e.
interstitial intestinal e.
interstitial lung e.
intestinal e.
intramural gastric e.
irregular e.
linear e.
liquefactive e.
lobar e.
localized obstructive e.
lung e.
mediastinal e.
neck e.
necrotizing e.
neonatal cystic pulmonary e.
obstructive e.
orbital e.
oxygen-dependent e.
panacinar e.

panlobular e.
paracicatricial e.
paraseptal e.
pericicatricial e.
perifocal e.
postoperative e.
postsurgical e.
proximal acinar e.
pulmonary interstitial e. (PIE)
pulmonary subcutaneous
  encephalitis e.
restrictive pulmonary e.
scar e.
senile e.
skeletal e.
small-lunged e.
subcutaneous e.
surgical e.
traumatic e.
unilateral lobar e.
vesicular e.

emphysematosa
vaginitis e.

emphysematous
e. bleb
e. bulla
e. cholecystitis
e. COPD
e. cystitis
e. enterocolitis
e. expansion
e. gastritis
e. lung
e. pyelitis
e. pyelonephritis (EPN)

empirical method

empty
e. collapsed lung
e. delta sign
e. gestational sac
e. heart
e. sella
e. sella syndrome
e. uterus

emptying
complete bladder e.
delayed gastric e.
gastric e. (GE)
incomplete bladder e.
oropharyngeal e.
e. time
tortuous e.

empyema
brain e.
chest e.
CNS e.
epidural e.
gallbladder e.
Hawkins accordion-type e.
interlobar e.
intracranial e.
latent e.
left-sided e.
loculated e.
metapneumonic e.
pericardial e.
pleural e.
pulsating e.
right-sided e.
spinal e.
subdural e.
synpneumonic e.
thoracic e.
tuberculous e.

E-MRI
extremity MRI

emu
electromagnetic unit

emulsion
e. film
nuclear e.

Emulsoil bowel preparation

en
en bloc excision
en bloc resection
en face
en face view
en passage feeder artery

enalaprilat

enalaprilat-enhanced renography

enamel
e. crypt
e. lamella

enantiomer

enarthrosis

encapsulated
e. brain abscess
e. fat-containing lesion
e. fat necrosis
e. fluid
e. gas bubble
e. mass
e. neoplasm

NOTES

307

encapsulated *(continued)*
    e. radioactive seed
    e. subdural hematoma
encased heart
encasement
    vascular e.
    ventricular e.
encephali
    arachnoidea mater e.
encephalic
    e. angioma
    e. vesicle
encephalitis, pl. **encephalitides**
    brainstem e.
    bronzed sclerosing e.
    CMV e.
    cytomegalovirus e.
    herpes simplex virus type 1 e.
    HIV e.
    HSV1 e.
    listeria e.
    e. periaxialis concentrica
    postinfectious e.
    primary HIV e.
    Rasmussen e.
    subacute e.
    toxoplasmosis e.
encephaloarteriography
encephalocele
    frontoethmoidal e.
    frontosphenoidal e.
    occipital e.
    parietal e.
    sphenoethmoidal e.
    sphenoidal e.
    sphenomaxillary e.
    sphenoorbital e.
    sphenopharyngeal e.
    transethmoidal e.
encephaloclastic
    e. lesion
    e. porencephaly
encephalocystocele
encephaloduroarteriomyosynangiosis (EDAMS)
encephaloduroarteriosynangiosis (EDAS)
encephalodysplasia
encephalogram
encephalograph
encephalography
    air e.
    A-mode e.
    fractional e.
    gamma e.
    positive contrast e.
encephaloid carcinoma
encephalolith
encephaloma

encephalomalacia
    inherited cavernous angioma–related posthemorrhage e.
    macrocystic e.
    microcystic e.
    multicystic e.
    neonate e.
encephalomeningocele
encephalometry
encephalomyelitis
    acute disseminated e. (ADEM)
    enteroviral e.
    postinfectious e. (PIE)
encephalomyelopathy
    subacute necrotizing e.
encephalomyopathy
    mitochondrial e.
encephalopathia subcorticalis progressiva
encephalopathy
    AIDS e.
    anoxic e.
    Binswanger e.
    HIV e.
    hypertensive e.
    hypoxic ischemic e.
    ischemic e.
    lead e.
    subcortical arteriosclerotic e.
    subcortical atherosclerotic e.
encephalotrigeminal
    e. angiomatosis
    e. syndrome
encerclage
enchondral
    e. bone formation
    e. ossification
enchondroma
enchondromatosis
    multiple e.
enchondrosarcoma
encode
    frequency e. (FE, FR)
encoded
    sensitivity e. (SENSE)
encoded-Fourier
encoding
    amplitude of phase e.
    centrally ordered phase e.
    coil sensitive e.
    1-dimensional phase e.
    3D spatial e.
    frequency e.
    gradient e.
    ordered phase e.
    phase e. (PE)
    position e.
    reordering of phase e.
    respiratory ordered phase e. (ROPE)

respiratory sorted phase e.
sensitivity e. (SENSE)
spatial e.
wavelet e.
encroaching endothelial cell
encroachment
bony e.
foraminal e.
luminal e.
soft tissue canal e.
stenosis e.
encrustation
bile e.
encryption algorithm
encysted
e. calculus
e. pleurisy
end
e. of atrial systole
bone e.
e. bud
e. bulb
e. exhalation
e. expiration
fimbriated e.
e. inhalation
e. organ resistance
e. plate
e. point
e. of saturated bombardment
(EOSB)
seen on e.
e. systole (ES)
e. systolic pressure to end systolic
volume
endarterectomy
carotid e. (CEA)
extraluminal e.
femoral e.
e. graft
surgical e.
transluminal e.
endarteritis obliterans
end-diastolic
e.-d. aortic-left ventricular pressure
gradient
e.-d. imaging
e.-d. polar map
e.-d. pressure-volume relation
e.-d. velocity measurement
e.-d. volume
e.-d. volume index

Endeavor drug-eluting stent
end-expiratory lung volume
end-fire transducer
end-hole introducer
endoanal
e. coil
e. MR imaging
e. sonography
e. ultrasound
Endobile
endobiliary stenting
EndoBlade
endobrachyesophagus
endobronchial
e. carcinoma
e. hamartoma
e. Kaposi sarcoma
e. lesion
e. metastasis
e. obstruction
e. sarcoidosis
e. tube
e. tuberculosis
e. tumor
endocardial, endocardiac
e. activation mapping
e. catheter mapping
e. centroid
e. cushion
e. cushion defect (ECD)
e. cushion development
e. cushion malformation
e. cushion ventricular septal defect
e. dysplasia
e. fibroelastosis
e. fibrosis
e. plaque
e. pressure
e. sclerosis
e. trabeculation
e. volume
endocarditis
aortic valve e.
atypical verrucous e.
bacterial e.
Löffler fibroplastic e.
maranti e.
marantic e.
subacute bacterial e.
thrombotic e.

E

NOTES

endocardium
    disc of e.
    wafer of e.
endocatheter ruler
endocervical
    e. canal
    e. canal coloscopy
    e. mucosa
endochondral
    e. bone
    e. bone deposit
endochondroma
endocranium
endocrine
    e. ablative therapy
    e. gland
    e. imaging
    e. tumor
endocyst
endodermal
    e. cyst
    e. pouch
    e. sinus
    e. sinus ovarian tumor
    e. sinus testis tumor
endodiascope
endodiascopy
endoergic reaction
endoesophageal MRI coil
endofluoroscopic technique
endofluoroscopy
    flexible e.
    percutaneous e.
    rigid e.
endogenous
    e. adenosine contrast medium
    e. callus formation
    e. contrast agent
    e. lipid pneumonia
Endografin
endograft
    AneuRx e.
endografting
    transluminal e.
endolaser venous therapy (ELVT)
endoleak
    e. graft
    type 1, 2 e.
    type I e. (T1EL)
    type II e. (T2EL)
    type III e.
    type IV e.
endoluminal
    e. density
    e. fly through
    e. MRI
    e. radiofrequency electrocautery
    e. sonography

    e. view
    e. visualization
endolymphatic
    e. duct
    e. hydrops
    e. sac
    e. sac tumor
    e. stromal myosis
endometria (*pl. of* endometrium)
endometrial
    e. adenocanthoma
    e. anatomy
    e. canal fluid
    e. carcinoma
    e. cavity
    e. cyst
    e. echo
    e. fluid in canal
    e. hyperplasia
    e. implant
    e. island
    e. polyp
    e. secretory adenocarcinoma
    e. stripe
    e. stromal sarcoma
    e. surface deformity
    e. thickness
endometrioid
    e. cystadenoma
    e. ovarian carcinoma
    e. tumor
endometrioma
endometriosis
    bladder e.
    colonic involvement of e.
    GI tract e.
    gynecologic e.
    e. interna
    sciatic e.
    ureteral e.
endometriotic cyst
endometritis
    inflammatory e.
endometrium, pl. **endometria**
    decidualized e.
    FIGO staging of adenocarcinoma
      of e.
    inactive e.
    postmenopausal e.
    proliferative phase e.
    secretory phase e.
    thickened irregular e.
endometry
endomyelography
endomyocardial
    e. fibroplasia
    e. fibrosis (EMF)
endoneural
endoneurium

endoneurosonography
end-on vessel
endopelvic fascia
endophlebitis
Endo-P-Probe
endoprobe
> rotating e.
> single-crystal e.

endoprosthesis
> biliary e.
> Carey-Coons soft stent biliary e.
> constrained Wallgraft e.
> double-lumen e.
> double-pigtail e.
> Hemobahn e.
> IntraCoil e.
> large-bore bile duct e.
> metallic biliary e.
> self-expanding metallic e.
> Viabahn e.
> Viabil biliary e.
> VIATORR E.
> Wallgraft e.
> Wallstent biliary e.

endopyelotomy
> percutaneous e.

endorectal
> e. coil
> e. ileal pouch
> e. surface-coil MR imaging
> e. ultrasound (ERU, ERUS, EUS)

end-organ response
endosaccular packing
endosalpingosis
endoscope
> double-channel e.
> Olympus EVIS Q-200V e.
> Olympus TJF-100 e.
> virtual e.
> Zeiss EndoLive e.

endoscopic
> e. cholangiography (ERC)
> e. coronary artery bypass graft (E-CABG)
> e. decompression
> e. laser
> e. laser cholecystectomy
> e. laser dacryocystorhinostomy
> e. lithotripsy
> e. optical coherence tomography (EOCT)
> e. percutaneous cholangiopancreatography
> e. procedure
> e. quadrature radiofrequency coil
> e. retrograde cholangiogram (ERC)
> e. retrograde cholangiopancreatography (ERCP)
> e. retrograde pancreatic duct cannulation
> e. retrograde pancreatography
> e. retrograde parenchymography (ERP)
> e. sonography
> e. surveillance
> e. ultrasound (EUS)
> e. ultrasound-guided fine needle aspiration (EUS-FNA)
> e. washing pipe

endoscopy
> colorectal cancer e.
> digital high-speed e.
> gastrointestinal e.
> laser-assisted spinal e. (LASE)
> M2A imaging capsule e.
> percutaneous e.
> upper gastrointestinal e.
> velolaryngeal e.
> virtual arterial e.
> wireless capsule e.

endoskeleton
endosonographic image
endosonography
> 3D e.
> hydrogen peroxide-enhanced anal e.
> rectal e.
> transduodenal e.
> transgastric e.
> vaginal e.

endosonoscopy
Endosound endoscopic ultrasound catheter
endosseous implant
Endostaple device
endosteal
> e. callus
> e. chondrosarcoma
> e. revascularization
> e. scalloping
> e. surface

endosteoma
endosteum
endothelia (*pl. of* endothelium)

NOTES

endothelial
  e. damage
  e. hypoplasia
  e. injury
  e. leukocyte
  e. myeloma
  e. surface
endothelialization
endothelialized vascular graft
endotheliomatous meningioma
endothelium, pl. **endothelia**
  arterial e.
  capillary e.
  pulmonary capillary e.
endothoracic fascia
endothorax
  tension e.
endotracheal (ET)
  e. intubation
  e. tube
endovaginal
  e. coil
  e. sonography
  e. ultrasound (EVUS)
endovascular
  e. aneurysm repair (EVAR)
  e. aortic graft
  e. brachytherapy
  e. coil
  e. embolization femoral approach
  e. exclusion
  e. flow wire study
  e. photo acoustic recanalization
   (EPAR)
  e. recanalization
  e. repair
  e. stent-graft
  e. system
  e. technique
  e. ultrasonography
  e. ultrasound
EndoVasix EPAR laser system
endovenous laser treatment (EVLT)
endplate
  cartilage e.
  cartilaginous e.
  hyaline cartilage e.
  e. sclerosis
  vertebral body e.
endpoint
  clear e.
  measurable e.
  stress e.
end-pressure artifact
end-stage
  e.-s. adult cardiac decompensation
  e.-s. cardiomyopathy
  e.-s. cirrhosis
  e.-s. fetal cardiac decompensation

  e.-s. lung disease
  e.-s. renal disease
  e.-s. renal failure (ESRF)
end-systolic
  e.-s. polar map
  e.-s. pressure (ESP)
  e.-s. pressure-end-systolic volume
   ratio (ESP-ESV)
  e.-s. pressure-volume relation
  e.-s. residual volume
  e.-s. reversal
  e.-s. volume (ESV)
  e.-s. volume index (ESVI)
  e.-s. wall index:end-systolic volume
   ratio
end-to-side biliary-enteric anastomosis
end-viewing transducer
**Enecat CT concentrated rectal
  suspension**
enema
  air-contrast barium e. (ACBE)
  analeptic e.
  barium e. (BE)
  blind e.
  cleansing e.
  contrast e.
  Cortenema retention e.
  double-contrast barium e. (DCBE)
  full-column barium e.
  Gastrografin e.
  Harris flush e.
  hydrocortisone e.
  hydrogen peroxide e.
  Hypaque e.
  hypertonic e.
  mesalamine e.
  methylene blue e.
  nuclear e.
  oil-retention e.
  opaque e.
  phosphate e.
  phosphosoda e.
  retention e.
  Rowasa e.
  saline e.
  self-administered cleansing e.
  single-contrast barium e.
  small bowel e.
  soap suds e.
  tap water e.
  therapeutic barium e.
  water-soluble contrast e.
enemas until clear
energetic positron
energy
  atomic e.
  average positron e.
  beam e.
  binding e.

chemical potential e.
e. decay
electrical potential e.
electromagnetic e.
e. fluence
e. flux density
e. frequency
gravitational potential e.
kinetic e.
laser e.
e. level
e. level diagram (ELD)
low-photon e.
mechanical potential e.
nuclear e.
photon e.
potential e.
quadrant e.
quantum e.
radiant e.
radiation e.
radiofrequency e.
recoil e.
e. resolution
e. spectrum
e. subtraction
thermal e.
e. transfer
e. transfer process
treatment e.
variable e.
e. wave
e. wavelength
e. window
x-ray e.

energy-dispersive x-ray fluorescence (EDXRF)

enforcer
Cook e.

Engel alkalinity

Engelmann
E. disc
E. disease

engine
Kodak Mammography CAD e.

engorged
e. collateral venous channel
e. tissue
e. vein

enhanced
e. CT
e. CT scan

e. fast gradient echo (efgre)
e. glycolysis
e. imaging

enhancement
acoustic e.
arterylike pattern of e.
bolus contrast e.
bright contrast e.
cocurrent flow-related e.
contrast e.
countercurrent flow-related e.
Doppler flow signal e.
Doppler signal e.
dynamic e.
echo e.
edge e.
evanescent e.
exercise-induced contrast e.
e. factor
flip-flop e.
flow-related e.
focal nodular e.
gadolinium e.
gyral brain e.
heterogeneous isodense e.
homogeneous e.
hybrid rapid acquisition with
  relaxation e. (HRARE)
inhomogeneous contrast e.
inhomogeneous moderate e.
internal e.
isodense e.
meningeal e.
microbubble contrast e.
e. morphology
multislice flow-related e.
nodular e.
nonhomogeneous e.
nuclear magnetic resonance
  relaxation rate e.
paradoxic e.
paramagnetic contrast e.
parenchymal e.
e. pattern
e. pattern type I–IV
peak of maximum e. (PME)
peripheral lesion e.
peritoneal e.
peritumoral e.
portal vein e.
posterior acoustic e.
proton relaxation e. (PRE)

NOTES

enhancement *(continued)*
    pulmonary nodule e.
    punctate e.
    radiation e.
    rapid acquisition with relaxation e.
      (RARE)
    real-time e.
    rim e.
    ring e.
    scan with contrast e.
    serpentine e.
    signal e.
    sulcal e.
    temporal peritumoral e.
    time-of-flight e.
    T2 proton relaxation e. (T2 PRE)
    transient peritumoral e.
    vascular MR contrast e.
enhancer
    vein contrast e. (VCE)
enhancing
    e. brain lesion
    e. mass
    e. nodule
    e. septa
    e. ventricular margin
enlarged
    e. cardiac silhouette
    e. frontal horn
    e. gallbladder
    e. heart
    e. kidney
    e. liver
    e. presacral space
    e. pulmonary vessel
    e. thyroid gland
    e. vascular channel
    e. vertebral foramen
    e. vestibular vascular aqueduct
      syndrome
enlargement
    airspace e.
    azygos vein e.
    biventricular e.
    bony e.
    bulbous e.
    cardiac silhouette e.
    cervical e.
    chamber e.
    compensatory e.
    diffuse hepatic e.
    diffuse liver e.
    diffuse thymic e.
    diffuse uterine e.
    e. of epididymis
    epiglottic e.
    extraocular muscle e.
    gastric fold e.
    global renal e.

    iliopsoas compartment e.
    e. of lacrimal gland
    left atrial e. (LAE)
    lymph node e.
    masseteric e.
    mediastinal lymph node e.
    optic nerve e.
    panchamber e.
    papilla of Vater e.
    e. of parotid gland
    pituitary gland e.
    placenta e.
    right atrial e. (RAE)
    right ventricular e. (RVE)
    sella e.
    e. of subarachnoidal space
    sulcal e.
    thymic e.
    e. of uterus
    e. of ventricle
    ventricular e.
    e. of vertebral body
    e. of vertebral foramen
    e. with low-density lymph node
      center
enostosis
ensemble contrast imaging (ECI)
ensheathing callus
ensiform
    e. appendix
    e. cartilage
    e. process
EnSite 3000 imaging system
eNTEGRA workstation
enteric
    e. coated
    e. duplication cyst
    e. exocrine drainage
    e. fistula
    e. plexus
    e. stricture
enteric-drained pancreas transplant
enteritis
    candida e.
    Crohn granulomatous e.
    Crohn regional e.
    eosinophilic e.
    e. follicularis
    radiation e.
    regional e.
enterobiliary
enterocele sac
enterocleisis
enteroclysis
    computed tomographic e.
enterococcus, pl. **enterococci**
enterocolic fistula
enterocolitis
    emphysematous e.

granulomatous e.
Hirschsprung-associated e. (HAEC)
necrotizing e.
neutropenic e.
enterocutaneous fistula
enterocystoma
enterocytic processing
enteroenteral fistula
enterogenous cyst
enterohepatic
enteroinsular axis
enterolith
enteropathica
acrodermatitis e.
enteropathy
exudative e.
gluten-sensitive e.
protein-losing e.
radiation e.
enteropathy-associated T-cell lymphoma
enteroperitoneal abscess
enteroptosis
enteroscope
Olympus SIF-100 video e.
enteroscopy
small bowel e. (SBE)
virtual e.
enterospinal fistula
enterostomal therapist
enterourethral fistula
enterovaginal fistula
enterovesical fistula
enteroviral encephalomyelitis
Entero Vu contrast medium
"entertainment" ultrasound
enthesis
enthesitis
enthesopathic transformation
enthesophyte
plantar calcaneal e.
subacromial e.
entity
tumor e.
entorhinal cortex
entrance
e. block
e. skin exposure
entrapment
artery e.
gas e.
guidewire e.
lateral e.

median nerve e.
nerve e.
e. neuropathy
patellar e.
posterior interosseous nerve e.
scar tissue e.
soft tissue e.
suprascapular nerve e.
ulnar nerve e.
entrapped
e. ovarian cyst
e. plantar sesamoid bone
EntroEase oral radiopaque contrast medium
entry
capacitative calcium e.
e. flap
e. point
e. slice phenomenon artifact
e. tear
e. zone
envelope
capsuloperiosteal e.
fascial e.
soft tissue e.
synovial e.
environment
echo-poor areas of e.
high-tech-low-touch examination e.
environmental
e. factor
e. plutonium
Envision CT power injector
Envoy 6F guiding catheter
enzyme
angiotensin-converting e. (ACE)
e. replacement therapy
e. supplementation therapy
enzyme-multiplied immunoassay technique
EOCT
endoscopic optical coherence tomography
EOSB
end of saturated bombardment
eosinophilia
tumor-associated tissue e.
eosinophilic
e. brain adenoma
e. enteritis
e. granuloma
e. infiltrate
e. leukocyte

E

NOTES

eosinophilic *(continued)*
    e. lung disease
    e. pneumonia
Eovist contrast agent
EP
    ectopic pregnancy
    electrophysiology
    excretory phase
      HearTwave EP
EP2000 electrophysiology imaging system
epactal bone
EPAR
    endovascular photo acoustic recanalization
      EPAR laser system
EPB
    extensor pollicis brevis
      EPB muscle
EPBF
    effective pulmonary blood flow
EPC
    echo phase correction
ependyma
ependymal cyst
ependymitis
    bacterial e.
    e. granularis
ependymoblastoma
ependymoma
    anaplastic e.
    brain e.
    brainstem e.
    e. cord
    intracranial e.
    intramedullary e.
    malignant e.
    myxopapillary e.
    spinal cord e.
    subcutaneous sacrococcygeal myxopapillary e.
ephemeral pneumonia
EPI
    echo-planar imaging
      spiral EPI (SEPI)
epiarterial bronchus
epiarticular osteochondromatous dysplasia
epiblast
epicardial
    e. attachment
    e. centroid
    e. coronary artery
    e. Doppler echocardiography
    e. Doppler flow sector transducer
    e. fat pad
    e. imaging
    e. implantation
    e. mapping

    e. space
    e. surface
    e. tension
    e. volume
epicardium
epicenter
    eccentric e.
epicolic lymph node
epicondylar
    e. fracture
    e. fracture of humerus
    e. ridge
epicondyle
    humeral e.
    medial e.
epicondylitis
    lateral e.
    medial e.
epicondyloolecranon ligament
Epic ophthalmic 3-in-1 laser
epicortical lesion
epicranial aponeurosis
epidermal
    e. carcinoma
    e. inclusion cyst
    e. ridge
epidermoid
    acquired e.
    black e.
    cerebellar e.
    e. lung carcinoma
    e. mediastinum
    e. spine
    e. tumor
    white e.
epidermoidoma
    incisural e.
    intradural e.
    prepontine white e.
epididymal
    e. cyst
    e. descent
    e. fibrosarcoma
epididymis, pl. **epididymides**
    appendix of e.
    body of e.
    edema of e.
    enlargement of e.
    inflammation of e.
    interstitial congestion of e.
    e. lesion
    ligament of e.
    lobule of e.
    postvasectomy change in e.
    sinus of e.
    tail of e.
epididymitis
epididymography imaging
epididymoorchitis

epididymovesiculography
epidural
   e. abscess
   e. angiolipoma
   e. anular fibrosis
   e. arachnoid cyst
   e. blood
   e. blood patch
   e. cavernous hemangioma
   e. cavity
   e. effusion
   e. empyema
   e. extramedullary lesion
   e. fat
   e. hematoma (EDH)
   e. hemorrhage
   e. implant
   e. infusion
   e. lipoma
   c. lipomatosis
   e. lymphoma
   e. mass
   e. pneumatosis
   e. space
   e. steroid injection
   e. venography
   e. venous plexus
epidurogram
epidurography
   magnetic resonance e.
epigastric
   e. angle
   e. fold
   e. fossa
   e. hernia
   e. lymph node
   e. vein
epigastrium
epiglottic
   e. carcinoma
   e. cartilage
   e. disruption
   e. enlargement
   e. fold
   e. tubercle
epiglottitis
   bacterial e.
epignathus
epihyal
   e. bone
   e. ligament

epihyoid bone
epilarynx
EpiLaser
epilation dose
epilepsy
   chronic partial e.
   drug-resistant extratemporal e.
   extratemporal e.
   idiopathic e.
   structural e.
   temporal lobe e. (TLE)
epileptic focus
epileptogenic
   e. center
   e. focus
   e. lesion
   e. zone
Epimed spring guide catheter
epipericardial ridge
epiphora
epiphrenic bulge
epiphyseolysis
   femoral head e.
   idiopathic e.
   juvenile e.
epiphysial, epiphyseal
   e. arrest
   e. cartilage
   e. cartilage plate
   e. chondroblastic growth
   e. chondrocyte
   e. coxa vara
   e. disc
   e. dysgenesis
   e. dysostosis
   e. dysplasia
   e. exostosis
   e. fetal bone center
   e. growth plate
   e. hematopoietic marrow
   e. hyperplasia
   e. hypertrophy
   e. ischemic necrosis
   e. lesion
   e. line
   e. ossification center
   e. osteochondroma
   e. overgrowth
   e. plate fracture
   e. plate injury
   e. slip fracture

E

NOTES

epiphysial *(continued)*
    e. slippage
    e. tibial fracture
epiphysis, pl. **epiphyses**
    anular e.
    atavistic e.
    e. avulsion
    ball-and-socket e.
    balloon e.
    e. bone
    bone lesion e.
    capital e. (CE)
    capital femoral e.
    capitular e.
    cartilaginous e.
    cone e.
    congenital stippled e.
    familial avascular necrosis of
      phalangeal e.
    femoral capital e.
    humeral e.
    ossifying e.
    osteochondrotic separation of
      epiphysis
    Perthes e.
    pressure e.
    ring e.
    slipped capital femoral e. (SCFE)
    slipped upper femoral e. (SUFE)
    tibial e.
    traction e.
epiphysitis
    juvenile e.
    vertebral e.
epiploia
epiploic
    e. appendage
    e. appendix
    e. foramen
epiploica
    appendix e.
epipteric bone
epirenal septum
episcleral
    e. plaque brachytherapy
    e. space
    e. vein
episode
    ischemic e.
    mitochondrial encephalomyopathy
      with lactic acidosis and stroke-
      like e.'s (MELAS)
    silent ischemic e.
epispadia exstrophy complex
EPISTAR
    E. Diode Laser System
    E. perfusion technique
    E. subtraction angiography
episternal bone

epitendineum
epithalamus
epithelia (*pl. of* epithelium)
epithelial
    e. cell
    e. colon
    e. colonic polyp
    e. degenerative change
    e. hyperplasia
    e. inclusion cyst
    e. malignancy
    e. neoplasm
    e. ovarian carcinoma
    e. spleen
    e. tumor
epithelialization
    creeping e.
epithelial-myoepithelial carcinoma
epithelioid
    e. angiomatosis
    e. granuloma
    e. hemangioendothelioma
    e. hemangioma
    e. leiomyoma
    e. malignant mesothelioma
    e. osteosarcoma
    e. sarcoma
epithelioma
    calcifying Malherbe e.
epitheliosis
    infiltrating breast e.
epitheliotropism
epithelium, pl. **epithelia**
    atypical e.
    Barrett e.
    e. crypt
    ductal e.
    normal ovarian surface e. (NOSE)
    papilla of columnar e.
    squamous metaplasia white e.
    surface e.
    tumor of surface e.
    white e.
epithermal neutron
EpiTouch laser
epitrochlear lymph node
epituberculous infiltrate
epitympanic
    e. recess (EPR)
    e. space
epitympanum
EPL
    effective path length
    extensor pollicis longus
      EPL muscle
EPN
    emphysematous pyelonephritis
epoch
    VNS e.

eponychium
epoophoron
Eppendorf pO$_2$ histograph
EPR
    electron paramagnetic resonance
    epitympanic recess
epsilon m
    TDE-derived epsilon p and e.
EPSS
    E point to septal separation
EPT-Dx steerable diagnostic catheter
eptifibatide
epulofibroma
EQP
    extensor quinti proprius
equal in intensity
equalization
    histogram e.
    pressure e.
equalized diastolic pressure
equation
    Bernoulli e.
    bio-heat e.
    Bloch e.
    Bohr e.
    Boltzmann e.
    Bragg e.
    Carter e.
    continuity e.
    decay e.
    Derenzo e.
    Doppler e.
    Fick e.
    hamiltonian e.
    Kety e.
    Larmor e.
    linear-quadratic e.
    modified Bernoulli e.
    Nernst e.
    Schroedinger e.
    Solomon-Bloembergen e.
    Stewart-Hamilton e.
    Teichholz e.
    tracer concentration e.
    transformer e.
equilibration
equilibrium
    e. dissociation constant
    e. dose constant
    e. factor
    e. magnetization
    e. MUGA imaging

    e. MUGA scan
    e. phase
    e. point
    radioactive e.
    e. radionuclide angiocardiography
    e. radionuclide angiocardiography
        technique
    e. radionuclide angiography
    secular e.
    state e.
    thermal e.
    transient e.
    e. view
equina
    cauda e.
    nerve roots of cauda e.
equinovalgus
    e. deformity
    pes e.
equinovarus
    e. hindfoot deformity
    pes e.
    talipes e.
Equinox
    20-mm E. balloon microcatheter
    E. occlusion balloon catheter
equinus
    e. deformity
    pes e.
equipment
    e. artifact
    Digitron Koordinat angiography e.
    Polytron DSA e.
    RapidScreen RS-2000 x-ray e.
equivalence
    mass energy e.
equivalent
    chance e.
    dose e. (DE)
    meconium ileus e.
    total effective dose e. (TEDE)
    total organ dose e. (TODE)
    e. treatment
equivalent-physical
    roentgen e.-p. (REP)
equivocal finding
ER
    estrogen-receptor
    ER positive
erase
    background e.

NOTES

Erb
    E. disease
    E. injury
    E. point
Erb-Duchenne-Klumpke injury
erbium
    e. 171
    e. chromium:yttrium-aluminum-garnet
    (ErCr:YAG)
    2040 e. SilkLaser
erbium:YAG infrared laser
ERC
    endoscopic cholangiography
    endoscopic retrograde cholangiogram
ERCP
    endoscopic retrograde
    cholangiopancreatography
      ERCP catheter
      ERCP imaging
      ERCP manometry
ErCr:YAG
    erbium chromium:yttrium-aluminum-
    garnet
      ErCr:YAG laser
Erdheim
    E. cystic medial necrosis
    E. tumor
Erdheim-Chester disease
ERE
    estrogen-response element
    external rotation in extension
erect
    e. fluoro spot projection
    e. lateral flexion/extension
    radiograph
    e. position
    e. view
erector spinae
ERF
    edge response function
    external rotation in flexion
ERFP
    effective renal plasma flow
ERG
    electroretinogram
ergometer
    bicycle e.
    Cybex e.
ergonomics
    hands-up e.
Erichsen sign
Erlenmeyer
    E. flask
    E. flask appearance
Erlenmeyer-flask-like deformity
Ernst angle
erosion
    articular e.
    e. of articular surface

    bony e.
    bronchial e.
    duodenal e.
    e. of epiphysial bone
    focal cartilage e.
    gastric antral e.
    graft-enteric e.
    infraspinatus insertion e.
    linear e.
    marginal e.
    mouse ear e.
    odontoid e.
    osteoclastic e.
    pedicle e.
    plaque e.
    rat-bite e.
    salt-and-pepper duodenal e.
    stomach varioliform e.
    tumor e.
    varioliform e.
erosive
    e. duodenitis
    e. gastritis
    e. gingivitis
    e. osteoarthritis
ERP
    effective refractory period
    endoscopic retrograde parenchymography
ERPF
    effective renal plasma flow
erratum
    anatomic moment e.
error
    ADC quantization e.
    analog-to-digital conversion
    quantization e.
    CT imaging e.
    darkroom e.
    data clipping detection e.
    data spike detection e.
    e. diffusion method
    dorsal induction e.
    duplex ultrasound e.
    flow-related phase e.
    generalized compensation for
    resonance offset and pulse
    length e.'s (GROPE)
    Hausdorff e.
    interobserver e.
    intraobserver e.
    isocenter placement e.
    magnification e.
    mean-square e.
    photoreceptor fractional velocity e.
    positioning e.
    preparation e.
    quantization e.
    random e.
    raster spacing e.

relative e.
sampling e.
sensing e.
size estimation e.
spatial frequency e.
systematic e.
error-sum criterion
ERU
endorectal ultrasound
gray-scale ERU
eruption
rhythmic paradoxic e.
ERUS
endorectal ultrasound
ERV
expiratory reserve volume
erythema
e. dose
e. of joint
radiation e.
e. threshold
erythrocyte
e. iron turnover
technetium-99m heat-denatured e.
erythropoietin
e. assay
e. bioassay
ES
end systole
Es
einsteinium
^{255}Es
einsteinium 255
Esaote extremity scanner
escalation
escape
e. of air into lung connective
tissue
e. beat
e. interval
escape-capture rhythm
escape-peak ratio
ESIN
elastic stable intramedullary nailing
Esmarch bandage
EsophaCoil stent
esophageal
e. achalasia pattern
e. aperistalsis
e. apple-core lesion
e. atresia
e. balloon technique

e. body
e. carcinoma
e. carcinosarcoma
e. choriocarcinoma
e. contraction
e. degeneration
e. dilatation
e. displacement
e. dissection
e. diverticulum
e. duplication
e. duplication cyst
e. dysmotility
e. dysphagia
e. electrogram
e. fibroadenoma
e. filling defect
e. fold
e. functional disorder
e. function imaging
e. graft
e. groove
e. hernia
e. hiatus
e. impression
e. inflammation
e. inlet
e. leiomyoma
e. leiomyomatosis
e. leiomyosarcoma
e. lipomatosis
e. lumen
e. manometry
e. margin serration
e. morphologic disorder
e. motility
e. motility disorder
e. mucosal nodule
e. mucosal ring
e. muscular ring
e. narrowing
e. neoplasm
e. obstruction
e. obturator airway
e. opening
e. peptic stricture
e. perforation
e. peristalsis
e. peristaltic pressure
e. pill electrode
e. plaque
e. plexus

E

NOTES

esophageal *(continued)*
  e. pseudosarcoma
  e. reflux
  e. rupture
  e. shiver
  e. shunt
  e. spasm
  e. sphincter relaxation
  e. stenosis
  e. stent
  e. tear
  e. transition zone
  e. transit time
  e. tumor
  e. ulcer
  e. variceal sclerosis
  e. varix
  e. vein
  e. vestibule
  e. web
  e. window
esophageal-pleural stripe
esophagectomy
  Ivor Lewis e.
  transhiatal e.
  transthoracic e.
esophagi (*pl. of* esophagus)
esophagitis
  acute e.
  AIDS-related e.
  candida e.
  caustic e.
  chronic e.
  corrosive e.
  cytomegalovirus e.
  drug-induced e.
  herpes e.
  HIV e.
  peptic e.
  pill e.
  reflux e. (RE)
  Sonnenberg classification of
    erosive e.
  stasis e.
  viral e.
esophagogastrectomy
esophagogastric (EG)
  e. fat pad
  e. intubation
  e. junction
  e. orifice
  e. region
  e. tamponade
esophagogastroduodenoscopy (EGD)
esophagogastrostomy
esophagogram (*var. of* esophagram)
esophagography
  double-contrast e.
  e. imaging

esophagojejunostomy
esophagorespiratory fistula
esophagoscopy
esophagospasm
esophagostomy
  cervical e.
  palliative e.
esophagotracheal fistula
esophagram, esophagogram
  air e.
  barium e.
  barium-water e.
  contrast e.
  pullback e.
  radionuclide e.
esophagraphy
esophagus, pl. **esophagi**
  abnormal peristaltic e.
  achalasia of e.
  A level of e.
  aperistaltic e.
  A ring of e.
  atonic e.
  Barrett e.
  bird-beak e.
  B level of e.
  B ring of e.
  cervical e.
  cobblestone appearance e.
  columnar-lined e.
  congenitally short e.
  corkscrew appearance of e.
  curling e.
  diffuse dilation of e.
  diffuse spasm of e.
  dilated e.
  discrete segment of normal e.
  double-barrel e.
  double-ring e.
  dysmotile e.
  extrinsic impression of e.
  foamy e.
  foreign body in e.
  intramural rupture of e.
  long smooth narrowing e.
  middle third of thoracic e.
  muscular ring e.
  nutcracker e.
  polypoid lesion of lower e.
  rat-tail e.
  rosary beading e.
  scleroderma of e.
  shaggy e.
  shish kabob e.
  short-segment Barrett e. (SSBE)
  spastic e.
  submerged segment of e.
  thoracic e.
  tortuous e.

upper thoracic e.
Z-line of e.

ESP
early systolic peak
end-systolic pressure

ESP-ESV
end-systolic pressure-end-systolic volume
ratio

ESR
electron spin resonance

ESRF
end-stage renal failure

essential
e. osteolysis
e. tumor

Essex-Lopresti
E.-L. calcaneal fracture
classification
E.-L. joint depression fracture
E.-L. lesion

ester
iodipamide ethyl e.

esthesioneuroblastoma
esthesioneurocytoma
esthesioneuroepithelioma
estimated fetal weight (EFW)
estimation
bayesian image e. (BIE)
fractional moving blood volume e.
frequency e.
magnetic resonance volume e.
stereologic method of volume e.
volume e.

estradiol
estrogen-producing tumor
estrogen-receptor (ER)
e.-r. positive

estrogen-response element (ERE)
ESV
end-systolic volume

ESVI
end-systolic volume index

ESWL
extracorporeal shock wave lithotripsy

ET
ejection time
endotracheal
etiology

etching
track e.

ETF
extension teardrop fracture

ethanol (EtOH)
e. ablation
e. injection

Ethiodane
ethiodized
e. oil
e. oil contrast medium

Ethiodol imaging agent
ethmocephaly
ethmoid
e. air cell
e. bone
e. canal
e. sinus
e. sinus carcinoma

ethmoidal
e. artery
e. bulla
e. crest
e. foramen
e. groove
e. labyrinth
e. meningoencephalocele
e. notch
e. process
e. vein

ethmoidolacrimal suture
ethmoidomaxillary suture
ethmovomerine plate
ethyl
e. cysteinate dimer (ECD)
^{18}F-labeled polyfluorinated e.

ethylenediaminetetramethylene
phosphonic acid (EDTMP)
ethyliodophenylundecyl contrast medium
etidronate
e. disodium imaging agent
rhenium-186 e.
technetium-99m e.

etiology (ET)
fever of unknown e. (FUE)
multifactorial e.'s

etiopathogenetic
ETL
echo-train length

E-to-F
E-t.-F slope
E-t.-F slope of valve

E-TOF detecting module

E

NOTES

EtOH
  ethanol
ETT
  exercise tolerance test
EU
  excretory urography
euchromatin
eukinesis
Euler number
Eureka collimator
europium-activated barium fluorohalide
EUS
  endorectal ultrasound
  endoscopic ultrasound
    depth of tumor invasion assessed by EUS
EUS-FNA
  endoscopic ultrasound-guided fine needle aspiration
eustachian
  e. canal
  e. tonsil
  e. tube
  e. valve
eV, ev
  electron volt
ev3
    ev3 premounted balloon expandable stent
    ev3 self-expanding stent
    ev3 unmounted balloon expandable stent
Evac-Q-Kwik bowel preparation
evacuation
  colonic e.
  digital rectal e.
  e. disorder
  e. pouchography
  precipitate e.
  e. proctography
evaluation
  e. of glucose metabolism
  e. of mass mammography
  shunt e.
evanescent enhancement
Evans
  E. blue albumin
  E. blue imaging agent
  E. intertrochanteric fracture classification
  E. ratio
Evans-D'Angio staging system
EVAR
  endovascular aneurysm repair
EVD
  external ventricular drain
even distribution of echoes
even-echo rephasing

event
  cardinal e.
  cerebral ischemic e.
  coincidence e.
  e. counter
  embolic e.
  inciting e.
  ischemic e.
  main timing e. (MTE)
  major adverse cardiac e. (MACE)
  precipitating e.
  random coincidence e.
  scattered coincidence e.
  true e.
eventration
  e. of diaphragm
  diaphragmatic e.
event-related paradigm
everolimus
eversion
  e. of ankle
  cervical e.
  e. position
  e. sprain
eversion-external rotation deformity
evidence
  scintigraphic e.
EVLT
  endovenous laser treatment
  EVLT laser
evolution
  E. CT scanner
  stroke in e. (SIE)
  E. XP scanner
evolving
  e. hematoma
  e. myocardial infarct
EVS mechanical closure device
evulsion
EVUS
  endovaginal ultrasound
Ewald
  E. node
  E. test meal
Ewart sign
Ewing
  E. sarcoma
  E. sarcoma-Wilms tumor 1 (EWS-WT1)
  E. tumor
EWS-WT1
  Ewing sarcoma-Wilms tumor 1
EX
  Filter Wire EX
ex
  ex vacuo ventriculomegaly
  ex vivo magnetic resonance imaging
ExAblate 2000 ultrasound system

exacerbation
exact framing
exaggerated
    e. craniocaudal lateral (XCCL)
    e. craniocaudal view
exametazime imaging agent
examination
    barium follow-through e.
    contrast-enhanced radiographic e.
    Doppler venous e.
    double-contrast eversion e.
    first-pass e.
    ^{67}Ga e.
    gated exercise e.
    gray-scale e.
    image-acquisition gated e.
    limited e.
    neuroradiologic e.
    postglucose loading e.
    proton brain e. (PROBE)
    reinjection thallium stress e.
    rest redistribution e.
    single-voxel proton brain e.
    1-stop-shop e.
    stress-gated blood pool cardiac e.
    stress-redistribution e.
    stress-rest reinjection e.
    suboptimal e.
    transcranial e.
    transforaminal e.
    unsuppressed e.
    venous Doppler e.
    in vivo e.
    volumetric interpolated breath-hold e. (VIBE)
    whole-body nuclear physical e.
    whole-body screening e.
excavation
    saucer-shaped e.
excavatum
    pectus e.
Excel-14 microcatheter
Excelart short-bore MRI
Excelsior microcatheter
excessive
    e. callus formation
    e. lateral pressure syndrome (ELPS)
exchange
    air e.
    coupling e.
    e. guidewire

    half-time of e.
    intestinal gas e.
    narrowing e.
    proton-proton magnetization e.
    pulmonary gas e.
    rapid e. (RX)
    spin e.
excimer
    e. laser
    e. laser coronary angioplasty (ELCA)
    e. laser system
    XeCl e.
excision
    CT-guided percutaneous e.
    en bloc e.
    large loop e.
excisional biopsy
excitation
    delay alternating with nutation for tailored e. (DANTE)
    fast acquisition multiple e.
    e. function
    e. function measurement
    magnetization-prepared rapid gradient echo-water e. (MP-RAGE-WE)
    nonuniform e.
    number of e. (NEX, NOX)
    e. profile
    quadrature e.
    rebound e.
    selective e.
    slice-selective e.
    spatial and chemical-shift encoded e. (SPACE)
    e. spectrum
    supernormal e.
    tailored e.
    tilted optimized nonsaturating e. (TONE)
    uniform TR e.
    variable-angle uniform signal e. (VUSE)
    variable flip-angle e.
    volume-selective e.
    wave of e.
excitation-spoiled fat-suppressed T1-weighted SE image
excitatory
    e. lesion

NOTES

E

excitatory (continued)
  e. neurotransmitter
  e. pulse characteristic
excited
  e. atom
  e. electron
  e. proton
excitotoxic
  e. cord injury
  e. mechanism
Excluder stent-graft
exclusion
  endovascular e.
  subtotal gastric e.
exclusion-HPLC technique
excrescence
  bony e.
  papillary e.
excrescentic thickening of optic nerve
excretion
  ammonium e.
  colonic mucosal e.
  contrast media e.
  ^{67}Ga e.
  e. pyelography
  uptake and e.
  urinary e.
  e. urography
  vicarious contrast e.
excretory
  e. cystogram
  e. duct
  e. intravenous pyelography
  e. phase (EP)
  e. urethrogram drip infusion
    urography
  e. urogram
  e. urography (EU)
  e. urography imaging
excursion of diaphragm
exencephaly
exenteration
  anterior e.
  pelvic e.
exercise
  e. echocardiography
  e. first-pass LVEF
  flexion and extension e.'s
  e. image
  e. index
  e. load
  e. LV function
  modified stage e.
  e. myocardial perfusion scintigraphy
  e. radionuclide angiocardiography
  e. radionuclide ventriculogram
  e. renography
  e. strain gauge venous
    plethysmography

  e. stress-redistribution scintigraphy
  e. thallium scintigraphy
  e. thallium-201 stress imaging
  e. thallium-201 tomography
  e. tolerance test (ETT)
exercise-induced
  e.-i. bronchoconstriction
  e.-i. contrast enhancement
  e.-i. transient myocardial ischemia
exertion
  Borg scale of treadmill e.
exertional rhabdomyolysis
exhalation
  end e.
exit
  e. block
  e. dose
  e. wound
Exner plexus
exocardia
exoccipital
  e. bone
  e. part of occipital bone
exoergic reaction
Exogen
  E. 2000+ low-intensity, ultrasound
    fracture healing system
  E. 2000+ noninvasive ultrasound
    therapy
  E. 2000 SAFHS
exogenous
  e. glucose rate
  e. invasion
  e. lipoid pneumonia
exon-specific primer pair
exophthalmic goiter
exophytic
  e. adenocarcinoma
  e. carcinoma
  e. fibroid
  e. mass
  e. neoplasia
exoskeleton
exostosis, pl. **exostoses**
  blocker's e.
  bony e.
  cartilage-capped e.
  epiphysial e.
  hereditary multiple exostoses
    (HME)
  hereditary multiple cartilaginous
    exostoses
  hypertrophic e.
  impingement e.
  marginal e.
  multiple cartilaginous exostoses
  multiple hereditary exostoses
  osteocartilaginous e.
  pelvic e.

retrocalcaneal e.
tackler's e.
traction e.
turret e.

exostotica
bursa e.

exostotic chondrosarcoma
expandable Gianturco metallic stent
expanded
e. lung
e. polytetrafluoroethylene-covered
nitinol TIPS stent graft
e. polytetrafluoroethylene graft

expanded-disability status scale (EDSS)
expanding
e. cavernous sinus brain lesion
e. intracranial mass

expansile
e. aneurysmal bone cyst
e. aortic segment
e. configuration
e. lytic lesion
e. mass
e. multilocular bone lesion
e. osteoblastoma
e. osteolysis
e. rib lesion
e. unilocular well-demarcated bone
lesion

expansion
air e.
bone e.
complete stent e.
emphysematous e.
fluid e.
infarct e.
localized e.
lung e.
passive chest e.
peripheral e.
rapid fluid e.
stent e.
uneven air e.

expenditure
resting energy e.

experimental protocol
Expert-XL densitometer
expiration
end e.
flow-limited e.
quantitative CT during e.
e. view

expiratory
e. attenuation
e. chest
e. computed tomography
e. CT
e. film
e. flow
e. image
inspiratory to e.
e. phase
e. reserve volume (ERV)
e. resistance
e. view

exploration
common bile duct e. (CBDE)

explorer
E. 360-degree rotational diagnostic
catheter
E. ST fixed curve diagnostic
catheter
E. X70 intraoral radiography
system

explosion fracture
explosive follicular hyperplasia
exponential
e. decay
e. kinetics
e. shape
e. weighting

Export catheter
exposure
e. angle
anthrax e.
asbestos e.
bioterrorism e.
bone-tendon e.
e. data recognizer (EDR)
DES e.
e. dose
electromagnetic radiation e.
entrance skin e.
index of e.
intraperitoneal e.
ionizing radiation e.
magnetic radiation e.
e. meter
operator e.
overcouch e.
radiation e.
uneven e.
e. variation
zero e.

E

NOTES

expoSURE
express
> E. balloon-expanded stent
> E. biliary LD premounted stent
> system
> E. biliary LD stent
> E. PTCA catheter

expression
> antigen e.
> AQP4 e.
> catheter-based inducible enhancers
> of gene e.
> e. cystourethrography
> receptor e.
> upregulated AQP4 e.
> e. vector

exquisite detail
exsanguinating hemorrhage
exstrophy
> bladder e.
> cloacal e.
> closed e.
> urinary bladder e.

extended
> e. field of view
> e. pattern

extended-field
> e.-f. irradiation therapy
> e.-f. radiotherapy

extended-field-of view technique (EFOV)
extension
> angle of greatest e. (AGE)
> basal e.
> Buck e.
> capital e.
> Codivilla e.
> external rotation in e. (ERE)
> extraaxial e.
> extracapsular e. (ECE)
> extranodal tumor e.
> extrascleral e.
> hilar e.
> e. injury
> e. injury of spine
> internal rotation in e. (IRE)
> intracavitary e.
> medial e.
> metaphysial e.
> parenchymal e.
> parietal e.
> e. position
> radiolucent operating room table e.
> subligamentous e.
> supradiaphragmatic e.
> suprasellar e.
> e. teardrop fracture (ETF)
> thrombus e.
> tumor e.
> e. view

extensive
> e. anterior myocardial infarct
> e. bilateral pneumonia
> e. dissection
> e. head injury
> e. intraductal carcinoma (EIC)
> e. intraductal component (EIC)

extensor
> e. apparatus
> e. carpi radialis brevis (ECRB)
> e. carpi radialis brevis muscle
> e. carpi radialis brevis tendon
> e. carpi radialis longus (ECRL)
> e. carpi radialis longus muscle
> e. carpi radialis longus tendon
> e. carpi ulnaris (ECU)
> e. carpi ulnaris muscle
> e. carpi ulnaris sheath
> e. carpi ulnaris tendon
> e. compartment
> e. digiti longus (EDL)
> e. digiti minimi tendon
> e. digiti quinti (EDQ)
> e. digiti quinti muscle
> e. digiti quinti tendon
> e. digitorum
> e. digitorum brevis (EDB)
> e. digitorum brevis muscle
> e. digitorum brevis tendon
> e. digitorum communis (EDC)
> e. digitorum communis muscle
> e. digitorum communis tendon
> e. digitorum longus
> e. digitorum longus muscle
> e. digitorum longus tendon
> e. hallucis longus (EHL)
> e. hallucis longus muscle
> e. hallucis longus tendon
> e. indicis
> e. indicis proprius (EIP)
> e. indicis proprius muscle
> e. indicis proprius tendon
> e. mechanism
> e. pollicis brevis (EPB)
> e. pollicis brevis muscle
> e. pollicis brevis tendon
> e. pollicis longus (EPL)
> e. pollicis longus muscle
> e. pollicis longus tendon
> e. quinti tendon
> e. retinaculum
> ulnar e.

extensor-supinator group
extensus
> hallux e.

extent
> anular tear e.

exteriorization

externa
    theca e.
external
    e. absorption
    e. acoustic foramen
    e. anal sphincter
    e. artifact
    e. auditory canal atresia
    e. auditory canal dysplasia
    e. auditory meatus
    e. band
    e. beam irradiation
    e. beam radiation
    e. beam radiation therapy (EBRT)
    e. beam radiotherapy
    e. beam with tandem
    e. biliary drainage catheter
    e. biliary fistula
    e. callus
    e. capsule
    e. carotid
    e. carotid artery (ECA)
    e. condyle
    e. ear mass
    e. ear neoplasm
    e. elastic lamina
    e. fiducial marker
    e. fixation
    e. fixation device
    e. gamma dose reconstruction
    e. heat generating source
    e. hemorrhage
    e. hernia
    e. iliac artery
    e. iliac lymph node
    e. iliac stenosis
    e. inguinal ring
    e. jugular vein (EJV)
    e. looping technique
    e. nose
    e. oblique aponeurosis
    e. oblique muscle
    e. orthovoltage irradiation
    e. os
    e. pneumatic calf compression
    e. pudendal vein
    e. retractor
    e. ring apex
    e. rotation in extension (ERE)
    e. rotation in flexion (ERF)
    e. rotation view
    e. scanning

    e. snapping hip
    e. table of calvaria
    e. tibial torsion
    e. urethral orifice
    e. urethral sphincter
    e. ventricular drain (EVD)
    e. wire fixation
    e. x-ray therapy
external-internal drainage
externe
    horizontal toit e. (HTE)
externum
    os tibiale e.
externus
    obturator e.
extinction phenomenon
extirpation
    e. of saphenous vein
    tumor e.
extraabdominal desmoid
extraadrenal
    e. chromaffin tissue
    e. paraganglioma
    e. site
extraalveolar
    e. air (EAA)
    e. air collection
extraarachnoid
    e. injection
    e. myelography
extraarticular
    e. debris
    e. fracture
    e. hip fusion
    e. posterior ossification
    e. resection
extraaxial
    e. cavernous hemangioma
    e. CNS lesion
    e. extension
    e. fluid collection
    e. low-attenuation lesion
    e. space
    e. tumor
extracapsular
    e. ankylosis
    e. dissection
    e. extension (ECE)
    e. fracture
    e. ligament
    e. metastasis

NOTES

extracardiac
   e. anomaly
   e. collateral circulation
   e. focal uptake
   e. mass
extracavitary
   e. infected graft
   e. prosthetic arterial graft
extracellular
   e. compartment
   e. contrast agent
   e. domain
   e. fluid
   e. fluid volume
   e. matrix
   e. matrix component
   e. space
extracerebral
   e. aneurysm
   e. cavernous angioma
   e. fluid collection
   e. hematoma
   e. intracranial glioneural hamartoma
   e. soft tissue uptake
extrachorial placenta
extracolonic
   e. disease
   e. structure
extracompartmental tumor
extracorporeal
   e. circulation
   e. irradiation
   e. liver
   e. membrane oxygenation
   e. membrane oxygenator
   e. photochemotherapy
   e. shock wave
   e. shock wave lithotripsy (ESWL)
extracranial
   e. aneurysm
   e. carotid artery atherosclerosis
   e. carotid artery occlusive disease
   e. carotid circulation
   e. carotid system
   e. cerebral circulation
   e. cerebral vasculature
   e. course
   e. mass lesion
   e. meningioma
   e. pneumatocele
   e. vertebral artery
   e. vessel
extracranial-intracranial bypass
extraction
   anatomy-based e. (ABE)
   automatic e.
   e. catheter atherectomy
   e. column
   contour e.

   disphenoid e.
   first-pass thallium e.
   fringe skeleton e.
   e. generator
   e. method
   stone e.
   vacuum e.
   vascular segmentation and e.
extradural
   e. abscess
   e. anastomosis
   e. arachnoid cyst
   e. artery
   e. brain hematoma
   e. compartment
   e. defect
   e. hemorrhage
   e. space
   e. tumor
   e. venography
   e. vertebral plexus
   e. vertebral plexus of vein
extraembryonic mesoderm
extrafascial hysterectomy
extragastric placement
extragonadal seminoma
extrahepatic
   e. bile duct
   e. bile duct carcinoma
   e. biliary atresia (EBA)
   e. biliary cystic dilatation
   e. binary obstruction
   e. cholangiectasis
   e. cholangiocarcinoma
   e. lesion
   e. metastasis (EHM)
   e. portal hypertension
   e. portal vein tributary
   e. primary malignant tumor
   e. pseudoaneurysm
   e. stone
extraintestinal
extralobar sequestration
extralobular
   e. connective tissue
   e. stroma
   e. terminal duct
extraluminal
   e. air
   e. contrast medium
   e. endarterectomy
   e. gas
   e. hemorrhage
extramammary Paget disease
extramedullary
   e. compressive lesion
   e. hemangioma
   e. hematopoiesis
   e. involvement

e. plasmacytoma (EMP)
e. tumor
extramural hemorrhage
extraneous material
extranodal
e. follicular lymphoma
e. proliferation
e. site
e. tumor extension
extraoctave fracture
extraocular
e. muscle
e. muscle enlargement
extraoral radiograph
extraosseous
e. angioma
e. Ewing sarcoma
e. mass
e. osteosarcoma
e. uptake
extraovarian mass
extraparenchymal cyst
extrapelvic malignancy
extrapericardial dissection
extraperitoneal
e. bladder rupture
e. fascia
e. fat
e. implant
e. organ
extrapleural
e. drainage
e. hemorrhage
e. mass
e. pneumothorax
e. sign
e. space
extrapolate
extrapolation
half-scan with e. (HE)
extrapontine myelinolysis
extrapulmonary
e. activity
e. bronchus
e. sequestration
e. small cell carcinoma
e. tuberculosis
extrapyramidal
e. reaction
e. system
e. tract
extrarenal renal pelvis

extrascleral extension
extraskeletal
e. chondroma
e. mesenchymal chondrosarcoma
e. osteosarcoma
e. uptake
extrasphincteric anal fistula
extraspinal neurofibroma
extra stiff guidewire
extrasynovial
extratemporal
e. epilepsy
e. structural lesion
extratesticular
e. lesion
e. tumor
extrathecal nerve root
extrathoracic
e. disease
e. lesion
e. metastasis
e. obstruction
extrauterine
e. gestation
e. pelvic mass
e. pregnancy
extravaginal testicular torsion
extravasated
e. blood
e. contrast agent
extravasation
bile e.
contrast e.
e. of contrast agent
e. detection accessory
dye e.
fluid e.
intravascular content e.
joint fluid e.
radiopaque fluid e.
renal transplant urine e.
secondary e.
spontaneous urinary e.
urinary e.
extravascular
e. compartment
e. fluid
e. granuloma
e. mass
e. pressure
extraventricular obstructive hydrocephalus

NOTES

331

extravesical
    e. infrasphincteric ectopic ureter
    e. opacification
extravital ultraviolet
E³xtreme Access
extremely
    e. low frequency (ELF)
    e. low-frequency field
extreme micromelia
extremity
    e. coil
    e. CT angiography
    e. gigantism
    e. hemangioma
    left lower e. (LLE)
    lower e. (LE)
    e. malformation
    e. MRI (E-MRI)
    e. osteosarcoma
    e. rhabdomyosarcoma
    upper e. (UE)
extrinsic
    e. allergic alveolitis
    e. bladder compression
    e. cellular parameter
    e. esophageal impression
    e. field uniformity
    e. filling defect
    e. foot muscle
    e. impression of esophagus
    e. intraabdominal inflammation
    e. lesion
    e. ligament
    e. malignant obstruction
    e. neoplasia
    e. sphincter
    e. stomach impression
    e. ureteral defect
extrude
extruded
    e. disc
    e. disc fragment
extrusion
    disc e.
    joint fluid e.

extubate
extubation
exuberant
    e. atheroma formation
    e. callus
    e. granulation tissue
    e. synovium
    e. tumor
exudative
    e. bronchiolitis
    e. consolidation
    e. enteropathy
    e. pleural effusion
    e. pleurisy
    e. tuberculosis
eye
    conus e.
    e. exposure limit
    fetal e.
    hamartoma of e.
    intraconal portion of e.
    e. myositis
    e. trauma
eyebrow ring artifact
eye-ear plane
eyelet
    rod e.
eyepiece
    Huygens e.
eye-view 3D conformal radiation therapy
E-Z-CAT
    E-Z-C. Dry barium sulfate
    E-Z-C. Dry contrast agent
E-Z-EM
    E-Z-EM barium powder
    E-Z-EM cut biopsy needle
E-zero offset
E-Z-Guar mouthpiece
E-Z-Paque barium suspension

F

    female
    fluorine
        F point of cardiac apex
        F T line

5F

        5F minipuncture sheath
        5F Pinnacle sheath

^{18}F, F-18

    fluorine 18
        ^{18}F 2-deoxyglucose uptake
        ^{18}F L-DOPA imaging agent
        ^{18}F estradiol imaging agent
        ^{18}F FDG-negative imaging
        ^{18}F fludeoxyglucose imaging agent
        ^{18}F fluorodeoxyglucose imaging
          agent
        ^{18}F fluoro-DOPA imaging agent
        ^{18}F fluoroisonidazole imaging agent
        ^{18}F fluorotamoxifen imaging agent
        ^{18}F N-methylspiperone imaging
          agent
        ^{18}F sodium fluoride imaging agent
        ^{18}F spiperone imaging agent

^{19}F, F-19

    fluorine 19

f

    farad
    frequency

F-1200, 2000, 4500 fluorescence spectrophotometer

F-15 renogram

FA

    fractional anisotropy

FAA

    flavone acetic acid

Fab

    ^{131}I-labeled monoclonal Fab

fabella

    os f.

fabellofibular

    f. complex
    f. ligament

Fabian stent

Fabricius

    bursa of F.

FAcE

    FID-acquired echo

face

    congenital infiltrating lipomatosis of
      the f.
    en f.
    f. presentation

faceless kidney

facet

    f. arthropathy
    articular f.
    atlas f.
    bilateral locked f.'s
    capitate f.
    f. capsule disruption
    f. cartilage
    clavicular f.
    corneal f.
    costal f.
    f. degeneration
    f. dislocation
    flat f.
    f. fusion
    hamate f.
    inferior medial f.
    f. joint
    f. joint arthritis
    f. joint capsule
    f. joint incongruity
    f. joint injection
    f. joint vacuum
    jumped f.
    Lenoir f.
    locked f.
    lunate f.
    occlusal f.
    scaphoid f.
    squatting f.
    superior articular f.
    superior costal f.
    f. surface of vertebra
    f. syndrome
    transverse costal f.
    f. tropism

facetal imbrication

facetectomy

faceted gallstone

faceting

facial

    f. abnormality
    f. artery
    f. asymmetry
    f. bipartition
    f. bone
    f. cleft
    f. colliculus
    f. eminence
    f. fracture
    f. hemangioma
    f. nerve
    f. nerve anatomy
    f. nerve canal
    f. plane

F

facial *(continued)*
    f. plexus
    f. root
    f. schwannoma
    f. thickening
    f. triangle
    f. vein
faciale
facialis
facies
    f. ossea
    Potter f.
facioauriculovertebral syndrome
faciostenosis
FACScan
    fluorescence-activated cell sorter
    FACScan flow cytometer
FACSVantage cell sorter
FACT
    focused appendix computed tomography
factitious
    f. clinodactyly
    f. regurgitation
factor
    accelerator f.
    activation f.
    adherence f.
    f. analysis of dynamic series (FADS)
    f. analysis of dynamic study
    angiogenic f.
    anisotropy f.
    automotility f.
    backscatter f. (BSF)
    blocking f.
    breast cancer risk f.
    calibration f.
    contrast-improvement f.
    decay-activating f.
    diffusion f.
    dose/dose-rate effective f. (DDREF)
    enhancement f.
    environmental f.
    equilibrium f.
    filling f.
    Fletcher f.
    gamma f.
    geometry f.
    granulocyte colony stimulating f.
    growth f.
    Hageman f. (HF)
    inciting f.
    incremental risk f.
    intensification f.
    intrinsic f.
    kerma-to-dose conversion f.
    magnification f. (MF)
    Mayneord F f.
    net magnetization f.

    off-axis f. (OAF)
    overrelaxation f.
    peak scatter f.
    protection f.
    quality f. (QF)
    radiation weighting f.
    relative conversion f.
    releasing f.
    rheumatoid f.
    scatter degradation f.
    screen-intensifying f. (IF)
    therapeutic gain f.
    tissue inhomogeneity f.
    tissue weighting f.
    tumor-angiogenesis f.
    f. VIII
    wedge f.
factorial design
FADS
    factor analysis of dynamic series
Fahr disease
failed
    f. back surgery syndrome (FBSS)
    f. back syndrome (FBS)
    f. pregnancy
    f. valve
failure
    acute heart f.
    acute renal f. (ARF)
    acute respiratory f. (ARF)
    adrenal f.
    backward heart f.
    bypass f.
    cardiac f.
    chronic heart f.
    chronic renal f. (CRF)
    circulation f.
    compensated congestive heart f.
    congestive heart f. (CHF)
    contrast-induced renal f.
    decompensated congestive heart f.
    diastolic heart f.
    end-stage renal f. (ESRF)
    fetal heart f.
    forward heart f.
    frank congestive heart f.
    fulminant hepatic f. (FHF)
    functional classification of congestive heart f.
    graft f.
    heart f. (HF)
    hepatic f.
    high-output heart f.
    intractable heart f.
    intrauterine cardiac f.
    intrauterine heart f.
    irreversible organ f.
    kidney f.
    left-sided heart f.

left ventricular f.
liver f.
low-output heart f.
Mamm-Aire heart f.
multiple organ f.
neonatal cardiac f.
neonatal heart f.
ovulatory f.
pituitary f.
posttransplant acute renal f.
prerenal f.
pulmonary f.
refractory congestive heart f.
renal f.
respiratory f.
right-sided heart f.
right ventricular f.
systolic heart f.
time-to-distant f.
time-to-local f.
time-to-treatment f. (TTF)
TIPS f.
ventilatory f.
ventricular f.
failure-free survival
FAIR
flow-sensitive alternating inversion recovery
Fairbank disease
falces (*pl. of* falx)
falciform
f. cartilage
f. crest
f. fold
f. ligament
f. ligament sign
f. process
falcine meningioma
falcotentorial meningioma
falcula
falcular
fallen-fragment sign
fallen lung sign
fallopian
f. canal
f. ligament
f. pregnancy
f. tube
f. tube carcinoma
f. tube diverticulum
f. tube mass

f. tube occlusion
f. tube recanalization
falloposcopy
Fallot
pentalogy of F.
F. syndrome
F. tetrad
tetralogy of F. (TOF)
trilogy of F.
fallout
radioactive f.
signal f.
false
f. aneurysm
f. aneurysmal chamber
f. ankylosis
f. bundle-branch block
f. channel
f. colonic obstruction
f. color scale
f. cord carcinoma
f. diverticulum
f. emphysema
f. frequency
f. hypoechogenicity
f. knot
f. localizing sign
f. lumen
f. pelvis
f. pregnancy
f. rib
f. sac
f. splenic cyst
f. steal
f. suture
f. vertebra
f. vocal cord
false-negative
f.-n. correlation
f.-n. mammogram
f.-n. ratio
f.-n. result
f.-n. test
false-positive
f.-p. ratio
f.-p. result
f.-p. test
falx, pl. **falces**
f. artery
f. calcification
f. cerebelli
f. cerebri

NOTES

F

falx (*continued*)
- f. cerebri lesion
- f. fenestration
- f. increased density

FAME
- fast acquisition with multiphase efgre

familial
- f. adenomatous polyposis (FAP)
- f. adenomatous polyposis syndrome
- f. aortic dissection
- f. arterial fibromuscular dysplasia
- f. atresia
- f. avascular necrosis of phalangeal epiphysis
- f. cavernous malformation
- f. cerebral ferrocalcinosis
- f. chondrocalcinosis
- f. colorectal polyposis
- f. dysautonomia
- f. fibromuscular dysplasia of artery
- f. gastrointestinal polyposis
- f. goiter
- f. hypertrophic cardiomyopathy (FHC)
- f. hypertrophy (FHC)
- f. idiopathic hyperphosphatasia
- f. intestinal polyposis
- f. intestinal pseudoobstruction
- f. juvenile polyposis
- f. multiple polyposis
- f. myxoma
- f. onychoosteodysplasia
- f. polyposis coli
- f. varicose vein

fan
- f. angle
- f. beam
- f. sign

fan-beam
- f.-b. collimator
- f.-b. formula
- offset f.-b.
- f.-b. projection
- f.-b. reconstruction

Fanconi-Hegglin syndrome
Fanconi syndrome
fanning
- f. of the interspinous distance
- f. of the spinous process

fan-shaped
- f.-s. mesentery
- f.-s. view

FAP
- familial adenomatous polyposis

farad (f)
Faraday
- F. cage
- F. law

- F. shield
- F. shielded resonator

far field
farmer's lung
FAS
- fetal alcohol syndrome
- MAS in FAS

fascia, pl. **fasciae, fascias**
- anal f.
- antebrachial f.
- anterior rectus f.
- axillary f.
- bicipital f.
- brachial f.
- f. of breast
- broad f.
- buccopharyngeal f.
- Buck f.
- Camper f.
- cervical f.
- clavipectoral f.
- Cloquet f.
- Colles f.
- cremasteric f.
- cribriform f.
- crural f.
- Cruveilhier f.
- deep f.
- deltoid f.
- Denonvilliers f.
- dentate f.
- diaphragmatic f.
- endopelvic f.
- endothoracic f.
- extraperitoneal f.
- Gerota f.
- iliac f.
- infraspinous f.
- investing f.
- Laimer f.
- f. lata
- lateral conal f.
- lateral oblique f.
- lateroconal f.
- lumbar f.
- medial geniculate f.
- obturator internus f.
- palmar f.
- parietal pelvic f.
- pelvic f.
- perineal f.
- pharyngobasilar f.
- prepectoral f.
- prevertebral f.
- psoas f.
- quadratus femoris f.
- rectal f.
- renal f.
- retromammary f.

rim of f.
Scarpa f.
Sibson f.
spigelian f.
subcutaneous f.
superficial temporalis f.
superficial temporoparietal f.
supraanal f.
thoracolumbar f.
transversalis f.
umbilicovesical f.
vesical f.
visceral pelvic f.
Waldeyer f.
Zuckerkandl f.

fasciagram
fasciagraphy
fascial
f. band
f. envelope
f. incisor
f. margin necrosis
f. plane
f. rent
f. sheath
f. stranding
f. tract

fascias (*pl. of* fascia)
fascicle
synovium-lined f.
tibioligamentous f.
triquetroscaphoid f.
triquetrotrapezoid f.

fascicular
f. block
f. bundle
f. sarcoma

fasciculata
zona f.

fasciculation
tongue f.

fasciculus, pl. **fasciculi**
arcuate f. (AF)
Gowers f.
lenticular f.
longitudinal f.
longitudinalis medialis f.
mamillothalamic f.
medial longitudinal f. (MLF)
occipitofrontal f.
superior longitudinal f.
superior occipitofrontal f.

fasciitis
fulminant f.
necrotizing f.
f. ossificans
palmar f.
plantar f.
pseudosarcomatous f.
scrotal f.

fasciogram
fasciolar gyrus
fascioliasis
fashion
snapshot f.

fasiculoventricular bypass tract
FAST
focused abdominal sonography for
trauma
Fourier-acquired steady state
contrast-enhanced FAST
FAST pulse sequence
reduced-acquisition matrix FAST
RF-spoiled FAST
FAST technique
T1-weighted FAST

fast
f. acquisition multiple excitation
f. acquisition with multiphase efgre
(FAME)
f. adiabatic trajectory in steady
state (FATS)
f. cardiac phase contrast cine
imaging
f. dynamic volumetric x-ray CT
f. exchange-cellular suspension
f. exchange-soft tissue
f. FLAIR sequence
f. fluid-attenuation inversion
recovery image
f. Fourier flow (FFF)
f. Fourier imaging
f. Fourier projection (FFP)
f. Fourier spectral analysis
f. Fourier transform (FFT)
f. Fourier transform image
f. fractionation
f. gradient-echo sequence
F. Imaging Employing Steady-State
Acquisition technique
f. imaging with steady-state
precession (FISP)
f. inversion-recovery Fourier
transform (FIRFT)

NOTES

fast *(continued)*

    f. low-angle shot (FLASH)
    f. multiplanar inversion recovery imaging
    f. multiplanar spoiled gradient-recalled imaging
    f. neutron
    f. neutron radiotherapy
    f. PC cine MR sequence with echo-planar gradient
    f. routine production
    f. scan magnetic resonance imaging
    f. short tau inversion recovery
    f. spin-echo (FSE)
    f. spin-echo acquisition
    f. spin-echo black blood imaging
    f. spin-echo and fast inversion recovery imaging
    f. spin-echo MR imaging
    f. spin-echo T2-weighted image
    f. spin-echo view
    f. spoiled gradient-recalled echo (FSPGR)
    f. spoiled gradient-recalled MR imaging
    f. STIR

fast-array processor
fast-breeder reactor
Fastcard
Fast-Cath introducer catheter
FastCINE
FASTER

    field echo acquisition with short repetition time and echo reduction
        3D FASTER

fast-field echo (FFE)
fast-FLAIR technique
fast-flow

    f.-f. lesion
    f.-f. malformation
    f.-f. vascular anomaly

fast-neutron radiation therapy
FasTracker catheter
fast-scan magnetic resonance
fast-twitch muscle
fat

    abdominal f.
    f. absorption test
    anterior epidural f.
    bony glenoid marrow f.
    f. density
    f. density mass
    digital process of f.
    dirty f.
    f. embolism syndrome (FES)
    f. embolus
    epidural f.
    extraperitoneal f.

    herniated preperitoneal f.
    intraabdominal f.
    f. island
    isointense background f.
    lipid content of storage f.
    f. lobule
    f. and long T_2 suppressed ultrashort echo time (FLUTE)
    f. lung herniation
    mediastinal f.
    mesocolonic f.
    f. metabolism
    microvesicular f.
    mistiness of pericolonic f.
    muckiness of pericolonic f.
    f. necrosis
    f. pad
    f. pad sign
    parametrial f.
    peribursal f.
    pericolonic f.
    perigastric f.
    perihilar f.
    perinephric f.
    perineural f.
    perirectal f.
    perirenal f.
    f. plane
    posterior epidural f.
    preperitoneal f.
    prerenal f.
    properitoneal f.
    protruding f.
    radiolucent f.
    renal sinus f.
    retrobulbar f.
    retromammary f.
    f. saturation
    f. signal intensity
    f. signal suppression
    f. stranding
    f. stripe
    subcutaneous f.
    subdiaphragmatic f.
    subepicardial f.
    f. suppression
    f. suppression pulse
    f. suppression technique
    tumoral f.
    ventral epidural f.

fatal dose of radiation
fat-blood

    f.-b. interface (FBI)
    f.-b. interface sign

fat-containing

    f.-c. breast lesion
    f.-c. lesions
    f.-c. mass

fat-density
> f.-d. area
> f.-d. line

fat-fluid
> f.-f. density interface
> f.-f. level

fat-fraction measurement

fatigue
> f. damage
> f. fracture

FATS
> fast adiabatic trajectory in steady state

fat-saturated
> f.-s. axial image
> f.-s. spin-echo proton density-
> weighted image
> f.-s. T2-weighted fast spin-echo
> image

fat-selective presaturation

fat-spared
> f.-s. area in fatty liver
> f.-s. area in pancreas

fat-suppressed
> f.-s. acquisition with TE and TR
> times shortened
> f.-s. body coil
> f.-s. 3D spoiled gradient-echo
> FLASH MR imaging
> f.-s. 3D spoiled gradient-recall
> echo imaging
> f.-s. gadolinium-enhanced imaging
> f.-s. spin echo
> f.-s. T1-weighted 3D spoiled
> gradient-echo image
> f.-s. T2-weighted fast spin-echo
> sequence
> f.-s. T2-weighted FSE technique
> f.-s. ultrashort echo time (FUTE)

fat-suppressing content

fat-suppression pulse sequence

fatty
> f. acid metabolism
> f. cirrhosis
> f. degeneration
> f. filum
> f. filum terminale
> f. halo
> f. heart
> f. infiltrate
> f. intima streak
> f. kidney
> f. liver

> f. marrow
> f. meal
> f. meal sonogram (FMS)
> f. meal sonography
> f. mesentery
> f. metastatic lesion
> f. necrosis
> f. plaque
> f. prostatic tissue
> f. renal capsule
> f. soft tissue tumor
> f. sparing
> f. streak atherosclerosis

fat-water
> f.-w. chemical shift imaging
> f.-w. interface
> f. w. out of phase
> f.-w. signal cancellation
> f.-w. signal separation

fat- and water-suppressed T2-weighted image

fauces
> anterior pillar of f.
> arch of f.

faucial
> f. pillar
> f. tonsil

fault
> sagittal plane f.

faulty
> f. radiofrequency shielding
> f. radiofrequency shielding artifact
> f. union

faveolate

Favre disease

FB
> foreign body

FBI
> fat-blood interface
> FBI sign

FBM
> fetal breathing movement

FBP
> filtered back projection
> FBP method

FBS
> failed back syndrome

FBSS
> failed back surgery syndrome

FC
> flow compensation

F

NOTES

FCMD
Fukuyama congenital muscular disease
Fukuyama congenital muscular dystrophy
FCPA2 laser
FCS
full cervical spine
FCS · series
FCS view
FD
fractal dimension
FDDNP
fluorine-18 2-dialkylamino-6-
acylmalononitrile substituted
naphthalenes
FDDNP PET scan contrast medium
FDG
^{18}F-fluoro-2-deoxyglucose
fluorodeoxyglucose
FDG myocardial imaging
FDG positron emission tomography
FDG SPECT
FDG uptake
FDG-blood flow mismatch
FDG-labeled positron imaging
FDG-PET
fluorodeoxyglucose positron emission
tomography
positron emission tomography with
fluorodeoxyglucose
FDG-PET scan
^{18}FDG-PET
^{18}F-fluorodeoxyglucose positron emission
tomography
^{18}FDG-PET scan
FDG-6-phosphate
FDI
first digital interosseous
frequency domain imaging
FDI ultrasound
FDL muscle
FDQB
flexor digiti quinti brevis
FDQB muscle
FDS
flexor digitorum sublimis
flexor digitorum superficialis
FDS muscle
FE
field echo
frequency encode
^{52}Fe
iron 52
^{55}Fe
iron 55
^{59}Fe
iron 59
feasibility of image registration
FeatherTouch CO_2 laser

feathery
f. appearance
f. pattern
feature
clinical f.
differential diagnostic lung mass f.
geriatric f.
mammographic f.
mongoloid f.
proctographic f.
featureless appearance
fecal
f. concretion
f. diversion colostomy
f. fistula
f. impaction
f. incontinence
f. material
f. obstruction
f. residue
f. stone
f. tumor
fecal-filled colon
fecalith
fecaloid
fecaloma
fecaluria
feces
impacted f.
inspissated f.
semiliquid f.
feculence
feculent
Fédération Internationale de
Gynécologie Obstétrique (International
Federation of Obstetric Gynecology)
(FIGO)
feedback
breathing f.
real-time respiratory f.
feeder
f. artery
f. vein
feeding
f. artery of aneurysm
f. branch
f. branch of artery
f. mean arterial pressure (FMAP)
f. tube
f. vessel
f. vessel sign
FEER
field-echo sequence with even-echo
rephasing
field-even echo rephasing
feet (*pl. of* foot)
Fe-Ex orogastric tube magnet
Feigenbaum echocardiography
feign tumor

Feiss line
Feist-Mankin position
Feldkamp algorithm
fellow
>F. of the American College of
>Nuclear Medicine
>F. of the American College of
>Nuclear Physicians

Felson
>silhouette sign of F.

felt enforcing ring
Felty syndrome
female (F)
>f. genital tract calcification
>f. genital tract rhabdomyosarcoma
>intersex f.
>f. pelvis
>f. pseudohermaphroditism
>f. urethra

feminine aorta
feminization
>testicular f.

feminizing
>f. adrenal tumor
>f. testes syndrome

femora (*pl. of* femur)
femoral
>f. access
>f. antetorsion
>f. anteversion
>f. artery
>f. artery approach
>f. artery pseudoaneurysm
>f. articulation
>f. bone
>f. capital epiphysis
>common f. (CF)
>f. condylar shaving
>f. condyle
>f. cortex
>f. endarterectomy
>f. fossa
>f. head
>f. head amputation
>f. head deformity
>f. head epiphyseolysis
>f. head vascularity
>f. hernia
>f. intertrochanteric fracture
>f. leak
>f. ligament
>f. medullary canal

f. neck
f. neck fracture
f. nerve
f. ossification center
f. physial scar
f. plate
f. plexus
f. pulsatility index (FPI)
f. pulse
f. retrotorsion
f. retroversion
f. ring
f. runoff angiography
f. runoff arteriography
f. septum
f. shaft
f. shaft axis
f. shaft fracture
f. sheath
f. supracondylar fracture
f. torsion V angle
f. triangle
f. triangular content
f. tuberosity
f. varus derotational osteotomy
f. vein
f. vein percutaneous insertion
f. venous approach
f. view

femorale
>calcar f.

femoris
>quadratus f.
>quadriceps f.
>rectus f.

femorocerebral catheter angiography
femorocrural graft
femorodistal popliteal bypass graft
femorofemoral
>f. bypass graft
>f. cross-over

femorofemoropopliteal
femoropatellar joint
femoroperoneal in situ vein bypass graft
femoropopliteal
>f. artery
>f. atheromatous stenosis
>f. bypass graft
>f. Gore-Tex graft
>f. system

F

NOTES

femoropopliteal *(continued)*
    f. thrombosis
    f. vessel
femorotibial
    f. angle (FTA)
    f. bypass graft
FemoStop compression device
femtocurie
femtoliter
femtosecond
    f. laser keratome
    f. laser system
femur, pl. **femora**
    apex of f.
    body of f.
    distal f.
    greater trochanter of f.
    head of f.
    isthmus of f.
    f. length (FL)
    f. length to abdominal
      circumference
    lesser trochanter of f.
    neck of f.
    NSA of f.
    nutrient artery of f.
    proximal f.
fencer's bone
fender fracture
fenestra, pl. **fenestrae**
fenestral otosclerosis
fenestram
    fissula ante f.
fenestrated
    f. alphanumeric compression
    f. compression plate
    f. sheath
    f. tube
    f. vessel
fenestration
    aortopulmonary f.
    apical f.
    arterial f.
    balloon f.
    balloon catheter f.
    f. of basilar artery
    catheter-directed f.
    cusp f.
    f. of dissecting aneurysm
    falx f.
    interchordal space f.
    middle cerebral artery f.
    vertebral artery f.
fenoldopam mesylate
fentanyl citrate
Fe$_3$O$_4$
    magnetite
Ferguson
    F. angle

    F. method
    F. method for measuring scoliosis
    F. view
Feridex IV MRI contrast agent
fermium (Fm)
fermium 255 (^{255}Fm)
fernlike pattern
ferpentetate
    technetium-99m f.
Ferrein
    F. canal
    F. foramen
    F. ligament
ferric ammonium citrate-cellulose paste
ferrite
ferritin-labeled yttrium
ferrocalcinosis
    familial cerebral f.
ferroelectric relaxor
ferrokinetic data
ferromagnetic
    f. artifact
    f. implant
    f. material
    f. microembolization
    f. microembolization treatment
    f. microsphere
    f. relaxation
    f. tamponade
ferrous citrate
ferruginous body
Fertinex
ferucarbotran MR imaging agent
feruglose contrast agent
ferumoxide imaging agent
ferumoxsil imaging agent
ferumoxtran-enhanced
    f.-e. echo-planar GRE T2*-weighted
      imaging
    f.-e. echo-planar SE T2-weighted
      and echo-planar GRE
    f.-e. echo-planar SE T2-weighted
      imaging
ferumoxtran imaging agent
FES
    fat embolism syndrome
    flame emission spectroscopy
    fluoroestradiol
fetal
    f. abdominal circumference
    f. abdominal cystic mass
    f. abdominal wall
    f. abdominal wall defect
    f. abnormality
    f. adenoma
    f. age
    f. alcohol syndrome (FAS)
    f. amputation
    f. aortic flow volume

f. ascites
f. asphyxia
f. attitude
f. biometry
f. biometry ulna
f. biophysical profile score
f. bowel obstruction
f. BPS
f. breathing movement (FBM)
f. cardiac anomaly
f. cardiosplenic syndrome
f. cerebellum
f. chest anomaly
f. circulation
f. CNS anomaly
f. cranium
f. cystic adenomatoid malformation
f. cystic fibrosis
f. death
f. death in utero
f. detail
f. dystocia
f. echocardiographic view
f. echocardiography
f. echocardiography in utero
f. ectopia cordis
f. epiphysial bone center
f. eye
f. femoral length
f. foot length measurement
f. fracture
f. gallbladder
f. gastrointestinal anomaly
f. goiter
f. growth acceleration
f. growth retardation
f. hand malformation
f. head circumference
f. heart
f. heart anomaly
f. heart failure
f. hydrops
f. hypomineralization
f. incarceration
f. intraabdominal calcification
f. kidney lobation
f. lie
f. liver biopsy
f. liver magnetic resonance imaging
f. lobe
f. lobulation
f. long bone measurement

f. lung hypoplasia
f. lymphoid tissue
f. mesenchymal tumor
f. mesenchymal tumor of kidney
f. midface
f. movement (FM)
f. musculoskeletal dysplasia
f. musculoskeletal system
f. neck anomaly
f. neck pseudomembrane
f. period
f. placenta
f. pleural effusion
f. pole
f. position
f. pyelectasis
f. renal function
f. renal hamartoma
f. renal obstruction
f. scalp edema
f. skin biopsy
f. small part
f. sonography
f. spine
f. stress test
f. swallowing
f. thoracic circumference
f. ultrasound
f. urinary tract anomaly
f. urogenital tract
f. uterus
f. ventricular heart disproportion
f. ventriculomegaly
f. weight

fetalis
  chondrodystrophia f.
  hydrops f.
  nonimmune hydrops f.
fetal-pelvic
  f.-p. disproportion
  f.-p. index
feticide
fetogram
fetography
fetoliter
fetometry
fetus, pl. **fetuses**
  amorphous f.
  calcified f.
  cephalic presentation of f.
  demise of f.
  disappearing f.

F

NOTES

fetus *(continued)*
    growth-retarded f.
    impacted f.
    intrauterine f.
    malpositioned f.
    maturity of f.
    multiple fetuses
    nonviable f.
    paper-doll f.
    f. papyraceus
    parasitic f.
    postterm f.
    previable f.
    retained dead f.
    small for gestational age f.
    small part of f.
    stunted f.
    syndactyly in f.
    tissue of f.
    trisomic f.
    viable f.
fetus-in-fetu (FIF)
Feuerstein-Mims syndrome
fever
    f. of unknown etiology (FUE)
    f. of unknown origin (FUO)
FF
    filtration fraction
FFA
    free fatty acid
FFD
    focal film distance
^{18}F-FDG
    2-[fluorine-18]fluoro-2-deoxy-D-glucose
FFE
    fast-field echo
FFF
    fast Fourier flow
^{18}F-fluoro-6-thia-heptadecanoic acid (FTHA)
18F-fluorocholine
    radiation dosimetry of -f.
^{18}F-fluoro-2-deoxyglucose (FDG)
^{18}F-fluorodeoxyglucose positron emission tomography (^{18}FDG-PET)
FFP
    fast Fourier projection
FFT
    fast Fourier transform
FG-36UX scanning echoendoscope
FHC
    familial hypertrophic cardiomyopathy
    familial hypertrophy
FHF
    fulminant hepatic failure
FHI
    frontal horn index
FI
    fusion inhibitor

    FI method
    FI projection
fiber
    anular f.
    asbestos f.
    association f.
    atrio-His f.
    Bergman f.
    cardiac muscle f.
    cerebellar f.
    climbing f.
    differencing f.
    gastric sling f.
    Herxheimer f.
    long f.
    Mahaim and James f.
    mossy f.
    Müller f.
    muscle f.
    myocardial f.
    nodoventricular bypass f.
    notch from gastric sling f.
    obliquely oriented f.
    onionskin configuration of collagenous f.
    parasympathetic f.
    pontocerebellar f.
    postganglionic gray f.
    postganglionic sympathetic f.
    precharred f.
    Purkinje f.
    radial glial f.
    f. retraction
    Sharpey f.
    skeletal muscle f.
    sling muscle f.
    type I, II muscle f.
    unmyelinated nerve f.
fiber-bundle striation
fibered
    2 (x) 3, 4, 5, 6 f. Guglielmi detachable coil
fiberglass pneumoconiosis
Fiberlase laser
fiberoptic
    f. bronchogram
    f. bronchoscopy (FOB)
    f. bundle
    f. conductor
    f. light source
    f. probe
    f. taper
    f. video glasses
FiberScan laser
fiberscopic
fiber-shortening velocity
4-fiber therapy
fiber-type disproportion
fibrillary

fibrillation
   atrial f.
   chondromalacia with f.
Fibrimage diagnostic imaging agent
fibrin
   f. mass
   f. platelet embolus
   f. polymerization
   f. sleeve stripping
fibrinogen
   f. degradation
   iodinated I-125 f.
   labeled f.
   radiolabeled f.
fibrinoid necrosis
fibrinolytic
   f. therapy
   f. treatment
fibrinoma
fibrinopeptide A
fibrinopeptide B
fibrinopurulent pleurisy
fibrinous
   f. calculus
   f. degeneration
   f. inflammation
   f. pleurisy
   f. pneumonia
   f. polyp
fibrinous calculus
fibrin-split product
fibroadenolipoma
   breast f.
fibroadenoma
   breast f.
   calcified f.
   cellular f.
   degenerated f.
   esophagcal f.
   giant breast f.
   hyalinized breast f.
   involuting f.
   juvenile f.
   noncalcified f.
fibroadenomatosis
   breast f.
fibroadipose tissue
fibroareolar tissue
fibroblastic
   f. meningioma
   f. osteosarcoma

fibroblastoma
   perineural f.
fibroblast radiosensitivity
fibrocalcific
   f. cusp
   f. residual
fibrocalcification
fibrocartilage
   avascular f.
   circumferential f.
   f. complex
   intraarticular plate of f.
   labral f.
   triangular f. (TFC)
fibrocartilaginous
   f. disc
   f. labrum
   f. meniscus
   f. nodule
   f. overgrowth
   f. pad
   f. ridge
   f. scar
   f. tissue
   f. volar plate
fibrocaseous
fibrocavitary infiltrate
fibrochondrogenesis
fibrocollagenous
   f. connective tissue
   f. stroma
fibrocongestive splenomegaly
fibrocystic
   f. breast
   f. breast disease
   f. breast syndrome
   f. change
   f. lung disease
   f. residual
fibrodysplasia ossificans progressiva
fibroelastic
   f. band
   f. cartilage
fibroelastoma
   f. of heart valve
   papillary f.
fibroelastosis
   endocardial f.
fibroepithelial
   f. papilloma
   f. urethral polyp

NOTES

F

fibroepithelioma
    urinary tract f.
fibrofatty
    f. breast tissue
    f. layer
    f. plaque
fibrogenesis imperfecta ossium
fibrogenic pneumoconiosis
fibroglandular
    f. density
    f. element
    f. tissue
fibrohistiocytic lesion
fibrohistiocytoma
fibrohistiocytosis
fibroid
    f. adenoma
    calcified f.
    f. curvature
    f. degeneration
    f. embolization
    exophytic f.
    f. heart
    intramural f.
    f. lung
    f. myocarditis
    pedunculated uterine f.
    f. polyp
    submucosal f.
    subserosal f.
    f. tumor
    uterine f.
    f. uterus
fibrointimal hyperplasia
fibrolamellar
    f. HCC
    f. hepatocarcinoma
    f. hepatocellular carcinoma
fibroleiomyoma
    metastasizing f.
fibrolipoma
    filum terminale f.
    neural f.
fibrolipomatosis
    pelvic f.
    renal pelvic f.
fibrolipomatous nerve hamartoma
fibroma
    ameloblastic f.
    aponeurotic f.
    benign pleural f.
    calcified f.
    cardiac f.
    cementifying f.
    cementoossifying f.
    central cementifying f.
    central ossifying f.
    chondromyxoid f. (CMF)
    concentric f.

    desmoplastic f.
    giant cell f.
    heart f.
    irritation f.
    juvenile aponeurotic f.
    juvenile ossifying f.
    f. of lung
    meningeal f.
    f. molle
    f. molle gravidarum
    f. molluscum
    musculoaponeurotic f.
    f. myxomatodes
    nonossifying f.
    nonosteogenic f.
    ossifying bone f.
    ossifying skull f.
    osteogenic bone f.
    ovarian f.
    periosteal f.
    peripheral ossifying f.
    periungual f.
    polypoid f.
    psammomatoid ossifying f.
    recurrent digital f.
    scrotal f.
    senile f.
    Shope f.
    sinonasal psammomatoid
      ossifying f.
    soft tissue f.
    subcutaneous f.
    subungual f.
    telangiectatic f.
    ungual f.
fibroma-thecoma tumor of ovary
fibromatogenic
fibromatoid
fibromatosis
    abdominal f.
    aggressive f.
    aggressive infantile f.
    f. colli
    congenital diffuse f.
    congenital generalized f.
    infantile digital f.
    juvenile f.
    mesenteric f.
    multicentric f.
    multiple congenital f.
    musculoaponeurotic f.
    palmar f.
    penile f.
    plantar f.
fibromatous
fibromuscular
    f. band
    f. dysplasia
    f. lesion

f. pelvic floor
f. renal artery stenosis
f. ridge
f. subaortic stenosis
f. tissue
fibromyoma, pl. **fibromyomata**
fibromyositis
fibromyxoma
    kidney f.
    odontogenic f.
    pleural f.
fibronodular infiltrate
fibronuclear
fibroosseous
    f. attachment
    f. lesion
    f. pseudotumor of digit
    f. tunnel
fibroosteoma of tooth
fibroplasia
    adventitial f.
    endomyocardial f.
    intimal f.
    medial f.
    perimedial f.
    retrolental f.
fibroplastic
    f. process
    f. proliferation
fibroproductive tuberculosis
fibroretractive
fibrosa
    f. disseminata
    hepatica f.
    osteitis f.
    osteodystrophia f.
    pseudoaneurysm of mitral-aortic f.
fibrosarcoma
    ameloblastic f.
    bone f.
    cardiac f.
    central f.
    congenital kidney f.
    epididymal f.
    infantile f.
    inflammatory f.
    nonmetastasizing f.
    periosteal f.
    f. variant
fibrosclerotic
fibrosed muscle

fibrosing
    f. arachnoiditis
    f. colonopathy
    f. cryptogenic alveolitis
    f. inflammation
    f. inflammatory pseudotumor
    f. mediastinitis
    f. mesenteritis
    f. mesothelioma
    f. piecemeal necrosis
    f. tissue
fibrosis
    acute diffuse interstitial f.
    alcoholic f.
    anular f.
    arachnoid f.
    asbestos-induced pleural f.
    basilar f.
    benign meningeal f.
    bone marrow f.
    brachytelephalangic type of
      cystic f.
    breast f.
    cerebellar vermis hypoplasia,
      oligophrenia, congenital ataxia,
      ocular coloboma, hepatic f.
      (COACH)
    cirrhosis-related f.
    confluent f.
    congenital hepatic f. (CHF)
    congenital liver f.
    cystic f.
    Davies endocardial f.
    Davies endomyocardial f.
    diffuse interstitial pulmonary f.
      (DIPF)
    endocardial f.
    endomyocardial f. (EMF)
    epidural anular f.
    fetal cystic f.
    focal f.
    hepatic f.
    horseshoe f.
    hyalinized fibroadenoma with f.
    idiopathic interstitial f.
    idiopathic pulmonary f. (IPF)
    inflammatory f.
    interstitial diffuse pulmonary f.
    interstitial prematurity f.
    interstitial pulmonary f. (IPF)
    intimal f.
    intraalveolar f.

F

NOTES

fibrosis *(continued)*
    intralobular f.
    leptomeningeal f.
    f. of lung
    massive f.
    mediastinal f.
    meningeal f.
    mesenteric f.
    mural endomyocardial f.
    nodal f.
    nodular subepidermal f.
    noncirrhotic portal f. (NCPF)
    nonnodular f.
    pancreatic cystic f.
    parietal lobe gray-matter cytosolic choline pathogenetic mechanism of myocardial f.
    periadventitial f.
    perialveolar f.
    periaortic f.
    peribronchial f.
    pericentral f.
    periductal f.
    peridural f.
    perihilar f.
    perimuscular f.
    perineural f.
    periportal f.
    periureteral f.
    perivascular f.
    perivenular f.
    pipestem f.
    portal f.
    portal-to-portal f.
    postinflammatory pulmonary f.
    postradiation f.
    posttraumatic f.
    primary retroperitoneal f.
    progressive interstitial pulmonary f.
    progressive massive f. (PMF)
    progressive nodular pulmonary f.
    pulmonary idiopathic f.
    pulmonary interstitial idiopathic f.
    pulmonary vein f.
    radiation-induced f. (RIF)
    reactive f.
    replacement f.
    retroperitoneal f. (RPF)
    secondary retroperitoneal f.
    subadventitial f.
    subintimal f.
    subserosal f.
    Symmers f.
    transmural f.

fibrosum
    adenoma f.
    molluscum f.
    pericardium f.

fibrosus
    anulus f.
fibrothorax
fibrotic
    f. cavitating pattern
    f. change
    f. honeycombing
    f. island
    f. kidney
    f. plaque
    f. residual
    f. resolution
    f. scarring
    f. tissue
fibrous
    f. ankylosis
    f. attachment
    f. band
    f. bar
    f. bone lesion
    f. cap
    f. cartilage
    f. coalition
    f. connective tissue
    f. connective tissue tumor
    f. cord
    f. cortical defect
    f. dysplasia ossificans progressiva
    f. GI tract polypoid lesion
    f. goiter
    f. hamartoma
    f. histiocytoma
    f. hood
    f. intima plaque
    f. mastopathy
    f. medullary defect
    f. meningioma
    f. metaphysial-diaphysial defect
    f. nodular pattern
    f. nodule
    f. nonunion
    f. obliterative cholangitis
    f. osteodystrophy
    f. osteoma
    f. pericardium
    f. plaque atherosclerosis
    f. pleural adhesion
    f. pneumonia
    f. renal capsule
    f. ring
    f. ring of disc
    f. scar tissue
    f. septum
    f. sheath
    f. skeleton
    f. temporal bone dysplasia
    f. tissue hyperplasia
    f. trigone
    f. tubercle

f. tumor pleura
f. union
f. urinary tract polyp
f. web
fibrovascular
f. core
f. polyp
f. stalk
f. tissue
fibroxanthoma
malignant f.
multiple f.'s
pediatric f.
fibroxanthosarcoma
fibula, pl. **fibulae**
apex of f.
capitulum fibulae
inferior tip of f.
malleolus fibulae
nutrient artery of f.
proximal f.
fibular
f. articular surface
f. collateral ligament
f. fracture
f. hallux sesamoid
f. lymph node
f. notch
f. physis
f. sesamoid bone
f. vein
fibulotalar ligament
fibulotalocalcaneal (FTC)
f. ligament
Ficat
F. and Axlet staging system
F. stage of avascular necrosis
F. staging
Fick
F. cardiac index
F. equation
F. first law of diffusion
F. law
F. method
F. method for measuring cardiac output
F. position
F. principle
Ficoll gradient

FID
flexion interspinous distance
free-induction decay
FID-acquired echo (FAcE)
fiducial
f. alignment system
f. movement
f. skin marker
field
f. alignment
blocked vertex f.
Brodmann cytoarchitectonic f.
f. cancerization
collapsed lung f.
3D deformation f.
f. defect
dipole f.
disc-to-magnetic f.
f. drift
f. echo (FE)
electromagnetic f.
electromagnetic focusing f. (EFF)
electronic focusing f.
f. emission tube
f.-even echo rephasing (FEER)
extremely low-frequency f.
far f.
fringe f.
Gibbs random f.
gonion gradient magnetic f.
f. gradient
gradient magnetic f.
harmonic f.
helmet f.
high-powered f. (hpf)
insonifying wave f.
involved f.
large hinge angle electron f.
f. lock
lower lung f.
lung f.
magnetic fringe f.
mantle f.
Markov random f.
midlung f.
near f.
oscillating magnetic f.
parietal eye f. (PEF)
perturbing magnetic f.
radiofrequency electromagnetic f.
rotational f.
skimming of magnetic f.

NOTES

F

field *(continued)*
    spade f.
    static magnetic f.
    stationary f.
    stippling of lung f.
    stray neutron f.
    f. strength
    tangential breast f.
    Tesla f.
    time-varying magnetic f.
    f. uniformity
    upper lung f.
    f. variation
    f. of view (FOV)
    Z axis f.
4-field
    4-f. technique
    4-f. x-ray dosimetry
field-echo
    f.-e. difference
    f.-e. imaging
    f.-e. pulse sequence
    f.-e. sequence with even-echo
      rephasing (FEER)
    f.-e. sum
field-even echo rephasing (FEER)
field-fitting
    f.-f. analysis
    f.-f. technique
Fielding-Magliato subtrochanteric
  fracture classification
field-of-view
    f.-o.-v. imaging
    f.-o.-v. information
field-profiling coil
Fiessinger-Leroy-Reiter syndrome
Fiessinger-Leroy syndrome
FIESTA
    Formation Internationale en
      Epidémiologie et Statistique de Terrains
      Approfondies
      FIESTA imaging technique
      micro-MRI with FIESTA
FIF
    fetus-in-fetu
fifth
    f. compartment
    f. cranial nerve
    f. intercostal space
    f. rib
    f. ventricle
fighter's fracture
FIGO
    Fédération Internationale de Gynécologie
      Obstétrique (International Federation of
      Obstetric Gynecology)
      FIGO stage carcinoma
      FIGO staging of adenocarcinoma
       of endometrium

figure
    acetabular teardrop f.
    teardrop f.
figure-3 sign
figure-4 position
figure-8 appearance
filament
    f. emission
    f. transformer
filament-nonfilament count
filarial infection
file
    Indian f.
filiform
    f. appendix
    f. polyp
    f. polyposis
filigree pattern
filipuncture
fill-and-spill of dye
filler block
filling
    augmented f.
    capillary f.
    compensatory capillary f.
    f. defect
    early venous f.
    f. factor
    late venous f.
    passive f.
    peak f.
    f. pressure
    rapid f. (RF, rf)
    reduced f.
    retrograde f.
    subintimal f.
    ureteral f.
    ventricular f.
    vessel f.
    zero f.
film *(See* projection, radiograph, scan,
  view, x-ray)
    f. alternator
    anteroposterior f.
    f. badge
    biplane axial f.
    bitewing f.
    Bucky f.
    f. changer
    chest f.
    cine f.
    comparison f.
    corner f.
    cross-table lateral f.
    Curix Ultra UV-L f.
    cut and cine f.
    decubitus f.
    delayed f.
    f. density calibration

f. diameter
digital subtraction f.
f. dispenser
drain-out f.
dual-emulsion mammography f.
DuPont Cronex x-ray f.
emulsion f.
expiratory f.
flat plate f.
f. fog
gamma f.
GLP7 f.
f. graininess
grid f.
f. hanger
high-contrast f.
horizontal beam f.
in-department f.
intraoperative f.
kidneys, ureter, and bladder f.
Knuttsen bending f.
Kodak Min-R f.
Kodak X-OMAT f.
late f.
lateral cervical spine f.
lateral decubitus f.
latitude f.
limited f.
low-contrast f.
low-dose f.
manual subtraction f.
mobility f.
nitrocellulose f.
normal chest f.
oblique f.
occlusal f.
overhead f.
overpenetrated f.
f. oxygenator
PA and lateral f.'s
panoramic x-ray f.
photo plotter f.
plain f.
Polaroid f.
port f.
portable chest f.
posteroanterior chest f.
postevacuation f.
postexercise f.
postreduction f.
postvoiding f.
preliminary f.

prone f.
radiochromic f.
right or left lateral decubitus f.
runoff f.
Scopix Laser f.
scout f.
f. screen cassette
f. screen contact test
screenless mammography f.
screen type f.
semierect f.
sequential f.'s
serial subtraction f.
shoot-through lateral x-ray f.
silver halide f.
simulation f.
skull f.
f. slippage
f. speed
spot f.
stress f.
suboptimal f.
subtraction f.
supine f.
survey f.
f. tube distance
UP7 f.
upright chest f.
upright compression spot f.
weightbearing f.
wide latitude f.
working f.
x-ray f.

film-based
f.-b. screening mammogram
f.-b. viewing
FilmFax teleradiology system
film-focus distance
filmless
f. imaging
f. radiography
film-screen
f.-s. magnification
f.-s. mammography
f.-s. radiography
filter
bandpass f.
bird's nest f.
Butterworth f.
caval f.
compensating f.
density equalization f.

NOTES

F

filter *(continued)*
    differencing f.
    flattening f.
    Greenfield vena cava f.
    Günther Tulip vena cava MReye f.
    Hann f.
    helix f.
    high-pass f.
    inherent f.
    Kalman f.
    K-edge f.
    Keeper vena cava f.
    low-pass f.
    Metz f.
    Metz spatially varying f.
    Mobin-Uddin vera cava f.
    f. mold
    nitinol inferior vena cava f.
    OptEase permanent vena cava f.
    over-the-wire Greenfield f.
    10-pole Butterworth f.
    prophylactic IVC f.
    ramp f.
    Recovery f.
    Recovery Nitinol f.
    retrievable IVC f.
    rhodium f.
    SafeFlo IVC f.
    sigma f.
    Simon Nitinol f.
    Simon Nitinol IVC f.
    Simon Nitinol vena cava f.
    software-controlled internal
      hardware f.
    spatial f.
    stainless-steel Greenfield f.
    Tempofilter vena cava f.
    temporal f.
    Thoreau f.
    titanium Greenfield f.
    translation-invariant f.
    TrapEase inferior vena cava f.
    TrapEase permanent IVC f.
    TrapEase vena cava f.
    vena caval f.
    Vena Tech LGM f.
    Vena Tech LGM vena cava f.
    Vena Tech low-profile f.
    Vena Tech LP vena cava f.
    wall f.
    wedge f.
    Weiner spatially varying f.
    Wiener MRI f.
    F. Wire distal protection device
    F. Wire EX
    Wratten 6B f.
filtered
    f. back projection (FBP)

    f. back-projection algorithm
    f. back-projection method
filtering
    3D low pass f.
    3D post f.
    dynamic f.
    low-pass f.
    morphologic f.
    phase f.
filtration
    beam f.
    copper f.
    dynamic beat f.
    f. fraction (FF)
    glomerular f.
    postbeat f.
    supplemental beam f.
filum
    fatty f.
    f. terminale
    f. terminale fibrolipoma
fimbriated end
finding
    angiographic f.
    atypical f.
    auscultatory f.
    cardinal f.
    characteristic f.
    concomitant f.
    concordance of MR f.'s
    constellation of f.'s
    discordant f.
    equivocal f.
    focal lateralizing f.
    incidental f.
    lateralizing f.
    no discernible f.
    nonspecific f.
    pathognomonic f.
    roentgenographic f.
    secondary sonographic f.
    specious f.
    spurious f.
    ultrasonographic f.
fine
    f. calcification
    f. detail
    f. injection
    f. peripheral reticular pattern
    f. reticular pattern
fine-needle
    f.-n. aspiration
    f.-n. aspiration biopsy
    f.-n. puncture
    f.-n. transhepatic cholangiogram
      (FNTC)
fine-speckled appearance
finger
    base of f.

baseball f.
bolster f.
bony tuft of f.
clubbed f.
Dawson f.
drop f.
football f.
f. fracture
hippocratic f.
index f.
jammed f.
jersey f.
little f.
long f.
f. lucent lesion
mallet f.
middle f.
overlapping f.
pedicle f.
pulley of f.
pulp of f.
replantation of f.
ring f.
sausage f.
spade f.
speck f.
spider f.
stoved f.
f. sweep
tapered f.
trigger f.
f. of tumor
f. web
webbed f.

finger-in-glove pattern
fingerlike
f. mucous plug
f. projection
f. villus
fingerprint
f. edema
f. image compression
f. mark artifact
f. pattern
fingertip
f. amputation
f. calcification
f. lesion
Finkelstein sign
fire
side f.
firearm injury

FIRFT
fast inversion-recovery Fourier transform
firing
f. of ectopic atrial focus
f. temperature
firm
f. mass
f. neoplasm
Firooznia
threshold of F.
first
f. branchial arch
f. branchial cleft cyst
f. carpal row
f. cuneiform bone
f. diagonal branch artery
f. digital interosseous (FDI)
f. duodenal sphincter
f. major diagonal branch
f. metatarsal angle
f. metatarsal head (FMH)
f. obtuse marginal artery
f. parallel pelvic plane
f. portion of duodenum
f. ray instability
f. reader
f. rib
f. septal perforator branch
f. temporal gyrus
f. trimester gestational trophoblastic disease
f. ventricle of cerebrum
f. visceral cleft
first-degree
f.-d. AV block
f.-d. heart block
first-fifth intermetatarsal angle
first-line therapy
first-order
f.-o. chorda
f.-o. reaction
first-pass
f.-p. acquisition
f.-p. cardiac perfusion
f.-p. effect
f.-p. examination
f.-p. MUGA
f.-p. myocardial perfusion imaging
f.-p. myocardial perfusion MR
f.-p. radionuclide angiography (FPRNA)

NOTES

F

first-pass *(continued)*
    f.-p. radionuclide exercise
        angiocardiography
    f.-p. radionuclide ventriculography
    f.-p. study
    f.-p. technique
    f.-p. thallium extraction
    f.-p. view
first-second intermetatarsal angle
first-trimester
    f.-t. bleeding
    f.-t. hemorrhage
    f.-t. nuchal translucency
    f.-t. placenta
Fischer sign
Fischgold
    F. bimastoid line
    F. biventer line
Fisher grade 1–4
fish flesh appearance
fishmeal worker's lung
fishmouth
    f. amputation
    f. configuration of mitral valve
    f. cusp
    f. fracture
    f. mitral stenosis
    f. mitral valve configuration
    f. vertebra
fishnet appearance
fish-scale gallbladder
fishtail
    f. tear
    f. vertebra
FISP
    fast imaging with steady-state precession
    true fast imaging and steady progression
    mirrored FISP (mFISP)
    FISP pulse sequence
fission
    nuclear f.
    f. product
    f. track analysis
fissula ante fenestram
fissuration
fissure
    abdominal f.
    accessory f.
    anal f.
    f. in ano
    anterior interhemispheric f.
    anterior median f.
    antitragohelicine f.
    f. of anulus
    auricular f.
    azygos f.
    brain f.
    bulging lung f.
    calcarine f.

    callosomarginal f.
    central cerebellar f.
    cerebral f.
    choroidal f.
    chronic f.
    collateral f.
    cutaneous f.
    decidual f.
    dentate f.
    displacement of interhemispheric f.
    f. fracture
    glaserian f.
    hepatic f.
    hippocampal f.
    horizontal f.
    incomplete pulmonary f.
    inferior accessory f.
    inferior orbital f.
    interhemispheric f. (IHF)
    interlobar f.
    lateral f.
    ligamentum venosum f.
    liver f.
    longitudinal f.
    lung f.
    main f.
    major f.
    minor f.
    nasopalatal f.
    oblique f.
    occipital f.
    oral f.
    orbital f.
    palpebral f.
    portal f.
    rolandic f.
    f. of Rolando
    f. sign
    studded f.
    superior orbital f.
    supraorbital f.
    sylvian f.
    transitional zone f.
    umbilical f.
    widened superior orbital f.
fissured atheromatous plaque
fisting
    rectal f.
fistula, pl. **fistulae, fistulas**
    abdominal f.
    aerodigestive f.
    anal f.
    f. in ano
    anorectal f.
    anovaginal f.
    aorta-left ventricular f.
    aorta-right ventricular f.
    aortic-enteric f.
    aortic sinus to right ventricle f.

aortocaval f.
aortoduodenal f.
aortoenteric f.
aortoesophageal f.
aortojejunal f.
aortopulmonary f.
aortosigmoid f.
arterial-arterial f.
arterial-portal f.
arteriobiliary f.
arterioportobiliary f.
arteriosinusoidal penile f.
arteriovenous f. (AVF)
autogenous hemodialysis f.
biliary f.
biliary-cutaneous f.
biliary-duodenal f.
biliary-enteric f.
bilioenteric f.
Blom-Singer tracheoesophageal f.
BP f.
branchial f.
Brescia-Cimino f.
bronchobiliary f.
bronchocavitary f.
bronchocutaneous f.
bronchoesophageal f.
bronchopleural f.
bronchopulmonary f.
cameral f.
caroticocavernous f.
carotid-cavernous f. (CCF)
carotid-cavernous sinus f.
carotid-dural f.
carotid-jugular f.
cavernous sinus f.
cecocutaneous f.
cerebral arteriovenous f.
cerebrospinal fluid f.
cholecystenteric f.
cholecystenteric f.
cholecystocholedochal f.
cholecystocolic f.
cholecystocutaneous f.
cholecystoduodenal f.
cholecystoduodenocolic f.
choledochal-colonic f.
choledochoduodenal f.
chyle f.
chylous f.
coil closure of coronary artery f.
colocolic f.

colocutaneous f.
colonic f.
colovaginal f.
colovesical f.
communicating f.
complex anorectal f.
congenital pulmonary
  arteriovenous f.
congenital tracheobiliary f.
coronary arteriosystemic f.
coronary arteriovenous f.
coronary artery cameral f.
coronary artery-pulmonary artery f.
coronary artery to right
  ventricular f.
cystic f.
dialysis f.
digestive-respiratory f.
dorsal enteric f.
duodenocolic f.
duodenopancreatic f.
dural arteriovenous f. (DAVF)
dural carotid cavernous f. (DCCF)
durocutaneous f.
dysfunctional autogenous
  hemodialysis f.
Eck f.
enteric f.
enterocolic f.
enterocutaneous f.
enteroenteral f.
enterospinal f.
enterourethral f.
enterovaginal f.
enterovesical f.
esophagorespiratory f.
esophagotracheal f.
external biliary f.
extrasphincteric anal f.
fecal f.
f. formation
gastric f.
gastrocolic f.
gastrocutaneous f.
gastroduodenal f.
gastrointestinal f.
gastrojejunocolic f.
genitourinary f.
graft-enteric f.
hepatic arteriovenous f.
hepatic artery-portal vein f.
hepatopleural f.

F

NOTES

fistula *(continued)*
    hepatoportal biliary f.
    high-flow arteriovenous f.
    horseshoe f.
    H-type tracheoesophageal f.
    hyperdynamic AV f.
    iatrogenic iliocaval f.
    ileosigmoid f.
    infralevator f.
    intersphincteric anal f.
    intracranial arteriovenous f.
    intradural retromedullary
      arteriovenous f.
    intrahepatic arterial-portal f.
    intrahepatic AV f.
    intrapulmonary arteriovenous f.
    jejunocolic f.
    labyrinthine f.
    Mann-Bollman f.
    mediastinal f.
    mesenteric f.
    metroperitoneal f.
    microvenoarteriolar f.
    mucous f.
    orofacial f.
    f. ostium
    pancreatic cutaneous f.
    pancreaticopleural f.
    paraprosthetic-enteric f.
    parietal f.
    periareolar f.
    perineovaginal f.
    persistent bronchopleural f.
    pilonidal f.
    pleural f.
    pleurocutaneous f.
    postbiopsy renal AV f.
    premedullary arteriovenous f.
    pulmonary arteriovenous f.
    radial artery to cephalic vein f.
    radiation f.
    radiculomeningeal f.
    rectal f.
    rectovaginal f.
    rectovesical f.
    respiratory-esophageal f.
    retroperitoneal f.
    spinal dural arteriovenous f.
    splanchnic AV f.
    splenic AV f.
    splenobronchial f.
    supralevator f.
    suprasphincteric f.
    TE f.
    thoracic duct-cutaneous f.
    tracheobiliary f.
    tracheobronchial f.
    tracheobronchoesophageal f.
    tracheoesophageal f. (TEF)
    f. tract study
    transdural f.
    transsphincteric anal f.
    trigeminal cavernous f.
    type A carotid cavernous f.
    ureteral f.
    ureterocutaneous f.
    ureterointestinal f.
    ureteroperitoneal f.
    ureterovaginal f.
    urethrovaginal f.
    urinary f.
    vaginal f.
    venobiliary f.
    vertebrojugular f.
    vertebrovertebral f.
    vesical f.
    vesicocolic f.
    vesicovaginal f.
    vitelline f.

fistulogram
    cine f.
    venous f.

fistulography

fistulous
    f. gas communication
    f. tract

fit
    smoothed curve f.

fitting
    peak f.

Fitz-Hugh and Curtis syndrome

fixation
    f. articulation
    atlantoaxial rotary f.
    bowel loop f.
    catheter f.
    f. disc
    external f.
    external wire f.
    intramedullary f.
    intrapedicular f.
    metallic rod f.
    open reduction and internal f.
      (ORIF)
    plate and screw f.
    f. of scoliosis
    screw f.
    spinal f.
    suprasyndesmotic f.
    transsyndesmotic screw f.
    triangular external ankle f.
    wire f.

fixator
    dynamic axial f.
    f. muscle

fixed
    f. airway obstruction
    f. coronary obstruction

f. flexion contracture
f. gantry
f. intracavitary filling defect
f. mass
f. perfusion defect
f. pulmonary valvular resistance
f. segment of bowel
f. shaped coplanar or nonplanar radiation beam bouquet
f. third-degree AV block
fixed-orifice aortic stenosis
fixer
fixing time
FL
femur length
flabby heart
¹⁸F-labeled
fluorine-18-labeled
¹⁸F-labeled fatty acid
¹⁸F-labeled HFA-134a
¹⁸F-labeled polyfluorinated ethyl
Flack sinuatrial node
flag
Rudick red f.
flail
f. air
f. chest
f. digit
f. foot
f. joint
f. mitral valve
f. shoulder
FLAIR
fluid-attenuated inversion recovery
FLAIR echo-planar imaging
FLAIR image
FLAIR-FLASH imaging
FLAK
flow artifact killer
FLAK technique
flake
f. fracture
f. fracture of hamate
flake-shaped injury
flaking of cartilage
flaky calcification
flame
f. appearance
f. emission spectroscopy (FES)
f. ionization detector
Flamingo stent

flange
shaft f.
flank
f. bone
f. stripe
flap
bone f.
bursal f.
entry f.
foramen ovale f.
intimal f.
Karapandzic f.
liver f.
localized intimal f.
lytic area bone f.
necrotic f.
osteoplastic f.
pedicle f.
pericardial f.
pleural f.
f. positioning
postangioplasty intimal f.
rotary door f. (RDF)
scapular f.
scimitar-shaped f.
subclavian f.
f. tear
TRAM f.
f. valve ventricular septal defect
flaplike valve
flap-valve mechanism
flare
condylar f.
metaphysial f.
f. phenomenon
f. reaction
tibial f.
trochanteric f.
flared ilium
FLASH
fast low-angle shot
FLASH acquisition
diffusion/perfusion snapshot FLASH (DPSF)
FLASH image
FLASH magnetic resonance imaging
flashlamp-pulsed dye laser
flashlamp-pumped pulsed dye laser
flash photolysis
FlashPoint image-guided surgical instrument

NOTES

F

flask
    Erlenmeyer f.
    vascular f.
flask-shaped
    f.-s. heart
    f.-s. ulcer
flat
    f. adenoma
    f. bone
    f. colorectal carcinoma
    f. diastolic slope
    f. electroencephalogram
    f. facet
    f. neck vein
    f. pelvis
    f. plate
    f. plate of abdomen
    f. plate film
    f. suture
    f. time-intensity profile
    f. vertebral body
Flatau-Schilder disease
flat-field imaging
flatfoot
    calcaneovalgus f.
    f. deformity
    Durham f.
flat-hand test
flat-panel megavoltage imager
flat-plate detector
flattened
    f. arch
    f. duodenal fold
    f. E-to-F slope
    f. longitudinal arch of foot
flattening
    cortical f.
    f. of diaphragm
    f. filter
    f. filter beam
    f. of gyrus
    f. of normal lordotic curvature
    f. of normal lumbar curve
    f. ratio (FR)
flat-top
    f.-t. bladder
    f.-t. talus
flaval ligament
flavone acetic acid (FAA)
flavum, pl. **flava**
    ligamentum f.
    pleating of ligamentum f.
flawed
    f. image
    f. imaging
flax-dresser disease
Flechsig bundle
Fleckinger view
fleck sign

fleecy mass
Fleet
    F. Phospho-Soda bowel preparation
    F. Prep Kit 1, 2, 3
fleeting lung infiltrate
Fleischmann bursa
Fleischner
    F. line
    F. position
    F. sign
Fletcher
    F. afterloader
    F. factor
    F. projection
    F. rule of irradiation tolerance
Fletcher-Delclos dome cylinder
Fletcher-Suit-Delclos (FSD)
    F.-S.-D. tandem
Fletcher-Suit system for radium therapy
fleur-de-lis pattern
flexa
    coxa f.
Flexart MRI scanner
flexible
    f. biopsy needle
    f. endofluoroscopy
    f. nephroscope
    f. over-wire system
    f. radiofrequency coil
    f. spastic equinovarus deformity
    f. surface coil
    f. surface-coil-type resonator
    (FSCR)
flexible-tip guidewire
Flexiflo
Flexima biliary drainage catheter
flexion
    angle of greatest f. (AGF)
    f. contracture
    f. deformity
    f. and extension exercises
    f. and extension views
    external rotation in f. (ERF)
    internal rotation in f. (IRF)
    f. interspinous distance (FID)
    f. maneuver
    f. position
    f. teardrop fracture
flexion-adduction contracture
flexion-burst fracture
flexion-compression fracture
flexion-distraction
    f.-d. fracture
    f.-d. injury
flexion-extension
    f.-e. plane
    f.-e. projection
    f.-e. radiography
flexion-rotation injury

Flexi-Tip ureteral catheter
Flexlase 600 laser
flexor
  f. bursa
  f. canal
  capital f.
  f. carpi radialis
  f. carpi radialis muscle
  f. carpi radialis tendon
  f. carpi ulnaris
  f. carpi ulnaris aponeurosis
  f. carpi ulnaris tendon
  f. digiti minimi
  f. digiti minimi brevis
  f. digiti quinti brevis (FDQB)
  f. digiti quinti brevis muscle
  f. digitorum brevis
  f. digitorum communis tendon
  f. digitorum longus
  f. digitorum longus muscle
  f. digitorum longus tendon
  f. digitorum profundus
  f. digitorum profundus muscle
  f. digitorum profundus tendon
  f. digitorum sublimis (FDS)
  f. digitorum sublimis tendon
  f. digitorum superficialis (FDS)
  f. digitorum superficialis muscle
  f. digitorum superficialis tendon
  f. hallucis brevis
  f. hallucis brevis muscle
  f. hallucis brevis tendon
  f. hallucis longus
  f. hallucis longus tendon
  F. introducer
  f. plate
  f. pollicis brevis
  f. pollicis brevis tendon
  f. pollicis longus
  f. pollicis longus tendon
  f. profundus tendon
  f. retinaculum
  f. sublimis tendon
  f. tendon sheath
  f. tenosynovitis
flexor-pronator muscle group
FlexStent
  Gianturco-Roubin F.
FlexStrand cable
Flex-T guidewire
flexure
  caudal f.

  cephalic f.
  cerebral f.
  cervical f.
  colonic f.
  cranial f.
  duodenojejunal f. (DJF)
  hepatic f.
  inferior duodenal f. (IDF)
  left colonic f.
  right colonic f.
  sigmoid f.
  splenic f.
flicker electroretinogram
Flint colon injury scale
flip
  f. angle
  spin f.
  tristimulus value f.
  value f.
flip-angle image
flip-flop
  f.-f. enhancement
  f.-f. pattern
flipped meniscus sign
floating
  f. arch fracture
  f. cartilage
  f. elbow
  f. endocardial centroid
  f. epicardial centroid
  f. gallbladder
  f. gallstone
  f. image
  f. kidney
  f. knee
  f. leaflet
  f. ligament
  f. liver
  f. organ
  f. osteophyte
  f. patella
  f. prostate
  f. rib
  f. spleen
  f. teeth
  f. thumb
  f. villus
  f. viscera sign
floccular fossa
flocculation of barium
flocculent focus of calcification

F

NOTES

flocculonodular
- f. lobe
- f. lobe of cerebellum
- f. tumor

flocculus, pl. **flocculi**

Flocks and Kadesky system

flood
- F. ligament
- f. phantom
- f. section
- f. source

floor
- bladder f.
- fibromuscular pelvic f.
- inguinal f.
- f. of orbit
- pelvic f.
- sellar f.
- f. of ventricle

floppy
- f. mitral valve
- f. valve syndrome

floppy-thumb sign

Flo-Rester vessel occluder

florid
- f. callus
- f. cardiac tamponade
- f. duct lesion
- f. follicular hyperplasia
- f. plaque
- f. reactive periostitis

flow
- absolute blood f.
- f. acceleration
- aliased f.
- altered blood f.
- anatomic shunt f.
- antegrade bile f.
- antegrade blood f.
- antegrade diastolic f.
- aortic f. (AF)
- f. arrest
- f. artifact killer (FLAK)
- autoregulation of cerebral blood f.
- azygos blood f.
- backward f.
- bile f.
- blood f.
- capillary blood f.
- cephalization of blood f.
- cerebral blood f. (CBF)
- cerebral xenon-enhanced blood f. (X-CBF)
- chronic reserve f.
- collateral blood f.
- f. compensation (FC)
- compromised f.
- f. of contrast material
- coronary blood f.

- coronary reserve f. (CRF)
- f. cytometric DNA measurement
- f. cytometry
- f. cytometry sample preparation
- f. cytometry technique
- dampened pulsatile f.
- 2D color-coded imaging of blood f.
- decreased cerebral blood f.
- diastolic zero f.
- Doppler study of blood f.
- f. effect artifact
- effective pulmonary blood f. (EPBF)
- effective renal plasma f. (ERFP, ERPF)
- electron f.
- expiratory f.
- fast Fourier f. (FFF)
- fluid f.
- flush f.
- forward f.
- Ganz formula for coronary sinus f.
- global intracranial blood f.
- great cardiac vein f. (GCVF)
- hepatofugal f.
- hepatopetal f.
- high-velocity f.
- hyperemic f.
- f. imaging
- inspiratory f.
- intercoronary collateral f.
- internal carotid systolic peak f. (ICSPF)
- intrarenal arterial f.
- intrasac f.
- jet f.
- laminar f.
- left-to-right f.
- local bone blood f.
- low-velocity f.
- lung-volume loop f.
- maintenance of f.
- f. mapping technique
- maximum midexpiratory f. (MMEF)
- microcirculatory blood f.
- midexpiratory tidal f.
- mitral valve f.
- mixed petal-fugal f.
- f. mode ultrafast computed tomography
- myocardial blood f. (MBF)
- peak expiratory f. (PEF)
- peak flush f.
- peak velocity of blood f.
- peripheral blood f.
- petal-fugal f.
- f. phenomenon
- physiologic shunt f.

plug f.
Poiseuille f.
portal f.
f. portion of bone scan
preferential f.
protodiastolic reversal of blood f.
pulmonary blood f. (PBF)
pulmonic output f.
pulmonic versus systemic f.
f. quantification
f. rate
real-time phase-contrast f.
real-time quantitative f.
f. redistribution
regional cerebral blood f. (rCBF)
regional myocardial blood f.
regurgitant pandiastolic f.
regurgitant systolic f.
relative cerebral blood f.
relative regional blood f. (rrBF)
relative shunt f.
resistance blood f.
f. respiratory artifact obliteration
   with directed orthogonal pulses
   (FRODO)
resting regional myocardial blood f.
restoration of f.
retrograde systolic f.
reversed vertebral blood f.
F. Rider microcatheter
sluggish f.
stasis of blood f.
straight-line f.
f. study
supratentorial cerebral blood f.
systemic blood f. (SBF)
systemic output f.
through-plane f.
time-averaged f.
tissue f.
to-and-fro f.
total cerebral blood f. (TCBF)
f. tract
transmitral f.
tricuspid valve f.
turbulent blood f.
turbulent intraluminal f.
unequal pulmonary blood f.
uterine blood volume f.
f. velocity
f. velocity profile
f. velocity signal

f. velocity waveform
f. void
f. void effect
f. volume
zero net f.
flow-compensated
   f.-c. gradient-echo sequence
   f.-c. image
flow-compromising lesion
flow-controlled valve
flow-dependent obstruction
flow-directed approach
flow-encoding gradient
flow-function mismatch
flow-induced artifact
flowing
   f. anterior vertebra ossification
   f. spin
FloWire
   F. Doppler ultrasound
   F. ultrasound device
flow-limited expiration
flow-limiting
   f.-l. lesion
   f.-l. stenosis
flowmeter
   Doppler f.
   Gould electromagnetic f.
   Parks bidirectional Doppler f.
   pulsed Doppler f.
flowmetry
   blood f.
   Doppler f.
   laser Doppler f. (LDF)
   Narcomatic f.
   Parks 800 bidirectional Doppler f.
   Statham electromagnetic f.
flow-on gradient-echo image
flow-related
   f.-r. artifact
   f.-r. enhancement
   f.-r. enhancement effect
   f.-r. phase error
   f.-r. phase shift
flow-sensitive
   f.-s. alternating inversion recovery
      (FAIR)
   f.-s. MR imaging
flow-time curve
flow-volume loop
fluctuant mass

F

NOTES

fluctuation
>Poisson noise f.

fluence
>energy f.
>photon f.
>f. profile

fluffy
>f. and amorphous calcification
>f. infiltrate
>f. margin
>f. periosteal reaction
>f. pulmonary nodule
>f. rarefaction

fluid
>abdominal collection of f.
>f. accumulation
>amnionic f. (AF)
>anechoic f.
>articular f.
>ascitic f.
>bloodless f.
>bursal f.
>cavitary f.
>cerebrospinal f. (CSF)
>f. collection
>cystic f.
>dammed-up cerebrospinal f.
>f. density
>edema f.
>encapsulated f.
>endometrial canal f.
>f. expansion
>extracellular f.
>f. extravasation
>extravascular f.
>f. flow
>free abdominal f.
>free cul-de-sac f.
>free peritoneal f.
>high-signal intratendinous collection of f.
>increased interstitial f.
>f. intake
>f. interface
>interstitial f.
>intestinal f.
>intraperitoneal f.
>joint f.
>f. level
>loculated pleural f.
>f. overload
>pelvic f.
>pericardial f.
>pericerebral f.
>pericholecystic f.
>pericolonic f.
>periesophageal f.
>perigraft f.
>peritoneal cavity f.

>pleural f.
>prostatic f.
>f. resorption
>retained fetal lung f.
>f. retention
>f. sequestration
>serohemorrhagic f.
>serosanguineous f.
>f. signal
>silicone f.
>f. space
>spinal f.
>subgaleal cerebrospinal f.
>subphrenic f.
>subpulmonic f.
>synovial f.
>transudation of f.
>transudative pericardial f.
>f. volume
>f. wave

fluid-attenuated
>f.-a. inversion recovery (FLAIR)
>f.-a. inversion recovery-fast low-angle shot

fluid-blood layer

fluid-filled
>f.-f. bronchogram
>f.-f. catheter
>f.-f. cyst
>f.-f. kidney mass
>f.-f. loop of bowel
>f.-f. sac

fluid-flow artifact

fluid-fluid level

fluke
>liver f.
>lung f.
>Oriental lung f.

Fluoratec imaging agent

fluorescein
>f. angiogram
>f. angiography
>f. sodium
>f. uptake

fluorescence
>energy-dispersive x-ray f. (EDXRF)
>f. microscopy
>f. spectroscopy

fluorescence-activated cell sorter (FACScan)

fluorescent
>f. phosphor
>f. ray
>f. scan
>f. screen

Fluorescite injection

fluoride
>barium f.

f. ion-positron emission tomography (F-18-PET)
lithium f. (LiF)
neodymium:yttrium-lithium f. (Nd:YLF)
yttrium lithium f. (YLF)

fluorine (F)
 f. 18 (^{18}F, F-18)
 f. 19 (^{19}F, F-19)
 f. imaging agent

fluorine-18
 f.-18 2-dialkylamino-6-acylmalononitrile substituted naphthalenes (FDDNP)
 f.-18 fluorodeoxyglucose-positron emission tomography

fluorine-19 spectroscopy
2-[fluorine-18]fluoro-2-deoxy-D-glucose (^{18}F-FDG, ^{18}F-FDG-PET)
fluorine-18-labeled (^{18}F-labeled)
Fluor-I-Strip
Fluor-I-Strip-AT
fluorocaptopril
fluorocarbon-based ultrasound contrast agent
fluorochloride
 barium f.
fluorochrome
fluorodeoxyglucose (FDG)
 f. F-18 injection
 f. imaging agent
 positron emission tomography with f. (FDG-PET)
2-fluoro 2-deoxyglucose (FDG)
fluorodeoxyglucose-6-phosphate
fluorodeoxyuridine
fluoro-DOPA
fluoroestradiol (FES)
fluorography
 digital f.
 spot film f.
fluorohalide
 europium-activated barium f.
fluorometer
 96-well scanning f.
fluorometry
 image intensification f.
 2-plane f.
fluoromibolerone
fluoromisonidazole
Fluoroplex

FluoroPlus
 F. angiography
 F. Cardiac digital fluoroscopy
 F. Cardiac digital imaging system
 F. real-time digital imaging system
fluoropropylepidepride
fluoroptic thermometry system
fluoropyrimidine
fluororoentgenography
FluoroScan C-arm fluoroscopy
fluoroscope
 Edison f.
fluoroscopic
 f. assistance
 f. control
 f. gantry
 f. guidance
 f. image
 f. imaging
 f. localization
 f. observation
 f. pushing technique
 radiographic and f. (R&F)
 f. road-mapping technique
 f. triggering
 f. view
fluoroscopy
 airway f.
 biplane f.
 C-arm f.
 chest f.
 computed tomography f. (CTF)
 computerized f.
 digital f.
 digital pulsed f. (DPF)
 electric joint f.
 FluoroPlus Cardiac digital f.
 FluoroScan C-arm f.
 high-resolution f.
 image-amplified f.
 mobile f.
 Orca C-arm f.
 orthogonal C-arm f.
 portable C-arm image intensifier f.
 real-time CT f.
 region of interest f.
 simultaneous f.
 f. time
fluoroscopy-guided
 f.-g. condylar lift-off imaging
 f.-g. subarachnoid phenol block therapy

F

NOTES

fluorosis
> osteophytosis in f.

fluorotamoxifen

Fluoro Tip cannula

FluoroTrak fluoroscopy-based surgical navigation system

fluorotropapride

fluorotyrosine

FluoroVision

flush
> f. angiogram
> f. aortogram imaging
> f. aortography
> cervical f.
> f. flow
> saline solution f.

flush-tank sign

FLUTE
> fat and long T_2 suppressed ultrashort echo time

flutter
> atrial fetal f.

flux, pl. **fluxes**
> electron f.
> improved photon f.
> magnetic f.
> photon f.

fluxionary hyperemia

flying
> f. focal spot
> f. spot excimer laser
> f. spot excimer laser system

fly-through
> f.-t. viewing
> virtual f.-t.

FM
> fetal movement

Fm
> fermium

^{255}Fm
> fermium 255

FMAP
> feeding mean arterial pressure

FMH
> first metatarsal head

F-misonidazole

fMR
> functional magnetic resonance
> fMR tube

fMRA
> functional magnetic resonance angiography

fMRI
> functional magnetic resonance imaging
> cognitive fMRI
> integrated fMRI
> fMRI signal change
> VNS-synchronized BOLD fMRI

FMS
> fatty meal sonogram

FNH
> focal nodular hyperplasia
> follicular nodular hyperplasia

FNTC
> fine-needle transhepatic cholangiogram

foam
> f. cushion
> f. embolus
> minimally attenuating medical-grade f.
> f. vacuum pillow

foam-padded Velcro restraint

foamy esophagus

FOB
> fiberoptic bronchoscopy

focal
> f. alimentary tract calcification
> f. alveolar infiltrate
> f. area of hemorrhage
> f. area of hypometabolism
> f. articular cartilage lesion
> f. asymmetric density
> f. asymmetry
> f. atrophy
> f. attenuation
> f. bacterial nephritis
> f. biliary cirrhosis
> f. bone sclerosis
> f. caliectasis
> f. cartilage erosion
> f. cecal apical thickening
> f. cerebellar dysplasia
> f. cerebral ischemia
> f. cold liver lesion
> f. colitis
> f. cortical dysplasia
> f. cortical hyperplasia
> f. damage
> f. decreased radiotracer uptake
> f. deficit
> f. degenerative change
> f. and diffuse lung texture analysis
> f. disc herniation
> f. distortion
> f. eccentric stenosis
> f. edema
> f. endocardial hemorrhage
> f. esophageal narrowing
> f. fat necrosis
> f. fatty infiltration of liver
> f. fibrocartilaginous dysplasia of tibia
> f. fibrosis
> f. film distance (FFD)
> f. gallbladder wall thickening
> f. gigantism
> f. hemispheric lesion

f. hepatic necrosis
f. high-intensity zone
f. hot liver lesion
f. hydronephrosis
f. hyperinflation
f. indentation
f. inflammation
f. interstitial infiltrate
f. intimal thickening
f. ischemic lesion
f. lateralizing finding
f. length
f. limb abnormality
f. liver hot spot
f. liver scintigraphic defect
f. lobular carcinoma
f. lung disease
f. malformation
f. mass
f. metabolic abnormality
f. myometrial contraction
f. neurologic sign
f. nodular enhancement
f. nodular hyperplasia (FNH)
f. nuclear herniation
f. organizing pneumonia
f. osseous offset
f. pancreatitis
f. parenchymal brain lesion
f. parenchymal cryptococcoma
f. pattern
f. perihepatitis
f. perivascular infiltrate
f. plane tomography
f. plaquelike defect
f. pleural plaque
f. pool
f. pooling of tracer
f. pulmonary hemorrhage
f. pulmonary uptake
f. pyloric hypertrophy
f. renal hypertrophy
f. small-bowel disease
f. splenic lesion
f. spot (FS)
f. spot blur
f. spot-to-film angle
f. spot-to-object distance
f. spot tracking
f. subluxation of vertebrae
f. tumor
f. ulcer

f. wall motion abnormality
f. white matter signal abnormality
f. zone (FZ)
focal-dust emphysema
focally
f. decreased renal neoplasm
f. dilated duct
f. increased renal echogenicity
focus, pl. foci
Assmann f.
atrial f.
basal ganglia echogenic f.
bright cystic f.
brightly echogenic f.
f. of calcification
f. detection
discrete hyperintense f.
echogenic f.
ectopic f.
epileptic f.
epileptogenic f.
firing of ectopic atrial f.
Ghon f.
hemorrhagic f.
hyperechoic f.
hypermetabolic activity f.
inflammatory f.
junctional f.
linear f.
mesial frontal f.
metastatic f.
midline parasagittal f.
multifocal residual f.
multiple foci
multizone transmit-receive f.
nodular hyperintense f.
f. object distance (FOD)
occipital f.
punctate hyperintense f.
radiolucent f.
residual f.
satellite cartilaginous f.
Simon f.
stationary f.
subependymal/subpial f.
f. of tumor
focused
f. abdominal sonography for
trauma (FAST)
f. appendix computed tomography
(FACT)
f. grid

NOTES

focused (*continued*)
    f. nuclear magnetic resonance
    f. segmented ultrasound machine
    f. ultrasound
focusing
    f. collimator
    dynamic f.
    zone f.
focus-skin distance (FSD)
FOD
    focus object distance
fog
    f. artifact
    base f.
    film f.
Fogarty
    F. Adherent Clot catheter
    F. balloon embolectomy catheter
    Edwards F.
    F. maneuver
    F. Thru-Lumen catheter
fogging phenomenon
foil
    scattering f.
Foix-Alajouanine syndrome
Foix-Chavany-Marie syndrome
fold
    abnormal esophageal f.
    abnormal small bowel f.
    accordion f.
    adipose f.
    alar f.
    amnionic f.
    aryepiglottic f.
    blunted mucosal f.
    caval f.
    cecal f.
    cholecystoduodenocolic f.
    circular f.
    costocolic f.
    crescentic submucosal f.
    distorted mucosal f.
    Douglas f.
    duodenojejunal f.
    duodenomesocolic f.
    dural f.
    effaced mucosal f.
    epigastric f.
    epiglottic f.
    esophageal f.
    falciform f.
    flattened duodenal f.
    fragmented mucosal f.
    gastric f.
    gastropancreatic f.
    genital f.
    giant gastric f.
    glossoepiglottic f.
    glossopalatine f.

gluteal f.
Guérin f.
haustral f.
Hensing f.
hepatopancreatic f.
hidebound small bowel f.
ileocecal f.
ileocolic f.
inferior transverse rectal f.
inframammary f.
inguinal f.
irregular mucosal f.
Kerckring f.
Kohlrausch f.
lateral umbilical f.
longitudinal esophageal f.
medical umbilical f.
mucosal f.
Nélaton f.
palatopharyngeal f.
paraduodenal f.
f. pattern
pericardial f.
peritoneal f.
pleuroperitoneal f.
prepyloric f.
rectal f.
rectouterine f.
rugal f.
sacrogenital f.
semilunar f.
sentinel f.
sickle-shaped f.
sigmoid f.
skin f.
smooth thickened mucosal f.
spiral f.
stack-of-coins mucosal f.
submucosal circular f.
superior duodenal f.
superior transverse rectal f.
tethered small bowel f.
thickened duodenal f.
thickened esophageal f.
thickened gastric f.
thickened nodular irregular small
  bowel f.
thickened stomach f.
thickened straight small bowel f.
transverse esophageal f.
uteric f.
Vater f.
ventriculoinfundibular f.
vestigial f.
folded
    f. fundus of gallbladder
    f. lung
    f. step ramp
folding potential analysis

foldover
>f. artifact
>image f.

folia
>cerebellar f.
>disorganized f.
>shrunken f.

folial pattern
folium vermis
Folius muscle
follicle
>aggregated lymphatic f.
>anovular ovarian f.
>ascendant f.
>atretic ovarian f.
>dominant f.
>gastric lymphatic f.
>geographic f.
>graafian f.
>intestinal f.
>inverse f.
>luteinized unruptured f.
>lymphoid f.
>f. lysis
>malpighian f.
>nabothian f.
>primordial f.
>ruptured f.
>thyroid f.
>unruptured f.

follicular
>f. bronchiectasis
>f. bronchiolitis
>f. bronchitis
>f. center-cell lymphoma
>f. gastritis
>f. involution
>f. mixed small cleaved lymphoma
>f. nodular hyperplasia (FNH)
>f. ovarian cyst
>f. pattern
>f. phase
>f. predominantly large cell lymphoma
>f. predominantly small cell lymphoma
>f. salpingitis
>f. thyroid adenoma
>f. thyroid carcinoma

folliculare
>oophoroma f.

follicularis
>enteritis f.

follow-through
>barium meal and f.-t. (BaFT)
>small-bowel f.-t. (SBFT)
>upper GI with small bowel f.-t.
>f.-t. view

follow-up duplex Doppler sonography
fomes, pl. **fomites**
FONAR-360 MRI scanner
FONAR Standing Ovation MRI system
Fong disease
Fontana canal
fontanelle, fontanel
>anterior f.
>anterolateral f.
>bregmatic f.
>bulging f.
>closed f.
>cranial f.
>frontal f.
>fused f.
>Gerdy f.
>mastoid f.
>occipital f.
>open f.
>overriding sutures of f.
>posterior f.
>posterolateral f.
>sagittal f.
>sphenoid f.
>tense f.
>triangular f.

Fontan operation
food
>f. bolus obstruction
>cholecystokinetic f.
>retention of f.

foot, pl. **feet**
>abnormal position of f.
>arch of f.
>f. architecture
>ball of f.
>calcaneocavus f.
>Charcot f.
>f. deformity
>digital artery of f.
>drop f.
>f. dysplasia
>flail f.
>flattened longitudinal arch of f.
>f. fracture

NOTES

F

foot *(continued)*
    Friedreich f.
    hollow f.
    large-vessel disease of diabetic f.
    lateral spring ligament of f.
    Madura f.
    march f.
    phalanges of f.
    planovalgus f.
    f. plate
    f. revascularization
    rocker-bottom f.
    valgus f.
    varus f.
foot-ankle complex
football
    f. finger
    f. player shoulder
    f. sign
footling presentation
footplate
    intraluminal polymeric f.
footprint analysis
foot-progression angle (FPA)
foramen, pl. **foramina**
    alveolar f.
    anterior condyloid f.
    anterior palatine f.
    anterior sacral f.
    aortic f.
    apical f.
    arachnoidal f.
    base of skull f.
    Bichat f.
    blind f.
    Bochdalek f.
    Botallo f.
    brain mass in jugular f.
    carotid f.
    cecal f.
    cervical neural f.
    conjugate f.
    costotransverse f.
    cranial f.
    Duverney f.
    emissary sphenoidal f.
    enlarged vertebral f.
    enlargement of vertebral f.
    epiploic f.
    ethmoidal f.
    external acoustic f.
    Ferrein f.
    Froesch f.
    frontal f.
    greater palatine f.
    greater sciatic f.
    great sacrosciatic f.
    Huschke f.
    Hyrtl f.

    intertransverse f.
    interventricular f.
    intervertebral f.
    jugular f.
    f. lacerum
    lesser sciatic f.
    f. of Luschka
    Magendie f.
    f. magnum
    f. magnum decompression
    f. magnum herniation
    mandibular f.
    mastoid f.
    f. of Monro
    Morgagni f.
    neural f.
    nutrient f.
    obturator f.
    optic f.
    f. ovale
    f. ovale flap
    ovale skull base of f.
    f. ovale valve
    palatine f.
    parietal f.
    petrosal f.
    restrictive bulboventricular f.
    Retzius f.
    f. rotundum
    sacral f.
    sacrosciatic f.
    skull-base f.
    sphenopalatine f.
    f. spinosum
    spinous f.
    Stensen f.
    stylomastoid f.
    sublabral f.
    superior maxillary f.
    supraorbital f.
    thebesian f.
    f. transversarium
    f. venosum
    vertebral f.
    f. of Vesalius
    Weitbrecht f.
    f. of Winslow
    zygomaticofacial f.
foraminal
    f. encroachment
    f. node
    f. space
    f. stenosis
force
    chronic outward f.
    coulomb f.
    electromotive f. (emf)
    magnetic lines of f.
    nuclear f.

pascals of f.
radial resistive f.
reserve f.
rotational f.
shearing f.
stroke f.
tensile f.
torsion impaction f.
transverse plane f.

forced
f. expiratory volume
f. flexion injury
force-frequency relation
forceful parasternal motion
force-length relation
force-velocity relation
forearm
f. amputation
f. fracture
forebrain
forefoot
f. abduction deformity
f. angulation
narrowing of f.
foregut
bronchopulmonary f.
f. cyst
f. duplication
foreign
f. body (FB)
f. body embolus
f. body in esophagus
f. body granuloma
f. body upper airway obstruction
f. debris
f. material artifact
Forel
H field of F.
foreshortened image data set
foreshortening
anular f.
Forestier disease
forking
aqueductal f.
f. of sylvian aqueduct
form
ring-shaped f.
Formad kidney
format
cylindrical f.
2D f.
3D f.

DICOM f.
DICOM-3 compatible digital
computer f.
hemodynamic f.
slice f.
tag image file f. (TIFF)
formation
abscess f.
batwing f.
beaklike osteophyte f.
bone f.
bony callus f.
brainstem reticular f.
bulla f.
bunion f.
callosal f.
callus f.
cellule f.
Chiari f.
cloacal f.
degenerative microcystic f.
eddy f.
enchondral bone f.
endogenous callus f.
excessive callus f.
exuberant atheroma f.
fistula f.
geode f.
glomeruloid f.
Gothic arch f.
hematoma f.
heterotopic bone f.
hippocampal f. (HF)
honeycomb f.
hooklike osteophyte f.
image f.
F. Internationale en Epidémiologie
et Statistique de Terrains
Approfondies (FIESTA)
intracavitary clot f.
lateral reticular f.
marginal osteophyte f.
mesencephalic reticular f.
microcystic f.
midbrain reticular f. (MRF)
mural thrombus f.
mycetoma f.
myelin ball f.
neointima f.
new bone f.
nipplelike osteophyte f.
osteoid f.

F

NOTES

formation *(continued)*
    osteophyte f.
    palisade f.
    pannus f.
    paramedian pontine reticular f.
    (PPRF)
    periosteal new bone f.
    pontine reticular f.
    pseudoaneurysm f.
    pseudogland f.
    pseudointimal f.
    pseudopod f.
    reticular f. (RF, rf)
    reticular activating f.
    ruffled border f.
    saccular f.
    scar f.
    semilunar bone f.
    sparsity of bone f.
    spur f.
    thrombin f.
    thrombus f.
    tophus f.
    vesical stone f.
formatter
former
    low-risk single-stone f.
formic aldehyde
formula, pl. **formulas, formulae**
    autotransformer f.
    bayesian f.
    Boyd f.
    cigarroa f.
    configurational f.
    fan-beam f.
    Poisson-Pearson f.
    projection f.
    rapid dissolution f.
Forney syndrome
fornicatus
    gyrus isthmus f.
forniceal rupture
fornicis
    corpora f.
fornix, pl. **fornices**
    f. cerebri
    vaginal f.
forward
    f. flow
    f. heart failure
    f. positioning of head
    f. stroke volume (FSV)
    f. subluxation
    f. transport
    f. velocity
forward-angle light scattering
fossa, pl. **fossae**
    acetabular f.
    adipose f.

amygdaloid f.
anconal f.
antecubital f.
anterior recess of ischiorectal f.
articular f.
axillary f.
biloma in gallbladder f.
bony f.
cardiac f.
condylar f.
coronoid f.
cranial f.
crural f.
cubital f.
digastric f.
digital f.
duodenal f.
duodenojejunal f.
epigastric f.
femoral f.
floccular f.
gallbladder f.
glenoid f.
Gruber f.
hepatorenal f.
hyaloid f.
hypoglossal f.
hypophysial f.
iliac f.
infraspinous f.
infrasternal f.
infratemporal f.
intercondylar f.
intercondyloid f.
interpeduncular f.
intratemporal f.
ischiorectal f.
Jobert f.
Landzert f.
malleolar f.
mandibular f.
meningioma of posterior f.
mesentericoparietal f.
middle cranial f.
f. navicularis
olecranon f.
f. ovalis
f. ovalis cordis
ovarian f.
paraduodenal f.
pararectal f.
paravesical f.
patellar f.
pituitary f.
popliteal f.
posterior cranial f.
posterior pituitary f.
pterygoid f.
pterygopalatine f.

radial f.
rectouterine f.
retroappendiceal f.
rhomboid f.
Rosenmüller f.
sphenoidal f.
subscapular f.
supraclavicular f.
Sylvius f.
temporal f.
Treitz f.
uterovesical f.
valve of navicular f.
Waldeyer f.
fourchette
Fourier
F. analysis
F. coefficient
F. 2-dimensional imaging
F. 2-dimensional projection
reconstruction
F. direct transformation imaging
F. discrete transformation
F. domain
F. imaging technique
F. multislice modified KWE direct
imaging
F. optical theory
F. pulsatility index
F. transfer
F. transform (FT)
F. transformation reconstruction
F. transformation zeugmatography
F. transform imaging
F. transform infrared spectroscopy
F. transform NMR spectrometry
F. transform Raman spectroscopy
Fourier-acquired
F.-a. steady state (FAST)
F.-a. steady state technique
Fourier-encoded
Fourmentin thoracic index
fourth
f. branchial arch
f. branchial cleft pouch
f. compartment
f. cranial nerve
f. intercostal space
f. mogul
f. parallel pelvic plane
f. turbinated bone
f. ventricle (V4)

f. ventricle diverticulum
f. ventricle tumor
fourth mogul
FOV
field of view
FOV imaging
fovea
f. capitis
f. centralis
f. inferior
foveal fat pad
foveated chest
foveola
gastric f.
Fowler position
FP
frontopolar
FP artery
FPA
foot-progression angle
F-18-PET
fluoride ion-positron emission
tomography
FPI
femoral pulsatility index
FPRNA
first-pass radionuclide angiography
FR
flattening ratio
frequency encode
fractal
f. analysis
f. dimension (FD)
fractal-based method
fraction
absorbed f.
active emptying f.
area-length method for ejection f.
blood flow extraction f.
blunted ejection f.
branching f.
cardiac scintigraphy ejection f.
computed ejection f.
depressed ejection f.
digital ejection f.
Dodge method for ejection f.
drug f.
ejection f. (EF)
filtration f. (FF)
gallbladder ejection f.
global ejection f.
globally depressed ejection f.

NOTES

F

fraction *(continued)*
 interval ejection f.
 Kennedy method for calculating
  ejection f.
 left atrial active-emptying f.
 left ventricular ejection f. (LVEF)
 Maddahi method of calculating
  right ventricular ejection f.
 MB f.
 myofibril volume f.
 one-third ejection f.
 oxygen extraction f. (OEF)
 packing f.
 penetration f.
 photopeak f.
 radionuclide ejection f.
 regional ejection f.
 regional oxygen extraction f.
  (rOEF)
 regurgitant f.
 resting left ventricular ejection f.
 right ventricular ejection f. (RVEF)
 scatter f.
 shortening f.
 shunt f.
 S-phase f.
 systolic ejection f.
 Teichholz ejection f.
 thermodilution ejection f.
 thickening f.
 unattached f.
 ventricular ejection f.
 well-preserved ejection f.

fractional
 f. anisotropy (FA)
 f. area
 f. encephalography
 f. moving blood volume
 f. moving blood volume estimation
 f. myocardial shortening
 f. pneumoencephalography
 f. shortening (FS)
 f. shortening of left ventricle
 f. vascular volume
 f. volumetric analysis

fractionated
 f. dose
 f. dose-survival curve
 f. external beam irradiation
 f. external beam radiation therapy
 f. radiation
 f. stereotactic radiation therapy
 f. stereotactic radiotherapy (FSR)

fractionation
 accelerated f.
 fast f.
 quasiaccelerated f.

 f. of radiation dose
 S-phase f.

fracture (fx) *(See* fracture-dislocation)
 abduction f.
 abduction-external rotation f.
 acetabular posterior wall f.
 acetabular rim f.
 acute avulsion f.
 acute on chronic f.
 adduction f.
 adult-type III TIE f.
 agenetic f.
 Aitken classification of
  epiphysial f.
 alveolar bone f.
 anatomic f.
 Anderson-Hutchins tibial f.
 angulated f.
 ankle mortise f.
 anterior column f.
 anteroinferior corner f.
 anterolateral compression f.
 anular f.
 AO classification of ankle f.
 apophysial f.
 arch f.
 articular mass separation f.
 articular pillar f.
 artificial f.
 Ashhurst-Bromer classification of
  ankle f.
 f. of astragalus
 Atkin epiphysial f.
 atlas f.
 atrophic f.
 avulsion chip f.
 avulsion stress f.
 axial compression f.
 axial load 3-part, 2-plane f.
 axial load teardrop f.
 axis f.
 backfire f.
 banana f.
 Bankart f.
 Barton f.
 Barton-Smith f.
 basal neck f.
 basal skull f.
 baseball finger f.
 basicervical f.
 basilar femoral neck f.
 basilar skull f.
 bayonet f.
 beak f.
 bedroom f.
 bending f.
 Bennett comminuted f.
 bicondylar T-shaped f.
 bicondylar Y-shaped f.

bicycle spoke f.
bimalleolar ankle f.
bipartite f.
f. blister
blow-in f.
blowout f.
bone f.
boot-top f.
Bosworth f.
both-bone f.
both-column f.
bowing f.
boxer's f.
Boyd type II f.
f. bracing
bronchial f.
bucket-handle pattern of f.
bucket-handle pelvic f.
buckle f.
bumper f.
bunk-bed f.
Burkhalter-Reyes method of
 phalangeal f.
burst f.
bursting f.
butterfly f.
buttonhole f.
calcaneal avulsion f.
calcaneal displaced f.
calcaneal stress f.
f. callus
f. callus loading
calvarial f.
capitate f.
capitellar f.
capitulum radiale humeri f.
carpal bone stress f.
carpal navicular f.
carpal scaphoid bone f.
carpometacarpal joint f.
cartwheel f.
Cedell f.
cemental f.
central f.
cephalomedullary nail f.
cerebral palsy pathological f.
cervical spine f.
cervicotrochanteric f.
Chance spinal f.
Chaput f.
Charcot f.
chauffeur's f.

chevron f.
childhood f.
chip f.
chisel f.
chondral f.
Chopart f.
circumferential f.
f. classification
clavicular birth f.
clay shoveler's f.
cleavage f.
f. in close apposition
closed f.
closed-break f.
coccyx f.
Colles f.
collicular f.
combined flexion-distraction injury
 and burst f.
combined radial-ulnar-humeral f.
comminuted bursting f.
comminuted intraarticular f.
comminuted teardrop f.
complete f.
complex simple f.
complicated f.
composite f.
compound comminuted f.
compound complex f.
compound skull f.
compression f.
condylar split f.
congenital f.
Conrad-Bugg trapping of soft
 tissue in ankle f.
contrecoup f.
coracoid f.
corner f.
coronoid process f.
cortical f.
Cotton ankle f.
crack f.
craniofacial dysjunction f.
crush f.
crushed eggshell f.
cuboid f.
cuneiform f.
dancer's f.
Danis-Weber f.
Darrach-Hughston-Milch f.
dashboard f.
decompression of f.

F

NOTES

fracture *(continued)*
 f. deformity
 Denis classification of spinal f.
 dens f.
 dentate f.
 depressed skull f.
 depression-type intraarticular f.
 de Quervain f.
 derby hat f.
 Desault f.
 f. deviation
 diacondylar f.
 diametric pelvic f.
 diaphysial f.
 f. diastasis
 diastatic f.
 dicondylar f.
 die-punch f.
 direct f.
 dishpan f.
 f. dislocation
 displaced f.
 distal femoral epiphysial f.
 distal humoral f.
 distal radial f.
 distraction of f.
 dome f.
 dorsal rim distal radial f.
 dorsal wing f.
 double f.
 Dupuytren f.
 Duverney f.
 dye punch f.
 dyscrasic f.
 El-Ahwany classification of humeral
  supracondylar f.
 elbow f.
 elementary f.
 Ellis technique for Barton f.
 f. en coin
 f. en rave
 epicondylar f.
 epiphysial plate f.
 epiphysial slip f.
 epiphysial tibial f.
 Essex-Lopresti joint depression f.
 explosion f.
 extension teardrop f. (ETF)
 extraarticular f.
 extracapsular f.
 extraoctave f.
 facial f.
 fatigue f.
 femoral intertrochanteric f.
 femoral neck f.
 femoral shaft f.
 femoral supracondylar f.
 fender f.
 fetal f.

 fibular f.
 fighter's f.
 finger f.
 fishmouth f.
 fissure f.
 flake f.
 flexion-burst f.
 flexion-compression f.
 flexion-distraction f.
 flexion teardrop f.
 floating arch f.
 foot f.
 forearm f.
 f. fragment
 f. fragment separation
 f. frame
 Freiberg f.
 frontal f.
 Frykman classification of hand f.
 Frykman radial f.
 fulcrum f.
 Gaenslen f.
 Galeazzi f.
 f. gap
 Gartland classification of humeral
  supracondylar f.
 glenoid rim f.
 Gosselin f.
 greater trochanteric femoral f.
 greater tuberosity f.
 greenstick f.
 grenade thrower's f.
 gross f.
 growth plate f.
 Guérin f.
 gunshot f.
 Gustilo-Anderson open clavicular f.
 gutter f.
 hairline f.
 hamate tail f.
 hand f.
 hangman's f.
 Hawkins classification of talar f.
 head-splitting humeral f.
 healing f.
 heat f.
 hemicondylar f.
 hemitransverse f.
 Henderson f.
 Herbert scaphoid bone f.
 Hermodsson f.
 hickory-stick f.
 Hill-Sachs posterolateral
  compression f.
 hip f.
 hockey-stick f.
 Hoffa f.
 Holstein-Lewis f.
 hook of hamate f.

hoop stress f.
horizontal maxillary f.
humeral condylar f.
humeral head-splitting f.
humeral physial f.
humeral supracondylar f.
Hutchinson f.
hyperextension teardrop f.
hyperflexion teardrop f.
ice skater's f.
idiopathic f.
ileofemoral wing f.
impacted subcapital f.
impacted valgus f.
implant f.
impression f.
incomplete f.
indented f.
indirect f.
inflammatory f.
infraction f.
insufficiency f.
intercondylar femoral f.
intercondylar humeral f.
intercondylar tibial f.
internally fixed f.
interperiosteal f.
intertrochanteric 4-part f.
intraarticular calcaneal f.
intraarticular proximal tibial f.
intracapsular femoral neck f.
intraoperative f.
intraperiosteal f.
intrauterine f.
inverted-Y f.
ipsilateral femoral neck f.
ipsilateral femoral shaft f.
irreducible f.
ischioacetabular f.
isolated hook f.
Jefferson burst f.
Jefferson cervical f.
Jeffery classification of radial f.
joint depression f.
Jones classification of diaphysial f.
juvenile Tillaux f.
juxtaarticular f.
juxtacortical f.
Kapandji radical f.
Key-Conwell classification of
  pelvic f.

Kilfoyle classification of
  condylar f.
knee f.
Kocher f.
labral and anterior inferior glenoid
  rim f.
LaGrange classification of humeral
  supracondylar f.
laryngeal f.
lateral column calcaneal f.
lateral condylar humeral f.
laterally displaced f.
lateral malleolar f.
lateral tibial plateau f.
lateral wedge f.
Laugier f.
lead pipe f.
Le Fort fibular f.
Le Fort I, II, and III f.
Le Fort mandibular f.
Le Fort-Wagstaffe f.
lesser trochanteric f.
f. line
linear skull f.
f. line of consolidation
Lisfranc f.
local compression f.
local decompression f.
long bone f.
longitudinal tibial fatigue f.
long oblique f.
loose f.
lorry driver's f.
low-energy f.
low-T humerus f.
lumbar spine f.
lunate f.
Maisonneuve fibular f.
malar f.
Malgaigne pelvic f.
malignant vertebral compression f.
malleolar f.
mallet f.
malunited f.
mandibular f.
march f.
marginal f.
Marmor-Lynn f.
Mathews classification of
  olecranon f.
maxillary f.
maxillofacial f.

F

NOTES

fracture *(continued)*

medial column calcaneal f.
medial epicondyle f.
medial malleolar f.
metacarpal f.
metaphysial f.
metatarsal f.
midfacial f.
midfoot f.
midshaft f.
midwaist scaphoid f.
Milch classification of humeral f.
milkman's f.
minimally displaced f.
Moberg-Gedda f.
molar tooth f.
monomalleolar f.
Monteggia f.
Montercaux f.
Moore f.
Mouchet f.
multangular ridge f.
multipartite f.
multiple f.'s
multiray f.
nasal f.
nasomaxillary f.
nasoorbital f.
navicular body f.
navicular hand f.
naviculocapitate f.
f. of necessity
neck f.
Neer classification of shoulder f.
Neer-Horowitz classification of
  humeral f.
neoplastic f.
neural arch f.
neurogenic f.
neuropathic f.
neurotrophic f.
Newman classification of radial
  neck and head f.
nightstick f.
nonarticular radial head f.
noncontiguous f.
nondisplaced f.
nonphysial f.
nonrotational burst f.
f. nonunion
nonunited f.
nutcracker f.
oblique spiral f.
O'Brien classification of radial f.
obturator avulsion f.
occipital condyle f.
occult osseous f.
odontoid condyle f.

Ogden classification of
  epiphysial f.
olecranon tip f.
open f.
open-book f.
open-break f.
orbital blowout f.
orbital floor f.
osteochondral slice f.
osteoporotic compression f.
overlapping f.
Pais f.
panfacial f.
Papavasiliou classification of
  olecranon f.
paratrooper's f.
parry f.
pars interarticularis f.
1-part f.
2-part f.
3-part f.
4-part f.
patellar sleeve f.
pathologic f.
pedicle f.
pelvic insufficiency f.
pelvic rim f.
pelvic ring f.
pelvic straddle f.
penetrating f.
perforating f.
periarticular f.
peripheral f.
periprosthetic f.
peritrochanteric f.
pertrochanteric f.
phalangeal diaphysial f.
physial plate f.
Piedmont f.
pillar f.
pillion f.
pillow f.
pilon ankle f.
ping-pong f.
pisiform f.
plafond f.
plaque f.
plastic bowing f.
plateau tibia f.
pond f.
Posada f.
posterior arch f.
posterior element f.
posterior ring f.
posterior wall f.
postirradiation f.
Pott ankle f.
pressure f.
pronation-abduction f.

pronation-eversion f.
proximal femoral f.
proximal humeral f.
proximal tibial metaphysial f.
pseudo-Jefferson f.
puncture f.
pyramidal f.
Quinby classification of pelvic f.
radial head f.
radial neck f.
radial styloid f.
radiographically occult f.
f. reduction
resecting f.
retrodisplaced f.
reverse Barton f.
reverse Colles f.
reverse Monteggia f.
reverse Segond f.
rib f.
ring f.
ring-disrupting f.
Rolando f.
rotational burst f.
Ruedi-Allgower tibial plafond f.
f. running length of bone
sacral insufficiency f. (SIF)
sacroiliac f.
Sakellarides classification of
  calcaneal f.
Salter-Harris classification of
  epiphysial f. groups 1–5
sandbagging f.
scaphoid hand f.
scottie dog f.
seatbelt f.
secondary f.
segmental bronchus f.
Segond f.
Seinsheimer classification of
  femoral f.
senile subcapital f.
sentinel f.
SER-IV f.
shaft f.
shear f.
Shepherd f.
short oblique f.
sideswipe f.
silver fork f.
f. simple and depressed full-scale
  deflection (FSD)

simple skull f.
f. site
skier's f.
Skillern f.
skull f.
sleeve f.
slice f.
Smith f.
snowboarder f.
sphenoid bone f.
spinal f.
spinous process f.
spiral oblique f.
splintered f.
split compression f.
split-heel f.
splitting f.
spontaneous f.
sprain f.
Springer f.
sprinter's f.
stability of f.
stable f.
stairstep f.
stellate skull f.
stellate undepressed f.
stepoff of f.
Stieda f.
straddle f.
strain f.
stress f.
strut f.
subcapital f.
subchondral f.
subcutaneous f.
subperiosteal f.
subtrochanteric f.
supination-adduction f.
supination-eversion f.
supination, external rotation type
  IV f.
supracondylar femoral f.
supracondylar humeral f.
supracondylar Y-shaped f.
surgical neck f.
T f.
talar avulsion f.
talar dome f.
talar neck f.
talar osteochondral f.
T condylar f.
teacup f.

F

NOTES

fracture *(continued)*
    teardrop burst f.
    teardrop-shaped flexion-
      compression f.
    temporal bone f.
    tension f.
    testis f.
    thalamic f.
    thoracic spine f.
    thoracolumbar burst f.
    thoracolumbar junction f.
    f. threshold
    through-and-through f.
    thrower's f.
    Thurston Holland f.
    tibial bending f.
    tibial condyle f.
    tibial diaphysial f.
    tibial open f.
    tibial pilon f.
    tibial plafond f.
    tibial plateau f.
    tibial shaft f.
    tibial triplane f.
    tibial tuberosity f.
    tibiofibular f.
    Tillaux f.
    Tillaux-Chaput f.
    Tillaux-Kleiger f.
    toddler's f.
    tongue f.
    tongue-type intraarticular f.
    torsion f.
    torus f.
    total condylar depression f.
    trabecular f.
    tracheal f.
    traction f.
    trampoline f.
    transcaphoid f.
    transcapitate f.
    transcervical femoral f.
    transchondral talar f.
    transcondylar f.
    transepiphysial f.
    transhamate f.
    transiliac f.
    transsacral f.
    transscaphoid dislocation f.
    transtriquetral f.
    transverse comminuted f.
    transversely oriented endplate
      compression f.
    transverse maxillary f.
    transverse process f.
    trapezium f.
    traversing the f.
    trimalleolar ankle f.
    triplanar f.

    triplane f.
    tripod f.
    triquetral f.
    trophic f.
    T-shaped f.
    tuft f.
    ulnar f.
    uncinate process f.
    undepressed skull f.
    undisplaced f.
    unicondylar f.
    unilateral f.
    unimalleolar f.
    unstable f.
    ununited f.
    upper thoracic spine f.
    vertebral body f.
    vertebral compression f. (VCF)
    vertebral plana f.
    vertebral wedge compression f.
    vertical shear f.
    volar rim distal radial f.
    Volkmann f.
    V-shaped f.
    Wagstaffe f.
    Walther f.
    Weber C f.
    wedge compression f.
    wedge flexion-compression f.
    western boot in open f.
    willow f.
    Wilson f.
    Y f.
    Y-T f.
    ZMC f.
    f. zone
    zygomaticomaxillary f.
fractured
    f. bronchus
    f. kidney
    f. vertebra
fracture-dislocation
    Chopart f.-d.
    cuneiform f.-d.
    Galeazzi f.-d.
    intermediate cuneiform f.-d.
    Monteggia f.-d.
    pedicolaminar f.-d.
    perilunate f.-d.
    posterior f.-d.
fragilitas ossium
fragility
    acquired f.
fragment
    alignment of fracture f.
    anteroinferior triangular f.
    apoptic nuclear f.
    articular f.
    avulsed fracture f.

bayoneting of fracture f.
bone f.
butterfly fracture f.
calcified free f.
capital f.
chondral f.
cortical f.
f. depression
disc f.
displaced fracture f.
displaced osteochondral f.
extruded disc f.
fracture f.
free disc f.
free-floating cartilaginous f.
iodine-125-labeled f.
jagged bone f.
Klenow f.
loose osteochondral f.
LymphoScan Tc99m-labeled murine
   antibody f.
major fracture f.
malunion of fracture f.
metallic f.
nonunion of fracture f.
osteochondral fracture f.
overriding of fracture f.
retropulsed fracture f.
smear f.
Spengler f.
^{99m}Tc-labeled anti-E-selectin Fab f.
technetium-99m antimyosin Fab f.
torsion of fracture f.
union of fracture f.

fragmentation
   f. of apophysis
   f. of barium
   collagen f.
   electrohydraulic f.
   meniscal f.
   f. myocarditis
   f. therapy
   unilateral f.

fragmented
   f. mucosal fold
   f. pattern

fragmentocytosis

frame
   adduction f.
   adiabatic demagnetization in the
      rotating f. (ADRF)
   Balkan fracture f.

Brown-Roberts-Wells f.
CT/MRI-compatible stereotactic
   head f.
fracture f.
imaging compatible stereotactic
   coordinate f.
ISAH stereotactic immobilization f.
Komai stereotactic head f.
Laitinen stereotactic head f.
Leksell D-shaped stereotactic f.
Leksell-Elekta stereotactic f.
Malcolm-Lynn C-RXF cervical
   retractor f.
peak arterial f.
pelvic fracture f.
radiolucent spine f.
Radionics CRW stereotactic head f.
Reichert-Mundinger-Fischer
   stereotactic f.
robotics-controlled stereotactic f.
stereotactic head f.
stereotactic localization f.
Stryker f.

2-frame gated imaging

frameless
   f. stereotactic digital subtraction
      angiography
   f. stereotactic guidance
   f. stereotaxy

framing
   exact f.

frank
   f. breech presentation
   f. cerebral gumma
   f. cirrhosis
   f. congestive heart failure
   f. disc herniation
   f. dislocation
   f. hemorrhage
   f. lesion
   f. necrosis
   f. pulmonary edema
   f. rupture

Fränkel
   crossbar symptom of F.
   F. spinal cord injury classification
   F. typhus nodule
   F. white line

Frankfort
   F. horizontal plane
   F. line

F

NOTES

Frankfort *(continued)*
    F. mandibular incisor angle
    F. mandibular notch
Franklin changer
Frank-Starling
    F.-S. curve
    F.-S. mechanism
    F.-S. relation
Frank vectorcardiography
Franseen needle
fraternal twin
Fraunhofer zone
frayed
    f. disc
    f. metaphysis
frayed-string appearance
fraying
    chondromalacia with surface f.
Frederick-Miller tube
free
    f. abdominal fluid
    f. air passage
    f. air under diaphragm
    f. band of colon
    f. band of colon band
    f. body
    f. body calcification
    f. breathing
    f. cul-de-sac fluid
    f. disc fragment
    f. electron
    f. fatty acid (FFA)
    f. fibered coil
    f. flap of cartilage
    f. gas bubble
    f. hepatic venography
    f. induction decay signal
    f. induction delay curve
    f. intraperitoneal air
    f. intraperitoneal gas
    f. knee joint
    f. pericardial space
    f. peritoneal air
    f. peritoneal fluid
    f. pleural effusion
    f. precession
    f. precession sequence steady state
    f. radical
    f. reflux
    f. subphrenic gas
FreeDop Doppler monitor
FreeFlo
    F. proximal Nitinol stent
    F. stent-graft
free-floating
    f.-f. cartilaginous fragment
    f.-f. loop of bowel
    f.-f. meniscus
    f.-f. retinaculum

free-fragment disc herniation
freehand
    f. interventional sonography
    f. interventional ultrasound
    f. probe
free-induction decay (FID)
freely movable mass
Freeman calcaneal fracture classification
free-radical dosimetry
freestanding workstation
Freiberg
    F. disease
    F. fracture
    F. infraction
French
    F. tip catheter
    F. T-tube
9-French guiding catheter
8-French guiding catheter
2.1-French microcatheter
1.8-French microcatheter
frenulum of valve
frequency (f)
    f. analysis
    angular f.
    f. component
    disappearance f.
    f. domain
    f. domain image
    f. domain imaging (FDI)
    Doppler shift f.
    f. encode (FE, FR)
    f. encoding
    energy f.
    f. estimation
    extremely low f. (ELF)
    false f.
    halftone f.
    f. intensification
    Larmor f.
    Nyquist f.
    offset f.
    pelvic mass f.
    precessional f.
    pulse repetition f.
    f. range
    raster f.
    resonance f.
    resonant f.
    respiratory f.
    rotational f.
    f. separation
    spatial f.
    f. spectrum
    f. synthesizer
    vibration f.
frequency-encoding gradient
frequency-related peak

frequency-selective
    f.-s. fat saturation
    f.-s. inversion
    f.-s. pulse
Fresnel
    F. zone
    F. zone plate
Freund anomaly
friability
friable
    f. anulus
    f. artery
    f. lesion
    f. mass
    f. mucosa
    f. thickened degenerated intima
    f. tumor
    f. vegetation
    f. wall
Fricke
    F. dosimetry
    F. gel
friction-fit
friction neuritis
Friedländer pneumonia
Friedman
    F. method
    F. position
Friedreich
    F. ataxia
    F. ataxic cardiomyopathy
    F. disease
    F. foot
    F. phenomenon
    F. sign
Fries score for rheumatoid arthritis classification
fringe
    f. field
    moiré f.
    f. of osteophyte
    f. skeleton extraction
    synovial f.
    f. thinning algorithm
FRODO
    flow respiratory artifact obliteration with directed orthogonal pulses
    FRODO technique
Froesch foramen
frogleg
    f. lateral projection
    f. lateral view

    f. position
    f. view of hips
froglike appearance
Frohse
    arcade of F.
    F. ligamentous arcade
Froment sign
frond
    villous f.
frondlike
    f. appearance
    f. filling defect
frondy lesion
frontal
    f. abscess
    f. arteriovenous malformation
    f. artery
    f. biauricular plane
    f. bone
    f. bossing
    f. bossing of Parrot
    f. cephalometric radiograph
    f. cortex
    f. crest
    f. defect
    f. eminence
    f. fontanelle
    f. foramen
    f. fracture
    f. gyrus
    f. horn
    f. horn asymmetry
    f. horn index (FHI)
    f. horn of lateral ventricle
    f. horn Mickey Mouse ear
    f. lobe
    f. lobe contusion
    f. lobe dysfunction
    f. lobe infarct
    f. lobe lesion
    f. lobe sign
    f. lobe tumor
    f. nerve
    f. notch
    f. plane loop
    f. plane vectorcardiography
    f. plate
    f. pole
    f. process
    f. section
    f. sinus
    f. sinus mucocele

F

NOTES

frontal *(continued)*
    f. sulcus
    f. suture
    f. vein
    f. view
frontalis
    apertura sinus f.
    f. sinus
frontier ulcer
frontocentral convexity
frontoethmoidal
    f. encephalocele
    f. giant cell reparative granuloma
    f. mucocele
    f. suture
frontolacrimal suture
frontomalar suture
frontomaxillary suture
frontomental diameter
frontonasal
    f. duct
    f. dysplasia
    f. dysplasia malformation complex
    f. process
    f. suture
frontooccipital diameter
frontoorbital advancement
frontoparallel plane
frontoparietal
    f. arteriovenous malformation
    ascending f. (ASFP)
    f. parasagittal cortex
    f. suture
frontopolar (FP)
    f. artery
    f. point
frontopontine tract
frontosphenoidal
    f. encephalocele
    f. process
frontosphenoid suture
frontotemporal (FT)
    f. atrophy
    f. muscle
    f. tract
frontozygomatic suture
Frostberg sign
frosted liver
frothy colonic mucosa
Frouin
    quadrangulation of F.
frozen
    f. hemithorax
    f. joint
    f. pelvis
    f. shoulder
FRP
    functional refractory period

Frykman
    F. classification of hand fracture
    F. distal radius fracture
      classification
    F. radial fracture
FS
    focal spot
    fractional shortening
    FS burst MR imaging
**FS-069 sterile injectable sonography
    contrast agent**
F-scan
FSCR
    flexible surface-coil-type resonator
FSD
    Fletcher-Suit-Delclos
    focus-skin distance
    fracture simple and depressed full-scale
      deflection
FSE
    fast spin-echo
FSE-T2 with fat suppression
FSPGR
    fast spoiled gradient-recalled echo
    FSPGR technique
FSR
    fractionated stereotactic radiotherapy
FSU
    functional subunit
FSV
    forward stroke volume
FT
    Fourier transform
    frontotemporal
FTA
    femorotibial angle
FTC
    fibulotalocalcaneal
    FTC ligament
FTHA
    ^{18}F-fluoro-6-thia-heptadecanoic acid
Fuchs
    F. adenoma
    F. odontoid view
    F. position
    F. principle
fucose
fucosidosis
FUE
    fever of unknown etiology
fugax
    amaurosis f.
    coxitis f.
Fuji
    F. AC2 storage phosphor computed
      radiology system
    F. FCR9000 computed radiology
      system
    F. QA 771 workstation

Fukuyama
    F. congenital muscular disease
    (FCMD)
    F. congenital muscular dystrophy
    (FCMD)
fulcrum
    f. fracture
    joint f.
fulguration
    nephroscopic f.
full
    f. bladder ultrasound
    f. cervical spine (FCS)
    f. cervical spine series
    f. cervical spine view
    f. column view
    f. lateral position
    f. length view
    f. ring scanner
    f. scan with interpolation
    f. scan with interpolation projection
    f. thickness
    f. three-dimensional mode
    f. width at half maximum
    (FWHM)
full-blown cardiac tamponade
full-body
    f.-b. CT scan
    f.-b. echo-planar system imager
full-column
    f.-c. barium enema
    f.-c. technique
full-energy peak efficiency
Fuller earth pneumoconiosis
full-field
    f.-f. digital mammography
    f.-f. digital mammography system
full-intensity needle
full-line scanning
full-scan
    f.-s. method
    f.-s. projection
full-thickness
    f.-t. button of aortic wall
    f.-t. Carrel button
    f.-t. chondral lesion
    f.-t. cleft
    f.-t. infarct
    f.-t. tear
full-to-empty VAD mode
full-volume loop spirometry

full-wave
    f.-w. rectification
    f.-w. rectifier
full-width
    f.-w. at half-maximum
    f.-w. at half-maximum of
    lorentzian curve
fully automated segmentation algorithm
fulminant
    f. cerebral lymphoma
    f. colitis
    f. fasciitis
    f. hepatic failure (FHF)
    f. hydrocephalus
    f. pulmonary edema
    f. tuberculosis
fulminating ulcerative colitis
function
    abnormal tubular f.
    arterial input f. (AIF)
    atrial-phase volumetric f.
    autocorrelation f.
    brain f.
    bundle f.
    cerebrospinal fluid shunt f.
    commissural f.
    compromised ventricular f.
    contractile f.
    depressed right ventricular
    contractile f.
    edge response f. (ERF)
    excitation f.
    exercise LV f.
    fetal renal f.
    gaussian f.
    global ventricular f.
    gonadal f.
    harmonic f.
    impaired renal f.
    Kaiser-Bessel window f.
    leaflet f.
    left atrial f.
    left ventricular systolic/diastolic f.
    left ventricular systolic pump f.
    line spread f. (LSF)
    midbrain f.
    mitochondrial f.
    modulation transfer f. (MTF)
    myocardial contractile f.
    nasal mucociliary clearance f.
    pharyngoesophageal f.
    point-spread f. (PSF)

NOTES

F

function (*continued*)
    rectosigmoid f.
    regional left ventricular f.
    regional myocardial f.
    reserve cardiac f.
    rest left ventricular f.
    rest right ventricular f.
    right and left atrial phasic volumetric f.
    right ventricular systolic/diastolic f.
    Shepp-Logan filter f.
    sinusoid reference f.
    stress perfusion and rest f.
    swallowing f.
    systolic f.
    time correlation f. (TCF)
    tubular f.
    velocity distribution f. (F(v))
    ventricular contractility f. (VCF)
    volumetric f.
    Zeeman hamiltonian f.

functional
    f. abnormality
    f. aerobic impairment
    f. anatomical mapping
    f. bladder capacity
    f. bowel syndrome
    f. brain imaging
    f. classification of congestive heart failure
    f. correlation
    f. data
    f. diffusion anisotropy
    f. disorder
    f. diverticulum
    f. hyperlordosis
    f. hypertrophy
    f. ileus
    f. imaging
    f. immaturity of bowel
    f. magnetic resonance (fMR)
    f. magnetic resonance angiography (fMRA)
    f. magnetic resonance imaging (fMRI)
    f. map
    f. marrow
    f. MRI
    f. MR tube
    f. neuroimaging
    f. ovarian cyst
    f. paraganglioma
    f. radioiodine scintigraphy
    f. reentry
    f. refractory period (FRP)
    f. residual capacity
    f. scoliosis
    f. sphincter
    f. spin-echo imaging

    f. subunit (FSU)
    f. units of spine
    f. ureteral obstruction
functional imaging
functioning
    f. neoplasm
    f. nodule
    f. pituitary adenoma
FuncTool software
fundal
    f. leiomyoma
    f. placenta
fundamental Doppler mode
fundic-antral junction
fundic metaphysis
fundiform ligament
fundoplication
    Nissen f.
fundus, pl. **fundi**
    f. of aneurysm
    aneurysmal f.
    bald gastric f.
    bladder f.
    gallbladder f.
    gastric f.
    saddle-shaped uterine f.
    stomach f.
    urinary bladder f.
    f. uteri
    uterine f.
    vaginal f.
Funduscein injection
fungal
    f. hypha
    f. infection
    f. meningitis
    f. plaque
    f. pneumonia
fungating tumor
fungoides
    tumeur d'emblée mycosis f.
fungus ball
funic souffle
funicular inguinal hernia
funiculus
    f. cuneatus
    f. dorsalis
    f. gracilis
    f. medullae spinalis
    f. ventralis
funnel
    f. chest
    f. chest deformity
funnellike cardiomegaly
funnel-shaped
    f.-s. cavity
    f.-s. pelvis
FUO
    fever of unknown origin

furosemide imaging agent
furrier's lung
fused
    f. ankle
    f. colliculi
    f. commissure
    f. fontanelle
    f. image technology
    f. kidney
    f. papillary muscle
    f. physis
    f. rib
    f. vertebrae
fusiform
    f. aneurysm
    f. bronchiectasis
    f. defect
    f. dilatation
    f. enlargement of optic nerve
    f. gyrus
    f. high signal intensity
    f. malformation
    f. narrowing of artery
    f. shadow
    f. swelling
    f. syrinx
    f. thickening
    f. widening of duct
fusion
    ankle f.
    anterior cervical f. (ACF)
    anterior spine f. (ASF)
    atlantooccipital f.
    bony f.
    calcaneotibial f.
    carpometacarpal f.
    CAT-MIBI image f.
    cervical interbody f.
    cervical spine f.
    cervicooccipital f.
    chevron f.
    f. of cusp
    f. defect
    diaphysial-epiphysial f.
    extraarticular hip f.
    facet f.
    Hatcher-Smith cervical f.

    image f.
    f. inhibitor (FI)
    interbody f.
    interphalangeal f.
    intersegmental laminar f.
    interspinous process f.
    intraarticular knee f.
    joint f.
    Kellogg-Speed lumbar spinal f.
    metatarsocuneiform joint f.
    metatarsophalangeal joint f.
    multilevel f.
    nuclear f.
    occipitoatlantoaxial f.
    occipitocervical f.
    pantalar f.
    f. plate
    posterior lumbar interbody f.
      (PLIF)
    posterior spine f. (PSF)
    sacroiliac joint f.
    spinal f.
    splenogonadal f.
    2-stage f.
    talar body f.
    talocrural f.
    tibiocalcaneal f.
    tibiotalocalcaneal f.
    transfibular f.
    vertebral f.
FUTE
    fat-suppressed ultrashort echo time
fuzzy
    f. clustering algorithm
    f. echo
    f. logic contrast correction
    f. set theory
F(v)
    velocity distribution function
FWHM
    full width at half maximum
fx
    fracture
FX-wire
    Cragg FX-w.
FZ
    focal zone

NOTES

385

γ (*var. of* gamma)

G
>gauss

GA
>gestational age

Ga
>gallium

^{67}Ga
>gallium 67
>>^{67}Ga bone scan
>>^{67}Ga citrate scintigraphy
>>^{67}Ga examination
>>^{67}Ga excretion
>>^{67}Ga GABA uptake carrier
>>^{67}Ga higher dose
>>^{67}Ga SPECT

Ga-67 uptake
^{68}Ga, Ga-68
>gallium 68

GABA
>gamma-aminobutyric acid

gadobenate dimeglumine (Gd-BOPTA, Gd-BOPTA imaging agent, Gd-BOPTA imaging agent)
gadobenic acid imaging agent
gadobutrol imaging agent
gadodiamide (Gd-DTPA-BMA)
>g. imaging agent

gadofosveset trisodium
gadolinium (Gd)
>g. chelate
>g. complex
>g. diethylenetriamine pentaacetic acid (Gd-DTPA)
>g. diethylenetriamine-penta-acetic acid (Grl-DTPA)
>g. diethylenetriamine pentaacetic acid bismethylamide (Gd-DTPA-BMA)
>g. enhanced imaging group
>g. enhancement
>g. ethoxybenzyl diethylenetriamine pentaacetic acid (Gd-EOB-DTPA)
>g. fast multiplanar spoiled gradient (Gd-FMPSPGR)
>g. Gd 159 hydroxycitrate intraarticular g.
>g. iron
>g. oxide imaging agent
>g. oxyorthosilicate sandwiched g.
>g. scan
>g. sucralfate

>g. tetraazacyclododecanetetraacetic acid (Gd-DOTA)
>g. texaphyrin (Gd-Tex)

gadolinium 153 (^{153}Gd, Gd-153)
gadolinium-based contrast agent
gadolinium-DTPA
gadolinium-enhanced
>g.-e. elliptically reordered three-dimensional MR angiography
>g.-e. MR imaging
>g.-e. subtracted MR angiography
>g.-e. subtracted MR angiography, 3D
>g.-e. T1-weighted axial image
>g.-e. T1-weighted image
>g.-e. T1-weighted MRI image
>g. e. venographic technique

Gadolite oral suspension contrast agent
gadopentetate
>g. contrast agent
>g. dimeglumine (Gd-DTPA)
>g. dimeglumine imaging agent

gadopentetic acid
gadopentolate-polylysine
gadoterate meglumine
gadoterate-enhanced digital subtraction angiography
gadoteridol (Gd-DO3A, Gd-HP-DO3A)
>g. imaging agent

gadoversetamide
>g. contrast agent
>g. imaging agent

gadoxetate
gadoxetic acid
Gaeltec catheter-tip pressure transducer
Gaenslen
>G. fracture
>G. sign

Gaertner (*var. of* Gärtner)
Gaffney joint
GAG
>glycosaminoglycan

gain
>accelerated phase g.
>brightness g.
>color g.
>Doppler g.
>phase g.
>power g.
>quadratic phase g.
>time-compensated g.
>time-varied g. (TVG)

Gaisböck syndrome
galactocele

G

galactogram
    mammary g.
galactography
galactophoritis
galactophorous
    g. canal
    g. duct
galactose-based suspension
galactose contrast medium
galactosyl human serum albumin (GSA)
Galassi arachnoidal cyst classification
galea aponeurotica
galeal extension of tumor
Galeazzi
    G. fracture
    G. fracture-dislocation
    G. sign
Galen
    great cerebral vein of G.
    G. Scan scanner
    G. teleradiology system
    G. vein aneurysm
    G. ventricle
galenic venous malformation
Galileo intravascular radiotherapy
  system
gallbladder
    g. adenoma
    g. agenesis
    g. bed
    bilobed g.
    blunt trauma g.
    body of g.
    g. calculus
    g. carcinoma
    comet-tail artifact g.
    contracted g.
    Courvoisier g.
    dilated g.
    displaced g.
    distended g.
    g. diverticulum
    double g.
    g. duplication
    ectopic g.
    edematous g.
    g. ejection fraction
    g. empyema
    enlarged g.
    fetal g.
    g. filling defect
    fish-scale g.
    floating g.
    folded fundus of g.
    g. fossa
    g. function test
    g. fundus
    gangrene of g.
    g. gravel

    hourglass constriction of g.
    g. hydrops
    g. hypoplasia
    g. ileus
    g. imaging
    g. infundibulum
    g. lift
    mobile g.
    multiseptated g.
    neck of g.
    nonfunctioning g.
    nonvisualization of g.
    pearl necklace g.
    g. perforation
    g. polyp
    porcelain g.
    porcine g.
    g. septation
    g. series (GBS)
    shrunken g.
    g. size
    g. sludge
    small g.
    S-shaped g.
    stasis g.
    g. stone
    strawberry g.
    g. study
    thick-walled g.
    thin-walled g.
    g. torsion
    g. trauma
    g. ultrasound
    g. villus
    g. wall
    g. wall abscess
    wandering g.
gallbladder-gastrointestinal (GB-GI)
    g.-g. series
gallbladder-vena cava line
gall duct
galli
    ala cristae g.
    crista g.
Gallie H-graft
gallium (Ga)
    g. 67 (^{67}Ga)
    g. 68 (^{68}Ga, Ga-68)
    g. bone scintigraphy
    g. imaging agent
    g. lung imaging
    g. lung scintigraphy
    radioactive g.
    g. scan
    g. titrate
    g. tumor scintigraphy
    g. uptake
gallium-67-avid lesion
gallium-67 citrate

gallium-67-labeled leukocyte
gallium-arsenide laser
gallium-avid thymic hyperplasia
gallium-transferrin complex
gallstone
    asymptomatic g.
    cholesterol g.
    dissolution of g.
    g. dissolution therapy
    ectopic intraluminal g.
    faceted g.
    floating g.
    gas-containing g.
    g. ileus
    innocent g.
    intraluminal g.
    laminated g.
    layered g.
    layering of g.'s
    g. migration
    mulberry g.
    opacifying g.
    radiolucent g.
    retained g.
    silent g.
    solitary g.
    symptomatic g.
GALT
    gut-associated lymphoid tissue
galvanometer
gamekeeper's thumb
gamma, γ
    g. aminobutyrate
    g. camera
    g. cascade
    g. emission
    g. emitter
    g. encephalography
    g. factor
    g. film
    g. heating
    g. irradiation
    g. knife radiosurgery
    g. nail
    g. photon
    g. probe
    g. probe radiation detector
    g. radiation
    g. radiography
    g. ray
    g. ray attenuation
    g. ray capture

    g. ray counter
    g. ray level indicator
    g. ray scanner
    g. ray spectrometer
    g. ray spectrum
    g. ray therapy
    g. scan
    g. scanning
    g. signal
    g. spectrometric analysis
    g. tocopherol (gamma-T, γ-T)
    g. transverse colon loop
    g. unit
    g. well counter
gamma-aminobutyric acid (GABA)
gamma-detection probe
gamma-emitting isotope
gammagram
gamma-irradiated plug
GammaPlan software
gamma-ribbon radiation therapy
gamma-T
    gamma tocopherol
Gammex
    G. RBA-5 radiation beam analyzer
    G. RMI DAP meter
    G. RMI scanner
gammography
    cerebral g.
gammopathy
    monoclonal g.
Gamna-Gandy nodule
Gamna nodule
Gandy-Nanta disease
ganglia (*pl. of* ganglion)
gangliocytic paraganglioma
gangliocytoma
    dysplastic cerebellar g.
ganglioglioma
    cystic g.
    infantile g.
    intracerebral g.
gangliolysis
    radiofrequency g.
ganglioma
    intracerebral g.
ganglion, pl. **ganglia**
    aberrant g.
    acousticofacial g.
    Acrel g.
    aorticorenal g.
    auditory g.

G

NOTES

ganglion *(continued)*
    auricular g.
    basal g.
    calcification of basal g.
    cardiac g.
    carotid g.
    celiac g.
    g. cell tumor
    cervical g.
    cervicothoracic g.
    coccygeal g.
    g. cyst
    diffuse g.
    dorsal root g. (DRG)
    gasserian g.
    geniculate g.
    g. impar block
    intraarticular g.
    intraosseous g.
    ipsilateral basal g.
    otic g.
    palmar g.
    paravertebral g.
    periosteal g.
    petrosal g.
    posterior root g.
    prevertebral g.
    pterygopalatine g.
    radiocapitellar joint g.
    g. ridge
    Scarpa g.
    sensory g.
    soft tissue g.
    sphenopalatine g.
    spinal g.
    submandibular g.
    superior cervical g.
    superior mesenteric g.
    sympathetic g.
    trigeminal g.
    uterine cervical g.
    vestibular g.
    Wrisberg cardiac g.
ganglioneuroblastoma (GNB)
ganglioneurofibromatosis
    mucosal g.
ganglioneuroma
    adrenal g.
ganglionic
    g. canal
    g. crest
gangliosidosis
    GM_1/GM_2 g.
gangrene
    bowel g.
    g. of gallbladder
    g. of lung
gangrenous
    g. cholecystitis

    g. emphysema
    g. pneumonia
    g. tissue
Gans
    incisura dextra of G.
Ganser diverticulum
gantry
    g. angulation
    CT scan g.
    fixed g.
    fluoroscopic g.
    g. rotation
    g. rotation time
    g. tilt
gantry-free gamma camera
Gantzer muscle
Ganz formula for coronary sinus flow
gap
    air g.
    artifactual g.
    Bochdalek g.
    g. calculation
    distraction g.
    fracture g.
    intersection g.
    interslice g.
GARD
    glenoid articular rim disruption
    GARD lesion
garden
    G. angle
    G. femoral neck fracture
       classification
    g. spade deformity
Gardner bone syndrome
Gardray dosimeter
garland
    g. sign
    G. triad
    G. triangle
GARP
    globally optimized alternating-phase
    rectangular pulse
Garré
    G. disease
    G. sclerosing osteomyelitis
Garren-Edwards
    G.-E. gastric (GEG)
    G.-E. gastric bubble
Garth view
Gartland classification of humeral
    supracondylar fracture
Gartner
    G. canal
    G. duct
    G. duct cyst
Gärtner, Gaertner
    G. phenomenon
gas, pl. **gases**

abdominal g.
accumulation of g.
aneurysmal wall g.
g. angiocardiography
bile duct g.
biliary tree g.
bowel g.
g. bubble
g. collection
coursing of g.
crescent of g.
g. CT cisternography
g. cupula
g. density line
displacement of bowel g.
g. entrapment
extraluminal g.
free intraperitoneal g.
free subphrenic g.
g. gangrene of uterus
genital tract g.
hyperpolarized ^{129}Xe g.
g. insufflation
intestinal g.
intrahepatic portal vein g.
intramural g.
intrauterine g. (IUG)
g. mediastinography
natural neon g.
noble g.
overlying bowel g.
g. pattern
paucity of bowel g.
portal venous g.
pulmonary g.
radioactive g.
radiopaque xenon g.
scrotal g.
small bowel g.
soft tissue g.
subcutaneous tissue g.
superimposed bowel g.
g. target
g. trapping
urinary tract g.
g. ventilation imaging
g. ventilation study
g. volume
gas-bloat syndrome
gas-containing
g.-c. gallstone
g.-c. stone

gaseous
g. cholecystitis
g. dilatation
g. distention
g. drainage
g. injection
g. mediastinography
g. oxygen artifact
gas-filled detector
gas-fluid level
gasless
g. abdomen
g. laparoscopic system
gas-liquid phase chromatography (GLPC)
gasserian ganglion
Gasser syndrome
gastric
g. adenopapillomatosis
g. air bubble
g. antral erosion
g. antrum
g. artery
g. atony
g. atrophy
g. bypass surgery (GBS)
g. canal
g. capacity
g. cardia
g. channel
g. chloroma
g. content
g. decompression
g. diaphragm
g. dilatation
g. distention
g. diverticulum
g. duplication cyst
g. emphysema
g. emptying (GE)
g. emptying imaging
g. emptying scan
g. fistula
g. fold
g. fold enlargement
g. foveola
g. fundus
Garren-Edwards g. (GEG)
g. groove
g. hamartomatous polyposis
g. hemic calculus
g. hemorrhage

NOTES

G

gastric (*continued*)
   g. hernia
   g. heterotopia
   g. hypersecretion
   g. impression
   g. insufficiency
   g. interposition
   g. intramural-extramucosal lesion
   g. leiomyoma
   g. leiomyosarcoma
   g. lumen
   g. lymphatic follicle
   g. lymph node
   g. lymphoma
   g. metastasis
   g. motor disorder
   g. mucosa (GM)
   g. mucosa imaging
   g. mucosal pattern
   g. narrowing
   g. omentum
   g. outlet obstruction
   g. outline
   g. parietography
   g. partition
   g. pit
   g. plexus
   g. pneumatosis
   g. polyp
   g. pool
   g. pouch
   g. pseudolymphoma
   g. pull-through procedure
   g. pull-up
   g. reflux of bile
   g. remnant
   g. remnant carcinoma
   g. remnant filling defect
   g. residual
   g. rugae
   g. sclerosis
   g. secretion
   g. sling fiber
   g. stump
   g. stump carcinoma
   g. surface
   g. thumbprinting
   g. transit time
   g. transposition
   g. ulcer (GU)
   g. varices
   g. varix
   g. vein
   g. volvulus
   g. wall deformity
   g. wall thickening
   g. window
   g. xanthoma

gastrica
   area g.
gastricae
gastrinoma
   duodenal g.
gastritis
   acute erosive g. (AEG)
   antral g.
   atrophic g.
   bile reflux g.
   chronic g.
   cirrhotic g.
   corrosive g.
   emphysematous g.
   erosive g.
   follicular g.
   giant hypertrophic g.
   hypertrophic g.
   necrotizing g.
   phlegmonous g.
   pseudomembranous radiation g.
   radiation g.
   reflux g.
   zonal g.
gastrocardiac syndrome
gastrocnemial ridge
gastrocnemius
   g. bursa
   g. muscle
   g. tendon
gastrocnemius-semimembranosus bursa
gastrocnemius-soleus
   g.-s. complex
   g.-s. contracture
   g.-s. junction
   g.-s. muscle group
   g.-s. tendon
gastrocolic
   g. fistula
   g. ligament
   g. omentum
gastrocutaneous fistula
gastrodiaphragmatic ligament
gastroduodenal
   g. artery
   g. artery complex
   g. fistula
   g. junction
   g. lumen
   g. lymph node
   g. mucosal prolapse
   g. orifice
gastroduodenitis
gastroduodenoscopy
gastroduodenostomy
   Billroth I, II g.
gastroenteric anastomosis

gastroenteritis
    cobblestone appearance
    eosinophilic g.
gastroenterocolitis
gastroenteroptosis
gastroenterostomy
    percutaneous g.
    g. stoma
gastroepiploic
    g. arcade
    g. artery
    g. lymph node
    g. vein
    g. vessel
gastroesophageal (GE)
    g. angle
    g. collateral
    g. incompetence
    g. junction
    g. junction carcinoma
    g. junction stricture
    g. junction tumor
    g. reflux (GER)
    g. reflux disease (GERD)
    g. variceal plexus
Gastrografin
    G. enema
    G. imaging agent
    G. swallow
gastrohepatic
    g. bare area
    g. ligament
    g. ligament node
    g. omentum
gastrointestinal (GI)
    g. adverse effect
    g. bleeding
    g. carcinoma
    g. cyst
    g. endoscopic ultrasound
    g. endoscopy
    g. fetal anomaly
    g. fibrous tumor (GIFT)
    g. fistula
    g. glial/schwannoma tumor (GIGT)
    g. leiomyogenic tumor (GILT)
    g. lymphoma
    g. malignancy
    g. motility imaging
    g. plaque
    g. protein loss test
    g. renal transplant hemorrhage

    g. scintigraphy
    g. series
    g. stoma
    g. stromal tumor (GIST)
    g. tract
    g. tract adenocarcinoma
    g. tract obstruction
    g. ulcer
    upper g. (UGI)
gastrointestinal-associated lymphoid tissue
gastrojejunal mucosal prolapse
gastrojejunocolic fistula
gastrojejunostomy
    Billroth I, II g.
    g. catheter
gastrolienal ligament
GastroMARK oral imaging agent
gastroomental lymph node
gastropancreatic
    g. fold
    g. ligament
gastroparesis
    diabetic g.
gastropathy
    hyperplastic g.
gastropexy
gastrophrenic ligament
gastroplasty (GP)
Gastroport
gastroptosis
gastrorenal shunt
gastroschisis
gastroscope
    Olympus XQ230 g.
    Pentax ELLB 6000, 6500
    ultrasound g.
gastroscopy
gastrosphincteric pressure gradient
gastrosplenic
    g. ligament
    g. omentum
gastrostomy
    g. catheter
    CT-guided percutaneous
      endoscopic g.
    percutaneous endoscopic g. (PEG)
    radiologic percutaneous g.
    g. tube
gastrotomy
Gastroview imaging agent
Gastrovist imaging agent

G

NOTES

gate array
gated
    g. blood pool angiography
    g. blood pool scan
    g. blood pool scintigraphy
    g. blood pool ventriculogram
    g. cardiac blood pool imaging
    g. cine imaging
    g. CT scanner
    g. 3D reconstruction
    g. equilibrium blood pool scanning
    g. equilibrium cardiac blood pool
      imaging
    g. equilibrium radionuclide
      angiography
    g. exercise examination
    g. image
    g. imaging study
    g. inflow magnetic resonance
    g. inflow technique
    g. magnetic resonance imaging
    g. nuclear angiography
    g. nuclear ventriculogram
    g. planar study
    g. radionuclide angiocardiography
    g. radionuclide ventriculogram
    g. RNA
    g. single-photon emission-computed
      tomography (GSPECT)
    g. SPECT myocardial perfusion
      imaging
    g. stress myocardial perfusion
      (GMP)
    g. stress myocardial perfusion slice
    g. system
    g. view
gating
    cardiac g.
    diastolic g.
    echocardiographic g.
    electrocardiographic g.
    heartbeat g.
    peripheral pulse g.
    respiratory g.
    retrospective respiratory g.
    spirometric g.
    systolic g.
Gaucher
    G. disease
    G. splenomegaly
gauge
    x-ray thickness g.
gauss (G)
gaussian
    g. curve
    g. distribution
    g. dose-volume histogram
    g. function
    g. line

    g. line saturation
    g. line shape
    g. mode profile laser beam
    g. noise
    g. radiofrequency
    g. smoothing
Gavard muscle
Gaynor-Hart method
GB-GI
    gall bladder-gastrointestinal
      GB-GI series
GBM
    glioblastoma multiforme
    glomerular basement membrane
GBS
    gallbladder series
    gastric bypass surgery
GCH
    giant cavernous hemangioma
GCVF
    great cardiac vein flow
Gd
    gadolinium
^{153}Gd, Gd-153
    gadolinium 153
Gd-153 imaging agent
Gd-BOPTA
    gadobenate dimeglumine
      Gd-BOPTA imaging agent
        gadobenate dimeglumine
Gd-BOPTA/Dimeg imaging agent
GDC
    Guglielmi detachable coil
      3/6-cm 3D GDC
      2/3-cm UltraSoft GDC
      2/6-cm UltraSoft GDC
      UltraSoft GDC
GDC-18
GDC-10 soft coil
Gd-DO3A
    gadoteridol
Gd-DOTA
    gadolinium
      tetraazacyclododecanetetraacetic acid
      Gd-DOTA contrast medium
Gd-DOTA-enhanced subtraction dynamic
study
Gd-DTPA
    gadolinium diethylenetriamine
      pentaacetic acid
    gadopentetate dimeglumine
      Gd-DTPA PGTM imaging agent
      Gd-DTPA radioisotope
      Gd-DTPA with mannitol contrast
        agent
Gd-DTPA-BMA
    gadodiamide
    gadolinium diethylenetriamine
      pentaacetic acid bismethylamide

Gd-DTPA-enhanced turbo FLASH MRI
Gd-DTPA-labeled
   Gd-DTPA-l. albumin
   Gd-DTPA-l. dextran
Gd-enhanced
   Gd-e. imaging agent
   Gd-e. MR angiography
Gd-EOB-DTPA
   gadolinium ethoxybenzyl
     diethylenetriaminepentaacetic acid
   Gd-EOB-DTPA imaging agent
Gd-FMPSPGR
   gadolinium fast multiplanar spoiled
     gradient
   Gd-FMPSPGR imaging
Gd-HIDA chelate
Gd-HP-DO3A
   gadotcridol
   Gd-HP-DO3A imaging agent
Gd-Tex
   gadolinium texaphyrin
GDx
   Nerve Fiber Analyzer GDx
GE
   gastric emptying
   gastroesophageal
   General Electric
     GE 400AC/T; STAR II camera
     GE Advance PET scanner
     GE Advantage 1.5T imager
     GE CT Advantage scanner
     GE CT HiSpeed Advantage CT
      system
     GE CTI 9800 scanner
     GE CTI single detector scanner
     GE CT Max scanner
     GE CT Pace scanner
     GE CT/T 8800 scanner
     GE CT/T7 scanner
     GE 8800 CT/T scanner
     GE detector
     GE EchoSpeed 1.5T whole-body
      MR imager
     GE gamma camera
     GE Genesis CT scanner
     GE GN 500-MHz scanner
     GE GN300 7.05-T/89-mm bore
      multinuclear spectrometer
     GE 9800 high-resolution CT
      scanner
     GE HiSpeed Advantage helical CT
      scanner

     GE HiSpeed single detector
      scanner
     GE Lightspeed CT scanner
     GE MR Max scanner
     GE MR Signa scanner
     GE MR Vectra scanner
     GE Neurocam camera
     GE NMR spectrometer
     GE Omega 500-MHz scanner
     GE Pace CT scanner
     GE proton head coil probe
     GE QE 300-MHz scanner
     GE Senographe 2000D digital
      mammography system
     GE Signa 5.4 Genesis MR imager
     GE Signa 5.5 Horizon EchoSpeed
      MR imager
     GE Signa 4.7 MRI scanner
     GE Signa 0.5T double doughnut
     GE Signa 1.5-T magnet
     GE Signa 1.5-T scanner
     GE Signa 5.2 with SR-230 3-axis
      EPI gradient upgrade scanner
     GE single-detector SPECT-capable
      camera
     GE SPECT
     GE Spiral CT scanner
     GE Starcam single-crystal
      tomographic scintillation camera
     GE Vectra MR scanner
     GE Viewer software
     GE Voluson 730 4D ultrasound
      system
GE-Amersham merger signal
Gee-Herter disease
Gee-Thaysen disease
GEG
   Garren-Edwards gastric
     GEG bubble
Gehan methodology
Geiger counter
Geiger-Müller (G-M)
   G.-M. counter
   G.-M. detector
   G.-M. survey meter
   G.-M. tube
gel
   acoustic g.
   g. bleed
   coupling g.
   cross-linked silicone g.
   Fricke g.

NOTES

G

gel (continued)
    methylcellulose g.
    ultrasound g.
gelatin
    g. phantom
    g. sponge
    g. sponge particle
    g. sponge pledget
    g. sponge powder
gelatinous
    g. ascites
    g. brain pseudocyst
    g. carcinoma
    g. debris
    g. hematoma
    g. tissue
Gelbfish-Endovasc device
gemellary pregnancy
gemellus, pl. **gemelli**
gemistocytic astrocytoma
gemistocytoma
gene
    BRCA2 g.'s
    g. therapy
general
    G. Electric (GE)
    g. pattern matching
generalisata
    platyspondyly g.
generalized
    g. angiofollicular lymph node hyperplasia
    g. arteriosclerosis
    g. autocalibrating partially parallel acquisition (GRAPPA)
    g. breast hyperplasia
    g. calcinosis
    g. capillary leak
    g. compensation for resonance offset and pulse length errors (GROPE)
    g. cortical hyperostosis
    g. cortical hyperstasis
    g. emphysema
    g. hamartomatosis
    g. hazy opacity
    g. increased liver echogenicity
    g. interferography using spin echoes and stimulated echoes (GINSEST)
    g. lymphadenopathy syndrome
    g. lymphangiectasis
    g. nephrographic (GNG)
    g. osteoarthritis
    g. pulmonary edema
    g. seizure
    g. SENSE (GSENSE)

generation
    g. echo
    g. 6 integrated radiotherapy system
generator
    anterior current (AC) g.
    carbon dioxide g.
    g. characteristic
    CO_2 g.
    CORI computerized endoscopic report g.
    deuterium-tritium g.
    direct current g.
    ^{166}Dy g.
    dysprosium-holmium (^{166}Dy-166Ho) in vivo g.
    electric g.
    electrostatic g.
    extraction g.
    high-voltage g.
    ^{166}Ho in vivo g.
    molybdenum-99 g.
    molybdenum-technetium g.
    nuclide g.
    3-phase g.
    pizoelectric g.
    polyphase g.
    6-pulse, 3-phase g.
    12-pulse, 3-phase g.
    radiofrequency g.
    radionuclide g.
    resonance g.
    spark gap g.
    Super 50 CP high-voltage g.
    supervoltage g.
    g. system
    technetium-99m g.
    Triphasix g.
    Van de Graaf g.
    video signal g.
    VNUS radiofrequency g.
    waveform g.
    x-ray g.
generator-produced ^{188}**Re**
Genesis
    G. 2000 carbon dioxide laser
    G. stent
Genesys camera
genetically
    g. engineered oncolytic adenovirus
    g. homogeneous
    g. significant dose
genial
    g. tubercle
    g. tubercle of mandible
geniculate
    g. body
    g. branch
    g. ganglion
    g. ganglion schwannoma

geniculocalcarine tract
geniculocalvarium
geniculum
genioglossus muscle
genital
    g. blood pooling
    g. canal
    g. carcinoma
    g. duct
    g. eminence
    g. fold
    g. groove
    g. ligament
    g. ridge
    g. tract
    g. tract calcification
    g. tract embryology
    g. tract gas
    g. visualization
genitalia
    ambiguous g.
genitalis
genitoinguinal ligament
genitourinary (GU)
    g. adverse effect
    g. anomaly
    g. carcinoma
    g. fistula
    g. injury
    g. reflex
    g. rhabdomyosarcoma
    g. tract
    g. tract trauma
    g. tuberculosis
Gennari
    G. band
    line of G.
    G. stripe
genome
    mitochondrial g.
    nuclear g.
genomic instability
genotype
GentleLASE
    G. Plus laser
    G. Plus laser system
gentle lordosis
genu, pl. **genua**
    g. of corpus callosum
    g. recurvatum
    g. valgum

    g. valgum deformity
    g. varum
    g. varum deformity
geode formation
geographic
    g. bone destruction
    g. follicle
    g. lesion
    g. pattern
    g. skull
geography
    brain g.
geometric
    g. blur
    g. distortion
    g. distribution
    g. efficiency
    g. optimization algorithm
    g. unsharpness
geometrical efficiency
geometry
    beam g.
    coil g.
    coronary vessel g.
    g. factor
    g. factor map
    Golay g.
    scintillation camera g.
    slice g.
geophagia artifact
GER
    gastroesophageal reflux
GERD
    gastroesophageal reflux disease
Gerdy
    G. fontanelle
    G. interatrial loop
    G. interauricular loop
    G. ligament
    G. tubercle
Gerhardt
    G. sign
    G. triangle
geriatric
    g. configuration
    g. feature
germanate 68
    bismuth g.
German horizontal plane
germanium
    high-purity g. (HPGe)

NOTES

G

germinal
    g. bleed matrix
    g. pole
germinate
    bismuth g.
germinolysis
    subependymal g.
germinoma
    intracranial g.
    mediastinum g.
    multicentric g.
    pineal g.
    suprasellar hemorrhagic g.
Gerota
    G. capsule
    G. fascia
    G. method
Gerstmann-Sträussler-Scheinker disease
Gerstmann syndrome
Gertzbein seatbelt injury classification
gestalt impression on CT
gestation
    extrauterine g.
    intrauterine g.
    multiple g.'s
    nonviable g.
    normal g.
    triplet g.
gestational
    g. age (GA)
    g. choriocarcinoma
    g. diabetes
    g. sac (GS)
    g. sac abnormality
    g. sac diameter
    g. sac measurement
    g. trophoblastic disease (GTD)
    g. trophoblastic neoplasm
    g. trophoblastic tumor
    g. week
geyser sign
GFR
    glomerular filtration rate
GGO
    ground-glass opacification
GHA
    glucoheptonate acid
GHCH
    giant hepatic cavernous hemangioma
Ghon
    G. complex
    G. focus
    G. node
    G. primary lesion
    G. tubercle
Ghon-Sachs complex
ghost
    g. image
    red cell g.

    g. reduction by equalized
      acquisition triplets (GREAT)
    separation of g.'s
ghosting artifact
GHz
    gigahertz
GI
    gastrointestinal
    GI bleed
    Imagent GI
    Innerview GI
    GI tract
    GI tract amyloidosis
    GI tract endometriosis
    GI tract lipoma
    GI tract lymphoid hyperplasia
    GI tract mastocytosis
    GI tract scintigraphy
    GI tract trauma
    GI tract tuberculosis
Gianotti-Crosti syndrome
giant
    g. brain aneurysm
    g. breast fibroadenoma
    g. bullous emphysema
    g. cavernous hemangioma (GCH)
    g. cell adenocarcinoma
    g. cell astrocytoma
    g. cell carcinoma of thyroid gland
    g. cell fibroma
    g. cell interstitial pneumonia (GIP)
    g. cell lung carcinoma
    g. cell pneumonitis
    g. cell reparative granuloma
    g. cell sarcoma
    g. cell tumor
    g. cell tumor of the tendon sheath
    g. cell-type MFH
    g. colon
    g. duodenal ulcer
    g. follicle lymphoma
    g. follicular hyperplasia
    g. gastric fold
    g. hepatic cavernous hemangioma
      (GHCH)
    g. hyperplasia lymph node
    g. hypertrophic gastritis
    g. left atrium
    g. myofibroblastoma
    g. osteoid osteoma
    g. peptic ulcer
    g. saccular aneurysm
    g. serpentine aneurysm
    g. sigmoid diverticulum
    g. villous adenoma
Gianturco
    G. biliary Z-stent
    G. occlusion coil
    G. stent

G. wool-tufted wire coil
G. Z-stent
Gianturco-Rosch biliary stent
Gianturco-Roubin FlexStent
Gianturco-Wallace-Anderson coil
Gianturco-Wallace-Chuang coil
gibbous deformity
Gibbs
G. random field
G. ringing
G. sampling
Gibbs-Donnan law
gibbus
thoracic g.
Gierke respiratory bundle
GIFT
gastrointestinal fibrous tumor
gigahertz (GHz)
gigantiform cementoma
gigantism
cerebral g.
extremity g.
focal g.
GIGT
gastrointestinal glial/schwannoma tumor
Gilchrist disease
gill
g. arch skeleton
g. cleft
G. lesion
Gillette
G. joint
G. suspensory ligament
Gillies suture
GILT
gastrointestinal leiomyogenic tumor
Gimbernat ligament
gingival
g. carcinoma
g. crest
g. curvature
g. septum
g. space
gingivitis
erosive g.
necrotizing ulcerative g. (NUG)
gingivobuccal groove
gingivodental ligament
gingivolabial groove
GINSEST
generalized interferography using spin
echoes and stimulated echoes

GIP
giant cell interstitial pneumonia
girdle
limb g.
pectoral g.
pelvic g.
shoulder g.
girth
abdominal g.
Gissane
G. angle
crucial angle of G.
GIST
gastrointestinal stromal tumor
Given
G. Diagnostic imaging system
G. imaging capsule/M2A capsule
GK-SRS boost
glabella
glabelloalveolar line
glabellomeatal line
glabrous cirrhosis
GLAD
glenolabral articular cartilage disruption
GLAD lesion
gladiolus
gladiomanubrial
gland
absorbent g.
accessory thyroid g.
admaxillary g.
adrenal g.
Albarran g.
alveolar g.
anteprostatic g.
aortic g.
apical g.
apocrine sweat g.
aporic g.
artcrial g.
arteriococcygeal g.
axillary sweat g.
Bartholin g.
Bruch g.
Brunner g.
bulbocavernous g.
bulbourethral g.
calcified pineal g.
carotid g.
coccygeal g.
Duverney g.
ectopic g.

NOTES

G

gland *(continued)*
    endocrine g.
    enlarged thyroid g.
    enlargement of lacrimal g.
    enlargement of parotid g.
    giant cell carcinoma of thyroid g.
    globate g.
    glomiform g.
    haversian g.
    hilar g.
    interscapular g.
    lacrimal g.
    Littre g.
    lymph g.
    mammary g.
    Montgomery g.
    mucosal g.
    ovary g.
    pancreas g.
    paramediastinal g.
    paraurethral g.
    parotid g.
    periurethral g.
    pineal g.
    pituitary g.
    prostate g.
    salivary g.
    Stensen g.
    subaortic g.
    sublingual g.
    submandibular g.
    submaxillary g.
    substernal thyroid g.
    supernumerary parathyroid g.
    suprarenal g.
    testicular g.
    thymus g.
    thyroid g.
    urethral g.
    Virchow g.
    g. volume
    Wharton g.
glandular
    g. carcinoma
    g. dose
    g. proliferation
glans
    g. carcinoma
    g. penis
glare
    imaging chain veiling g.
    scatter and veiling g. (SVG)
    veiling g.
glaserian fissure
Glasgow
    G. outcome scale
    G. sign
glass, pl. **glasses**
    g. blower's emphysema

    g. eye artifact
    fiberoptic video glasses
    hepatic test of G.
    quartz g.
    g. ray
    g. thermometer
    g. tract detector
    vita g.
    wine g.
Glasscock-Jackson classification
glaze consistency
Glazunov tumor
Gleason grade
Glénard disease
Glenn
    G. anastomosis
    G. procedure
    G. shunt
glenohumeral
    g. dislocation
    g. instability
    g. joint
    g. ligament
glenoid
    g. articular rim disruption (GARD)
    g. articular rim disruption lesion
    g. cavity
    g. fossa
    g. labral ovoid body
    g. labrum
    g. labrum capsule
    g. labrum injury
    g. ligament
    g. ovoid mass
    g. point
    g. process
    g. rim
    g. rim fracture
    g. surface
glenolabral
    g. articular cartilage disruption
     (GLAD)
    g. articular disruption lesion
    g. ovoid mass (GLOM)
Gliadel wafer
glial
    g. brain tumor
    g. limiting membrane
    g. nodule
    g. rest
    g. scarring
    g. stranding
    g. tumor calcification
GliaSite radiotherapy system
Glidecath
    Radifocus G.
Glidecatheter
Glide Cobra catheter

Glidewire
> angled G.
> 0.035-inch G.
> long taper stiff shaft G.
> Radifocus G.

gliding joint
glioblast
glioblastoma
> butterfly g.
> multicentric g.
> g. multiforme (GBM)

glioma
> anaplastic cerebral g.
> brainstem g.
> butterfly g.
> cerebral g.
> cystic g.
> high-grade g.
> hypothalamic g.
> intracranial g.
> low-grade g.
> malignant g.
> multicentric malignant g.
> nonanaplastic g.
> optic nerve g.
> pontine g.
> pontocerebellar g.
> recurrent high-grade malignant g.
> rolandoparietal g.
> spinal cord g.
> supratentorial g.
> tectal g.
> temporooccipital g.
> thalamic g.

gliomatosis
> arachnoidal g.
> g. cerebri
> g. peritonei

glioneural hamartoma
gliosarcoma
> cerebellar g.

gliosis
> astrocytic g.
> ischemic g.
> progressive subcortical g.
> reactive g.
> secondary g.
> g. of sylvian aqueduct

gliosis-induced microcystic degeneration
Glisson capsule
global
> g. cavus

> g. cerebral hypoperfusion
> g. cerebral ischemia
> g. cortical defect
> g. ejection fraction
> g. hypokinesis
> g. hypometabolism
> g. intracranial blood flow
> g. myocardial ischemia
> g. phantogeusia
> g. renal enlargement
> g. tissue loss
> g. ventricular function
> g. wall motion abnormality

globally
> g. depressed ejection fraction
> g. optimized alternating-phase rectangular pulse (GARP)
> g. optimized alternating phase rectangular pulse

globate gland
globe
> optic g.

globe-orbit relationship
globoid heart
globular
> g. cardiomegaly
> g. chest
> g. configuration
> g. meningioma
> g. tumor
> g. valve

globulin
> technetium-99m human immune g.

globulus, pl. **globuli**
globus
> g. major
> g. minor
> g. pallidus

Glofil-125 injection
GLOM
> glenolabral ovoid mass
> GLOM lesion

glomangioma
glomera
> choroid g.

glomerular
> g. basement membrane (GBM)
> g. filtration
> g. filtration agent
> g. filtration rate (GFR)
> g. lesion

G

NOTES

glomerular *(continued)*
    g. mesangial cell
    g. nephritis
glomeruli *(pl. of* glomerulus)
glomerulocytoma
glomeruloid formation
glomerulonephritis
    acute g.
    chronic g.
    crescent-shaped g.
    membranous g.
    necrotizing g.
    proliferative g.
    segmental necrotizing g.
glomerulopathy
glomerulosa
    zona g.
glomerulosclerosis
glomerulus, pl. **glomeruli**
    renal g.
glomiform gland
glomus
    body g.
    g. body tumor
    g. bone tumor
    g. choroideum
    g. of choroid plexus
    g. jugulare
    g. jugulare tumor
    g. jugulotympanicum tumor
    g. neck tumor
    g. tympanicum
    g. vagale
glomus-type arteriovenous malformation
glossoepiglottic
    g. fold
    g. ligament
glossopalatine fold
glossopharyngeal nerve
glottic
    g. carcinoma
    g. larynx
    g. narrowing
glottis, pl. **glottides**
glove
    optic g.
    g. phenomenon
    g. phenomenon artifact
    radiation-attenuating surgical g.'s
gloved-finger
    g.-f. shadow
    g.-f. sign
glow
    cathode g.
    g. curve
    g. modular tube
GLP7 film
GLPC
    gas-liquid phase chromatography

glucagon imaging agent
glucagonoma
glucamoma
glucarate imaging agent
glucaric acid-labeled contrast medium
gluceptate
    TechneScan G.
Glucoband electronic scanning device
glucoheptanoate
    ^{99m}Tc g.
glucoheptonate acid (GHA)
glucose water
glucosyl-galactosyl-pyridinoline
    urinary g.-g.-p.
glue
    Technovit 7210 VLC contact g.
    TruFill n-BCA surgical g.
glutamate spectroscopy
glutaric aciduria type I, II
gluteal
    g. bonnet
    g. fold
    g. line
    g. lymph node
    g. ridge
gluten-sensitive enteropathy
gluteus
    g. maximus
    g. medius
    g. minimus
glycerolphosphorylcholine (GPC)
glycogenic acanthosis
glycogen-rich pancreatic cystadenoma
glycol
    isoosmotic polyethylene g.
    polyethylene g. (PEG)
glycolysis
    enhanced g.
glycoprotein-secreting adenoma
glycosaminoglycan (GAG)
glycoside
    cardiac g.
GM
    gastric mucosa
    GM segmentation
G-M
    Geiger-Müller
    G-M counter
GM₁/GM₂ gangliosidosis
GMN
    gradient moment nulling
GMP
    gated stress myocardial perfusion
GMR
    gradient moment reduction
    gradient moment rephasing
    gradient motion rephasing
gnathic osteosarcoma

GNB
  ganglioneuroblastoma
GNG
  generalized nephrographic
  GNG phase imaging
goblet-shaped pelvis
Godwin tumor
Goethe bone
goggles
  Avotec MR-compatible liquid
  crystal display g.
goiter
  adenomatous g.
  Basedow g.
  colloid g.
  congenital g.
  cystic g.
  diffuse toxic g.
  diving g.
  exophthalmic g.
  familial g.
  fetal g.
  fibrous g.
  intrathoracic g.
  iodide g.
  iodine-deficiency g.
  lingual g.
  multinodular g.
  nodular g.
  parenchymous g.
  retrotracheal g.
  retrovascular g.
  simple g.
  substernal g.
  suffocative g.
  thyroid g.
  toxic multinodular g.
  toxic nodular g.
  vascular g.
  wandering g.
goitrogen
Golay
  G. coil
  G. geometry
gold (Au)
  g. Au-198 imaging agent
  g. particle
  g. radioactive source
  g. seed
Goldblatt kidney

golden
  motility of G.
  S sign of G.
Goldenhar syndrome
gold-195m
  g. radionuclide
  g. tracer
gold-marked stent
Goldsmith and Woodburne classification
Goldthwait sign
Gold-tip micro guidewire
golfer's elbow
Golgi tendon
GoLYTELY bowel preparation
gonad
  indifferent g.
gonadal
  g. artery
  g. dose
  g. dysgenesis
  g. function
  g. neoplasm
  g. shielding
  g. stroma
  g. stromal tumor
  g. vein reflux
  g. venography
  g. venous ectasia
gonadoblastoma
gonadotroph cell adenoma
gonadotropin
  chorionic g.
gonadotropin-secreting adenoma
gonecystic calculus
gonial angle
goniometer
  Sceratti g.
gonion
  g. gradient coil
  g. gradient magnetic field
gonion-gnathion plane
goodness-of-match criteria
Goodpasture syndrome
Good Samaritan law
goose foot tendon
gooseneck
  g. concept
  g. outflow tract deformity
  g. shape
Gordon-Brostrom single-contrast arthrography
Gordon sign

G

NOTES

Gore
  G. covered biliary stent-graft
  G. 1.5T torso array MRI surface
    coil
Gorham disease
Gorlin
  G. formula for aortic valve area
  G. formula for mitral valve area
  G. method for measuring cardiac
    output
  G. syndrome
Gorlin-Goltz syndrome
Gosling pulsatility index
Gosselin fracture
Gosset
  spiral band of G.
gossypiboma
Gothic arch formation
Gottron sign
gouge defect
Gould
  G. electromagnetic flowmeter
  G. Statham pressure transducer
gout
  articular g.
  spinal tophaceous g.
  tophaceous g.
gouty
  g. arthritis
  g. arthropathy
  g. node
  g. tophus
Gowers
  G. bundle
  G. bundle in cerebellum
  G. column
  G. fasciculus
  G. sign
GP
  gastroplasty
GPC
  glycerolphosphorylcholine
g-probe localization
graafian
  g. follicle
  g. vesicle
**Grace method of ratio of metatarsal
  length**
gracile
  g. bone
  g. habitus
gracilis
  funiculus g.
  g. tendon
gradation
  subtle g.
grade
  Fisher g. 1–4
  Gleason g.

histologic g.
Hunt and Hess aneurysm g. I–V
Hunt and Kosnik (grade 0–V)
  aneurysmal g.
g. 0, 2 insonation condition
osteoarthritis g.
placental g.
Scharff-Bloom-Richardson g.
Severin g.
g. 1–3 signal intensity
subarachnoid hemorrhage Fisher g.
  1–4
thrombolysis in brain ischemia
  flow g.
graded
  g. compression sonography
  g. compression sonography
    technique
  g. compression ultrasound
  g. infusion
gradient
  g. acquisition
  g. across valve
  g. amplifier
  g. amplitude
  aortic outflow g.
  aortic valve g. (AVG)
  aortic valve peak instantaneous g.
  aortic valve pressure g.
  arteriovenous pressure g.
  atrioventricular g.
  balanced g.
  biliary-duodenal pressure g.
  bipolar g.
  brain-core g.
  g. compensation
  conjugate g.
  coronary perfusion g.
  dephasing g.
  3D Fourier transform gradient-echo
    sequence with spoiler g.
  diastolic g.
  diffusion g.
  diffusion-sensitizing g.
  discontinuous density g.
  g. drive current
  duodenobiliary pressure g.
  g. echo MR with magnetization
    transfer
  echo-speed g.
  electric field g. (EFG)
  elevated g.
  g. encoding
  end-diastolic aortic-left ventricular
    pressure g.
  fast PC cine MR sequence with
    echo-planar g.
  Ficoll g.
  field g.

flow-encoding g.
frequency-encoding g.
gadolinium fast multiplanar
  spoiled g. (Gd-FMPSPGR)
gastrosphincteric pressure g.
hepatic venous pressure g.
holosystolic g.
imaging g.
instantaneous g.
left ventricular outflow pressure g.
linear g.
g. linearity
magnetic field g. (MFG)
g. magnetic field
maximal estimated g.
mean mitral valve g.
mean systolic g.
mitral valve g.
g. moment nulling (GMN)
g. moment reduction (GMR)
g. moment rephasing (GMR)
motion-nulling g.
g. motion rephasing (GMR)
negligible pressure g.
nonisotropic g.
oscillating g.
osmotic g.
outflow tract g.
peak diastolic g.
peak instantaneous g.
peak pressure g.
peak right ventricular-right atrial
  systolic g.
peak systolic g.
peak-to-peak pressure g.
perfusion g.
phase-encoding g.
portosystemic g.
potential g.
Power Trak 6000 g.
pressure-flow g.
pre-TIPS g.
pullback pressure g.
pulmonary artery to right ventricle
  diastolic g.
pulmonary outflow g.
pulmonic valve g.
g. pulse
g. pump
readout g.
rephasing g.
residual g.

g. reversal
right ventricular to main pulmonary
  artery pressure g.
g. scheme
g. selection
sensitizing g.
g. sheet coil
g. slew rate
slice select g. (SS)
Stejskal-Tanner g.
stenotic g.
g. subsystem in MRI
subvalvular g.
g. switching noise
g. system
systolic g.
thoracoabdominal g.
g. timing
transaortic systolic g.
transjugular intrahepatic
  portosystemic shunt g.
translesional g.
transmitral g.
transpulmonic g.
transstenotic g.
transtricuspid valve diastolic g.
transvalvular pressure g.
tricuspid valve g.
twister g.
velocity g.
ventricular g.
voxel g.
washout g.
g. waveform
X g.
Z g.

gradient-echo
g.-e. axial image
g.-e. cine technique
g.-e. coronal image
g.-e. 3-dimensional Fourier
  transform volume imaging
g.-e. flow imaging
g.-e. imaging sequence
g.-e. method
g.-e. MR imaging
g.-e. phase imaging
g.-e. pulse sequence
g.-e. recall technique
g.-e. sequence imaging
spin lock g.-e. (SL-GRE)
g.-e. T2-weighted image

NOTES

gradient-encoded image
gradient-induced phase dispersion
gradient-recalled
>   g.-r. acquisition in steady state (GRASS)
>   g.-r. echo
>   g.-r. echo image
>   spoiled g.-r.

gradient-refocused echo (GRE)
gradient-spin echo
gradient-to-noise imaging
grading
gradually tapering border
Graf
>   G. alpha angle
>   G. beta angle
>   G. hip dysplasia classification
>   G. method

graft
>   Ancure tube g.
>   aorticorenal g.
>   aortic tube g.
>   aortofemoral bypass g. (AFBG)
>   aortoiliac bypass g.
>   aortoplasty with patch g.
>   arterial bypass g.
>   autogenous vein bypass g.
>   autologous patch g.
>   autologous vein g.
>   axillary-axillary bypass g.
>   axillary-brachial bypass g.
>   axillary-femoral bypass g.
>   axillary-femorofemoral bypass g.
>   axillobifemoral bypass g.
>   bifemoral g.
>   bifurcation g.
>   bilateral myocutaneous g.
>   bone g.
>   bone-tendon-bone g.
>   Brescia-Cimino g.
>   bypass g.
>   carotid-carotid venous bypass g.
>   Cloward bone g.
>   coronary artery bypass g. (CABG)
>   Corvita endoluminal g.
>   custom-fabricated g.
>   Dacron-covered stent g.
>   disc-shaped bone g.
>   donor g.
>   dowel-shaped bone g.
>   elephant trunk g.
>   endarterectomy g.
>   endoleak g.
>   endoscopic coronary artery bypass g. (E-CABG)
>   endothelialized vascular g.
>   endovascular aortic g.
>   esophageal g.
>   expanded polytetrafluoroethylene g.

expanded polytetrafluoroethylene-covered nitinol TIPS stent g.
extracavitary infected g.
extracavitary prosthetic arterial g.
g. failure
femorocrural g.
femorodistal popliteal bypass g.
femorofemoral bypass g.
femoroperoneal in situ vein bypass g.
femoropopliteal bypass g.
femoropopliteal Gore-Tex g.
femorotibial bypass g.
H g.
Hemobahn stent g.
hepatorenal saphenous vein bypass g.
iliac-renal bypass g.
ilioprofunda bypass g.
infected thrombosed g.
infrainguinal arterial bypass g.
infrainguinal vein bypass g.
inlay g.
interbody bone g.
internal thoracic artery g.
interposition g.
g. interstice
intraabdominal arterial bypass g.
ITA g.
Jostent Peripheral Stent G.
jump vein g.
g. kinking
limb of bifurcation g.
loop g.
modular stent g.
occluded g.
g. occlusion
onlay g.
osseous g.
g. patency
patency of vein g.
pedicle bone g.
polytetrafluoroethylene g.
prosthetic femoral distal g.
g. revascularization
reversed vein g.
g. roof impingement
saphenous vein bypass g.
Sauvage filamentous velour g.
self-expanding stent g.
sequence bypass g.
g. shrinkage
in situ g.
Smith-Robinson bone g.
snake g.
splenorenal arterial bypass g.
g. stenosis
straight interposition g.
subcutaneous arterial bypass g.

suprailiac aortic mesenteric g.
synthetic vascular bypass g.
Talent bifurcated abdominal aortic
stent g.
Talent stent g.
transluminally placed stented g.
Varivas loop g.
vascular bypass g.
vein g.
venous bypass g.
venous interposition g.
VIATORR transjugular intrahepatic
portosystemic shunt stent g.
Zenith AAA endovascular g.

graft-enteric
g.-e. erosion
g.-e. fistula

graft-related complication
graft-versus-host disease of liver
graft-versus-tumor response
Graham-Burford-Mayer syndrome
Graham-Cole cholecystogram
grain handler's lung
graininess
film g.

grand mal seizure
Granger
G. line
G. projection
G. view

Grantham femur fracture classification
granular
g. breast-cell myoblastoma
g. calcification
g. infiltrate
g. kidney
g. leukocyte
g. lung-cell myoblastoma
g. microcalcification
g. opacity
g. sella-cell myoblastoma

granularis
ependymitis g.

granulation
arachnoid g.
Bayle g.
pacchionian g.
g. stenosis
g. tissue

granule
neurosecretory g.

granulocyte
antibody labeled circulating g.
g. colony stimulating factor

granulocytic sarcoma
granuloma, pl. **granulomata**
actinic g.
apical g.
aspergillotic g.
beryllium g.
bilharzial g.
button sequestrum eosinophilic g.
calcified g.
calcified cysticercus g.
caseating g.
ceroid gallbladder g.
cholesterol ear g.
coalescent g.
cysticercus g.
dental g.
eosinophilic g.
epithelioid g.
extravascular g.
foreign body g.
frontoethmoidal giant cell
reparative g.
giant cell reparative g.
Hodgkin g.
hyalinizing g.
inguinal g.
lethal midline g.
lung g.
malarial g.
mediastinal g.
midline g.
Mignon g.
miliary g.
noncaseating g.
paracoccidioidal g.
periapical g.
plasma cell g.
pseudopyogenic g.
pulmonary hyalinizing g.
reparative giant cell g.
reticulohistiocytic g.
rheumatic g.
root end g.
sarcoid g.
sea urchin g.
silicone g.
sperm g.
stellate g.
swimming pool g.

G

NOTES

granuloma *(continued)*
 thorium dioxide g.
 tracheal g.
 tuberculous g.
 umbilical g.
 xanthomatous g.
 zirconium g.
granulomatosis
 allergic g.
 bronchocentric g.
 lipoid g.
 lymphomatoid g.
 mainline g.
 Miescher g.
 necrotizing respiratory g.
 organic g.
 pulmonary mainline g.
 Wegener g.
granulomatous
 g. brain abscess
 g. enterocolitis
 g. ileitis
 g. inflammation of bronchus
 g. lesion of sinus
 g. lymphoma
 g. myositis
 g. pneumonia
 g. pneumonitis
 subacute g.
 g. transmural colitis
 g. uveitis
granulomonocyte
granulosa
 g. cell carcinoma
 pyoderma g.
 g. theca neoplasm
granulosa-theca cell tumor
granulovacuolar degeneration
grapelike
 g. cluster
 g. multilocular cystic lesion
 g. vesicle
grape-skin lung cavity
graph
 scatter g.
 spin-phase g.
 velocity-time g.
graphics
 Reality Engine g.
graphite fibrosis of lung
GRAPPA
 generalized autocalibrating partially
  parallel acquisition
Graser diverticulum
Grashey
 G. method
 G. position
 G. shoulder view
grasping technique

GRASS
 gradient-recalled acquisition in steady
  state
 GRASS MR imaging
 GRASS pulse sequence
 spoiled GRASS (SPGR)
 GRASS system
Gratiolet
 G. convolution
 radiation of G.
gravel
 gallbladder g.
Graves disease
gravidarum
 fibroma molle g.
gravid uterus
gravis
 colitis ulcerosa g.
gravitational
 g. edema
 g. potential energy
gravity
 center of g.
Grawitz tumor
gray (Gy)
 g. commissure
 g. horns in spinal canal
 g. lung
 g. matter
 g. matter abnormality
 g. matter degeneration
 g. matter heterotopia
 g. matter–white matter
  differentiation
 periventricular g. (PVG)
 g. radiation absorbed dose
 g. reticular
 g. scale
 g. unit
gray-level
 g.-l. histogram
 g.-l. spacing
 g.-l. thresholding
gray-scale
 g.-s. baseline imaging
 g.-s. Doppler
 g.-s. endorectal ultrasound
 g.-s. ERU
 g.-s. examination
 g.-s. image
 g.-s. imaging
 g.-s. inversion
 g.-s. monitor
 g.-s. range
 g.-s. sonography
 g.-s. ultrasound
Grayson ligament
gray-to-white
 g.-t.-w. matter activity ratio

g.-t.-w. matter contrast ratio
g.-t.-w. matter interface
g.-t.-w. matter utilization ratio
gray-white
  g.-w. differentiation
  g.-w. matter junction
GRE
  gradient-refocused echo
  GRE breath-hold hepatic imaging
  3D GRE
  ferumoxtran-enhanced echo-planar
    SE T2-weighted and echo-planar
    GRE
  GRE gadolinium-chelate enhanced
    imaging
  GRE magnetic resonance imaging
  GRE technique
GREAT
  ghost reduction by equalized acquisition
    triplets
great
  g. cardiac plexus
  g. cardiac vein
  g. cardiac vein flow (GCVF)
  g. cerebral vein of Galen
  g. cistern
  g. sacrosciatic foramen
  g. terminal vertebra
  g. toe sesamoid bone
  g. vein of cerebrum
  g. vessel
  g. vessel transposition
  g. vessel view
greater
  g. arc injury
  g. circulation
  g. curvature of stomach
  g. curvature ulcer
  g. multangular bone
  g. omentum
  g. palatine canal
  g. palatine foramen
  g. pelvis
  g. peritoneal sac
  g. petrosal
  g. sac of peritoneal cavity
  g. saphenous system
  g. saphenous vein
  g. sciatic foramen
  g. sciatic notch
  g. sigmoid notch
  g. sphenoid wing

g. sphenoid wing lesion
g. superficial petrosal nerve
g. trochanter
g. trochanter of femur
g. trochanteric femoral fracture
g. tubercle
g. tuberosity
g. tuberosity fracture
green
  iodocyanine g. (ICG)
Greene
  G. biopsy set
  G. needle
Greenfield
  G. catheter
  G. vena cava filter
greenstick fracture
GRE-in
  GRE-i. image
  GRE-i. imaging
grenade thrower's fracture
grenz ray
GRE-out
  GRE-o. image
  GRE-o. imaging
Greullch
  G. and Pyle atlas
  G. and Pyle method
Grey Turner sign
grid
  antiscatter g.
  Bucky g.
  cross-hatch g.
  g. film
  focused g.
  localization g.
  Lysholm g.
  megavoltage g.
  oscillating g.
  Potter-Bucky g.
  g. ratio
  scatter g.
  g. technique
  g. therapy
Griesinger sign
griffe
  simian g.
Griffith point
Grisel syndrome
Grl-DTPA
  gadolinium diethylenetriamine-penta-
    acetic acid

NOTES

G

Grocco sign
Grocott methenamine silver
groin
    g. dissection
    g. mass
Grollman pigtail catheter
groove
    alveolingual g.
    alveolobuccal g.
    alveololabial g.
    anal intersphincteric g.
    anterior interventricular g.
    anterolateral g.
    anteromedian g.
    arterial g.
    atrioventricular g.
    auriculoventricular g.
    basilar g.
    bicipital g.
    bronchial g.
    buccal g.
    carotid g.
    carpal g.
    caudothalamic g.
    cavernous g.
    central g.
    chiasmatic g.
    coronary g.
    costal g.
    deltopectoral g.
    dental g.
    developmental g.
    digastric g.
    ectodermal g.
    esophageal g.
    ethmoidal g.
    gastric g.
    genital g.
    gingivobuccal g.
    gingivolabial g.
    Harrison g.
    infraorbital g.
    interatrial g.
    intercollicular g.
    intercondylar g.
    intertubercular g.
    interventricular g.
    labial g.
    lacrimal g.
    Liebermeister g.
    meningeal artery g.
    middle meningeal artery g.
    neural g.
    paravertebral g.
    patellar g.
    posterior coronary g.
    posterior interventricular g.
    proximal trochlear g.
    radial neck g.
    Ranvier g.
    retromalleolar g.
    sagittal g.
    Sibson g.
    spindle colonic g.
    striatothalamic g.
    supraorbital g. (SOG)
    trochlear g.
    trochleocapitellar g.
    ulnar g.
    urethral g.
    vascular g.
    venous g.
    Verga lacrimal g.
    vertebral g.
    Waterston g.
grooved director
grooving of articular surface
GROPE
    generalized compensation for resonance
    offset and pulse length errors
Groshong
    G. distal-valve catheter
    G. NXT PICC
gross
    g. fracture
    g. lesion
    g. tumor
    g. tumor volume (GTV)
Grossman
    G. principle
    G. scale for regurgitation
ground
    g. plate
    g. state
ground-glass
    g.-g. appearance
    g.-g. attenuation
    g.-g. definition
    g.-g. density
    g.-g. infiltrate
    g.-g. lesion
    g.-g. nodule
    g.-g. opacification (GGO)
    g.-g. opacity
    g.-g. osteoporosis
    g.-g. pattern
    g.-g. texture
group
    Dodd perforating vein g.
    Eisenmenger g.
    extensor-supinator g.
    flexor-pronator muscle g.
    gadolinium enhanced imaging g.
    gastrocnemius-soleus muscle g.
    interosseous muscle g.
    iodinated tyrosine g.
    thalamogeniculate g. (TGG)
    g. viewing

growth
- g. acceleration
- g. arrest line
- g. center of bone
- g. center closure
- g. disc
- ectopic bone g.
- epiphysial chondroblastic g.
- g. factor
- g. hormone-producing adenoma
- g. impairment
- lepidic g.
- morphologic g.
- nutrient artery g.
- papillomatous g.
- g. parameter
- g. plate
- g. plate abscess
- g. plate arrest
- g. plate complex
- g. plate fracture
- g. plate injury
- g. plate widening
- g. retardation
- spinal g.
- targetoid g.
- twin pregnancy discordant g.
- Virchow law of skull g.

growth-retarded fetus

Gruber
- G. fossa
- petrosphenooccipital suture of G.
- G. suture

grumous
- g. debris
- g. tissue

Grüntzig
- G. balloon dilatation catheter
- G. PTCA technique

Grynfeltt triangle

GS
- gestational sac
- GS diameter

GSA
- galactosyl human serum albumin
- GSA imaging agent

Gsell-Erdheim syndrome

GSENSE
- generalized SENSE

GSPECT
- gated single-photon emission-computed tomography

GSW
- gunshot wound

GTD
- gestational trophoblastic disease

GTF-A
- Olympus Gastrocamera GTF-A

GTV
- gross tumor volume

GU
- gastric ulcer
- genitourinary
- GU tract cholesteatoma
- GU tract tuberculosis

GuardWire
- G. distal balloon
- G. Plus

gubernacular canal

Gubler
- G. line
- G. tumor

Guérin
- G. fold
- G. fracture
- G. sinus

Guglielmi
- G. detachable coil (GDC)
- G. detachable coil embolization

guidance
- active biplanar MR imaging g.
- angioscopic g.
- biplanar MR imaging g.
- computerized tomography g.
- fluoroscopic g.
- frameless stereotactic g.
- indirect ultrasound g.
- mammographic g.
- puncture g.
- radiologic g.
- sonographic g.
- g. system selection
- ultrasonic g.

Guidant
- G. Ancure endograft procedure
- G. Megalink peripheral stent

guide
- Brown-Roberts-Wells CT stereotactic g.
- BRW CT stereotaxic g.
- CT stereotactic g.
- side-exiting g.

guide-catheter

G

NOTES

guided
> g. biopsy
> g. drainage

guideline
> Mallinckrodt Institute of
>   Radiology g.
> MIR g.'s
> string g.

guidewire, guide wire, guide-wire
> Amplatz Super Stiff g.
> Athlete GT coronary g.
> color-coded g.
> Cope mandril g.
> g. entrapment
> exchange g.
> g. exchange technique
> extra stiff g.
> flexible-tip g.
> Flex-T g.
> Gold-tip micro g.
> Hi-Torque Floppy g.
> Hi-Torque Modified J-GW g.
> Hi-Torque steerable g.
> hydromer-coated micro g.
> hydrophilic-coated g.
> 0.016-inch Headliner g.
> 0.016-inch hydrophilic g.
> 0.035-inch hydrophilic angulated g.
> InQwire g.
> intracoronary Doppler flow g.
> J-tipped g.
> Katzen infusion g.
> Lunderquist exchange g.
> Lunderquist-Ring g.
> movable core g.
> Newton g.
> nitinol g.
> Nitrex ev3 g.
> Nitrex Nitinol g.
> Platinum Plus g.
> platinum tip g.
> Radifocus hydrophilic coated g.
> Ring g.
> Roadrunner NaviGuide g.
> Rosen curved g.
> Silver Speed 0.010-inch g.
> Sniper Elite hydrophilic g.
> Sniper Elite hydrophilic Ni-Ti
>   alloy g.
> standard fixed core g.
> stiff g.
> straight g.
> super-stiff g.
> SV-5 g.
> TAD steerable g.
> tapered core g.
> tapered-tip g.
> Teflon-coated g.
> torqueable g.

> Transend steerable g.
> V18 g.
> variable stiffness g.
> V18 Control Wire g.
> V18 micro g.
> WaveWire angioplasty g.
> x-shaped g.

guiding
> g. sheath
> g. shot

guillotine rib

guilt screen

Gumley seatbelt injury classification

gumma, pl. **gummas, gummata**
> frank cerebral g.
> g. of rib

gun
> automated biopsy g.
> Biopty biopsy g.
> electron g.

Gunn crossing sign

gunshot
> g. fracture
> g. wound (GSW)

gunstock deformity

Günther Tulip vena cava MReye filter

Günzberg ligament

gurgling cyst

Gustilo-Anderson
> G.-A. open clavicular fracture
> G.-A. tibial plafond fracture
>   classification

gut
> aging g.
> blind g.
> g. edema
> large g.
> primitive g.
> g. signature
> small g.

gut-associated lymphoid tissue (GALT)

Guthrie muscle

gutter
> anterolateral g.
> g. fracture
> lateral g.
> left g.
> paracolic g.
> parapelvic g.
> paravertebral g.
> peritoneal g.
> right g.
> sacral g.
> synovial g.

Guyon
> G. amputation
> G. canal

Gy
> gray

gymnast's wrist
Gynecare Versascope hysteroscope
gynecography
gynecoid pelvis
gynecologic endometriosis
gynecomastia
　　dendritic g.
gynecophoric canal
gynogram
gynography
gyral
　　g. abnormality
　　g. brain enhancement
　　g. crest
　　g. infarct
gyration
Gyratome
gyriform
　　g. calcification
　　g. pattern
gyromagnetic ratio
Gyroscan
　　G. ACS-NT
　　G. ACS-NT MRI scanner
　　G. ACS-NT MR unit
　　G. ACS-NT 1.5 T MR scanner
　　G. Interna scanner
　　G. NT 10 magnet
　　G. S15 scanner
　　G. 1.5T superconducting magnet
gyrus, pl. **gyri**
　　angular g. (AG)
　　ascending parietal g.
　　Broca g.
　　callosal g.
　　central g.
　　g. cerebelli
　　cingulate g.
　　contiguous supramarginal g.
　　dentate g.
　　G. endourology system
　　fasciolar g.
　　first temporal g.
　　flattening of g.

frontal g.
fusiform g.
Heschl transverse g.
hippocampal g.
inferior frontal g.
inferior temporal g.
infracalcarine g.
insular g.
g. isthmus fornicatus
lamination of g.
lateral occipitotemporal g.
lingual g.
marginal g.
medial occipitotemporal g.
middle frontal g.
middle temporal g.
occipital g.
occipitotemporal g.
olfactory g.
orbital g.
paracentral g.
parahippocampal g.
paraterminal g.
parietal g.
postcentral g.
posterior central g.
precentral g.
preinsular g.
quadrate g.
g. recti
sensorimotor g.
short insular g.
subcallosal g.
subcollateral g.
superior frontal g.
superior parietal lobule g.
superior temporal g.
supracallosal g.
supramarginal g.
temporal g.
transverse temporal g.
Turner marginal g.
uncal g.
uncinate g.

NOTES

G

413

H
   henry
   Holzknecht unit
   Hounsfield unit
   hydrogen
      H band
      H and D curve
      H disc
      H field of Forel
      H graft
      H ray
H-1
      H-1 MR spectroscopic imaging
      H-1 MR spectroscopy
H2
      H2 150-positron emission
         tomography
      H2 Score office-based diagnostic
         device
hν
   photon
H1 catheter
Haas
      H. method
      H. position
habenula, pl. **habenulae**
habenular commissure calcification
habitus
      body h.
      gracile h.
      large h.
      twisted body h.
HADD
   hydroxyapatite deposition disease
hadron therapy
HAEC
   Hirschsprung-associated enterocolitis
Hageman factor (HF)
Hagie pin
HAGL
   humeral avulsion of the glenohumeral
      ligament
   HAGL lesion
Haglund
      H. deformity
      H. syndrome
Hahn
      H. cleft
      H. spin-echo sequence
Hahn-Steinthal capitellum fracture
   classification
HAI
   hepatic arterial infusion
Haifa camera

Haines-McDougall medial sesamoid
   ligament
hair artifact
hairbrush pattern
hairline
      h. crack
      h. fracture
hair-on-end
      h.-o.-e. appearance
      h.-o.-e. periosteal reaction
      h.-o.-e. of skull
hairpin vessel
hairy heart
Hajdu-Cheney syndrome
half-axial
      h.-a. anteroposterior projection
      h.-a. view
half-body radiation therapy
half-dose enhanced MRI with MT
half-Fourier
      h.-F. acquisition single-shot turbo
         spin-echo (HASTE)
      h.-F. 3-dimensional technique
      h.-F. imaging (HFI)
      h.-F. RARE image
      h.-F. transformation technique
half-intensity needle
half-life (HL)
      antibody h.-l.
      biologic h.-l.
      biological h.-l.
      effective h.-l.
      elimination h.-l.
      h.-l. layer
      positronium h.-l.
      radioactive h.-l.
      short h.-l.
half-maximum
      full-width at h.-m.
half-moon
      h.-m. artifact
      h.-m. patella
      h.-m. shape
      h.-m. sign
half-Nex imaging
half-scan (HS)
      h.-s. with extrapolation (HE)
      h.-s. with extrapolation projection
half-thickness
      narrow-beam h.-t.
half-time
      blood clearance h.-t.
      clearance h.-t.
      h.-t. of exchange
      pressure h.-t.

H

415

halftone
    h. banding
    h. frequency
halftoning
    iterative h.
half-value layer (HVL)
half-wedged field technique
Hallermann-Streiff-François syndrome
hallmark
    radiofrequency radiographic h.
hallucal pronation
hallucis
    adductor h.
    hyperdynamic abductor h.
hallux
    h. abductovalgus
    h. dorsiflexion angle (DFA)
    h. elevatus
    h. extensus
    h. flexus deformity
    h. interphalangeal joint
    h. interphalangeus angle (HIA)
    intrinsic minus h.
    h. limitus (HL)
    h. malleus deformity
    h. migration
    h. rigidus
    h. rigidus deformity
    h. saltans
    h. sesamoid bone
    h. sesamoid complex
    h. valgus (HV)
    h. valgus angle (HVA)
    h. valgus deformity
    h. valgus interphalangeus angle
    h. valgus-metatarsus primus varus
      complex
    h. varus
    h. varus deformity
halo
    h. crown
    h. device
    h. effect
    fatty h.
    hypoechoic h.
    lucent h.
    nodule h.
    pericardial h.
    perinuclear h.
    periventricular h.
    radiolucent fat h.
    h. ring
    h. sign
    signal h.
    h. sign of hydrops
    sonolucent h.
    subendometrial h.
    h. vest
halofuginone probucol

halogenated
    h. phenolphthalein dye
    h. pyrimidine
    h. thymidine analog
    h. thymidine analog radiosensitizer
hamartoma, pl. **hamartomata**
    angiomatous lymphoid h.
    astrocytic h.
    benign fetal h.
    bile duct multiple h.
    brain h.
    breast h.
    cardiac h.
    cartilaginous h.
    chest wall h.
    chondromatous h.
    CNS cortical h.
    cortical h.
    duodenal wall h.
    eccrine angiomatous h.
    elevated retinal h.
    endobronchial h.
    extracerebral intracranial
      glioneural h.
    h. of eye
    fetal renal h.
    fibrolipomatous nerve h.
    fibrous h.
    glioneural h.
    hypothalamic h.
    h. of kidney
    leiomyomatous kidney h.
    lung h.
    lymphoid h.
    mesenchymal liver h.
    multiple bile duct hamartomas
    myoid h.
    pancreatic h.
    pigmented iris h.
    pulmonary h.
    renal h.
    retrorectal cystic h.
    h. spleen
    splenic h.
    subcortical CNS h.
    subependymal h.
    tuber cinereum h.
    vascular h.
    ventromedial hypothalamic h.
hamartomatosis
    generalized h.
hamartomatous
    h. gastric polyp
    h. lesion
hamate
    h. bone
    h. facet
    flake fracture of h.
    h. tail fracture

hamiltonian equation
Hamilton-Stewart formula for measuring cardiac output
Hamman-Rich syndrome
Hamman sign
hammered-brass appearance
hammered-silver
    h.-s. appearance
    h.-s. skull
hammer-marked skull
hammertoe deformity
hammocking of mitral valve leaflet
hammock ligament
Hampson unit
Hampton
    H. hump
    H. line
    H. maneuver
    H. technique
    H. view
hamstring tendon
hamulus
    pterygoideus h.
Hanafy piano-concave transducer design
hand
    h. angiography
    apelike h.
    bear's paw h.
    bipenniform muscles of h.
    Breuerton view of h.
    calcium pyrophosphate dihydrate h.
    chiasm of digit of h.
    CPPD arthritis of h.
    digital artery of h.
    h. and forearm artery scoring level I–V
    h. fracture
    hypothenar muscle groups of h.
    h. injection
    h. injection of contrast medium
    h. motor deficit
    opera-glass h.
    h. osteoarthritis
    phalanges of h.
    spadelike h.
    tangential layer of h.
    trident h.
    ulnar h.
    h. vascularization
    windswept h.
hand-agitated imaging agent

hand-carried ultrasound-guided pericardiocentesis
hand-held
    h.-h. exploring electrode probe
    h.-h. mapping probe
    h.-h. 8-MHz Doppler probe
handle
    Amplatz radiolucent h.
hand-shaped bend
hands-up ergonomics
hand/wrist arthritis
hanging
    h. heart
    h. hip
hanging-block technique
hanging-fruit pattern
hangman's fracture
Hann filter
Hannover canal
Hanot cirrhosis
Hansen fracture classification
HAP
    hepatic arterial phase
Hapad metatarsal arch
HAPE
    high-altitude pulmonary edema
HARC-C wavelet compression technique
hard
    h. disc herniation
    h. palate carcinoma
    h. papilloma
    h. ray
hard-copy image
hardened
    h. lung
    h. pelvis
hardening
    h. artifact
    beam h.
    bone h.
Hardy-Clapham sesamoid classification
Hare syndrome
Harken valve
harlequin sign
harmonic
    h. field
    h. function
    h. imaging
harmonics
    simultaneous acquisition of spatial h. (SMASH)
    spatial h.

NOTES

H

Harms cage
harness-shaped distribution
Harrington
    H. rod
    H. rod insertion
Harris
    H. band
    H. flush enema
    H. line
    H. tube
    H. view
Harris-Beath axial hindfoot view
Harrison
    H. curve
    H. groove
    H. sulcus
HART
    hyperfractionated accelerated radiation
      therapy
Hartmann
    H. closure of rectum
    H. point
    H. pouch
    H. solution
Harvard multidetector scanner
harvested vein
harvester's lung
Hashimoto thyroiditis
hashing
    image h.
HASTE
    half-Fourier acquisition single-shot turbo
      spin-echo
      magnetic resonance cholangiography
        with HASTE
      HASTE MRI
HAT
    head-arms-trunk
    HAT-transformed imaging
Hatcher-Smith cervical fusion
hatchet
    h. defect
    h. sign
hatchet-head deformity
**Hatle method to calculate mitral valve
area**
Hausdorff
    H. error
    H. measurement
haustral
    h. blunting
    h. fold
    h. indentation
    h. marking
    h. pattern
    h. pouch

haustration
haustrum, pl. **haustra**
    colonic haustra
Haut-Einheits-Dosis (HED)
    H.-E.-D. unit skin dose
haversian
    h. canal
    h. canaliculus
    h. channel
    h. fat pad
    h. gland
Hawkin hookwire
Hawkins
    H. accordion catheter drainage set
    H. accordion-type empyema
    H. breast lesion localization needle
    H. classification of talar fracture
    H. inside-out nephrostomy set
    H. line
    H. method
    H. sign
    H. 1-stick needle
    H. talar neck fracture classification
Hawkins-Akins needle
hay-fork sign
Haygarth node
hazard
    sandbag h.
haze
    hilar h.
haziness
    diffuse h.
    subtle h.
hazy
    h. density
    h. infiltrate
    h. opacity
hazy-opaque lung
HBCT
    helical biphasic contrast-enhanced CT
    HBCT imaging
HBE
    His bundle electrogram
HBI
    hemibody irradiation
    human blood index
HC
    head circumference
HC-AC
    head circumference-to-abdominal
     circumference
      HC-AC ratio
HCC
    hepatocellular carcinoma
      HCC chemoembolization
      fibrolamellar HCC
HCM
    hypertrophic cardiomyopathy

HCS
hematocystic spot
HCTA
helical computed tomographic
angiography
HCTE
helical CT-enteroclysis
H and D
Hurter and Driffield
HD
heart disease
Hirschsprung disease
Hodgkin disease
HDI
high-definition imaging
HDI 1000, 3000, 3500, 4000,
5000 ultrasound imaging system
HDIC
hepatodiaphragmatic interposition of
colon
HDR
high-dose rate
HE
half-scan with extrapolation
⁴He
helium 4
³He
helium 3
³He MRI
head
h. of barium column
cartilaginous cap of phalangeal h.
h. of caudate nucleus
h. circumference (HC)
circumference of fetal h.
h. circumference-to-abdominal
circumference (HC-AC)
h. coil
femoral h.
h. of femur
first metatarsal h. (FMH)
forward positioning of h.
h. of humerus
h. injury (HI)
ischemic necrosis of femoral h.
(INFH)
large fetal h.
long h.
metatarsal h.
h. and neck carcinoma
h. of pancreas
pancreatic h.

radial h.
radial facing of metacarpal h.
h. of rib
h. shape
short h.
strawberry-shaped h.
terminal h.
transillumination of h.
h. trauma
ulnar h.
ulnar facing of metacarpal h.
ureter cobra h.
3-head
3-h. gamma camera-based SPECT
system
3-h. scan
head-arms-trunk (HAT)
4-head camera
Headhunter catheter
Headisc
Headliner
headphones
Avotec MR-compatible h.
head-splitting humeral fracture
Heaf test
healed gastric ulcer
healing
bony h.
h. flare response
h. fracture
h. infarct
resorption phase of h.
h. ulcer
heart
abdominal h.
air-driven artificial h.
alcoholic h.
h. amyloidosis
angioreticuloendothelioma of h.
angiosarcoma of h.
h. anomaly
anterior border of h.
aortic opening of h.
apex of h.
apical surface of h.
armored h.
artificial h.
athlete's h.
axis of h.
balloon-shaped h.
base of h.
Baylor total artificial h.

NOTES

H

heart *(continued)*
beer h.
beriberi h.
h. block
boat-shaped h.
bony h.
booster h.
boot-shaped h.
h. border
bread-and-butter h.
h. bulb
cardiogenic shock h.
cervical h.
chamber of h.
3-chambered h.
chaotic h.
cloudy swelling of h.
conical h.
coronary artery of h.
h. count-mediastinum count ratio
  (H-M)
crisscross h.
H. CT scan
h. decortication
h. degeneration
dextroversion of h.
diaphragmatic surface of h.
h. disease (HD)
dome-shaped h.
donor h.
double density h.
drop h.
dynamite h.
dysrhythmia of fetal h.
egg-on-its-side h.
electrocardiogram-gated multislice
  spiral CT of h.
elongated h.
empty h.
encased h.
enlarged h.
h. failure (HF)
fatty h.
fetal h.
fibroid h.
h. fibroma
flabby h.
flask-shaped h.
globoid h.
h. and great vessels
hairy h.
hanging h.
Holmes h.
horizontal h.
hyperdynamic h.
hyperkinetic h.
hyperthyroid h.
hypertrophied h.
hypokinesis of h.

hypoplastic right h.
hypothermic h.
inferior border of h.
inflammation of h.
intermediate h.
irritable h.
ischemic h.
H. Laser
left border of h.
L-loop h.
malpositioned h.
massively enlarged h.
mesoversion of h.
mildly enlarged h.
movable h.
h. muscle necrosis
myxedema of h.
h. myxoma
myxoma of h.
ovoid h.
ox h.
paracorporeal h.
parasternal view of h.
parchment h.
pear-shaped h.
pectoral h.
pendulous h.
h. position
posterior border of h.
h. pseudoaneurysm
pulmonary h.
Quain fatty degeneration of h.
h. rate reserve mechanism
h. remnant
resting h.
rhabdomyoma of h.
right border of h.
right ventricle of h.
round h.
sabot h.
h. sac
h. scintigraphy
semihorizontal h.
semivertical h.
h. shadow
shift of h.
shoulder of h.
h. silhouette
single-outlet h.
snowman appearance of h.
soldier's h.
h. sound
spastic h.
squared-off h.
sternocostal surface of h.
stone h.
h. stroke volume
superior border of h.
superoinferior h.

suspended h.
swinging h.
systemic h.
h. tamponade
Taussig-Bing congenital
  malformation of h.
teardrop h.
thrush breast h.
thymoma of h.
tobacco h.
total artificial h.
h. transplant
transverse h.
Traube h.
triatrial h.
trilocular h.
h. tumor
univentricular h.
upstairs-downstairs h.
h. valve
h. valve calcification
h. valve leaflet
h. valve vegetation
venting of h.
1-ventricle h.
vertical h.
wandering h.
water-bottle h.

heartbeat gating
heart-lung
  h.-l. ratio (HLR)
  h.-l. transplant
heart-shaped
  h.-s. collimator
  h.-s. pelvis
  h.-s. uterus
heart-to-background ratio
heart-to-lung ratio (HLR)
heart-to-thorax volume
HeartView
  H. cardiac reconstruction software
  H. CT
  H. CT cardiac monitor
HearTwave EP
heat
  h. fracture
  h. shape
  h. shaping
  h. unit (HU)
heat-damaged ^{99m}**Tc-RBC**
heat-denatured autologous RBC SPECT
  imaging

heater
  resistance wire h.
heat-generating source
heating
  gamma h.
  hot-source h.
  interstitial conductive h.
  nonablative h.
heave
  h. and lift
  sustained left ventricular h.
heavily penetrated view
heaving precordial motion
heavy
  h. chain
  h. charged particle
  h. hydrogen
  h. ion imaging
  h. ion irradiation
  h. metal injection
  h. particle therapy
  h. water
heavy-chain disease
heavy-charged particle Bragg peak
  radiosurgery
heavy-duty standard exchange wire
heavy-particle irradiation
Heberden
  H. disease
  H. node
Hecht pneumonia
Hector
  tendon of H.
HED
  Haut-Einheits-Dosis
HEDP
  hydroxyethylidene-1,1-diphosphonic acid
heel
  black-dot h.
  h. bone
  h. effect
  h. fat pad
  h. pad thickening
  Sorbol h.
  h. spur
  h. tendon
  varus h.
Hegglin syndrome
Heidelberg
  H. protocol
  H. retina tomograph II (HRT II)

NOTES

H

Heidenhain
    H. pouch
    H. variant
height
        disc space h.
        intervertebral disc space h.
        knee joint space h.
        radial h.
        relative peak h.
        vertebral body h.
Heim-Kreysig sign
Heimlich MicroTrach
Heineke-Mikulicz maneuver
Heinig view
Heister
        valve of H.
helical
    h. biphasic computed tomography
    h. biphasic contrast-enhanced CT
      (HBCT)
    h. computed tomographic
      angiography (HCTA)
    h. CTA
    h. CT angiography
    h. CT-enteroclysis (HCTE)
    h. CT holography
    h. CT scanner
    h. CT scanning protocol
    h. hydro-CT
    h. pattern
    h. technique
    h. thin-section CT
    h. thin-section CT scan
helices (*pl. of* helix)
helicine artery
helicoid
Helios
    H. diagnostic imaging
    H. laser system
Helioseal
helium
    h. 3 (^{3}He)
    h. 4 (^{4}He)
    hyperpolarized h.
    h. ion beam
    h. magnetic resonance imaging
      (He-MRI)
helium-cadmium laser
helium-filled balloon catheter
helium-neon (HeNe)
    h.-n. laser
helix, pl. **helices, helixes**
    H. camera
    h. filter
helmet
    collimator h.
    h. field
Helmholtz
    H. axis ligament

    H. coil
    H. configuration
helminth
helminthic infestation
helminthoma
heloma
    h. durum
    h. molle
hemal
    h. arch
    h. canal
    h. node
hemangioblastoma
    capillary h.
    cerebelloretinal h.
    craniospinal h.
    cystic h.
    retinal h.
    spinal capillary h.
    third ventricular h.
hemangioblastomatosis
    cerebelloretinal h.
hemangioendothelial
    h. bone sarcoma
    h. liver sarcoma
hemangioendothelioma
    capillary h.
    epithelioid h.
    infantile h.
    kaposiform h. (KHE)
    malignant h.
    osseous h.
hemangioepithelioma
hemangiofibroma
hemangiolymphangioma
hemangioma, pl. **hemangiomata**
    arteriovenous h.
    bone capillary h.
    brain calcification h.
    capillary h.
    cardiac h.
    cavernous brain h.
    choroidal h.
    epidural cavernous h.
    epithelioid h.
    extraaxial cavernous h.
    extramedullary h.
    extremity h.
    facial h.
    giant cavernous h. (GCH)
    giant hepatic cavernous h. (GHCH)
    hepatic h.
    infantile hepatic h.
    intraarticular h.
    intramuscular h.
    liver capillary h.
    lung h.
    orbital capillary h.
    osseous h.

pediatric h.
pulmonary sclerosing h.
sclerosing h.
small bowel h.
soft tissue h.
splenic h.
subcutaneous h.
subglottic h.
synovial h.
trigeminal h.
umbilical cord h.
urinary bladder h.
vascular h.
venous h.
verrucous h.
vertebral h.
hemangiomatosis
pulmonary capillary h.
hemangiopericytoma
meningeal h.
primary pulmonary h.
renal h.
hemangiosarcoma
liver h.
hemarthrosis
hematobilia
hematocele
scrotal h.
hematocrit effect
hematocystic spot (HCS)
hematogenous
h. dissemination
h. embolus
h. osteomalacia
h. route
h. spread
h. tuberculosis
hematologic parameter
hematoma
acute intramural h.
acute subdural h.
adrenal h.
aneurysmal h.
aortic intramural h.
axillary h.
balancing subdural h.
basal ganglia h.
bladder flap h.
bowel wall h.
brain h.
breast h.
carotid plaque h.

chronic subdural h. (CSDH)
corpus luteum h.
delayed traumatic intracerebral h.
  (DTICH)
dissecting aortic h.
dissecting intramural h.
dural h.
encapsulated subdural h.
epidural h. (EDH)
evolving h.
extracerebral h.
extradural brain h.
h. formation
gelatinous h.
hemispheral h.
infected pelvic h.
interhemispheric subdural h.
intermuscular h.
interstitial loculated h.
intracerebral h.
intracranial h.
intramural h.
intraparenchymal h.
intrarenal h.
intraventricular h.
isodense subdural h.
mediastinal h.
mural h.
nasal septum h.
nasopharyngeal h.
organized h.
parenchymal h.
perianal h.
periaortic mediastinal h.
pericardial h.
peridiaphragmatic h.
perigraft h.
perinephric h.
perirenal h.
posterior fossa h.
postoperative breast h.
primary intracerebral h.
rectal sheath h.
retromembranous h.
retroperitoneal h.
retropharyngeal h.
retroplacental h.
scalp h.
spontaneous h.
subacute subdural h.
subcapsular renal h.
subchorionic h.

NOTES

H

hematoma *(continued)*
    subdural interhemispheric h.
    subfascial h.
    subgaleal h.
    submembranous placental h.
    subperiosteal h.
    umbilical cord h.
hematomediastinum
hematometra
hematomyelia
hematopericardium
hematopoiesis
    extramedullary h.
hematopoietic
    h. bone marrow
    h. reticulum
hematopoietically active bone marrow
hematoporphyrin derivative
  photosensitizing agent (HpD)
hematosalpinx
hematoxylin and eosin stain
hemiagenesis
hemianopsia
    altitudinal h.
hemiarch
hemiatrophy
    cerebral h.
hemiaxial view
hemiazygos vein
hemiballismus
hemiblock
    left anterosuperior h. (LASH)
    left bundle branch h.
hemibody
    h. irradiation (HBI)
    h. radiotherapy
hemicardium
hemic calculus
hemicolon
hemicondylar fracture
hemicord
hemicranium
hemidecortication
    cerebral h.
hemidesmosome
hemidiaphragm
    accessory h.
    h. attenuation
    h. depression
    h. rupture
    tenting of h.
hemidiaphragmatic
hemifacial
    h. microsomia
    h. spasm
hemihypertrophy
hemimegalencephaly
    ipsilateral h.
hemimelia

hemimelica
    bilateral dysplasia epiphysialis h.
    dysplasia epiphysialis h.
hemimyelocele
hemiparkinsonism
hemipelvis
hemiplegia
    congenital h.
    infantile h.
    spinal h.
hemiscrotum
hemisection
    spinal cord h.
hemisensory syndrome
hemispheral
    h. hematoma
    h. mass effect
hemisphere
    h. atrophy
    cerebellar h.
    cerebral h.
    h. damage
    dominant h.
    left h.
    h. lesion
    mesial h.
    right h.
    h. stroke
    swollen brain h.
hemispheric
    h. demyelinating lesion
    h. infarct
    h. regional lateralization difference
    h. vein
hemithorax, pl. hemithoraces
    frozen h.
    h. opacification
hemitransverse fracture
hemitruncus
hemivertebra
    balanced h.
    unbalanced h.
hemivertebral
hemizygosity
Hemobahn
    H. endoprosthesis
    H. PTFE-covered stent-graft
    H. stent
    H. stent graft
Hemochron
HemoCue photometer
hemodialysis catheter
hemodialysis-related venous stenosis
hemodynamic
    h. alteration
    h. assessment
    h. decompensation
    h. effect
    h. format

h. impotence
h. index
h. pattern
h. penumbra
h. reserve impairment
h. response
hemodynamically
  h. significant lesion
  h. significant stenosis
  h. weighted echo-planar MR
    imaging
hemolymph node
hemolytic splenomegaly
hemolyticuremic syndrome
hemomediastinum
hemoperfusion
hemopericardium
hemoperitoneum
hemophilic pseudotumor
hemopneumothorax
hemorrhage
  abdominal h.
  acute subarachnoid h.
  adrenal h.
  alveolar h.
  anastomotic h.
  aneurysmal h.
  antepartum h.
  arterial h.
  8-ball h.
  basilar intracerebral h.
  bladder h.
  brainstem h.
  brain stenosis h.
  bulbar intracerebral h.
  capillary h.
  carotid h.
  catheter-induced pulmonary
    artery h.
  cerebellar h.
  cerebral h.
  cerebromeningeal intracerebral h.
  choroid plexus h.
  chronic parenchymal h.
  colonic diverticular h.
  colorectal h.
  concealed h.
  h. consolidation
  cortical intracerebral h.
  delayed traumatic intracerebral h.
  diffuse pulmonary alveolar h.
  diffuse subarachnoid h.

Duret h.
epidural h.
exsanguinating h.
external h.
extradural h.
extraluminal h.
extramural h.
extrapleural h.
first-trimester h.
focal area of h.
focal endocardial h.
focal pulmonary h.
frank h.
gastric h.
gastrointestinal renal transplant h.
hypertensive brain h.
hypothalamic h.
infant gastrointestinal h.
internal capsule intracerebral h.
interstitial h.
intertrabecular h.
intraabdominal arterial h.
intracerebral h. (ICH)
intracranial subarachnoid h.
intradural h.
intraluminal h.
intramural arterial h.
intramural gastrointestinal tract h.
intraparenchymal h.
intraplaque h. (IPH)
intrapleural h.
intrapontine intracerebral h.
intrapulmonary h.
intrathecal h.
intratumoral h.
intraventricular h. (IVH)
intraventricular neonate h.
labyrinthine h.
life-threatening h.
lobar intracerebral h.
lower gastrointestinal h.
lung h.
massive exsanguinating h.
mediastinal h.
meningeal h.
multifocal h.
neonatal choroid plexus h.
neonatal intracerebellar h.
neonatal intracranial h.
neonatal intraventricular h.
neonatal subdural h.

NOTES

H

hemorrhage *(continued)*
  nonaneurysmal perimesencephalic subarachnoid h.
  nondominant putaminal h.
  nontraumatic epidural h.
  obstetrical h.
  old h.
  pancreatic h.
  periaqueductal h.
  peribronchial h.
  perigestational h.
  perimesencephalic nonaneurysmal subarachnoid h.
  perinephric space h.
  perirenal h.
  placental h.
  plaque h.
  pontine h.
  postoperative mediastinal h.
  posttraumatic h.
  preplacental h.
  pulmonary artery h.
  putaminal h.
  retrobulbar h.
  retroperitoneal h.
  retropharyngeal h.
  retroplacental h.
  salmon-patch h.
  sentinel transoral h.
  slit h.
  small bowel h.
  spinal epidural h. (SEH)
  spinal subarachnoid h.
  spinal subdural h. (SSH)
  spontaneous renal h.
  striate h.
  subacute h.
  subarachnoid h. (SAH)
  subchorionic h.
  subcortical intracerebral h.
  subdural h. (SDH)
  subependymal h.
  subgaleal h.
  submassive h.
  submucosal h.
  subperiosteal h.
  subserosal h.
  thalamic h.
  traumatic meningeal h.
  upper gastrointestinal h.
  variceal h.
  venous h.
  ventricular intracerebral h.
  vitreous h.

hemorrhagic
  h. brain infarct
  h. bronchopneumonia
  h. consolidation of lung
  h. corpus luteum cyst
  h. duodenitis
  h. focus
  h. hereditary telangiectasia
  h. lesion
  h. lung nodule
  h. mediastinal adenopathy
  h. metastasis
  h. necrosis
  h. ovarian cyst
  h. pericarditis
  h. pleural effusion
  h. pleurisy
  h. pneumonia
  h. pulmonary edema
  h. salpingitis
  h. stroke
  h. transformation

hemorrhagicum
  corpus h.

hemorrhoidal plexus

hemosiderosis
  idiopathic pulmonary h.

hemostatic puncture closure device

hemosuccus pancreaticus

hemothorax, pl. **hemothoraces**

hemp seed calculus

He-MRI
  helium magnetic resonance imaging
  dynamic ventilation He-MRI

Henderson fracture

Henderson-Jones chondromatosis

HeNe
  helium-neon
  HeNe laser

Henke
  H. triangle
  H. trigone

Henle
  H. canal
  jejunal interposition of H.
  jejunal loop interposition of H.
  H. ligament
  loop of H.
  H. sheath
  trapezoid bone of H.

Hennekam syndrome

Henoch-Schönlein syndrome

henry (H)
  master knot of H.
  vertebral artery of H.

Henschke
  H. afterloader
  H. seed applicator

Hensen
  H. canal
  H. node
  H. plane

Hensing
    H. fold
    H. ligament
hen worker's lung
hepar lobatum
hepatic
    h. abscess
    h. adenoma
    h. anaplastic sarcoma
    h. angiography
    h. angiomyolipoma
    h. angiosarcoma
    h. angle
    h. architecture
    h. arterial anastomosis
    h. arterial dominant
    h. arterial infusion (HAI)
    h. arterial phase (HAP)
    h. arteriography
    h. arteriovenous fistula
    h. artery
    h. artery anatomy
    h. artery aneurysm
    h. artery-portal vein fistula
    h. artery pseudoaneurysm
    h. artery stenosis
    h. artery system
    h. artery thrombosis
    h. bed
    h. bleeding
    h. calcification
    h. calculus
    h. capsular rupture
    h. capsule
    h. carcinoma
    h. chemoembolization
    h. cirrhosis
    h. congestion
    h. cord
    h. cyst
    h. degeneration
    h. diverticulum
    h. duct
    h. ductal system
    h. duct bifurcation
    h. echo pattern
    h. failure
    h. fibrosis
    h. fissure
    h. flexure
    h. fungal infection
    h. hemangioma

    h. hilum
    h. hydrothorax
    h. insufficiency
    h. ligament
    h. lipoma
    h. lobe
    h. lymph node
    h. metabolism
    h. metastasis
    h. necrosis
    h. neoplasm
    h. nerve plexus
    h. outflow tract
    h. parenchyma
    h. pattern echo
    h. resistive artery index
    h. sarcoidosis
    h. sclerosis
    h. sinusoid
    h. steatosis
    h. test of Glass
    h. transplant
    h. trauma
    h. tumor
    h. vein
    h. vein disease
    h. vein thrombosis
    h. venography
    h. venoocclusive disease
    h. venous outflow
    h. venous outflow obstruction
    h. venous pressure gradient
    h. venous system
    h. web
    h. web dilatation
    h. wedge pressure (HWP)
hepatica fibrosa
hepaticojejunostomy
    percutaneous h.
hepatis
    parenchymal peliosis h.
    phlebectatic peliosis h.
    porta h.
    sagittal porta h.
hepatitis, pl. hepatitides
    acute h.
    chronic h.
    neonatal h.
    radiation h.
    recurrent pyogenic h.
hepatization
    lung h.

NOTES

hepatobiliary
  h. carcinoma
  h. contrast agent
  h. disease
  h. ductal system imaging
  h. pathway
  h. scan
  h. scintigraphy
  h. tree
hepatoblastoma
hepatocarcinogenesis
hepatocarcinoma
  fibrolamellar h.
hepatocellular
  h. adenoma
  h. carcinoma (HCC)
  h. dysfunction
hepatocerebral
  h. degeneration
  h. disease
hepatocholescintigraphy
hepatoclavicular view
hepatocolic ligament
hepatocystocolic ligament
hepatocyte tracer uptake
hepatodiaphragmatic
  h. interposition
  h. interposition of colon (HDIC)
hepatoduodenal ligament
hepatoesophageal ligament
hepatofugal flow
hepatogastric ligament
hepatogastroduodenal ligament
hepatogram
  emission h.
hepatography
hepatoid adenocarcinoma
hepatoiminodiacetic
  h. acid (HIDA)
  h. acid scan
hepatojejunal anastomosis
hepatojugular reflux
hepatolenticular degeneration
hepatolienography
Hepatolite
  H. imaging agent
  technetium-99m H.
hepatolithiasis
hepatoma
hepatomalacia
hepatomegaly
hepatopancreatic
  h. ampulla
  h. fold
hepatopancreatica
  ampulla h.
hepatopathy
hepatopetal flow
hepatophlebography

hepatophrenic ligament
hepatopleural fistula
hepatoportal
  h. biliary fistula
  h. sclerosis
hepatoportoenterostomy
hepatoptosis
hepatorenal
  h. angle
  h. fossa
  h. ligament
  h. pouch
  h. recess
  h. saphenous vein bypass graft
  h. syndrome (HRS)
hepatoscan
hepatosplenic
hepatosplenography
hepatosplenomegaly (HSM)
hepatoumbilical ligament
herald
  h. bleed
  h. patch lesion
Herbert-Fisher fracture classification
Herbert scaphoid bone fracture
Hercules
  H. 7000 mobile x-ray unit
  H. power injector
hereditary
  h. amyloidosis
  h. flat adenoma syndrome
  h. multiple cartilaginous exostoses
  h. multiple exostoses (HME)
  h. nonpolyposis colorectal cancer
    (HNPCC)
  h. nonpolyposis colorectal
    carcinoma (HNPCC)
  h. predisposition
  h. stenosis of the aqueduct of
    Sylvius (HSAS)
Hering canal
Hermansky-Pudlak syndrome
hermaphroditism
  true h.
HERMES system
Hermodsson
  H. fracture
  H. tangential projection
Herndon hump
hernia, pl. **herniae**
  abdominal wall h.
  axial hiatal h.
  Barth h.
  Beclard h.
  Bochdalek h.
  broad ligament h.
  h. canal
  cecal h.
  concentric h.

congenital diaphragmatic h.
h. defect
diaphragmatic h.
direct inguinal h.
duodenal h.
epigastric h.
esophageal h.
external h.
femoral h.
funicular inguinal h.
gastric h.
hiatal h.
Holthouse h.
incarcerated h.
incisional h.
incomplete h.
indirect inguinal h.
inguinal h.
internal h.
interstitial h.
intrapericardial diaphragmatic h.
Lesgaft h.
lesser sac h.
Littre h.
lumbar h.
mediastinal h.
mixed h.
Morgagni h.
obturator h.
ovarian h.
pantaloon h.
paraduodenal h.
paraesophageal h.
parahiatal h.
paraileostomal h.
h. paralysis
parastomal h.
peritoneal h.
peritoneopericardial diaphragmatic h.
h. pouch
properitoneal h.
Richter h.
Rieux h.
rolling hiatal h.
h. rupture
h. sac
scrotal h.
short esophagus–type hiatal h.
sliding hiatal h.
spigelian h.
strangulated inguinal h.
transient hiatal h.

traumatic diaphragmatic h.
Treitz h.
tubular hiatal h.
ultrasound-guided reduction of a
　spigelian h.
umbilical h.
ventral h.
hernial aneurysm
herniated
　h. abdominal content
　h. bowel
　h. bowel loop
　h. intervertebral disc (HID)
　h. nucleus pulposus (HNP)
　h. preperitoneal fat
herniation
　brain tissue h.
　central h.
　cerebral h.
　cervical disc h.
　cingulate h.
　cisternal h.
　concentric h.
　diencephalic h.
　disc h.
　fat lung h.
　focal disc h.
　focal nuclear h.
　foramen magnum h.
　frank disc h.
　free-fragment disc h.
　hard disc h.
　hippocampal h.
　impending h.
　intercervical disc h.
　internal disc h.
　intradural disc h.
　intraspongy nuclear disc h.
　lateral disc h.
　lumbosacral intervertebral disc h.
　nuclear h.
　nucleus pulposus h.
　pancreatic h.
　phalangeal h.
　physiologic h.
　h. pit
　posterolateral disc h.
　soft disc h.
　subfalcine h.
　subligamentous disc h.
　supraligamentous disc h.
　temporal lobe h.

NOTES

herniation *(continued)*
  tentorial notch h.
  thoracic disc h.
  tonsillar h.
  transtentorial h.
  uncal h.
herniography
heroin vapor leukoencephalopathy
herophili
  torcular h.
herpes
  h. esophagitis
  h. simplex virus (HSV)
  h. simplex virus 1 (HSV1)
  h. simplex virus 1 kinase (HSV1-tk)
  h. simplex virus type 1 encephalitis
herpesvirus (HV)
  human h. (HHV)
  h. pneumonia
herpetic whitlow
herringbone pattern
Herring tube
hertz (Hz)
Herxheimer fiber
Heschl
  H. convolution
  H. transverse gyrus
Hesselbach
  H. ligament
  H. triangle
herocladic anastomosis
heterocyclic free radical
heterogeneity
heterogeneous
  h. appearance
  h. breast mass
  h. carotid plaque
  h. color speckling
  h. hyperattenuation
  h. internal echo pattern
  h. isodense enhancement
  h. microdistribution
  h. perfusion pattern
  h. radiation
  h. signal intensity
  h. uptake
heterogenicity
heterophilic leukocyte
heterotaxia, heterotaxy
  abdominal h.
  visceral h.
heterotopia
  band h.
  cerebellar h.
  gastric h.
  gray matter h.
  subependymal h.

heterotopic
  h. bone
  h. bone formation
  h. gray matter
  h. nodule
  h. pancreas
  h. pregnancy
  h. scar ossification
  h. white matter island
Heubner
  H. artery
  recurrent artery of H.
Hewlett-Packard (HP)
  H.-P. color flow imager
  H.-P. phased-array ultrasound imaging system
  H.-P. scanner
  H.-P. ultrasound
Hexabrix imaging agent
hexadactyly
hexafluoride
  sulfur h. (SF_6)
hexagonal configuration
hexametazime (HMPAO)
hexamethylpropyleneamine oxime (HMPAO)
hexokinase reaction
Hey
  H. amputation
  H. ligament
HF
  Hageman factor
  heart failure
  hippocampal formation
  HF infrared laser
HFA-134a
  ^{18}F-labeled H.
HFD
  high-frequency Doppler
HFI
  half-Fourier imaging
H-graft
  Gallie H-g.
HGSIL
  high-grade squamous intraepithelial lesion
HHV
  human herpesvirus
HI
  head injury
HIA
  hallux interphalangeus angle
5-HIAA
  5-hydroxyindoleacetic acid
hiatal hernia
hiatus
  adductor h.
  aortic h.
  crus h.

diaphragmatic esophageal h.
esophageal h.
patulous h.
popliteal h.
h. semilunaris
Hibbs metatarsocalcaneal angle
hibernating myocardium
hibernation
myocardial h.
hibernoma
Hickey
H. method
H. position
Hickman
H. line
H. long-term catheter
H. tunneled indwelling catheter
hickory-stick fracture
HID
herniated intervertebral disc
HIDA
hepatoiminodiacetic acid
HIDA imaging
HIDA scan
TechneScan HIDA
hidebound small bowel fold
hierarchical
h. information
h. scanning pattern
Hieshima microcatheter
HIFU
high-intensity focused ultrasound
high
h. arch
h. brachial artery catheterization
h. cervical spinal cord lesion
h. defect
h. endothelial venule
h. filling pressure
h. Fowler position
h. frame rate
H. Frequency Induced Thermo-Treatment (HiTT)
h. gradient field strength
h. hydrophilicity
h. interstitial pressure
h. jugular bulb (HJB)
h. lateral wall myocardial infarct
h. left main diagonal artery
h. linear energy transfer radiation
h. normal
h. pitch

h. pontine lesion
h. pulse repetition frequency Doppler
h. reflectivity
h. right atrial electrogram (HRA)
h. right atrium (HRA)
h. signal intensity
h. small bowel obstruction
h. spatial frequency reconstruction algorithm
h. spatial resolution algorithm
h. spatial resolution cine computed tomography (HSRCCT)
h. spatial resolution cine CT
h. spatial resolution mode
h. spin
h. takeoff
h. temporal resolution
h. temporal resolution mode
h. tibial osteotomy
h. torque
h. velocity
h. wedge pressure
high-altitude pulmonary edema (HAPE)
high-amplitude
h.-a. echo
h.-a. impulse
high-attenuation stone
high-caliber, low-velocity handgun injury
high-contrast film
high-definition
h.-d. 3-dimensional analysis
h.-d. imaging (HDI)
high-density
h.-d. barium
h.-d. barium imaging agent
h.-d. lesion
h.-d. linear array
h.-d. rim
h.-d. structure
high-dose
h.-d. film dosimeter
h.-d. film dosimetry
h.-d. radiotherapy
h.-d. rate (HDR)
h.-d. therapy
high-dose-rate
h.-d.-r. intracavitary radiation therapy
h.-d.-r. remote afterloading

NOTES

high-energy
  h.-e. bent-beam linear accelerator
  h.-e. imaging
  511-keV h.-e. imaging
  h.-e. laser
  h.-e. proton
  h.-e. trauma
high-field
  h.-f. open MRI scanner
  h.-f. system
high-field-strength
  h.-f.-s. MR imaging
  h.-f.-s. scanner
Highflex large stone retrieval basket
high-flow arteriovenous fistula
high-frame-rate run
high-frequency
  h.-f. Doppler (HFD)
  h.-f. Doppler ultrasound
  h.-f. Doppler ultrasound imaging
  h.-f. miniature probe
  h.-f. therapeutic ultrasound
  h.-f. transducer
high-grade
  h.-g. AV block
  h.-g. glioma
  h.-g. infiltrative astrocytoma
  h.-g. malignancy
  h.-g. narrowing
  h.-g. obstruction
  h.-g. obstructive lesion
  h.-g. partial tear
  h.-g. proximal stenosis
  h.-g. signal intensity
  h.-g. squamous intraepithelial lesion (HGSIL)
  h.-g. surface osteogenic sarcoma
  h.-g. surface osteosarcoma
  h.-g. tumor
high-heat-capacity x-ray tube
high-impedance circulation
high-intensity
  h.-i. focused ultrasound (HIFU)
  h.-i. focus ultrasound
  h.-i. lesion
  h.-i. signal
  h.-i. transient signal (HITS)
  h.-i. zone (HIZ)
high-kV technique
highly
  h. mobile echo
  h. reflective echo
  h. vascular tumor
high-lying patella
high-minute ventilation

Highmore
  antrum of H.
  H. antrum
high-osmolar contrast agent (HOCA)
high-osmolarity contrast medium (HOCM)
high-output
  h.-o. heart failure
  h.-o. state
high-pass filter
high-performance
  h.-p. liquid chromatography
  h.-p. size-exclusion chromatography
high-pitched signal
high-powered field (hpf)
high-pressure
  h.-p. Blue Max balloon
  h.-p. liquid chromatography
  h.-p. mercury arc lamp
high-probability lesion
high-pulse repetition frequency Doppler echocardiography
high-purity germanium (HPGe)
high-quality pitch
high-rate
  h.-r. detect interval
  h.-r. ventricular response
high-resolution
  h.-r. B-mode imaging
  h.-r. bone algorithm technique
  h.-r. collimator
  h.-r. computed tomography (HRCT)
  h.-r. coronal cut
  h.-r. CT imaging
  h.-r. CT mammography
  h.-r. 3DFT MR imaging
  h.-r. diffraction
  h.-r. 3D microcomputed tomography
  h.-r. 3D spoiled-GRASS image
  h.-r., fan-beam collimator
  h.-r. fluoroscopy
  h.-r. infrared (HRI)
  h.-r. infrared imaging
  h.-r. linear array transducer
  h.-r., low-speed radiography
  h.-r. magnetic resonance (HR-MR)
  h.-r. magnification
  h.-r. MRI (HR-MRI)
  h.-r. multileaf collimator
  h.-r. multisweep (HRMS)
  h.-r. storage phosphor imaging
  h.-r. storage phosphor managing
  h.-r. transverse view image
  h.-r. ultrasound
  h.-r. ultrasound scanning
  h.-r. volumetric sequence
high-riding
  h.-r. patella
  h.-r. scapula

h.-r. third ventricle
h.-r. variant
high-sensitivity measurement
high-signal
   h.-s. abnormality
   h.-s. intratendinous collection of
    fluid
   h.-s. lesion
   h.-s. mass
high-signal-intensity
   h.-s.-i. ischemic change
   h.-s.-i. yellow marrow
   h.-s.-i. zone
high-speech pitch
high-speed
   h.-s. gradient coil
   h.-s. imaging
HighSpeed CT scanner
high-tech-low-touch examination
   environment
high-temperature diffraction
high-temporal-resolution cine computed
   tomography (HTRCCT)
high-velocity
   h.-v. flow
   h.-v. gunshot wound
   h.-v. jet
   h.-v. signal loss
high-voltage
   h.-v. generator
   h.-v. pulsed galvanic stimulation
    (HVPGS)
   h.-v. radiotherapy
   h.-v. roentgen therapy
   h.-v. stimulation (HVS)
   h.-v. transformer
hila (*pl. of* hilum)
   h. measurement
Hilal
   H. embolization apparatus
   H. microcoil
hilar
   h. adenopathy
   h. area
   h. artery
   h. cap
   h. cell tumor of ovary
   h. cholangiocarcinoma
   h. displacement
   h. extension
   h. gland
   h. haze

h. height ratio
h. kidney lip
h. lipoma
h. lymph node
h. mass
h. obstruction
h. plate
h. prominence
h. reaction
h. shadow
h. sign
h. structure
h. tumor
h. vessel
Hildreth sign
Hilgenreiner
   H. acetabular index
   H. epiphysial angle
   H. line
HiLight Advantage System CT scanner
Hillock arch
Hill-Sachs
   H.-S. defect (HSD)
   H.-S. deformity
   H.-S. dislocation
   H.-S. posterolateral compression
    fracture
   H.-S. shoulder lesion
Hill sign
Hilton
   H. law
   H. muscle
hilum, pl. **hila**
   central fatty h.
   hepatic h.
   kidney h.
   lip of h.
   lung h.
   pruned h.
   pulmonary h.
   renal h.
   splenic h.
   waterfall h.
hilus of tendon
Hinchey classification
hindbrain
   h. deformity
   h. dysgenesis
   h. malformation
hindfoot
   h. deformity
   h. instability

NOTES

hindfoot *(continued)*
  h. joint complex
  h. valgus
hindgut
  h. duplication
  primitive h.
Hine-Duley phantom
hinged implant
hinge joint
hip
  h. bone
  h. bump
  h. capsule joint
  congenital dislocation of h. (CDH)
  congenital dysplasia of h.
  developmental dysplasia of h.
    (DDH)
  h. disarticulation
  dislocated h.
  h. dislocation
  h. dysplasia
  external snapping h.
  h. flexion contracture
  h. fracture
  frogleg view of h.'s
  hanging h.
  h. hump
  h. joint space
  h. muscle cross section
  h. pinning
  h. pointer
  h. protrusion
  h. replacement
  snapping h.
  transient osteoporosis of h.
  transient synovitis of h.
Hipper twist release coil
hippocampal
  h. atrophy
  h. fissure
  h. formation (HF)
  h. gyrus
  h. head, body, and tail
  h. herniation
  h. infarct
  h. magnetic resonance volumetry
  h. sclerosis
  h. sulcus
  h. volume
hippocampal-amygdaloid complex
hippocampus
  electronic atlas of h.
hippocratic finger
hippuran
  I h.
Hippuran imaging agent
hip-to-ankle view
Hirschberg sign

Hirschfeld canal
**Hirschsprung-associated enterocolitis
  (HAEC)**
Hirschsprung disease (HD)
His
  H. angle
  H. band
  H. bundle
  H. bundle electrogram (HBE)
  H. canal
  H. line
  H. spindle
His-Haas muscle transfer
**HiSonic ultrasonic bone conduction
  hearing device**
HiSpeed
  H. Advantage helical scanner
  H. Advantage System CT scanner
Hi-Star MRI system
histiocyte
  sinusoidal h.
histiocytic
  h. bone lymphoma
  h. bone tumor origin
  h. brain lymphoma
  h. chest lymphoma
histiocytoma
  angiomatoid malignant fibrous h.
  atypical benign fibrous h.
  benign fibrous h.
  fibrous h.
  malignant fibrous h. (MFH)
  malignant fibrous osseous h.
  myxoid malignant fibrous h.
  primary pulmonary malignant
    fibrous h.
  scrotal h.
  storiform-pleomorphic malignant
    fibrous h.
histiocytosis
  diffuse cerebral h.
  Langerhans lung cell h.
  sinus h.
  h. X
Histoacryl
  30–50% H.
  H. embolic agent
histogenesis
histogram
  average diffusivity h.
  dose-surface h.
  dose-volume h. (DVH)
  h. equalization
  h. equalization algorithm
  gaussian dose-volume h.
  gray-level h.
  hose-volume h.
  integrated optical density h.

multisectional dose-volume h.
volume h.
histogram-derived metrics
histograph
Eppendorf pO$_2$ h.
histologic
h. correlation
h. grade
histology
bone h.
histomorphometric
h. image
h. measurement
histomorphometry
bone h.
plaque h.
histopathologic
h. comparison
h. CT correlation
histopathology
ischemic h.
histoplasmoma
histoplasmosis
disseminated CNS h.
lung h.
pulmonary h.
historadiography
history
problem-focused h.
Hitachi
H. Altaire Open MRI system
H. CT scanner
H. EUB-555 diagnostic ultrasound
system
H. four-head system
H. MR scanner
H. Open MRI system scanner
H. rotating detector array system
H. SPECT 2000H-40 camera
H. 0.3-T unit scanner
H. ultrasound
hitch-hiker's thumb
Hi-Torque
H.-T. Floppy guidewire
H.-T. Modified J-GW guidewire
H.-T. steerable guidewire
HITS
high-intensity transient signal
HiTT
High Frequency Induced Thermo-
Treatment

HIV
human immunodeficiency virus
HIV encephalitis
HIV encephalopathy
HIV esophagitis
HIV nephropathy
HIV-related TB
HIZ
high-intensity zone
HJB
high jugular bulb
HL
half-life
hallux limitus
HLA
human leukocyte antigen
HLA imaging
HLA-A3 histocompatibility antigen
HLA-B14 histocompatibility antigen
HLA-B7 histocompatibility antigen
HLHS
hypoplastic left heart syndrome
HLR
heart-lung ratio
heart-to-lung ratio
H-M
heart count-mediastinum count ratio
HMD
hyaline membrane disease
HME
hereditary multiple exostoses
H-mode echocardiography
HMPAO
hexametazime
hexamethylpropyleneamine oxime
^{99m}Tc HMPAO
1H-MRS
single voxel proton MR spectroscopy
HN
Huckman number
HNP
herniated nucleus pulposus
HNPCC
hereditary nonpolyposis colorectal cancer
hereditary nonpolyposis colorectal
carcinoma
Hobb view
hobnail liver
HOC
hypertrophic obstructive cardiomyopathy
HOCA
high-osmolar contrast agent

NOTES

H

hockey-stick
    h.-s. appearance of catheter tip
    h.-s. appearance of ureter
    h.-s. catheter
    h.-s. deformity of tricuspid valve
    h.-s. fracture
    h.-s. guiding sheath
    h.-s. tricuspid valve deformity
HOCM
    high-osmolarity contrast medium
    hypertrophic obstructive cardiomyopathy
Hodge plane
Hodgkin
    H. disease (HD)
    H. granuloma
    H. lymphoma
    H. tumor
Hodgson
    H. aneurysmal dilatation of aorta
    H. disease
Hodson-type kidney
Hoffa
    H. disease
    H. fat pad
    H. fracture
Hoffmann
    H. atrophy
    H. sign
Hofmeister
    H. anastomosis
    H. procedure
Hohl tibial condylar fracture classification
hold
    single breath-h.
Holdaway ratio
holder
    limb h.
    Vogele-Bale-Hohner head h.
Holdsworth spinal fracture classification
holdup in flow of barium
hole
    black h.
    h. pattern
hole-within-hole
    h.-w.-h. appearance
    h.-w.-h. bone lesion
holiday heart syndrome
Holl ligament
hollow
    h. albumin microsphere
    h. bone
    h. chest
    h. foot
    h. organ
    h. ribbon
    h. structure
    h. viscus
    h. viscus injury

hollow-point bullet
holly leaf appearance
Holmes
    H. cortical cerebellar degeneration
    H. heart
    H. syndrome
holmium
    h. 166
    h. imaging agent
    h. laser
holmium-YLF
holmium-yttrium-aluminum-garnet (Ho:YAG)
    h.-y.-a.-g. laser
holoacardia
holocord
    h. hydromyelia
    h. syringohydromyelia
Hologic
    H. 2000 densitometer
    H. QDR 1000W dual-energy x-ray absorptiometry scanner
    H. 2000 scanner
holography
    computerized tomographic h. (CTH)
    helical CT h.
    h. imaging
    medical h.
    multiple-exposure volumetric h.
    volumetric multiplexed transmission h.
    Voxgram multiple-exposure h.
holoprosencephaly
    alobar h.
    lobar h.
    microform of h.
    semilobar h.
holosystolic
    h. gradient
    h. mitral valve prolapse
holoventricle
Holstein-Lewis fracture
Holthouse hernia
Holt-Oram syndrome
Holzknecht
    H. space
    H. unit (H)
Holz phlegmon
home infusion care
homeostasis
    brain h.
Homer
    H. Mammalok needle
    H. needle/wire localizer
Homerlok needle
homing
    h. mechanism
    h. molecule
homogeneity

homogeneous
    h. appearance
    h. carotid plaque
    h. echo
    h. echo pattern
    h. enhancement
    genetically h.
    h. intrasellar mass
    h. lesion
    h. MR pattern
    h. opacity
    h. perfusion
    h. positive charge
    h. radiation
    h. signal intensity
    h. soft tissue density
    h. susceptibility distribution
    h. thallium distribution
homogeneously
homogenous echogenic uterine content
homograft
    aortic root h.
homology mapping
homonuclear spin system
homophilic Purkinje cell
homospoil
homovanillic acid (HVA)
Honda sign appearance
honeycomb
    h. appearance
    h. cyst
    h. degeneration
    h. formation
    h. lung
    h. pattern
    h. vertebra
honeycombing
    fibrotic h.
    subpleural h.
hood
    fibrous h.
hood-shaped ureter
hooked
    h. acromion
    h. bone
    h. vertebra
hook of hamate fracture
hooklike osteophyte formation
hookwire
    Hawkin h.
    Kopans spring h.

hoop
    h. strength
    h. stress
    h. stress fracture
hoop-shaped loops of bowel
Hoover sign
Hopkins
    H. hook-guiding catheter
    H. rod
Hopmann
    H. papilloma
    H. polyp
horizon
    H. LX scanner
    H. LX 1.5-T superconducting
      magnet
horizontal
    h. beam film
    h. beam study
    h. boundary
    h. dipole configuration
    h. fissure
    h. heart
    h. lie
    h. long axial
    h. long axis
    h. long axis slice
    h. long axis SPECT image
    h. maxillary fracture
    h. overframing
    h. plane
    h. plane loop
    h. position
    h. segment of middle cerebral
      artery
    h. striping
    h. toit externe (HTE)
    h. toit externe angle
horizontal-beam radiography
hormesis
    radiation h.
hormone
    adrenocorticotropic h. (ACTH)
    mediobasal hypothalamus luteinizing
      hormone-releasing h.
hormone-receptor negative carcinoma
hormone-resistant prostate carcinoma
horn
    Ammon h.
    anterior h.
    central h.
    dorsal spinal cord h.

NOTES

437

H

horn (*continued*)
    H. endootoprobe laser
    enlarged frontal h.
    frontal h.
    iliac h.
    lateral h.
    meniscal h.
    occipital h.
    posterior gray h.
    posterior spinal cord h.
    projectile h.
    spinal dorsal h.
    splaying of frontal h.
    temporal h.
    uterine h.
    h. of uterus
    ventral h.
    ventricular h.
Horner
    H. muscle
    H. sign
    H. syndrome
horseshoe
    h. abscess
    h. appearance
    h. configuration
    h. configuration of brain
    h. fibrosis
    h. fistula
    h. kidney
    h. lung
    h. osteophyte
    h. placenta
    h. shape
Horsley anastomosis
Horton disease
hose-pipe appearance of terminal ileum
hose-volume histogram
hot
    h. area
    h. cathode x-ray tube
    h. caudate lobe
    h. defect
    h. laser
    h. lesion
    h. light
    h. nose sign
    h. quartz lamp
hot-cross
    h.-c. bun appearance
    h.-c. bun skull
hot-source heating
hot-spot
    h.-s. artifact
    h.-s. heart imaging
    h.-s. myocardial imaging
hot-tipped laser probe

Hough
    H. transform (HT)
    H. transform mapping
Hounsfield
    H. calcium density measurement unit
    H. number
    H. unit (H, HU)
4-hour delayed thallium imaging
hourglass
    h. bladder
    h. chest
    h. configuration
    h. constriction
    h. constriction of gallbladder
    h. deformity
    h. membrane
    h. pattern
    h. phalanx
    h. shape
    h. stenosis
    h. stomach
    h. tumor
    h. ventricle
    h. vertebra
hour-glass constriction of hip capsule
hourglass-shaped lesion
House grading system
housemaid's knee
housing
    x-ray tube h.
Houston
    H. muscle
    valve of H.
^{166}Ho in vivo generator
Howell-Evans syndrome
Howship-Romberg sign
Howtek Scanmaster DX scanner
Ho:YAG
    holmium-yttrium-aluminum-garnet
    Ho:YAG laser
Hoyeraal-Hreidarsson syndrome
HP
    Hewlett-Packard
    Profasi HP
    ScleroPLUS HP
    HP SONOS 5500 ultrasound echocardiography system
    HP SONOS 5500 ultrasound imaging system
HPA
    hypothalamic-pituitary-adrenal
    HPA axis
HpD
    hematoporphyrin derivative photosensitizing agent
hpf
    high-powered field

HPGe
  high-purity germanium
    HPGe detector
HPS
  hypertrophic pyloric stenosis
HPV
  human papillomavirus
    HPV16-associated tumor
    HPV18-associated tumor
H&R
  hysterectomy and radiation
HRA
  high right atrial
  high right atrium
HRARE
  hybrid rapid acquisition with relaxation
    enhancement
HRCT
  high-resolution computed tomography
    cystic airspace HRCT
    inhomogeneous lung attenuation
      HRCT
    interstitial nodule HRCT
    noncontiguous expiratory HRCT
    volumetric expiratory HRCT
HRI
  high-resolution infrared
    HRI imaging
HR-MR
  high-resolution magnetic resonance
    sagittal HR-MR
HR-MRI
  high-resolution MRI
HRMS
  high-resolution multisweep
HRS
  hepatorenal syndrome
HRT II
  Heidelberg retina tomograph II
HS
  half-scan
  Hurler syndrome
H/S
  hysterosalpingogram
  hysterosalpingography
    H/S Elliptosphere balloon catheter
HSA
  human serum albumin
    ^{99m}Tc HSA
HSAS
  hereditary stenosis of the aqueduct of
    Sylvius

H2 Score office-based diagnostic device
HSD
  Hill-Sachs defect
HSG
  hysterosalpingogram
  hysterosalpingography
  hysterosonography
    HSG catheter
H-shaped
    H-s. vertebra
    H-s. vertebral body
HSM
  hepatosplenomegaly
HSRCCT
  high spatial resolution cine computed
    tomography
HSSG
  hysterosalpingosonography
HSV
  herpes simplex virus
HSV1
  herpes simplex virus 1
    HSV1 encephalitis
HSV1-tk
  herpes simplex virus 1 kinase
HT
  Hough transform
HTE
  horizontal toit externe
    HTE angle
HTRCCT
  high-temporal-resolution cine computed
    tomography
H-type tracheoesophageal fistula
HU
  heat unit
  Hounsfield unit
Huckman number (HN)
Hudson attachment
Hueck ligament
Hughes-Stovin syndrome
Hughston
    H. Clinic injury classification
    H. view
Huguier canal
Huisman percutaneous drainage set
Huldshinsky radiation
Hulten variance
human
    h. albumin microphere
    h. aortic smooth muscle cell
    h. blood index (HBI)

NOTES

H

human (*continued*)
    h. herpesvirus (HHV)
    h. immunodeficiency virus (HIV)
    h. leukocyte antigen (HLA)
    h. papillomavirus
    h. serum albumin (HSA)
    h. serum albumin imaging agent
    h. thrombin
    h. visual sensitivity weighting
HumaSPECT imaging agent
humeral
    h. avulsion of the glenohumeral
      ligament (HAGL)
    h. bone
    h. capitellum
    h. circumflex
    h. condylar fracture
    h. epicondyle
    h. epiphysis
    h. head-splitting fracture
    h. length
    h. line
    h. mechanism
    h. metaphysis
    h. physial fracture
    h. ridge
    h. supracondylar fracture
humeroradial articulation
humeroulnar articulation
humerus, pl. **humeri**
    capitulum humeri
    epicondylar fracture of h.
    head of h.
    surgical neck of h.
humidifier lung
hump
    buffalo h.
    diaphragmatic h.
    dowager's h.
    dromedary h.
    Hampton h.
    Herndon h.
    hip h.
    Kumpe h.
humpback deformity
Humphry ligament
hunchback
    Kokopelli h.
hundredth-normal solution
hunger
    air h.
Hunner ulcer
Hunt
    H. and Hess aneurysm grade I–V
    H. and Hess aneurysm grading
      system
    H. and Hess subarachnoid
      hemorrhage scale

    H. and Kosnik (grade 0–V)
      aneurysmal grade
Hunter
    H. aneurysm ligation
    H. canal
    H. disease
    H. ligament
hunterian ligation of aneurysm
Hunter-Schreger band
Hunter-Sessions
Hunt-Kosnik
    H.-K. classification
    H.-K. classification of aneurysm
Huppert disease
Hurler-Scheie syndrome
Hurler syndrome (HS)
Hurst phenomenon
Hurter
    H. and Driffield (H and D)
    H. and Driffield curve
Hürthle cell adenoma
Huschke
    H. canal
    H. foramen
    H. ligament
Hutch diverticulum
Hutchinson
    H. fracture
    H. plaque
    H. syndrome
    H. teeth
Hutchinson-Gilford syndrome
Hutchinson-type neuroblastoma
Hutinel-Pick syndrome
Hutson loop
Huygens
    H. eyepiece
    H. principle
HV
    hallux valgus
    herpesvirus
HVA
    hallux valgus angle
    homovanillic acid
HVL
    half-value layer
HVPGS
    high-voltage pulsed galvanic stimulation
HVS
    high-voltage stimulation
HWP
    hepatic wedge pressure
hyaline
    h. arteriosclerosis
    h. articular cartilage
    h. cartilage endplate
    h. cartilage plate
    h. degeneration

h. membrane disease (HMD)
h. necrosis
hyalinized
h. breast fibroadenoma
h. fibroadenoma with fibrosis
h. fibrocollagenous tissue
hyalinizing granuloma
hyalocapsular ligament
hyaloid
h. artery
h. canal
h. canal of Cloquet
h. fossa
hyaloserositis pleura
Hyams grading of esthesioneuroblastoma classification
hybrid
h. approach
h. detector configuration
h. imaging
h. magnet
h. MRI imaging agent
h. PET/SPECT camera
h. probe
h. rapid acquisition with relaxation enhancement (HRARE)
h. subtraction technique
hybridization probe
hybridization-subtraction technique
hybrid-RARE imaging
hydatid
alveolar h.
h. heart cyst
h. lung cyst
h. mediastinum cyst
Morgagni h.
h. polyp
h. pregnancy
sessile h.
Virchow h.
hydatidosis
cardiac h.
osseous h.
Hydradjust IV table
hydramnios, hydramnion
hydrated pyelogram
hydraulic
h. chamber
h. distention
vascular h.'s
Hydra Vision Plus DR, ES, HP urological imaging system

hydrencephaly
hydrocalycosis
hydrocalyx
hydrocele
congenital h.
idiopathic h.
infantile h.
primary h.
secondary h.
hydrocephalic obstruction
hydrocephalocele
hydrocephalus
acquired h.
acute h.
asymptomatic h.
bilateral h.
chronic communicating h.
communicating h.
compensated h.
congenital h.
corpus callosum hypoplasia, retardation, adducted thumbs, spastic paraparesis, and h. (CRASH)
delayed h.
extraventricular obstructive h.
h. ex vacuo
fulminant h.
hyperdynamic h.
idiopathic h.
infantile h.
intraventricular obstructive h.
low-pressure h.
mass-effect h.
noncommunicating h.
nonobstructive h.
normal-pressure h.
normotensive h.
obstructive h.
occult h.
posthemorrhagic h.
postinfectious h.
posttraumatic h.
primary h.
progressive h.
secondary h.
shunted h.
symptomatic obstructive h.
unilateral h.
unshunted h.
HydroCoil Embolic System
hydrocolpocele

NOTES

H

hydrocolpos
hydrocortisone enema
hydro-CT
    helical h.-CT
hydrodynamic
    h. potential of disc
    h. thrombectomy system
hydroencephalocele
hydroencephalomeningocele
hydrogel plug
hydrogen (H)
    heavy h.
    hydrogen atom-# radioactive h.
    h. peroxide enema
    h. peroxide-enhanced anal
      endosonography
    h. peroxide imaging agent
    h. proton imaging
    h. spin density
hydrogen-1, -2, -3 MR spectroscopy
hydrography
    MR h.
Hydrolyser hydrodynamic thrombectomy
  catheter
hydrolysis in vivo
hydrolyzed technetium
hydromer-coated micro guidewire
hydrometra
hydrometrocolpos
hydro-MRI
hydromyelia
    holocord h.
hydromyoma
hydronephrosis
    acute h.
    chronic h.
    congenital h.
    focal h.
hydronephrotic
    h. kidney
    h. sac
hydropericardium
hydroperitoneum
hydrophilic
    h. contrast agent
    h. guidewire
    h. nonflocculating barium
hydrophilic-coated
    h.-c. guidewire
    h.-c. guiding catheter
hydrophilicity
    high h.
hydrophone
    needle h.
hydrophthalmos
hydropic
    h. change
    h. composition

    h. degeneration
    h. villus
hydropneumothorax
    loculated h.
hydrops
    h. canal
    endolymphatic h.
    fetal h.
    h. fetalis
    gallbladder h.
    halo sign of h.
    labyrinthine h.
    nonimmune fetal h.
    semicircular canal h.
    transient gallbladder h.
    h. tubae profluens
hydropyonephrosis
hydrosalpinx
Hydro-Sil coating
hydrosoluble contrast agent
hydrostatic
    h. decompression
    h. pressure of blood
hydrosyringomyelia
hydrotherapy
hydrothorax
    hepatic h.
    refractory hepatic h.
hydroureter
hydroureteronephrosis
hydroxide
    iron h.
hydroxyapatite
    air plasma spray h.
    calcium h.
    h. deposition disease (HADD)
    h. implant
    h. rheumatism
hydroxycitrate
    gadolinium Gd 159 h.
hydroxyethylidene-1,1-diphosphonic acid
  (HEDP)
5-hydroxyindoleacetic acid (5-HIAA)
hygroma, pl. hygromata
    cystic neck h.
    cystic orbital h.
    pseudocystic h.
    subdural h.
hyoepiglottic ligament
hyoglossus muscle
hyoid
    h. arch
    h. bar
    h. bone
hyopharyngeal carcinoma
hyoscine butylbromide imaging agent
Hypaque
    H. enema
    H. Meglumine imaging agent

H. myelography
H. Sodium imaging agent
H. swallow
Hypaque-76 imaging agent
Hypaque-Cysto imaging agent
Hypaque-M imaging agent
hyparterial bronchus
hyperabduction
  h. maneuver
  h. syndrome
hyperactive peristalsis
hyperacute
  h. ischemic brain infarct
  h. myocardial infarct
  h. stroke
hyperaeration
hyperattenuated
  h. blood
  h. intrasellar mass
hyperattenuation
  heterogeneous h.
hypercalcemic supravalvular aortic stenosis
hypercellular reconverted bone marrow
hyperconcentration of contrast medium
hypercycloidal tomography
hyperdense
  h. brain lesion
  h. mass
  h. middle cerebral artery sign
  h. sinus secretion
  h. spleen
hyperdontia
hyperdynamic
  h. abductor hallucis
  h. AV fistula
  h. fourth ventricle
  h. heart
  h. hydrocephalus
  h. right ventricular impulse
hyperechogenicity
hyperechoic
  h. area
  h. breast mass
  h. focus
  h. region
  h. renal medulla
  h. renal nodule
  h. splenic spot
  h. structure with shadowing
  uniformly h.
hyperechoicity

hyperemia
  active h.
  arterial h.
  collateral h.
  diffuse h.
  fluxionary h.
  mucous membrane h.
  passive h.
  reactive h.
  subchondral marrow h.
  venous h.
hyperemic flow
hyperexpanded lobe
hyperexpansion
  compensatory lobe h.
hyperextensibility
  joint h.
hyperextension
  h. dislocation
  h. injury
  h. of neck
  h. teardrop fracture
hyperfine coupling
hyperfixation
  ^{99m}Tc HMPAO h.
hyperflexion
  spine h.
  h. teardrop fracture
hyperflexion/hyperextension cervical injury
hyperflexion/rotation injury
hyperfractionated
  h. accelerated radiation therapy (HART)
  h. radiation
  h. radiotherapy
  h. total body irradiation
hyperfractionation
hyperfunction
  adrenocortical h.
hypergastrinemia
hyperglycinemia
hypergonadotropic hypogonadism
hyperinflation
  congenital lobar h.
  dynamic pulmonary h.
  focal h.
  pulmonary h.
hyperintense
  h. marrow space
  h. mass
  h. muscle

NOTES

H

hyperintense *(continued)*
    h. periventricular brain lesion
    h. signal
hyperintensity
    cortical h.
    diffuse signal h.
    incidental punctate white matter h.
    localized h.
    multifocal area of h.
    muscle h.
    pulvinar h.
    punctate white matter h.
    sacral h.
    white matter signal h.
Hyperion
    H. LTK laser
    H. LTK system
hyperkinesia
hyperkinesis
hyperkinetic
    h. heart
    h. segmental wall motion
    h. segmental wall motion
      abnormality
hyperlordosis
    functional h.
hyperlucency
hyperlucent
    h. lung
    h. rib
hypermaturation
hypermetabolic
    h. activity focus
    h. nodule
    h. region
hypermobile
    h. first ray
    h. joint
    h. kidney
hypermotility
hypermyelination
hypernephroid carcinoma
hypernephroma
hyperosmolar
hyperosmotic solution
hyperostosis
    ankylosing h.
    bony h.
    Caffey h.
    chronic infantile h.
    cortical h.
    diffuse idiopathic skeletal h.
      (DISH)
    h. frontalis interna
    generalized cortical h.
    idiopathic cortical h. (ICH)
    infantile cortical h.
    h. of Morgagni
    senile ankylosing h.

    skeletal h.
    skull h.
    sternoclavicular h.
    vertebral h.
HyperPACS teleradiology system
hyperparathyroidism
    brown tumor of h.
    persistent h.
    primary h.
    recurrent h.
    secondary h.
    tertiary h. (tHPT)
hyperperfusion
    h. abnormality of liver
    ictal h.
    mesial h.
    septal h.
hyperperistalsis
hyperpermeability
    contrast medium–induced pulmonary
      vascular h.
hyperphenylalaninemia
hyperphosphatasia
    familial idiopathic h.
hyperplasia
    adaptive h.
    adenomatous h.
    adrenal h.
    adrenocortical h.
    alveolar epithelial h.
    angiofibroblastic h.
    angiofollicular lymph node h.
    angiolymphoid h.
    antral G-cell h.
    atypical ductal h.
    atypical lobular h. (ALH)
    atypical lobular breast h.
    atypical regenerative h.
    benign prostatic h. (BPH)
    bone marrow lymphoid h.
    breast h.
    Brunner gland h.
    compensatory h.
    congenital adrenal h. (CAH)
    congenital adrenocortical h.
    cortical nodular h.
    cystic endometrial h.
    cystic glandular h.
    desquamated epithelial breast h.
    diffuse pulmonary neuroendocrine
      cell h.
    ductal epithelial h.
    endometrial h.
    epiphysial h.
    epithelial h.
    explosive follicular h.
    fibrointimal h.
    fibrous tissue h.
    florid follicular h.

focal cortical h.
focal nodular h. (FNH)
follicular nodular h. (FNH)
gallium-avid thymic h.
generalized angiofollicular lymph
  node h.
generalized breast h.
giant follicular h.
GI tract lymphoid h.
intimal h. (IH)
intravascular papillary endothelial h.
lipoid adrenal h.
localized angiofollicular lymph
  node h.
lung lymphoid h.
lymphoid h.
lymphonodular h.
medial h.
mucosal h.
myointimal h.
neointimal h.
neoplastic h.
nodular adrenal h.
nodular lymphoid h.
nodular regenerative h. (NRH)
paracortical h.
parathyroid h.
physiologic h.
pituitary h.
plantar h.
polypoid lymphoid h.
prostatic h.
pseudoangiomatous stromal h.
  (PASH)
pseudointimal h.
pulmonary neuroendocrine cell h.
reactive follicular h.
reactive lymphoid h.
sclerosing duct h.
sinus h.
smooth h.
splenic h.
subadventitial h.
tenocyte h.
thymic h.
thyroid h.
torus h.
unicentric angiofollicular lymph
  node h.
hyperplastic
  h. adenomatous polyp
  h. bone

h. cholecystosis
h. colon polyp
h. gastric polyp
h. gastropathy
h. inflammation
h. lesion
h. stomach polyp
h. synovium
h. tissue
hyperpolarized
  h. ^{3}He imaging agent
  h. helium
  h. ^{129}Xe gas
  h. ^{129}Xe imaging agent
hyperpressure
hyperreactivity
  airway h. (AHR)
hyperreflexia
  detrusor h.
hyperreninemic hypertension
hyperrugosity
hypersecretion
  gastric h.
  mucous h.
hypersegmentation
  manubrium h.
hypersensitivity
  alveolar h.
  carotid sinus h.
  h. lung
  h. pneumonia
  h. pneumonitis
  h. reaction
  tracheobronchial h.
hypersplenism
hyperstasis
  generalized cortical h.
hyperstereoroentgenography
hyperstimulation of ovary
hypertelorism
hypertension
  acute thromboembolic pulmonary
    arterial h.
  arterial h.
  benign intracranial h.
  extrahepatic portal h.
  hyperreninemic h.
  hypoxic pulmonary h.
  idiopathic intracranial h.
  idiopathic noncirrhotic portal h.
  idiopathic portal h. (IPH)
  h. injury

NOTES

H

hypertension *(continued)*
    intracranial h.
    isolated systolic arterial h. (ISAH)
    obstructive pulmonary arterial h.
    persistent pulmonary h.
    portal h.
    precapillary lung h.
    primary pulmonary h. (PPH)
    pulmonary h.
    pulmonary arterial h. (PAH)
    pulmonary venous h.
    refractory h.
    renal artery h.
    renal transplant h.
    renal vascular h. (RVH)
    renovascular h.
    secondary intracranial h. (SIH)
    segmental portal h.
    sinistral portal h.
    suprahepatic h.
    systemic arterial h.
    systemic venous h.
    systolic h.
    venous h.
hypertensive
    h. arteriosclerosis
    h. brain hemorrhage
    h. cardiovascular disease
    h. contrast concentration
    h. diathesis
    h. encephalopathy
    h. ischemic ulcer
    h. left ventricular hypertrophy
    h. lower esophageal sphincter
    h. renal disease
    h. stroke
    h. vascular degeneration
    h. vascular disease
hyperthermia
    anular phased-array h.
    interstitial h.
    locoregional h.
    microwave h.
    h. probe
    radiofrequency h.
    radiotherapy with h.
    radiotherapy without h.
    volumetric interstitial h.
hyperthyroid heart
hyperthyroidism
    neonatal h.
hypertonic
    h. airway
    h. enema
    h. solution
hypertransradiancy
hypertrophic
    h. asymmetry
    h. bladder

    h. cardiomyopathy (HCM)
    h. cirrhosis
    h. duct network
    h. exostosis
    h. gastritis
    h. inflammation
    h. infundibular subpulmonic stenosis
    h. marginal spurring
    h. nonunion
    h. obstructive cardiomyopathy
      (HOC, HOCM)
    h. olivary degeneration
    h. pulmonary osteoarthropathy
    h. pyloric stenosis (HPS)
    h. pyloric string sign stenosis
    h. pyloric target sign stenosis
    h. pylorus
    h. subaortic stenosis
    h. tissue
hypertrophied
    h. heart
    h. intima
    h. myocardium
    h. trigone
hypertrophy
    adaptive h.
    asymmetric septal h. (ASH)
    asymptomatic h.
    benign prostatic h. (BPH)
    biatrial h.
    biventricular h.
    bladder h.
    bone h.
    Brunner gland h.
    cardiac h.
    4-chamber h.
    compensatory nodular kidney h.
    complementary h.
    concentric heart h.
    contralateral h.
    dilatation and h.
    eccentric left ventricular h.
    epiphysial h.
    familial h. (FHC)
    focal pyloric h.
    focal renal h.
    functional h.
    hypertensive left ventricular h.
    interatrial septal h.
    left atrial h.
    left ventricular h. (LVH)
    ligamentous-muscular h.
    lipomatous h.
    muscular h.
    myocardial cellular h.
    olivary h.
    panchamber h.
    physiologic h.
    pyloric h.

right atrial h.
right ventricular h. (RVH)
Romhilt-Estes score for left
   ventricular h.
scalenus anticus muscle h.
septal h.
septate h.
smooth muscle h.
symmetric heart h.
trigeminal trigonal h.
trigonal h.
type A–C right ventricular h.
unilateral h.
ventricular h.
villous h.
Wigle scale for ventricular h.

hypervariable
h. region
h. sequence

hypervascular
h. arterialization
h. granulation tissue
h. hepatocellular carcinoma
h. liver metastasis
h. mediastinal mass
h. pancreatic tumor

hypervascularity
hypervolemia of pregnancy
hypervolemic pulmonary edema
hypha
fungal h.

hyphidrosis
hypoacousia
hypoaeration
hypoattenuating mass
hypoattenuation
hypocellular marrow
hypochordal arch
hypocycloidal tomography
hypodense
h. area
h. basal ganglion brain lesion
h. mass
h. mesencephalic low-density brain
   lesion

hypodensity
periventricular h.
white matter h.

hypodiploid tumor
hypodiploidy
hypodontia

hypoechogenic
h. retroplacental myometrial zone
h. tumor

hypoechogenicity
false h.

hypoechoic
h. area
h. area of ultrasound
h. band
h. fluid collection
h. halo
h. layer
h. liver
h. mantle
h. plaque
h. renal sinus
h. rim
h. solid tumor
h. structure
h. testis
h. tissue
h. zone

hypofractionated radiation therapy
hypofrontality
hypoganglionosis of colon
hypogastric
h. artery
h. plexus

hypogastrium
hypogenetic lung
hypoglossal
h. canal
h. fossa
h. nerve
h. trigone

hypogonadism
hypergonadotropic h.

hypoInflation of lung
hypointense
h. fibrous capsule
h. marrow signal
h. nodule
h. sella lesion
h. signal
h. signal inhomogeneity
h. signal shadowing

hypointensity
cortical h.

hypokinesis, hypokinesia
apical h.
cardiac h.
diffuse ventricular h.

NOTES

H

hypokinesis *(continued)*
    global h.
    h. of heart
    inferior wall h.
    h. on echocardiography
    regional h.
    septal h.
    wall h.
hypokinetic
    h. left ventricle
    h. myocardium
    h. segment
    h. segmental wall motion
    h. segmental wall motion
      abnormality
hypolordosis
hypolucency of lung
hypometabolic area
hypometabolism
    bilateral superior parietal h.
    biparietotemporal h.
    focal area of h.
    global h.
    lesion h.
hypomineralization
    fetal h.
hypoparathyroidism
    idiopathic h.
    secondary h.
hypoperfused state
hypoperfusion
    acute alveolar h.
    apical h.
    cerebellar h.
    cerebral h.
    h. complex
    global cerebral h.
    peripheral h.
    pulmonary h.
    resting regional myocardial h.
    septal h.
    systemic h.
hypoperistalsis
hypopharyngeal
    h. carcinoma
    h. diverticulum
    h. tumor
hypopharynx
hypophosphatemic osteomalacia
hypophysial
    h. fossa
    h. pouch
    h. Rathke duct
hypophysis
    h. cerebri
    infundibulum of h.
hypophysitis
    lymphocytic h.
    lymphoid h.

hypopituitarism
    hypothalamic h.
hypoplasia
    anular h.
    aortic tract complex h.
    ascending aorta h.
    basiocciput h.
    biliary h.
    bone marrow h.
    cartilage hair h.
    cerebellar h.
    cerebral white matter h.
    condylar skull h.
    congenital renal h.
    conus h.
    h. of dens
    endothelial h.
    fetal lung h.
    gallbladder h.
    isolated cerebellar h.
    left ventricular h.
    lung h.
    mandible h.
    maxillary sinus h.
    medullaris h.
    occipital condyle h.
    optic nerve h.
    pontocerebellar h.
    pulmonary h.
    radius h.
    seminal vesicle h.
    sinus h.
    skeletal h.
    transverse h.
    tubular aortic h.
    uterine h.
    vermian h.
    vermian-cerebellar h.
    vermis h.
hypoplastic
    h. aortic arch
    h. disc interval
    h. emphysema
    h. heart ventricle
    h. horizontal rib
    h. left heart syndrome (HLHS)
    h. left parietal syndrome
    h. left ventricle
    h. lung
    h. penis
    h. right heart
    h. right heart syndrome
    h. right ventricle
    h. subpulmonic outflow
    h. thumb
    h. tricuspid orifice
    h. valve
hypopnea
    obstructive h.

hyposensitization
hyposmia
hyposplenism
hypostatic
  h. bronchopneumonia
  h. congestion
  h. pneumonia
  h. pulmonary insufficiency
hypotelorism
hypotension
  arterial h.
  cerebral h.
  spontaneous intracranial h.
hypothalamic
  h. glioma
  h. hamartoma
  h. hemorrhage
  h. hypopituitarism
  h. hypothyroidism
  h. infundibulum
  h. lesion
  h. sulcus
hypothalamic-pituitary-adrenal (HPA)
  hypothalamic-pituitary-adrenal axis
hypothalamic-pituitary axis
hypothalamic-pituitary-gonadal axis
hypothalamohypophysial tract
hypothalamoneurohypophysial axis
hypothalamus
  anterior h.
  rostral h.
  h. tumor
hypothenar
  h. eminence
  h. muscle groups of hand
hypothermia
  scalp h.
hypothermic
  h. heart
  h. perfusion
hypothyroidism
  hypothalamic h.
  primary h.
  secondary h.
  tertiary h.
hypotonia
hypotonic
  h. bladder
  h. duodenography
  h. duodenography imaging
hypovascular zone
hypoventilation

hypovolemia trauma
hypovolemic
  h. complex
  h. shock
hypoxemia
hypoxia
  ischemic h.
  relative h.
  tumor h.
hypoxia-ischemia
hypoxic
  h. brain damage
  h. injury
  h. ischemic encephalopathy
  h. ischemic insult
  h. pulmonary hypertension
  h. pulmonary vasoconstriction
Hyrtl foramen
hysterectomy
  abdominal h.
  extrafascial h.
  h. and radiation (H&R)
  h. and radiation therapy
  supracervical h.
  Wertheim h.
hysteresis
Hysterocath hysterosalpingography
  device
hysterogram
hysterograph
hysterography
  conventional h.
  ultrasonic h.
hysterometry
hysteromyoma
hysterosalpingo-contrast sonography
hysterosalpingogram (H/S, HSG)
hysterosalpingography (H/S, HSG)
  h. catheter
  h. imaging
  ultrasonic h.
hysterosalpingosonography (HSSG)
hysteroscope
  Gynecare Versascope h.
hysteroscopy
hysterosonography (HSG)
  transvaginal h. (TVHS)
hysterotubogram
hysterotubography
Hz
  hertz
440-Hz tone

NOTES

I
  iodine
  isoleucine
  I hippuran
I-123 (*var. of* ^{123}I)
I-125 (*var. of* ^{125}I)
I-127 (*var. of* ^{127}I)
I-131 (*var. of* ^{131}I)
I-132 (*var. of* ^{132}I)
^{111}**I**
  iodine 111
^{123}**I, I-123**
  iodine 123
    ^{123}I BMIPP imaging
    ^{123}I brain imaging spectamine
    ^{123}I heptadecanoic acid
    ^{123}I iodoamphetamine
    ^{123}I isopropyl iodoamphetamine
      (IMP)
    ^{123}I metaiodobenzylguanidine
    ^{123}I metaiodobenzylguanidine
      scintigraphy
    ^{123}I OIH
^{125}**I, I-125**
  iodine 125
    ^{125}I fibrinogen scan
    ^{125}I interstitial radiation implant
^{127}**I, I-127**
  iodine 127
^{131}**I, I-131**
  iodine 131
    ^{131}I-mIB6
    ^{131}I radioactive iodine
    ^{131}I therapy
^{132}**I, I-132**
  iodine 132
    ^{132}I radioactive iodine
IA
  interbronchial angle
  intraarterial
IAB
  intraabdominal
IABP
  intraaortic balloon pump
IADSA
  intraarterial digital subtraction
    angiography
IAR
  instantaneous axis of rotation
IAS
  interatrial septum
iatrogenic
    i. avulsion
    i. cardiomegaly
    i. dural tear

    i. esophageal perforation
    i. iliocaval fistula
    i. pseudoaneurysm
    i. ureteral injury
IAVB
  incomplete atrioventricular block
**I-B1 radiolabeled antibody injection
  radiation therapy**
IBC
  inflammatory breast carcinoma
IBM
    IBM field-cycling research
      relaxometer
    IBM NMR spectrometer
IBTR
  ipsilateral breast tumor recurrence
ICA
  internal carotid artery
  intracranial aneurysm
    juxtasellar ICA
    petrous ICA
    supraclinoid ICA
ICE
  intracardiac echocardiography
ice
    i. cream cone shape
    i. skater's fracture
iceberg
    i. lesion
    i. radiotherapy
ice-pick view
ICEUS
ice-water swallow
ICG
  iodocyanine green
ICH
  idiopathic cortical hyperostosis
  intracerebral hemorrhage
ichorous pleurisy
ICIS
  integrated clinical information system
ICON
    Siemens ICON
ICP
  intracranial pressure
ICP-AES
  inductively coupled plasma atomic
    emission spectrometry
    ICP-AES detection
ICRT
  intracoronary radiation therapy
ICRU
  International Commission on Radiation
    Units
    ICRU reference point

ICS
improved Chen-Smith
    ICS coder

ICSPF
internal carotid systolic peak flow

ictal
    i. hyperperfusion
    i. PET scan
    i. phase study
    i. ^{99m}Tc HMPAO brain SPECT

ICUS
intracoronary ultrasound

ICV
internal cerebral vein
intracerebroventricular
    ICV reservoir

ICW
intracranial width

ID
internal diameter
interscan delay

IDA
image display and analysis
    IDA scanning

IDC
idiopathic dilated cardiomyopathy
interlocking detachable coil
intraductal carcinoma

IDD
intraluminal duodenal diverticulum

identification
    particle i.
    peak i.
    phase i.
    topographic i.

IDET
intradiscal electrothermal therapy

IDF
inferior duodenal flexure

idiopathic
    i. amyloidosis
    i. avascular necrosis
    i. cortical hyperostosis (ICH)
    i. diffuse cerebellar dysplasia
    i. dilated cardiomyopathy (IDC)
    i. dilated pulmonary artery
    i. edema
    i. epilepsy
    i. epiphyseolysis
    i. fibrous mediastinitis
    i. fracture
    i. gastric perforation
    i. hydrocele
    i. hydrocephalus
    i. hypertrophic subaortic sclerosis (IHSS)
    i. hypertrophic subaortic stenosis
    i. hypoparathyroidism
    i. interstitial fibrosis
    i. interstitial pneumonia
    i. interstitial pneumonitis
    i. intestinal pseudoobstruction
    i. intracranial hypertension
    i. megacolon
    i. multicentric osteolysis
    i. mural endomyocardial disease
    i. noncirrhotic portal hypertension
    i. obstruction
    i. osteolysis
    i. pleural calcification
    i. portal hypertension (IPH)
    i. pulmonary arteriosclerosis (IPA)
    i. pulmonary artery dilatation
    i. pulmonary fibrosis (IPF)
    i. pulmonary hemosiderosis
    i. restrictive cardiomyopathy
    i. right atrial dilatation
    i. scoliosis
    i. unilateral hyperlucent lung
    i. unilobar emphysema
    i. varicocele

idiosyncratic anaphylactoid reaction

idioventricular rhythm (IVR)

IDIS angiography system

IDK
internal derangement of knee

IDP
imidodiphosphonate

IDSA
intraoperative digital subtraction angiography

IDSI
internodular difference in signal intensity
    IDSI scanner

IDXrad radiology information system

I-E
inspiratory to expiratory ratio

IES
inferior esophageal sphincter

IF
screen-intensifying factor

IFT
inverse Fourier transform

IgG
immunoglobulin G
    ^{111}In IgG
    indium-111-labeled IgG

Iglesias fiberoptic resectoscope

IGLLC
inferior glenohumeral ligament labral complex

IGRT
image-guided radiation therapy

IH
intimal hyperplasia

IHA
intrahepatic atresia

IHF
    interhemispheric fissure
^{192}I high-dose-rate remote afterloader
IHSA
    iodinated human serum albumin
IHSS
    idiopathic hypertrophic subaortic
        sclerosis
IJV
    internal jugular vein
I-labeled
        I-l. cholesterol
        I-l. macroaggregated albumin
        I-l. rose bengal
^{131}I-labeled
        ^{131}I-l. human MoAb
        ^{131}I-l. monoclonal Fab
^{123}I-labeled Z-MIVE
ILBBB
    incomplete left bundle-branch block
ileal
        i. atresia
        i. conduit
        i. crypt
        i. inflow tract
        i. jejunization
        i. loop
        i. loopography
        i. motility
        i. neobladder
        i. obstruction
        i. pouch-anal anastomosis
        i. spill
        i. S pouch
        i. stenosis
ileitis
        backwash i.
        Crohn i.
        distal i.
        granulomatous i.
        obstructive dysfunctional i.
        prestomal i.
        reflux i.
        regional i.
        terminal i.
ileoanal pouch
ileocecal
        i. cystoplasty
        i. edema
        i. fat pad
        i. fold
        i. insufficiency

        i. junction
        i. orifice
        i. pouch
        i. recess
        i. syndrome
        i. valve
        i. valve abnormality
ileococcygeus muscle
ileocolic
        i. anastomosis
        i. artery
        i. disease
        i. fold
        i. intussusception
        i. lymph node
        i. plexus
        i. vein
        i. vessel
ileocolitis
        Crohn i.
ileocolostomy
ileoentectropy
ileofemoral wing fracture
ileogram
ileoileal intussusception
ileorectal anastomosis (IRA)
ileosacral (IS)
ileosigmoid
        i. fistula
        i. knot
ileostogram
ileostomy
ileotransverse colon anastomosis
ileum
        antimesenteric border of distal i.
        cobblestone i.
        collapsed distal i.
        hose-pipe appearance of terminal i.
        jejunization of i.
        neoterminal i.
        terminal i.
ileus
        adhesive i.
        adynamic i.
        adynamic/paralytic i.
        cecal i.
        chronic duodenal i.
        colonic i.
        dynamic i.
        functional i.
        gallbladder i.
        gallstone i.

NOTES

453

ileus *(continued)*
   localized i.
   mechanical i.
   meconium i.
   nonobstructive i.
   occlusive i.
   paralytic i.
   postoperative i.
   reflex i.
   spastic i.
Ilfeld-Holder deformity
ilia (*pl. of* ilium)
iliac
   i. apophysitis
   i. artery
   i. artery aneurysm
   i. artery stenosis
   i. artery stenting
   i. artery stent placement
   i. bifurcation
   i. canal
   i. cancellous bone
   i. circumflex lymph node
   i. colon
   i. crest
   i. dowel
   i. fascia
   i. fossa
   i. fossa abscess
   i. horn
   i. index
   i. lesion
   i. plaque
   i. PTA category 1–4
   i. spine
   i. tubercle
   i. tuberosity
   i. vein
   i. vein compression syndrome
   i. vein obstruction
   i. venography
   i. vessel
   i. wing
iliac-renal bypass graft
iliacus
iliocaval
   i. disease
   i. junction
   i. thrombus
   i. tree
iliocostal muscle
iliofemoral
   i. artery
   i. crossover bypass
   i. ligament
   i. thrombosis
   i. triangle
   i. vein
   i. venous stenosis

ilioinguinal lymph node
ilioischial line
iliolumbar ligament
iliopectineal
   i. eminence
   i. ligament
   i. line
ilioprofunda bypass graft
iliopsoas
   i. abscess
   i. bursa
   i. bursitis
   i. compartment
   i. compartment enlargement
   i. impingement
   i. muscle
   i. muscle shadow
   i. sign
   i. tendon
iliopubic
   i. eminence
   i. ligament
iliotibial (IT)
   i. band
   i. band friction syndrome
   i. ligament
   i. tract
iliotrochanteric ligament
ilium, pl. **ilia**
   flared i.
Ilizarov
   I. device
   I. ring
ill-defined
   i.-d. appearance
   i.-d. breast density
   i.-d. consolidation
   i.-d. margin
   i.-d. mass
   i.-d. multifocal lung density
illuminator
   Mammo Mask i.
ILUS
   intraluminal ultrasound
     ILUS catheter
IM
   intramedullary
     IM joint
     IM rod
     IM rodding
IMA
   inferior mesenteric artery
   intermetatarsal angle
   internal mammary artery
image (*See* imaging, film, projection, radiograph, radiography, scanning, scan, view, x-ray)
   acetazolamide dual-isotope i.
   i. acquisition

i. acquisition-gated scan imaging
Add-On Bucky radiographer
  detector i.
i. aliasing
alignment and registration of 3D i.
i. amplifier
amplitude i.
i. analysis system
anatomic i.
arm-down i.
arm-up i.
arterial flow-phase i.
artifact i.
attenuated i.
attenuation-corrected i.
axial fat-suppressed T2-weighted i.
axial gradient echo i.
axial proton-density-weighted i.
axial transabdominal i.
binarized i.
binary i.
black blood cardiac i.
bolus chase i.
bone phase i.
breath-hold fast spin-echo i.
bull's eye i.
calculated i.
cervicothoracic sagittal scout i.
i. chain
cine-encoded i.
cine magnetic resonance function i.
color-scale i.
column mode sinogram i.
i. compression
computer-generated i.
computerized transverse axial i.
cone-beam i.
confocal i.
contact i.
contiguous i.
i. contrast
contrast-enhanced MR i.
contrast-enhanced T1-weighted fat-
  suppressed i.
i. control
conventional transverse cross-
  sectional i.
i. converter
i. coregistration
coronal ECD brain SPECT i.
coronal GRE MR i.
coronal planar i.

coronal proton-density-weighted fast
  spin-echo i.
coronal SPIR i.
coronal T1-weighted i.
cross-sectional ultrasonographic i.
CTA i.
CT/MRI-defined tumor slice i.
CT/MRI-defined tumor volume i.
CT reconstruction i.
i. cytometry
3D-DSA i.
deformation-based surface-
  rendered i.
degradation of i.
delayed phase i.
2D gradient-encoded i.
diffusion-weighted i.
digitally fused CT and radiolabeled
  monoclonal antibody SPECT i.
digitized film i.
4-dimensional i.
3-dimensional Fourier transform
  volume i.
i. display
i. display and analysis (IDA)
i. distortion
Dixon quantitative chemical shift i.
2D portal i.
DSA i.
3D volume-rendering
  reconstruction i.
dynamic i.
ECG-triggered i.
ECG-triggered, flow-compensated
  gradient echo i.
echo i.
echo-planar i.
endosonographic i.
excitation-spoiled fat-suppressed T1-
  weighted SE i.
exercise i.
expiratory i.
fast fluid-attenuation inversion
  recovery i.
fast Fourier transform i.
fast spin-echo T2-weighted i.
fat-saturated axial i.
fat-saturated spin-echo proton
  density-weighted i.
fat-saturated T2-weighted fast spin-
  echo i.

NOTES

image *(continued)*
fat-suppressed T1-weighted 3D spoiled gradient-echo i.
fat- and water-suppressed T2-weighted i.
FLAIR i.
FLASH i.
flawed i.
flip-angle i.
floating i.
flow-compensated i.
flow-on gradient-echo i.
fluoroscopic i.
i. foldover
i. formation
frequency domain i.
i. fusion
gadolinium-enhanced T1-weighted i.
gadolinium-enhanced T1-weighted axial i.
gadolinium-enhanced T1-weighted MRI i.
gated i.
ghost i.
gradient-echo axial i.
gradient-echo coronal i.
gradient-echo T2-weighted i.
gradient-encoded i.
gradient-recalled echo i.
gray-scale i.
GRE-in i.
GRE-out i.
half-Fourier RARE i.
hard-copy i.
i. hashing
high-resolution 3D spoiled-GRASS i.
high-resolution transverse view i.
histomorphometric i.
horizontal long axis SPECT i.
imaginary i.
immediate postflow i.
inhomogeneous i.
in-phase T1-weighted i.
i. intensification
i. intensification fluorometry
i. intensifier
i. intensifier system
i. intensifier tube
intercondylar sagittal i.
intermediate i.
inversion recovery i.
inversion recovery-weighted i.
IR i.
large-field-of-view i.
late-phase i.
lateral sagittal i.
localizing i.
longitudinal i.

magnetic resonance multispectral color I.
magnetic susceptibility-weighted i.
magnetization transfer gradient-echo i.
magnitude i.
matrix i.
maximum intensity projection and source i.
midcoronal oblique i.
midplane sagittal i.
midsagittal MR i.
minimum intensity projection i.
MIP i.
mirror i.
misleading i.
i. modulation
modulus i.
motion-triggered cine kinematic MR i.
multiecho axial i.
multiecho coronal i.
multiplanar volume-reformatted i.
multiple planar gradient-recalled i.
native i.
near-isotropic reformatted i.
negative i.
i. noise
nonattenuation-corrected i.
nonmagnetization transfer gradient-refocused echo i.
nonmagnified i.
nonsubtracted i.
nonsubtraction i.
nuclear magnetic resonance i.
opposed GRE i.
opposed-phase T1-weighted i.
overlapping i.
panoramic i.
parallel-tagged MR i.
parametric i.
parasagittal i.
parenchymal phase i.
phantom i.
phase i.
phase-corrected GRE i.
phase-velocity i.
pinhole i.
plain-paper i.
planar left anterior oblique i.
postexercise i.
post fire i.
postintraarticular paramagnetic contrast injection T1-weighted i.
i. postprocessing
i. postprocessing error artifact
poststress i.
prefire i.
i. processing workstation

projectional i.
proton-density axial i.
proton-density-weighted fast spin-
  echo i.
pulse-echo i.
PVP i.
i. quality
i. quality degradation
quasiradiographic i.
radiographic i.
rapid half-Fourier T2-weighted i.
real-time echo-planar i.
reconstructed i.
i. reconstruction
i. reconstruction algorithm
i. reconstruction computer
i. recording system
recovery time i.
reference i.
i. reformation
reformatted T1 magnetic
  resonance i.
i. registration
registration and alignment of 3D i.
renal i.
respiratory triggered fat-saturated
  axial i.
i. restoration algorithm
sagittal fat-suppressed T1-weighted
  3D spoiled gradient-echo i.
sagittal scout i.
sagittal T1-weighted MR i.
saturation recovery i.
scout i.
scrambled i.
second-echo i.
see-through i.
SE proton-density weighted i.
sequential postcontrast MR i.
i. set
i. shading
i. sharpness
short axis i.
short tau inversion recovery i.
single section 2D i.
single-slice gradient-echo i.
i. slice thickness
sliding thin-slab maximum intensity
  projection i.
smoked glass i.
spatial modulation of
  magnetization i.

i. spatial resolution
spectral-spatial i.
spin-echo pilot i.
spin-echo T1-weighted i.
spin-lock-induced T1-rho
  weighted i.
SPIR-FLAIR i.
spot compression i.
spot-magnification i.
standard-dose enhanced conventional
  T1 weighted i.
static i.
stop-action i.
stress-and-rest i.
stress thallium i.
striation across i.
stroke count i.
stroke volume i.
subtracted i.
subtraction i.
T2 i.
tensor diffusion-weighted MR i.
T2-gradient refocused i.
thick slab 3D multiplanar
  reformatted i.
thin-collimation i.
thin-cut axial CT i.
thin-section axial i.
transaxial fat-saturated 3D i.
transcoronal STIR i.
transient punctate cortical
  hyperintensities on T1-weighted i.
transverse ECD brain SPECT i.
transverse-plane PET i.
trauma register i.
TSE i.
turboSTIR i.
T1-weighted i. (T1WI)
T2-weighted i. (T2WI)
T1-weighted axial i.
T2-weighted axial i.
T1-weighted coronal i.
T1-weighted fat-suppressed i.
  (T1FS)
T1-weighted fat-suppressed
  gadolinium-enhanced SE i.
T1-weighted gadolinium-enhanced
  SE i.
T2-weighted sagittal oblique i.
T2-weighted spin-echo i.
T2-weighted turbo SE i.
ultrasonic tomographic i.

NOTES

image *(continued)*
underexposed i.
i. uniformity
unopposed i.
variance i.
velocity-encoded i.
ventilation i.
ventricular function equilibrium i.
i. volume
volume-rendered 3D i.
volumetric i.
x-ray i.
zebra stripe i.
image-acquisition
i.-a. gated examination
i.-a. time
image-amplified fluoroscopy
Imagecast imaging system
**ImageChecker CT CAD software
system**
image-degrading scattering
image-forming system
image-guided
i.-g. injection technique
i.-g. radiation therapy (IGRT)
i.-g. radiofrequency tumor ablation
i.-g. radiosurgery
i.-g. surgery
i.-g. therapy
i.-g. tumor ablation
image-intensifier node
ImageMASTER
Imagent
I. BP
I. GI
I. GI, US imaging agent
I. LN
image-processing software
imager
Acuson 128EP i.
Agfa LR 3300 laser i.
DaTSCAN i.
Digirad 2020tc i.
Digirad 2020 TC i.
digital fundus i.
Drystar dry i.
flat-panel megavoltage i.
full-body echo-planar system i.
GE Advantage 1.5T i.
GE EchoSpeed 1.5T whole-body
MR i.
GE Signa 5.4 Genesis MR i.
GE Signa 5.5 Horizon EchoSpeed
MR i.
Hewlett-Packard color flow i.
I. II catheter
Integris V3000 i.
IRIS III i.

Kodak Digital Science 1200, 3600
distributed medical i.
laser i.
Lorad digital breast i.
MAGNETOM SP MRI i.
NeuroScan 3D i.
Sonata i.
Tesla magnetic resonance i.
Voxar Plug n View 3D i.
image-reconstruction time
imager/spectrometer
1.5T Signa whole body i.
**image-selected in vivo spectroscopy
(ISIS)**
imaginary
i. image
i. mode
i. number
i. signal
imagine
4D US i.
imaging *(See* image, MRI)
3DFT gradient-echo MR i.
3DFT volume i.
3D magnetic source i.
3D processed ultrafast
computerized i.
3D turbo SE i.
3D ultrasound reconstruction i.
acetazolamide challenge brain
SPECT i.
acoustic i.
AC-PC referenced MR i.
acute cerebral infarct i.
adenosine stress i.
adrenal i.
A-FAIR i.
i. agent
agent detection i.
air-contrast i.
air enema fluoroscopic i.
Aloka i.
amplitude i.
AMT-25-enhanced MR i.
angiography i.
anisotropically rotational diffusion i.
anisotropic 3D i.
annotated i.
antegrade pyelography i.
anthropometric i.
antifibrin antibody i.
aortography i.
aperiodic functional MR i.
AquariusBLUE 3D i.
arteriovenous shunt i.
arthrography i.
Artoscan MRI i.
A-scan i.
ascending contrast phlebography i.

attenuation i.
axial breath-hold gradient-echo cine magnetic resonance i.
axial echo planar diffusion weighted i.
axial grade echo i.
axial plane i.
axial 0.2T T1-weighted spin-echo i.
balloon expulsion i.
balloon test occlusion i.
barium enema i.
barium swallow i.
bile duct i.
biliary tract CT scan i.
binary i.
bird-cage coil designed for wrist i.
black blood T2-weighted inversion-recovery MR i.
blipped echo planar i. (bEPI)
blood flow i.
blood oxygenation level-dependent-functional magnetic resonance i. (BOLD-fMRI)
blood oxygen level-dependent contrast i.
blood pool i.
blush on i.
BMIPP SPECT scan i.
B-mode i.
body coil i.
body section radiography i.
BOLD contrast i.
bolus challenge i.
bone age i.
bone density i.
bone length i.
bone marrow edema pattern on MR i.
bone mineral content i.
bone phase i.
bone scintiscan i.
brain scan i.
breath-hold i.
breath-hold segmented k-space gradient-echo i.
breath-hold T1-weighted gradient echo i.
breath-hold T1-weighted MP-GRE MR i.
breath-hold ungated i.
breath-hold velocity-encoded cine MR i.

bright-field i.
bronchial provocation i.
bronchogram i.
B-scan i.
bull's eye i.
captopril-stimulated renal i.
cardiac blood pool i.
cardiac catheterization i.
cardiac positron emission tomography i.
cardiac radiography i.
cardiac wall motion i.
Cardiolite scan i.
cardiotocography i.
cardiovascular radioisotope scan and function i.
carotid duplex i.
carotid sinus i.
CAS i.
CEA-Scan diagnostic i.
cephalogram i.
cerebral perfusion SPECT i.
Ceretec brain i.
i. chain veiling glare
chemical-selective fat-saturation i.
chemical shift i. (CSI)
cholangiography i.
Chopper-Dixon fat suppression i.
i. chronology
cine CT i.
cine-gated i.
cine gradient-echo MR i.
cine gradient magnetic resonance i.
Cine Memory with color flow Doppler i.
cine phase contrast i.
cineradiography i.
cine view i.
cisternography i.
CKG i.
CMJ i.
coded-aperture i.
cognitive functional MR i.
coincidence i.
cold spot myocardial i.
collimation i.
color amplitude i.
color-coded Doppler flow i. (CDFI)
color-coded pulmonary blood flow i.
color Doppler i. (CDI)
color encoded brain MR i.

NOTES

imaging *(continued)*

color-flow i. (CFI)
color-flow Doppler i.
color-flow Doppler real-time 2D
 blood flow i.
color-flow duplex i.
color velocity i.
column-mode sinogram i.
combined leukocyte-marrow i.
combined Myoscint/thallium i.
combined thallium-Tc-HMPAO i.
i. compatible stereotactic coordinate
 frame
Compuscan Hittman computerized i.
computed transmission
 tomography i.
computer fusion i.
continuous i. (CI)
continuous moving bed (MR) i.
 (COMBI)
continuous-wave Doppler i.
contrast-enhanced fundamental i.
contrast-enhanced magnetic
 resonance i.
contrast-enhanced T1-GRE i.
contrast-enhanced T1-weighted spin-
 echo high-field-strength MR i.
contrast enhancement of computed
 tomographic i.
contrast-enhancing parametric i.
conventional planar i. (CPI)
conventional spin-echo i.
convergent color Doppler i.
coronary artery scan i.
corpus cavernosonography i.
corrected gradient echo phase i.
correlative diagnostic i.
correlative pertechnetate thyroid i.
cross-sectional i.
CSF-suppressed T2-weighted 3D
 MP-RAGE MR i.
CTAT i.
CT/SPECT fusion i.
cystography i.
cystourethroscopy i.
dacryocystography i.
darkfield i.
3D echo planar i.
delayed bone i.
DentaScan i.
DEXA bone density scan i.
dexamethasone suppression test i.
3D fast low-angle shot i.
3D fast spin-echo magnetic
 resonance i.
2D Fourier transformation i.
diagnostic i. (DI)
DIET fast SE i.
diffraction-enhanced i. (DEI)

diffusion magnetic resonance i.
diffusion tension i. (DTI)
diffusion tensor i. (DTI)
diffusion tensor MR i.
diffusion-weighted i. (DWI)
diffusion-weighted echo planar i.
diffusion-weighted magnetic
 resonance i.
diffusion-weighted MR i.
digital chest i.
digitally fused CT and
 radiolabeled i.
digital radiography i.
digital vascular i. (DVI, DVI
 mode)
4-dimensional i.
1-dimensional chemical-shift i. (1D-
 CSI)
dipyridamole echocardiography i.
dipyridamole handgrip i.
dipyridamole infusion i.
dipyridamole thallium-201 i.
dipyridamole thallium stress i.
direct Fourier transformation i.
discontinuous i.
displacement field-fitting MR i.
diuretic renal i.
2D KWE direct Fourier i.
3D KWE direct Fourier i.
2D modified KWE direct
 Fourier i.
Doppler color-flow i.
Doppler tissue i. (DTI)
Doppler ultrasonography i.
Doppler venous i.
double-dose gadolinium i.
double-helical CT i.
double-phase technetium-99m
 sestamibi i.
double pulse interlaced echo i.
3D projection reconstruction i.
dry laser i.
DSC MR i.
DT MR i.
3D T1-weighted gradient-echo i.
dual-coil i.
dual-echo DIET fast spin-echo i.
dual-echo and DT MR i.
dual-echo interleaved spiral out-
 in i.
dual-energy i.
dual isotope i.
dual-phase ^{99m}Tc-sestamibi i.
dual-tracer i.
duodenography i.
duplex carotid i.
duplex Doppler i.
dynamic contrast-enhanced magnetic
 resonance i. (DCE-MRI)

dynamic contrast-enhanced subtraction MR i.
dynamic liver i.
dynamic magnetic resonance i.
dynamic renal i.
dynamic scintigraphy i.
dynamic susceptibility contrast magnetic resonance i.
dynamic volume i.
dynamic weightbearing cervical magnetic resonance i.
ECG-gated multislice MR i.
ECG-gated spin-echo MR i.
echo i.
echocardiogram planar i.
echocardiography i.
echo-planar i. (EPI)
echo-planar diffusion-weighted i.
echo-planar FLAIR i.
echo-planar GRE T2*-weighted i.
echo plane i.
echo time chemical shift i.
elastic i.
electric joint fluoroscopy i.
electrocardiogram-gated MRI i.
electrocardiography-gated echo-planar i.
electrodiagnostic i.
electromagnetic blood flow i.
electronic portal i.
electron paramagnetic resonance spatial i.
electron radiography i.
electrostatic i.
end-diastolic i.
endoanal MR i.
endocrine i.
endorectal surface-coil MR i.
enhanced i.
ensemble contrast i. (ECI)
epicardial i.
epididymography i.
equilibrium MUGA i.
ERCP i.
esophageal function i.
esophagography i.
excretory urography i.
exercise thallium-201 stress i.
ex vivo magnetic resonance i.
fast cardiac phase contrast cine i.
fast Fourier i.

fast multiplanar inversion recovery i.
fast multiplanar spoiled gradient-recalled i.
fast scan magnetic resonance i.
fast spin-echo black blood i.
fast spin-echo and fast inversion recovery i.
fast spin-echo MR i.
fast spoiled gradient-recalled MR i.
fat-suppressed 3-dimensional spoiled gradient-echo FLASH MR i.
fat-suppressed 3D spoiled gradient-recall echo i.
fat-suppressed gadolinium-enhanced i.
fat-water chemical shift i.
FDG-labeled positron i.
FDG myocardial i.
ferumoxtran-enhanced echo-planar GRE T2*-weighted i.
ferumoxtran-enhanced echo-planar SE T2-weighted i.
fetal liver magnetic resonance i.
^{18}F FDG-negative i.
field-echo i.
field-of-view i.
filmless i.
first-pass myocardial perfusion i.
FLAIR echo-planar i.
FLAIR-FLASH i.
FLASH magnetic resonance i.
flat-field i.
flawed i.
flow i.
flow-sensitive MR i.
fluoroscopic i.
fluoroscopy-guided condylar lift-off i.
flush aortogram i.
Fourier 2-dimensional i.
Fourier direct transformation i.
Fourier multislice modified KWE direct i.
Fourier transform i.
FOV i.
2-frame gated i.
frequency domain i. (FDI)
FS burst MR i.
functional i.
functional brain i.

NOTES

imaging *(continued)*

functional magnetic resonance i. (fMRI)
functional spin-echo i.
gadolinium-enhanced MR i.
gallbladder i.
gallium lung i.
gastric emptying i.
gastric mucosa i.
gastrointestinal motility i.
gas ventilation i.
gated cardiac blood pool i.
gated cine i.
gated equilibrium cardiac blood pool i.
gated magnetic resonance i.
gated SPECT myocardial perfusion i.
Gd-FMPSPGR i.
GNG phase i.
i. gradient
gradient-echo 3-dimensional Fourier transform volume i.
gradient-echo flow i.
gradient-echo MR i.
gradient-echo phase i.
gradient-echo sequence i.
gradient-to-noise i.
GRASS MR i.
gray-scale i.
gray-scale baseline i.
GRE breath-hold hepatic i.
GRE gadolinium-chelate enhanced i.
GRE-in i.
GRE magnetic resonance i.
GRE-out i.
i. guided catheter drainage
half-Fourier i. (HFI)
half-Nex i.
harmonic i.
HAT-transformed i.
HBCT i.
heat-denatured autologous RBC SPECT i.
heavy ion i.
Helios diagnostic i.
helium magnetic resonance i. (He-MRI)
hemodynamically weighted echo-planar MR i.
hepatobiliary ductal system i.
HIDA i.
high-definition i. (HDI)
high-energy i.
high-field-strength MR i.
high-frequency Doppler ultrasound i.
high-resolution B-mode i.
high-resolution CT i.

high-resolution 3DFT MR i.
high-resolution infrared i.
high-resolution storage phosphor i.
high-speed i.
HLA i.
H-1 MR spectroscopic i.
holography i.
hot-spot heart i.
hot-spot myocardial i.
4-hour delayed thallium i.
HRI i.
hybrid i.
hybrid-RARE i.
hydrogen proton i.
hypotonic duodenography i.
hysterosalpingography i.
^{123}I BMIPP i.
image acquisition-gated scan i.
infarct-avid i.
infection i.
infrared i.
initial i.
in-phase GRE i.
integrated functional magnetic resonance i.
intermediate i.
interventional i.
interventional magnetic resonance i. (I-MRI)
intracoronary i.
intracranial i.
intraoperative i.
intraperitoneal technetium sulfur colloid i.
intrathecal i.
intravascular ultrasound i.
intravenous fluorescein angiography i.
inversion recovery echo planar i. (IR-EPI)
^{111}In white blood cell i.
iodine fluorescence i.
iodomethyl-norcholesterol scintigraphy i.
irreversible compression of MR i.
Isocam scintillation i.
isotope colloid i.
isotope hepatobiliary i.
isotope-labeled fibrinogen i.
isotope shunt i.
isotopic 3D i.
isotropic diffusion-weighted i.
IVFA i.
KCD i.
511-keV high-energy i.
kidney function i.
kidney radionuclide i.
kidneys, ureter, and bladder i.
kinematic magnetic resonance i.

kinestatic charge detector i.
KUB i.
laser-polarized helium MR i.
laser projection i. (LPI)
limitation of MR i.
limited i.
line i.
linear scan i.
lipid-polarized helium MR i.
lipid-sensitive MR i.
liver-spleen i.
localizing i.
longitudinal section i.
loopogram i.
lower extremity i.
lower limb venography i.
low-field-strength MR i.
low-flip-angle gradient-echo i.
low-resolution i.
lung i.
lymphangiography i.
lymphatic i.
lymph node i.
macromolecular contrast-enhanced
  MR i.
magic-angle spinning i.
Magnes 2500 whole-head i.
magnetic resonance i. (MRI)
magnetic resonance catheter i.
magnetic resonance diffusion i.
magnetic resonance perfusion i.
magnetic resonance spectroscopic i.
  (MRSI)
magnetic source i. (MSI)
magnetization and spin-lock
  transfer i.
magnetization transfer weighted i.
magnetoacoustic i.
malignant melanoma gallium i.
mammary ductogram i.
mammary galactogram i.
mangafodipir trisodium-enhanced
  MR i.
i. manifestation
marker transit i.
mass i.
material spin echocardiogram total
  volume i.
Matrix LR3300 laser i.
maxillofacial i.
maximum intensity projection i.
MCD i.

mediastinal cross-sectional i.
micro-CT i.
microscopic i.
microwave i.
middle-field-strength MR i.
midsagittal MR i.
miniature i.
minimum intensity projection i.
mirror i.
misleading i.
M-mode echocardiogram i.
morphologic i.
motion-free i.
moving tabletop MR i.
MRA i.
MR echo-planar i.
MR enteroclysis i.
MRI-guided laser-induced
  interstitial i.
MUGA cardiac blood pool i.
multiecho i.
multiformatted i.
multigated i.
multigated spectral Doppler i.
  (MSDI)
multimodality i.
multiorgan i.
multiphase-multisection T2-weighted
  MR i.
multiplanar MR i.
multiplanar reformatted radiographic
  and digitally reconstructed
  radiographic i.
multiple-echo i.
multiple-gated blood pool i.
multiple line scan i. (MLSI)
multiple-plane i.
multiple slice i.
multisection diffuse-weighted
  magnetic resonance i.
multisection gradient-echo echo-
  planar i.
multishot echo-planar i. (MS-EPI)
multishot spin-echo echo-planar i.
multislice first-pass myocardial
  perfusion i.
multislice modified KWE direct
  Fourier i.
multitime point i.
multitracer i.
musculoskeletal i.
MUSTPAC ultrasound i.

NOTES

imaging *(continued)*

myelography i.
myocardial I-123 MIBG i.
myocardial infarct i.
myocardial perfusion i. (MPI)
myocardial thallium i.
Myoscint i.
^{23}Na magnetic resonance i.
native tissue harmonic i. (NTHI)
navigated spin-echo diffusion-
  weighted MR i.
nephrostogram i.
nephrotomography i.
neurodiagnostic i.
neuroradiologic i.
neurotransmitter i.
NMR i.
nonattenuation-corrected SPECT i.
nonavid infarct i.
noninvasive i.
nonsubtraction i.
nuclear bone i.
nuclear cardiovascular i.
nuclear gated blood pool i.
nuclear hepatobiliary i.
nuclear magnetic resonance i.
nuclear medicine i.
nuclear perfusion i.
oblique axial MR i.
oblique magnetic resonance i.
oblique sagittal EKG-gated spin-
  echo magnetic resonance i.
OCG i.
octreotide i.
off-resonance saturation pulse i.
on-line portal i.
opposed-phase GRE, MR i.
optic surface i. (OSI)
optimal angle i.
oral cholecystogram i.
organ-specific scintigraphic i.
orthopantogram i.
orthoroentgenogram i.
out-of-phase GRE i.
oxygenation-sensitive functional
  MR i.
oxygen-enhanced lung MR i.
PACS PathSpeed MR i.
pancreas ultrasonography i.
pancreatography i.
panoramic i.
parallel i.
parallel hole i.
paramagnetic enhancement
  accentuation by chemical shift i.
parathyroid ultrasonography i.
partial Fourier i.
PASTA i.
pediatric nuclear medicine i.

percutaneous intracoronary
  angioscopy i.
perfusion MR i.
perfusion and ventilation lung i.
perfusion-weighted i. (PWI)
perineogram i.
peripheral vascular i.
peritoneogram i.
Persantine thallium i.
PET lung i.
PET metabolic i.
PET myocardial fatty acid i.
PET perfusion metabolism i.
PETT i.
3-phase i.
2-phase computed tomographic i.
2-phase computed tomographic i.
2-phase CT i.
phased-array body coil MR i.
phased-array multicoil i.
phased-array surface coil MR i.
phase-dependent spectroscopic i.
phase-encode time-reduced
  acquisition sequence i.
phase inversion harmonic i.
phase-sensitive gradient-echo MR i.
phase velocity i.
3-phase whole-body bone i.
  (TPWBBI)
photostimulable phosphor digital i.
physiologic i.
PIPIDA hepatobiliary i.
plain film i.
planar radionuclide i.
planar spin i.
planar thallium i.
i. plane
point i.
polarity-altered spectral-selective
  acquisition i.
POMP i.
portal venous phase i.
postcontrast MR i.
postdrainage i.
postexercise i.
postinjection i.
postmetrizamide CT i.
postoperative cholangiography i.
power Doppler i. (PDI)
precontrast i.
preoperative i.
pressure perfusion i.
pretherapy i.
projection reconstruction i.
projection tract i.
protodensity MR i.
proton chemical shift i.
proton-density-weighted i.

proton-electron double-resonance i.
  (PEDRI)
proton MR spectroscopic i.
pseudodynamic MR i.
pullback i.
pulmonary perfusion i.
pulmonary ventilation i.
pulsed electron paramagnetic i.
pulsed magnetization transfer
  MR i.
pulse-echo i.
pulse-inversion i.
pulse-inversion harmonic i. (PIHI)
pulse sequence echo-planar i.
PunctSURE vascular access i.
pyelography i.
PYP i.
pyrophosphate i.
QCT i.
quantitative brain i.
quantitative chemical shift i.
  (QCSI)
quantitative fluorescence i.
quantitative lung perfusion i.
quantitative magnetic resonance i.
  (qMRI, QMRI)
quantitative spirometrically
  controlled CT i.
radioactive fibrinogen i.
radiographically normal i.
radioisotope cisternography i.
radioisotope gallium i.
radioisotope indium-labeled white
  blood cell i.
radioisotope technetium i.
radiolabeled antibody i.
radionuclide-gated blood pool i.
radionuclide milk i.
radionuclide renal i.
radionuclide renography i.
radionuclide thyroid i.
rapid axial MR i.
rapid-excitation MR i.
rapid-sequence i.
^{82}Rb-based cardiac i.
real-time color Doppler i.
real-time 2D blood flow i.
receptor i.
reconstructed radiographic i.
reconstruction from projections i.
reconstructive i.
rectilinear bone scan i.

redistribution thallium-201 i.
renal angiography i.
renal CT i.
renal cyst i.
renal duplex i.
renal ultrasonography i.
renogram i.
respiratory gated i.
resting MUGA i.
rest myocardial perfusion i.
rest redistribution i.
rest thallium-201 myocardial i.
reticuloendothelial i.
ring-type i.
rose bengal sodium I-131 biliary i.
rotating delivery of excitation off-
  resonance MR i.
rotating frame i.
rotationally invariant i.
row-mode sinogram i.
R-to-R i.
sagittal fast spin-echo T2-weighted
  MR i.
sagittal gradient-echo i.
sagittal oblique i.
sagittal transabdominal i.
saline-enhanced MR i.
scanogram i.
3-Scape real-time 3D i.
scintigraphic scan i.
scintillation i.
scout i.
second-harmonic i.
sector-scan echocardiography i.
segmental k-space turbo gradient-
  echo breath-hold sequence i.
segmented echo-planar i. (SEPI)
segmenting dual-echo MR i.
selective excitation projection
  reconstruction i.
selenium-labeled bile acid i.
Senographe 2000D digital
  mammography i.
sensitive plane projection
  reconstruction i.
sequence echo-planar i.
sequence quantitative MR i.
sequential first pass i.
sequential line i.
sequential plane i.
sequential point i.
sequential quantitative MR i.

NOTES

imaging *(continued)*

serial contrast MR i.
serial duplex i.
serial dynamic i.
serialography i.
sestamibi stress scan i.
shaded surface display i.
short-echo-time chemical shift i.
short inversion recovery i.
short TI inversion recovery i.
1-shot echo-planar i.
shuntogram i.
sialography i.
silhouette i.
simultaneous volume i.
single-dose gadolinium i.
single-echo diffusion i.
single-shot gradient echo-planar i.
single voxel proton brain
  spectroscopy i.
sinus tract i.
slip-ring i.
small field-of-view MR i.
SmartScore CT i.
sodium i.
SonoCT real-time compound i.
Sonoline Antares 4-D ultrasound i.
source i.
spastic electron paramagnetic
  resonance i.
SPECT i.
spectamine brain i.
spectral Doppler i.
spike-related functional MR i.
spin-echo cardiac i.
spin-echo magnetic resonance i.
spin-echo T1-weighted transaxial
  MR i.
spin-lock and magnetization
  transfer i.
spin-warp i.
SPIO-enhanced MR i.
splanchnic vascular i.
spleen ultrasonography i.
splenoportography i.
split-brain i.
SSD i.
stacked-scan i.
static 3D FLASH i.
static liver i.
steady-state free precession i.
steady-state gradient-echo i.
STIR i.
stop-action i.
storage phosphor i.
strain-rate MR i.
stress-only perfusion i.
stress-redistribution i.
stress thallium-201 myocardial i.

i. study
subsecond FLASH i.
subtraction i.
superparamagnetic iron oxide
  MR i.
i. surveillance
susceptibility-weighted MR i.
target-to-nontarget ratio for
  myocardial i.
^{99m}Tc-HMPAO cerebral perfusion
  SPECT i.
^{99m}Tc-labeled denatured autologous
  RBC i.
^{99m}Tc Myoview myocardial
  perfusion i.
technetium-99m anti-CEA Fab
  murine monoclonal antibody i.
technetium-99m Infecton i.
technetium-99m pyrophosphate i.
technetium-99m tetrofosmin
  exercise-rest SPECT myocardial
  perfusion i.
technetium stannous
  pyrophosphate i.
technetium-thallium subtraction i.
thallium-201 i.
thallium myocardial perfusion i.
thallium myocardial scan with
  SPECT i.
thallium rest-redistribution i.
thallium scintography i.
thallium stress i.
thick-slice i.
thin-collimation i.
thin-slice i.
thoracic duct i.
ThromboScan i.
through-transfer i.
thyroid ultrasonography i.
i. time
timed i.
time-of-flight echo-planar i.
i. timing artifact
TIPS i.
tissue Doppler i.
tissue harmonic i. (THI)
TOF i.
tomographic i.
Toshiba Aspire continuous i.
total body scan i.
transabdominal i.
transaxial i.
transcervical catheterization of
  fallopian tube i.
transcranial real-time color
  Doppler i.
transesophageal Doppler color
  flow i.
transfer i.

transform i.
transjugular intrahepatic
  portosystemic shunt i.
transthoracic i.
transverse breath-hold gradient-echo
  cine magnetic resonance i.
transverse section i.
triple-dose gadolinium i.
triple-phase bone scan i.
true dynamic joint i.
TSPP i.
tumor i.
turboFLAIR i.
turboFLASH i.
T1-weighted coronal i.
T1-weighted sagittal i.
UBM i.
ultrafast CT i.
ultrasonic tomographic i.
ultrasound backscatter microscopy i.
ultrasound-based strain rate and
  strain i.
unenhanced MR i.
unsuppressed i.
urethrocystography i.
urography i.
vagus nerve stimulated functional
  magnetic resonance i. (VNS-
  fMRI)
vascular flow i.
vectorcardiography i.
velocity i.
velocity-density i.
velocity-encoded cine i. (VEC)
velocity-encoded cine MR i.
venography i.
venous i.
ventilation-perfusion i.
vesiculography i.
videofluoroscopic i.
virtual reality i.
Vitrea 3D i.
in vivo He-3 MR i.
volume i.
volumetric i.
V/Q i.
VScore with AutoGate cardiac i.
wall motion i.
water selective spin-echo i.
wavelet-encoded magnetic
  resonance i.
wet laser i.

white blood cell i.
whole-body echo-planar MR i.
whole-body scan i.
whole-body thallium i.
i. workstation
xenon-133 SPECT i.
imaging-anatomic correlation
imaging-based stereotaxis
**imaging-directed 3D volumetric
  information**
imaging-pathologic correlation
Imagopaque contrast medium
Imagyn microlaparoscope
Imatron
  I. C-100 EBT scanner
  I. C-150L EBCT scanner
  I. C-1000 UFCT scanner
  I. C-100 Ultrafast CT scanner
  I. C-150XL CT scanner
  I. C-100XP CT scanner
  I. Fastrac C-100 cine x-ray CT
    scanner
  I. Ultrafast CT scanner
imbalance
  biomechanical i.
  i. of gain artifact
  i. of phase artifact
  ventilatory capacity-demand i.
imbrication
  capsular i.
  facetal i.
**IMED Gemini PC-2 volumetric
  controller**
IMI
  inferior myocardial infarct
imidoacetic acid imaging agent
imidodiphosphonate (IDP)
immature
  i. bone
  i. lung
  i. lung syndrome
  i. ovarian teratoma
  skeletally i.
immaturity
  structural pulmonary i.
immediate
  i. postflow image
  i. postictal period
immediately detachable coil
immersion
  i. B-scan ultrasound
  i. technique

NOTES

imminent
- i. death
- i. demise

immobilization
- bone mineral i.

immobilizer
- Angle-Iron skull i.
- ankle i.
- AP-PA skull i.
- i. board
- cross-table leg i.
- dual leg i.
- molded i.
- Pigg-O-Stat mechanical i.
- sheet i.
- shoulder i.
- tomographic skull i.
- Velcro strap i.
- waist i.

immobilizing vest
immovable joint
immune
- i. electron microscopy
- i. response

immunity
- acquired i.
- active acquired i.
- artificial active acquired i.
- artificial passive acquired i.
- natural active acquired i.
- passive acquired i.

immunoblastic large-cell lymphoma
immunocytic amyloidosis
immunocytochemical staining
immunofluorimetric assay
immunoglobulin
- i. G (IgG)
- indium-111-labeled human nonspecific i. G
- ^{111}In-labeled human nonspecific i. G

immunologic injury
immunolymphoscintigraphy
immunomagnetic
- i. bead
- i. purging

Immuno-mini NJ-2300 microplate reader
immunoprecipitate
immunoproliferative small intestine disease (IPSID)
immunoradioassay
immunoreactivity
immunoscintigraphy
immunoscintimetry
immunostained surface
ImmuRAID antibody imaging agent
IMN
- intramammary node

IMO
- in my opinion

IMP
- ^{123}I isopropyl iodoamphetamine
- iodoamphetamine

impacted
- i. calculus
- i. feces
- i. fetus
- i. subcapital fracture
- i. urethral stone
- i. valgus fracture

impaction
- anteromedial superior humeral head i.
- fecal i.
- lateral compartment i.
- i. lesion
- mucoid i.
- stone i.

impact velocity
impaired
- i. renal function
- i. renal perfusion
- i. tubular transit
- i. venous return
- i. ventilation-perfusion

impairment
- axonal transport i.
- circulatory i.
- functional aerobic i.
- growth i.
- hemodynamic reserve i.
- inspiratory muscle function i.
- motor i.
- posterior cingulate functional i.
- renal function i.
- sensory i.

IMPAX PACS system
impedance
- acoustic i.
- aortic i.
- diastolic notch i.
- i. matching
- i. MR phlebogram
- i. phlebography
- i. plethysmography (IPG)
- pulmonary arterial input i.
- pulmonary vascular bed i.
- respiratory modulation of vascular i.
- vascular i.
- i. venography

impeller basket catheter
impending
- i. herniation
- i. myocardial infarct

imperfecta
- amelogenesis i.

dentinogenesis i.
osteogenesis i. (OI)
Sillence classification of
osteogenesis i.
imperfect regeneration
imperforate anus
impingement
anterolateral i.
chronic friction and i.
dural i.
i. exostosis
graft roof i.
iliopsoas i.
lateral i.
ligamentous i.
nerve root i.
outlet i.
posterior i.
posterosuperior glenoid i.
shoulder i.
sidewall i.
i. spur
syndesmotic i.
i. syndrome
talar i.
talofibular i.
triquetral i.
ulnolunate i.
impinging osteophyte
implant
Baerveldt glaucoma drainage i.
biodegradable i.
bone i.
bowel serosal endometrial i.
BrachySeed i.
BrachySeed PD-103 i.
carcinomatous i.
cesium i.
cobalt-chromium-molybdenum alloy
metal i.
cobalt-chromium-tungsten-nickel
alloy metal i.
cochlear i.
Co-Cr-Mo alloy metal i.
collapsed subpectoral i.
i. collar
double-lumen breast i.
double-stem silicone lesser MP i.
electrically activated i.
endometrial i.
endosseous i.
epidural i.

extraperitoneal i.
ferromagnetic i.
i. fracture
hinged i.
hydroxyapatite i.
^{125}I interstitial radiation i.
interstitial low-dose-rate iridium-192
needle i.
intracavitary i.
iridium-192 endobronchial i.
iridium-192 wire i.
i. irradiation
Joseph valve i.
Krupin-Denver eye valve-to-disc i.
malignant pleural i.
mammary i.
mechanically activated i.
metallic otologic i.
methyl methacrylate bead i.
ocular i.
open-cord tendon i.
otologic i.
palladium i.
^{103}Pd prostatic i.
penile i.
peritoneal metastatic i.
permanent interstitial i.
polymethyl methacrylate i.
prostate i.
prosthetic i.
retropectoral mammary i.
saline i.
serosal endometrial i.
silicone elastomer rubber ball i.
silicone wrist i.
single-lumen silicone breast i.
subglandular i.
subpectoral i.
synthetic bone i.
temporary interstitial i.
total knee i.
transperineal i.
transvaginal i.
tumor i.
VDS i.
implantable
i. access catheter
i. drug delivery system
i. infusion port
i. infusion pump
i. vascular access device

NOTES

implantation
  cornual i.
  i. cyst
  epicardial i.
  percutaneous transperineal seed i.
  peroral i.
  radon seed i.
  i. site
  2-staged stent i.
  subxiphoid i.
  transluminal aortic endograft i.
  transluminal endograft i.
  transvenous i.
implanted
  i. imaging opaque marker
  i. NCP
  i. pacemaker
impotence
  arteriogenic i.
  hemodynamic i.
  vasogenic i.
impression
  basilar i.
  cardiac i.
  colic i.
  convolutional i.
  digastric i.
  duodenal i.
  esophageal i.
  extrinsic esophageal i.
  extrinsic stomach i.
  i. fracture
  gastric i.
  liver i.
  renal i.
  suprarenal i.
imprint
  tissue i.
improved
  i. Chen-Smith (ICS)
  i. Chen-Smith coder
  i. photon flux
improvement
  interval i.
impulse
  apical i.
  bifid precordial i.
  double systolic apical i.
  downward displacement of apical i.
  ectopic i.
  high-amplitude i.
  hyperdynamic right ventricular i.
  jugular venous i.
  nodal i.
  prolonged left ventricular i.
  sustained apical i.
  systolic i.
  undulant i.

I-MRI
  interventional magnetic resonance
  imaging
IMRT
  intensity-modulated radiation therapy
  intensity-modulated radiotherapy
  treatment
    SmartBeam IMRT
IMT
  intimal-medial thickness
In
  indium
In-111
    In-111 oxine WBCs
    In-111 pentetreotide scan
^{111}In
  indium 111
    ^{111}In antimyosin scintigraphy
    ^{111}In chloride
    ^{111}In DTPA
    ^{111}In IgG
    ^{111}In imciromab pentetate
    ^{111}In labeling
    ^{111}In murine monoclonal antibody
      Fab to myosin
    ^{111}In octreotide
    ^{111}In oxine
    ^{111}In pentetreotide
    ^{111}In satumomab pendetide
    ^{111}In WBCs
    ^{111}In white blood cell imaging
in
  i. my opinion (IMO)
  i. situ
  i. situ graft
  i. situ pinning
  i. toto
  i. utero
  i. utero detection of cardiac
    anomaly
  i. utero MRI
  i. vitro evaluation of coil
  i. vitro labeling
  i. vivo
  i. vivo balloon pressure
  i. vivo correlation
  i. vivo disposition study
  i. vivo examination
  i. vivo He-3 MR imaging
  i. vivo labeling
  i. vivo method
  i. vivo microscopy
  i. vivo MR spectroscopy
  i. vivo optical spectroscopy
    (INVOS)
  i. vivo 31-P MR spectroscopy
  i. vivo 31P MR spectroscopy
  i. vivo proton MR spectroscopy

i. vivo stereologic assessment
i. vivo technique
inactivator
inactive
i. endometrium
i. mode
inadequate
i. bowel preparation
i. calvarial calcification
i. cardiac output
i. cranial calcification
i. runoff
i. visualization
inadvertent arterial injection
incarcerated
i. hernia
i. omentum
i. placenta
incarceration
fetal i.
incessant ovulation
0.016-inch
0.016-i. Headliner guidewire
0.016-i. hydrophilic guidewire
0.035-inch
0.035-i. Glidewire
0.035-i. hydrophilic angulated
guidewire
incidence
incident
i. angle
i. ray
incidental
i. finding
i. lung uptake
i. punctate white matter
hyperintensity
incidentaloma
adrenal i.
brain i.
incision
Brödel bloodless line of i.
incisional hernia
incisive
i. bone
i. canal
i. suture
incisor
fascial i.
i. teeth
incisura, incisure, pl. **incisurae**
i. angularis

aortic i.
cardiac i.
i. defect
i. dextra of Gans
i. scapulae
stomach defect i.
incisural
i. epidermoidoma
i. sclerosis
inciting
i. event
i. factor
inclination
radial i.
ulnar i.
urethral i. (UI)
i. verse
volar i.
inclinometer
inclusion cyst
incoherence
magnetic resonance spin i.
incoherent
i. motion
i. spin
incompetence
aortic valvular i.
chronotropic i.
communicating vein i.
deep venous i.
gastroesophageal i.
mitral valve i.
myocardial i.
postphlebitic valvular i.
pulmonary i.
saphenous vein i.
sphincter i.
traumatic tricuspid i.
tricuspid i. (TI)
valvular i.
incompetent
i. blood-brain barrier
i. cervix
i. ileocecal valve
i. perforator
incomplete
i. atrioventricular block (IAVB)
i. bladder emptying
i. closure
i. dislocation
i. fracture
i. fracture of bone

NOTES

incomplete *(continued)*
    i. heart block
    i. hernia
    i. left bundle-branch block
      (ILBBB)
    i. lower esophageal sphincter
      relaxation
    i. neurofibromatosis
    i. obstruction
    i. placenta previa
    i. pulmonary fissure
    i. resolution of pneumonia
    i. right bundle-branch block
      (IRBBB)
    i. stroke
    i. tumor
    i. unfolding
    i. ureteral duplication
incongruency
    patellofemoral i.
incongruity
    angle of i.
    facet joint i.
    joint i.
incontinence
    bladder i.
    bowel i.
    fecal i.
    motor urge i.
    stress i.
increased
    i. airway
    i. anteroposterior diameter
    i. attenuation
    i. basilar cistern
    i. bone density
    i. carrying angle
    i. central venous pressure
    i. cerebrovascular resistance
    i. density spleen
    i. echogenicity
    i. echo signal
    i. extracellular fluid volume
    i. interstitial fluid
    i. interstitial marking
    i. intracranial pressure
    i. intrapericardial pressure
    i. isotope uptake
    i. lateral joint space
    i. left ventricular ejection time
    i. marking of emphysema
    i. myocardial oxygen requirement
    i. outflow resistance
    i. peripheral resistance
    i. peristalsis
    i. prominence of pulmonary vessel
    i. pulmonary arterial pressure
    i. pulmonary obstruction
    i. pulmonary vascularity

    i. pulmonary vascular marking
    i. pulmonary vascular resistance
    i. pulmonary vasculature
    i. renal echogenicity cortex
    i. skull thickness
    i. splenic density
    i. thyroid uptake
    i. tracer activity
    i. tracer uptake
    i. uptake of radiotracer
    i. ventricular afterload
increase in intensity
increasingly dense nephrogram
increment
    i. in luminal diameter
    i. of perfusion
incremental
    i. dose
    i. risk factor
incrementation
    time-proportional phase i. (TPPI)
increta
    placenta i.
incus, pl. incudes
    i. bone
indemnity
    crown i.
indentation
    anterior central i.
    central i.
    focal i.
    haustral i.
    irregular extrinsic i.
    i. of myelography dye
    posterior central i.
    semilunar i.
indented
    i. fracture
    i. fracture of skull
in-department film
independent jaw
indeterminate age
indeterminatus
index, pl. indices, indexes
    acceleration i. (AI)
    acetabular i.
    acetabular head i. (AHI)
    amnionic fluid i. (AFI)
    angiographic muscle mass i.
    ankle-arm i. (AAI)
    ankle-brachial i. (ABI)
    apnea-hypopnea i. (AHI)
    arch length i.
    Ashman i.
    axial acetabular i. (AAI)
    Benink tarsal i.
    bicaudate i. (BCI)
    bifrontal i. (BFI)
    biliary saturation i.

NOTES

index *(continued)*
    resistive i. (RI)
    resting ankle pressure i. (RAPI)
    right and left ankle i.
    right ventricular stroke work i.
        (RVSWI)
    Ritchie i.
    i. of runoff resistance
    runoff resistance i.
    saturation i. (SI)
    scoliosis i.
    i. of sensitivity
    short-increment sensitivity i.
    Singh osteoporosis i.
    stroke i. (SI)
    stroke volume i. (SVI)
    stroke-work i. (SWI)
    superior-medial acetabular i.
        (SMAI)
    systemic arteriolar resistance i.
    systemic output i.
    systemic vascular resistance i.
        (SvO$_2$, SVRI)
    systolic pressure-time i.
    systolic toe/brachial i.
    talocalcaneal i.
    tension-time i. (TTI)
    therapeutic i.
    thoracic i.
    thymic i.
    thymidine labeling i. (TLI)
    tritiated thymidine labeling i.
    truncated arch i.
    tubular fertility i.
    ulnar styloid process i. (USPI)
    valgus i.
    venous distensibility i. (VDI)
    ventricular i. (VI)
    vertebral body i.
    wall motion score i.
    water perfusable tissue i.
    weighted-CT-dose i.
    widened anterior meningeal i.
    Wood unit i.
india ink artifact
Indian
    I. childhood cirrhosis
    I. file
Indiana pouch
indicator
    i. dilution curve
    i. dilution method of perfusion
        assessment
    i. dilution therapy
    i. fractionation principle
    gamma ray level i.
    xylol pulse i.
**indicator-dilution method for cardiac
    output measurement**

indicis
    extensor i.
Indiclor
indifferent gonad
indigo
    i. calculus
    I. LaserOptic
    I. LaserOptic treatment system
indirect
    i. blood supply
    i. computed tomography
    i. computed tomography
        lymphography
    i. CT
    i. fracture
    i. hernia sac
    i. inguinal hernia
    i. laryngoscopy
    i. MR arthrography
    i. MR arthrography of knee
    i. placentography
    i. ray
    i. ultrasound guidance
indirect-contract transmission
indiscernible
indiscrete
indiscriminate lesion
indistinct
    i. endometrial margin
    i. interface
indium (In)
    i. 111 (^{111}In)
    cistern i.
    i. imaging agent
    i. transferrin
indium-111-labeled
    i.-111-l. human nonspecific
        immunoglobulin G
    i.-111-l. IgG
    i.-111-l. leukocyte
    i.-111-l. white blood cell scan
indocyanine
    i. dilution curve
    i. green angiography
    i. green dye
    i. green imaging agent
indoleamine
indolent
    i. lesion
    i. myeloma
    i. radiation-induced rectal ulcer
Indomitable scanner
induced
    i. acoustic emission
    i. biopotential
    i. pneumothorax
    i. radioactivity
    i. thrombosis of aortic aneurysm
inducibility basal state

inducible
inductance
inductance-capacitance (LC)
induction
> dorsal i.
> electric i.
> electromagnetic i.
> magnetic i.
> neuromuscular system electric i.
> ovulation i.
> i. therapy

inductively coupled plasma atomic emission spectrometry (ICP-AES)
inductive reactance (XL)
indurated
> i. mass
> i. tissue

indurativa
> tuberculosis cutis i.

indurative
> i. necrosis
> i. pleurisy
> i. pneumonia

indwelling
> i. cannula
> i. Foley catheter
> i. nonvascular shunt
> i. stent

inelastic pericardium
inequality
> limb-length i.
> ventilation-perfusion i.

inert
> i. dust pneumoconiosis
> i. pneumoconiosis

inexorable progression
infant
> i. cranial Doppler ultrasonography
> i. gastrointestinal hemorrhage

infantile
> i. arteriosclerosis
> i. cardiomyopathy
> i. coarctation
> i. coarctation of aorta
> i. cortical hyperostosis
> i. digital fibromatosis
> i. embryonal carcinoma
> i. fibrosarcoma
> i. ganglioglioma
> i. hemangioendothelioma
> i. hemangioendothelioma of liver
> i. hemiplegia

> i. hepatic hemangioma
> i. hydrocele
> i. hydrocephalus
> i. lobar emphysema
> i. myofibromatosis
> i. pneumonia
> i. polycystic kidney disease
> i. pylorospasm
> i. thoracic dystrophy
> i. tibia vara
> i. uterus

infantilism
> intestinal i.

infarct
> acute ischemic brain i.
> acute myocardial i.
> acute nonhemorrhagic i.
> acute renal i.
> age-indeterminate i.
> anemic i.
> anterior communicating artery distribution i.
> anterior myocardial i.
> anterior septal myocardial i.
> anterior wall myocardial i.
> anteroinferior myocardial i.
> anterolateral myocardial i.
> anteroseptal myocardial i.
> apical-lateral wall myocardial i.
> apical myocardial i.
> arrhythmic myocardial i.
> atherothrombotic brain i.
> atrial i.
> basal ganglia i.
> bicerebral i.
> bilateral i.
> bland i.
> bone i.
> bowel i.
> brain i.
> brainstem i.
> capsular i.
> capsulocaudate i.
> capsuloputaminal i.
> capsuloputaminocaudate i.
> cardiac i.
> cerebellar i.
> cerebral artery i.
> chronic ischemic brain i.
> chronic renal i.
> concomitant i.
> cortical bone i.

NOTES

infarct (*continued*)
- diaphragmatic myocardial i. (DMI)
- digital livedo reticularis i.
- dominant hemisphere i.
- dural sinus thrombosis i.
- embolic cerebral i.
- evolving myocardial i.
- i. expansion
- extensive anterior myocardial i.
- frontal lobe i.
- full-thickness i.
- gyral i.
- healing i.
- hemispheric i.
- hemorrhagic brain i.
- high lateral wall myocardial i.
- hippocampal i.
- hyperacute ischemic brain i.
- hyperacute myocardial i.
- impending myocardial i.
- inferior myocardial i. (IMI)
- inferolateral wall myocardial i.
- inferoposterior wall myocardial i.
- inferoposterolateral myocardial i.
- intestinal i.
- ischemic brainstem i.
- kidney i.
- lacunar brain i.
- lateral myocardial i.
- lobar renal i.
- marrow i.
- medullary bone i.
- mesencephalic i.
- mesenteric i.
- middle cerebral artery i.
- multifocal i.
- multiple cortical i.'s
- muscle i.
- myocardial i. (MI)
- nonarrhythmic myocardial i.
- nonembolic i.
- nonhemorrhagic i.
- nonseptic embolic brain i.
- nontransmural myocardial i.
- occipital lobe i.
- occlusive mesenteric i.
- old myocardial i.
- omental i.
- papillary muscle i.
- paramedian i.
- parenchymal i.
- periventricular hemorrhagic i.
- pituitary i.
- placental i.
- i. of pons
- pontine i.
- posterior cerebral territory i.
- posterior wall myocardial i.
- posterobasal wall myocardial i.
- posteroinferior myocardial i.
- posterolateral wall myocardial i.
- postmyocardial i.
- postmyocardiotomy i.
- pulmonary i.
- Q-wave myocardial i.
- red i.
- renal i.
- right ventricular i.
- rule out myocardial i. (ROMI)
- i. scan
- segmental bowel i.
- segmental omental i.
- septal myocardial i.
- septic pulmonary i.
- silent myocardial i. (SMI)
- sinuatrial node i.
- i. size limitation
- small bowel i.
- small, deep, recent i. (SDRI)
- spinal cord i.
- splenic i.
- subacute ischemic brain i.
- subacute myocardial i.
- subcortical i.
- subendocardial i. (SEI)
- subendocardial myocardial i.
- temporal lobe i.
- testicular i.
- thalamic i.
- thromboembolic pontine i.
- Thrombolysis in Myocardial I. (TIMI)
- thrombotic i.
- transmural myocardial i.
- traumatic i.
- uncomplicated myocardial i.
- uninfected i.
- venous i.
- ventral pontine i.
- watershed brain i.
- wedge-shaped i.
- white matter i.

infarct-avid imaging
infarcted
- i. heart muscle
- i. lung segment
- i. myocardium
- i. scar
- i. testis

infarction
- diffuse multinodular i.

infarct-localized asynergy
infected
- i. aneurysm
- i. bone
- i. pelvic hematoma
- i. thrombosed graft

infection
    alveolar i.
    aortic graft i.
    buccal space i.
    diffuse i.
    discovertebral i.
    disc space i.
    filarial i.
    fungal i.
    hepatic fungal i.
    i. imaging
    interstitial i.
    intraabdominal i.
    intracranial opportunistic i.
    intravascular catheter-related i.
    masticator space i.
    mycotic lung i.
    nosocomial i.
    opportunistic lung cavity i.
    orbital i.
    pelvic i.
    pneumocystic i.
    pulmonary parenchymal i.
    renal fungal i.
    respiratory tract i.
    retroperitoneal i.
    rickettsial lung i.
    sacroiliac i.
    salivary gland i.
    spinal i.
    subperiosteal i.
    superimposed fungal i.
    temporal space i.
    tendon sheath space i.
    vessel displacement brain i.

infectious
    i. aortitis
    i. arthritis
    i. bubbly bone lesion
    i. cardiomyopathy
    i. heart disease
    i. pulmonary disorder
    i. splenomegaly

infective
    i. embolus
    i. thrombosis

inferior
    i. accessory fissure
    apertura pelvis i.
    i. apical aspect of myocardium
    i. aspect
    i. beaking

    i. border
    i. border of heart
    i. cardiac branch
    i. cerebellar peduncle
    i. colliculus
    i. dental canal
    i. displacement
    i. dorsal radioulnar ligament
    i. duodenal flexure (IDF)
    i. duodenal recess
    i. epigastric artery
    i. esophageal sphincter (IES)
    i. extensor retinaculum
    fovea i.
    i. frontal gyrus
    i. gemellus muscle
    i. glenohumeral ligament labral
      complex (IGLLC)
    i. jugular vein bulb
    i. lobe
    i. lobe bronchus
    i. lobe of lung
    i. longitudinal diameter
    i. margin of superior rib
    i. medial facet
    i. mediastinum
    i. mesenteric artery (IMA)
    i. mesenteric plexus
    i. mesenteric vein
    i. myocardial infarct (IMI)
    i. olive
    i. ophthalmic vein
    i. orbital fissure
    i. parietal lobule
    i. peroneal retinaculum
    i. pole
    i. pubic ramus
    i. pulmonary ligament
    i. pulmonary vein
    i. quadriceps retinaculum
    i. rectal vein
    i. sagittal sinus (ISS)
    i. spur
    i. syndrome of red nucleus
    i. temporal gyrus
    i. temporal lobule
    i. thyroid vein
    i. tip of fibula
    i. tip of scapula
    i. transverse rectal fold
    i. turbinated bone
    i. vena cava (IVC)

NOTES

inferior *(continued)*
    i. vena cava diaphragm
    i. vena cava duplication
    i. vena cavagram
    i. vena caval obstruction
    i. vena cava orifice
    i. vena cava syndrome
    i. vena cava transposition
    i. venacavography (IVCV)
    i. wall
    i. wall akinesis
    i. wall branch
    i. wall hypokinesis
    i. wall MI
    i. wall motion
    zygapophysis i.
inferior-anterior count ratio
inferiormost
inferoapical
    i. defect
    i. segment
    i. wall
inferobasal segment
inferolateral
    i. displacement of apical beat
    i. surface of prostate
    i. wall myocardial infarct
inferolaterally
inferomedial
inferoposterior
    i. segment
    i. wall myocardial infarct
inferoposterolateral myocardial infarct
inferred presence
infestation
    helminthic i.
INFH
    ischemic necrosis of femoral head
infiltrate
    active i.
    acute alveolar i.
    aggressive interstitial i.
    aggressive perivascular i.
    alveolar i.
    apical i.
    Assmann tuberculous i.
    basilar zone i.
    benign i.
    bilateral interstitial pulmonary i.
    bilateral upper lobe cavitary i.
    bone marrow i.
    brachial plexus i.
    bronchocentric inflammatory i.
    butterfly pattern of i.
    calcareous i.
    calcium i.
    cavitary i.
    chronic alveolar i.
    circumscribed i.

    confluent i.
    consolidated i.
    diffuse aggressive polymorphous i.
    diffuse alveolar interstitial i.
    diffuse bilateral alveolar i.
    diffuse fatty liver i.
    diffuse perivascular i.
    diffuse reticulonodular i.
    eosinophilic i.
    epituberculous i.
    fatty i.
    fibrocavitary i.
    fibronodular i.
    fleeting lung i.
    fluffy i.
    focal alveolar i.
    focal interstitial i.
    focal perivascular i.
    granular i.
    ground-glass i.
    hazy i.
    interstitial nonlobar i.
    invasive angiomatous interstitial i.
    linear i.
    lingular i.
    lung base i.
    lymphoplasmacytic i.
    marrow i.
    massive i.
    meningeal i.
    micronodular i.
    migratory patchy i.
    mottled i.
    multifocal aggressive i.
    mural i.
    parasitic i.
    patchy migratory i.
    peribronchial i.
    pericapsular fat i.
    perihilar batwing i.
    peripheral i.
    perivascular i.
    pneumonic i.
    pulmonary parenchymal i.
    pulmonic i.
    punctate i.
    recurrent fleeting i.
    reticular i.
    reticulonodular i.
    retrocardiac i.
    reverse peripheral bat-wing i.
    soft i.
    subcutaneous i.
    sulfasalazine-induced pulmonary i.
    transient symmetric pulmonary i.
    tuberculous i.
infiltrating
    i. adenocarcinoma
    i. breast epitheliosis

i. ductal carcinoma
i. esophageal carcinoma
i. lesion
i. lipoma
i. lobular carcinoma
i. plaque
infiltration
dose i.
marrow i.
myocardial i.
pathologic marrow i.
i. pattern
i. suture
infiltrative
i. astrocytoma
i. cardiomyopathy
i. hemorrhagic element
i. lymphoma
infinitesimal Z spectrum
inflamed
i. bronchus
i. pleura
inflammation
abdominal i.
acute phase of i.
adhesive i.
alveolar septal i.
aortic i.
atrophic i.
i. of bone
i. of brain
bronchial i.
bursal i.
calcaneal bursa i.
cardiac muscle i.
chronic abdominal i.
cirrhotic i.
i. of colon
diffuse i.
disseminated i.
i. of epididymis
esophageal i.
extrinsic intraabdominal i.
fibrinous i.
fibrosing i.
focal i.
i. of heart
hyperplastic i.
hypertrophic i.
interstitial i.
intrinsic intraabdominal i.
lung i.

meningeal i.
mucosal i.
myocardial i.
necrotic i.
obliterative i.
parenchymatous i.
pill-induced i.
polyarticular symmetric tophaceous
  joint i.
proliferative i.
pseudomembranous i.
radionuclide i.
renal i.
retrodiscal temporomandibular joint
  pad i.
sclerosing i.
spinal i.
spleen i.
subacute i.
suppurative i.
tendon i.
thyroid gland i.
transmural i.
tumor i.
vein i.
inflammatoria
dysphagia i.
inflammatory
i. adhesion
i. aortic aneurysm
i. bowel disease
i. bowel disease arthritis
i. breast carcinoma (IBC)
i. carotid pseudotumor
i. cholesteatoma
i. colonic polyp
i. edema
i. element
i. endometritis
i. esophagogastric polyp
i. fibroid polyp
i. fibrosarcoma
i. fibrosis
i. focus
i. fracture
i. heart block
i. idiopathic orbital pseudotumor
i. intestinal pseudotumor
i. joint effusion
i. lesion
i. MFH
i. myofibroblastic tumor

NOTES

inflammatory *(continued)*
  i. osteoarthritis
  i. polypoid mass
  i. reaction
  i. spleen
  i. stomach polyp
  i. synovial process
inflation
  air i.
  balloon i.
  delivered by balloon i.
  sequential balloon i.
  simultaneous balloon i.
inflow
  aortic i.
  blood i.
  i. cuff
  i. disease progression
  i. MRA
  third i.
  i. tract of left ventricle
inflow/outflow method
influence
  paramagnetic i.
information
  field-of-view i.
  hierarchical i.
  imaging-directed 3D volumetric i.
infraapical
infraaxillary
infracalcaneal bursitis
infracalcarine gyrus
infracardiac-type total anomalous venous return
infraclavicular
  i. area
  i. node
  i. pocket
infraclusion *(var. of* infraocclusion)
infracolic
  i. compartment
  i. midline
infracostal
infracristal ventricular septal defect
infraction
  i. fracture
  Freiberg i.
infradiaphragmatic
  i. application
  i. totally anomalous pulmonary venous drainage
  i. vein
infragastric infragenicular popliteal artery
infragenicular
  i. position
  i. revascularization
infrageniculate popliteal artery

infraglenoid
  i. recess
  i. tuberosity
infraglottic
  i. larynx
  i. space
infragluteal crease
infrahepatic
  i. arteriography
  i. inferior vena cava anastomosis
  i. vena cava
infrahilar area
infra-His block
infrahyoid lymph node
infrainguinal
  i. arterial bypass graft
  i. bypass stenosis
  i. DSA
  i. percutaneous transluminal angioplasty
  i. revascularization
  i. vein bypass graft
infralevator fistula
inframammary
  i. crease
  i. fold
inframammillary
inframesocolic space
infranuclear lesion
infraocclusion, infraclusion
infraorbital
  i. canal
  i. groove
  i. line
  i. margin (IOM)
  i. suture
infraorbitomeatal line (IOML)
infrapatellar
  i. aspect
  i. bursa
  i. contracture syndrome (IPCS)
  i. ligament
  i. plica
  i. tendon
  i. view
infrapopliteal
  i. artery occlusion
  i. vessel
infrapulmonary position
infrared
  i. camera
  high-resolution i. (HRI)
  i. imaging
  i. light
  i. light-emitting diode
  i. navigational system
  near i. (NIR)
  i. radiation
  i. ray

i. spectrum
i. thermography
infrarenal
i. abdominal aorta
i. abdominal aortic aneurysm
i. stenosis
infraroentgen ray
infrascapular
infraspinatus
i. insertion erosion
i. muscle
i. tendon
infraspinous
i. fascia
i. fossa
infrasternal
i. angle
i. fossa
infratemporal fossa
infratentorial
i. compartment
i. gray matter
i. Lindau tumor
infraumbilical
i. mound
i. omphalocele
infravesical obstruction
infundibular
i. atresia
i. chamber
i. pulmonary stenosis
i. septum
i. stalk
i. subpulmonic stenosis
i. systolic/diastolic ratio
i. tilt
i. tumor
i. ventricular septal defect
infundibular-bulb ratio
infundibuloovarian ligament
infundibulopelvic ligament
infundibuloventricular crest
infundibulum, pl. **infundibula**
i. of bile duct
bile duct i.
cerebral i.
ductus i.
gallbladder i.
i. of hypophysis
hypothalamic i.
junctional i.
i. of kidney

os i.
pituitary i.
right ventricular i.
tumor of i.
i. widening
Infuse-a-Port catheter
infuser
IVAC P4000 i.
Ohio i.
infusion
arterial i.
balloon-occluded arterial i.
i. catheter
circadian continuous i.
continuous intravenous i. (CIVI)
epidural i.
graded i.
hepatic arterial i. (HAI)
intralymphatic i.
intraportal i.
intrathrombus i.
intravenous i.
isolated hepatic i.
isoproterenol i.
local streptokinase i.
i. nephrotomography
pericardial i.
prostaglandin i.
protective cold saline i.
protracted venous i. (PVI)
pulse spray i.
i. pyelogram
i. pyelography
regional i.
regional intraarterial i.
retrograde coronary sinus i.
stepwise i.
subcutaneous i.
superselective i.
systemic intravenous i.
i. transcatheter therapy
viral i.
infusothorax
Ingenor silicone mixture
ingrowth
bone i.
peripheral perimeniscal capillary i.
porous i.
inguinal
i. bulge
i. canal
i. crease

NOTES

inguinal *(continued)*
 i. floor
 i. fold
 i. granuloma
 i. hernia
 i. ligament
 i. ligament syndrome
 i. lymph node
 i. lymph node metastasis
 i. pseudoaneurysm
 i. ring
 i. triangle
 i. trigone
inguinale
 papilloma i.
inhalation
 i. anthrax
 i. bronchopneumonia
 end i.
 i. of krypton-77
 i. pneumonia
 radioactive xenon gas i.
 i. study
 i. technique
 tin oxide i.
 i. tuberculosis
inhaled
 i. oxygen imaging agent
 i. radionuclide
inherent
 i. density
 i. filter
inherited cavernous angioma–related posthemorrhage encephalomalacia
inhibited
 atrial i. (AAI)
inhibition
 competitive i.
inhibitor
 efflux i.
 fusion i. (FI)
 thrombin-activatable fibrinolysis i. (TAFI)
inhibitory
 i. neurotransmitter
 i. syndrome
inhomogeneities
 shim i.
inhomogeneity
 contrast i.
 i. correction
 hypointense signal i.
 metaphysial-diaphysial low-signal-intensity red marrow i.
 off-axis dose i.
 signal intensity i.
inhomogeneous
 i. attenuation
 i. contrast enhancement

 i. echo
 i. echo pattern
 i. echo texture
 i. image
 i. lung attenuation HRCT
 i. moderate enhancement
 i. perfusion
 i. tracer distribution
iniencephaly
inion bump
initial
 i. atelectasis
 i. imaging
initiative
 private finance i. (PFI)
injectable procoagulant mixture
injectate
injection
 accidental intradural i.
 air i.
 barium i.
 bismuth i.
 bolus intravenous i.
 coarse i.
 contrast i.
 Definity suspension for IV i.
 double i.
 epidural steroid i.
 ethanol i.
 extraarachnoid i.
 facet joint i.
 fine i.
 Fluorescite i.
 fluorodeoxyglucose F-18 i.
 Funduscein i.
 gaseous i.
 Glofil-125 i.
 hand i.
 heavy metal i.
 inadvertent arterial i.
 intraamniotic i.
 intraarterial i.
 intracavernosal i.
 intradermal i.
 intradiscal i.
 intramuscular fetal i.
 intraperitoneal fetal i.
 intratumoral 90Y glass microsphere i.
 intravascular i.
 intravenous bolus i.
 intravenous fetal i.
 iobenguane I-123 i.
 iodinated I-131 albumin aggregated i.
 ipsilateral i.
 kit for preparation of technetium ^{99m}Tc depreotide i.
 machine i.

manual i.
i. mass
Miraluma i
Omnipaque i.
opacifying i.
paratumoral i.
percutaneous ethanol i. (PEI)
percutaneous thrombin i.
percutaneous ultrasound-guided
  thrombin i.
perinephric air i.
i. port
power i.
prostaglandin E_1 i.
radionuclide i.
rest i.
retrograde i.
i. scan interval (ISI)
sclerosing i.
selective arterial i.
serial i.
silicone i.
straight AP pelvic i.
subarachnoid i.
subcutaneous i.
subdural contrast i.
subureteric Teflon i. (STING)
test i.
transduodenal fiberscopic duct i.
ultrasonographically guided i.
ultrasound-guided methotrexate i.
venous i.

injector

Cordis i.
double-power i.
Envision CT power i.
Hercules power i.
Injectron CT2 power i.
Mark V Plus automatic i.
Medrad automated power i.
Medrad contrast medium i.
Medrad power angiographic i.
MR-compatible power i.
Optistat power i.
power i.
pressure i.
Pulse-Spray i.
Renovist II i.
single-power i.
Spectris MR-compatible i.
Spectris power i.
Taveras i.

Injectron CT2 power injector

injury

acute radiation i.
acute stretch i.
acute thoracic aortic i.
acute traumatic aortic i. (ATAI)
ankle inversion i.
anterior cruciate ligament i.
anterior urethral i.
aortic-brachiocephalic i.
apophysial i.
axial compression i.
axial loading i.
ballistic i.
barked i.
bilateral incomplete ureteral i.
blunt i.
bony trabecular i.
brachial plexus birth i.
burst i.
cervical spine i.
chronic ligamentous i.
closed head i. (CHI)
clothesline i.
cocking i.
2-column i.
3-column i.
compression flexion i.
compressive hyperextension i.
concomitant tracheal i.
contrecoup i.
crush i.
decelerative i.
diffuse axonal i. (DAI)
diffuse white matter i.
distraction hyperflexion i.
endothelial i.
epiphysial plate i.
Erb i.
Erb-Duchenne-Klumpke i.
excitotoxic cord i.
extension i.
extensive head i.
firearm i.
flake-shaped i.
flexion-distraction i.
flexion-rotation i.
forced flexion i.
genitourinary i.
glenoid labrum i.
greater arc i.
growth plate i.

NOTES

injury *(continued)*
    head i. (HI)
    high-caliber, low-velocity
      handgun i.
    hollow viscus i.
    hyperextension i.
    hyperflexion/hyperextension
      cervical i.
    hyperflexion/rotation i.
    hypertension i.
    hypoxic i.
    iatrogenic ureteral i.
    immunologic i.
    intercostal nerve i.
    intraoperative gastrointestinal i.
    intraperitoneal i.
    inversion i.
    irradiation i.
    ischemic i. (SE)
    ischemic reperfusion i.
    isolated airway i.
    Klumpke brachial plexus i.
    Kulkarni i.
    labral i.
    lateral bending i.
    lateral compartment traumatic
      bony i.
    lateral talar dome i.
    lesser arc i.
    lethal myocardial i.
    Lisfranc i.
    low back i.
    Maisonneuve i.
    matrix i.
    mechanism of i.
    medial talar dome i.
    medial talar osteochondral i.
    meniscal i.
    metatarsal i.
    midtarsal i.
    mild head i.
    mild traumatic brain i.
    motor vehicle i.
    multiple recurrent inversion i.'s
    muscle crushing i.
    myocardial reperfusion i.
    nerve i.
    nonlethal myocardial ischemic i.
    occult osseous i.
    osseous cervical spine i.
    osteochondral i.
    penetrating lung i.
    pericarinal i.
    perinatal i.
    peripheral nerve i.
    peroneal tendon i.
    phrenic nerve i.
    physial i.
    plexus i.

    posterior cruciate ligament i.
    posterior urethral i.
    posterolateral corner i.
    postnatal i.
    prenatal i.
    pronation-abduction i.
    pronation-external rotation i.
    proximity i.
    pulmonary parenchymal i.
    radial vascular thermal i.
    radiation i.
    radiation-induced skin i.
    radiocontrast-induced i.
    rapid deceleration i.
    rectal radiation i.
    renal i.
    repetitive strain i. (RSI)
    repetitive stress i. (RSI)
    rotation-shearing i.
    Sage-Salvatore classification of
      acromioclavicular joint i.
    seatbelt i.
    sesamoid i.
    i. severity scale (ISS)
    i. severity score (ISS)
    shearing white matter i.
    skier's i.
    softball sliding i.
    soft tissue i.
    solid viscus i.
    spinal cord i. (SCI)
    straddle i.
    stress i.
    subendocardial i.
    superior labral anterior-posterior i.
    supination-adduction i.
    supination-external rotation i.
    supination-outward rotation i.
    talar dome osteochondral i.
    talofibular ligament i.
    tensile i.
    through-and-through i.
    throwing arm i.
    tracheobronchial i. (TBI)
    transcutaneous crush i.
    traumatic aortic i. (TAI)
    traumatic brain i. (TBI)
    traumatic head i.
    ultrasonic assessment of i.
    unilateral locked facet i.
    urethral straddle i.
    valgus-external rotation i.
    vesical i.
    wafer-shaped i.
    weightbearing rotational i.
    whiplash i.
    white matter shearing i.
    windup i.
inking the margin

^{111}In-labeled
  ^{111}In-l. human nonspecific immunoglobulin G
  ^{111}In-l. white blood cell
inlay graft
inlet
  esophageal i.
  pelvic i.
  i. position
  thoracic i.
  transaxial thoracic i.
inner
  i. adrenal cortex
  i. bright layer
  i. ear
  i. ear anatomy
  i. ear atresia
  i. ear mass
  i. ear vestibule
  i. stripe of Baillinger
  i. table
  i. table of frontal bone
  i. table of skull
  i. table thickening
innermost intercostal muscle
InnerVasc vascular access system
innervation
  sympathetic i.
Innerview GI
Innervision MR scanner
innocent gallstone
innocuous
innominate
  i. absence of line
  i. aneurysm
  i. angiography
  i. artery
  i. artery buckling
  i. artery compression syndrome
  i. artery kinking
  i. artery stenosis
  i. artery stenting
  i. bone
  i. canaliculus
  i. vein
inoperable brain tumor
inorganic phosphorus
^{111}In-oxime-labeled leukocyte
In-pentetreotide scintigraphy
in-phase
  i.-p. GRE imaging
  i.-p. sequence
  i.-p. T1-weighted image
in-plane
  i.-p. spatial resolution
  i.-p. vessel
InQwire guidewire
Insall ratio
Insall-Salvati
  I.-S. index
  I.-S. ratio
insertion
  anomalous i.
  Bosworth bone peg i.
  capsular i.
  catheter i.
  femoral vein percutaneous i.
  Harrington rod i.
  ligamentous i.
  percutaneous pin i.
  percutaneous tube i.
  sartorius i.
  tendinous i.
  velamentous i.
inside-out x-ray
inside-to-outside segmentation
InSightec
Insight Millennium scan
InSite Her-2/neu kit
insoluble
insonation
  angle of i.
  i. condition
  Doppler i.
  transforaminal i.
  transtemporal i.
insonifying wave field
Inspec-100
inspection
  surgical i.
  visual i.
inspiration
  degree of i.
  i. and expiration views
  shallow i.
  suspended i.
inspiratory
  i. effort
  i. to expiratory
  i. to expiratory ratio (I-E)
  i. flow
  i. flow rate
  i. increase in venous pressure

NOTES

inspiratory *(continued)*
  i. muscle function impairment
  i. phase
  i. reserve volume (IRV)
  i. retraction
  i. spasm
  i. view
inspired air
inspissated
  i. feces
  i. material
  i. secretion
instability
  alveolar i.
  ankle i.
  anterolateral rotary knee i.
  articular i.
  atlantoaxial i.
  atraumatic, multidirectional, bilateral
    radial i. (AMBRI)
  chronic functional i.
  degenerative spinal i.
  detrusor i.
  dissociative i.
  dorsal intercalated segmental i.
    (DISI)
  first ray i.
  genomic i.
  glenohumeral i.
  hindfoot i.
  inversion i.
  ischemic i.
  joint i.
  lateral rotatory ankle i.
  ligamentous i.
  microsatellite i.
  midcarpal i.
  nondissociative i.
  osseous i.
  perilunar i.
  perilunate i.
  phase i.
  posterolateral rotatory i.
  postlaminectomy i.
  rotary ankle i.
  rotational i.
  rotatory i.
  shoulder joint i.
  sonographic measurement of
    subtalar joint i.
  spinal i.
  subtalar i.
  sympathetic vascular i.
  truncal i.
  varus-valgus i.
  ventricular electrical i.
  volar-flexed intercalated segment i.
  volar intercalated segment i. (VISI)

instantaneous
  i. axis of rotation (IAR)
  i. enhancement rate
  i. gradient
InstaScan scanner
in-stent
  i.-s. restenosis
  i.-s. stenosis
instillation
  contrast material i.
  percutaneous ethanol i.
  subarachnoid i.
institute
  National Heart, Lung, and
    Blood I. (NHLBI)
instrument
  Bard Monoply reusable core
    biopsy i.
  FlashPoint image-guided surgical i.
  ionization i.
  Magnum biopsy i.
  i. output
  Sabouraud-Noire i.
  single-headed i.
instrumentation
  advanced breast biopsy i. (ABBI)
  interspinous segmental spinal i.
    (ISSI)
  long-term venous i.
insufficiency
  acute cerebrovascular i.
  acute coronary i.
  adrenal i.
  aortic valvular i.
  arterial i.
  autonomic i.
  basilar artery i.
  brachial-basilar i.
  cardiac i.
  cardiopulmonary i.
  cerebrovascular i.
  chronic venous i.
  congenital pulmonary valve i.
  coronary i.
  deep venous i. (DVI)
  i. fracture
  gastric i.
  hepatic i.
  hypostatic pulmonary i.
  ileocecal i.
  mesenteric vascular i.
  mitral i. (MI)
  muscular i.
  myocardial i.
  nonocclusive mesenteric arterial i.
  nonrheumatic aortic i.
  pad sign of aortic i.
  parathyroid i.
  postirradiation vascular i.

posttraumatic pulmonary i.
primary adrenal i.
pulmonary arterial flow i.
pulmonary valve i.
pulmonic i. (PI)
pyloric i.
renal i.
respiratory i.
rheumatic aortic i.
secondary venous i.
Sternberg myocardial i.
subchondral i.
thyroid i.
transient ischemic carotid i.
tricuspid i. (TI)
uterine i.
uteroplacental i.
valvular aortic i.
vascular i.
velopharyngeal i.
venous i.
vertebrobasilar i. (VBI)
insufficient
i. acoustic penetration
i. cochlear turn
i. venous opacification
insufflation
air i.
CO_2 i.
gas i.
mechanical i.
perirenal i.
retroperitoneal gas i.
tubal i.
insufflator
Protoco₂l automated CO_2 i.
insula, pl. **insulae**
roof of i.
i. root
insular
i. gyrus
i. lobe
i. region
i. region of brain
i. ribbon sign
i. segment of middle cerebral
artery
i. triangle
insulinase
insulin-iodine
insulinoma

insult
aortic i.
bihemispheral i.
cerebrovascular i.
hypoxic ischemic i.
mechanical i.
myocardial i.
notable cerebral i.
occlusive cerebrovascular i.
thermal i.
vascular i.
Insyte Autoguard Shielded IV catheter
intact
i. valve cusp
i. ventricular septum
intake
fluid i.
integral
Choquet fuzzy i.
i. dose
systolic velocity-time i.
time velocity i.
i. uniformity scintillation camera
integrated
i. clinical information system
(ICIS)
i. fMRI
i. functional magnetic resonance
imaging
i. optical density (IOD)
i. optical density histogram
i. parallel acquisition technique
(iPAT)
i. reference air kerma (IRAK)
Integrilin
Integris
I. 3D RA
I. III-V DSA system
I. 3000 scanner
I. V-3000 DDSA
I. V 3000 digital subtraction
system
I. V3000 imager
integrity
spinal i.
Intelect Legend Combo stimulator and
ultrasound unit
intense uptake
intensification
i. factor

NOTES

487

intensification *(continued)*
    frequency i.
    image i.
intensified radiographic imaging system
  (IRIS)
intensifier
    image i.
    portable C-arm i.
intensifying
    i. screen
    i. screen artifact
intensity
    absolute dose i. (ADI)
    amorphous high signal i.
    beam i.
    bright signal i.
    calcified sequestra of low signal i.
    central fat signal i.
    central intrasubstance signal i.
    dark signal i.
    decreased i.
    diminished marrow signal i.
    discrete hyperintense signal i.
    equal in i.
    fat signal i.
    fusiform high signal i.
    grade 1–3 signal i.
    heterogeneous signal i.
    high-grade signal i.
    high signal i.
    homogeneous signal i.
    increase in i.
    intermediate signal i.
    internodular difference in signal i.
      (IDSI)
    intrameniscal signal i.
    intravascular signal i.
    juxtaarticular low signal i.
    linear degenerative signal i.
    linear high signal i.
    low signal i.
    marrow fat signal i.
    maximal i.
    nuclear magnetic resonance
      signal i.
    ovoid high signal i.
    pedicle signal i.
    photostimulable luminescence i.
    radiation i.
    reduced signal i.
    reverse pattern of signal i.
    scene i.
    signal i. (SI)
    single photon/maximum i.
    site of maximal i.
    spatial average-pulse average i.
    spatial average-temporal average i.
    spatial peak-temporal average i.
    symmetric confluent high signal i.

    temporal average i.
    temporal peak i.
    time-to-peak i. (TTP)
    variable i.
    vertebral body marrow signal i.
    water-like signal i.
    i. windowing
intensity-modulated
    i.-m. arc therapy
    i.-m. photon beam
    i.-m. radiation therapy (IMRT)
    i.-m. radiotherapy treatment (IMRT)
intentional reversible thrombosis
interaction
    capacitive i.
    Compton i.
    dipolar i.
    dipole-dipole i.
    effector/target cell i.
    electric i.
    magnetic i.
    mind-body i.
    photoelectric i.
    proton dipole-dipole i.
interactive
    i. electronic scalpel
    i. gradient optimization
    i. MR-guided biopsy
    i. volume rendering
interactive volume rendering
interaorticobronchial diverticulum
interarch distance
interarticular
    i. cartilage
    i. disc
    i. ridge
interarticularis
    pars i.
interatrial
    i. baffle leak
    i. communication
    i. groove
    i. septal defect
    i. septal hypertrophy
    i. septum (IAS)
    i. transposition of venous return
interbody
    i. bone graft
    i. bone plug
    i. fusion
interbronchial
    i. angle (IA)
    i. diverticulum
    i. mass
intercalary defect
intercalated segment
intercalating agent
intercalation
intercapital ligament

intercarpal
   i. angle
   i. articular
   i. articulation
   i. coalition
   i. joint
   i. ligament
intercartilaginous rim
intercaudate distance
intercaval band
intercavernous
   i. anastomosis
   i. sinus
intercellular
   i. edema
   i. space
Intercept
   I. esophagus microcoil
   I. prostate microcoil
   I. urethra microcoil
   I. Vascular 0.030^2 internal MR coil
intercervical disc herniation
interchondral joint
interchordal space fenestration
interclavicular
   i. ligament
   i. notch
interclinoid ligament
intercollicular groove
intercomparison
   i. measurement
   i. measurement technique
intercondylar
   i. eminence
   i. femoral fracture
   i. fossa
   i. groove
   i. humeral fracture
   i. joint space
   i. notch
   i. process
   i. roof
   i. sagittal image
   i. tibial fracture
   i. tubercle
intercondyloid fossa
intercornual ligament
intercoronary collateral flow
intercostal
   i. artery
   i. artery angiography
   i. lymph node

   i. muscle
   i. nerve
   i. nerve block
   i. nerve injury
   i. neuromuscular bundle
   i. retraction
   i. space
   i. vein
   i. vessel
intercostobrachial nerve
intercristal diameter
intercuneiform ligament
interdigital
   i. clavus
   i. ligament
   i. neoplasm
   i. neuroma
interdigitation
   cerebral gyri i.
   i. of vastus lateralis
interecho spacing
interest
   region of i. (ROI)
   volume of i. (VOI)
interface
   acetabular-prosthetic i.
   acoustic i.
   air i.
   air-soft tissue i.
   bidirectional i.
   body i.
   bone-air i.
   bone-implant i.
   catheter-skin i.
   common gateway i. (CGI)
   dermal-subcutaneous fat i.
   disc-thecal sac i.
   fat-blood i. (FBI)
   fat-fluid density i.
   fat-water i.
   fluid i.
   gray-to-white matter i.
   indistinct i.
   joint i.
   lumen-intimal i.
   Magnetic Resonance User I.
    (MRUI)
   media-adventitia i.
   muscle-fat i.
   reactive i.
   shear i.
   i. sign

NOTES

interface *(continued)*
    socket-stump i.
    tissue-air i.
    transducer-skin i.
interfacetal dislocation
interfacial canal
interference
    i. dissociation
    electromagnetic i. (EMI)
    i. phenomenon
    i. screw
    slice i.
interferential current therapy
interferometry
    phase-shifting i.
interfibrosis
interfollicular Hodgkin disease
interfoveolar ligament
interfraction interval
interfragmental compression
interfragmentary plate
intergluteal cleft
interhaustral septum
interhemispheric
    i. asymmetry
    i. cyst
    i. fissure (IHF)
    i. pathway
    i. subdural hematoma
    i. transfer
interictal
    i. brain SPECT
    i. normalization
    i. PET FDG study
    i. phase
    i. SPECT scan
    i. SPECT study
    i. spiking
interiliac
    i. lymph node
    i. plane
interinnominoabdominal cleft
interior surface of pancreas
interlacing
interlaminar distance
interleaved
    i. axial slab
    i. BOLD-fMRI scanning
    i. GRE sequence
    i. image acquisition
    i. imaging pass
    i. inversion-readout segment
    i. k-space coverage
    i. phase contrast technique
interligamentous bursa
interlobar
    i. artery
    i. empyema
    i. fissure

    i. pleurisy
    i. septal line
    i. septum
    i. space
interlobular
    i. bile duct
    i. emphysema
    i. lung septum
    i. septal thickening
    i. tissue
    i. vasculature
    i. vessel
interlocking detachable coil (IDC)
interloop abscess
intermaxillary
    i. bone
    i. spine
    i. suture
intermediate
    i. bronchus
    i. bursa
    i. callus
    i. coronary artery
    i. coronary syndrome
    i. CT slice
    i. cuneiform bone
    i. cuneiform fracture-dislocation
    i. fetal death
    i. heart
    i. image
    i. imaging
    i. nerve of Wrisberg
    i. ray
    i. signal intensity
    i. signal intensity layer
    i. signal intensity mass
    i. signal striation
intermediolateral
    i. gray column
    i. tract
intermedius
    bronchus i.
    nervus i.
    vastus i.
intermesenteric
    i. abscess
    i. plexus
intermetacarpal articulation
intermetatarsal
    i. angle (IMA)
    i. bursitis
    i. joint
    i. ligament
    i. space
intermetatarsophalangeal
    i. bursa
    i. bursitis
intermittent
    i. diffuse esophageal spasm

i. obstruction
i. occlusion
i. sinus arrest
i. third-degree AV block
intermodality image registration
intermuscular
i. hematoma
i. septum
interna
endometriosis i.
theca i.
internal
i. abdominal ring
i. aberrant carotid artery
i. architecture
i. auditory canal
i. auditory canal anatomy
i. auditory canal enhancing lesion
i. auditory meatus
i. band
i. biliary drainage
i. biliary stent
i. caliber
i. capsule
i. capsule intracerebral hemorrhage
i. carotid
i. carotid angiography
i. carotid artery (ICA)
i. carotid artery aneurysm
i. carotid artery occlusion
i. carotid balloon test
i. carotid system
i. carotid systolic peak flow (ICSPF)
i. cerebral vein (ICV)
i. cervical os
i. clot
i. collateral ligament
i. conjugate diameter
i. conversion
i. conversion electron
i. cyclotron target
i. degeneration
i. derangement
i. derangement of knee (IDK)
i. diameter (ID)
i. disc herniation
i. echo
i. echogenicity
i. echotexture
i. enhancement
i. and external rotation views

i. femoral rotation
i. fixation device
i. hernia
i. iliac artery
i. inguinal ring
i. intercostal muscle
i. intermuscular septum
i. jugular bulb
i. jugular triangle
i. jugular vein (IJV)
i. mammary artery (IMA)
i. mammary artery pedicle
i. mammary lymphatic chain
i. mammary lymph node
i. mammary lymphoscintigraphy
i. oblique aponeurosis
i. oblique radiograph
i. pudendal artery
i. pudendal vessel
i. radiation therapy
i. retention mechanism
i. rotation deformity
i. rotation in extension (IRE)
i. rotation in flexion (IRF)
i. table of calvaria
i. thoracic artery (ITA)
i. thoracic artery graft
i. thoracic vein
i. tibial torsion (ITT)
i. tibiofibular torsion
i. ureteral stent
i. urethral orifice
i. urethrotomy
internal/external catheter
internally fixed fracture
internasal suture
international
I. Commission on Radiation Units (ICRU)
i. reference preparation
i. standard (IS)
internervous plane
internodular difference in signal intensity (IDSI)
internuclear distance
internus
obturator i.
interobserver
i. error
i. variation
interopercular distance
interorbital distance

NOTES

interossei
    dorsal i.
    palmar i.
    plantar i.
interosseous
    i. border
    i. cyst
    first digital i. (FDI)
    i. membrane (IOM)
    i. muscle
    i. muscle group
    i. nerve
    i. ridge
    i. sacroiliac ligament
    i. space
    i. talocalcaneal ligament
    i. tendon
interpalatine suture
interparietal
    i. bone
    i. suture
interpectoral lymph node
interpedicular
    i. distance
    i. distance widening
interpediculate
interpeduncular
    i. cistern (IPC)
    i. fossa
    i. notch
    i. space
interperiosteal fracture
interphalangeal (IP)
    i. articulation
    i. dislocation
    distal i. (DIP)
    i. fusion
    i. joint
    i. osteoarthritis
    proximal i. (PIP)
interpleural space
interpolation
    i. algorithm
    color space i.
    cubic convolution i.
    80-degree linear i.
    full scan with i.
    i. kernel
    linear i.
    object-based i.
    prism i.
    scene-based i.
    sinc i.
    trilinear i.
    zero-fill i. (ZIP)
interpolator
    color space i.
Interpore bone replacement material

interposed
    i. colon segment
    i. colon segment obstruction
interposition
    colonic i.
    gastric i.
    i. graft
    hepatodiaphragmatic i.
    soft tissue i.
interpretation
    mirror-image i.
    radiographic i.
interpretive
    i. criterion
    i. variability
interpulse
    i. interval
    i. time
interpupillary line
interridge distance
interrogation
    color duplex i.
    deep Doppler velocity i.
    Doppler i.
    pulse Doppler i.
    radiation i.
interrupted
    i. duct sign
    i. periosteal reaction
interruption
    aortic arch i.
    bony cortex i.
    juxtahilar bronchus i.
    pulmonary artery i.
    surgical venous i.
intersacral canal
interscalene approach
interscan delay (ID)
interscapular gland
interscapulothoracic amputation
intersection gap
intersegmental
    i. aberration
    i. laminar fusion
    i. tract
intersesamoid ligament
intersex
    i. female
    true i.
intersigmoid recess
interslice
    i. distance
    i. gap
interspace
    ballooning of vertebral i.
    disc i.
    vertebral disc i.
    wedging of vertebral i.

Interspec Apogee RX400 diagnostic ultrasound system
intersperse
interspersed lucency
intersphincteric
    i. abscess
    i. anal fistula
    i. plane
    i. region
intersphincteric region
interspinal
    i. muscle
    i. plane
interspinous
    i. distance (ISD)
    i. ligament
    i. plane
    i. process
    i. process fusion
    i. segmental spinal instrumentation (ISSI)
    i. widening
interstice, pl. **interstices**
    bone i.
    graft i.
interstitial
    i. abnormality
    i. absorption
    i. afterloading nylon tube
    i. atrophy
    i. boost
    i. brachytherapy
    i. calcinosis
    i. change
    i. conductive heating
    i. congestion of epididymis
    i. cystitis
    i. diffuse pulmonary fibrosis
    i. ectopic pregnancy
    i. fibrotic lung disease
    i. fluid
    i. fluid hydrostatic pressure
    i. fluid space
    i. heat-generating source
    i. hemorrhage
    i. hernia
    i. hyperthermia
    i. hyperthermia treatment
    i. infection
    i. inflammation
    i. intestinal emphysema
    i. laser photocoagulation

    i. loculated hematoma
    i. low-dose-rate iridium-192 needle implant
    i. lung disease distribution
    i. lung disease with increased lung volume
    i. lung emphysema
    i. lung pattern
    i. marking
    i. meniscal tear
    i. nephritis
    i. nodule
    i. nodule HRCT
    i. nonlobar infiltrate
    i. organizing pneumonia
    i. plasma cell pneumonia
    i. pneumonia air leak
    i. pneumonitis
    i. prematurity fibrosis
    i. probe
    i. prominence
    i. pulmonary edema
    i. pulmonary fibrosis (IPF)
    i. radiation
    i. radiation therapy
    i. radioactive colloid therapy
    i. radioelement application
    i. radiosurgery
    i. radiotherapy
    i. radium therapy
    i. salpingitis
    i. scarring
    i. shadowing
    i. tear pattern
    i. template irradiation
    i. thickening
    i. tissue
    i. water proton
interstitium
    lung i.
    pulmonary i.
    renal i.
intertarsal
interthalamic bridge
intertrabecular
    i. hemorrhage
    i. soft tissue
intertransverse
    i. foramen
    i. ligament
    i. muscle

NOTES

intertrochanteric
- i. crest
- i. 4-part fracture
- i. plate
- i. ridge

intertubercular
- i. bursitis
- i. diameter
- i. groove
- i. plane

intertumoral variability
intertwin membrane
interuncal distance (IUD)
interureteric ridge
interval
- acromiohumeral i. (AHI)
- i. articulation
- atlantoaxial i.
- atlantodens i. (ADI)
- basion axial i. (BAI)
- basion dens i. (BDI)
- i. change
- confidence i. (CI)
- i. development
- i. ejection fraction
- escape i.
- high-rate detect i.
- hypoplastic disc i.
- i. improvement
- injection scan i. (ISI)
- interfraction i.
- interpulse i.
- i. intraatrial conduction
- lucent i.
- preejection i.
- i. progression
- prolonged i.
- QRS i.
- reconstruction i.
- i. resolution
- rotator i.
- supracricoid i.
- upper rate i.
- ventriculoatrial i.

intervention
- magnetic-assisted i. (MAI)
- percutaneous nonvascular abdominal i.
- stage-matched i.
- i. study
- therapeutic i.

interventional
- i. angiography
- i. catheterization
- i. imaging
- i. magnetic resonance imaging (I-MRI)
- i. neuroradiology
- i. procedure
- i. radiography
- i. reference point (IRP)
- i. vascular angiogram

interventionalist
interventricular
- i. block
- i. foramen
- i. groove
- i. septal defect (IVSD)
- i. septal rupture
- i. septal thickness (IVST)
- i. septum

intervertebral
- i. cartilage calcification
- i. disc
- i. disc calcification
- i. disc index
- i. disc narrowing
- i. discogram
- i. disc space
- i. disc space height
- i. disc space uniformity
- i. foramen
- i. joint
- i. ligament
- i. notch
- i. osteochondrosis

intervillous
- i. circulation
- i. lacuna
- i. placental thrombosis

interzone
intestinal
- i. atony
- i. Behçet syndrome
- i. bypass procedure
- i. calculus
- i. canal
- i. carcinoid tumor
- i. conduit
- i. congenital atresia
- i. content
- i. decompression
- i. dilatation
- i. distention
- i. diverticulum
- i. duplication
- i. emphysema
- i. fluid
- i. follicle
- i. gas
- i. gas exchange
- i. gas pattern
- i. hypoperistalsis syndrome
- i. infantilism
- i. infarct
- i. intussusception
- i. kinking
- i. lipodystrophy

i. loop
i. lumen
i. lymphangiectasis
i. mesentery
i. metaphysis
i. metaplasia
i. necrosis
i. obstruction
i. perforation
i. polyposis
i. prolapse
i. tract
i. tract malrotation
i. tube
i. ulcer
i. ureter
i. villous architecture
i. villus
i. wall
i. web

intestinalis
pneumatosis cystoides i.

intestine
blind i.
bullous emphysema of i.
coils of i.
congenital lymphangiectasia of i.
kink in i.
large i.
malrotation of i.
papillary adenoma of large i.
small i.

intima
arterial i.
friable thickened degenerated i.
hypertrophied i.
pulmonary artery i.
tunica i.

intimal
i. arteriosclerosis
i. atherosclerosis
i. attachment of diseased vessel
i. debris
i. degeneration
i. fibroplasia
i. fibrosis
i. flap
i. hyperplasia (IH)
i. irregularity
i. proliferation
i. remodeling

i. tear
i. thickening

intimal-medial
i.-m. dissection
i.-m. thickness (IMT)

intimate attachment

intraabdominal (IAB)
i. abscess
i. arterial bypass graft
i. arterial hemorrhage
i. calcification
i. fat
i. fetal calcification
i. infection
i. mass
i. viscus

intraacetabular

intraacinar pulmonary artery

intraalveolar fibrosis

intraamniotic injection

intraaneurysmal
i. flow circulation
i. inflow pattern
i. outflow pattern
i. thrombus

intraaortic
i. balloon assist
i. balloon counterpulsation
i. balloon pump (IABP)
i. endovascular sonography

intraarterial (IA)
i. chemotherapy
i. chemotherapy catheter
i. chemotherapy pump
i. digital subtraction angiography (IADSA)
i. filling defect
i. injection
i. stereotactic digital subtraction angiography
i. superselective nimodipine
i. therapy
i. thrombosis
i. thrombus

intraarticular
i. adhesion
i. calcaneal fracture
i. contrast
i. debris
i. gadolinium
i. ganglion
i. hemangioma

NOTES

495

intraarticular *(continued)*
  i. knee fusion
  i. ligament
  i. localized nodular synovitis
  i. loose body
  i. plate of fibrocartilage
  i. proximal tibial fracture
  i. radiopharmaceutical therapy
intraatrial
  i. block
  i. electrogram
  i. filling defect
  i. reentry
  i. thrombus
intraauricular muscle
intraaxial
  i. brain lesion
  i. brain tumor
  i. varix
Intrabeam intraoperative radiotherapy system
intracanalicular
  i. irradiation
intracapsular
  i. ankylosis
  i. fat-fluid level
  i. fat pad
  i. femoral neck fracture
  i. osteoid osteoma
intracardiac
  i. calcification
  i. calcium
  i. echocardiography (ICE)
  i. electrogram
  i. lead
  i. mass
  i. mixing
  i. pressure
  i. pressure waveform analysis
  i. thrombus
IntraCardiac Echocardiography IVUS catheter
intracartilaginous
  i. bone
  i. ossification
Intracath catheter
intracaval
  i. endovascular ultrasonography
  i. fat mass
intracavernosal injection
intracavernous internal carotid artery
intracavitary
  i. afterloading applicator
  i. application brachytherapy
  i. clot formation
  i. delivery
  i. extension
  i. extension of tumor
  i. filling defect

  i. hyperthermia treatment
  i. implant
  i. irradiation
  i. radiation source
  i. radiation therapy
  i. radioactive colloid therapy
  i. radioelement application
  i. radiotherapy
  i. radium
intracavity mass
intracellular
  i. adhesion molecule
  i. water
intracerebral
  i. aneurysm
  i. arteriovenous malformation
  i. artery
  i. blood
  i. ganglioglioma
  i. ganglioma
  i. hematoma
  i. hemorrhage (ICH)
  i. lesion
  i. lymphoma
  i. thrombolysis
  i. tumor
  i. vascular malformation
intracerebroventricular (ICV)
intrachondral bone
IntraCoil
  I. endoprosthesis
  I. self-expanding peripheral stent
  I. self-expanding stent
  I. stent
intracompartmental
  i. edema
  i. ischemia
  i. tumor
intraconal
  i. lesion
  i. portion of eye
intracondyloid
intracoronary
  i. artery radiation
  i. contrast echocardiography
  i. Doppler flow guidewire
  i. imaging
  i. radiation therapy (ICRT)
  i. stenting
  i. stent placement
  i. thrombolytic therapy
  i. ultrasound (ICUS)
intracorporeal liver
intracortical
  i. osteogenic sarcoma
  i. osteosarcoma
intracranial
  i. air
  i. aneurysm (ICA)

i. arteriovenous fistula
i. arteriovenous malformation
i. berry aneurysm
i. carotid artery atherosclerosis
i. cavernous angioma
i. circulation
i. cryptococcosis
i. dermoid cyst
i. electroencephalography
i. embolus
i. empyema
i. ependymoma
i. fat prolapse
i. germinoma
i. glioma
i. hematoma
i. hypertension
i. imaging
i. leptomeningeal vascular anomaly
i. lipoma
i. mass
i. mass lesion
i. metastasis
i. MR angiography
i. neoplasm
i. neuroblastoma
i. opportunistic infection
i. physiologic calcification
i. pneumatocele
i. pneumocephalus
i. pressure (ICP)
i. pulse pressure
i. saccular aneurysm
i. seeding
i. shift
i. sinus thrombosis
i. stenoocclusive disease
i. structure
i. subarachnoid hemorrhage
i. tuberculoma
i. tumor
i. vascular abnormality
i. vascular lesion
i. vascular occlusion
i. vertebral artery
i. vessel
i. volume
i. width (ICW)
intractable
i. bleeding disorder
i. heart failure
i. ulcer

intracystic
i. bleeding
i. breast carcinoma
i. breast papillary carcinoma in situ
i. solid mass
intracytoplasmic
intradecidual sign
intradermal
i. angioma
i. injection
i. neurilemoma
intradiaphragmatic aortic segment
intradiscal, intradiskal
i. administration of gadolinium followed by MRI
i. electrothermal therapy (IDET)
i. injection
intraductal
i. breast filling defect
i. breast papillomatosis
i. bridge
i. calcification
i. carcinoma (IDC)
i. mucin-producing tumor
i. papillary carcinoma
i. papillary-mucinous neoplasm (IPMN)
i. papillary mucinous tumor (IPMT)
i. papillary mucinous tumor of pancreas
i. papilloma
i. pressure
i. solid mass
i. ultrasonography
intraduodenal choledochal cyst
intradural
i. abscess
i. arachnoid cyst
i. disc herniation
i. epidermoidoma
i. extramedullary lesion
i. extramedullary mass
i. extramedullary tumor
i. hemorrhage
i. intramedullary tumor
i. lipoma
i. nerve root
i. retromedullary arteriovenous fistula
i. rootlet

NOTES

intradural *(continued)*
   i. spinal AVM
   i. vessel
intraforaminal vein
intragastric
   i. bubble
   i. placement
intragraft stenosis
intrahepatic
   i. abscess
   i. arterial-portal fistula
   i. atresia (IHA)
   i. AV fistula
   i. bile duct
   i. biliary atresia
   i. biliary calculus
   i. biliary carcinoma
   i. biliary cystic dilatation
   i. biliary ductal dilatation
   i. biliary neoplasm
   i. biliary stasis
   i. biliary tract
   i. biliary tract dilatation
   i. biliary tree
   i. biloma
   i. cholangiocarcinoma
   i. cholestasis
   i. portal vein branch
   i. portal vein gas
   i. sclerosing cholangitis
   i. stone
   i. umbilical vein
intra-His block
intrahisian block
intralabyrinthine
intralaminar thalamus
intralesional chemotherapy
intraligamentary pregnancy
intraligamentous bursa
intralobar sequestration
intralobular
   i. connective tissue
   i. fibrosis
   i. interstitial thickening
   i. terminal duct
intraluminal
   i. adenocarcinoma
   i. air
   i. attenuation decrease
   i. brachytherapy
   i. debris
   i. dephasing
   i. detail
   i. dilatation
   i. dimension
   i. duodenal diverticulum (IDD)
   i. electrocoagulation
   i. embolus
   i. esophageal pressure

   i. filling defect
   i. foreign body
   i. gallstone
   i. hemorrhage
   i. intubation
   i. membrane
   i. plaque
   i. polymeric footplate
   i. polyp
   i. stomach mass
   i. stone
   i. thrombus
   i. ultrasound (ILUS)
   i. ultrasound catheter
intralymphatic
   i. infusion
   i. radioactivity administration
intramammary
   i. lesion
   i. lymph node
   i. node (IMN)
intramedullary (IM)
   i. arteriovenous malformation
   i. canal
   i. compartment neoplasm
   i. cord lesion
   i. demyelination
   i. ependymoma
   i. epidermoid cyst
   i. fixation
   i. fixation device
   i. lipoma
   i. marrow involvement
   i. nail
   i. osteosarcoma
   i. rodding
   i. skeletal kinetic distractor (ISKD)
   i. skeletal kinetic distractor system
   i. space-occupying lesion
   i. spinal cord tumor
   i. spinal lesion
   i. tumor biopsy
intramembranous
   i. bone
   i. ossification
intrameniscal
   i. cyst
   i. mucoid degeneration
   i. signal intensity
intramesenteric abscess
intramural
   i. air in colon
   i. arterial hemorrhage
   i. clot
   i. colonic air
   i. coronary artery aneurysm
   i. diverticulum
   i. esophageal diverticulosis
   i. esophageal pseudodiverticulosis

i. esophageal rupture
i. fibroid
i. filling defect
i. gas
i. gastric emphysema
i. gastrointestinal tract hemorrhage
i. hematoma
i. hematoma of aorta
i. leiomyosarcoma
i. mapping
i. mechanics
i. myoma
i. portion of distal ureter
i. rupture of esophagus
i. thrombus
i. tumor
i. tunnel
intramural-extramucosal stomach lesion
intramuscular
i. aortic segment
i. fetal injection
i. fluid pressure
i. hemangioma
i. hemosiderin deposit
i. venous malformation
intramyocardial
intranasal microbubble
intraneural ganglion cyst
intraneuronal neurofibrillary tangle
intranodal
i. architecture
i. block
i. myofibroblastoma
in-transit metastasis
intranuclear
i. cleft
i. discogram
intraobserver
i. error
i. variation
intraoccipital
anterior synchondrosis i.
intraocular
i. calcification
i. foreign body
i. lesion
i. spread
Intra-Op autotransfusion system
intraoperative
i. arteriography
i. cardioplegic contrast
echocardiography

i. cholangiogram
i. cholangiography
i. device
i. digital subtraction angiography
(IDSA)
i. Doppler
i. electrocortical stimulation
i. electrocortical stimulation
mapping
i. film
i. fracture
i. gamma probe
i. gastrointestinal injury
i. high dose rate (IOHDR)
i. imaging
i. laser photocoagulation
i. lymphatic mapping
i. MIBG scanning
i. pancreatography
i. radiation therapy
i. radiography
i. radiolymphoscintigraphy
i. radiotherapy
i. red light therapy (IRLT)
i. scanning technique
i. sonography (IOS)
i. ultrasound (IOUS)
i. ventriculogram
i. view
i. x-ray visualization
intraoral
i. cone irradiation
i. periapical radiography
i. projection
i. radiograph
i. radiology
i. roentgentherapy
intraorbital air
intraosseous
i. abscess
i. arteriovenous malformation
i. bone lesion
i. desmoid tumor
i. edema
i. ganglion
i. hemophilic pseudotumor
i. keratin cyst
i. lipoma
i. loculation
i. low-grade osteosarcoma
i. meningioma
i. osteosarcoma

NOTES

intraosseous (*continued*)
   i. vascular malformation
   i. venography
   i. wiring
intrapancreatic obstruction
intrapapillary terminus
intraparenchymal
   i. bleed
   i. blood
   i. cyst
   i. hematoma
   i. hemorrhage
   i. lung tumor
   i. lymph node
   i. meningioma
   i. metastasis
   i. microvessel
   i. tuberculoma
intrapatellar fat pad
intrapedicular fixation
intrapericardial
   i. bleeding
   i. diaphragmatic hernia
   i. patch lead placement
   i. portion
   i. pressure
intraperiosteal fracture
intraperitoneal
   i. abscess
   i. air
   i. cavity
   i. chemohyperthermia
   i. drug administration
   i. exposure
   i. fetal injection
   i. fluid
   i. hyperthermic perfusion (IPHP)
   i. injury
   i. lesion
   i. pregnancy
   i. rupture
   i. rupture of bladder
   i. technetium sulfur colloid imaging
   i. viscus
intraperitoneal chemohyperthermia
intrapixel sequential processing (IPSP)
intraplacental venous lake
intraplaque hemorrhage (IPH)
intrapleural
   i. hemorrhage
   i. pressure
intrapontine intracerebral hemorrhage
intraportal
   i. endovascular ultrasonography
     (IPEUS)
   i. infusion
intrapulmonary
   i. arteriovenous fistula
   i. barotrauma

   i. bronchogenic cyst
   i. bronchus
   i. hemorrhage
   i. lymph node
   i. pressure
intrarectal
   i. coil
   i. ultrasound
intrarenal
   i. arterial flow
   i. collecting system
   i. hematoma
   i. pelvis
   i. reflux
   i. stenosis
intrarun realignment
intrasac
   i. flow
   i. spectral Doppler flow velocity
intrascapular ligament
intrascrotal abscess
intrasellar
   i. brain mass
   i. lesion
   i. Rathke cleft cyst
   i. tumor
intrasinus air-fluid level
Intrasound
   Medtronic Pulsor I.
intraspinal
   i. adenoma
   i. dermoid cyst
   i. enteric cyst
   i. epidermoid cyst
   i. lesion
   i. neurenteric cyst
   i. tumor
intraspongy nuclear disc herniation
IntraStent
   I. balloon-expanded stent
   I. biliary stent
   I. DoubleStrut biliary stent
   I. DoubleStrut ParaMount
     premounted stent-biliary system
   I. DoubleStrut ParaMount XS
     premounted stent-biliary system
   I. DS balloon-expanded stent
   I. LD balloon-expanded stent
   I. LP balloon-expanded stent
intrastitial radiation source
intrasubstance cleavage tear
intrasynovial disease
intratemporal fossa
intratendinous
   i. bursa
   i. fluid collection
   i. rupture
intratendon sheath
intratentorial lipoma

intratesticular
   i. band
   i. cyst
intrathecal (IT)
   i. hemorrhage
   i. imaging
   i. root
   i. space
intrathoracic
   i. catheter drainage
   i. cyst
   i. dimension
   i. dislocation of shoulder
   i. fetal mass
   i. goiter
   i. Kaposi sarcoma
   i. low-attenuation mass
   i. pressure
   i. stomach
   i. thyroid
   i. trachea
   i. upper airway obstruction
intrathrombus infusion
intratracheal
intratumoral
   i. accumulation
   i. agent
   i. calcification
   i. cyst
   i. hemorrhage
   i. necrosis
   i. structure
   i. variability
   i. 90Y glass microsphere injection
intrauterine
   i. cardiac failure
   i. demise
   i. fetus
   i. fracture
   i. gas (IUG)
   i. gestation
   i. growth restriction
   i. growth retardation (IUGR)
   i. heart failure
   i. membrane
   i. pregnancy (IUP)
   i. sac
intravaginal
   i. roentgentherapy
   i. torsion
intravasation
   venous i.

intravascular
   i. angiogenesis gene delivery
   i. catheter-related infection
   i. clotting process
   i. coil
   i. congestion
   i. consumption coagulopathy
   i. content
   i. content extravasation
   i. contrast-enhanced computed tomography
   i. contrast-enhanced CT
   i. contrast medium
   i. filling defect
   i. foreign body
   i. injection
   i. leiomyosarcoma
   i. mass
   i. MRI catheter-based technique
   i. papillary endothelial hyperplasia
   i. radiopharmaceutical therapy
   i. sickling
   i. signal intensity
   i. space
   i. stent
   i. stent artifact
   i. stenting
   i. thrombosis
   i. tumor thrombus
   i. ultrasound (IVUS)
   i. ultrasound catheter
   i. ultrasound imaging
   i. volume depletion
intravenous (IV, I.V., i.v.)
   i. access (IVAC)
   i. accurate control (IVAC)
   i. administration of contrast material
   i. angiocardiography
   i. aortography
   i. block
   i. bolus
   i. bolus injection
   i. cholangiogram (IVC)
   i. cholangiography
   i. cholecystography
   i. contrast medium
   i. digital subtraction angiography (IVDSA)
   i. fetal injection
   i. fluorescein angiography (IVFA)
   i. fluorescein angiography imaging

NOTES

intravenous *(continued)*
  i. infusion
  i. infusion line
  i. injection of isotope
  i. microbubble contrast agent
  i. pyelography (IVP)
  i. renal angiography
  i. stereotactic digital subtraction angiography
  i. urography (IVU)
intravenously
  i. enhanced CT scan
  i. enhanced MRI
intraventricular
  i. aberration
  i. block (IVB)
  i. blood
  i. brain tumor
  i. conduction block
  i. conduction delay
  i. cryptococcal cyst
  i. heart block
  i. hematoma
  i. hemorrhage (IVH)
  i. mass
  i. meningioma
  i. neonate hemorrhage
  i. neuroblastoma
  i. neurocytoma
  i. obstructive hydrocephalus
  i. right ventricular obstruction
  i. septum
  i. systolic tension
intravertebral body vacuum cleft
intravesical
  i. obstruction
  i. stone
  i. ureter
intravital ultraviolet
intravoxel
  i. coherent motion
  i. dephasing
  i. incoherent motion (IVIM)
  i. phase dispersion
intrinsic
  i. cellular parameter
  i. compression
  i. deflection
  i. efficiency
  i. energy resolution
  i. factor
  i. field uniformity
  i. field uniformity test
  i. filling defect
  i. foot muscle
  i. intraabdominal inflammation
  i. ligament
  i. minus deformity
  i. minus hallux

  i. plus deformity
  i. spatial linearity
  i. stenotic lesion
  i. stomach wall lesion
  i. vein graft stenosis
introducer
  Desilets-Hoffman i.
  end-hole i.
  Flexor i.
  Tuohy-Borst i.
introduction
  single-stick catheter i.
Intropaque
intubated small bowel series
intubation
  endotracheal i.
  esophagogastric i.
  intraluminal i.
  nasal i.
  nasogastric i.
  nasotracheal i.
  oral i.
  orotracheal i.
intussusception
  appendiceal i.
  bowel i.
  colocolic i.
  ileocolic i.
  ileoileal i.
  intestinal i.
  jejunoduodenogastric i.
  jejunogastric i.
  pneumatic reduction of i.
  rectal i.
  rectorectal i.
  retrograde jejunoduodenogastric i.
  stomal i.
  transient i.
  vein i.
  venous i.
intussusceptum
intussuscipiens
Inutest
invagination
  basilar i.
  i. skull base
invasion
  arterial i.
  blood vessel i.
  capillary lymphatic space i.
  deep myometrial i.
  early stromal i.
  exogenous i.
  mediastinal i.
  neoplastic i.
  occipital condyle i.
  perineural i.
  seminal vesicle i. (SVI)
  transmural i.

tumoral i.
vascular i.

invasive
i. angiomatous interstitial infiltrate
i. assessment
i. breast carcinoma
i. lesion
i. lobular carcinoma
i. malignant sheath tumor
i. papillomatosis
i. pulmonary aspergillosis (IPA)
i. radiological vascular procedure
i. surgical staging (ISS)
i. thermometry

inverse
i. cerebellum
i. comma appearance
i. follicle
i. follicle pattern
i. Fourier transform (IFT)
i. inspiratory-expiratory time ratio
i. radiotherapy technique
i. square law
i. symmetry

inversion
i. ankle stress view
cardiac i.
frequency-selective i.
gray-scale i.
i. injury
i. injury of ankle
i. instability
isolated ventricular i.
magnetic i.
i. position
i. pulse
i. recovery (IR)
i. recovery echo planar imaging (IR-EPI)
i. recovery image
i. recovery sequence
i. recovery spin-echo (IRSE)
i. recovery spin-echo sequence
i. recovery-weighted image
selective population i. (SPI)
i. sprain
terminal i.
i. time (TI)
torcular-lambdoid i.
i. transfer
ventricular i.

inversion-eversion

inversion-prepared
basis imaging with selective i.-p.

inversion-recovery
selective partial i.-r. (SPIR)
i.-r. technique

inversum
duodenum i.

inversus
abdominal situs i.
complete situs i.
situs i.
situs viscerum i.

inverted
i. left atrial appendage
i. Meckel diverticulum
i. papilloma
i. pelvis
i. teardrop sign
i. umbrella defect
i. Y field irradiation
i. Y field radiotherapy

inverted-T appearance
inverted-T-appearance mainstem bronchus
inverted-V sign
inverted-Y
i.-Y. block
i.-Y. complex
i.-Y. configuration
i.-Y. fracture

invertus
cardiac situs i.

investing fascia
invisible
i. light
i. main pulmonary artery
i. spectrum

involucrum, pl. **involucra**
involuting fibroadenoma
involution
i. of duct
follicular i.
spontaneous i.

involutional breast calcification
involved
i. field
i. field irradiation

involved-region irradiation
involvement
arcuate fiber i.
axillary node i.
contiguous organ i.

NOTES

involvement *(continued)*
    cranial nerve i.
    extramedullary i.
    intramedullary marrow i.
    lymph node i.
    metastatic axillary i.
    pagetoid epidermal i.
    supraclavicular node i.
    thalamotegmental i.

INVOS
    in vivo optical spectroscopy
    INVOS 3100, 3100A cerebral
      oximeter monitoring system
    INVOS 2100 optical spectroscopy

inwardly displaced calcification
iobenguane I-123 injection
iobenzamic acid
iobitridol imaging agent
iocarmate meglumine
iocarmic acid
iocetamic
    i. acid
    i. acid imaging agent

IOCM
    isosmolar contrast medium

IOD
    integrated optical density
iodamine imaging agent
iodide
    i. contrast medium
    i. goiter
    potassium i.
    propidium i.
    silver i.
    sodium i. (NaI)
    thallium-activated sodium i.
    i. transport

iodinated
    i. CM-induced cardiac depression
    i. contrast material
    i. contrast material-induced cardiac
      depression
    i. human serum albumin (IHSA)
    i. I-131 aggregated albumin
    i. I-131 albumin aggregated
      injection
    i. I-125 fibrinogen
    i. imaging agent
    i. intravascular CM
    i. intravascular contrast medium
    i. I-125 serum albumin
    i. I-131 serum albumin
    i. nanoparticle
    i. radiologic contrast medium
      (IRCM)
    i. tyrosine group

iodination
iodine (I)
    i. 111 (^{111}I)
    i. 123 (^{123}I, I-123)
    i. 125 (^{125}I, I-125)
    i. 127 (^{127}I, I-127)
    i. 131 (^{131}I, I-131)
    i. 132 (^{132}I, I-132)
    i. allergy
    butanol-extractable i. (BEI)
    i. dose
    i. fluorescence imaging
    i. 131–induced cellulitis
    ^{131}I radioactive i.
    ^{132}I radioactive i.
    i. load
    protein-bound i. (PBI)
    radioactive i.
    i. radioactive source
    i. scintigraphy
    i. uptake

iodine-123
    i.-123 iodophenyl pentadecanoic
      acid (IPPA)
    i.-123 orthoiodohippurate (OIH)

**iodine-123-MIBG radioactive imaging
agent**
iodine-123, -131 thyroid
iodine-131
    i.-131 antiferritin treatment
    i.-131 isotope
    i.-131 metaiodobenzylguanidine
    i.-131 OIH
    i.-131 orthoiodohippurate
    i.-131 outcome analysis
    i.-131 triolein
    i.-131 whole-body scan
    i.-131 whole-body scintigraphy

**iodine-131-MIBG radioactive imaging
agent**
iodine-containing contrast medium
iodine-deficiency goiter
iodine-125-labeled fragment
iodine-labeled product
iodine-particle ratio
iodipamide
    i. ethyl ester
    i. meglumine
    i. meglumine imaging agent
    i. methylglucamine

iodixanol contrast medium
iodized
    i. oil imaging agent
    i. oil study
    i. poppy seed oil

iodo
5-iodo-2-deoxyuridine imaging agent
iodoalphionic acid
iodoamphetamine (IMP)
    ^{123}I i.
    ^{123}I isopropyl i. (IMP)
iodobenzamide

iodocholesterol
iodocyanine green (ICG)
iododeoxyuridine (IUdR)
    i. labeling
Iodo-gen imaging agent
iodohippurate
    i. sodium
    i. sodium imaging agent
iodomethamate
iodomethyl-norcholesterol-59 scintigraphy
iodomethyl-norcholesterol scintigraphy
  imaging
iodopanoic acid
iodophendylate contrast medium
iodophenyl pentadecanoic acid (IPPA)
Iodotope imaging agent
iodovinylestradiol
iodoxamate meglumine
ioglunide contrast medium
ioglycamic acid contrast medium
ioglycamide
IOHDR
  intraoperative high dose rate
    IOHDR brachytherapy
iohexol
    i. CT ventriculogram
    i. imaging agent
IOM
  infraorbital margin
  interosseous membrane
iomeprol
Iomeron 150, 250, 300, 350 contrast
  medium
IOML
  infraorbitomeatal line
ion
  amphoteric dipolar i.
  calcium i.
  i. chamber
  i. pump
ion-bound water
ion-exchange chromatography
ionic
    i. binding
    i. dimer contrast medium
    i. hexaiodinated dimer
    i. monomer
    i. monomeric contrast medium
    i. paramagnetic contrast medium
    i. paramagnetic imaging agent
    i. polar valence
    i. potassium

iON IntraOperative Navigation System
ionization
    i. chamber
    i. counter
    i. current
    i. density
    i. detector
    i. instrument
    i. potential
    i. radiation
    i. track
ionized atom
ionizing
    i. radiation
    i. radiation exposure
ionograph
ionography
iopamidol imaging agent
Iopamiron 310, 370 imaging agent
iopanoic
    i. acid
    i. acid imaging agent
iopentol nonionic imaging agent
iophendylate
    i. imaging agent
    i. oil
iopromide
    i. contrast medium
    i. nonionic imaging agent
iopydol
IOS
  intraoperative sonography
iosefamic acid imaging agent
iothalamate
    i. meglumine imaging agent
    i. sodium
    i. sodium imaging agent
iothalamic acid
iotrol, iotrolan
iotroxamide contrast medium
iotroxic acid imaging agent
IOUS
  intraoperative ultrasound
ioversol imaging agent
ioxaglate
    i. meglumine
    i. meglumine imaging agent
    i. sodium
    i. sodium imaging agent
ioxaglic
    i. acid
    i. acid contrast medium

NOTES

ioxilan imaging agent
ioxithalamate contrast medium
ioxithalamic acid contrast agent
IP
> interphalangeal
> > IP joint

IPA
> idiopathic pulmonary arteriosclerosis
> invasive pulmonary aspergillosis

iPAT
> integrated parallel acquisition technique

IPC
> interpeduncular cistern

IPCS
> infrapatellar contracture syndrome

IPEUS
> intraportal endovascular ultrasonography

IPF
> idiopathic pulmonary fibrosis
> interstitial pulmonary fibrosis

IPG
> impedance plethysmography

IPH
> idiopathic portal hypertension
> intraplaque hemorrhage

IPHP
> intraperitoneal hyperthermic perfusion

I-Plant brachytherapy seeds
IPMN
> intraductal papillary-mucinous neoplasm

IPMT
> intraductal papillary mucinous tumor
> > IPMT of branch duct type

ipodate
> i. calcium imaging agent
> i. sodium
> i. sodium imaging agent

ipodic acid contrast agent
ipomeanol
IPPA
> iodine-123 iodophenyl pentadecanoic
> acid
> iodophenyl pentadecanoic acid

IP-plus image processing software
IPSID
> immunoproliferative small intestine
> disease

ipsilateral
> i. antegrade arteriography
> i. antegrade site
> i. basal ganglion
> i. breast tumor recurrence (IBTR)
> i. bundle-branch block
> i. cortical diaschisis
> i. downstream artery
> i. femoral neck fracture
> i. femoral shaft fracture
> i. hemimegalencephaly
> i. hemispheric carotid TIA

> i. injection
> i. jugular lymphatic bed
> i. lateral ventricle
> i. lung volume
> i. margin
> i. pleural effusion

IPSP
> intrapixel sequential processing
> > IPSP neuron evaluation method

IR
> inversion recovery
> arrhythmia-insensitive flow-sensitive
> > alternating IR
> IR image

Ir
> iridium

^{192}Ir, Ir-192
> iridium 192
> > ^{192}Ir ribbon
> > ^{192}Ir seed therapy
> > ^{192}Ir wire

^{194}Ir, Ir-194
> iridium 194

IRA
> ileorectal anastomosis

IRA-400 resin
IRAK
> integrated reference air kerma

IRBBB
> incomplete right bundle-branch block

IRCM
> iodinated radiologic contrast medium

IRE
> internal rotation in extension

IR-EPI
> inversion recovery echo planar imaging

Irex
> I. Exemplar ultrasound
> I. Exemplar ultrasound scanner

IRF
> internal rotation in flexion

Iriditope
iridium (Ir)
> i. imaging agent
> i. needle
> i. wire

iridium-192
> i.-192 endobronchial implant
> i.-192 wire implant

iridium 192 (^{192}Ir, Ir-192)
iridium 194 (^{194}Ir, Ir-194)
IRIS
> intensified radiographic imaging system
> IRIS III imager
> IRIS scanner

irislike stenosis
^{192}Ir-loaded stent
IRLT
> intraoperative red light therapy

iron
    i. 52 (^{52}Fe)
    i. 55 (^{55}Fe)
    i. 59 (^{59}Fe)
    i. accumulation in kidney
    i. dextran
    gadolinium i.
    i. hydroxide
    i. overload artifact
    radioactive i.
iron-ascorbate-DTPA
    technetium-99m i.-a.-D.
iron-transporting protein mechanism
IRP
    interventional reference point
irradiating
irradiation
    i. chamber
    convergent beam i. (CBI)
    i. injury
    i. phenomenon
    i. pneumonia
    stereotactic external-beam i. (SEBI)
    i. tolerance
irradiator
    MDS-2000 microwave i.
irreducible
    i. dorsal dislocation
    i. fracture
irregular
    i. block
    i. bone
    i. border
    i. calcification
    i. emphysema
    i. enchondral ossification
    i. extrinsic indentation
    i. gallbladder wall thickening
    i. hazy luminal contour
    i. kidney
    i. mass
    i. mucosal fold
    i. shape
    i. tapered appearance
irregularity
    avulsive cortical i.
    diffuse i.
    intimal i.
    luminal i.
    margin i.
    nodular i.

    sinus i. (SI)
    tendon i.
irregularly
    i. layered astrocytic component
    i. layered neuronal component
    i. shaped lesion
irreversible
    i. airway obstruction
    i. compression
    i. compression of MR imaging
    i. ischemia
    i. narrowing of bronchiole
    i. organ failure
irrigoradioscopy
irrigoscopy
irritability
    atrial i.
    cardiac i.
    muscle i.
    myocardial i.
    nerve root i.
    ventricular i.
irritable
    i. bowel syndrome
    i. colon
    i. heart
    i. stricture
irritant
    i. bronchitis
    primary i.
irritation
    chronic i.
    i. fibroma
IRSE
    inversion recovery spin-echo
    IRSE sequence
IRV
    inspiratory reserve volume
IS
    ileosacral
    international standard
ISAH
    isolated systolic arterial hypertension
    ISAH stereotactic immobilization
    frame
    ISAH stereotactic immobilizing
    mask
ischemia
    acute mesenteric i. (AMI)
    anoxic i.
    balanced i.
    brachiocephalic i.

NOTES

ischemia *(continued)*
> brain i.
> brainstem i.
> cardiac i.
> carotid artery i.
> cerebral i.
> chronic cerebral i.
> chronic mesenteric i. (CMI)
> coronary i.
> cortical i.
> exercise-induced transient
>   myocardial i.
> focal cerebral i.
> global cerebral i.
> global myocardial i.
> intracompartmental i.
> irreversible i.
> limb-threatening i.
> mesenteric i.
> myocardial i.
> neonatal intracranial i.
> nonhemorrhagic i.
> nonlocalized i.
> nonocclusive mesenteric i. (NOMI)
> organ i.
> periinfarction i.
> provocable i.
> radiation-induced i.
> radiation-related i.
> regional myocardial i.
> regional transmural i.
> remote i.
> reversible myocardial i.
> rostral brainstem i.
> segmental bronchus i.
> silent myocardial i.
> stress-induced i.
> subendocardial i.
> talar dome i.
> testicular i.
> transient cerebral i.
> transient myocardial i.
> vertebrobasilar i.

ischemic
> i. area
> i. bowel
> i. bowel disease
> i. brain damage
> i. brainstem infarct
> i. change
> i. colitis
> i. complication
> i. congestive cardiomyopathy
> i. contracture
> i. core
> i. decompensation
> i. defect
> i. encephalopathy
> i. episode

> i. event
> i. gliosis
> i. heart
> i. histopathology
> i. hypoxia
> i. index
> i. injury (SE)
> i. instability
> i. lesion
> i. mesentery
> i. necrosis
> i. necrosis of femoral head (INFH)
> i. nephropathy
> i. penumbra
> i. reperfused myocardium
> i. reperfusion injury
> i. segment
> i. time
> i. ulcer
> i. viable myocardium
> i. zone

ischemically mediated mitral
> regurgitation

ischial
> i. bone
> i. bursitis
> i. spine
> i. tuberosity

ischioacetabular fracture
ischiocapsular ligament
ischiocavernosus muscle
ischiofemoral ligament
ischiogluteal
> i. bursa
> i. bursitis

ischiopagus twin
ischiopubic ramus
ischiorectal
> i. abscess
> i. fat pad
> i. fossa
> i. fossa lesion
> i. fossa plane

ischiospongiosus muscle of penis
ischium
> ascending ramus of i.
> ramus of i.
> transverse diameter between i.'s

ISD
> interspinous distance

ISG medical imaging workstation
ISI
> injection scan interval

ISIS
> image-selected in vivo spectroscopy

ISKD
> intramedullary skeletal kinetic distractor
> ISKD system

island

    bone i.
    bony i.
    cartilage i.
    compact i.
    endometrial i.
    fat i.
    fibrotic i.
    heterotopic white matter i.
    mucosal i.
    Pander i.
    i. of red marrow
    Reil i.
    sclerotic calvarium bone i.
    tissue i.
    i. of tissue

islet cell tumor
isoattenuating
isoattenuation
isobaric transition
isobar nuclide
isobutyl

    dipyridamole technetium-99m-2-methoxy i.

Isocam

    I. scintillation imaging
    I. scintillation imaging system
    I. SPECT imaging system

isocapnic hyperventilation-induced bronchoconstriction
isocenter

    i. placement error
    i. shift method
    shoulder i.
    single i.

isochromat
isoclosed curve
isocon camera
isodense

    i. appearance
    i. enhancement
    i. mass
    i. subdural hematoma

isodose

    i. contour
    i. curve
    i. line
    i. plan
    i. shift method
    i. width

isoechoic

    i. breast mass
    i. clot

isoefamate contrast medium
isoeffect dose
isoeffective bronchial mucosa
isoelectric

    i. electroencephalogram
    i. line
    i. period

isoflurane
isoform

    CSF 14-3-3 i.

isoimmunization

    rhodium i.

isointense

    i. background fat
    i. lesion
    i. signal
    i. soft tissue

isointensity
Isolar rod
isolated

    i. airway injury
    i. cerebellar hypoplasia
    i. clustered calcifications
    i. dislocation
    i. focal cerebellar cortical dysplasia
    i. hepatic infusion
    i. hook fracture
    i. systolic arterial hypertension (ISAH)
    i. ventricular inversion

isolation

    i. perfusion
    protective i.
    reverse i.
    strict i.

isoleucine (I)
isomer

    i. nuclide
    optic i.

isomeric

    i. decay
    i. transition

isomerism

    atrial i.

isonitrile

    dipyridamole technetium-99m-2-methoxy isobutyl i.
    methoxyisobutyl i.

isoosmotic polyethylene glycol

NOTES

Isopaque contrast medium
isophil
isoporosis
isopotential line
isoproterenol infusion
isosceles triangular configuration
isosexual precocity
isosmolar contrast medium (IOCM)
isosmotic water solution
isotone nuclide
isotonicity
isotope
> beta-emitting i.
> i. bone scan
> i. calibrator
> carrier-free i.
> cistern i.
> i. clearance
> i. colloid imaging
> daughter i.
> i. decay
> i. dilution analysis
> i. effect
> gamma-emitting i.
> i. hepatobiliary imaging
> intravenous injection of i.
> iodine-131 i.
> isotope hepatobiliary imaging
>   radioactive i.
> labeling of the i.
> i. meal
> i. nephrography
> neutron-deficient short-lived i.
> i. nuclide
> parent i.
> ^{103}Pd i.
> phosphorus i.
> poorly concentrated i.
> radioactive i.
> i. renogram
> rhenium i.
> i. scintigraphy
> short-range i.
> i. shunt imaging
> stable i.
> strontium i.
> i. uptake
> i. venography
> i. ventriculography
> i. voiding cystourethrography
>   (IVCU)

isotope-labeled fibrinogen imaging
isotope-tagged marker
isotopic
> i. cisternography
> i. dilution
> i. 3D imaging
> i. 3D study
> i. lung scan

> i. ratio
> i. skeletal survey
> i. volume study

isotretinoin
isotropic
> i. dataset
> i. diffusion-weighted imaging
> i. disc
> i. motion
> i. resolution
> i. tissue
> i. voxel

isotropy
isotype
isovolumetric
> i. contraction time
> i. period
> i. relaxation

isovolumic relaxation time (IVRT)
Isovue
> I. nonionic imaging agent
> I. prefilled syringe

Isovue-200, -250, -300, -370 imaging agent
Isovue-370 prefilled syringe
Isovue-M 200, 300 imaging agent
Israel camera
ISS
> inferior sagittal sinus
> injury severity scale
> injury severity score
> invasive surgical staging

ISSI
> interspinous segmental spinal
>   instrumentation

isthmic
> i. coarctation
> i. organizer
> i. region
> i. spondylolisthesis

isthmus, pl. isthmi, isthmuses
> aortic i.
> i. of corpus callosum
> i. of femur
> pontine i.
> renal i.
> stenotic i.
> temporal i.
> thyroid i.
> uterine i.
> i. of uterus
> i. of Vieussens

IT
> iliotibial
> intrathecal
>   IT band

ITA
> internal thoracic artery
>   ITA graft

iterative
    i. algorithm
    i. halftoning
    i. reconstruction
    i. sweep
ITT
    internal tibial torsion
IUD
    interuncal distance
IUdR
    iododeoxyuridine
IUG
    intrauterine gas
IUGR
    intrauterine growth retardation
      asymmetric IUGR
      late flattening IUGR
      low-profile IUGR
      mixed IUGR
      symmetric IUGR
IUP
    intrauterine pregnancy
IV, I.V., i.v.
    intravenous
      supination-external rotation IV
      (SER-IV)
IVAC
    intravenous access
    intravenous accurate control
      IVAC P4000 infuser
Ivalon
    I. particle
    I. plug
    I. sponge
IVB
    intraventricular block
      renal cell carcinoma stage I, II,
      IIIA, IIIB, IIIC, IVA, IVB
IVC
    inferior vena cava
    intravenous cholangiogram
    IVC to portal vein shunt
    solitary left IVC
IVCU
    isotope voiding cystourethrography
IVCV
    inferior venacavography
IVDSA
    intravenous digital subtraction
    angiography
Ivemark CHD syndrome
IVFA
    intravenous fluorescein angiography
    IVFA imaging
IVH
    intraventricular hemorrhage
IVIM
    intravoxel incoherent motion
Ivor Lewis esophagectomy
ivory
    i. osteoma
    i. phalanx
    i. vertebra
IVP
    intravenous pyelography
    rapid-sequence IVP
IVR
    idioventricular rhythm
IVRT
    isovolumic relaxation time
IVSD
    interventricular septal defect
IVST
    interventricular septal thickness
IVU
    intravenous urography
IVUS
    intravascular ultrasound
    IVUS catheter
    2D IVUS
    3D IVUS

NOTES

J

joule
- J chain
- J junction
- J loop
- J point

Jaboulay amputation

Jaccoud
- J. arthritis
- J. arthropathy
- J. sign

JACE-Stim electrotherapy unit

jackknife position

Jackson
- J. coil
- J. and Huber classification of bronchial segments
- J. sign
- J. staging system

Jacobson canal

Jadassohn-Lewandowsky syndrome

Jaffe-Campanacci syndrome

Jaffe-Lichtenstein disease

jagged
- j. bone fragment
- j. osteophyte

Jahss dislocation classification

jail-bar
- j.-b. appearance
- j.-b. chest
- j.-b. rib

James bundle

jammed finger

Janeway lesion

Jansen
- J. disease
- J. metaphysial dysplasia

Jansen-type metaphysial chondrodysplasia

Jansky-Bielschowsky disease

Jaquet apparatus

Jarcho-Levin syndrome

Jarjavay ligament

Jatene transposition

javelin thrower's elbow

jaw
- ameloblastoma of the j.
- j. bone
- claudication of j.
- independent j.
- osteosarcoma of j.

JB1 catheter

Jefferson
- J. burst fracture
- J. cervical fracture

Jeffery classification of radial fracture

jejunal
- j. diverticulosis
- j. diverticulum
- j. interposition of Henle
- j. leiomyosarcoma
- j. loop
- j. loop interposition of Henle
- j. motility
- j. obstruction
- j. pouch
- j. ulcer

jejunitis
- Crohn j.
- ulcerative j.

jejunization
- j. of colon
- ileal j.
- j. of ileum
- vascular j.

jejunocolic fistula

jejunoduodenogastric intussusception

jejunogastric intussusception

jejunoileal (JI)
- j. bypass (JIB)
- j. diverticulum
- j. shunt

jejunoileitis
- ulcerative j.

jejunostomy catheter

jejunum
- proximal j.

jelly-belly appearance

jeopardized myocardium

jersey finger

jet
- aqueductal j.
- j. flow
- high-velocity j.
- j. length (JL)
- j. lesion
- pressurized fluid j.
- regurgitant j.
- ureteral j.
- ureteric j.

Jeune syndrome

Jewett nail

JGA
- juxtaglomerular apparatus

J-hook
- J-h. deformity
- J-h. deformity of distal ureter

JI
- jejunoileal
- JI shunt

JIB
    jejunoileal bypass
JL
    jet length
J-modulation
JNPA
    juvenile nasopharyngeal angiofibroma
Jobert fossa
Jod-Basedow phenomenon
Jography angiographic catheter
Johnson-Jahss classification of posterior
    tibial tendon tear
Johnson position
joint
    acromioclavicular j.
    ankle j.
    j. ankylosis
    apophysial j.
    j. arthrography
    j. articular surface
    j. articulation
    atlantoaxial j.
    atlantooccipital j.
    bail-lock knee j.
    ball-and-socket j.
    basal j.
    Budin j.
    calcaneocuboid j.
    j. calculus
    capitate hamate j.
    capitolunate j.
    j. capsule
    j. capsule defect
    j. capsule thickening
    carpometacarpal j. (CMC)
    carpophalangeal j.
    j. cavity
    Charcot j.
    j. chondroma
    Chopart j.
    Clutton painful j.
    computed tomography-guided
        percutaneous radiofrequency
        denervation of the sacroiliac j.
    condyloid j.
    j. contracture
    coracoclavicular j.
    costochondral j.
    costotransverse j.
    costovertebral j.
    Cruveilhier j.
    cubonavicular j.
    cuneiform j.
    j. cyst
    j. debris
    j. deformity
    j. depression fracture
    diarthrodial intervertebral j.
    DIP j.

j. dislocation
distal interphalangeal j.
distal radioulnar j. (DRUJ)
j. distraction
j. effusion
elbow j.
ellipsoid j.
erythema of j.
facet j.
femoropatellar j.
flail j.
j. fluid
j. fluid extravasation
j. fluid extrusion
free knee j.
frozen j.
j. fulcrum
j. fusion
Gaffney j.
Gillette j.
glenohumeral j.
gliding j.
hallux interphalangeal j.
hinge j.
hip capsule j.
j. hyperextensibility
hypermobile j.
IM j.
immovable j.
j. incongruity
j. instability
intercarpal j.
interchondral j.
j. interface
intermetatarsal j.
interphalangeal j.
intervertebral j.
IP j.
j. kinematics
knee j.
j. laxity
lesser metatarsophalangeal j.
j. line
Lisfranc j.
loss of parallelism of facet j.
lunotriquetral j.
Luschka j.
manubriosternal j.
metacarpophalangeal j. (MCPJ)
metatarsal j.
metatarsocuneiform j.
metatarsophalangeal j.
midcarpal j.
middle facet of the subtalar j.
midtarsal j.
j. morphology
mortise j.
MTP j.
naviculocuneiform j.

near-anatomic position of j.
neuropathic tarsometatarsal j.
neurotrophic j.
occipitoaxial j.
osteolysis on both sides of j.
parallelism of facet j.
patellofemoral j.
perched facet j.
PIP j.
pisotriquetral j.
pivot j.
j. play
primary cartilage j.
proximal interphalangeal j. (PIPJ)
proximal radioulnar j.
pseudoneuropathic j.
pulvinar hip j.
radiocapitellar j.
radiocarpal j.
radioscaphoid j.
radioulnar j.
Regnauld degeneration of MTP j.
sacrococcygeal j.
sacroiliac j.
saddle j.
scaphocapitate j.
scapholunate j.
scaphotrapeziotrapezoid j.
scapulothoracic j.
seagull j.
secondary cartilaginous j.
j. segment
sesamoidometatarsal j.
shoulder j.
SI j.
signal j.
silastic finger j.
SL j.
j. space
j. space narrowing
j. space pseudowidening
sternal j.
sternoclavicular j.
sternocostal j.
sternomanubrial j.
STT j.
subluxed facet j.
subtalar j.
j. survey
Swanson finger j.
j. swelling
symphysis cartilage j.

synovial diarthroidal j.
talocalcaneal j.
talocalcaneonavicular j.
talocrural j.
talofibular j.
talonavicular j.
tarsal j.
tarsometatarsal j.
temporomandibular j. (TMJ)
thoracic j.
tibiofibular j.
tibiotalar j.
j. tissue
transverse tarsal j.
trapeziometacarpal j.
trapezioscaphoid j.
trapeziotrapezoid j.
triquetrohamate j.
j.'s of trunk
uncovertebral j.
unstable j.
weightbearing j.
widened sacroiliac j.
j. widening
wrist j.
xiphisternal j.
zygapophysial j.

Joliot method
Jomed
    J. Flexmaster stent
    J. peripheral stent
    J. peripheral stent-graft
Jones
    J. classification
    J. classification of diaphysial
      fracture
    J. criterion
    J. view
Jones-Mote reaction
Joseph valve implant
Jostent
    J. covered stent
    J. Peripheral Stent Graft
    J. SelfX Nitinol stent
Joubert
    J. focal cerebellar dysplasia
    J. malformation
    J. syndrome
joule (J)
    j. radiation-absorbed dose
    J. shock

NOTES

JPA
>juvenile pilocytic astrocytoma

J-pouch
>small colonic J-p.

JPS
>juvenile polyposis syndrome

JRA
>juvenile rheumatoid arthritis

J-sella deformity

J-shaped
>J-s. anastomosis
>J-s. sella
>J-s. stomach
>J-s. tube
>J-s. ureter

J-tipped
>J-t. guidewire
>J-t. wire

Jude
>J. pelvic view
>J. pelvic x-ray

Judet
>J. epiphysial fracture classification
>J. view

Judkins
>J. coronary arteriography
>J. 4 diagnostic catheter
>J. left coronary catheter
>J. right coronary catheter
>J. selective left coronary cinearteriography
>J. technique

jugal
>j. ligament
>j. suture

jugular
>j. bulb anomaly
>j. bulb tumor
>j. catheter
>j. compression maneuver
>j. foramen
>j. foramen schwannoma
>j. foramen syndrome
>j. foraminal mass
>j. lymph node
>j. megabulb
>j. node metastatic carcinoma
>j. process
>j. technique
>j. tubercle
>j. vein
>j. vein thrombosis
>j. venous access
>j. venous distention
>j. venous impulse
>j. venous oxygen saturation
>j. venous pressure
>j. venous pressure collapse

jugulare
>glomus j.

jugulodigastric
>j. chain
>j. node

juguloomohyoid lymph node

jumped facet

jumper's knee

jumping
>bite j.

jump vein graft

junction
>anomalous craniovertebral j.
>anorectal j. (ARJ)
>aortic sinotubular j.
>arch-isthmic j.
>atlantooccipital j.
>atriocaval j.
>atrioventricular j.
>beaked cervicomedullary j.
>bird-beak taper at esophagogastric j.
>bulbous costochondral j.
>caniocervical j.
>cardioesophageal j.
>cardiophrenic j.
>cavoatrial j.
>CE j.
>cervicomedullary j.
>cervicothoracic j.
>choledochopancreatic ductal j.
>chondrosternal j.
>competence of ureterovesical j.
>corticomedullary j. (CMJ)
>costochondral j.
>craniocervical j.
>craniovertebral j.
>cystic-choledochal j.
>duodenojejunal j. (DJJ)
>esophagogastric j.
>fundic-antral j.
>gastrocnemius-soleus j.
>gastroduodenal j.
>gastroesophageal j.
>gray-white matter j.
>ileocecal j.
>iliocaval j.
>J j.
>lateral margin of the esophagogastric j.
>meniscocapsular j.
>meniscosynovial j.
>metaphysial-diaphysial j.
>midbrain-hindbrain j.
>mucocutaneous j.
>musculotendinous j.
>myoneural j.
>myotendinous j.
>neuromuscular j.

occipitocervical j.
pancreaticobiliary ductal j.
pelviureteric j. (PUJ)
phrenovertebral j.
pontomedullary j.
pontomesencephalic j.
prostaticovesical j.
pyloroduodenal j.
rectosigmoid j.
saphenofemoral j.
sinotubular j.
splenoportal j.
sternochondral j.
supraspinatus musculotendinous j.
sylvian-rolandic j.
temporooccipital j.
temporoparietooccipital j.
tracheoesophageal j.
ureteropelvic j. (UPJ)
ureterorenal j.
ureterovesical j.
uterovesical j.
venous j.

junctional
j. cortical defect
j. dilatation
j. epidermolysis bullosa
j. focus
j. infundibulum
j. nest
j. parenchymal kidney defect
j. zone

Junghans pseudospondylolisthesis

juvenile
j. ankylosing spondylitis
j. aponeurotic fibroma
j. autosomal recessive polycystic
disease
j. breast papillomatosis
j. calcific discitis
j. chronic polyarthritis
j. cirrhosis
j. embryonal carcinoma
j. epiphyseolysis
j. epiphysitis
j. fibroadenoma
j. fibromatosis
j. idiopathic scoliosis
j. laryngeal papillomatosis
j. nasopharyngeal angiofibroma
(JNPA)
j. nephronophthisis

j. orbital pilocytic astrocytoma
j. ossifying fibroma
j. osteoporosis
j. Paget disease
j. pelvis
j. pilocytic astrocytoma (JPA)
j. polyp
j. polyposis
j. polyposis syndrome (JPS)
j. rheumatoid arthritis (JRA)
j. spondyloarthropathy
j. Tillaux fracture
j. T-wave pattern
j. xanthogranuloma

juvenilis
kyphosis dorsalis j.
osteochondrosis deformans j.

juxtaanastomotic stenosis
juxtaarterial ventricular septal defect
juxtaarticular
j. fracture
j. low signal intensity
j. osteoid osteoma

juxtaarticulation
juxtacortical
j. bone lesion
j. chondroma
j. chondrosarcoma
j. fracture
j. osteogenic sarcoma
j. osteosarcoma

juxtacrural
juxtadiaphragmatic location
juxtaductal
j. aortic coarctation
j. coarctation of aorta

juxtaepiphysial
juxtaglomerular
j. apparatus (JGA)
j. tumor

juxtahilar bronchus interruption
juxtaintestinal node
juxtapapillary diverticulum
juxtaphrenic peak
juxtaposition
atrial appendage j.

juxtapyloric ulcer
juxtarenal
j. aortic aneurysm
j. aortic atherosclerosis
j. cava

juxtarestiform body

NOTES

517

juxtasellar ICA
juxtaspinal

juxtatricuspid ventricular septal defect
juxtavesical

K

potassium
K capture
K electron
K radiation
K shell

^{38}**K**

potassium 38

^{39}**K**

potassium 39

^{40}**K**

potassium 40

^{42}**K**

potassium 42

^{43}**K**

potassium 43

Kadish

K. staging
K. staging system

Kager triangle
Kahler disease
Kaiser-Bessel window function
Kalamchi-Dawe congenital tibial deficiency classification
Kallmann syndrome
Kalman filter
Kanavel sign
Kantor string sign
kaolin pneumoconiosis
Kapandji radical fracture
Kaplan

K. PenduLaser 115
K. PenduLaser 115 laser system

kaposiform hemangioendothelioma (KHE)
Kaposi sarcoma (KS)
Karapandzic flap
Karplus

K. relationship
K. sign
K. sign of pleural effusion

Kartagener

K. syndrome
K. triad

Kasabach-Merritt syndrome
Kasai procedure
Kast syndrome
Katayama syndrome
Katzen infusion guidewire
Katzman infusion of radionuclide cisternography
Katz-Wachtel phenomenon
Kauppi method
Kawasaki disease
Kayser-Fleischer ring

Kazangia and Converse facial fracture classification
KBR

kidney length to body height ratio

K-capture
KCC

Kulchitsky cell carcinoma

KCD

kinestatic charge detector
KCD imaging

kCi

kilocurie

Kearns-Sayre syndrome
K-edge filter
keel

laryngeal k.

keeled chest
Keeper vena cava filter
Kehr sign
Keinböck disease
Keith

K. node
K. sinuatrial bundle

Keith-Flack sinuatrial node
Kellgren arthritis
Kellock

K. sign
K. sign of pleural effusion

Kellogg-Speed lumbar spinal fusion
Kelly-Goerss Compass stereotactic system
Kempe series
Kendall sequential compression device
Kennedy method for calculating ejection fraction
Kensey-Nash lithotrite
Kent

bundle of K.

Kent-His bundle
keratectomy

phototherapeutic k. (PTK)

keratin

k. pearl
k. plug
k. testicular cyst
k. urinary tract ball

keratinizing squamous metaplasia
keratocyst

odontogenic k.

keratoma
keratome

femtosecond laser k.

keratoplasty

laser thermal k. (LTK)

keratosis
    actinic k.
Kerckring
    K. fold
    K. nodule
    K. ossicle
Kerley A, B, C lines
kerma
    kinetic energy released per unit mass and
    kinetic energy released in medium
    air kerma
    integrated reference air kerma
    (IRAK)
    total reference air kerma (TRAK)
kerma-to-dose conversion factor
kernel
    dose k.
    interpolation k.
    large k.
    noise reconstruction k.
    k. size
    soft tissue k.
    spheric k.
kernel-of-corn appearance
Kernig sign
Kernohan brain tumor classification
Keshan disease
ketamine
ketanserin
ketene
ketoacidosis
    diabetic k.
ketone body
Kety equation
Kety-Schmidt method
keV, kev
    kiloelectron volt
    keV gamma ray
Key-Conwell
    K.-C. classification of pelvic
    fracture
    K.-C. pelvic fracture classification
keyhole
    k. deformity
    k. method
keystone
    k. of calcar arch
    k. wedging
kg
    kilogram
KHE
    kaposiform hemangioendothelioma
kHz
    kilohertz
kick
    atrial k.
Kidner lesion
kidney
    abdominal k.

k. abscess
absent k.
k. adenocarcinoma
k. adenoma
k. amyloidosis
k. anatomy
k. aneurysm
k. angiomyolipoma
k. anomaly
k. arteriosclerosis
arteriosclerotic k.
Ask-Upmark k.
atrophic k.
k. atrophy
bilateral large k.
bilateral small k.
blunt trauma k.
cake k.
k. calcification
k. calculus
k. carcinoma chromophobe
k. chloroma
cicatricial k.
congenital absence of k.
congested k.
contracted k.
contralateral k.
cortical scarring of k.
cross-ectopic k.
crush k.
cyanotic k.
k. cyst
cystic k.
k. disc
discoid k.
distended k.
double k.
doughnut k.
duplication of left k.
duplication of right k.
dysfunctional k.
dysgenetic k.
k. dyskeratosis
dysplastic k.
ectopic k.
edematous k.
enlarged k.
k. extraction efficiency
faceless k.
k. failure
fatty k.
fetal mesenchymal tumor of k.
k. fibromyxoma
fibrotic k.
floating k.
Formad k.
fractured k.
k. function imaging
k. function study

k. fungus ball
fused k.
Goldblatt k.
granular k.
hamartoma of k.
k. hilum
Hodson-type k.
horseshoe k.
hydronephrotic k.
hypermobile k.
k. infarct
infundibulum of k.
iron accumulation in k.
irregular k.
k. leiomyoma
k. length to body height ratio
  (KBR)
lobe of k.
lobulated k.
long axis of k.
lower pole of k.
lumbar k.
lump k.
k. lymphoma
k. malrotation
k. mass growth pattern
medullary sponge k.
mesonephric k.
k. metastasis
movable k.
multicystic k. (MCK)
multicystic dysgenetic k.
multicystic dysplastic k. (MCDK)
mural k.
k. mycetoma
native k.
k. neurofibromatosis
nonfunctioning k.
k. oxalosis
Page k.
pancake k.
k. papillary blush
partially polycystic k.
pelvis of k.
k. pole
pole-to-pole length of k.
polycystic k.
porous k.
Potter type IV k.
k. pseudotumor
ptotic k.

putty k.
k. radionuclide imaging
Rose-Bradford k.
sacciform k.
k. scan
scarred k.
sclerotic k.
k. shadow
shattered k.
shriveled k.
sigmoid k.
single functioning k.
k. sinus mass
k. size
sponge k.
k. stone
supernumerary k.
suspension of k.
thoracic k.
k. tomography
k. transplant
k. trauma
tree-barking k.
unicaliceal k.
unilateral large smooth k.
unilateral small k.
unipapillary k.
up-sloping curve of k.
k.'s, ureter, and bladder film
k.'s, ureter, and bladder imaging
k.'s, ureters, bladder (KUB)
k. vessel
wandering k.
k. washout
kidney-pancreas transplant
kidney-shaped
  k.-s. distended cecum
  k.-s. placenta
kidney-to-background ratio
**Kiel non-Hodgkin lymphoma
  classification**
Kienböck
  K. dislocation
  K. unit (X)
Kienböck-Adamson point
Kikuchi disease
Kikuchi-Fujimoto disease
Kilfoyle
  K. classification of condylar
    fracture
  K. condylar fracture classification

NOTES

Kilian
   K. line
   K. pelvis
killer
   flow artifact k. (FLAK)
   natural k. (NK)
Killian's dehiscence
kilocurie (kCi)
kiloelectron volt (keV, kev)
kilogram (kg)
kilohertz (kHz)
kilomegacycle
kilovolt (kV)
   k. peak (kVp)
kilovoltage (kV)
Kimmelstiel-Wilson syndrome
Kimura classification
Kimura-type choledochal cyst
kinase
   k. C antiglioma monoclonal
     antibody imaging agent
   herpes simplex virus 1 k. (HSV1-
     tk)
kindling phenomenon
kinematic
   joint k.'s
   k. magnetic resonance imaging
   k. MR cholangiopancreatography
   k. MRCP
   k. MRI study
   k. MR technique
   k. wrist device
kineradiography
kinesis
   color k.
kinestatic
   k. charge detector (KCD)
   k. charge detector imaging
kinetic
   k. cervical spine
   k. curve
   elimination k.'s
   k. energy
   k. energy released per unit mass
     and kinetic energy released in
     medium (kerma)
   exponential k.'s
   k. parameter analysis
   k. perfusion parameter
   sorption k.'s
   time-resolved imaging of
     contrast k.'s (TRICKS)
   washout k.'s
kinetics
   Elliptical Centric-Time Resolved
     Imaging of Contrast K. (EC-
     TRICKS)
kinetocardiogram
kinetoscopy

Kinevac imaging agent
King classification of thoracic scoliosis
King-Moe
   K.-M. classification
   K.-M. scoliosis
kinin
kininogen
kininogenase
kink
   k. artifact
   cervicomedullary k.
   k. in intestine
   Lane k.
kinked
   k. aorta
   k. bowel
   k. ureter
kinking
   aortic k.
   arterial k.
   blood vessel k.
   bronchial k.
   carotid artery k.
   catheter k.
   colon k.
   graft k.
   innominate artery k.
   intestinal k.
   limb k.
   patch k.
   ureteric k.
Kinnier-Wilson disease
Kinsbourne syndrome
Kirchner diverticulum
Kirk distal thigh amputation
Kirklin meniscal complex
Kirner deformity
Kirsch laser
Kirschner wire (K-wire)
kissing
   k. artifact
   k. atherectomy technique
   k. balloon
   k. contraction
   k. lesion
   k. sequestrum
   k. spine
   k. stent
   k. ulcer
kissing-balloon technique
Kistler subarachnoid hemorrhage
   classification
Kistner tracheal button
kit
   ARROWgard Blue Plus multilumen
     central venous catheter k.
   A·S·KMerit safety access k.
   Banyan emergency k.
   Fleet Prep K. 1, 2, 3

InSite Her-2/neu k.
k. preparation
k. for preparation of technetium
    99mTc depreotide injection
Pyrolite k.
Ultra Tag k.
vascular access safety k.
kite angle
Klatskin
    K. tumor
    K. tumor classification
kleeblatschädel deformity
kleeblattschadel
Kleffner-Landau syndrome
Klein
    K. muscle
    K. technique
Klemm sign
Klenow fragment
Klippel-Feil
    K.-F. deformity
    K.-F. sequence
    K.-F. syndrome
Klippel-Trenaunay syndrome
Klippel-Trenaunay-Weber syndrome
Klumpke
    K. brachial plexus injury
    K. paralysis
K-means
    K-m. cluster
    K m. clustering algorithm
knee
anterior cruciate deficit of k.
k. arthrography bolster
breaststroker's k.
Brodie k.
collateral ligament of k.
corner of k.
dislocated k.
double camelback sign of k.
k. flexion contracture
floating k.
k. fracture
housemaid's k.
indirect MR arthrography of k.
internal derangement of k. (IDK)
k. joint
k. joint effusion
k. joint space height
jumper's k.
k. knob
locked k.

medial and lateral support
    structures of k.
medial plica of k.
motorcyclist's k.
reefing of medial retinaculum
    of k.
k. rest
runner's k.
spontaneous osteonecrosis of k.
    (SONK)
tricompartmental chondromalacia of
    the k.
k. view
wrenched k.
kneecap
kneelike bend
Kniest dysplasia
knife, pl. **knives**
Leksell 201-source cobalt-60
    Gamma k.
roentgen k.
UltraCision ultrasonic k.
knob
absent aortic k.
aortic k.
blurring of aortic k.
knee k.
notched aortic k.
knobby process
knocked-down shoulder
knock-knee deformity
knot
false k.
ileosigmoid k.
lovers' k.
surfer's k.
true umbilical cord k.
known primary carcinoma
knuckle
aortic k.
k. bone
boxer k.
k. of colon
knuckle-shaped
Knuttsen bending film
Koch
    K. sinuatrial node
    K. triangle
    K. triangle apex
Kocher
    K. anastomosis
    K. dilatation ulcer

K

NOTES

Kocher *(continued)*
   K. fracture
   K. maneuver
Kocher-Lorenz capitellum fracture classification
Kock pouch
Kodak
   K. Digital Science 1200, 3600 distributed medical imager
   K. Mammography CAD engine
   K. Min-R film
   K. Min-R screen
   K. RP X-OMAT processor
   K. software
   K. X-OMAT film
Koeppe nodule
Köhler
   K. disease
   K. line
Kohlrausch fold
Kokopelli hunchback
Köllicker nucleus
Komai stereotactic head frame
Kommerell
   K. diverticulum
   ductus of K.
Konica scanner
Konstram angle
Kopans
   K. needle
   K. spring hookwire
Korányi-Grocco triangle
Kormed liver biopsy needle
Korotkoff test for collateral circulation
Kostuik-Errico spinal stability classification
Kovalevsky canal
Kr
   krypton
Krabbe
   K. diffuse sclerosis
   K. disease
K-radiation
Krause
   K. ligament
   transverse suture of K.
Krebs cycle
Kretztechnik ultrasound system
Krigel staging system
kringle
Kromayer lamp
Krönlein orbitotomy
Krukenberg tumor
Krupin-Denver eye valve-to-disc implant
Kruskal-Wallis test
krypton (Kr)
   k. laser
   k. laser photocoagulation
   k. scan

krypton 77
   inhalation of k. 77
krypton 81, 81m
KS
   Kaposi sarcoma
K-shell
k-space
   k-s. matrix
   k-s. trajectory
   k-s. traversal
   k-s. velocity mapping
k-t BLAST
KTP
   potassium-titanyl-phosphate
   KTP laser
KUB
   kidneys, ureters, bladder
   KUB imaging
   KUB view
Kubelka-Munk theory
Kugel
   K. anastomosis
   K. artery
Kugelberg-Welander disease
Kulchitsky
   K. cell
   K. cell carcinoma (KCC)
Kulkarni injury
Kumar, Welti and Ernst method
Kumeral diverticulum
Kumpe
   K. catheter
   K. hump
Kupffer cell sarcoma
Kürner septum
Kussmaul-Maier disease
Kussmaul sign
kV
   kilovolt
   kilovoltage
kVp
   kilovolt peak
   kVp meter
kwashiorkor
KWE method
K-wire
   Kirschner wire
kx-ky plane
Ky
   sliding interleaved Ky (SLINKY)
Kyle fracture classification
kyllosis
kymograph
kymography
   roentgen k.
kymoscopy
kyphoplasty
kyphoscoliosis

kyphoscoliotic
    k. heart disease
    k. pelvis
kyphosis
    Cobb method of measuring k.
    k. dorsalis juvenilis
    loss of thoracic k.
    lumbar k.
    lumbosacral k.

    postlaminectomy k.
    Scheuermann juvenile k.
    thoracic k.
    thoracolumbar k.
kyphotic
    k. angulation
    k. curvature
    k. pelvis
    k. view

NOTES

K

Λ
    Avogadro number
    Ostwald solubility coefficient
    radioactive constant
    wavelength

L
    lumbar vertebra
      L electron
      L shell

L5-S1 projection

LA
    left atrium

L/A
    liver-aorta

LAA
    left atrial appendage
    left auricular appendage

LA-AR
    left atrium-aortic root ratio

LABA
    laser-assisted balloon angioplasty

Labbé
    L. triangle
    L. vein

label
    double l.
    long wave-length photo l.
    radioactive l.
    radionuclide l.
    single l.
    triple l.

labeled
    l. atom
    l. fibrinogen
    l. free fatty acid scintigraphy
    l. leukocyte scan
    l. phosphorus
    l. positron
    l. RBC
    l. red blood cell sequestration

labeling
    l. abnormality
    antibody l.
    ^{111}In l.
    iododeoxyuridine l.
    l. of the isotope
    microglobulin l.
    pulse l.
    pulsed arterial spin l.
    radioactive l.
    radioisotope l.
    site-specific l.
    technetium-99m antibody l.
    technetium-tagged RBC l.

    in vitro l.
    in vivo l.

labial
    l. groove
    l. vein

labile blood pressure

labor dystocia

labral
    l. and anterior inferior glenoid rim
      fracture
    l. capsular complex
    l. fibrocartilage
    l. injury
    l. variant

labral-ligamentous complex

labrum, pl. labra
    acetabular l.
    anterior glenoid l. (AGL)
    articular l.
    fibrocartilaginous l.
    glenoid l.

labrum-ligament complex

labyrinth, labyrinthus
    artery of l.
    bony l.
    cochlear l.
    ethmoidal l.
    membranous l.
    osseous l.
    renal l.
    vestibular l.

labyrinthine
    l. artery
    l. fistula
    l. hemorrhage
    l. hydrops
    l. structure

labyrinthitis ossificans

LACD
    left apexcardiogram, calibrated
    displacement

lacelike
    l. appearance
    l. trabecular pattern

laceration
    bladder l.
    brain l.
    liver l.
    lung l.
    parenchymal l.
    spinal cord l.
    spleen l.
    tendon l.

lacerum
    foramen l.

L

Lachman sign
laciniate
    l. ligament
    l. ligament of ankle
lack of acoustic penetration
lacrimal
    l. artery
    l. bone
    l. canal
    l. duct
    l. gland
    l. gland lesion
    l. groove
    l. mass
    l. nerve
    l. recess
    l. sac
    l. scan
    l. scintigraphy
lacrimoconchal suture
lacrimoethmoidal suture
lacrimomaxillary suture
lacrimoturbinal suture
lactate
    l. proton
    l. resonance
lactating adenoma
lacteal
    l. calculus
    l. vessel
lactiferous
    l. duct
    l. sinus
lactobezoar
lactoferrin production
lacuna, pl. **lacunae, lacunas**
    bone l.
    cartilage l.
    intervillous l.
    Morgagni l.
    osseous l.
    resorption l.
lacunaire
lacunar
    l. abscess
    l. brain infarct
    l. ligament
    l. node
    l. skull
    l. stroke
LAD
    left anterior descending
    left axis deviation
LADARVision excimer laser
Ladd band
Ladder diagram
ladderlike pattern
Lady Windermere syndrome

LAE
    left atrial enlargement
LAFB
    left anterior fascicular block
LAG
    lymphangiogram
lag
    l. effect
    l. screw
Lagios classification system
LaGrange classification of humeral
    supracondylar fracture
LAID
    left anterior internal diameter
Laimer
    L. fascia
    triangle of L.
LAIS excimer laser
Laitinen
    L. CT guidance system
    L. stereotactic head frame
lake
    bile l.
    capillary l.
    intraplacental venous l.
    lipid l.
    maternal l.
    mucous l.
    venous intraplacental l.
    venous skull l.
lambda, λ
    L. Plus PDL1, PDL2 laser
    white matter l.
lambdoid
    l. suture
    l. synostosis
lambdoidal cranial suture
Lambert
    L. canal
    L. channel
    L. projection
Lambert-Eaton myasthenic syndrome
lamella, pl. **lamellae**
    anular lamellae
    articular l.
    basal l.
    circumferential l.
    concentric l.
    enamel l.
lamellar
    l. body
    l. body density (LBD)
    l. bone
    l. periosteal reaction
lamina, pl. **laminae**
    l. dura
    external elastic l.
    medullary l.
    osseous spiral l.

l. papyracea
l. propria
vertebral l.
laminagraphy (*var. of* laminography)
laminar
l. brain necrosis
l. flow
laminated
l. calcification
l. gallstone
l. intraluminal thrombus
lamination of gyrus
laminectomy
laminogram, laminagram
laminograph, laminagraph
laminography, laminagraphy
cardiac l.
laminoplasty
laminotomy
lamp
cold quartz lamp germicidal l.
high-pressure mercury arc l.
hot quartz l.
Kromayer l.
mercury arc l.
mercury vapor l.
quartz l.
sun l.
ultraviolet l.
Wood l.
xenon arc l.
lanceolate deformity
Lancet
Laser L.
Lancisi
L. muscle
L. sign
Landau diamagnetism
Landau-Kleffner syndrome
landmark
anatomic l.
bony skull l.
l. registration
Landolfi sign
Landry vein light Venoscope
landscape
anatomic l.
Landsmeer ligament
Landzert fossa
Lane
L. band
L. kink

Lanex medium screen
Langenbeck triangle
Langerhans lung cell histiocytosis
Langer line
Lannelongue ligament
lanthanide
l. metal
l. shift reagent (LSR)
lanthanide-induced shift
lanthanum
Lanz
L. line
L. point
LAO
left anterior oblique
LAO position
LAO projection
LAP
left atrial pressure
laparoscope
3D l.
3-Dscope l.
EL2-LS2 flexible video l.
EL2-TF410 l.
Surgiview l.
laparoscopic
l. contact ultrasonography (LCU)
l. intracorporeal ultrasound (LICU)
l. laser
l. probe
l. ultrasound (LapUS, LUS)
l. ultrasound probe
laparoscopy
laparotomy
radioguided l.
L-A peak ratio
Laplace
L. effect
L. mechanism
LapUS
laparoscopic ultrasound
large
l. airway
l. airway narrowing
l. bowel
l. bowel obstruction
l. cell neuroendocrine carcinoma (LCNEC)
l. cell undifferentiated carcinoma
l. cleaved cell lymphoma
l. clothing artifact
l. colloidal particle

L

NOTES

large *(continued)*
    l. duct papilloma
    l. fetal head
    l. field of view (LFV)
    l. field of view gamma camera
    l. for gestational age
    l. gut
    l. habitus
    l. hinge angle electron field
    l. intestine
    l. kernel
    l. loop excision
    l. obtuse marginal branch
    l. solid adrenal mass
    l. spleen
    l. susceptibility artifact
    l. thymus shadow
    l. utricle
    l. venous tributary
    l. vestibule
    l. volume joint effusion

large-bore
    l.-b. bile duct endoprosthesis
    l.-b. catheter
    l.-b. magnet
    l.-b. 0.6-T, 1,5-T imaging system scanner

large-caliber tube
large-core
    l.-c. technique
    l.-c. ultrasound-guided biopsy

large-droplet fatty liver
large-fiber demyelination
large-field
    l.-f. radiation therapy
    l.-f. radiotherapy
    l.-f. x-ray dosimetry

large-field-of-view image
large-for-dates uterus
larger-caliber cutting needle
large-vessel
    l.-v. disease of diabetic foot
    l.-v. thrombosis

Larkin position
Larmor
    L. equation
    L. frequency
    L. precession

Larsen syndrome
laryngeal
    l. atresia
    l. carcinoma
    l. cartilage
    l. edema
    l. fracture
    l. keel
    l. musculature fluorodeoxyglucose uptake
    l. nerve

    l. nodule
    l. papilloma
    l. papillomatosis
    l. part of pharynx
    l. polyp
    l. skeleton
    l. ventricle
    l. vestibule
    l. web

laryngectomy
    supraglottic l.
    vertical partial l.

larynges (*pl. of* larynx)
laryngitis
laryngocele
laryngogram
laryngography
    contrast l.
    double-contrast l.

laryngomalacia
laryngopharyngography
laryngopyocele
laryngoscope
    Benjamin binocular slimline l.
    Benjamin pediatric l.
    Bullard l.
    Olympus ENF-P2 l.

laryngoscopy
    indirect l.

larynx, pl. **larynges**
    appendix of ventricle of l.
    glottic l.
    infraglottic l.
    supraglottic l.
    ventricle of l.
    vestibule of l.

LASE
    laser-assisted spinal endoscopy

Lasègue sign
laser
    AccuLase excimer l.
    acupuncture l.
    alexandrite l.
    AlexLAZR l.
    Apex Plus excimer l.
    ArF excimer l.
    argon l.
    argon/krypton l.
    argon-pumped dye l.
    Aura desktop l.
    Aurora diode soft-tissue l.
    l. beam
    l. biliary lithotripsy
    biocavity l.
    BriteSmile l.
    Candela 405-nm pulsed dye l.
    carbon dioxide l.
    CHRYS CO_2 l.
    Clearview CO_2 l.

CO_2 l.
l. coagulation
Coherent CO_2 surgical l.
Coherent UltraPulse 5000C l.
CoolGlide l.
copper-vapor pulsed l.
l. correlational spectroscopy (LCS)
coumarin pulsed dye l.
CTE:YAG l.
Derma 20 l.
Derma K l.
DermaLase l.
l. desiccation of thrombus
DIAGNOdent l.
l. diffraction scanning
l. digitizer
diode l.
Diomed EVLT l.
l. Doppler flowmetry (LDF)
l. Doppler velocimetry
dye l.
Eclipse TMR l.
ELCA l.
endoscopic l.
l. energy
l. energy absorption
Epic ophthalmic 3-in-1 l.
EpiTouch l.
erbium:YAG infrared l.
ErCr:YAG l.
EVLT l.
excimer l.
FCPA2 l.
FeatherTouch CO_2 l.
Fiberlase l.
FiberScan l.
flashlamp-pulsed dye l.
flashlamp-pumped pulsed dye l.
Flexlase 600 l.
flying spot excimer l.
gallium-arsenide l.
Genesis 2000 carbon dioxide l.
GentleLASE Plus l.
Heart l.
helium-cadmium l.
helium-neon l.
HeNe l.
HF infrared l.
high-energy l.
holmium l.
holmium-yttrium-aluminum-garnet l.
Horn endoootoprobe l.

hot l.
Ho:YAG l.
Hyperion LTK l.
l. imager
Kirsch l.
krypton l.
KTP l.
LADARVision excimer l.
LAIS excimer l.
Lambda Plus PDL1, PDL2 l.
L. Lancet
L. Lancet laser device
laparoscopic l.
Laserscope l.
LaserSonics EndoBlade l.
LaserSonics Nd-YAG Laserblade l.
LaserSonics Surgiblade l.
Laserthermia l.
LaserTripter MDL 3000 l.
Lasertrolysis l.
Lastec System angioplasty l.
LightSheer SC diode l.
Lightstic 180, 360 fiberoptic l.
low-energy l. (LEL)
LX 20 l.
Lyra l.
Mainster retina l.
Maloney endootoprobe l.
Microlase transpupillary diode l.
Microlight 830 l.
Microprobe l.
microsecond pulsed flashlamp
   pumped dye l.
midinfrared l.
Nd:YLF l.
Nidek EC-5000 excimer l.
NovaLine excimer l.
NovaLine Litho-S DUV excimer l.
NovaPulse CO_2 l.
Nuvolase 660 l.
OcuLight SL diode l.
OmniPulse-MAX holmium l.
Opmilas CO_2 multipurpose l.
Optical Biopsy System l.
OptiVision l.
OtoLAM l.
Pegasus PIV l.
PhotoGenica V-Star l.
PhotoPoint l.
Polaris 1.32 Nd:YAG l.
Prima l.
l. projection imaging (LPI)

L

NOTES

laser *(continued)*
    pulsed-dye l.
    pulsed infrared l.
    pulsed metal vapor l.
    PulseMaster l.
    Pulsion FS l.
    Pulsolith l.
    Q-switched Nd:YAG l.
    Q-switched ruby l.
    Revitalase erbium cosmetic l.
    l. scanning cytometry (LSC)
    l. sclerosis
    Selecta 7000 l.
    Sharplan SilkTouch Flashscan
      surgical l.
    SilkLaser aesthetic carbon
      dioxide l.
    Skinlight erbium YAG l.
    SLS l.
    Smoothbeam l.
    SoftLight l.
    Softscan l.
    Spectranetics excimer l.
    SPTL-1b vascular lesion l.
    STATLase-SDL diode l.
    Surgilase 150 high-powered CO_2 l.
    Surgilase Nd:YAG l.
    l. system
    TEC-2100 postioning l.
    THC:YAG l.
    l. thermal ablation (LTA)
    l. thermal keratoplasty (LTK)
    Topaz CO_2 l.
    TruPulse CO_2 l.
    UltraPulse CO_2 l.
    Urolase fiber l.
    l. uterosacral nerve ablation
      (LUNA)
    Vbeam pulsed dye l.
    VersaLight l.
    VersaPulse holmium l.
    Versatome l.
    Visulas Nd:YAG l.
    VISX excimer l.
    VISX Star 3 excimer l.
    VISX Star S2 excimer l.
    Vitesse Cos l.
    l. welding
    Xanar 20 Ambulase CO_2 l.
    XeCl l.
      xenon-chloride laser
    xenon-chloride l. (XeCl laser)
    XTRAC l.
    YAG l.
    yttrium-aluminum-garnet l.
    Zeiss Visulas 690s l.
laser-assisted
    l.-a. balloon angioplasty (LABA)
    l.-a. microvascular anastomosis

    l.-a. spinal endoscopy (LASE)
    l.-a. uvulopalatoplasty (LAUP)
laser-Doppler flowmetry probe
laser-induced
    l.-i. interstitial thermotherapy
      (LITT)
    l.-i. thermography (LITT)
    l.-i. thermotherapy (LITT)
LaserOptic
    Indigo L.
laser-polarized
    l.-p. helium MRI
    l.-p. helium MR imaging
Laserprobe-PLR Plus
Laserscope
    L. laser
LaserSonics
    L. EndoBlade laser
    L. Nd-YAG Laserblade laser
    L. Surgiblade laser
laserthermia
Laserthermia laser
LaserTripter MDL 3000 laser
Lasertrolysis laser
LaserTweezers
LASH
    left anterosuperior hemiblock
Lasix renography
Lastec System angioplasty laser
last normal vertebra (LNV)
lata
    fascia l.
    snapping fascia l.
latae
    tensor fasciae l.
Latarjet
    nerve of L.
LATC
    lateral talocalcaneal
late
    l. effect analysis
    l. effect of normal tissue (LENT)
    l. effect toxicity score
    l. false aneurysm
    l. fetal death
    l. film
    l. flattening IUGR
    l. graft occlusion
    l. normal tissue sequela
    l. phase
    l. systolic bulge
    l. systolic retraction
    l. venous filling
latent
    l. coccidioidomycosis
    l. empyema
    l. pleurisy
late-onset dwarfism

late-phase
    l.-p. image
    l.-p. termination
lateral
    l. aneurysm
    l. anterior drawer stress view
    l. arcuate ligament
    l. aspect
    l. band
    l. basal segmental bronchus
    l. bending injury
    l. bending view
    l. border
    l. cephalometric radiograph
    l. cervical spine film
    l. collateral ligament (LCL)
    l. collateral ligament complex
    l. column calcaneal fracture
    l. compartment
    l. compartment impaction
    l. compartment traumatic bony
      injury
    l. conal fascia
    l. condylar humeral fracture
    l. condyle
    l. corticospinal tract
    l. costotransverse ligament
    l. crus
    l. cystourethrogram
    l. decubitus film
    l. decubitus position
    l. decubitus radiograph
    l. decubitus view
    l. disc herniation
    l. divergence angle (LDA)
    l. entrapment
    l. epicondylar bursa
    l. epicondylitis
  exaggerated craniocaudal l. (XCCL)
    l. extension view
    l. facial cleft
    l. femoral notch
    l. femoral sulcus
    l. fissure
    l. flexion/extension radiograph
    l. flexion view
    l. geniculate body
    l. gutter
    l. horn
    l. hypopharyngeal pouch (LHP)
    l. impingement
    l. joint line

    l. joint space
    l. left anterior oblique position
    l. lemniscus tract
    l. lobe of prostate
    l. lumbar meningocele
    l. lumbar support
    l. malleolar fracture
    l. malleolus
    l. margin of the esophagogastric
      junction
    l. mass
    l. meniscal uncovering
    l. myocardial infarct
    l. oblique axial projection
    l. oblique fascia
    l. oblique jaw radiograph
    l. oblique view
    l. occipital sulcus
    l. occipitotemporal gyrus
    l. opposed beam
    l. part of occipital bone
    l. patellofemoral angle
    l. placenta previa
    l. plantar metatarsal angle
    l. posterior choroidal (LPCh)
    l. precordium
    l. process of the talus
    l. pterygoid muscle
    l. pterygoid tendinous attachment
    l. pyelography
    l. ramus radiograph
    l. recess
    l. recess stenosis
    l. recess syndrome
    l. rectus muscle
    l. recumbent position
    l. reflection of colon
    l. resolution
    l. reticular formation
    l. root
    l. rotatory ankle instability
    l. sagittal image
    l. semicircular canal
    l. sesamoid bone
    l. shelf
    l. sinus
    l. skull radiograph
    l. spinothalamic tract
    l. spring ligament of foot
    l. subluxation
    l. talar dome
    l. talar dome injury

L

NOTES

lateral *(continued)*
l. talar process
l. talocalcaneal (LATC)
l. talocalcaneal angle
l. talocalcaneal ligament
l. talometatarsal angle
l. tarsometatarsal angle
l. temporal epileptogenic lesion
l. thoracic meningocele
l. tibial plateau fracture
l. tilt stress ankle view
l. tomography
l. transcranial projection
l. transfacial projection
l. tug
l. ulnar collateral ligament (LUCL)
l. umbilical fold
l. ventricle
l. ventricle of cerebrum
l. ventricle trigone
l. wall refractive shadowing
l. web
l. wedge fracture

lateralis
interdigitation of vastus l.
meniscus l.
proboscis l.
sinus l.
vastus l.

laterality
lateralization deficit
lateralizing
l. finding
l. sign

laterally displaced fracture
laterocervical region
lateroconal fascia
lateromedial
l. oblique projection
l. oblique view

latex
Spli-Prest l.

LaTIS endovascular laser system
latissimus dorsi muscle
latitude film
lattice
l. index
l. relaxation time
l. vibration
l. work

Laubry-Pezzi syndrome
Laue pattern
Lauge-Hansen ankle fracture classification
Laugier fracture
LAUP
laser-assisted uvulopalatoplasty

Laurin
L. angle
L. x-ray view

Lauth ligament
lavage
cavity l.
oral colonic l. (OCL)

law
Angström l.
Avogadro l.
Beer l.
Bergonie-Tribondeau l.
Bragg l.
Coulomb l.
Courvoisier l.
Curie l.
Doerner-Hoskins distribution l.
Faraday l.
Fick l.
Gibbs-Donnan l.
Good Samaritan l.
Hilton l.
inverse square l.
least square l.
Le Borgne l.
Lenz l.
Ohm l.
Poiseuille l.
L. position
Rayleigh scattering l.
transformer l.
L. view
Wolff l.

Lawrence
L. method
L. position
L. view

lawrencium (Lr, Lw)
laxative
bulk l.

laxity
chronic ligament complex l.
joint l.
ligamentous l.
varus stress l.

layer
basal l.
Bekhterev l.
boundary l.
bright l.
circumferential echo-dense l.
echo-dense l.
echo-free l.
fibrofatty l.
fluid-blood l.
half-life l.
half-value l. (HVL)
hypoechoic l.
inner bright l.

intermediate signal intensity l.
parietal l.
seromuscular l.
sonolucent l.
subserosal l.
tenth-value l.
visceral l.

layered gallstone

layering
l. calcification
calcium l.
l. of contrast material
l. debris
l. effusion
l. of gallstones

Lazarus sign

Lazorthes
posterior thalamic arteries of L.

L-B
lesion-brain ratio
L-B ratio

LBBB
left bundle-branch block

LBCD
left border of cardiac dullness

LBD
lamellar body density

LC
inductance-capacitance

L-C
lesion-countersite ratio

LCA
left coronary angiography
left coronary artery

LC-DCP
low-contact dynamic compression plate

LCDD
light chain deposition disease

LCF
left circumflex

LCIS
lobular carcinoma in situ

LCL
lateral collateral ligament

LCNEC
large cell neuroendocrine carcinoma

LCP
Legg-Calvé-Perthes disease

LCS
laser correlational spectroscopy

LCT
Leydig cell tumor
liquid crystal thermography

LCU
laparoscopic contact ultrasonography

LCX
left circumflex

LDA
lateral divergence angle
left descending artery

LDD
low-dose dobutamine
LDD-gated SPECT with ^{201}Tl

LDF
laser Doppler flowmetry

LE
lower extremity

Le
Lewis
Le Borgne law
Le Fort amputation
Le Fort fibular fracture
Le Fort I, II, and III fracture
Le Fort mandibular fracture
Le Fort-Wagstaffe fracture

lead (Pb)
bipolar l.
chest l.
intracardiac l.
pacemaker l.
pacing l.
precordial l.
radioactive l.

lead (Pb)
l. apron shield
l. collimation
l. encephalopathy
l. eye shield
l. gonad shield
l. line
l. pellet marker
l. pin
l. pipe fracture
l. point

leading edge

lead-pipe rigidity

lead-rubber apron

lead-time bias

leaf
l. of diaphragm
l. of mesentery

leafless tree appearance

NOTES

535

leaflet
  anterior motion of posterior mitral
    valve l.
  anterior tricuspid valve l.
  apposition of l.
  arching of mitral valve l.
  bowing of mitral valve l.
  coapted l.
  commissural l.
  doming of l.
  floating l.
  l. function
  hammocking of mitral valve l.
  heart valve l.
  mitral l.
  l. motion
  myxomatous valve l.
  noncalcified mitral l.
  posterior mitral l. (pML)
  posterior mitral valve l. (PMVL)
  pseudomitral l.
  redundant aortic valve l.
  redundant mitral valve l.
  l. retraction
  l. separation
  septal l.
  spoonlike protrusion of l.
  systolic prolapse of mitral valve l.
  valve l.
leaflike villus
leak
  air l.
  aortic paravalvular l.
  ascites due to bile l.
  baffle l.
  blood l.
  calibrated l.
  capillary l.
  cerebrospinal fluid l.
  chyle l.
  contained l.
  current l.
  femoral l.
  generalized capillary l.
  interatrial baffle l.
  interstitial pneumonia air l.
  light l.
  Luschka duct l.
  mitral l.
  paraprosthetic l.
  paravalvular l.
  periprosthetic l.
  perivalvular l.
  transient chyle l.
leakage
  anastomotic l.
  bile l.
  blood-tumor-barrier l.
  chylous l.

  contrast media l.
  paraprosthetic l.
  radiation l.
  silicone implant l.
leaking
  l. abdominal aortic aneurysm
  l. vein
leaky
  l. lung syndrome (LLS)
  l. valve
lean mass
LEAP
  Low Energy All Purpose
    LEAP collimator
least
  l. square (LS)
  l. square algorithm
  l. square analysis
  l. square law
leather bottle stomach
leave-alone lesion
Leclercq test
LE-CTV
  lower extremity CT venography
ledge
  eccentric l.
left
  l. anterior chest wall wall
  l. anterior descending (LAD)
  l. anterior descending artery
  l. anterior fascicular block (LAFB)
  l. anterior hemiblock block
  l. anterior internal diameter (LAID)
  l. anterior oblique (LAO)
  l. anterior oblique position
  l. anterior oblique projection
  l. anterior oblique projection
    ventriculogram
  l. anterior oblique view
  l. anterosuperior hemiblock (LASH)
  l. apexcardiogram, calibrated
    displacement (LACD)
  l. atrial active-emptying fraction
  l. atrial appendage (LAA)
  l. atrial cannulation
  l. atrial chamber
  l. atrial end-diastolic pressure
  l. atrial enlargement (LAE)
  l. atrial function
  l. atrial hypertrophy
  l. atrial maximal volume
  l. atrial myxoma
  l. atrial pressure (LAP)
  l. atrioventricular groove artery
  l. atrium (LA)
  l. atrium-aortic root ratio (LA-AR)
  l. auricle
  l. auricular appendage (LAA)
  l. axillary artery catheterization

l. axis deviation (LAD)
l. border of cardiac dullness (LBCD)
l. border of heart
l. brain
l. bundle branch
l. bundle-branch block (LBBB)
l. bundle branch hemiblock
l. circumflex (LCF, LCX)
l. circumflex coronary artery
l. colon
l. colonic flexure
l. common carotid artery
l. common femoral artery
l. coronary angiography (LCA)
l. coronary artery (LCA)
l. coronary cusp
l. coronary plexus
l. coronary sinus
l. crus
l. descending artery (LDA)
l. gastric artery
l. gutter
l. heart catheterization
l. heart syndrome
l. hemisphere
l. hepatic vein (LHV)
l. iliac system
l. intercostal space (LICS)
l. internal carotid artery (LICA)
l. internal mammary artery (LIMA)
l. internal mammary artery anastomosis
l. lateral projection
l. lobe of liver
l. lower extremity (LLE)
l. lower lobe (LLL)
l. lower lobe lesion
l. lower quadrant (LLQ)
l. main coronary artery (LMCA)
l. main stem bronchus
l. mediastinum
l. pleural apical hematoma cap
l. posterior oblique (LPO)
l. posterior oblique position
l. posterior oblique projection
l. primary bronchus
l. pulmonary artery (LPA)
l. pulmonary cusp
l. pulmonary vein (LPV)
l. respiratory nerve
l. retroaortic renal vein

l. sternal border (LSB)
l. subclavian central venous pressure (LSCVP)
l. upper lobe (LUL)
l. upper lobe lesion
l. upper quadrant (LUQ)
l. ventricle
l. ventricular afterload
l. ventricular aneurysm
l. ventricular angiography
l. ventricular apex
l. ventricular assist device (LVAD)
l. ventricular asynergy
l. ventricular cardiomyopathy
l. ventricular cavity pressure
l. ventricular chamber
l. ventricular chamber volume
l. ventricular configuration
l. ventricular contraction pattern
l. ventricular diastolic dimension (LVdd)
l. ventricular dilatation
l. ventricular dysfunction (LVD)
l. ventricular ejection fraction (LVEF)
l. ventricular ejection time (LVET)
l. ventricular end-diastolic dimension (LVEDD)
l. ventricular end-diastolic pressure (LVEDP)
l. ventricular end-diastolic volume
l. ventricular end-diastolic volume index (LVEDI)
l. ventricular end-systolic dimension (LVESD)
l. ventricular end-systolic volume index (LVESVI)
l. ventricular failure
l. ventricular fast filling time
l. ventricular filling pressure
l. ventricular fractional shortening index
l. ventricular free wall (LVFW)
l. ventricular functional shortening (LVFS)
l. ventricular function wall motion
l. ventricular gated blood pool scan
l. ventricular hypertrophy (LVH)
l. ventricular hypertrophy with strain
l. ventricular hypoplasia

L

NOTES

left (*continued*)
　　l. ventricular inflow tract
　　　obstruction
　　l. ventricular inflow volume
　　　(LVIV)
　　l. ventricular internal diameter
　　　(LVID)
　　l. ventricular internal diastolic
　　　dimension (LVIDd, LVIDD)
　　l. ventricular internal dimension at
　　　end systole (LVIDs)
　　l. ventricular internal end systole
　　l. ventricular loading
　　l. ventricular mass (LVM)
　　l. ventricular mass index (LVMI)
　　l. ventricular maximal volume
　　l. ventricular muscle
　　l. ventricular noncompaction
　　l. ventricular outflow pressure
　　　gradient
　　l. ventricular outflow tract (LVOT)
　　l. ventricular outflow tract
　　　obstruction (LVOTO)
　　l. ventricular outflow volume
　　　(LVOV)
　　l. ventricular peak systolic pressure
　　l. ventricular posterior superior
　　　process
　　l. ventricular posterior wall
　　　(LVPW)
　　l. ventricular preload
　　l. ventricular pressure (LVP)
　　l. ventricular regional wall motion
　　l. ventricular regional wall motion
　　　abnormality
　　l. ventricular slow filling time
　　l. ventricular strain pattern
　　l. ventricular stroke volume
　　l. ventricular stroke work (LVSW)
　　l. ventricular stroke work index
　　　(LVSWI)
　　l. ventricular support system
　　l. ventricular systolic (LVs)
　　l. ventricular systolic/diastolic
　　　function
　　l. ventricular systolic functional
　　　reserve
　　l. ventricular systolic pressure
　　l. ventricular systolic pump
　　　function
　　l. ventricular systolic time interval
　　　ratio
　　l. ventricular wall (LVW)
　　l. ventriculogram (LVG)
left-dominant coronary anatomy
left-handedness
　　ventricular l.-h.
left-right asymmetry

left-sided
　　l.-s. empyema
　　l.-s. heart failure
　　l.-s. heart pressure
　　l.-s. pleural effusion
left-sidedness
　　bilateral l.-s.
left-side-down
　　l.-s.-d. decubitus position
　　l.-s.-d. decubitus scan
left-to-right
　　l.-t.-r. flow
　　l.-t.-r. shift
　　l.-t.-r. shunting of blood
leg
　　l. axis
　　baker's l.
　　bayonet l.
　　bowed l.'s
　　champagne-bottle l.'s
　　deep vein system of l.
　　l. edema
　　postphlebitic l.
　　scissoring of l.'s
　　l. shortening
　　tennis l.
Legg-Calvé-Perthes disease (LCP)
Leggiero hydrophilic-coated
　　microcatheter
leg-length discrepancy (LLD)
Leichtenstern sign
Leigh
　　L. disease
　　L. syndrome
leiomyoblastoma
leiomyoma, pl. **leiomyomata, leiomyomas**
　　benign metastasizing l.
　　degenerated uterine l.
　　epithelioid l.
　　esophageal l.
　　fundal l.
　　gastric l.
　　kidney l.
　　multiple vascular leiomyomas
　　pedunculated l.
　　renal l.
　　small bowel l.
　　stomach l.
　　urinary bladder l.
　　uterine l.
　　vascular l.
leiomyomatosis
　　diffuse l.
　　esophageal l.
leiomyomatous kidney hamartoma
leiomyosarcoma
　　duodenal l.
　　esophageal l.
　　gastric l.

intramural l.
intravascular l.
jejunal l.
retroperitoneal l.
right atrial extension of uterine l.
small bowel l.
stomach l.

Leksell
L. D-shaped stereotactic frame
L. gamma unit
L. 201-source cobalt-60 Gamma
knife
L. stereotactic system

Leksell-Elekta stereotactic frame

LEL
low-energy laser

Lemierre syndrome

lemniscus, pl. **lemnisci**
medial l.

lemon sign

Lenard ray tube

length
basic cycle l. (BCL)
basic drive cycle l. (BDCL)
Beatson combined ankle l.
cervical l.
crown-heel l.
crown-rump l. (CR, CRL)
CSF systole l.
echo-train l. (ETL)
effective path l. (EPL)
femur l. (FL)
fetal femoral l.
focal l.
Grace method of ratio of
metatarsal l.
humeral l.
jet l. (JL)
limb l.
metacarpal l.
metacarpophalangeal l.
path l.
pulse l.
pyloric channel l.
radial l.
sinus cycle l. (SCL)
track cone l.
urethral l. (UL)

length-biased sampling

length-time bias

Lennox-Gastaut syndrome

Lenoir facet

lens
acoustic l.
right-angled telescopic l.
Thorpe plastic l.

lens-sparing external beam radiation therapy (LSRT)

LENT
late effect of normal tissue
LENT score
LENT scoring system

lenticular
l. area
l. bone
l. carcinoma
l. fasciculus
l. loop
l. nucleus

lenticulostriate
l. artery
l. supply
l. vasculopathy (LSV)
l. vessel

lentiform
l. bone
l. nucleus

lentigo, pl. **lentigines**

Lenz law

leontiasis ossea

leopard skin demyelination

lepidic growth

leptocyte

leptocytosis

leptofibril

leptomeningeal
l. anastomosis
l. angiomatosis
l. arachnoid cyst
l. artery
l. carcinoma
l. disease
l. fibrosis
l. ivy sign
l. metastasis
l. process

leptomeninges

leptomeningitis

leptomeningoencephalitis

leptomyelolipoma

lepton

Lequesne
center-edge angle of L.

NOTES

L

Leri
> melorheostosis of L.
> L. pleonosteosis
> L. sign

Leriche syndrome

Leri-Weill syndrome

LES
> lower esophageal sphincter

Lesch-Nyhan syndrome

Lesgaft
> L. hernia
> L. triangle

lesion
> acute cerebellar hemispheric l.
> admixture l.
> adrenal l.
> afferent nerve l.
> ALPSA l.
> anechoic l.
> angiocentric immunoproliferative l.
> angiocentric lymphoproliferative l.
> angulated l.
> anterior cranial base l.
> anterior labroligamentous periosteal sleeve avulsion l.
> anterior parietal l.
> anterochiasmatic l.
> Antopol-Goldman l.
> anular constricting l.
> aortic arch l.
> aortic valve l.
> apical l.
> apophysial l.
> appendiceal l.
> apple-core l.
> Armanni-Ebstein l.
> atheromatous l.
> atherosclerotic l.
> atrophic brain l.
> Baehr-Lohlein l.
> Bankart l.
> barrel-shaped l.
> basal hypodense ganglia l.
> benign fibrous bone l.
> benign lymphoepithelial l.
> benign lymphoproliferative l.
> benign vascular l.
> Bennett l.
> bifurcation l.
> bilateral l.
> bilobed polypoid l.
> biparietal l.
> bird's nest l.
> black star breast l.
> blastic l.
> bleeding l.
> blistering l.
> blowout bone l.
> Blumenthal l.

bone marrow l.
Bracht-Wachter l.
brain l.
brainstem l.
breast l.
Brown-Séquard l.
bubbling l.
bubbly bone l.
bulbourethral gland l.
bull's eye l.
butterfly l.
calcified l.
callosal l.
candidate l.
capsular drop l.
cardiac valvular l.
carinal l.
carpet l.
cartilaginous l.
cavernous sinus l.
caviar l.
cavitary lung l.
cavitary pulmonary l.
cavitary small bowel l.
central medullary bone l.
centrilobular l.
cerebral l.
cerebrospinal fluid-containing l.
cervical cord l.
chest wall l.
Chiari I–IV l.
chiasmal l.
cholesterol-containing brain l.
circular l.
circumscribed l.
cochlear l.
coin l.
cold l.
collar-button chest l.
colonic apple-core l.
colonic carpet l.
colonic saddle l.
complete nerve l.
complex sclerosing l. (CSL)
concentric l.
condylomatous atypia l.
congenital cystic neck l.
l. conspicuity
constricting esophageal l.
conus medullaris l.
convexity l.
cookie bite l.
cookie cutter l.
coordinates for target l.
cord epidural extramedullary l.
cord intramedullary l.
coronary artery l.
corpus callosum ring-enhancing l.
cortical bone l.

corticospinal pathway l.
Cowper gland l.
critical l.
culprit l.
cyclops l.
cystic epididymis l.
cystic intracranial fetal l.
cystic liver l.
cystic splenic l.
deep-seated l.
dendritic l.
de novo l.
dense enhancing brain l.
dense lung l.
desmoid l.
destructive bone l.
destructive discovertebral l.
l. detectability
diaphysial l.
Dieulafoy l.
differential diagnosis bone l.
difficult-to-treat vascular l.
diffuse ulcerative l.
disc l.
discrete l.
dominant hemisphere l.
"don't touch" l.
dorsal root entry zone l.
doughnut l.
DREZ l.
dumbbell l.
Duret l.
dysplasia-associated l.
Ebstein l.
eccentric medullary bone l.
eccentric restenosis l.
echogenic solid l.
ellipsoid l.
encapsulated fat-containing l.
encephaloclastic l.
endobronchial l.
enhancing brain l.
epicortical l.
epididymis l.
epidural extramedullary l.
epileptogenic l.
epiphysial l.
esophageal apple-core l.
Essex-Lopresti l.
excitatory l.
expanding cavernous sinus brain l.
expansile lytic l.

expansile multilocular bone l.
expansile rib l.
expansile unilocular well-demarcated
  bone l.
extraaxial CNS l.
extraaxial low-attenuation l.
extracranial mass l.
extrahepatic l.
extramedullary compressive l.
extratemporal structural l.
extratesticular l.
extrathoracic l.
extrinsic l.
falx cerebri l.
fast-flow l.
fat-containing l.'s
fat-containing breast l.
fatty metastatic l.
fibrohistiocytic l.
fibromuscular l.
fibroosseous l.
fibrous bone l.
fibrous GI tract polypoid l.
finger lucent l.
fingertip l.
florid duct l.
flow-compromising l.
flow-limiting l.
focal articular cartilage l.
focal cold liver l.
focal hemispheric l.
focal hot liver l.
focal ischemic l.
focal parenchymal brain l.
focal splenic l.
frank l.
friable l.
frondy l.
frontal lobe l.
full-thickness chondral l.
gallium-67-avid l.
GARD l.
gastric intramural-extramucosal l.
geographic l.
Ghon primary l.
Gill l.
GLAD l.
glenoid articular rim disruption l.
glenolabral articular disruption l.
GLOM l.
glomerular l.
grapelike multilocular cystic l.

NOTES

lesion (*continued*)
    greater sphenoid wing l.
    gross l.
    ground-glass l.
    HAGL l.
    hamartomatous l.
    hemisphere l.
    hemispheric demyelinating l.
    hemodynamically significant l.
    hemorrhagic l.
    herald patch l.
    high cervical spinal cord l.
    high-density l.
    high-grade obstructive l.
    high-grade squamous
      intraepithelial l. (HGSIL)
    high-intensity l.
    high pontine l.
    high-probability l.
    high-signal l.
    Hill-Sachs shoulder l.
    hole-within-hole bone l.
    homogeneous l.
    hot l.
    hourglass-shaped l.
    hyperdense brain l.
    hyperintense periventricular brain l.
    hyperplastic l.
    hypodense basal ganglion brain l.
    hypodense mesencephalic low-
      density brain l.
    hypointense sella l.
    l. hypometabolism
    hypothalamic l.
    iceberg l.
    iliac l.
    impaction l.
    indiscriminate l.
    indolent l.
    infectious bubbly bone l.
    infiltrating l.
    inflammatory l.
    infranuclear l.
    internal auditory canal enhancing l.
    intraaxial brain l.
    intracerebral l.
    intraconal l.
    intracranial mass l.
    intracranial vascular l.
    intradural extramedullary l.
    intramammary l.
    intramedullary cord l.
    intramedullary space-occupying l.
    intramedullary spinal l.
    intramural-extramucosal stomach l.
    intraocular l.
    intraosseous bone l.
    intraperitoneal l.
    intrasellar l.

    intraspinal l.
    intrinsic stenotic l.
    intrinsic stomach wall l.
    invasive l.
    irregularly shaped l.
    ischemic l.
    ischiorectal fossa l.
    isointense l.
    Janeway l.
    jet l.
    juxtacortical bone l.
    Kidner l.
    kissing l.
    lacrimal gland l.
    lateral temporal epileptogenic l.
    leave-alone l.
    left lower lobe l.
    left upper lobe l.
    lipomatous l.
    liver l.
    local l.
    local glomerular l.
    l. localization
    localized l.
    Löhlein-Baehr l.
    low-attenuation l.
    low-density mesencephalic l.
    lower motor neuron l.
    lucent finger l.
    lucent lung l.
    lumbar spine l.
    Lynch and Crues type 2 l.
    lytic bone l.
    macroorchidism l.
    macroscopic placental l.
    magnetic resonance-detected white
      matter l.
    malacic l.
    malignant osseous l.
    Mallory-Weiss l.
    mammographically suspicious l.
    mass l.
    masslike l.
    medial longitudinal fasciculus l.
    median nerve l.
    mediastinal l.
    melanocytic l.
    mesencephalic low-density brain l.
    mesencephalodiencephalic l.
    mesenteric vascular l.
    mesial temporal epileptogenic l.
    metabolic l.
    metachronous l.
    metastatic l.
    micro-crust formation l.
    micropapillary l.
    midbrain l.
    midline l.
    miliary l.

mixed fat-water density l.
mixed sclerotic and lytic bone l.
MLF l.
Mongolian spotlike l.
monomelic bone l.
Monteggia l.
mucosal l.
mulberry eye l.
multicentric lytic l.
multifocal enhancing brain l.
multilocular cystic l.
multiple lucent lung l.'s
multiple lytic bone l.'s
multiple osteosclerotic l.'s
multiple parotid gland l.'s
multiple stenotic l.'s
muscular l.
musculoskeletal l.
nail bed l.
napkin-ring anular l.
necrotic l.
needle localization of breast l.
neoplastic l.
neurogenic l.
neurologic bladder l.
neurovascular l.
nidus of l.
nodular l.
nondominant hemisphere l.
nonenhancing l.
nonexpansile multilocular bone l.
nonexpansile unilocular bone l.
noninvasive l.
nonmeningiomatous malignant l.
nonproliferative l.
nucleus ambiguus l.
nucleus basalis l.
obstructive l.
occipital l.
occlusive l.
occult l.
ocular l.
onionskin l.
optic nerve l.
organic l.
osseous l.
osteoblastic l.
osteocartilaginous l.
osteochondral l.
osteolytic l.
osteosclerotic l.
ostial l.

outcropping of l.
papillary l.
papular l.
papulonecrotic l.
paradiscal l.
paralabral l.
paraorbital l.
parasagittal l.
parasellar l.
parasellar region l.
parietal cortex l.
parietal lobe l.
parietooccipital l.
parosteal bone l.
partial l.
patch l.
pathologic l.
pedunculated l.
perforative l.
periapical l.
peripheral nerve l.
perisellar vascular l.
periventricular l.
permeative l.
Perthes l.
Perthes-Bankart l.
phlyctenule l.
phosphaturic intraosseous l.
photon-deficient bone l.
pinguecula l.
plaquelike l.
POLPSA l.
polyostotic bone l.
polypoid l.
pontine l.
popcornlike reticulated l.
portal vein l.
posterior column l.
posterior compartment l.
posterior fossa l.
posterior fossa-foramen magnum l.
posterior language area l.
posterior vertebral element
  blowout l.
prechiasmal optic nerve l.
presacral cystic l.
pretectal l.
primary l.
proliferative l.
prostate hypoechoic l.
pseudotumoral l.
pulmonary l.

NOTES

L

lesion *(continued)*
    punched-out lytic bone l.
    punctate l.
    purulent l.
    questionable l.
    radial sclerosing l.
    radiodense l.
    radiofrequency l.
    radiographic stability of l.
    radiolucent l.
    radiopaque l.
    reactive fibrous l.
    reactive lymphoid l.
    rectal l.
    rectosigmoid polypoid l.
    recurrent l.
    regurgitant l.
    remote lower motor neuron l.
    renal mass l.
    resectable l.
    retrochiasmal l.
    retroglandular l.
    reverse Hill-Sachs l.
    rheumatic l.
    rib l.
    right lower lobe l.
    right upper lobe l.
    rim-enhancing l.
    ring l.
    ring-enhancing brain l.
    ringlike l.
    ring-wall l.
    root entry-zone l.
    rotator cuff l.
    rounded l.
    round lucent l.
    saddle l.
    satellite l.
    scar l.
    scirrhous l.
    sclerosing l.
    sclerotic l.
    secondary l.
    segmental bronchus l.
    serial l.
    sessile l.
    shagreen l.
    sharply demarcated
      circumferential l.
    sinonasal l.
    sinusoidal l.
    skeletal l.
    skip l.
    SLAP l.
    slow-flow l.
    slowly developing l.
    small bowel cavitary l.
    solid splenic l.
    solid thymic l.

    solitary cold l.
    solitary osteosclerotic l.
    solitary rib l.
    solitary sternal l.
    sonolucent cystic l.
    space-occupying intracranial l.
    spheric l.
    spiculated scirrhous l.
    spinal cord l.
    spleen l.
    splenic l.
    spontaneous l.
    squamous intraepithelial l. (SIL)
    stacked ovoid l.
    stellate border breast l.
    Stener l.
    stenoobstructive l.
    stenotic l.
    sternal l.
    Sterner l.
    striatal l.
    structural l.
    subareolar l.
    subchondral l.
    subcortical intracranial l.
    subcortical low-intensity l.
    submucosal l.
    subtentorial l.
    subtotal l.
    superficial l.
    superior labral anterior-posterior l.
    supraaortic l.
    supranuclear l.
    suprasellar low-density l.
    supratentorial l.
    suspicious l.
    swan-neck tubular l.
    synchronous l.
    systemic l.
    tandem l.
    target lung l.
    teardrop-shaped l.
    tectal l.
    telangiectatic l.
    temporal lobe l.
    tentorium cerebelli l.
    testicular cystic l.
    thalamic l.
    thoracic inlet l.
    tight l.
    total l.
    trabeculated bone l.
    transfer l.
    transverse cord l.
    trophic l.
    true-negative l.
    tuberculous l.
    tubular l.
    tumorlike l.

tumor-mimicking breast l.
ulcerative l.
ulnar nerve l.
umbilical cord l.
uncommitted metaphysial l.
unilateral l.
unilocular cystic l.
unilocular well-demarcated bone defect expansile l.
unresectable l.
unstable l.
upper motor neuron l.
valvular regurgitant l.
vascular l.
vasculitic l.
vegetative l.
vertebral expansile l.
visceral l.
Waldeyer ring l.
wedge-shaped l.
well-circumscribed l.
well-defined l.
white matter l.
white star breast l.
wide field l.
wire-loop l.
Wolin meniscoid l.
X, Y, and Z coordinates for target l.

lesion-background ratio
lesion-brain ratio (L-B)
lesion-countersite ratio (L-C)
lesion-muscle ratio
lesion-nonlesion count ratio
lesion-normal tissue ratio
lesion-to-cerebrospinal fluid noise
lesion-to-white matter noise
LESP
lower esophageal sphincter pressure
lesser
l. arc injury
l. atrophy
l. curvature of stomach
l. curvature ulcer
l. metatarsophalangeal joint
l. muscle
l. omentum (LO)
l. pancreas
l. pelvis
l. peritoneal sac
l. petrosal
l. sac abscess

l. sac hernia
l. sac of peritoneal cavity
l. saphenous system
l. saphenous vein
l. sciatic foramen
l. sciatic notch
l. trochanter
l. trochanter of femur
l. trochanteric fracture
l. tubercle
l. tuberosity

Lester Jones bypass tube
LET
linear energy transfer
lethal
l. bone dysplasia
l. dose
l. dwarfism
l. midline granuloma
l. musculoskeletal dysplasia
l. myocardial injury
l. neoplasm
lettering artifact
leucine radical
leucotomy
LEUHR
low-energy ultra-high resolution
LEUHR fan beam collimator
LEUHR parallel-hole collimator
leukemia
acute lymphocytic l.
acute myeloid l.
chronic lymphocytic l.
chronic myeloid l.
Rieder cell l.
T-cell acute lymphoblastic l.
T-cell-type acute lymphoblastic l.
leukemic bone line
leukemid
leukemogenesis
leukemoid
leukocyte
agranular l.
autologous labeled l.
basophilic l.
endothelial l.
eosinophilic l.
gallium-67-labeled l.
granular l.
heterophilic l.
indium-111-labeled l.
^{111}In-oxime-labeled l.

NOTES

L

leukocyte *(continued)*
    mast l.
    motile l.
    neutrophilic l.
    nongranular l.
    nonmotile l.
    polymorphonuclear l.
    polynuclear neutrophilic l.
    technetium-99m l.
leukodystrophy
    congenital l.
leukoencephalitis
    acute hemorrhagic l.
leukoencephalopathy
    Cree l.
    diffuse necrotizing l.
    disseminated necrotizing l.
    heroin vapor l.
    multifocal l.
    periventricular l.
    postviral l.
    progressive multifocal l. (PML)
    radiation-induced l.
    spongiform l.
    toxic l.
leukomalacia
    periventricular l. (PVL)
leukopenia
    radiofrequency radiogenic l.
    radiogenic l.
LeukoScan
    L. imaging agent
    technetium-99m HMPAO mixed
      leukocyte L.
Leur-par collimator
LeuTech radiolabeled imaging agent
levator
    l. ani
    l. muscle
    l. palpebrae
    l. scapulae
    l. span
    l. veli palatini
LeVeen
    L. plaque cracker
    L. RF probe
level
    air-fluid l.
    attenuation l.
    contrast window l.
    C-reactive protein l.
    debris-fluid l.
    energy l.
    fat-fluid l.
    fluid l.
    fluid-fluid l.
    gas-fluid l.
    hand and forearm artery scoring l.
      I–V

    intracapsular fat-fluid l.
    intrasinus air-fluid l.
    l. I obstetric ultrasound
    pontine-medullary l.
    protein-fat fluid l.
    significance l.
    stairstep air-fluid l.
    supraventricular l.
    window l.
    zero reference l.
    Zielke derotation l.
level-dependent
    blood oxygenation l.-d. (BOLD)
3-level Haar wavelet decomposition
Levenberg-Marquardt method
Levine tube
levoangiocardiogram
levocardiogram
levogram
levoposition
levorotary scoliosis
levorotatory
levoscoliosis
levotransposition (L-transposition)
levoversion
Levovist
    L. imaging agent
    L. myocardial contrast
      echocardiography
Lewis (Le)
    L. angle
    L. position
Leydig
    L. cell adenoma
    L. cell tumor (LCT)
Leyla arm
LFUS
    low frequency ultrasound
LFV
    large field of view
LGL
    Lown-Ganong-Levine syndrome
LHBT
    long head of biceps tendon
    LHBT tenosynovitis
Lhermitte-Duclos-Cowden syndrome
Lhermitte-Duclos syndrome
LHP
    lateral hypopharyngeal pouch
LHV
    left hepatic vein
LI
    lumbar index
Libman-Sacks endocarditis disease
LICA
    left internal carotid artery
lichenoides
    tuberculosis l.
    tuberculosis cutis l.

Lichtenstein-Jaffe disease
licorice powder
LICS
    left intercostal space
LICU
    laparoscopic intracorporeal ultrasound
lidocaine-adrenaline solution
lidofenin
lie
    L. classification
    fetal l.
    horizontal l.
    longitudinal l.
    posterior l.
    transverse l.
    unusual fetal l.
Liebel-Flarsheim CT 9000 contrast
    delivery system
Lieberkühn crypt
Liebermeister groove
Liebow
    usual interstitial pneumonia of L.
        (UIP)
lienis
    sustentaculum l.
lienography
lienophrenic ligament
lienorenal ligament
Lieutaud trigone
LiF
    lithium fluoride
    LiF thermoluminescence dosimeter
    LiF thermoluminescence dosimetry
LifeJet catheter
LIFE-Lung fluorescence endoscopy
    system
Life-Pack 5 cardiac monitor
lifestyle-limiting claudication
life-threatening
    l.-t. hemorrhage
    l.-t. pneumothorax
lifetime regimen
lift
    gallbladder l.
    heave and l.
    sternal l.
ligament
    accessory atlantoaxial l.
    acromioclavicular l.
    acromiocoracoid l.
    adipose l.
    alar l.

anococcygeal l.
anterior cruciate l. (ACL)
anterior fibular l.
anterior inferior tibiofibular l.
anterior talofibular l. (ATF)
anterior tibiofibular l.
anterior tibiotalar l.
anular l.
apical l.
Arantius l.
arcuate l.
arterial l.
atlantal l.
attenuated l.
auricular l.
avulsed l.
axis l.
Bardinet l.
Barkow l.
beak l.
Bellini l.
Berry l.
Bertin l.
Bichat l.
bifurcated l.
Bigelow l.
Botallo l.
Bourgery l.
broad l.
Brodie l.
Burns l.
calcaneoclavicular l.
calcaneocuboid l.
calcaneofibular l. (CFL)
calcanconavicular l.
calcaneotibial l.
Caldani l.
Campbell l.
Camper l.
capsular l.
Carcassonne l.
cardinal l.
caroticoclinoid l.
carpometacarpal l.
Casser l.
casserian l.
caudal l.
ceratocricoid l.
cervical mover l.
checkrein l.
cholecystoduodenal l.
chondroxiphoid l.

L

NOTES

ligament *(continued)*
    ciliary l.
    Civinini l.
    Clado l.
    Cleland l.
    clinoid l.
    Cloquet l.
    coccygeal l.
    collateral l.
    Colles l.
    congenital laxity of l.
    conjugate l.
    conoid l.
    conus l.
    Cooper suspensory l.
    coracoacromial l.
    coracoclavicular l.
    coracohumeral l.
    corniculopharyngeal l.
    coronary l.
    costoclavicular l.
    costocolic l.
    costotransverse l.
    costoxiphoid l.
    cotyloid l.
    Cowper l.
    cricopharyngeal l.
    cricothyroid l.
    cricotracheal l.
    cross l.
    cruciate l.
    cruciatum cruris l.
    cruciform l.
    Cruveilhier l.
    cuboideonavicular l.
    cuneocuboid l.
    cuneonavicular l.
    cystoduodenal l.
    deep collateral l.
    deltoid l.
    Denonvilliers l.
    dentate l.
    denticulate l.
    diaphragmatic l.
    dorsal metacarpal l.
    dorsal wrist l.
    Douglas l.
    duodenal l.
    duodenorenal l.
    epicondyloolecranon l.
    l. of epididymis
    epihyal l.
    extracapsular l.
    extrinsic l.
    fabellofibular l.
    falciform l.
    fallopian l.
    femoral l.
    Ferrein l.

    fibular collateral l.
    fibulotalar l.
    fibulotalocalcaneal l.
    flaval l.
    floating l.
    Flood l.
    FTC l.
    fundiform l.
    gastrocolic l.
    gastrodiaphragmatic l.
    gastrohepatic l.
    gastrolienal l.
    gastropancreatic l.
    gastrophrenic l.
    gastrosplenic l.
    genital l.
    genitoinguinal l.
    Gerdy l.
    Gillette suspensory l.
    Gimbernat l.
    gingivodental l.
    glenohumeral l.
    glenoid l.
    glossoepiglottic l.
    Grayson l.
    Günzberg l.
    Haines-McDougall medial
      sesamoid l.
    hammock l.
    Helmholtz axis l.
    Henle l.
    l.'s of Henry and Wrisberg
    Hensing l.
    hepatic l.
    hepatocolic l.
    hepatocystocolic l.
    hepatoduodenal l.
    hepatoesophageal l.
    hepatogastric l.
    hepatogastroduodenal l.
    hepatophrenic l.
    hepatorenal l.
    hepatoumbilical l.
    Hesselbach l.
    Hey l.
    Holl l.
    Hueck l.
    humeral avulsion of the
      glenohumeral l. (HAGL)
    Humphry l.
    Hunter l.
    Huschke l.
    hyalocapsular l.
    hyoepiglottic l.
    iliofemoral l.
    iliolumbar l.
    iliopectineal l.
    iliopubic l.
    iliotibial l.

iliotrochanteric l.
inferior dorsal radioulnar l.
inferior pulmonary l.
infrapatellar l.
infundibuloovarian l.
infundibulopelvic l.
inguinal l.
intercapital l.
intercarpal l.
interclavicular l.
interclinoid l.
intercornual l.
intercuneiform l.
interdigital l.
interfoveolar l.
intermetatarsal l.
internal collateral l.
interosseous sacroiliac l.
interosseous talocalcaneal l.
intersesamoid l.
interspinous l.
intertransverse l.
intervertebral l.
intraarticular l.
intrascapular l.
intrinsic l.
ischiocapsular l.
ischiofemoral l.
Jarjavay l.
jugal l.
Krause l.
laciniate l.
lacunar l.
Landsmeer l.
Lannelongue l.
lateral arcuate l.
lateral collateral l. (LCL)
lateral costotransverse l.
lateral talocalcaneal l.
lateral ulnar collateral l. (LUCL)
Lauth l.
lienophrenic l.
lienorenal l.
limited proteoglycan matrix of l.
Lisfranc l.
Lockwood l.
longitudinal l.
lumbocostal l.
lunotriquetral interosseus l.
Luschka l.
Mackenrodt l.
macroscopic hemorrhage l.

Maissiat l.
Mauchart l.
Meckel l.
medial collateral l. (MCL)
median arcuate l.
median cruciate l.
median umbilical l.
meniscofemoral l.
meniscotibial l.
metacarpoglenoidal l.
metacarpophalangeal l.
microscopic hemorrhage of l.
mucosal suspensory l.
natatory l.
naviculocuneiform l.
nuchal l.
occipitoatlantoaxial l.
occipitoaxial l.
odontoid l.
opacification of posterior
    longitudinal l.
orbicular l.
Osborne l.
ossification of longitudinal l.
ossification of posterior
    longitudinal l. (OPLL)
ossified posterior longitudinal l.
ovarian suspensory l.
l. of ovary
palmar metacarpal l.
palmar radiocarpal l.
pectinate l.
pelvic ring l.
periodontal l.
peritoneal part of inguinal l.
Petit l.
Pétrequin l.
petroclinoid l.
phalangeal glenoidal l.
phrenicocolic l.
phrenicolienal l.
phrenicosplenic l.
phrenoesophageal l.
phrenogastric l.
phrenosplenic l.
pisohamate l.
pisometacarpal l.
pisounciform l.
pisouncinate l.
plantar l.
popliteal l.
posterior cruciate l. (PCL)

NOTES

L

ligament *(continued)*

posterior inferior tibiofibular l.
posterior longitudinal l. (PLL)
posterior oblique l.
posterior talofibular l.
posterior tibiotalar l.
Poupart inguinal l.
pterygomandibular l.
pterygospinous l.
PTF l.
pubocapsular l.
pubocervical l.
pubofemoral l.
puboprostatic l.
pubovesical l.
pulmonary l.
quadrate l.
radial collateral l.
radial metacarpal l.
radiate sternocostal l.
radiocarpal l.
radiolunotriquetral l.
radioscaphocapitate l.
radioscaphoid l.
radioscapholunate l.
reflected edge of Poupart l.
reflected inguinal l.
l. reflecting edge
retinacular l.
Retzius l.
rhomboid l.
right triangular l.
ring l.
Robert l.
round l.
Rouvière l.
sacrodural l.
sacrospinous l.
sacrotuberous l.
Santorini l.
Sappey l.
scapholunate l.
scaphotriquetral l.
l. of Scarpa
Schlemm l.
serous l.
sesamoid l.
sesamophalangeal l.
sheath l.
l. shelving edge
short radiolunate l.
Simonart l.
Soemmerring l.
sphenomandibular l.
spinoglenoid l.
spinous tarsus l.
spiral l.
splenocolic l.
splenorenal l.

spring l.
Stanley cervical l.
stellate l.
sternoclavicular l.
sternopericardial l.
stretched out l.
Struthers l.
stylohyoid l.
stylomandibular l.
stylomaxillary l.
superficial dorsal sacrococcygeal l.
superficial posterior
  sacrococcygeal l.
superficial transverse metacarpal l.
superficial transverse metatarsal l.
superior costotransverse l.
superior pubic l.
superior transverse scapular l.
suprascapular l.
supraspinous l.
suspensory l.
sutural l.
syndesmotic l.
synovial l.
talocalcaneal l.
talofibular l.
talonavicular l.
tarsal l.
tarsometatarsal l.
l. tear
tectoral l.
temporomandibular l.
Teutleben l.
Thompson l.
thyroepiglottic l.
thyrohyoid l.
tibial collateral l.
tibial sesamoid l.
tibiocalcaneal l.
tibiofibular l.
tibionavicular l.
torn meniscotibial l.
transverse atlantal l.
transverse carpal l.
transverse cervical l.
transverse crural l.
transverse genicular l.
transverse humeral l.
transverse intertarsal l.
transverse metacarpal l.
transverse metatarsal l.
transverse perineal l.
transverse tibiofibular l.
trapezoid l.
l. of Treitz
triangular l.
triquetrohamate l.
triquetroscaphoid l.
Tuffier inferior l.

ulnar collateral l. (UCL)
ulnocarpal l.
ulnolunate l.
ulnotriquetral l.
umbilical l.
urachal l.
uterine l.
uterosacral l.
uterovesical l.
vaginal l.
venous l.
ventral sacrococcygeal l.
ventral sacroiliac l.
ventricular l.
vertebropelvic l.
vesicosacral l.
vesicoumbilical l.
vesicouterine l.
vestibular l.
vocal l.
volar carpal l.
Walther oblique l.
Weitbrecht l.
Winslow l.
Wrisberg l.
xiphicostal l.
xiphoid l.
Y-shaped l.
Zaglas l.
Zinn l.

ligamentous
l. ankylosis
l. attachment
l. bouncing
l. box
l. calcification
l. complex
l. disruption
l. impingement
l. insertion
l. instability
l. laxity
l. luxation
l. strain
l. support
l. thickening
l. trauma

ligamentous-muscular hypertrophy
ligamentum, pl. **ligamenta**
l. arteriosum
l. flavum
l. flavum thickening

l. mucosum
l. nuchae
l. patellae
l. teres
l. venosum fissure

ligand
l. agent
^{99m}Tc-labeled l.

ligation
Doppler-guided hemorrhoid artery l. (DGHAL)
Hunter aneurysm l.
thoracic duct l.

light
l. bulb appearance
l. chain deposition disease (LCDD)
hot l.
infrared l.
invisible l.
l. leak
l. microscopy
l. pink lung
l. reflection rheography
l. scanning
l. sedation
structured l.
l. therapy
Wood l.

light-induced autofluorescence spectroscopy
LightSheer SC diode laser
LightSpeed
L. CT scanner
L. multidetector CT scanner
L. QXi CT scanner
L. QX/i scanner
L. Ultra CT system

Lightstic 180, 360 fiberoptic laser
Lightwood syndrome
likelihood ratio (LR)
LILI
low-intensity laser irradiation
Lilienfelds position
Liliequist membrane
LILT
low-intensity laser therapy
LIMA
left internal mammary artery
LIMA anastomosis
limb
l. absence
l. of anterior capsule

NOTES

L

limb *(continued)*
l. of bifurcation graft
l. bone length ratio
l. bud
chronic lymphedematous l.
l. girdle
l. holder
l. kinking
l. length
l. perfusion
l. reduction
l. reduction abnormality
l. reduction anomaly
Roux-en-Y l.
l. venography
vertebral, anal, cardiac, tracheal,
   esophageal, renal, l. (VACTERL)
limb-body wall complex
limb-girdle muscular dystrophy
limbic
l. lobe
l. region
l. system
limb-length
l.-l. asymmetry
l.-l. discrepancy (LLD)
l.-l. inequality
limb-lengthening procedure
limb-threatening ischemia
limbus
l. fossae ovalis
l. suture
l. vertebra
l. of Vieussens
limit
eye exposure l.
Nyquist l.
quantum l.
tracking l.
limitation
beam l.
biophysical l.
infarct size l.
l. of joint motion
l. of MR imaging
l. of ultrasound
limited
l. examination
l. film
l. imaging
l. oxidative capacity
l. proteoglycan matrix of ligament
Sirtex Medical L. (SIR)
l. view
limited-cut plane
limited-slice computed tomography
limited-stage
l.-s. diffuse large-cell lymphoma
l.-s. DLCL

limiting membrane
limitus
hallux l. (HL)
LINAC
linear accelerator
LINAC radiosurgery
Varian LINAC
Linac
X-band L.
Lindegaard ratio
line
absence of innominate l.
absorption l.
acanthiomeatal l.
acetabular l.
AC-PC l.
air-fluid l.
Andren-von Rosen l.
aneuploid cell l.
anorectal l.
anterior axillary l. (AAL)
anterior humeral l.
anterior junction l.
aortic vent suction l.
Arrow PICC l.
auricular l.
axillary l.
azygoesophageal l.
basilar l.
bimastoid l.
Blumensaat l.
Bolton-nasion l.
branching l.
calcification l.
Camper l.
canthomeatal l.
Cantlie l.
cement l.
central sacral l. (CSL)
central venous pressure l.
Chamberlain l.
Chaussier l.
clinoparietal l.
Conradi l.
Correra l.
costoclavicular l.
costophrenic septal l.
Crampton l.
crescent hip l.
curved radiolucent l.
curvilinear subpleural l.
Cyma l.
Daubenton l.
demarcation l.
dentate l.
digastric l.
displaced left paraspinal l.
divisionary l.
Ellis l.

Ellis-Garland l.
epiphysial l.
fat-density l.
Feiss l.
Fischgold bimastoid l.
Fischgold biventer l.
Fleischner l.
l. focus principle
fracture l.
Fränkel white l.
Frankfort l.
F T l.
gallbladder-vena cava l.
gas density l.
gaussian l.
l. of Gennari
glabelloalveolar l.
glabellomeatal l.
gluteal l.
Granger l.
growth arrest l.
Gubler l.
Hampton l.
Harris l.
Hawkins l.
Hickman l.
Hilgenreiner l.
His l.
humeral l.
ilioischial l.
iliopectineal l.
l. imaging
infraorbital l.
infraorbitomeatal l. (IOML)
innominate absence of l.
l. integral concept
interlobar septal l.
interpupillary l.
intravenous infusion l.
isodose l.
isoelectric l.
isopotential l.
joint l.
Kerley A, B, C l.'s
Kilian l.
Köhler l.
Langer l.
Lanz l.
lateral joint l.
lead l.
leukemic bone l.
linguine l.

Linton l.
Looser l.
lorentzian l.
lower lung l.
low-intensity l.
lucent l.
Mach l.
McGregor l.
McKee l.
McRae l.
medial joint l.
median l.
Mees l.
Merkel cell carcinoma cell l.
Meyer l.
midaxillary l.
midclavicular l. (MCL)
midhumeral l.
midscapular l.
midspinal l.
midsternal l.
Moyer l.
Nélaton l.
oblique prescription l.
obturator l.
Ogston l.
Ohngren l.
orbitomeatal l.
orthogonal tag l.
l. pair
parallel M l.
parallel pitch l.
paramedian l.
paraspinal l.
pectinate l.
peripheral intravenous infusion l.
peripherally inserted central
  catheter l.
Perkin l.
Perkins-Ombredanne l.
photon therapy beam l.
PICC l.
l. placement
pleural l.
pleuroesophageal l.
popliteal l.
posterior axillary l.
posterior cervical l.
posterior junction l.
posterior nipple l. (PNL)
pronator quadratus l.
properitoneal fat l.

L

NOTES

line *(continued)*
    psoas l.
    pubococcygeal l. (PCL)
    radiocapitellar l.
    radiolucent crescent l.
    raster l.
    reference l.
    Reid l.
    resonance l.
    l. of response (LOR)
    l. of Retzius
    Richter-Monroe l.
    Rolando l.
    sacrococcygeal inferior pubic
      point l.
    Sappey l.
    l. saturation
    l. scanning (LS)
    Schoemaker l.
    scorbutic white l.
    semilunar l.
    septal l.
    l. shadow
    l. shape
    Shenton l.
    Simpson white l.
    skin l.
    Skinner l.
    soleal l.
    spectral l.
    spinographic l.
    spinolaminar l. (SLL)
    l. spread function (LSF)
    subchondral fracture l.
    subclavian l.
    subcutaneous fat l.
    subpleural curvilinear l.
    suture l.
    transcondylar l.
    transverse lucent metaphysial l.
    trough l.
    Trümmerfeld l.
    twining l.
    Ullmann l.
    ventral venous pressure l.
    vertebral body l.
    visualization of the Z l.
    Wagner l.
    water density l.
    Wegner l.
    white l.
    l. width
    Z l.
    zero l.
linea, pl. **lineae**
    l. alba
    l. semilunaris
lineage
    M4-M5 l.

linear
    l. absorption coefficient
    l. accelerator (LINAC)
    l. accelerator isocenter motion
    l. accelerator unit
    l. actuator
    l. amplifier
    l. array echoendoscope
    l. array-hydrophone assembly
    l. array transducer
    l. array transrectal ultrasound probe
    l. artifact
    l. attenuation
    l. attenuation coefficient
    l. band of maximal radiolucency
    l. branching microcalcification
    l. calcification
    l. combination model software
    l. compartmental system
    l. defect
    l. degenerative signal intensity
    l. density
    l. echo
    l. electrode array
    l. emphysema
    l. energy transfer (LET)
    l. erosion
    l. focus
    l. focus within cyst wall
    l. gradient
    l. high signal intensity
    l. infiltrate
    l. interpolation
    l. interstitial disease pattern
    l. low signal
    l. lucency
    l. margin
    l. marking
    l. measure
    12- to 5-MHz l. array transducer
    7.5-MHz l. transducer
    l. opacity
    l. phased array
    l. phosphate
    l. photon
    l. polarization
    l. prediction (LP)
    l. prediction with singular value
      decomposition
    l. radiopacity
    l. regression analysis
    l. scan imaging
    l. scanning
    l. sebaceous nevus syndrome
    l. shadow
    l. skull fracture
    l. stenosis
    l. structure

l. tomography
l. ulcer

linearity
absolute l.
gradient l.
intrinsic spatial l.
lung l.
pulmonary l.
scintillation camera l.

linearization
perceptual l.

linearly polarized coil

linear-quadratic (LQ)
l.-q. equation

linebacker's arm

line-pair measurement

line-shape sensitivity

lingual
l. artery
l. bone
l. goiter
l. gyrus
l. nerve
l. root
l. thyroid
l. tonsil

linguine line

lingula, pl. **lingulae**
l. pulmonis
right middle lobe l.

lingular
l. bronchus
l. division of left lung
l. infiltrate
l. mandibular bony defect (LMBD)
l. nodule
l. orifice
l. pneumonia

lining
mucosal l.

linitis
l. plastica
l. plastica carcinoma

link
musculotendinous-osseous l.

Linsman water test

Linton line

Lintro-Scan

liothyronine sodium

LIP
lymphocytic interstitial pneumonia
lymphoid interstitial pneumonia

lip
hilar kidney l.
l. of hilum
l. of lateral sulcus
median cleft l.
osteophytic bone l.
posterior l.
rhombic l.
l. ring artifact

lipid
l. artifact
l. cholecystitis
l. content of storage fat
l. cyst
l. fraction relaxation rate
l. lake
l. signal
l. zone

lipid-laden
l.-l. foamy macrophage
l.-l. plaque

lipidosis
cerebroside l.
sphingomyelin l.

lipid-polarized helium MR imaging

lipid-rich material

lipid-sensitive
l.-s. MR
l.-s. MR imaging

Lipiodol
L. embolization
L. myelographic imaging agent
70–50% L. Ultra-Fluid

liplike projection of cartilage

lipoblastic meningioma

lipoblastoma

lipocalcinogranulomatosis

lipodystrophy
intestinal l.
mesenteric l.

lipofibroadenoma
breast l.

lipogenic tumor

lipogranuloma
sclerosing l.

lipogranulomatosis
disseminated l.

lipohemarthrosis

lipohyalinosis

lipoid
l. adrenal hyperplasia
l. dermatoarthritis

NOTES

lipoid *(continued)*
    l. endogenous pneumonia
    l. granulomatosis
    l. pneumonitis
lipoleiomyoma
lipoma
    l. arborescens
    bone l.
    brain l.
    breast l.
    cardiac l.
    corpus callosum l.
    diffuse synovial l.
    epidural l.
    GI tract l.
    hepatic l.
    hilar l.
    infiltrating l.
    intracranial l.
    intradural l.
    intramedullary l.
    intraosseous l.
    intratentorial l.
    liver l.
    l. macrodystrophia
    mediastinum l.
    pericallosal l.
    soft tissue l.
    spine l.
    subpial l.
    synovial diffuse l.
lipomatosa
    macrodystrophia l.
lipomatosis
    central sinus l.
    epidural l.
    esophageal l.
    mediastinal l.
    l. mediastinum
    multiple symmetric l.
    pancreatic l.
    pelvic l.
    peripelvic l.
    renal sinus l.
    sinus l.
    soft tissue l.
lipomatous
    l. hypertrophy
    l. hypertrophy of interatrial septum
    l. lesion
    l. polyp
    l. tissue
    l. tumor
lipomyelomeningocele
lipomyeloschisis
liponecrosis
    l. macrocystica calcificans
    l. microcystica calcificans

lipophilic
    l. cationic diphosphine
    l. compound
    l. dye
    l. imaging agent
    l. oxine-indium
    l. sequestration system
lipoplasty
    ultrasound-assisted l. (UAL)
LipoProfile
liposarcoma
    dedifferentiated l.
    metastatic pleomorphic l.
    myxomatous l.
    pleomorphic l.
    retroperitoneal l.
liposarcomatous differentiation
liposclerotic mesenteritis
liposculpture
    3D superficial l.
liposome
    antibody-conjugated paramagnetic l. (ACPL)
    mannan-coated l.
Lipowitz metal
Lippes loop
lipping
    osteophytic l.
Lippman-Cobb angle
LIQ
    lower inner quadrant
liquefaction
    l. degeneration
    l. necrosis
liquefactive emphysema
liquid
    l. barium suspension
    l. calcium
    l. crystal contact thermography
    l. crystal display projector
    l. crystal thermography (LCT)
    l. embolic agent
    l. food dysphagia
    l. nylon
    l. pleural effusion
    l. scintillation analysis
    l. scintillation spectrometer
    l. scintillation spectrometry
Lisch nodule
Lisfranc
    L. amputation
    L. dislocation
    L. fracture
    L. injury
    L. joint
    L. ligament
Lissauer
    L. column
    L. tract

lissencephaly, lissencephalia
  cobblestone l.
list
  l. mode data collection
  l. mode lithium
listeria encephalitis
Lister tubercle
lithiasis
  renal l.
lithium
  l. fluoride (LiF)
  list mode l.
lithium-7
lithoclast miniature pneumatic drill
lithogenic
  l. bile
  l. index
lithokelypedion
litholysis
litholytic agent
lithopedion
lithopedium
Lithostar nonimmersion lithotripter
lithotomy position
lithotripsy
  biliary l.
  candela l.
  electrohydraulic l. (EHL)
  electrohydraulic shockwave l.
  endoscopic l.
  extracorporeal shock wave l.
    (ESWL)
  laser biliary l.
  microexplosion l.
  pulsed-dye laser l.
  rotational contact l.
  ultrasonic l.
lithotripter, lithotriptor
  DoLi S extracorporeal shock
    wave l.
  Dornier compact l.
  Dornier HM3, HM4 l.
  Lithostar nonimmersion l.
  Modulith SL 20 l.
  Pulsolith laser l.
  Siemens Lithostar l.
  Sonolith Praktis l.
  Swiss lithoclast intracorporeal l.
  Wolf Piezolith 2200 l.
lithotrite
  Kensey-Nash l.
LithoTron

LITT
  laser-induced interstitial thermotherapy
  laser-induced thermography
  laser-induced thermotherapy
  LITT applicator
little
  l. finger
  L. Leaguer shoulder
Littre
  L. gland
  L. hernia
Litzmann obliquity
livedo reticularis
liver
  l. abscess
  l. agenesis
  alcoholic fatty l.
  amiodarone l.
  l. angiosarcoma
  l. bed
  biliary cirrhotic l.
  brimstone l.
  bronze l.
  l. calcification
  l. capillary hemangioma
  l. capsule
  cardiac impression on l.
  caudate lobe of l.
  l. cell adenoma
  centrilobular region of l.
  Chinese fluke l.
  l. cirrhosis
  cirrhotic l.
  l. coil
  l. cyst
  degenerative l.
  degraded l.
  diaphragmatic surface of l.
  l. dome
  l. echinococcosis
  echogenic l.
  l. edema
  l. edge
  enlarged l.
  extracorporeal l.
  l. failure
  fat-spared area in fatty l.
  fatty l.
  l. fissure
  l. flap
  floating l.
  l. fluke

NOTES

liver *(continued)*
    focal fatty infiltration of l.
    frosted l.
    graft-versus-host disease of l.
    l. hemangiosarcoma
    hobnail l.
    l. hydatid disease
    hyperperfusion abnormality of l.
    hypoechoic l.
    l. impression
    infantile hemangioendothelioma
      of l.
    intracorporeal l.
    l., kidneys, and spleen (LKS)
    l. laceration
    large-droplet fatty l.
    left lobe of l.
    l. lesion
    l. lipoma
    l. lymphoma
    l. mass
    l. metastasis
    nodular l.
    nodule-in-nodule l.
    noncirrhotic l.
    nutmeg appearance of l.
    l. parenchyma
    polycystic l.
    polylobar l.
    prominent l.
    pyogenic l.
    quadrate lobe of l.
    right lobe of l.
    l. scan
    l. scintigraphy
    l. scintiphotography
    l. segment
    shrunken l.
    small-droplet fatty l.
    l. span
    l. spoked-wheel pattern
    stasis l.
    l. steatosis
    tramline effect in l.
    l. transplant
    l. trauma
    undersurface of l.
    visceral surface of l.
    wandering l.
    waxy l.
liver-aorta (L/A)
liverlike lung
liverlung scan
Liverpool silicosis
liver-specific MRI contrast agent
liver-spleen
    l.-s. imaging
    l.-s. overlap
    l.-s. scan

liver-to-aorta peak ratio
liver-to-liver peak ratio
liver-to-muscle contrast ratio
Livierato sign
living donor liver transplantation
Livingston triangle
LKS
    liver, kidneys, and spleen
LL
    lower lobe
L-159, L-884
    ^{11}C L.
LLD
    leg-length discrepancy
    limb-length discrepancy
LLE
    left lower extremity
LLL
    left lower lobe
L-loop
    L-l. heart
    L-l. ventricular situs
L-looping
L-LP ratio
LLQ
    left lower quadrant
LLS
    leaky lung syndrome
L-malposition of aorta
LMBD
    lingular mandibular bony defect
LMCA
    left main coronary artery
L-methylmethionine
    ^{11}C L.-m.
LMR
    localized magnetic resonance
      Biosense-guided LMR
LN
    Imagent LN
LNV
    last normal vertebra
LO
    lesser omentum
load
    combination flow and pressure l.
    exercise l.
    iodine l.
    osmotic l.
    predominant flow l.
    rotatory l.
loading
    axial weight l.
    coil l.
    contrast l.
    fracture callus l.
    left ventricular l.
    longitudinal l.
    peripheral l.

spike l.
l. technique
uniform l.

lobar
l. breast anatomy
l. bronchus
l. cavitation
l. consolidation
l. dysmorphism
l. emphysema
l. holoprosencephaly
l. intracerebral hemorrhage
l. lung atrophy
l. nephronia
l. pneumonia
l. renal infarct
l. resorption atelectasis
l. sclerosis

lobation
fetal kidney l.
persistent cortical kidney l.
persistent renal l.

lobatum
hepar l.

lobatus
ren l.

lobe
accessory l.
anterior tip of temporal l.
association cortex of parietal l.
l. of azygos vein
calciform l.
caudate l.
collapsed l.
cuneiform l.
fetal l.
flocculonodular l.
frontal l.
hepatic l.
hot caudate l.
hyperexpanded l.
inferior l.
insular l.
l. of kidney
left lower l. (LLL)
left upper l. (LUL)
limbic l.
lower l. (LL)
medial temporal l.
middle l. (ML)
occipital l.
orbital aspect of frontal l.

parietal l.
polyalveolar l.
prominent pyramidal thyroid l.
pulmonary l.
pyramidal l.
ratio of caudate to right hepatic l.
Riedel l.
right lower l. (RLL)
right middle l. (RML)
right upper l. (RUL)
Rokitansky l.
sequestered l.
spigelian l.
succenturiate placental l.
superior l.
temporal l.
thyroid l.
uncus of temporal l.
upper l. (UL)
wedge-shaped l.

lobectomy
sleeve l.

lobster-claw deformity

lobular
l. alveolar pattern
l. architecture
l. atelectasis
l. breast calcification
l. breast microcalcification
l. bronchiole
l. carcinoma
l. carcinoma in situ (LCIS)
l. neoplasia
l. pneumonia

lobulated
l. border
l. contour
l. filling defect
l. kidney
l. mass
l. paratracheal mediastinum
l. saccular appearance
l. shape
l. tumor

lobulation
fetal l.

lobule
l. breast
l. of epididymis
fat l.
inferior parietal l.
inferior temporal l.

L

NOTES

lobule *(continued)*
lung l.
paracentral l.
primary pulmonary l.
Reid l.
secondary pulmonary l.
splenic l.

LOCA
low-osmolar contrast agent

local
l. bone blood flow
l. bulge of kidney contour
l. bulge renal contour
l. cavus
l. coil
l. compression fracture
l. decompression fracture
l. edema
l. glomerular lesion
l. gradient coil
l. lesion
l. metastasis
l. misregistration
l. nodal disease
l. recurrence (LR)
l. streptokinase infusion

LocaLisa cardiac navigation system
localization
anatomic l.
autologous white cell l.
autoradiographic l.
CT-directed hook-wire l.
fluoroscopic l.
g-probe l.
l. grid
lesion l.
magnetic resonance imaging-guided
wire l.
MRI-guided wire l.
needle l.
needle-hookwire l.
off-axis point l.
pelvic film for IUD l.
placental l.
point l.
preoperative l.
radiopharmaceutical l.
radiotherapy l.
sagittal l.
seizure l.
stereotactic l.
surface coil l.
l. technique
voxel l.
l. window
wire l.

localization-compression grid plate

localized
l. angiofollicular lymph node
hyperplasia
l. caliectasis
l. coarctation
l. edema
l. expansion
l. fibrous mesothelioma
l. fibrous tumor of pleura
l. H1 spectroscopy
l. hyperintensity
l. ileus
l. intimal flap
l. lesion
l. lucent lung
l. lymphangioma
l. magnetic resonance (LMR)
l. mass effect
l. myeloma
l. necrosis
l. obstructive emphysema
l. osteopenia
l. osteoporosis
l. pleura tumor
l. proton magnetic resonance
spectroscopy
l. pure ground-glass opacity
l. shimming
l. single-voxel proton spectrum
l. uptake

localizer
axial l.
breast l.
Homer needle/wire l.
Picket Fence stereotactic l.
T1-weighted axial l.

localizing
l. image
l. imaging
l. probe
l. sign

locally invasive tumor
location
juxtadiaphragmatic l.

loci (*pl. of* locus)
lock
field l.
suture l.

locked
l. facet
l. knee
l. nuclear magnetization

locked-in syndrome
locking
adiabatic off-resonance spin l.
l. disc

lock-washer configuration
Lockwood ligament

LOCM
  low-osmolar contrast medium
locomotor pattern
locoregional
  l. breast carcinoma
  l. control
  l. disease
  l. field radiotherapy
  l. hyperthermia
locular
loculated
  l. empyema
  l. hydropneumothorax
  l. pleural effusion
  l. pleural fluid
  l. ventricle
loculation
  dumbbell l.
  intraosseous l.
locule
loculus, pl. **loculi**
locus, pl. **loci**
  scanning l.
Loehlein diameter
Löffler, Loeffler
  L. fibroplastic endocarditis
  L. pneumonia
  L. syndrome
Löfgren syndrome
log
  l. amplifier
  l. roll
Logic 700 MR transducer
log-rank test
Löhlein-Baehr lesion
Löhlein diameter
loiasis
lollipop tree appearance
long
  l. axial oblique view
  l. axis
  l. axis acquisition
  l. axis of bone
  l. axis of kidney
  l. axis parasternal view
  l. axis ray
  l. axis of spleen
  l. bone
  l. bone fracture
  l. bone pseudoarthrosis
  l. bone survey
  l. dural tail

  l. fiber
  l. finger
  l. head
  l. head of biceps tendon (LHBT)
  l. oblique fracture
  l. segmental diaphysial uptake bone scintigraphy
  l. smooth esophageal narrowing
  l. smooth narrowing esophagus
  l. taper stiff shaft Glidewire
  l. TE MR spectroscopy
  l. tract
  l. tract sign
  l. TR-TE
  l. TR-TE sequence
  l. ultrashort T2-suppressed echo time (LUTE)
  l. wave-length photo label
long-axis slice
long-bore collimator
long-chain fatty acid
long-echo-train fast spin-echo sequence
longitudinal
  l. acoustic wave
  l. arch
  l. arteriography
  l. axis
  l. band
  l. blood supply
  l. B-mode
  l. esophageal fold
  l. esophageal stricture
  l. fasciculus
  l. fissure
  l. image
  l. lie
  l. ligament
  l. loading
  l. magnetization
  l. muscle
  l. narrowing
  l. oval pelvis
  l. raphe
  l. recovery time
  l. relaxation
  l. relaxation time
  l. relaxivity (R1)
  l. renal ectopia
  l. ridge
  l. scan
  l. section imaging
  l. section tomography

NOTES

longitudinal (*continued*)
    l. split biceps tendon
    l. suture
    l. taenia musculature
    l. tear of the brevis tendon
    l. tibial fatigue fracture
    l. transarticular derangement
    l. ultrasonic biometry
    l. ultrasound view
longitudinalis medialis fasciculus
long-scale
    l.-s. contrast
    l.-s. imaging agent
long-term
    l.-t. patency
    l.-t. venous instrumentation
longus
    abductor pollicis l. (APL)
    adductor l.
    l. colli muscle
    extensor carpi radialis l. (ECRL)
    extensor digiti l. (EDL)
    extensor digitorum l.
    extensor hallucis l. (EHL)
    extensor pollicis l. (EPL)
    flexor digitorum l.
    flexor hallucis l.
    flexor pollicis l.
    palmaris l.
    peroneus l.
loop
    access l.
    afferent l.
    air-filled l.
    alpha sigmoid l.
    bowel l.
    C l.
    capillary l.
    cervical l.
    cine l.
    closed conducting l.
    colonic l.
    conductive l.
    contiguous l.
    Cope l.
    Cordonnier ureteroileal l.
    dextro l. (D-loop)
    diathermic l.
    dilated bowel l.
    l. distribution
    double reverse alpha sigmoid l.
    duodenal l.
    duodenal C l.
    efferent l.
    flow-volume l.
    frontal plane l.
    gamma transverse colon l.
    Gerdy interatrial l.
    Gerdy interauricular l.

    l. graft
    l. of Henle
    herniated bowel l.
    horizontal plane l.
    Hutson l.
    ileal l.
    intestinal l.
    J l.
    jejunal l.
    lenticular l.
    Lippes l.
    malrotation of bowel l.
    matted bowel l.
    matted small-bowel l.
    Meyer l.
    Meyer-Archambault l.
    nonrotation of bowel l.
    N-shaped sigmoid l.
    l. ostomy bridge
    P l.
    peduncular l.
    pressure-volume l.
    puborectalis l.
    reentrant l.
    Roux l.
    rubber vessel l.
    sagittal plane l.
    sentinel l.
    separation of bowel l.
    sigmoid l.
    small bowel l.
    Stoerck l.
    subclavian l.
    T l.
    thickened bowel l.
    transverse colon l.
    unopacified bowel l.
    vector l.
    ventricular l.
    vessel l.
    Vieussens l.
    Waltman l.
2-loop ileal J pouch
loopless atenna
loopogram imaging
loopography
    ileal l.
loose
    l. fracture
    l. intraarticular body
    l. mesenchymal tissue
    l. osteochondral fragment
    l. shoulder
Looser
    L. line
    L. transformation zone
lopamidol
LOQ
    lower outer quadrant

LOR
    line of response
LORAD
    L. full-field digital mammography
        system
    L. StereoGuide
Lorad digital breast imager
Lorain-Lévi dwarfism
lordosis
    cervical l.
    gentle l.
    lumbar l.
    reversal of cervical l.
    spinal l.
    thoracic l.
lordotic
    l. aspect
    l. curve
    l. pelvis
    l. position
    l. view
lorentzian
    l. curve
    l. field mapping
    l. line
    l. line saturation
Lorenz position
lorry driver's fracture
LoSo Prep
loss
    l. of bone mass
    l. coincidence
    dead time l.
    l. of definition
    l. of distinction
    l. of elasticity of cartilage
    electron equilibrium l.
    global tissue l.
    high-velocity signal l.
    l. of parallelism of facet joint
    percentage signal intensity l.
    segmental bone l.
    l. of sigmoid curve
    signal l.
    single collision energy l.
    l. of thoracic kyphosis
    time-of-flight signal l.
    TOF signal l.
    transformer l.
    volume l.
lossless image data compression

lossy
    l. algorithm
    l. image data compression
lost intrauterine device
lotus position
Louis
    L. angle
    sternal angle of L.
Louis-Bar syndrome
lovers' knot
low
    l. attenuation
    l. attenuation pulsation artifact
    l. back injury
    l. back syndrome
    l. cardiac output
    l. conus medullaris
    l. density
    L. Energy All Purpose (LEAP)
    l. frame rate
    l. frequency ultrasound (LFUS)
    l. interobserver variation
    l. lung volume
    l. metastatic potential
    l. normal
    l. osmolality
    l. pitch
    l. right atrium (LRA)
    l. septal right atrium
    l. signal intensity
    l. signal intensity artifact
    l. signal intensity fibrous band
    l. signal intensity peripheral band
    l. signal intensity synchondrosis
    l. small bowel obstruction
    l. urethral pressure (LUP)
    l. yield
low-amplitude internal echo
low-angle
    l.-a. scattering
    l.-a. shot technique
low-attenuation
    l.-a. lesion
    l.-a. mediastinal mass
Low-Beers
    L.-B. position
    L.-B. projection
    L.-B. view
low-compliance, fixed diameter balloon
low-contact dynamic compression plate
    (LC-DCP)

NOTES

low-contrast
    l.-c. film
    l.-c. structure
low-density
    l.-d. mesencephalic lesion
    l.-d. rim
    l.-d. ring
    l.-d. structure
low-dose
    l.-d. dobutamine (LDD)
    l.-d. film
    l.-d. film mammographic technique
    l.-d. folic acid
    l.-d. mammography
    l.-d. screen-film technique
low-dose/high-dose protocol
Löwenberg canal
low-energy
    l.-e. collimator
    l.-e. fracture
    l.-e. laser (LEL)
    l.-e. photon attenuation
    measurement
    l.-e. radiofrequency conduction
    hyperthermia treatment
    l.-e. ultra-high resolution (LEUHR)
lower
    l. basilar aneurysm
    l. esophageal mucosal ring
    l. esophageal narrowing
    l. esophageal sphincter (LES)
    l. esophageal sphincter dysfunction
    l. esophageal sphincter pressure
    (LESP)
    l. extremity (LE)
    l. extremity arterial tree
    l. extremity CT venography (LE-
    CTV)
    l. extremity imaging
    l. field visual sector
    l. gastrointestinal hemorrhage
    l. inner quadrant (LIQ)
    l. limb venography
    l. limb venography imaging
    l. lobe (LL)
    l. lobe lung mass
    l. lobe pneumonia
    l. lobe reticulation
    l. lung field
    l. lung line
    l. moiety ureter
    l. motor neuron
    l. motor neuron lesion
    l. outer quadrant (LOQ)
    l. pole
    l. pole collecting system
    l. pole of kidney
    l. pole of patella
    l. pole ureter

    l. pulmonary lobe atelectasis
    l. right quadrant (LRQ)
    l. station
    l. sternal border (LSB)
    l. tract
Lower tubercle
low-field
    l.-f. magnetic resonance
    l.-f. MR angiography
    l.-f. MRI system
    l.-f. MR scanner
low-field-strength MR imaging
low-flip-angle gradient-echo imaging
low-flow syndrome
low-flux polysufone membrane
low-frame-rate run
low-frequency scatter
low-grade
    l.-g. astrocytoma
    l.-g. central osteogenic sarcoma
    l.-g. glioma
    l.-g. malignancy
    l.-g. neoplasm
low-intensity
    l.-i. laser therapy (LILT)
    l.-i. line
    l.-i. pulsed ultrasound
low-level echo
low-lying placenta
Lown-Ganong-Levine syndrome (LGL)
low-osmolar
    l.-o. contrast agent (LOCA)
    l.-o. contrast medium (LOCM)
low-output heart failure
low-pass
    l.-p. filter
    l.-p. filtering
    l.-p. three-dimensional postfiltering
low-photon energy
low-pressure
    l.-p. cardiac tamponade
    l.-p. hydrocephalus
    l.-p. mercury arc amp
low-profile
    l.-p. IUGR
    l.-p. mitral valve
low-resistance spectral waveform
low-resolution imaging
low-risk single-stone former
low-signal-intensity
    l.-s.-i. fibrous septum
    l.-s.-i. replacement
    l.-s.-i. tumor
low-signal mass
Lowsley lobar anatomy
low-temperature diffraction
low-T humerus fracture
low-velocity flow

LP
   linear prediction
   lumbar puncture
   lymphomatous polyposis
LPA
   left pulmonary artery
LPAM
   L-phenylalanine mustard
LPCh
   lateral posterior choroidal
L-phenylalanine mustard (LPAM)
LPI
   laser projection imaging
      LPI laser system
LPO
   left posterior oblique
      LPO position
LP² stainless steel delivery system
LPV
   left pulmonary vein
LQ
   linear-quadratic
      LQ ratio
LR
   likelihood ratio
   local recurrence
Lr
   lawrencium
LRA
   low right atrium
L-radiation
LRQ
   lower right quadrant
LS
   least square
   line scanning
   lumbosacral
   lumbosacral spine
LSB
   left sternal border
   lower sternal border
LSC
   laser scanning cytometry
LSCVP
   left subclavian central venous pressure
LSF
   line spread function
LSO
   cerium-doped lutetium oxyorthosilicate
      LSO crystal scintillator material
LSR
   lanthanide shift reagent

LSRT
   lens-sparing external beam radiation
      therapy
LSV
   lenticulostriate vasculopathy
LTA
   laser thermal ablation
      MRI-guided LTA
LTK
   laser thermal keratoplasty
L-transposition
   levotransposition
LTX3000 lumbar rehabilitation system
L-tyrosine imaging agent
Lu
   lutetium
lucency
      area of l.
      artifactual l.
      interspersed l.
      linear l.
      sandlike l.
      slitlike residual l.
lucent
      l. band
      l. calculus
      l. center
      l. defect
      l. finger lesion
      l. halo
      l. hilar notch
      l. interval
      l. line
      l. lung lesion
lucent-centered calcification
Lucite
      L. beam
      L. beam spoiler
LUCL
   lateral ulnar collateral ligament
Ludovici angle
Ludwig
      L. angle
      L. plane
luetic
      l. aortic aneurysm
      l. aortitis
      l. arteritis
      l. diaphysitis
luftsichel
      l. sign

NOTES

LUL
    left upper lobe
Luma cervical imaging system
lumazenil
    ^{11}C l.
lumbales
    vertebra l.
lumbar
    l. aortography
    l. arteriography
    l. artery
    l. curvature
    l. disc
    l. facet angle
    l. fascia
    l. flexion and extension study
    l. hernia
    l. index (LI)
    l. kidney
    l. kyphosis
    l. lordosis
    l. lordotic curve
    l. lymph node
    l. myelography
    l. nerve root
    l. part of diaphragm
    l. plexus
    l. pneumencephalography
    l. puncture (LP)
    l. rib
    l. root avulsion
    l. scoliosis
    l. spinal canal
    l. spinal stenosis
    l. spine
    l. spine dimension
    l. spine fracture
    l. spine lesion
    l. spine view
    l. sympathetic block
    l. synovial cyst
    l. transverse process
    l. vertebra (L)
    l. vertebral body index
lumbarization
lumbarized spine
lumbocostal ligament
lumbocostoabdominal triangle
lumboperitoneal shunting
lumborum
    quadratus l.
lumbosacral (LS)
    l. agenesis
    l. canal
    l. dermal sinus
    l. disc
    l. intervertebral disc herniation
    l. joint angle
    l. kyphosis

    l. lateral recess
    l. myelography
    l. plexus
    l. projection
    l. series
    l. spine (LS)
    l. spine depth
    l. spine strain
    l. trunk
lumbrical tendon
lumen, pl. **lumina, lumens**
    aortic l.
    arterial l.
    l. assessment
    attenuated l.
    bile duct l.
    bowel l.
    bronchial l.
    carotid l.
    clot-filled l.
    cloverleaf-shaped l.
    crescentic l.
    cystic duct l.
    l. delineation
    l. diameter
    double l.
    double-barrel l.
    D-shaped vessel l.
    duct l.
    duodenal l.
    eccentrically placed l.
    elliptic l.
    esophageal l.
    false l.
    gastric l.
    gastroduodenal l.
    intestinal l.
    midgroove portion of l.
    occluded l.
    patent l.
    scalloped bowel l.
    slitlike l.
    slit-shaped vessel l.
    star-shaped vessel l.
    tracheal l.
    true l.
    vascular l.
lumen-intimal interface
8-lumen manometric catheter
lumenogram (*var. of* luminogram)
luminal
    l. area
    l. caliber
    l. defect
    l. dimension
    l. distention
    l. encroachment
    l. irregularity
    l. narrowing

l. plaque
l. plug
l. silhouette
l. stenosis
l. thrombosis
l. wall

luminance
viewbox l.

Luminexx
L. biliary stent
L. self-expanding stent

luminogram, lumenogram
air l.

Lumiscan LS 85 scanner
Lumisys 20 digital x-ray scanner
lumpectomy bed
lump kidney
lumpy appearance of lung
LUNA
laser uterosacral nerve ablation

Lunar
L. DPX densitometer
L. Expert densitometer
L. scanner

lunate
avascular necrosis l.
l. bone
l. dislocation
l. facet
l. fracture
l. tilt

lunate-shaped trachea
lunate-triquetral coalition
lunatomalacia
Lunderquist exchange guidewire
Lunderquist-Ring guidewire
lung
l. abscess
acquired unilateral hyperlucent l.
l. adenocarcinoma
l. agenesis
air conditioner l.
air-filled l.
airless l.
l. airspace
amiodarone l.
l. amyloidosis
l. ankylosis spondylitis
l. apex
l. aplasia
l. arch
l. architecture

arc welder's l.
artificial l.
atelectatic l.
azygos lobe of l.
l. base
l. base infiltrate
bauxite fibrosis of l.
Bible printer's l.
bilateral hyperlucent l.
bird breeder's l.
bird fancier's l.
bird handler's l.
black l.
blunt border of l.
brown induration of l.
bubbly l.
budgerigar fancier's l.
l. calculus
l. capacity
l. carcinoma
l. cavity
cheese handler's l.
cheese washer's l.
chest fluke l.
cluster of grapes l.
coal miner's l.
coal worker's l.
l. coccidioidomycosis
coffee worker's l.
coin lesion of l.
collapsed l.
l. compliance
l. connectivity test
consolidated l.
contralateral l.
l. contusion
convexity of l.
corundum smelter's l.
l. count curve
l. cylindroma
l. cyst
dark l.
l. decortication
l. density
dependent l.
drowned l.
dynamic l.
l. echinococcosis
eclipse effect l.
l. edema
l. emphysema
emphysematous l.

NOTES

lung *(continued)*
    empty collapsed l.
    expanded l.
    l. expansion
    farmer's l.
    fibroid l.
    fibroma of l.
    fibrosis of l.
    l. field
    fishmeal worker's l.
    l. fissure
    l. fluke
    folded l.
    l. fungus ball
    furrier's l.
    gangrene of l.
    grain handler's l.
    l. granuloma
    graphite fibrosis of l.
    gray l.
    l. hamartoma
    hardened l.
    harvester's l.
    hazy-opaque l.
    l. hemangioma
    l. hemorrhage
    hemorrhagic consolidation of l.
    hen worker's l.
    l. hepatization
    l. hilum
    l. histoplasmosis
    honeycomb l.
    horseshoe l.
    humidifier l.
    hyperlucent l.
    hypersensitivity l.
    hypogenetic l.
    hypoinflation of l.
    hypolucency of l.
    l. hypoplasia
    hypoplastic l.
    idiopathic unilateral hyperlucent l.
    l. imaging
    immature l.
    inferior lobe of l.
    l. infiltrate distribution
    l. inflammation
    l. interstitium
    l. laceration
    light pink l.
    l. linearity
    lingular division of left l.
    liverlike l.
    l. lobule
    localized lucent l.
    lumpy appearance of l.
    l. lymphangiectasis
    l. lymphangioma
    l. lymphoid hyperplasia

    l. lymphoma
    malt worker's l.
    maple bark stripper's l.
    l. marking
    mason's l.
    l. mass
    meat wrapper's l.
    l. metastasis
    miller's l.
    miner's l.
    mottled gray l.
    mushroom worker's l.
    native l.
    l. necrosis
    l. nodularity
    l. nodule
    nondependent l.
    l. opacity
    l. overexpansion
    l. overinflation
    l. paragonimiasis
    parakeet fancier's l.
    l. parenchyma
    l. parenchyma consolidation
    partial collapse of l.
    l. perfusion
    l. perfusion defect
    l. perfusion radionuclide
    l. periphery
    physiologically immature l.
    pigeon fancier's l.
    polycystic l.
    l. popcorn calcification
    postperfusion l.
    l. pseudocavitation
    l. pseudolymphoma
    pump l.
    l. reexpansion
    reperfusion injury of
      postischemic l.
    right l.
    l. root
    rounded border of l.
    rudimentary l.
    l. sarcoid
    l. scan
    l. scintigraphy
    l. segmentation
    septic l.
    sequestered lobe of l.
    sharp border of l.
    l. shock
    shrunken l.
    silicotic fibrosis of l.
    silo-filler's l.
    silver finisher's l.
    silver polisher's l.
    smoker's l.
    solid edema of l.

l. starfish scar
static l.
l. stiffness
stiff noncompliant l.
l. stone
stretched l.
structurally immature l.
subsegment of l.
superior lobe of l.
surface tension of l.
l. talcosis
l. torsion
l. transplant
l. tuberculoma
l. tumor
l. underinflation
underventilated l.
unilateral hyperlucent l.
l. varix
l. volume (V)
l. washout
welder's l.
well-inflated l.
wet l.
white l.
l. window
l. zone
lung-heart ratio of thallium 201 activity
lung-volume loop flow
lunocapitate bone
lunohamate arthritis
lunotriquetral
l. interosseus ligament
l. joint
lunula, pl. **lunulae**
LUP
low urethral pressure
lupus
drug-induced erythematous l.
pernio l.
systemic erythematosus l.
LUQ
left upper quadrant
Luque rod
LUS
laparoscopic ultrasound
Luschka
L. bursa
L. crypt
L. duct leak
foramen of L.

L. joint
L. ligament
L. muscle
sinuvertebral nerve of L.
lusoria
arteria l.
dysphagia l.
LUTE
long ultrashort T2-suppressed echo time
luteal
l. cyst
l. phase
l. phase defect
luteinized
l. unruptured follicle
l. unruptured follicle syndrome
Lutembacher
L. complex
L. syndrome
luteoma
lutetium (Lu)
l. oxyorthosilicate-based PET scanner
l. tantalate
luxated bone
luxation
ligamentous l.
Luxtec fiberoptic system
luxury
l. perfusion
l. perfusion syndrome
Luys body
LVAD
left ventricular assist device
LVD
left ventricular dysfunction
LVdd
left ventricular diastolic dimension
LVEDD
left ventricular end-diastolic dimension
LVEDI
left ventricular end-diastolic volume index
LVEDP
left ventricular end-diastolic pressure
LVEF
left ventricular ejection fraction
exercise first-pass LVEF
LVESD
left ventricular end-systolic dimension
LVESVI
left ventricular end-systolic volume index

NOTES

LVET
  left ventricular ejection time
LVFS
  left ventricular functional shortening
LVFW
  left ventricular free wall
LVG
  left ventriculogram
LVH
  left ventricular hypertrophy
LVID
  left ventricular internal diameter
LVIDd, LVIDD
  left ventricular internal diastolic
    dimension
LVIDs
  left ventricular internal dimension at end
    systole
LVIV
  left ventricular inflow volume
LVM
  left ventricular mass
LVMI
  left ventricular mass index
LVOT
  left ventricular outflow tract
    LVOT flow rate
LVOTO
  left ventricular outflow tract obstruction
LVOV
  left ventricular outflow volume
LVP
  left ventricular pressure
LVPW
  left ventricular posterior wall
LVs
  left ventricular systolic
    LVs system
LVSW
  left ventricular stroke work
LVSWI
  left ventricular stroke work index
LVW
  left ventricular wall
Lw
  lawrencium
LX
    LX EchoSpeed 1.5T CV/i, NVi
      MR system
    LX 20 laser
    LX 8.3 software
Lyme carditis
lymph
  l. capillary
  l. duct
  l. gland
  l. node
  l. node eggshell calcification
  l. node enlargement

  l. node imaging
  l. node involvement
  l. node sinus
  l. node syndrome
  l. node tissue
  l. plexus
  l. vessel of prostate
lymphadenitis
  regional granulomatous l.
lymphadenography
lymphadenopathy
  angioblastic l.
  angioimmunoblastic l.
  axillary l.
  benign l.
  mesenteric l.
  peripancreatic l.
  persistent generalized l.
  reactive l.
  retrocrural l.
  retroperitoneal l.
  secondary axillary l.
  superficial l.
  l. syndrome
lymphangiectasis
  acquired intestinal l.
  congenital l.
  generalized l.
  intestinal l.
  lung l.
  primary pulmonary l.
  pulmonary cystic l.
  secondary l.
  submucosal l.
  subserosal l.
lymphangiogram (LAG)
lymphangiographic imaging agent
lymphangiography
  bipedal l.
  contrast l.
  l. imaging
  pedal l.
lymphangiohemangioma
lymphangioleiomyomatosis
lymphangioma
  capillary l.
  cardiac l.
  cavernous l.
  diffuse l.
  localized l.
  lung l.
  l. mesentery
  neck l.
  orbital l.
  pancreatic cystic l.
  retroperitoneal l.
  simple capillary l.
lymphangiomatosis
  pulmonary l.

lymphangiomyomatosis
lymphangiomyomatosis
lymphangitic
    l. carcinomatosis
    l. metastasis
lymphangitis
lymphatic
    l. canal
    l. carcinomatosis
    l. channel
    l. cortex
    l. development
    dilated l.
    l. drainage pattern
    l. duct
    l. edema
    l. imaging
    l. malformation
    l. mapping
    l. medulla
    l. metastasis
    l. needle disruption
    l. network
    l. obstruction
    paracervical l.
    prominent septal l.
    l. sac
    l. sarcoma
    subpleural l.
    l. tissue
    l. trunk
    l. tumor spread
    l. valve
    l. vessel
lymphatica
    pseudopolyposis l.
lymphaticovenous secondary edema
lymphatics
    thoracic l.
lymphaticum
    angioma l.
Lymphazurin imaging agent
lymphedema
    Meige l.
    Nonne-Milroy l.
    postmastectomy l.
lymphoblastic lymphoma
lymphoblastoma
lymphocapillary vessel
lymphocele
    renal transplant l.
lymphocyte-rich tumor

lymphocytic
    l. hypophysitis
    l. interstitial pneumonia (LIP)
    l. interstitial pneumonitis
    l. plasmacytoid lymphoma
    l. poorly-differentiated lymphoma
    l. well-differentiated lymphoma
lymphoepithelial parotid tumor
lymphoepithelioma
    salivary gland l.
lymphogenous
    l. dissemination
    l. embolus
    l. metastasis
lymphogranuloma venereum
lymphography
    computed tomographic l. (CT-LG)
    computed tomography l. (CT-LG)
    indirect computed tomography l.
    magnetic resonance l.
    MR l.
    pedal l.
    time-lapse quantitative computed
      tomography l.
lymphoid
    l. follicle
    l. hamartoma
    l. hyperplasia
    l. hypophysitis
    l. interstitial pneumonia (LIP)
    l. interstitial pneumonitis
    l. polyp
    l. tissue
    l. tumor
lymphoma
    acute lymphoblastic l.
    adult T-cell l.
    African Burkitt l.
    anaplastic large cell l. (ALCL)
    angioimmunoblastic
      lymphadenopathylike T-cell l.
    angiotropic large cell l.
    B-cell monocytoid l.
    bone l.
    brain l.
    breast l.
    Burkitt l.
    Burkitt-like l.
    butterfly l.
    B-zone small lymphocytic l.
    Castleman l.
    centroblastic l.

NOTES

L

lymphoma *(continued)*
    centrocytic l.
    cerebral l.
    cleaved cell l.
    cobblestone appearance l.
    colorectal l.
    convoluted T-cell l.
    cutaneous B-cell l. (CBCL)
    cutaneous T-cell l.
    diffuse aggressive l.
    diffuse intermediate lymphocytic l.
    diffuse large-cell l. (DLCL)
    diffuse mixed small- and large-cell l.
    diffuse small-cell lymphocytic l.
    dural arachnoid l.
    enteropathy-associated T-cell l.
    epidural l.
    extranodal follicular l.
    follicular center-cell l.
    follicular mixed small cleaved l.
    follicular predominantly large cell l.
    follicular predominantly small cell l.
    fulminant cerebral l.
    l. gallium scintigraphy
    gastric l.
    gastrointestinal l.
    giant follicle l.
    granulomatous l.
    histiocytic bone l.
    histiocytic brain l.
    histiocytic chest l.
    Hodgkin l.
    immunoblastic large-cell l.
    infiltrative l.
    intracerebral l.
    kidney l.
    large cleaved cell l.
    limited-stage diffuse large-cell l.
    liver l.
    lung l.
    lymphoblastic l.
    lymphocytic plasmacytoid l.
    lymphocytic poorly-differentiated l.
    lymphocytic well-differentiated l.
    macroglobulinemic l.
    MALT l.
    mantle cell l. (MCL)
    marginal zone l. (MZL)
    marginal zone B-cell l.
    mediastinal l.
    mesencephalic cerebral l.
    mesenterial Castleman l.
    mesenteric l.
    metastatic testicular l.
    mixed lymphocytic-histiocytic l.
    mixed small and large cell l.

    mucosa-associated lymphoid tissue l.
    multifocal l.
    noncleaved cell l.
    orbital l.
    osseous l.
    pancreatic l.
    peripheral l.
    perirenal l.
    plasmablastic l.
    pleomorphic T-cell l.
    polypoid l.
    primary adrenal l.
    primary bone l.
    primary brain l.
    primary CNS l.
    primary cutaneous large B-cell l. (PCLBCL)
    primary gastric non-Hodgkin l.
    primary refractory Burkitt l.
    pulmonary l.
    pyothorax-associated pleural l.
    recurrent l.
    renal l.
    retroperitoneal l.
    Revised European American L. (REAL)
    secondary brain l.
    secondary cutaneous large B-cell l. (SCLBCL)
    sinonasal l.
    skeletal l.
    small B-cell l.
    small lymphocytic T-cell l.
    spinal epidural l.
    splenic B-cell l.
    sporadic Burkitt l.
    l. staging
    systemic brain l.
    T-cell lymphoblastic l.
    thymic l.
    thyroid l.
    true histiocytic l.
    T-zone l.
    ulcerative l.
    undefined l.
    undifferentiated non-Hodgkin l.
    urinary bladder l.
    vitreous l.
    Waldeyer ring l.
lymphomatoid granulomatosis
lymphomatosis
lymphomatosum
    cystadenoma l.
    papillary cystadenoma l.
lymphomatous
    l. lymph node
    l. mass
    l. polyposis (LP)

lymphonodular hyperplasia
lymphoplasmacytic infiltrate
lymphopneumatosis
    peritoneal l.
lymphoproliferative disorder
lymphoreticular tissue
LymphoScan
    L. imaging agent
    L. nuclear imaging system
    L. nuclear imaging system scanner
    L. Tc99m-labeled murine antibody
      fragment
lymphoscintigraphy
    cutaneous l.
    internal mammary l.
    radiocolloid l.
lymphovascular
Lynch and Crues type 2 lesion
lyoluminescence
lyophilized
Lyra laser

lysate
Lyser
    trapezoid bone of L.
Lysholm
    L. grid
    L. method
lysis
    bony l.
    clot l.
    cystic l.
    follicle l.
    ultrasonic l.
lytic
    l. area
    l. area bone flap
    l. bone lesion
    l. change
    l. lesion of skull
    l. osteolysis
    l. osteosarcoma
    l. pattern

NOTES

L

μCi
  microcurie
μV
  microvolt
M
  M pattern
  M shell
m
  meter
113m
  tin with indium 113m
137m
  cesium with barium 137m
87m
  Sr 87m
99m
M1-M5 segment of middle cerebral artery
M1 segment aneurysm
M4-M5 lineage
M2A
  M2A capsule
  M2A imaging capsule endoscopy
  M2A Swallowable Imaging Capsule
MAA
  macroaggregated albumin
  MAA study
MACE
  major adverse cardiac event
maceration
  clot m.
Macewen sign
Mach
  M. band
  M. band effect
  M. line
machine
  Acoma portable x-ray m.
  Aestiva/5 MRI anesthesia m.
  cobalt megavoltage m.
  2D B-mode ultrasound m.
  Echospeed 1.5T MR m.
  focused segmented ultrasound m.
  m. injection
  neutron therapy m.
  panoramic rotating m.
  parallel virtual m. (PVM)
Mackenrodt ligament
Mackenzie point
Macklin effect
Macleod syndrome
macrencephaly, macrencephalia
macroadenoma
  pituitary m.
  prolactin-secreting pituitary m.

macroaggregated
  m. albumin (MAA)
  m. albumin imaging agent
macroangiography
macrocalcification
macrocephalia, macrocephaly
macrocirculation
macrocolon
macrocyst
  adrenocortical m.
macrocystic
  m. adenoma
  m. cystadenoma
  m. encephalomalacia
  m. neoplasm
  m. pilocytic cerebellar astrocytoma
macrodacryocystography
macrodystrophia
  lipoma m.
  m. lipomatosa
macrofistulous arteriovenous communication
macroglobulinemic lymphoma
macrolobular cirrhosis
macrolobulated
macromolecular
  m. content
  m. contrast-enhanced MR imaging
  m. contrast medium (MMCM)
  m. drug
  m. hydration effect
  m. imaging agent
macronodular pattern
macroorchidism lesion
macrophage
  m. inflammatory protein (MIP)
  lipid-laden foamy m.
MACRO-P solution
macroradiography
  Buckland-Wright m.
macroreentrant circuit
macroscopic
  m. hemorrhage ligament
  m. magnetic moment
  m. magnetization vector
  m. placental lesion
Macrotec imaging agent
macrovesicular steatosis
MacSpect real-time NMR workstation
macula, pl. maculae
macule
  coal m.
maculopathy bull's eye magnet
Maddahi method of calculating right ventricular ejection fraction

M

Madelung
    M. deformity
    M. neck
Madura foot
maduromycosis
Maffucci syndrome
MAG-3, MAG3
    mercaptoacetyltriglycine
magenblase
Magendie foramen
magenstrasse
Maggi biopsy needle
magic
    m. angle effect
    m. angle effect artifact
    m. angle phenomenon
    m. angle spinning NMR
    M. S/P Wallstent
magic-angle spinning imaging
MagicView workstation
Magilligan technique for measuring
    neutral anteversion
Maglinte catheter
magna
    abnormal cisterna m.
    arteria radicularis anterior m.
    chorda m.
    cisterna m.
    coxa m.
    mega cisterna m.
Magnascanner
    Picker M.
Magna-SL scanner
Magnes
    M. biomagnetometer
    M. biomagnetometer system
    M. 2500 whole-blood scanner
    M. 2500 whole-head imaging
magnesium
    m. chloride
    m. contrast medium
magnet
    air-core m.
    beam-bending m.
    m. compression anastomosis
    cryostable m.
    doughnut m.
    Eindhoven m.
    Fe-Ex orogastric tube m.
    GE Signa 1.5-T m.
    Gyroscan NT 10 m.
    Gyroscan 1.5T superconducting m.
    Horizon LX 1.5-T
      superconducting m.
    hybrid m.
    large-bore m.
    maculopathy bull's eye m.
    MAGNETOM SP4000 m.
    Magnex m.

    m. mode
    nonenclosed m.
    open m.
    Oxford m.
    pancake MRI m.
    passively shimmed
      superconducting m.
    permanent m.
    Philips Gyroscan ACS NT
      superconducting m.
    poor shimming of MRI m.
    m. rate
    resistive m.
    m. response
    shimmed m.
    short-bore m.
    m. stability
    superconducting m.
    superconductive m.
    1.0T, 1.5T superconducting m.
    tubular m.
    Walker m.
magnetic
    m. anisotropy
    m. bolus tracking
    m. circuit
    m. dipole
    m. dipole-dipole coupling
    m. dipole moment
    m. disc
    m. domain
    m. field gradient (MFG)
    m. field perturbation
    m. field strength
    m. flux
    m. flux density
    m. focal plane
    m. fringe field
    m. induction
    m. induction device
    m. interaction
    m. inversion
    m. iron oxide particle (MIOP)
    m. lines of force
    m. material
    m. nuclei
    m. particulate
    m. permeability
    m. pole
    m. radiation exposure
    m. resonance (MR)
    m. resonance angiography (MRA)
    m. resonance angiography-directed
      bypass procedure
    m. resonance arthrography
    m. resonance catheter imaging
    m. resonance cholangiogram (MRC)
    m. resonance cholangiography with
      HASTE

m. resonance
cholangiopancreatography (MRCP)

m. resonance dacryocystography

m. resonance depiction

m. resonance-detected white matter
lesion

m. resonance detection

m. resonance diffusion imaging

m. resonance digital subtraction
angiography (MRDSA)

m. resonance discriminator of
osseous metastasis

m. resonance elastography (MRE)

m. resonance enhancement pattern

m. resonance epidurography

m. resonance hydrographic
technique

m. resonance imaging (MRI)

m. resonance imaging–compatible
piezoelectric power drill

m. resonance imaging-guided
focused ultrasound sector
transducer

m. resonance imaging-guided wire
localization

m. resonance lymphography

m. resonance mammography
(MRM)

m. resonance multispectral color
images

m. resonance myelography

m. resonance needle tracking

m. resonance neurography (MRN)

m. resonance pancreatography
(MRP)

m. resonance pelvimetry

m. resonance perfusion imaging

m. resonance phase velocity
mapping

m. resonance phlebography

m. resonance receptor agent

m. resonance sialography

m. resonance signal

m. resonance simulator

m. resonance spectroscopic imaging
(MRSI)

m. resonance spectroscopy (MRS)

m. resonance spin incoherence

m. resonance tomography (MRT)

m. resonance urography (MRU)

M. Resonance User Interface
(MRUI)

m. resonance user interface
software

m. resonance venogram (MRV)

m. resonance venography (MRV)

m. resonance volume estimation

m. retentivity

m. servomotor

m. shielding

m. source imaging (MSI)

m. stimulation

M. Surgery System

m. susceptibility

m. susceptibility artifact

m. susceptibility-weighted image

m. tape storage

magnetic-assisted intervention (MAI)

magnetism

nuclear m.

magnetite (Fe_3O_4)

m. albumin imaging agent

magnetization

complementary spatial modulation
of m. (CSPAMM)

equilibrium m.

locked nuclear m.

longitudinal m.

net tissue m.

net transverse m.

m. precession angle

m. prepared (MP)

rephased transverse m.

residual m.

rest m.

spatial modulation of m. (SPAMM)

m. and spin-lock transfer imaging

SSFP m.

steady-state free precession m.

m. transfer (MT)

m. transfer contrast (MTC)

m. transfer effect

m. transfer gradient-echo image

m. transfer ratio (MTR)

m. transfer technique

m. transfer weighted imaging

transverse m.

magnetization-prepared

m.-p. rapid acquisition gradient
echo (MP-RAGE)

m.-p. rapid acquisition gradient-
echo sequence

m.-p. rapid gradient echo-water
excitation (MP-RAGE-WE)

M

NOTES

magnetoacoustic
    m. imaging
    m. MRI
magnetoencephalogram
magnetoencephalography (MEG)
magnetogyric ratio
magnetohydrodynamic effect
MAGNETOM
    M. Espree open MRI unit
    M. Open system
    M. Sonata 1.5T MR system
    M. SP4000 magnet
    M. SP MRI imager
    M. SP63 scanner
    M. Symphony MR scanner
    M. Trio 3T unlimited MRI system
    M. 1.5-T scanner
    1.5 T M. Symphony whole-body
      scanner
    M. Vision MR unit
    M. Vision scanner
    M. Vision 1.5T MR imaging
      system
magnetometer probe
magneton
    Bohr m.
magnetopharmaceutical
magnetoresistive sensor circuit
Magnevist
    M. gadopentate dimeglumine
    M. imaging agent
Magnex
    M. Alpha MR system
    M. magnet
    M. MR scanner
magnification (X)
    m. angiography
    electronic m.
    m. error
    m. factor (MF)
    film-screen m.
    m. hard copy
    high-resolution m.
    m. mammography
    m. radiography
    m. roentgenography
    signal m.
    spot m.
    m. and spot compression
    ultra-high m.
    m. view
magnitude
    m. calculation
    m. image
    m. of obliquity
    m. reconstruction
magnum
    M. biopsy instrument
    foramen m.

vertebra m.
visibility of the foramen m.
magnus
    adductor m.
Mahaim
    M. bundle
    M. and James fiber
MAI
    magnetic-assisted intervention
main
    m. bundle
    m. energy substrate
    m. fissure
    m. glow peak
    m. magnetic field inhomogeneity
      artifact
    m. pancreatic duct (MPD)
    m. papillary duct (MPD)
    m. portal vein peak velocity
      (MPPv)
    m. pulmonary artery (MPA)
    m. timing event (MTE)
    m. tumor
mainline granulomatosis
mainstem
    m. bronchus
    m. carina
    m. coronary artery
Mainster retina laser
maintenance of flow
Mainz pouch
Maisonneuve
    M. fibular fracture
    M. injury
    M. sign
Maissiat
    M. band
    M. ligament
Majestik shielded angiographic needle
major
    m. adverse cardiac event (MACE)
    m. aorticopulmonary collateral
      artery
    m. bronchus
    m. calyx
    m. duodenal papilla
    m. fissure
    m. fracture fragment
    globus m.
    m. muscle
    psoas m.
    rhomboid m.
    teres m.
majus, pl. **majora**
    omentum m.
malabsorption
Malacarne antrum
malacic lesion
maladie de Roger

malakoplakia, malacoplakia
    renal parenchymal m.
malaligned atrioventricular septal defect
malalignment
    patellar m.
    rotational m.
    subtle m.
malangulation
malar
    m. bone
    m. eminence
    m. fracture
    m. lymph node
malarial granuloma
Malcolm-Lynn C-RXF cervical retractor frame
maldescended testis
maldevelopment
    pubic bone m.
maldistribution of ventilation and perfusion
male
    m. genital tract calcification
    m. pelvis
    m. Turner syndrome
    m. urethra
Malecot nephrostomy catheter
malformation
    adenomatoid m.
    angiographically occult intracranial vascular m. (AOIVM)
    angiographically occult vascular m. (AOVM)
    angiographically visualized vascular m. (AVVM)
    anorectal m.
    aortic arch m.
    Arnold-Chiari m.
    arterial m. (AM)
    arteriovenous m. (AVM)
    arteriovenous brain m.
    arteriovenous colon m.
    arteriovenous cord m.
    arteriovenous kidney m.
    bronchopulmonary foregut m. (BPFM)
    capillary m.
    capillary-lymphatic m. (CLM)
    cardiovascular m.
    cavernous m.
    cerebral arteriovenous m.

cerebral microarteriovenous m. (micro-AVM)
cerebrovascular m.
Chiari I–II m.
cloacal m.
computer-assisted resection of cerebral arteriovenous m.
congenital cystic adenomatoid m. (CCAM)
congenital heart m.
congenital vascular m. (CVM)
coronary artery m.
cryptic vascular m. (CVM)
cystic adenomatoid m.
dancer's foot m.
Dandy-Walker m.
DeMyer system of cerebral m.
Dieulafoy vascular m.
diffuse m.
dural arteriovenous m.
Ebstein m.
endocardial cushion m.
extremity m.
familial cavernous m.
fast-flow m.
fetal cystic adenomatoid m.
fetal hand m.
focal m.
frontal arteriovenous m.
frontoparietal arteriovenous m.
fusiform m.
galenic venous m.
glomus-type arteriovenous m.
hindbrain m.
intracerebral arteriovenous m.
intracerebral vascular m.
intracranial arteriovenous m.
intramedullary arteriovenous m.
intramuscular venous m.
intraosseous arteriovenous m.
intraosseous vascular m.
Joubert m.
lymphatic m.
Michel m.
mixed venous-lymphatic m.
molar tooth m.
molar tooth midbrain-hindbrain m.
Mondini m.
mural-type vein of Galen m.
neural axis vascular m.
occult cerebral vascular m. (OCVM)

M

NOTES

malformation *(continued)*
    occult vascular brain m.
    pulmonary arterial m.
    pulmonary arteriovenous m.
     (PAVM)
    retromedullary arteriovenous m.
    saccular m.
    septal m.
    sink-trap m.
    slow-flow vascular m.
    spinal cord m. (SCM)
    spinal vascular m.
    split spinal cord m. (SSCM)
    subpial arteriovenous m.
    telencephalic m.
    valve m.
    vascular m.
    vein of Galen m.
    venous vascular m.
    Wyburn-Mason arteriovenous m.
malformed phlebectasia
Malgaigne pelvic fracture
malignancy
    aggressive m.
    borderline m.
    epithelial m.
    extrapelvic m.
    gastrointestinal m.
    high-grade m.
    low-grade m.
    metastatic m.
    mimicker of m.
    myeloid m.
    pelvic m.
    primary pulmonary m.
    secondary m.
    m. threshold
    uroepithelial m.
    urogenital m.
    vulvar m.
malignant
    m. acetabular osteolysis
    m. adrenal mass
    m. airway obstruction
    m. bone aneurysm
    m. brain edema
    m. breast calcification
    m. chondrosarcoma
    m. degeneration
    m. duodenal tumor
    m. ependymoma
    m. external otitis
    m. fibrous histiocytoma (MFH)
    m. fibrous histiocytoma of bone
     (MFH-B)
    m. fibrous osseous histiocytoma
    m. fibrous xanthoma
    m. fibroxanthoma
    m. gastric ulcer

    m. glioma
    m. hemangioendothelioma
    m. mediastinum teratoid tumor
    m. melanoma gallium imaging
    m. melanoma staging
    m. meningioma
    m. myeloid sarcoma
    m. nephrosclerosis
    m. osseous lesion
    m. osteoid
    m. osteopetrosis
    m. ovarian germ cell tumor
    m. ovarian teratoma tumor
    m. pleomorphic adenoma
    m. pleural effusion
    m. pleural implant
    m. pleural mesothelioma
    m. pulmonary mesothelioma
    m. small bowel tumor
    m. teratoma
    m. thymoma
    m. transformation
    m. urethral neoplasm
    m. vertebral compression fracture
malignum
    adenoma m.
Mallampati score
malleolar
    m. fossa
    m. fracture
malleolus, pl. **malleoli**
    m. bone
    m. fibulae
    lateral m.
    medial m.
    m. tibiae
mallet
    m. finger
    m. fracture
mallet-finger deformity
malleus, pl. **mallei**
Mallinckrodt
    M. Institute of Radiology guideline
    M. scanner
Mallory-Weiss
    M.-W. esophageal tear
    M.-W. lesion
    M.-W. mucosal tear
    M.-W. syndrome
Malmo mammographic screening trial
malocclusion
malomaxillary suture
Maloney endootoprobe laser
malperfused
malperfusion syndrome
malpighian
    m. body
    m. body of spleen

m. follicle
m. vesicle
malpositioned
m. fetus
m. heart
m. testis
malrotation
m. of bowel loop
complete small bowel m.
intestinal tract m.
m. of intestine
kidney m.
midgut volvulus with m.
partial small bowel m.
renal m.
small bowel m.
MALT
mucosa-associated lymphoid tissue
MALT lymphoma
malt worker's lung
malum perforans pedis
malunion of fracture fragment
malunited fracture
Malvern 2600 Sizer laser diffraction scanner
mamillary
m. body
m. suture
m. system
mamillothalamic fasciculus
Mamm-Aire heart failure
Mammalock needle
mammaplasty (*var. of* mammoplasty)
mammary
m. artery
m. calculus
m. cyst
m. duct
m. duct ectasia
m. duct obstruction
m. ductogram
m. ductogram imaging
m. dysplasia
m. galactogram
m. galactogram imaging
m. gland
m. implant
m. parenchyma
m. tissue
m. tumorigenesis
MAMMEX TR computer-aided mammography diagnosis system

Mammo
M. Mask dedicated viewer
M. Mask illuminator
M. Plus mammography system
M. QC mammography
mammogram
CAD-evaluated m.
digitized contact m.
false-negative m.
film-based screening m.
true-negative m.
mammographic
m. evaluation of breast mass
m. feature
m. guidance
m. measurement
m. phantom
m. technique
m. view box
mammographically
m. occult carcinoma
m. suspicious lesion
mammographic-histopathologic correlation
mammography
baseline m.
computed tomography laser m. (CTLM)
contoured tilting compression m.
contrast-enhanced near-infrared laser m.
contrast subtraction m.
diagnostic m.
digital m.
digital subtraction m. (DSM)
dual-energy m.
dynamic computed tomography m.
Egan m.
evaluation of mass m.
film-screen m.
full-field digital m.
high-resolution CT m.
low-dose m.
magnetic resonance m. (MRM)
magnification m.
Mammomat B m.
Mammo QC m.
microfocal spot m.
near-infrared optical m.
NIR optical m.
nonmagnified m.
orthogonal projection m.

M

NOTES

mammography *(continued)*
  positron emission m. (PEM)
  M. Quality Control Manual
  M. Quality Standards Act (MQSA)
  radionuclide m.
  screen-film m.
  screening m.
  Senographe 500T, 600T, 700T,
    800T m.
  single-view oblique m.
  spot compression magnification m.
  stage-matched intervention on
    repeat m.
  step-oblique m.
  stereo m.
  stereotactic m.
  m. technique
  ultra-high magnification m.
    (UHMM)
  ultrasound augmented m.
  2-view film-screen m.
  x-ray m.
Mammo-Lume
Mammomat B mammography
mammoplasia
mammoplasty, mammaplasty
  augmentation m.
  postreduction m.
MammoReader
  M. computer-aided dectection
    system
  M. mammogram device
  M. mammography system
Mammorex
MammoSite
  M. Radiation Therapy
  M. radiation therapy system
    catheter (MammoSite RTS catheter)
  M. RTS
  M. RTS catheter
Mammospot
Mammotest
  M. breast biopsy system
  M. unit
Mammotome
  Biopsys M.
  M. ultrasound system
Mammotrax
Mammoviewer
man
  roentgen equivalent m. (REM)
management
  real-time position m. (RPM)
managing
  high-resolution storage phosphor m.
Manchester
  M. LDR implant system
  M. ovoid

mandible
  alveolar border of m.
  genial tubercle of m.
  m. hypoplasia
  m. osteolysis
  symphysis of m.
mandibula, pl. **mandibulae**
  capitulum m.
  coronoid of m.
mandibular
  m. angle
  m. canal
  m. condyle
  m. disc
  m. division
  m. foramen
  m. fossa
  m. fracture
  m. lymph node
  m. nerve
  m. ramus
  m. triangle
mandibularis
  torus m.
mandibulofacial dysostosis
mandril
maneuver
  Adson m.
  circumduction-adduction shoulder m.
  costoclavicular m.
  flexion m.
  Fogarty m.
  Hampton m.
  Heineke-Mikulicz m.
  hyperabduction m.
  jugular compression m.
  Kocher m.
  manual Matas m.
  Müller m.
  Osler m.
  Phalen m.
  pull m.
  push m.
  Rivero-Carvallo m.
  scalene m.
  squatting m.
  temporal artery tap m.
  transabdominal left lateral
    retroperitoneal m.
  Valsalva m.
mangafodipir
  m. trisodium (MnDPDP)
  m. trisodium agent
  m. trisodium-enhanced MR imaging
mangafodipir-enhanced MRCP
manganese (Mn)
  m. chloride
  m. chloride contrast medium
  m. citrate

m. dipyridoxyl diphosphate
m. imaging agent
m. sulfate
m. tetrasodium-meso-tetra (Mn-TPPS₄)
manganese-BOPTA
manganese-containing contrast agent
manifestation
imaging m.
manifold
3-stopcock m.
manipulation
deformable m.
rigid m.
Mankin method
man-made environmental radiation
mannan-coated liposome
Mann-Bollman fistula
mannitol and saline imaging agent
Mannkopf sign
manofluorography (MFG)
manometer
mercury m.
manometric
m. measurement
m. pattern
manometry
anal m.
aneroid m.
anorectal m.
biliary m.
ERCP m.
esophageal m.
rectosigmoid m.
sphincter of Oddi m.
mantle
anechoic m.
m. block
brain m.
m. cell lymphoma (MCL)
cement m.
cerebral m.
m. complex
m. field
m. field irradiation
hypoechoic m.
m. radiotherapy
manual
m. compression
m. injection
Mammography Quality Control M.
m. Matas maneuver

m. pressure over carotid sinus
m. subtraction film
manubriosternalis
symphysis m.
synchondrosis m.
manubriosternal joint
manubrium, pl. **manubria**
m. hypersegmentation
manus
digiti m.
MAP
mean arterial pressure
map (*See* mapping)
acceleration m.
ADC m.
anisotropy m.
bladder m.
bull's eye polar m.
cerebral blood volume m.
cylindrical projection m.
decimalized variance m.
end-diastolic polar m.
end-systolic polar m.
functional m.
geometry factor m.
sestamibi polar m.
spheric m.
trace m.
MAPCA
multiple aortopulmonary collateral artery
map-guided partial endocardial ventriculotomy
maple
m. bark disease
m. bark stripper's lung
m. syrup urine disease
maplike skull
mapping
activation-sequence m.
advanced cardiac m.
m. algorithm
body surface laplacian m. (BSLM)
body surface potential m.
Bo field m.
brain electrical activity m. (BEAM)
cardiac m.
catheter m.
m. of cerebral sulcus
color-flow m.
contour m.
cortical m.
2D m.

M

NOTES

mapping *(continued)*
- m. of defect
- digital road m.
- direction-encoded color m. (DEC)
- Doppler color-flow m.
- 2D pulsatility index m.
- 2D resistance index m.
- eddy current m.
- electrophysiologic m.
- endocardial activation m.
- endocardial catheter m.
- epicardial m.
- functional anatomical m.
- homology m.
- Hough transform m.
- intramural m.
- intraoperative electrocortical stimulation m.
- intraoperative lymphatic m.
- k-space velocity m.
- lorentzian field m.
- lymphatic m.
- magnetic resonance phase velocity m.
- moving slice velocity m.
- MRI m.
- MR velocity m.
- pace m.
- parallel analog m.
- phase difference m.
- phase-shift velocity m.
- precordial m.
- quantitative multilevel m.
- radiocolloid m.
- retrograde atrial activation m.
- saphenous vein m.
- sinus rhythm m.
- spastic m.
- spatial m.
- susceptibility m.
- texture m.
- velocity m.
- volumetric magnetic resonance brain m.

marantic
- m. clot
- m. endocarditis

maranti endocarditis

marble
- m. bone
- m. bone disease

marbling of pancreatic parenchyma

Marcacci muscle

march
- m. foot
- m. fracture

Marchiafava-Bignami disease

Marchiafava-Micheli syndrome

Marconi/Elscint MxTwin CT

Marcus Gunn syndrome

Marex MRI system

Marfan syndrome

margin
- anterior vertebral body m.
- m. of apposition
- bandlike m.
- beveled m.
- blurring of disc m.
- cardiac m.
- circumscribed m.
- colon m.
- convex posterior m.
- cortical m.
- costal m.
- costodiaphragmatic m.
- depression of renal m.
- disc m.
- enhancing ventricular m.
- fluffy m.
- ill-defined m.
- indistinct endometrial m.
- infraorbital m. (IOM)
- inking the m.
- ipsilateral m.
- m. irregularity
- linear m.
- medial talar m.
- m. necrosis
- overhanging m.
- periarticular m.
- pleural m.
- posterior disc m.
- psoas m.
- m. of scapula
- scapular m.
- sclerotic m.
- sharp lateral m.
- spiculated m.
- stomach m.
- subcostal m.
- superomedial m.
- supraorbital m. (SOM)
- tumor m.
- vertebral body m.

marginal
- m. branch
- m. branch of left circumflex coronary artery
- m. branch of right coronary artery
- m. circumflex artery
- m. erosion
- m. exostosis
- m. fracture
- m. gyrus
- m. kidney depression
- obtuse m. (OM)
- m. osteophyte
- m. osteophyte formation

m. placenta
m. placenta previa
m. ridge
m. sclerosis
m. serration
m. sinus
m. spur
m. spurring
m. syndesmophyte
m. ulcer
m. vein
m. zone
m. zone B-cell lymphoma
m. zone lymphoma (MZL)
Marie-Bamberger disease
Marie-Strümpell disease
Marimastat
Marine-Lenhart syndrome
Marinesco-Sjögren syndrome
mark
    M. II Kodros radiolucent awl
    M. V Plus automatic injector
marked
    m. hypoechogenicity shadowing
    m. sclerosis
    m. shunting of blood
markedly accentuated pulmonic
  component
marker
    anatomic m.
    external fiducial m.
    fiducial skin m.
    implanted imaging opaque m.
    isotope-tagged m.
    lead pellet m.
    metallic m.
    MicroMark tissue m.
    molecular m.
    myocardial-specific m.
    needle m.
    nipple m.
    PINNACLE R/O II radiopaque m.
    radioactive string m.
    radiopaque m.
    radiopaque gold m.
    Sitzmarks radiopaque m.
    m. transit imaging
    m. transit study
    tumor m.
marker-channel diagram
marking
    absence of haustral m.

absence of vascular m.
accentuation of m.
bronchopulmonary m.
bronchovascular m.
bronchovesicular m.
coarse bronchovascular m.
confluence of vascular m.
convolutional m.
crowding of bronchovascular m.
digital m.
haustral m.
increased interstitial m.
increased pulmonary vascular m.
interstitial m.
linear m.
lung m.
peribronchial m.
perihilar m.
pullback arterial m.
pulmonary arterial m.
pulmonary vascular m.
sulcal m.
sutural m.
vascular m.
Markov
    M. chain
    M. chain Monte Carlo technique
    M. random field
Marlex band
Marmor-Lynn fracture
Maroteaux-Lamy syndrome
marrow
    aberrant bone m.
    m. agent bone scintigraphy
    m. blush
    bone m.
    bright fatty m.
    m. canal
    cancellous hematopoietic m.
    m. cavity
    central nidus of high-intensity m.
    m. dosimetry
    m. edema pattern
    epiphysial hematopoietic m.
    m. fat signal intensity
    fatty m.
    functional m.
    hematopoietically active bone m.
    hematopoietic bone m.
    high-signal-intensity yellow m.
    hypercellular reconverted bone m.
    hypocellular m.

M

NOTES

marrow *(continued)*
    m. infarct
    m. infiltrate
    m. infiltration
    island of red m.
    peripheral hematopoietic
      intermediate signal intensity m.
    shunting of tracer to bone m.
    m. signal change
    sternal m.
    m. transplant
    uptake in bone m.
Marshall vein
marshmallow bolus
Martin-Bell syndrome
Martin disease
Martorell
    M. aortic arch syndrome
    M. hypertensive ulcer
    M. sign
MAS
    midaortic syndrome
    MAS in FAS
masculine pelvis
masculinizing tumor
mask
    convolution m.
    m. data
    ISAH stereotactic immobilizing m.
    Orfit m.
    particle m.
    m. threshold
    m. ventilation
mask-based approach
masking
    unsharp m.
    white m.
Mason radial fracture classification
mason's lung
masquerading effect
mass
    abdominopelvic m.
    m. absorption coefficient
    adrenal cystic m.
    air-containing neck m.
    airless m.
    anechoic m.
    anterior mediastinal m.
    aortopulmonary window m.
    appendiceal m.
    apperceptive m.
    m. attenuation coefficient
    avascular brain m.
    avascular kidney m.
    avascular renal m.
    m. balance
    benign adrenal m.
    bilateral fetal chest m.
    bilateral renal m.

bilobed m.
brain m.
calcified brain m.
calcified intracranial m.
calcified kidney m.
calcified renal m.
cardiophrenic right-angle m.
carotid space m.
cavitary m.
cerebellar cystic m.
circumscribed m.
m. collision stopping power
complex solid and cystic m.
congenital nasal m.
conglomerate m.
conical m.
cord intradural extramedullary m.
cordlike m.
critical m.
cystic breast m.
cystic teratomatous m.
m. defect
dense brain m.
dense cerebral m.
dirty m.
discoid chest m.
discrete m.
doughy m.
dumbbell brain m.
dysplasia with associated lesion
  or m. (DALM)
echogenic m.
m. effect
elongated m.
encapsulated m.
m. energy equivalence
enhancing m.
epidural m.
exophytic m.
expanding intracranial m.
expansile m.
external ear m.
extracardiac m.
extraosseous m.
extraovarian m.
extrapleural m.
extrauterine pelvic m.
extravascular m.
fallopian tube m.
fat-containing m.
fat density m.
fetal abdominal cystic m.
fibrin m.
firm m.
fixed m.
fleecy m.
fluctuant m.
fluid-filled kidney m.
focal m.

freely movable m.
friable m.
glenoid ovoid m.
glenolabral ovoid m. (GLOM)
groin m.
heterogeneous breast m.
high-signal m.
hilar m.
homogeneous intrasellar m.
hyperattenuated intrasellar m.
hyperdense m.
hyperechoic breast m.
hyperintense m.
hypervascular mediastinal m.
hypoattenuating m.
hypodense m.
ill-defined m.
m. imaging
indurated m.
inflammatory polypoid m.
injection m.
inner ear m.
interbronchial m.
intermediate signal intensity m.
intraabdominal m.
intracardiac m.
intracaval fat m.
intracavity m.
intracranial m.
intracystic solid m.
intraductal solid m.
intradural extramedullary m.
intraluminal stomach m.
intrasellar brain m.
intrathoracic fetal m.
intrathoracic low-attenuation m.
intravascular m.
intraventricular m.
irregular m.
isodense m.
isoechoic breast m.
jugular foraminal m.
kidney sinus m.
lacrimal m.
large solid adrenal m.
lateral m.
lean m.
left ventricular m. (LVM)
m. lesion
liver m.
lobulated m.
loss of bone m.

low-attenuation mediastinal m.
lower lobe lung m.
low-signal m.
lung m.
lymphomatous m.
malignant adrenal m.
mammographic evaluation of
  breast m.
masticator space m.
mediastinal high-attenuation m.
mesenteric m.
middle ear m.
middle mediastinal m.
mixed attenuation m.
mixed density m.
mixed echogenic solid m.
mixed signal m.
mixed solid-cystic m.
mobile intraluminal gallbladder m.
molar m.
mulberrylike m.
multilobulated m.
multiloculated m.
mushroom-shaped m.
myocardial m.
nasal vault m.
nasopharyngeal m.
nodular m.
noncalcified nodular m.
nonhemorrhagic m.
nonhomogeneous hyperdense m.
nonopaque intraluminal m.
nonpulsatile abdominal m.
m. number
omental m.
orbital superolateral quadrant m.
ovarian m.
pancreatic m.
paraaortic m.
paracardiac m.
paranasal sinus m.
parasagittal intracranial m.
parasellar brain m.
paraspinal soft tissue m.
paravertebrally situated pelvic
  tumor m.
paravertebrally situated thoracic
  tumor m.
paucilocular cystic m.
pelvic cystic m.
periosseous soft tissue m.
perirenal m.

M

NOTES

mass *(continued)*
    peritoneal m.
    perivascular m.
    petrous apex dumbbell m.
    pharyngeal space m.
    phlegmonous m.
    phosphaturic m.
    pineal m.
    pleural m.
    polypoid calcified irregular m.
    porta hepatis low-density m.
    posterior mediastinal m.
    prepubertal testicular m.
    presacral m.
    prevertebral space m.
    promontory m.
    pulmonary m.
    pulsating m.
    red cell m. (RCM)
    relativistic m.
    renal sinus m.
    reniform m.
    retrobulbar m.
    retrocardiac m.
    retroperitoneal m.
    retropharyngeal space m.
    retrosternal m.
    right cardiophrenic angle m.
    right ventricular m. (RVM)
    ring-enhancing m.
    saccular m.
    scrotal m.
    soft tissue density m.
    solid m.
    solitary m.
    sonolucent cystic m.
    space-occupying m.
    m. spectrometer
    spheric m.
    spiculated m.
    stellate m.
    stony m.
    subareolar m.
    subinsular m.
    suprasellar m.
    suspicious m.
    teratomatous m.
    thalamic-hypothalamic m.
    thymic m.
    m. thymus
    thyroid m.
    tissue m.
    torsed ovarian m.
    tubal m.
    tuboovarian m.
    tubular fluid-density adnexal m.
    tumor m.
    umbilical m.
    uncinate process m.

    unilateral adrenal m.
    unilateral fetal chest m.
    unilateral kidney m.
    urinary bladder extrinsic m.
    urinary bladder wall m.
    uterine m.
    ventricular m.
    water-density m.
    wedge-shaped m.
    well-circumscribed breast m.
    well-defined m.
    woody m.
Massachusetts (General Hospital) Utility Multiprogramming System
mass-effect hydrocephalus
masseteric enlargement
masseter muscle
massive
    m. aortic regurgitation
    m. ascites
    m. embolus
    m. exsanguinating hemorrhage
    m. fibrosis
    m. hepatic necrosis
    m. herniated disc
    m. infiltrate
    m. osteolysis
    m. ovarian edema
    m. pleural effusion
    m. pneumonia
    m. pulmonary hemorrhagic edema
massively enlarged heart
masslike
    m. configuration
    m. lesion
Masson body
MAST
    military antishock trousers
    motion artifact suppression technique
        MAST suit
mast
    m. cell-enhancing activity
    m. cell reticulosis
    m. leukocyte
mastectomy
    non-skin-sparing m. (non-SSM)
master knot of Henry
masticator
    m. muscle
    m. space
    m. space infection
    m. space mass
mastitis
    m. fibrosa cystica
    m. obliterans
mastocytosis
    bone m.
    GI tract m.
    systemic m.

mastoid
    m. antrum
    m. bone
    m. canal
    m. complex
    m. fontanelle
    m. foramen
    m. lymph node
    m. polytomography
    m. process
    m. sinus
    m. suture
mastopathy
    diabetic m.
    fibrous m.
mastoplasia
    cystic m.
match
    nontransmural m.
    transmural m.
    triple m.
matched peripheral dose (MPD)
matching
    atlas m.
    electron-photon field m.
    general pattern m.
    impedance m.
    m. network
matchline wedge
material (*See* agent, contrast, medium)
    anthracotic m.
    atheromatous m.
    ballistic m.
    byproduct m.
    coffee grounds m.
    collection of contrast m.
    columnization of contrast m.
    contrast m.
    dental contrast m.
    embolic m.
    extraneous m.
    fecal m.
    ferromagnetic m.
    flow of contrast m.
    inspissated m.
    Interpore bone replacement m.
    intravenous administration of
      contrast m.
    iodinated contrast m.
    layering of contrast m.
    lipid-rich m.
    LSO crystal scintillator m.

    magnetic m.
    nonionic contrast m.
    opaque m.
    ^{103}Pd radioactive m.
    PET target m.
    phosphaturic m.
    radioactive m.
    m. spin echocardiogram total
      volume imaging
    superabsorbent polymer embolic m.
    target m.
    trophoblastic m.
    uptake of radioactive m.
    vessel cutoff of contrast m.
maternal
    m. lake
    m. placenta
**Mathews classification of olecranon
  fracture**
matrix, pl. **matrices**
    acquisition m.
    bone tumor m.
    calcific m.
    m. calculus
    cartilage m.
    chondroid m.
    decision m.
    demineralized bone m. (DBM)
    extracellular m.
    germinal bleed m.
    m. image
    m. injury
    k-space m.
    M. LR3300 laser imaging
    m. metalloprotease-3 (MMP-3)
    m. mineralization
    nuclear m.
    osteoid m.
    proteoglycan m.
    quantization m. (QM)
    reduced-acquisition m. (RAM)
    m. size
    solid m.
    m. stone
    stromal m.
    transformation m.
    tumor m.
matted
    m. bowel loop
    m. small-bowel loop
matter
    cortical gray m.

M

NOTES

matter *(continued)*
    cortical white m.
    cytotoxic edema of gray m.
    deep white ischemia m.
    gray m.
    heterotopic gray m.
    infratentorial gray m.
    normal-appearing white m.
      (NAWM)
    particulate m.
    Patient-Oriented Evidence that M.'s
      (POEM)
    periaqueductal gray m.
    perilesional white m.
    peritrigonal white m.
    periventricular gray m.
    periventricular white m.
    pulverized plaque particulate m.
    PVG m.
    scalloped appearance of white m.
    shearing of white m.
    supratentorial gray m.
    supratentorial white m.
    white m.

maturation
    bone m.
    disc m.
    m. index
    pulmonary structural m.
    skeletal m.

mature
    m. bone
    m. mediastinum teratoma
    m. ovarian cystic teratoma
    m. pancreatic pseudocyst
    m. pouch
    m. pseudocyst of pancreas
    skeletally m.
    m. vertebra

maturity
    m. of fetus
    skeletal m.

Mauchart ligament

MAVIS
    mobile artery and vein imaging system

Maxicamera

maxilla, pl. **maxillae**

maxillary
    m. antrum
    m. artery
    m. bone
    m. canal
    m. division
    m. fracture
    m. nerve anatomy
    m. process
    m. sinus
    m. sinus carcinoma
    m. sinus hypoplasia
    m. sinus opacification
    m. sinus puncture
    m. sinus radiograph
    m. spine

maxillofacial
    m. fracture
    m. imaging

Maxima II TENS unit

maximal
    m. estimated gradient
    m. intensity
    m. radiographic distention
    m. transaortic jet velocity
    m. volume of left atrium
    m. voluntary ventilation (MVV)

maximization
    ordered subset expectation m.
      (OSEM)

maximum
    m. amplitude constant
    m. anteroposterior diameter
    m. density (D_{max})
    m. diameter to minimum diameter
      ratio
    m. entropy processing
    full width at half m. (FWHM)
    m. inflation pressure
    m. inflation time
    m. intensity pixel (MIP)
    m. intensity projection (MIP)
    m. intensity projection algorithm
    m. intensity projection imaging
    m. intensity projection and source
      image
    m. likelihood algorithm
    m. midexpiratory flow (MMEF)
    m. midexpiratory flow rate
      (MMFR)
    m. permissible body burden
    m. permissible concentration
    m. predicted heart rate (MPHR)
    m. short-axis diameter (MSAD)
    m. slew rate ramp
    time delay between excitation and
      echo m. (TE)
    m. venous outflow (MVO)
    m. ventricular elastance

**maximum-intensity sliding thin slab
projection**

maximus
    gluteus m.

Max Plus MR scanner

Maxwell
    M. coil
    M. 3D field simulator
    M. pair
    M. theory of radiation

maxwellian distribution

Mayer
  M. position
  M. view
Mayer-Rokitansky-Küster-Hauser syndrome
May-Hegglin anomaly
Mayneord F factor
May-Thurner syndrome
Mazabraud syndrome
Mazur ankle evaluation classification
MB
  myocardial band
    MB fraction
M-band myeloma
MBF
  myocardial blood flow
MBS-MRA
  minimum basis set magnetic resonance angiography
MCA
  middle cerebral artery
  multichannel analyzer
  multiple congenital anomalies
MCAT
  myocardial contrast appearance time
McBurney point
McCabe-Fletcher classification
McCallum patch
McCune-Albright syndrome
MCD
  mean central dose
  molecular coincidence detection
  multicentric Castleman disease
    MCD imaging
MCDK
  multicystic dysplastic kidney
MCE
  myocardial contrast echocardiography
MCFSR
  mean circumferential fiber shortening rate
McGinn-White sign
McGregor line
MCi
  megacurie
mCi
  millicurie
mCi-hr
  millicurie-hour
McIlwain tissue chopper
MCK
  multicystic kidney

McKee line
McKusick-Kaufman syndrome
McKusick-type
  M.-t. metaphysial chondrodysplasia
  M.-t. metaphysial dysplasia
MCL
  mantle cell lymphoma
  medial collateral ligament
  midclavicular line
    MCL bursa
McLain-Weinstein spinal tumor classification
MCLC
  medial collateral ligament complex
MCLS
  mucocutaneous lymph node syndrome
McMurray test
McNamara coaxial catheter infusion set
MCP
  metacarpophalangeal
MCPJ
  metacarpophalangeal joint
MCPT
  Monte Carlo photon transport
    MCPT simulation
McRae line
MCS
  middle coronary sinus
MCT
  mean circulation time
MCTC
  metrizamide computed tomography cisternography
MCTD
  mixed connective-tissue disease
MCU
  micturating cystourethrogram
MDAC
  multiplying digital-to-analog converter
MDCT
  multidetector CT
  multidetector-row CT
MD-Gastroview imaging agent
MDP
  methylene diphosphonate
    TechneScan MDP
MDP-Bracco
MDS
  myelodysplastic syndrome
    MDS coil
MDS-2000 microwave irradiator

M

NOTES

MDT
    minimal deformation target
MEA
    microwave endometrial ablation
Meadows syndrome
meal
    barium m.
    Boyden test m.
    double-contrast barium m.
    Ewald test m.
    fatty m.
    isotope m.
    motor test m.
    opaque m.
    retention m.
    small bowel m.
    test m.
mean
    m. ankle-brachial systolic pressure
      index
    m. aortic flow velocity
    m. aortic pressure
    m. arterial pressure (MAP)
    m. blood pressure
    m. brachial artery pressure
    m. cardiac vector
    m. central dose (MCD)
    m. circulating time
    m. circulation time (MCT)
    m. circulatory filling pressure
    m. circumferential fiber shortening
      rate (MCFSR)
    m. corpuscular volume
    m. deviation
    m. diffusivity
    m. examination time
    m. free path
    m. gonad dose
    m. left atrial pressure
    m. mitral valve gradient
    m. perfusate temperature
    m. posterior wall velocity
    m. pulmonary artery pressure
      (MPAP)
    m. pulmonary artery wedge
      pressure
    m. pulmonary capillary pressure
      (MPCP)
    m. pulmonary flow velocity
    m. pulmonary transit time (MTT)
    m. right atrial pressure
    m. sac diameter (MSD)
    m. systolic gradient
    m. transit time (MTT)
    m. venous pulsation
    m. wall motion score
    m. wall motion score index
mean-diameter overframing
mean-square error

Meary metatarsotalar angle
measles pneumonia
measurable endpoint
measure
    linear m.
measurement
    ankle-brachial pressure m.
    antegrade perfusion pressure m.
      (APPM)
    appendicular bone mass m.
    attenuation m.
    automated cardiac flow m. (ACM)
    blood flow m.
    body composition m.
    bolus passage perfusion m.
    bone density m.
    breath pentane m.
    cardiac output m.
    cerebrospinal fluid flow m.
    Cerenkov m.
    Cobb m.
    densitometric m.
    diode m.
    Dixon fat-fraction m.
    end-diastolic velocity m.
    excitation function m.
    fat-fraction m.
    fetal foot length m.
    fetal long bone m.
    flow cytometric DNA m.
    gestational sac m.
    Hausdorff m.
    high-sensitivity m.
    hila m.
    histomorphometric m.
    indicator-dilution method for
      cardiac output m.
    intercomparison m.
    line-pair m.
    low-energy photon attenuation m.
    mammographic m.
    manometric m.
    microbubble concentration m.
    morphometric m.
    nondynamometric trunk strength m.
    nutation angle m.
    occlusion m.
    orbit m.
    phase-sensitive flow m.
    photon attenuation m.
    polarographic needle electrode m.
    pQCT m.
    pressure m.
    pulsatility m.
    pulse-echo distance m.
    quantitative regional myocardial
      flow m.
    regional washout m.
    renal length m.

rocking curve m.
root-mean-squared gradient m.
segmental correction using x-
ray m.
segmental pressure m.
semiquantitative m.
signal intensity m.
TCD m.
temperature distribution m.
thermodilution method of cardiac
output m.
thyroid uptake m.
time-of-flight flow m.
time-velocity m.
topographic m.
transcutaneous oxygen pressure m.
(tcPO$_2$)
true conjugate m.
U1-NA cephalometric m.
m. in vivo
whole-brain magnetization
transfer m.
Wits m.
xenon CT m.
Z-score in bone mineral
density m.
meatal segment
meatus
acoustic m.
external auditory m.
internal auditory m.
nasal m.
meat wrapper's lung
mebrofenin
mechanical
m. augmentation
m. axis
m. biliary obstruction
m. compound scan
m. counterpulsation
m. duct obstruction
m. extrahepatic obstruction
m. genu varus
m. ileus
m. insufflation
m. insult
m. intestinal obstruction
m. potential energy
m. respiratory tract obstruction
m. sector scanner
m. small bowel obstruction
m. thrombectomy

m. thrombolysis
m. valve
m. ventilation
mechanically
m. activated implant
m. detachable platinum coil
m. sealed
mechanics
body m.
intramural m.
mechanism
blood-clotting m.
central extensor m. (CEM)
check-valve m.
compensatory m.
contrecoup m.
deglutition m.
excitotoxic m.
extensor m.
flap-valve m.
Frank-Starling m.
heart rate reserve m.
homing m.
humeral m.
m. of injury
internal retention m.
iron-transporting protein m.
Laplace m.
osseous pinch m.
pinchcock m.
propulsive m.
sinus m.
sodium-potassium ATPase-dependent
exchange m.
sphincteric m.
swallowing m.
Taylor-Blackwood m.
ventricular escape m.
watershed m.
Mecholyl test
Meckel
M. band
M. cavity
M. diverticulitis
M. diverticulum
M. ligament
M. plane
M. scan
M. syndrome
Meckel-Gruber syndrome
meclofenamic acid

M

NOTES

meconium
- m. aspiration
- m. aspiration syndrome
- m. ileus
- m. ileus equivalent
- m. peristalsis
- m. peritonitis
- m. plug
- m. plug syndrome
- m. pseudocyst

Meddars cardiac catheterization analysis system

Medelec DMG 50 Teflon-coated monopolar electrode

Medgraphics body plethysmograph

media (*pl. of* medium)
- radiopaque contrast m. (ROCM)

media-adventitia interface

medial
- m. angle
- m. arch
- m. arteriosclerosis
- m. aspect
- m. basal segmental bronchus
- m. border
- m. calcific sclerosis
- m. carpal capsule
- m. collateral ligament (MCL)
- m. collateral ligament calcification
- m. collateral ligament complex (MCLC)
- m. column calcaneal fracture
- m. compartment
- m. condyle
- m. crus
- m. cuneiform bone
- m. cystic necrosis
- m. dissection
- m. eminence
- m. end of clavicle osteolysis
- m. epicondylar bursa
- m. epicondyle
- m. epicondyle fracture
- m. epicondylitis
- m. extension
- m. femoral buttressing
- m. fibroplasia
- m. geniculate body
- m. geniculate fascia
- m. hyperplasia
- m. joint line
- m. joint space
- m. and lateral support structures of knee
- m. lemniscus
- m. longitudinal fasciculus (MLF)
- m. longitudinal fasciculus lesion
- m. malleolar fracture
- m. malleolus

- m. malleolus periostitis
- m. oblique axial projection
- m. oblique view
- m. occipitotemporal gyrus
- m. papillary muscle
- m. physis
- m. plantar artery
- m. plica
- m. plica of knee
- m. posterior choroidal (MPCh)
- m. pterygoid muscle
- m. rotation
- m. sagittal plane
- m. sesamoid bone
- m. shelf
- m. supraclavicular node
- m. talar dome injury
- m. talar margin
- m. talar osteochondral injury
- m. temporal lobe
- m. tibial stress syndrome
- m. traction spur

medialis
- meniscus m.
- vastus m.

medially

median
- m. antebrachial vein
- m. arcuate ligament
- m. arcuate ligament of diaphragm
- m. bar
- m. cleft lip
- m. cruciate ligament
- m. facial cleft
- m. lethal dose
- m. level echo
- m. line
- m. lip cleft
- m. lobe of prostate
- multiples of the m.
- m. nerve
- m. nerve entrapment
- m. nerve lesion
- m. palatine suture
- m. raphe
- m. raphe plane
- m. sacral artery
- m. sagittal plane
- m. septum
- m. umbilical ligament

mediastinal
- m. abscess
- m. adenoma
- m. adenopathy
- m. air
- m. angiolipoma
- m. arterial variant
- m. border
- m. bronchogenic cyst

m. bulk
m. collagenosis
m. cross-sectional imaging
m. crunch
m. deviation
m. dorsal enteric cyst
m. duplication cyst
m. emphysema
m. fat
m. fat edema
m. fibrosis
m. fistula
m. granuloma
m. hematoma
m. hemorrhage
m. hernia
m. high-attenuation mass
m. invasion
m. lesion
m. lipomatosis
m. lung surface
m. lymph node enlargement
m. lymphoma
m. node
m. panniculitis
m. pleura
m. pleurisy
m. prominence
m. pseudomass
m. retraction
m. seminoma
m. septum
m. seroma
m. shift
m. structure
m. teratoid tumor
m. thickening
m. thyroid tissue
m. tube
m. uptake
m. vein
m. viscus
m. wedge
m. widening
m. window

mediastinitis
fibrosing m.
idiopathic fibrous m.
sclerosing m.

mediastinogram

mediastinography
gas m.

gaseous m.
opaque m.

mediastinoscopy

mediastinum
anterior m.
m. cerebelli
m. cerebri
m. dermoid
deviated m.
m. displacement
m. dysgerminoma
epidermoid m.
m. germinoma
inferior m.
left m.
m. lipoma
lipomatosis m.
lobulated paratracheal m.
middle m.
posterior m.
right m.
seminoma m.
superior m.
m. teratocarcinoma
teratoid m.
m. teratoma
m. testis
widened m.

medical
m. asepsis
BioSphere M.
m. cyclotron
m. holography
m. internal radiation dosimetry (MIRD)
M. Ultrasound Three-Dimensional Portable Advanced Communications (MUSTPAC)
m. umbilical fold

medicamentosa
thyrotoxicosis m.

medicine
complementary and alternative m. (CAM)
Digital Imaging and Communications in M. (DICOM)
Fellow of the American College of Nuclear M.
nuclear m.
photonic m.

Medigraphics analyzer

NOTES

Medilase angioscope-laser delivery system
MedImage scanner
Medinvent
mediobasal hypothalamus luteinizing hormone-releasing hormone
mediolateral
    m. aspect
    m. flow direction
    m. oblique (MLO)
    m. oblique projection
    m. oblique view
    m. radiocarpal angle
    m. stress
    m. view
medionecrosis
    cystic m.
medionodular cirrhosis
mediopatellar
MediPort catheter
Medison scanner
Medi-tech
    M.-t. catheter
    M.-t. ureteral stent system
medium, pl. **media** (*See* agent, contrast, material)
    barium sulfate contrast m.
    benzoic acid contrast m.
    bismuth contrast m.
    brominized oil contrast m.
    bullet kit culture m.
    m. caliber
    cerebral contrast m.
    contrast m. (CM)
    delayed excretion of contrast m.
    diatrizoic acid contrast m.
    endogenous adenosine contrast m.
    Entero Vu contrast m.
    EntroEase oral radiopaque contrast m.
    ethiodized oil contrast m.
    ethyliodophenylundecyl contrast m.
    extraluminal contrast m.
    FDDNP PET scan contrast m.
    galactose contrast m.
    Gd-DOTA contrast m.
    glucaric acid-labeled contrast m.
    hand injection of contrast m.
    high-osmolarity contrast m. (HOCM)
    hyperconcentration of contrast m.
    Imagopaque contrast m.
    intravascular contrast m.
    intravenous contrast m.
    iodide contrast m.
    iodinated intravascular contrast m.
    iodinated radiologic contrast m. (IRCM)
    iodine-containing contrast m.
    iodixanol contrast m.
    iodophendylate contrast m.
    ioglunide contrast m.
    ioglycamic acid contrast m.
    Iomeron 150, 250, 300, 350 contrast m.
    ionic dimer contrast m.
    ionic monomeric contrast m.
    ionic paramagnetic contrast m.
    iopromide contrast m.
    iotroxamide contrast m.
    ioxaglic acid contrast m.
    ioxithalamate contrast m.
    isoefamate contrast m.
    Isopaque contrast m.
    isosmolar contrast m. (IOCM)
    kinetic energy released per unit mass and kinetic energy released in m. (kerma)
    low-osmolar contrast m. (LOCM)
    macromolecular contrast m. (MMCM)
    magnesium contrast m.
    manganese chloride contrast m.
    meglumine salts contrast m.
    methylglucamine contrast m.
    Micropaque contrast m.
    MultiHance contrast m.
    nephrotoxic contrast m.
    Niopam contrast m.
    nonionic dimer contrast m.
    nonionic water-soluble contrast m.
    oil-soluble contrast m. (OSCM)
    opaque m.
    potassium bromide contrast m.
    ProHance contrast m.
    radiochromic dosimetry m.
    radiological contrast m.
    radiolucent m.
    radiopaque m.
    radiopaque contrast media (ROCM)
    rectal contrast m.
    Resovist MR contrast m.
    Solutrast 200, 250, 300, 370 contrast m.
    sonicated saline contrast m.
    tantalum-178 contrast m.
    Telebrix contrast m.
    tetraiodophenolphthalein contrast m.
    topical water-soluble contrast m.
    triiodobenzoic acid contrast m.
    Triosil contrast m.
    tunica m.
    Uromiro contrast m.
    water-soluble contrast m. (WSCM)
    Xenetix 250, 300, 350 contrast m.
medium-detachment-pressure
medium-energy collimator
medium-sized bronchus

medius
  digitus m.
  gluteus m.
  scalenus m.
MedNova
  M. Neuroshield
  M. stent
Medos Hakim programmable valve
Medrad
  M. automated power injector
  M. contrast medium injector
  M. MRInnervu endorectal colon
    probe coil
  M. power angiographic injector
medronate scan
Medsonic plethysmography
Medspec
  M. MR imaging system
  M. MR imaging system scanner
  M. 30/80 tesla MR scanner
**Med Tec Vac Loc immobilization
  system**
Medtronic
  M. catheter
  M. Minix
  M. Pulsor Intrasound
  M. radiofrequency receiver
  M. Talent prosthesis
medulla, pl. **medullae**
  adrenal m.
  hyperechoic renal m.
  lymphatic m.
  m. oblongata
  ovarian m.
  renal m.
  rostral m.
  spinal m.
medullare
  corpus m.
  osteoma m.
medullaris
  artery of conus m.
  conus arteriosus m.
  m. hypoplasia
  low conus m.
medullary
  m. artery
  m. bone
  m. bone infarct
  m. breast carcinoma
  m. calcification
  m. canal

  m. cavity
  m. cone
  m. cord
  m. cystic disease
  m. lamina
  m. nephrocalcinosis
  m. nephrogram
  m. pyramid
  m. rod
  m. sinus
  m. sponge
  m. sponge kidney
  m. tegmentum
  m. thyroid carcinoma
  m. vein
  m. venous anatomy
medullary-type adenocarcinoma
medulloblastoma
  m. metastasis
  vermian m.
medusae
  caput m.
Medusa hairlike opacity
Medweb clinical reporting system
MedX
  MedX camera
  MedX scanner
Mees line
mefenamic acid
MEG
  magnetoencephalography
megabulb
  jugular m.
megabulbus
  duodenum m.
megacalycosis
megacalyx
mega cisterna magna
megacolon
  acquired m.
  aganglionic m.
  congenital m.
  m. dilatation
  idiopathic m.
  toxic m.
megacurie (MCi)
megacystic microcolon
**megacystis-microcolon-intestinal
  hypoperistalsis syndrome**
megaduodenum
megaesophagus of achalasia
megahertz (MHz)

NOTES

megalencephaly
: unilateral m.

MEGALINK stent
megalocornea
megalocystis
megaloencephaly
megalosplenia
megalothymus
megaloureter
megalourethra
megarectum
megaureter
: primary m.
: primary congenital m.

megavolt (MeV, MV)
: m. therapy

megavoltage
: m. grid
: m. grid therapy
: m. radiation
: m. radiation therapy
: m. radiotherapy
: m. treatment beam
: m. x-ray therapy

meglumine
: m. acetrizoate
: Cholografin m.
: m. diatrizoate
: gadoterate m.
: iocarmate m.
: iodipamide m.
: m. iodipamide imaging agent
: iodoxamate m.
: m. iotroxate imaging agent
: ioxaglate m.
: m. salts contrast medium

megophthalmos
meibomian
: m. cyst
: m. gland carcinoma

Meiboom-Gill sequence
Meige lymphedema
Meigs
: M. capillary
: M. syndrome

Meigs-Cass syndrome
Meigs-Salmon syndrome
Meissner plexus
melanocytic lesion
melanoma
: vaginal malignant m.

melanosis coli
melanotic
: m. carcinoma
: m. neuroectodermal tumor
: m. whitlow

MELAS
: mitochondrial encephalomyopathy with lactic acidosis and stroke-like episodes

mellitus
: diabetes m., type 1
: diabetes m., type 2

Melnick-Needles syndrome
Melone distal radius fracture classification
melorheostosis
: m. of Leri
: soft tissue pathoanatomy in m.

Melrose solution
melting sign
Meltzer sign
memberment
membranacea
: placenta m.

membranaceous tendon
membranaceum
membrane
: amnionic m.
: atlantooccipital m.
: Bichat m.
: m. of bone
: m. closure time
: cricothyroid m.
: glial limiting m.
: glomerular basement m. (GBM)
: hourglass m.
: interosseous m. (IOM)
: intertwin m.
: intraluminal m.
: intrauterine m.
: Liliequist m.
: limiting m.
: low-flux polysufone m.
: microporous m.
: mucous m.
: obturator m.
: m. oxygenator
: m. permeability
: m. phosphate
: rolling m.
: serous m.
: Shrapnell m.
: synovial m.
: Transwell m.
: vernix m.

membranous
: m. bronchiole
: m. glomerulonephritis
: m. labyrinth
: m. obstruction of inferior vena cava
: m. pregnancy
: m. septum
: m. subaortic stenosis
: m. subvalvular aortic stenosis
: m. urethra
: m. ventricular septal defect
: m. viscerocranium

memory
> Aloka color Doppler real-time 2D
> blood flow imaging with cine m.
> thermal shape m.

memory-intensive algorithm
Memotherm Nitinol self-expandable stent
MEMP
> multiecho multiplane
> contiguous slice MEMP

MEN
> multiple endocrine neoplasia

Mendelson syndrome
Ménétrier disease
Mengert index
Menghini
Ménière
> M. disease
> M. syndrome

meningeal
> m. artery
> m. artery groove
> m. cell tumor
> m. enhancement
> m. fibroma
> m. fibrosis
> m. hemangiopericytoma
> m. hemorrhage
> m. infiltrate
> m. inflammation
> middle m.
> m. sarcoma
> m. tuberculosis
> m. vein

meninges (*pl. of* meninx)
meningioangiomatosis
meningioma
> angioplastic m.
> atypical m.
> cavernous sinus m.
> cerebellopontine angle m.
> clival m.
> convexity m.
> m. of cribriform plate
> cystic intraparenchymal m.
> ectopic m.
> endotheliomatous m.
> m. en plaque
> extracranial m.
> falcine m.
> falcotentorial m.
> fibroblastic m.

> fibrous m.
> globular m.
> intraosseous m.
> intraparenchymal m.
> intraventricular m.
> lipoblastic m.
> malignant m.
> meningothelial m.
> meningotheliomatous m.
> multicentric m.
> olfactory groove m.
> optic nerve sheath m.
> parasagittal m.
> perioptic m.
> posterior fossa m.
> m. of posterior fossa
> psammoma body m.
> psammomatous m.
> pulmonary m.
> sphenoid ridge m.
> sphenoid wing m.
> sphenoorbital m.
> spinal m.
> subfrontal m.
> suprasellar m.
> temporal m.
> tentorial m.
> transitional m.
> tuberculum sellae m.

meningiomatosis
meningitis, pl. **meningitides**
> cryptococcal m.
> fungal m.

meningocele
> anterior sacral m.
> anterior thoracic m.
> cervical m.
> cranial m.
> dorsal m.
> lateral lumbar m.
> lateral thoracic m.
> occipital m.
> occult intrasacral m.
> sacral m.
> simple m.
> traumatic m.

meningoencephalitis
meningoencephalocele
> ethmoidal m.
> sphenopharyngeal m.

meningofacial angiomatosis

NOTES

M

meningohypophysial
    m. artery
    m. trunk
meningomyelocele
meningotheliallike nodule
meningothelial meningioma
meningotheliomatous meningioma
meninx, pl. **meninges**
    m. of brain
    m. of spinal cord
meniscal
    m. cleft
    m. fragmentation
    m. horn
    m. injury
    m. ossicle
meniscocapsular
    m. attachment
    m. junction
    m. separation
meniscocondylar coordination
meniscofemoral
    m. attachment
    m. ligament
meniscosynovial junction
meniscotibial
    m. attachment
    m. ligament
    m. separation
meniscus, pl. **menisci**
    articular m.
    m. articularis
    discoid lateral m.
    diverging m.
    dysplastic m.
    fibrocartilaginous m.
    free-floating m.
    m. lateralis
    m. medialis
    radiohumeral m.
    m. sign
    m. tear
meniscus-shaped calcification
Menkes syndrome
Mennell sign
mensuration algorithm
mental
    m. canal
    m. spine
mentoanterior
mentooccipital diameter
mentoparietal diameter
Mentor prostatic biopsy needle
mentum
Menzel olivopontocerebellar degeneration
meralgia paresthetica

mercapto-acetyl-glycyl-glycyl-glycine
    technetium-99m m. (^{99m}Tc-MAG3)
mercaptoacetyltriglycine (MAG-3, MAG3)
    technetium-99m m.
Mercator
    M. atrial high-density array catheter
    M. projection
merchant
    M. angle
    M. view
Mercuhydrin
mercurihydroxypropane
1-mercuri-2-hydroxypropane (MHP)
mercury
    m. arc lamp
    m. artifact
    m. manometer
    millimeters of m. (mmHg, mm Hg)
    m. vapor lamp
mercury manometer
Meridian echocardiography
Merkel
    M. cell carcinoma
    M. cell carcinoma cell line
Merland perimedullary arteriovenous fistula classification
merlin
mermaid
    m. deformity
    m. syndrome
meroacrania
merosin
merosin-deficient congenital muscular dystrophy
mertiatide
    technetium-99m m.
mesalamine enema
mesatipellic pelvis
mesencephalic
    m. artery
    m. cerebral lymphoma
    m. cistern
    m. cistern effacement
    m. infarct
    m. low-density brain lesion
    m. reticular formation
    m. tract
    m. vein
mesencephalitis
mesencephalodiencephalic lesion
mesencephalon aqueduct
mesenchymal
    m. abnormality
    m. chondrosarcoma
    m. liver hamartoma
    m. neoplasm

m. tissue
m. tumor
mesenchymoma
atrial m.
benign m.
chest wall m.
mesenterial
m. Castleman lymphoma
m. sarcoma
mesenteric
m. adenitis
m. adenitis-ileitis complex
m. adenopathy
m. angiography
m. apoplexy
m. arterial thrombosis
m. arteriography
m. artery
m. artery occlusion
m. attachment
m. border
m. calcification
m. cyst
m. fat stranding
m. fibromatosis
m. fibrosis
m. fistula
m. infarct
m. ischemia
m. lipodystrophy
m. lymphadenopathy
m. lymph node pathology
m. lymphoma
m. mass
m. metastasis
m. node
m. panniculitis (MP)
m. phlegmon
m. pregnancy
m. rupture
m. sclerosis
superior m.
m. tear
m. thromboembolism (MTE)
m. tissue
m. triangle
m. tuberculosis
m. vascular insufficiency
m. vascular lesion
m. vascular occlusion
m. vasculitis (MV)
m. vein

m. venous thrombosis
m. vessel
m. Weber-Christian disease
mesentericoparietal fossa
mesenteritis
chronic fibrosing m.
fibrosing m.
liposclerotic m.
retractile m.
sclerosing m.
mesenterium commune
mesenteroaxial volvulus
mesentery
fan-shaped m.
fatty m.
intestinal m.
ischemic m.
leaf of m.
lymphangioma m.
root of m.
small intestine m.
ventral m.
Weber-Christian m.
mesh
stent m.
tantalum m.
tubular wire m.
mesial
m. aspect
m. frontal focus
m. hemisphere
m. hyperperfusion
m. temporal epileptogenic lesion
m. temporal sclerosis
mesial-frontal cortex
mesiodens
mesiodistal plane
mesoappendix
mesoblastic nephroma
mesocardia
mesocaval shunt
mesocephalic head shape
mesocolic
m. band
m. shelf
mesocolon
sigmoid m.
transverse m.
mesocolonic
m. fat
m. vessel
mesocuneiform bone

NOTES

mesoderm
> extraembryonic m.

mesodermal
> m. dysplasia
> m. sarcoma

mesomelia
mesomelic
> m. dwarfism
> m. dysplasia

mesometanephric carcinoma
mesonephric kidney
mesonephros, pl. **mesonephroi**
mesoporphyrine
> Bid-Gd m.

mesorectum
mesosigmoid colon
mesosternum
mesothelial cyst
mesothelioma
> asbestos-related m.
> atrioventricular nodal node m.
> benign m.
> cystic m.
> diffuse malignant peritoneal m.
> epithelioid malignant m.
> fibrosing m.
> localized fibrous m.
> malignant pleural m.
> malignant pulmonary m.
> peritoneal m.
> pleural m.

mesothorium
mesotympanum
mesoversion of heart
MESS
> multiple echo single shot

mesylate
> fenoldopam m.

metabolic
> m. alteration
> m. bone disease
> m. bone disorder
> m. bone series
> m. bone survey
> m. calculus
> m. cardiomyopathy
> m. cirrhosis
> m. lesion
> m. rate of oxygen
> m. response
> m. stone
> m. tracer uptake

metabolically inert area
metabolism
> calcium m.
> carbon m.
> cerebral m.
> evaluation of glucose m.
> fat m.

> fatty acid m.
> hepatic m.
> myocardial m.
> oxidative m.
> phosphorus m.

metacarpal
> base of m.
> m. bone
> m. fracture
> m. index
> m. length
> m. sign

metacarpoglenoidal ligament
metacarpophalangeal (MCP)
> m. articulation
> m. bone marrow development
> m. joint (MCPJ)
> m. length
> m. ligament

metacarpus
metachronous
> m. lesion
> m. metastasis
> m. transitional cell carcinoma

metadiaphysial
metadiaphysis
metaiodobenzylguanidine (MIBG)
> ^{123}I m.
> iodine-131 m.

metal
> m. chelate complex
> Co-Cr-W-Ni alloy implant m.
> lanthanide m.
> m. line-pair phantom
> Lipowitz m.
> m. oxide semiconductor (MOS)
> radioactive m.
> m. technetium target
> transition m.

metallic
> m. artifact
> m. biliary endoprosthesis
> m. cage
> m. debris
> m. density
> m. distal end of tube
> m. echo
> m. foreign body (MFB)
> m. fragment
> m. marker
> m. needle
> m. otologic implant
> m. pointer
> m. rod fixation
> m. screw
> m. staple
> m. stent
> m. suture

m. tip cannula
m. track of bullet

metalloporphyrin

metalloprotease
matrix m.-3 (MMP-3)

metanephric
m. diverticulum
m. vesicle

metanephros, pl. **metanephroi**

metaphysial, metaphyseal
m. abscess
m. chondrodysplasia
m. dysostosis
m. dysplasia
m. extension
m. fibrous defect
m. flare
m. fracture
m. lucent band
m. metaphysis

metaphysial-diaphysial
m.-d. angle
m.-d. junction
m.-d. low-signal-intensity red
marrow inhomogeneity

metaphysial-epiphysial angle

metaphysis, pl. **metaphyses**
agnogenic myeloid m.
autoparenchymatous m.
celomic m.
columnar m.
frayed m.
fundic m.
humeral m.
intestinal m.
metaphysial m.
myeloid m.
primary myeloid m.
secondary myeloid m.
squamous m.

metaplasia
agnogenic myeloid m.
apocrine m.
articular m.
cartilaginous m.
intestinal m.
keratinizing squamous m.
monarticular synovium-based
cartilage m.
osseous m.
osteocartilaginous m.
squamous m.

metaplastic
m. carcinoma
m. polyp

metapneumonic
m. empyema
m. pleurisy

metastable
m. radionuclide
m. state
m. trap

metastasis, pl. **metastases**
adnexal m.
adrenal m.
aortic node m.
axillary node m.
blastic m.
bone m.
brain m.
breast m.
calcareous m.
calcified ovarian metastases
calcifying m.
carcinomatous cavitary m.
cavitary m.
cavitating lung m.
celiac lymph node m.
cerebral m.
clivus m.
cystic m.
diffuse skeletal m.
distant m.
drop m.
echogenic liver m.
endobronchial m.
extracapsular m.
extrahepatic m. (EHM)
extrathoracic m.
gastric m.
hemorrhagic m.
hepatic m.
hypervascular liver m.
inguinal lymph node m.
intracranial m.
in-transit m.
intraparenchymal m.
kidney m.
leptomeningeal m.
liver m.
local m.
lung m.
lymphangitic m.
lymphatic m.

NOTES

M

metastasis *(continued)*
    lymphogenous m.
    magnetic resonance discriminator of osseous m.
    medulloblastoma m.
    mesenteric m.
    metachronous m.
    micronodular m.
    MR discriminator of osseous m.
    necrotic m.
    neuroendocrine hepatic m.
    nodal m.
    occult bone m.
    orbital m.
    osseous m.
    osteoblastic m.
    osteolytic m.
    osteolytic osseous m.
    ovarian m.
    "overcalling" m.
    m. to the pancreas
    pancreatic m.
    paracardiac m.
    parasellar m.
    parenchymal brain m.
    peritoneal m.
    placental m.
    pleura m.
    pulmonary m.
    pulsating m.
    renal m.
    satellite m.
    skeletal m.
    skip m.
    small bowel m.
    solitary sternal m.
    sphenoid sinus m.
    spinal cord m.
    splenic m.
    testicular m.
    uterine sarcoma m.
    Virchow m.
    white m.
    widespread m.
metastasizing fibroleiomyoma
metastatic
    m. adenocarcinoma
    m. adenopathy
    m. axillary involvement
    m. bone survey
    m. carcinoid syndrome
    m. disease
    m. focus
    m. lesion
    m. malignancy
    m. myocardial tumor
    m. osteosarcoma
    m. pleomorphic liposarcoma
    m. polyp

    m. renal neoplasm
    m. rhabdomyosarcoma
    m. seeding
    m. site
    m. soft tissue calcification
    m. testicular lymphoma
    m. urothelial carcinoma
metasynchronous tumor
metatarsal
    m. angle
    angle of declination of m.
    m. axis
    m. bone
    m. fracture
    m. head
    m. head width (MHW)
    m. injury
    m. joint
    m. length ratio
    m. parabola
    m. synostosis
metatarsocalcaneal angle
metatarsocuneiform
    m. joint
    m. joint fusion
metatarsophalangeal (MT, MTP)
    m. bone marrow development
    m. capsule
    m. joint
    m. joint arthritis
    m. joint fusion
metatarsotalar angle
metatarsus
    m. adductocavus deformity
    m. adductovarus deformity
    m. adductus
    m. adductus angle
    m. adductus deformity
    m. atavicus deformity
    m. latus deformity
    m. primus varus angle (MPVA)
    m. primus varus deformity
    m. valgus
    m. varus
    m. varus deformity
metatrophic
    m. dwarfism
    m. dysplasia
metencephalon
meter (m)
    analog rate m.
    counting rate m.
    dose-area product m.
    exposure m.
    Gammex RMI DAP m.
    Geiger-Müller survey m.
    kVp m.
    m.'s per second (MPS, mps, m/sec)

photovolt pH m.
rate m. (R-meter)
roentgen m.
roentgen(s) (per) hour (at one) m.
  (rhm, Rhm)
methemoglobin effect
methiodal sodium imaging agent
methionine
  ^{11}C m.
method
  acoustic reflection m.
  Agatston calcium scoring m.
  AIPH m.
  Andren m.
  Arelin m.
  attenuation in phantom m. (AIPH)
  autoattenuation correction m.
  automated airway tree
    segmentation m.
  Ball m.
  Bayler-Pinneau m.
  Benassi m.
  Benedict-Talbot body surface
    area m.
  Bertel m.
  Bigliani and Morrison m.
  black blood m.
  Blackett-Healy m.
  blood oxygen level-dependent
    fMRI m.
  border detection m. (BDM)
  Borell and Fernström m.
  Born m.
  Brasdor m.
  Bull m.
  Caldwell m.
  calibration m.
  Cameron m.
  CHESS m.
  chunk acquisition and
    reconstruction m. (CHARM)
  Clauss m.
  Cleaves m.
  Cobb m.
  Colbert m.
  column extraction m.
  computer m.
  deconvolution m.
  destroy and replace m.
  2DFT m.
  double-echo m.
  downstream sampling m.

dual-balloon m.
2-dye m.
echo-planar imaging m.
electrocardiographic trigger m.
ellipsoid m.
empirical m.
error diffusion m.
extraction m.
FBP m.
Ferguson m.
FI m.
Fick m.
filtered back-projection m.
fractal-based m.
Friedman m.
full-scan m.
Gaynor-Hart m.
Gerota m.
gradient-echo m.
Graf m.
Grashey m.
Greulich and Pyle m.
Haas m.
Hawkins m.
Hickey m.
inflow/outflow m.
in vivo m.
IPSP neuron evaluation m.
isocenter shift m.
isodose shift m.
Joliot m.
Kauppi m.
Kety-Schmidt m.
keyhole m.
KWE m.
Lawrence m.
Levenberg-Marquardt m.
Lysholm m.
Mankin m.
Meyerding m.
Monte Carlo m.
multiple-line scanning m.
multiple-sensitive-point m.
multisection m.
paddle wheel m.
parallax m.
Pearson m.
Pelizzari surface matching m.
m. of perpendiculars
Pfeiffer-Comberg m.
phase-inversion m.
phase-unwrapping m.

M

NOTES

method *(continued)*
    Pirie m.
    pixel count m.
    Porcher m.
    Powell m.
    pulse-echo m.
    radioimmunoassay m.
    radiotracer foil m.
    Ranawat m.
    ray-casting m.
    receiver operating characteristic m.
    ROC m.
    rotational m.
    Sansregret m.
    m. of Scarpa
    segmentation m.
    selective excitation m.
    selective saturation m.
    SENSE m.
    sensitivity encoding m.
    Settegast m.
    short-cannula coaxial m.
    simulated annealing m.
    spin-label m.
    spin-warp m.
    spiral imaging m.
    Strickler m.
    sum-peak m.
    surface coil m.
    surface normal overlap m.
    Sweet m.
    Thom m.
    thresholding m.
    time-of-flight m.
    triangulation m.
    TRICKS m.
    ultrashort m.
    under-scan m.
    Valdini m.
    vertebral body ratio m.
    volume-ratio m.
    Wolf m.
    Zimmer m.
methodology
    Gehan m.
methoxyisobutyl
    m. isonitrile
    m. isonitrile SPECT
methoxyisobutylisonitrile
    technetium-99m m. (^{99m}Tc-MIBI)
methoxystaurosporine
    ^{11}C m.
methyl
    m. methacrylate bead
    m. methacrylate bead implant
    m. methacrylate imaging agent
    m. proton
methyl-ABV
methylcellulose gel

methylene
    m. blue enema
    m. diphosphonate (MDP)
    m. diphosphonate (MDP) concentration
methylglucamine
    m. contrast medium
    m. diatrizoate
    iodipamide m.
***N*-methylspiperone**
***N*-methylspiroperidol (NMS)**
    ^{11}C *N*-m.
methylsulfate
    neostigmine m.
metopic suture
MET-PET
    ^{11}C-methionine positron emission tomography
    MET-PET scan
metrics
    histogram-derived m.
metrizamide
    m. computed tomography cisternography (MCTC)
    m. CT cisternogram
    m. imaging agent
    m. myelography
    m. ventriculogram
metrizamide-assisted computed tomography (CTMM)
metrizoate
    m. imaging agent
metrizoic acid
metrography
metroperitoneal fistula
metroplasty
metrosalpingography
mets
    metastases
Metz
    M. filter
    M. spatially varying filter
MeV
    megavolt
    million electron volt
Mewissen infusion catheter
Meyer
    M. dysplasia
    M. line
    M. loop
    supratubercular ridge of M.
Meyer-Archambault loop
Meyerding method
Meyer-McKeever tibial fracture classification
Meynet node
MF
    magnification factor

mf
  microfarad
MFB
  metallic foreign body
MFG
  magnetic field gradient
  manofluorography
MFH
  malignant fibrous histiocytoma
    giant cell-type MFH
    inflammatory MFH
    myxoid MFH
    postirradiation MFH
    storiform-pleomorphic MFH
MFH-B
  malignant fibrous histiocytoma of bone
mFISP
  mirrored FISP
MG
  Millenium MG
m/h
  midbrain-hindbrain
MHP
  1-mercuri-2-hydroxypropane
MH-908 slim ultrasonic probe
MHV
  middle hepatic vein
MHW
  metatarsal head width
MHz
  megahertz
  250 M. crossed-loop resonator
MI
  mitral insufficiency
  myocardial infarct
    inferior wall MI
MIBG
  metaiodobenzylguanidine
  MIBG scintigraphy
  MIBG SPECT scan
  MIBG washout
MIC
  MIC gastroenteric tube
  MIC jejunal tube
  MIC transgastric jejunal feeding
    tube
micaceous
mica pneumoconiosis
Michaelis
  M. complex
  rhomboid of M.
Michaelis-Gutmann body

Michel
  M. anomaly
  M. aplasia
  M. deformity
  M. malformation
Michels classification
Mickey
  M. Mouse appearance
  M. Mouse ears pelvis
MIC-Key low profile transgastric-jejunal feeding tube
Mick seed applicator
Mi-Cr
  myoinositol-creatine ratio
micrencephaly, micrencephalia
microabscess
  m. of spleen
  splenic m.
microadenoma
  adrenocorticotropin m.
  ectopic intracavernous pituitary m.
  pituitary m.
microaggregated albumin
microaneurysm
  Charcot-Bouchard intracerebral m.
  retinal m.
microangioarchitecture
microangiogram
microangiography
microangiopathy
  mineralizing m.
  thrombotic m.
microangioscopy
microarchitecture
  bone m.
microarteriography
microatelectasis
micro-AVM
  cerebral microarteriovenous malformation
  single-shot embolization of micro-AVM
microballoon
  Rand m.
microbubble
  m. concentration measurement
  m. contrast enhancement
  intranasal m.
  sonicated albumin m.
microbubble-based contrast agent
microbubble-enhanced CDUS
microcalcification
  breast m.

NOTES

M

microcalcification *(continued)*
    m. cluster
    coarse m.
    ductal breast m.
    granular m.
    linear branching m.
    lobular breast m.
    pleomorphic m.
    psammomatous m.
    sole cluster of m.
    subtle m.
microcalculus
microcardia
Micro-Cast collimator
microcatheter
    AngiOptic m.
    ball-tip m.
    Cardima Pathfinder m.
    Excel-14 m.
    Excelsior m.
    3F m.
    Flow Rider m.
    1.8-French m.
    2.1-French m.
    Hieshima m.
    Leggiero hydrophilic-coated m.
    Microferret m.
    20-mm Equinox balloon m.
    Rapidtransit m.
    Rapid Transit m.
    Renegade m.
    Renegade Hi-Flo m.
    Tracer m.
    Tracker 10 m.
microcavitation
microcinematography
microcirculation
    m. abnormality
    pulmonary m.
microcirculatory blood flow
microcluster
    biodegradable magnetic m.
microcoil
    complex platinum m.
    Dacron-coated m.
    Hilal m.
    Intercept esophagus m.
    Intercept prostate m.
    Intercept urethra m.
    platinum m.
microcolon
    megacystic m.
microcomputed tomography
microconidia
micro-crust formation lesion
microCT-20 scanner
micro-CT imaging
microcurie (μCi)

microcyst
    milk-of-calcium m.
microcystic
    m. adenoma
    m. degeneration
    m. encephalomalacia
    m. formation
    m. lumbar spine
    m. pancreatic tumor
    m. pilocytic cerebellar astrocytoma
microcystica
microcytosis
microdactylia
microdistribution
    heterogeneous m.
microdosimetry
microemboli (*pl. of* microembolus)
microembolism
    cerebral m.
microembolization
    ferromagnetic m.
microembolus, pl. **microemboli**
    showers of microemboli
microendoscope
    ophthalmic laser m. (OLM)
microenvironment
    bone marrow m.
microerosion
microexplosion lithotripsy
microextension
microfarad (mf)
Microferret microcatheter
microfibrillar collagen
microfixation plate
microfluidization
microfocal
    m. direct magnification in vitro x-ray tube
    m. spot mammography
microform of holoprosencephaly
microfracture
    subchondral m.
    trabecular m.
microgastria
microglandular adenosis
microglioma
microglobulin labeling
micrognathia
Micro-Guide
microhamartoma
    biliary m.
microimaging
microinfarct
microkymatotherapy
microlaparoscope
    Imagyn m.
Microlase transpupillary diode laser
microlattice
    cerebral vascular m.

microlesion
Microlight 830 laser
microlith
microlithiasis
    alveolar m.
    pulmonary alveolar m.
    testicular m.
microlobular cirrhosis
microlobulation
micromanometer-tipped catheter
MicroMark tissue marker
micromelia
    bowed m.
    extreme m.
micromelic
    m. dwarfism
    m. dysplasia
micrometallic artifact
micrometastasis
    systemic m.
micrometer
MicroMewi multiple sidehole infusion
  catheter
micro-MRI with FIESTA
micron
micronester platinum embolization coil
micronodular
    m. cirrhosis
    m. infiltrate
    m. metastasis
    m. pattern
micronodularity
micronodule
    centrilobular m.
    peribronchial m.
    subpleural m.
micron-resolution retinal image in vivo
micropapillary
    m. carcinoma
    m. DCIS
    m. lesion
    m. tumor
Micropaque contrast medium
microperforation
micropipette, micropipet
microplate reader
microporous membrane
Microprobe laser
microprolactinoma
micropuncture needle
microradiogram
microradiography

microreentrant circuit
microroentgen
microsatellite instability
microscintigraphy
microscope
    multimode imaging confocal
      optical m. (MIMCOM)
    projection x-ray m.
    scanning acoustic m. (SAM)
    scanning electron m. (SEM)
    video-rate two-photon laser
      scanning m.
    x-ray m.
    x-ray tomographic m. (XTM)
microscopic
    m. air bubble
    m. cortical dysplasia
    m. hemorrhage of ligament
    m. imaging
    m. polyangiitis
microscopy
    darkfield m.
    3D magnetic resonance m.
    electron m.
    fluorescence m.
    immune electron m.
    light m.
    polarized light m.
    ultrasound backscatter m. (UBM)
    in vivo m.
microsecond pulsed flashlamp pumped
  dye laser
microSelectron-HDR
microSelectron rapid delivery system
microsnare
microsomia
    hemifacial m.
microsphere
    acrylic m.
    calibrated tris-acryl gelatin m.
    Contour SE m.
    degradable starch m.
    EmboGold m.
    Embosphere m.
    ferromagnetic m.
    hollow albumin m.
    human albumin m.
    m. perfusion scintigraphy
    silicone m.
    sodium acrylate and vinyl alcohol
      copolymer m. (SAP-MS)
    stainless steel m.

M

NOTES

microsphere *(continued)*
    superabsorbent polymer m. (SAP-MS)
    superparamagnetic m.
    technetium-99m albumin m.
    technetium-99m human albumin m.
    tris-acryl gelatin m. (TAGM)
    trisacryl gelatin m.
    ^{90}Y m.
    ytterbium-90 m.
    yttrium-90 m.
microstructural architecture
microstructure
    3-dimensional trabecular bone m.
micro tear
Microtek ScanMaker 9600XL scanner
microtomography
    view m.
MicroTrach
    Heimlich M.
Microtrast
microtrauma
    repetitive m.
Microtron accelerator
microvascular
    m. circulation
    m. decompression
    m. disease
    m. retrieval
microvasculature
    pulmonary m.
microvenoarteriolar fistula
microvesicular fat
microvessel
    intraparenchymal m.
microvolt (μV)
microwave
    m. ablation
    m. cardiac ablation system
    m. coagulation therapy
    m. endometrial ablation (MEA)
    m. hyperthermia
    m. hyperthermia treatment
    m. imaging
    m. nonsurgical treatment
    m. therapy
    m. tumor coagulation
micturating
    m. cystourethrogram (MCU)
    m. cystourethrography
micturition cystourethrography
midabdominal wall
midaortic
    m. arch
    m. syndrome (MAS)
midarterial phase
midaxillary line
midbody of vertebra

midbrain
    m. aqueduct
    m. function
    m. lesion
    m. reticular formation (MRF)
    m. tegmentum
midbrain-hindbrain (m/h)
    m.-h. junction
midcarpal
    m. compartment
    m. dislocation
    m. instability
    m. joint
    m. joint cavity
midcircumflex
midclavicular
    m. line (MCL)
    m. plane
midcolon
midcoronal
    m. oblique image
    m. plane
middiastole
middistal
middle
    m. aortic syndrome
    m. cardiac vein
    m. cerebral artery (MCA)
    m. cerebral artery bifurcation
    m. cerebral artery fenestration
    m. cerebral artery infarct
    m. cerebral artery occlusion
    m. coronary sinus (MCS)
    m. cranial fossa
    m. cuneiform bone
    m. ear
    m. ear choristoma
    m. ear mass
    m. ear neoplasm
    m. extrahepatic bile duct
    m. facet of the subtalar joint
    m. finger
    m. fossa syndrome
    m. frontal gyrus
    m. hepatic vein (MHV)
    m. lobe (ML)
    m. lobe bronchus
    m. lobe syndrome
    m. mediastinal mass
    m. mediastinum
    m. meningeal
    m. meningeal artery
    m. meningeal artery groove
    m. muscle
    m. palatine suture
    m. perforating collagen bundle
    m. pole
    m. pulmonary lobe atelectasis
    m. rectal vein

m. temporal gyrus
m. third shaft
m. third of thoracic esophagus
m. turbinate bone
middle-caliber needle
middle-field-strength MR imaging
middorsal
midepigastrium
midesophageal diverticulum
midesophagus
midexpiratory tidal flow
midface
fetal m.
m. retrusion
midfacial fracture
midfemur
midfoot fracture
midfrontal
m. plane
m. plane coronal section
midget MRI scanner
midgraft stenosis
midgroove portion of lumen
midgut
m. volvulus
m. volvulus with malrotation
midhumeral line
midinfrared laser
midinguinal point
midlateral course
midleft sternal border
midline
m. of brain cyst
m. cerebellum
m. cystic structure
m. echoencephalograph
m. granuloma
m. herniation of disc
m. incense presentation
infracolic m.
m. lesion
m. longitudinal pontine cleft
m. malignant reticulosis
m. mucosa-sparing block
m. parasagittal focus
m. shift
midlung
m. field
m. zone
midmarginal branch

midpalmar
m. abscess
m. space
midpapillary short axis
midpatellar tendon
midpelvis
midplane
m. depth
m. sagittal image
midpole
midportion
midsagittal
m. diameter (MSD)
m. MR image
m. MR imaging
m. plane
midscapular line
midshaft fracture
midshunt peak velocity (MSPv)
midsigmoid colon
midspinal line
midsternal
m. area
m. line
midsternum
midsystolic
m. buckling of mitral valve
m. notching of velocity spectrum
m. retraction
midtarsal
m. injury
m. joint
midthalamic plane
midthigh amputation
midthoracic spine
midventricular short-axis slice
midwaist scaphoid fracture
midzonal necrosis
midzone
Miescher granulomatosis
Mignon granuloma
migrainous scintillation
migration
m. abnormality
m. of acetabular cup
bowel m.
catheter m.
coil m.
m. disorder
embolus m.
gallstone m.
hallux m.

M

NOTES

migration *(continued)*
  m. index
  neuronal m.
  placenta m.
  sesamoid m.
  stent m.
  tissue m.
migrational
  m. anomaly
  m. pattern
migratory
  m. patchy infiltrate
  m. pneumonia
Mikity-Wilson syndrome
Mikulicz
  M. angle
  M. disease
  M. syndrome
Milch
  M. classification of humeral
    fracture
  M. elbow fracture classification
mild
  m. edema
  m. head injury
  m. recess
  m. subcostal retraction
  m. traumatic brain injury
mildly enlarged heart
Miles operation
miliary
  m. aneurysm
  m. embolus
  m. granuloma
  m. lesion
  m. lung disease
  m. nodule
  m. parenchymal disease
  m. pattern
  m. pulmonary tuberculosis
military antishock trousers (MAST)
milk
  m. of calcium
  m. of calcium urinary tract cyst
  m. leg syndrome
  m. teeth
milk-alkali syndrome
milkmaid's
  m. elbow
  m. elbow dislocation
milkman's
  m. fracture
  m. pseudofracture
Milkman syndrome
milk-of-calcium
  m.-o.-c. calcification
  m.-o.-c. microcyst
milky effusion
Millar catheter-tip transducer

Millenium MG
millennium
  M. VG SPECT system
Miller
  M. double mushroom biliary stent
  M. index
  M. position
Miller-Abbott tube
Miller-Dieker syndrome
miller's lung
millicurie (mCi)
millicurie-hour (mCi-hr)
millimeter (mm)
  m.'s of mercury (mmHg, mm Hg)
millimole (mmol)
million electron volt (MeV)
millirad (mrad)
millirem (mrem)
milliroentgen (mR, mr)
millisecond (msec)
millivolt (mV)
Milroy disease
Milwaukee shoulder syndrome
MIMCOM
  multimode imaging confocal optical
    microscope
MIMIC
  multivane intensity modulation
    compensator
mimic
mimicked
mimicker of malignancy
mimicking
mimosa pattern
Minaar classification of coalition
minced rib
mind-body interaction
mineralization
  bone m.
  matrix m.
  stippled m.
mineralizing microangiopathy
mineralocorticoid secretion
mineral oil imaging agent
miner's lung
miniature
  m. imaging
  m. stomach
  m. uterine cavity
miniaturized mitral valve
Mini-Balloon system
Mini 6000 C-arm
minicholecystostomy
minicoil
minification
minimal
  m. deformation target (MDT)
  m. intensity projection (minIP)
  m. interstitial thickening

m. luminal diameter (MLD)
m. port diameter (MPD)
m. volume

minimally
m. attenuating medical-grade foam
m. displaced fracture
m. invasive access set
m. invasive endovascular stent
placement
m. invasive osteoplasty
m. invasive saline enhanced RFA

minimi
flexor digiti m.
opponens digiti m.

minimicroaggregated albumin colloid
minimizing bias
minimum
m. basis set magnetic resonance
angiography (MBS-MRA)
m. blood pressure
m. intensity projection image
m. intensity projection imaging
m. pixel density
m. tolerance dose

minimum-intensity sliding thin slab
projection
minimus
digitus m.
gluteus m.
scalenus m.
m. scalenus muscle

minIP
minimal intensity projection

Minix
Medtronic M.

Mink-Deutsch classification
Minnesota tube
minor
m. calyx
m. duodenal papilla
m. fissure
globus m.
m. muscle
rhomboid m.
M. sign
teres m.

Minot-von Willebrand syndrome
minus, pl. **minora**
omentum m.

minuscule
minus-density artifact

minute
m. bleeding ulcer
blood volume per m.
cycle per m. (cpm)
rotations per m. (rpm)
m. ventilation
m. vessel
m. volume

minute-sequence study
MION
monocrystalline iron oxide nanoparticle

MIOP
magnetic iron oxide particle

MIP
macrophage inflammatory protein
maximum intensity pixel
maximum intensity projection
MIP algorithm
MIP image
MIP image processing
MIP reconstruction

MIR
MIR guideline
MIR intrauterine tandem
MIR system

mirabile
rete m.

Miraluma
M. injection
M. nuclear scan of breast
M. scan

MIRD
medical internal radiation dose
medical internal radiation dosimetry

Mirizzi syndrome
mirror
beam-splitting m.
m. image
m. image aneurysm
m. image reversal
m. imaging
polygon m.

mirrored FISP (mFISP)
mirror-image
m.-i. artifact
m.-i. brachiocephalic branching
m.-i. interpretation

mirrorlike echo
misalign
misalignment
cytoskeletal m.
neurofilamentous m.

M

NOTES

miscible pool
miscommunication
    neural m.
Miser tube
misery perfusion
misinterpretation
misleading
    m. image
    m. imaging
mismapping
    phase m.
mismatch
    diffusion-perfusion m.
    FDG-blood flow m.
    flow-function m.
    perfusion-metabolism m.
    ventilation-perfusion m.
    V/Q m.
misplaced thoracentesis
misregistration
    anatomic m.
    m. artifact
    local m.
    oblique flow m.
missed
    m. bronchogenic carcinoma
    m. testicular torsion
missile
    m. effect
    m. wound
missing pulse steady-state free
  precession sequence
mistiness of pericolonic fat
Mitchell classification
Mitek bone anchor
mitochondrial
    m. ATP production
    m. encephalomyopathy
    m. encephalomyopathy with lactic
    acidosis and stroke-like episodes
    (MELAS)
    m. function
    m. genome
    m. uncoupler
mitosis-karyorrhexis index (MKI)
mitral
    m. apparatus
    m. arcade
    m. component
    m. configuration of cardiac shadow
    m. deceleration slope
    m. flow velocity index
    m. inflow velocity
    m. insufficiency (MI)
    m. leaflet
    m. leak
    m. orifice (MO)
    posterior m. (PM)
    m. regurgitant signal area

m. regurgitation (MR)
m. regurgitation artifact
m. ring calcification
m. stenosis (MS)
m. valve
m. valve of anulus
m. valve area (MVA)
m. valve atresia
m. valve calcification
m. valve commissure
m. valve cusp
m. valve deformity
m. valve echocardiography
m. valve echogram
m. valve flow
m. valve gradient
m. valve incompetence
m. valve leaflet systolic prolapse
m. valve leaflet tip
m. valve myxomatous degeneration
m. valve opening (MVO)
m. valve orifice (MVO)
m. valve prolapse (MVP)
m. valve regurgitation
m. valve replacement (MVR)
m. valve ring
m. valve septal separation
m. valve stenosis (MVS)
m. valve systolic anterior motion
mitralization
Mitsuyasu staging system
mixed
    m. aneurysm
    m. attenuation mass
    m. cell sarcoma
    m. connective-tissue disease
    (MCTD)
    m. density mass
    m. echogenic solid mass
    m. fat-water breast lesion density
    m. fat-water density lesion
    m. gonadal dysgenesis
    m. hernia
    m. IUGR
    m. lymphocytic-histiocytic
    lymphoma
    m. lytic and sclerotic pattern
    m. petal-fugal flow
    m. rheumatoid and degenerative
    arthritis
    m. sclerotic and lytic bone lesion
    m. sclerotic osteolysis
    m. signal mass
    m. small and large cell lymphoma
    m. solid-cystic mass
    m. venous blood
    m. venous-lymphatic malformation
    m. venous saturation
mixed-echo appearance

mixed-echoic
mixing
    intracardiac m.
mixture
    barium m.
    Ingenor silicone m.
    injectable procoagulant m.
MKI
    mitosis-karyorrhexis index
ML
    middle lobe
    ML 700 daylight processor
MLC
    multileaf collimator
MLD
    minimal luminal diameter
MLF
    medial longitudinal fasciculus
    MLF lesion
MLO
    mediolateral oblique
MLS
    multiple line scan
MLSI
    multiple line scan imaging
ML-Ultra balloon stent
mm
    millimeter
MMCM
    macromolecular contrast medium
MMEF
    maximum midexpiratory flow
MMFR
    maximum midexpiratory flow rate
mmHg, mm Hg
    millimeters of mercury
M-mode
    motion mode
    M-mode cardiography
    M-mode display
    M-mode echocardiogram imaging
    M-mode echocardiography
    M-mode echophonocardiography
    M-mode scanning
    M-mode sector transducer
    M-mode time motion scan
    M-mode ultrasound
mmol
    millimole
MMP-3
    matrix metalloprotease-3

MMR
    mobile mass x-ray
Mn
    manganese
MnDPDP
    mangafodipir trisodium
    MnDPDP enhanced MRI
Mn-TPPS$_4$
    manganese tetrasodium-meso-tetra
MO
    mitral orifice
Mo
    molybdenum
^{99}Mo
    molybdenum-99
MoAb
    ^{131}I-labeled human MoAb
    radiolabeled MoAb
Moberg-Gedda fracture
Mobetron
    M. electron beam system
    M. intraoperative radiation therapy
      treatment system
mobile
    m. artery and vein imaging system
      (MAVIS)
    cecum m.
    cor m.
    m. duodenum
    m. fat ball
    m. fluoroscopy
    m. gallbladder
    m. imaging procedure
    m. intraluminal gallbladder mass
    m. magnetic resonance
    m. mass x-ray (MMR)
    m. radiography
    m. spiral computed tomography
      scanner
    m. thrombus
    m. without recapture
    m. with recapture
mobility film
Mobin-Uddin umbrella endoluminal
    device
MobiTrak
    M. automated table
    M. moving table
MOD
    Multi-Operatory Dentalaser
modality
    cross-sectional m.

NOTES

M

modality (*continued*)
    diagnostic m.
    multislice m.
    neuroimaging m.
    optimal m.
    m. performed procedure step
      (MPPS)
    tomographic m.
modal velocity
mode
    AAI rate-responsive m.
    m. abandonment
    active m.
    asynchronous transfer m. (ATM)
    blink m.
    brightness m.
    byte m.
    cine m.
    coincidence detection m.
    continuous m.
    decay m.
    dispersion m.
    dual-demand pacing m.
    DVI m.
        digital vascular imaging
    electron-capture decay m.
    full three-dimensional m.
    full-to-empty VAD m.
    fundamental Doppler m.
    high spatial resolution m.
    high temporal resolution m.
    imaginary m.
    inactive m.
    magnet m.
    modified two-dimensional
      acquisition m.
    motion m. (M-mode)
    multiplanar m.
    multislice m.
    noncommitted m.
    pulsed m.
    road-mapping m.
    semicommitted m.
    sequential m.
    step-and-shoot m.
    stimulated echo acquisition m.
      (STEAM)
    stimulation m.
    triggered-flow m.
    triggered pacing m.
    underdrive m.
    unipolar pacing m.
    volume m.
    volume rendered m.
model
modeling
    compartmental m.
    3D m.
    electromagnetic m.

    Monte Carlo m.
    thermal m.
    ultrasonographic m.
    vascular and airway m.
moderately dilated ureter
moderate sedation
moderate-sized volume joint effusion
moderator band
modest caliber
Modic disc abnormality classification
modification
    thiol m.
modified
    m. Bernoulli equation
    m. bird-cage coil
    m. Blalock-Taussig shunt patency
    m. electron-beam CT scanner
    m. linear accelerator
    m. linear accelerator radiosurgery
    m. projection
    m. SENSE (mSENSE)
    m. Simpson rule
    m. stage exercise
    m. two-dimensional acquisition
      mode
    m. vessel image processor software
modiolus, pl. **modioli**
modular stent graft
modulation
    amplitude m. (A-mod)
    brightness m.
    image m.
    object m.
    off-center m.
    print reflectance m.
    specific m.
    m. transfer function (MTF)
module
    detecting m.
    E-TOF detecting m.
    tube geometry m.
Modulith SL 20 lithotripter
modulus image
mogul
    cardiac m.
    fourth m.
    third cardiac m.
Mohn-Wriedt brachydactyly
Mohr syndrome
moiety, pl. **moieties**
    upper pole m.
moiré
    m. fringe
    m. fringes artifact
    m. pattern
    m. photography
molal solution
molar
    m. mass

m. pregnancy
m. teeth
m. tooth appearance
m. tooth configuration
m. tooth fracture
m. tooth malformation
m. tooth midbrain-hindbrain
malformation
m. volume
mold
filter m.
molded immobilizer
molding
atheroma m.
m. of skull
molecular
m. coincidence detection (MCD)
m. diffusion
m. marker
m. recognition unit (MRU)
m. vibration
m. weight dependence of relaxation
molecule
accessory adhesion m.
costimulatory m.
homing m.
intracellular adhesion m.
signaling m.
molecule-1
vascular cell adhesion m.-1
(VCAM-1)
molle
fibroma m.
heloma m.
papilloma m.
molluscum, pl. **mollusca**
fibroma m.
m. fibrosum
Molnar disc
Molteno
M. double plate drainage device
M. single plate drainage device
molybdenum (Mo)
m. anode
m. target
m. target tube
molybdenum-99 (^{99}Mo)
m. breakthrough test
m. generator
molybdenum-molybdenum target filter combination (Mo-Mo)

molybdenum-rhodium target filter combination (Mo-Rh)
molybdenum-technetium generator
moment
macroscopic magnetic m.
magnetic dipole m.
nuclear magnetic m.
quadrupole m.
zeroth m.
momentum
angular m.
Mo-Mo
molybdenum-molybdenum target filter
combination
monarticular
m. process
m. synovium-based cartilage
metaplasia
Mönckeberg
M. arteriosclerosis
M. calcification
M. degeneration
Mondini
M. anomaly
M. dysplasia
M. malformation
Mondor disease
Mongolian spotlike lesion
mongoloid feature
moniliasis
moniliform ectasia
monitor
actocardiotocograph m.
Acuson V5M m.
air m.
Appraise m.
beam m.
Biotrack coagulation m.
blood perfusion m. (BPM)
Brilliance 109 MP PC m.
cardiac m.
Doppler blood flow m.
Doppler ultrasonic fetal heart m.
FreeDop Doppler m.
gray-scale m.
HeartView CT cardiac m.
Life-Pack 5 cardiac m.
MyoTrac EMG m.
MyoTrac 2 EMG m.
N-Cat N-500 tonometric blood
pressure m.
Nicolet Elite Doppler m.

M

NOTES

monitor *(continued)*
OnLine ABG m.
OxiFirst fetal oxygen m.
Polar Vantage XL heart rate m.
Propaq Encore vital signs m.
Pulse Pro heart rate m.
radiation beam m.
tonometric blood pressure m.
m. unit
monitoring
electrode m.
periprocedural m.
photoplethysmographic m.
ultrasound m.
video electroencephalography m.
whole-body dose m.
monoamine oxidase
monoarticular
monochorionic
m. diamniotic twin pregnancy
m. monoamniotic twin pregnancy
monochorionic-monoamniotic twin
monochromatic
m. synchrotron
m. synchrotron radiation
m. x-ray
m. x-ray beam
monochromatization
monoclonal
m. antibody imaging agent
m. gammopathy
monocrystalline iron oxide nanoparticle (MION)
monocuspid tilting disc valve
monocusp valve
monocyte
monodactylism
monodermal dermoid
monodisc
monodisperse iodinated macromolecular blood pool agent
monoenergetic radiation
Monoject hypodermic needle
monomalleolar fracture
monomelic bone lesion
monomer
ionic m.
nonionic triiodinated m.
monophasic
monophosphate
cyclic adenosine m.
cyclic guanosine m.
monopolar
m. electrode
m. radiofrequency electrocautery
Monopty
M. core biopsy
M. needle
monoradicular filling defect

Monorail
Carotid-Wallstent M.
M. Wallstent self-expanding stent
monorchia
monosomy X
monostotic
m. fibrous dysplasia
m. Paget disease
monotherapy
monoventricle
monoxide
carbon m.
^{11}C carbon m.
monozygotic twin
Monro
M. aqueduct
M. bursa
foramen of M.
Monroe-Kellie doctrine
mons pubis
Monte
M. Carlo calculation
M. Carlo method
M. Carlo modeling
M. Carlo photon transport (MCPT)
M. Carlo photon transport simulation
M. Carlo technique
Monteggia
M. dislocation
M. fracture
M. fracture-dislocation
M. lesion
Montercaux fracture
Montgomery gland
Moore fracture
morcellation
morcellator
Diva laparoscopic m.
morcellized bone
Morgagni
M. appendix
column of M.
M. crypt
M. foramen
M. hernia
M. hydatid
hyperostosis of M.
M. lacuna
M. nodule
sinus of M.
M. syndrome
tubercle of M.
M. ventricle
Morgagni-Adams-Stokes syndrome
morgagnian cyst
Mo-Rh
molybdenum-rhodium target filter combination

Morison pouch
morphine-augmented study
morphine sulfate scintigraphy
morphologic
    m. correlation
    m. criterion
    m. filtering
    m. growth
    m. imaging
    m. left ventricle
    m. and physiologic image
      coregistration
morphologically normal
morphologic imaging
morphology
    disc m.
    enhancement m.
    joint m.
    ovarian m.
    residuum m.
    spine m.
morphometric
    m. measurement
    m. x-ray absorptiometry
morphometry
    MRI m.
    pelvic m.
Morquio
    M. sign
    M. syndrome
Morquio-Brailsford syndrome
morrhuate
    sodium m.
Morris point
mortise
    ankle m.
    ball-and-socket ankle m.
    m. of bone
    cuneiform m.
    diaphysial cortical m.
    m. joint
    m. projection
    m. radiograph
    m. view
Morton
    M. neuroma
    M. plane
    M. toe
morula
morulalike epithelial cell

MOS
    metal oxide semiconductor
    MOS capacitator
mosaic
    m. artifact
    m. attenuation pattern
    m. detector configuration
    m. duodenal mucosal pattern
    m. jet signal
    m. oligemia
    m. perfusion
Moschcowitz test
Mossbauer spectrometer
Mosse syndrome
Moss gastrostomy tube
mossy fiber
Motarjeme catheter
moth-eaten
    m.-e. appearance
    m.-e. bone destruction
    m.-e. pattern
motile leukocyte
motility
    antroduodenal m.
    colonic m.
    m. disorder
    esophageal m.
    m. of Golden
    ileal m.
    jejunal m.
    small bowel m.
    m. study
motion
    akinetic segmental wall m.
    anterior wall m.
    apical wall m.
    m. artifact
    m. artifact suppression technique
      (MAST)
    m. averaging
    m. blur
    bowel m.
    brisk wall m.
    brownian water m.
    cardiac wall m.
    catheter tip m.
    chest wall paradoxic m.
    m. compensation gradient pulse
    CSF oscillatory m.
    cusp m.
    m. degradation
    discernible venous m.

M

NOTES

motion *(continued)*
    dyskinetic segmental wall m.
    forceful parasternal m.
    heaving precordial m.
    hyperkinetic segmental wall m.
    hypokinetic segmental wall m.
    incoherent m.
    inferior wall m.
    intravoxel coherent m.
    intravoxel incoherent m. (IVIM)
    isotropic m.
    leaflet m.
    left ventricular function wall m.
    left ventricular regional wall m.
    limitation of joint m.
    linear accelerator isocenter m.
    mitral valve systolic anterior m.
    m. mode (M-mode)
    nonoscillatory m.
    paradoxic leaflet m.
    paradoxic septal m.
    parasternal m.
    patient m.
    phantom simulating cardiac m.
    photoreceptor m.
    posterior wall m.
    posterolateral wall m.
    precessional m.
    random m.
    rapid oscillatory m.
    regional hypokinetic wall m.
    respiratory m.
    rocking precordial m.
    rotational m.
    scapulothoracic m.
    segmental wall m.
    septal wall m.
    stationary zero-order m.
    sustained anterior parasternal m.
    swirling m.
    systolic anterior m. (SAM)
    time m. (TM)
    translational m.
    trifid precordial m.
    m. unsharpness
    venous m.
    ventricular wall m.
    vibratory m.
    visible anterior m.
    wall m.
    within-view m.
motional narrowing
motion-compensating format converter
motion-free
    m.-f. imaging
    m.-f. positioning
motion-induced phase shift
motion-nulling gradient

motion-sensitive spin-echo sequence
    mechanical waves
motion-triggered cine kinematic MR image
motoneuron
motor
    m. area
    m. branch
    m. cortex
    m. impairment
    m. meal barium GI series
    m. nucleus
    programmable stepper m.
    m. reinnervation
    m. root
    m. test meal
    m. tract
    m. urge incontinence
    m. vehicle injury
    versive m.
motorcyclist's knee
MOTSA
    multiple overlapping thin-slab acquisition
Mott body
mottle
    photon m.
    quantum m.
    radiographic m.
mottled
    m. appearance
    m. calcification
    m. density
    m. distribution
    m. echotexture
    m. gas collection
    m. gray lung
    m. hepatic uptake
    m. infiltrate
    m. liver uptake
    m. pattern
    m. thickening
mottling
    diffuse m.
    m. of renal parenchyma
Mouchet fracture
mound
    infraumbilical m.
Mounier-Kuhn syndrome
Mountain View transducer
Mourits criteria (Graves ophthalmopathy)
mouse
    m. ear erosion
    peritoneal m.
"mouse-ear" appearance
mouth
    tapir m.
mouthpiece
    E-Z-Guar m.

movable
    m. core guidewire
    m. heart
    m. kidney
    m. vertebra
movement
    arcuate m.
    m. artifact
    bowel m.
    fetal m. (FM)
    fetal breathing m. (FBM)
    fiducial m.
    m. pattern
    pendulum m.
    propulsive m.
    spontaneous fetal m.
    systolic anterior m.
    table m.
movement-related cortical potential
mover
    smooth m.
moving
    m. platform posturography
    m. slice velocity mapping
    m. slot radiography
    m. table technique
    m. tabletop MR imaging
moving-bed infusion tracking MRA
moyamoya
    m. disease
    m. syndrome
    m. vascularity
Moyer line
Moynahan syndrome
MP
    magnetization prepared
    mesenteric panniculitis
    MP inversion pulse
MPA
    main pulmonary artery
MPAP
    mean pulmonary artery pressure
    multipurpose access port
MPCh
    medial posterior choroidal
MPCP
    mean pulmonary capillary pressure
MPD
    main pancreatic duct
    main papillary duct
    matched peripheral dose
    maximum permissible dose

    minimal port diameter
    multiplanar display
MPGR
    multiplanar gradient recall
    MPGR technique
MPHR
    maximum predicted heart rate
MPI
    myocardial perfusion imaging
mPower PET scanner
MPPS
    modality performed procedure step
MPPv
    main portal vein peak velocity
MPR
    multiplanar reconstruction
    multiplanar reformation
    myocardial perfusion reserve
    MPR view
MP-RAGE
    magnetization-prepared rapid acquisition
      gradient echo
    MP-RAGE protocol
    MP-RAGE technique
MP-RAGE-WE
    magnetization-prepared rapid gradient
      echo-water excitation
MPS
    mucopolysaccharidosis
    MPS types I–IV
mps, m/sec
    meters per second
MPVA
    metatarsus primus varus angle
MPVR
    multiplanar volume reformation
MQSA
    Mammography Quality Standards Act
MR
    magnetic resonance
    mitral regurgitation
    MR arthrography
    BP MR
    MR catheter imaging and
      spectroscopy system scanner
    chemical-selective fat-saturation MR
    MR colonographic technique
    MR colonography
    combined multisection diffuse-
      weighted and hemodynamically
      weighted echo-planar MR

M

NOTES

MR *(continued)*
    continuous arterial spin-labeling
      perfusion MR
    contrast-enhanced MR
    MR discriminator of osseous
      metastasis
    echo FLASH MR
    MR echo-planar imaging
    MR enteroclysis imaging
    first-pass myocardial perfusion MR
    MR flow quantification study
    MR hydrography
    MR imaging-guided endovascular
      device tracking
    lipid-sensitive MR
    MR lymphography
    oxygenation-sensitive functional MR
    MR proton spectroscopy
    renal artery stenosis screening MR
    MR SmartPrep
    MR velocity mapping

mR, mr
    milliroentgen

MRA
    magnetic resonance angiography
      body-coil-based contrast-enchanced
        MRA
      bolus-chase stepping-table 3D MRA
      contrast-enhanced MRA
      3D MRA
      MRA imaging
      inflow MRA
      moving-bed infusion tracking MRA
      multiphase MRA
      phase contrast MRA (PC-MRA)
      stepping-table MRA
      time-resolved CE MRA
      ultrafast contrast-enhanced MRA
      MRA using 3D k-space reordering

MRC
    magnetic resonance cholangiogram

MR-compatible power injector

MRCP
    magnetic resonance
     cholangiopancreatography
      breath-hold MRCP
      kinematic MRCP
      mangafodipir-enhanced MRCP
      secretin-enhanced dynamic MRCP
      MRCP using HASTE with a
        phased array coil

MRDSA
    magnetic resonance digital subtraction
     angiography
      2D MRDSA

MRE
    magnetic resonance elastography

mrem
    millirem

MRF
    midbrain reticular formation

MR-guided
    MR-g. laser-induced thermotherapy
    MR-g. lumbar sympathicolysis

MRI
    magnetic resonance imaging *(See*
     imaging)
     A-FAIR MRI
     body-coil MRI
     BOLD contrast functional MRI
     breath-hold contrast-enhanced MRI
     cardiac MRI
     catheter-based interventional MRI
     chondroitin sulfate iron colloid-
      enhanced MRI
     cine MRI
     coregistered MRI
     coronal FLAIR MRI
     MRI CSF flow study
     diffusion MRI
     digital reformatting knee MRI
     double-dose delayed-contrast MRI
     dual-echo chemical shift gradient-
      echo MRI
     dynamic-contrast MRI
     dynamic contrast-enhanced MRI
     electrocardiogram-gated MRI
     endoluminal MRI
     Excelart short-bore MRI
     extremity MRI (E-MRI)
     functional MRI
     Gd-DTPA-enhanced turbo FLASH
      MRI
     gradient subsystem in MRI
     HASTE MRI
     ^{3}He MRI
     high-resolution MRI (HR-MRI)
     intradiscal administration of
      gadolinium followed by MRI
     intravenously enhanced MRI
     laser-polarized helium MRI
     magnetoacoustic MRI
     MRI mapping
     MnDPDP enhanced MRI
     MRI morphometry
     multinuclear MRI
     multiplanar MRI
     nonaccelerated MRI
     nonproton MRI
     OPART MRI
     open MRI
     opposed-phase MRI
     OrthOne 1-tesla extremity MRI
     parallel MRI
     perfusion MRI
     perfusion-weighted MRI
     phase-contrast cine MRI
     phased-array MRI

MRI prescan
MRI probehead
PROPELLER MRI
proton-density-weighted MRI
MRI segmentation
selective partial inversion-recovery
 MRI (SPIR)
SENSE MRI
MRI Severity Scale score
Subtraction ictal SPECT
 coregistered to MRI (SISCOM)
susceptibility contrast-weighted MRI
3T MRI
MRI thermometry
T2 quantitative MRI
trueFISP MRI
ultrafast MRI
in utero MRI
vagus nerve stimulation-
 synchronized blood oxygen level-
 dependent functional MRI
velocity-encoded cine MRI
MRI-compatible electrode
MRI-guided
 MRI-g. breast biopsy
 MRI-g. focused ultrasound
 transducer
 MRI-g. laser-induced interstitial
 imaging
 MRI-g. laser-induced interstitial
 thermotherapy
 MRI-g. laser thermal ablation
 MRI-g. LTA
 MRI-g. periradicular nerve root
 infiltration therapy
 MRI-g. wire localization
MRM
 magnetic resonance mammography
MRN
 magnetic resonance neurography
MRP
 magnetic resonance pancreatography
MRS
 magnetic resonance spectroscopy
 slice-point MRS
MRSI
 magnetic resonance spectroscopic
 imaging
MRT
 magnetic resonance tomography
MR-trackable intramyocardial injection
 catheter

MRU
 magnetic resonance urography
 molecular recognition unit
 ThromboScan MRU
MRUI
 Magnetic Resonance User Interface
 MRUI software
MRV
 magnetic resonance venogram
 magnetic resonance venography
MS
 mitral stenosis
MS-325 contrast agent
MSA
 multiple system atrophy
 MSA syndrome
MSAD
 maximum short-axis diameter
 multiple scan average dose
MSCT
 multislice spiral CT
 aortic valve calcium quantification
 with MSCT
 MSCT technique
MSCTA
 multislice computed tomographic
 angiography
MSCV
 multislice cardiovolume
MSD
 mean sac diameter
 midsagittal diameter
MSDI
 multigated spectral Doppler imaging
 simultaneous MSDI
msec
 millisecond
mSENSE
 modified SENSE
MS-EPI
 multishot echo-planar imaging
M-shaped
 M-s. mitral valve pattern
 M-s. pattern of mitral valve
MSI
 magnetic source imaging
MSPv
 midshunt peak velocity
MT
 magnetization transfer
 metatarsophalangeal
 half-dose enhanced MRI with MT

M

NOTES

623

MT *(continued)*
    MT saturation
    triple-dose gadolinium-enhanced MR
      imaging without MT
MTC
    magnetization transfer contrast
MTC-Dox-Spheres
MTE
    main timing event
    mesenteric thromboembolism
MTF
    modulation transfer function
MTP
    metatarsophalangeal
      MTP joint
      semiflexed MTP
MTR
    magnetization transfer ratio
MTSA
    multiple thin slab acquisition
MTT
    mean pulmonary transit time
    mean transit time
m-tyrosine
mu, μ
    m. rhythm
mucicarmine stain
mucin-hypersecreting carcinoma
mucinous
    m. adenocarcinoma
    m. adenoma
    m. breast carcinoma
    m. bronchogram
    m. carcinoma
    m. cyst
    m. cystadenoma
    m. degeneration
    m. ductal ectasia of pancreas
    m. ductectatic tumor of pancreas
    m. ovarian cystadenocarcinoma
    m. ovarian tumor
    m. pancreatic cystic neoplasm
    m. tumor
mucin-producing
    m.-p. adenocarcinoma
    m.-p. carcinoma
muckiness of pericolonic fat
mucocele
    appendix m.
    breast m.
    bronchial m.
    frontal sinus m.
    frontoethmoidal m.
    orbital m.
    paranasal sinus m.
mucocutaneous
    m. junction
    m. lymph node syndrome (MCLS)

mucoepidermoid
    m. carcinoma
    m. carcinoma parotitis
mucoid
    m. degeneration of umbilical cord
    m. impaction
    m. impaction of bronchus
    m. plugging of airway
    m. umbilical cord degeneration
mucopolysaccharidosis types I–IV
mucopyocele
mucosa, pl. **mucosae**
    bowel m.
    bronchial m.
    buccal m.
    burned-out m.
    cobblestone m.
    colorectal m.
    endocervical m.
    friable m.
    frothy colonic m.
    gastric m. (GM)
    isoeffective bronchial m.
    muscularis m.
    m. muscularis
    outpocketing of m.
    polypoid m.
    prolapsed antral m.
    prolapsed gastric m.
    sloughed m.
mucosa-associated
    m.-a. lymphoid tissue (MALT)
    m.-a. lymphoid tissue lymphoma
mucosal
    m. abnormality
    m. bridge
    m. crinkling
    m. destruction
    m. esophageal nodule
    m. esophageal tumor
    m. fold
    m. fold pattern
    m. ganglioneurofibromatosis
    m. gland
    m. hyperplasia
    m. inflammation
    m. island
    m. lesion
    m. lining
    m. mass collecting system
    m. necrosis
    m. prolapse syndrome
    m. relief radiography
    m. relief roentgenography
    m. ring
    m. suspensory ligament
    m. thickening
    m. ulcer
mucosa-sparing block

mucosum
    ligamentum m.
mucous
    m. bronchogram
    m. carcinoma
    m. degeneration
    m. fistula
    m. hypersecretion
    m. lake
    m. lake of stomach
    m. membrane
    m. membrane hyperemia
    m. plug
    m. plugging
    m. polyp
    m. pseudomass
    m. retention cyst
mucus-filled small airway
mud
    biliary m.
MUGA
    multigated acquisition
    multiple gated acquisition
        MUGA cardiac blood pool imaging
        first-pass MUGA
        MUGA scan
Muir-Torre syndrome
mulberry
    m. calculus
    m. eye lesion
    m. gallstone
    m. ovary
mulberrylike mass
mulberry-type
    m.-t. calcification
    m.-t. classification
Mulder sign
Müller, Mueller
    M. canal
    M. fiber
    M. humerus fracture classification
    M. maneuver
    M. muscle
    M. sign
    M. test
    M. tray
müllerian
    m. duct
    m. duct anomaly
    m. duct cyst
    m. mucinous borderline tumor

multangular
    m. bone
    m. ridge fracture
multangulum
multiaccess catheter
multiarc LINAC radiosurgery
multiaxial classification
multibreath washout study
multicentric
    m. angiofollicular lymph node
    m. basal cell carcinoma
    m. carcinoid tumor
    m. Castleman disease (MCD)
    m. fibromatosis
    m. germinoma
    m. glioblastoma
    m. invasive lobular carcinoma
    m. lytic lesion
    m. malignant glioma
    m. meningioma
    m. osteogenic sarcoma
    m. osteosarcoma
    m. reticulohistiocytosis
multicentricity
multichannel analyzer (MCΛ)
multicoil
    phased-array m.
multicolor flow cytometry
multicompartment clearance
multicoupled loop-gap resonator
multicrystal
    m. BGO ring system
    m. gamma camera
multicystic
    m. acoustic neuroma
    m. dysgenetic kidney
    m. dysplasia
    m. dysplastic kidney (MCDK)
    m. encephalomalacia
    m. kidney (MCK)
multidetector
    m. computed tomography
    m. CT (MDCT)
    m. CTA
    m. CT scanner
    m. helical CT
    m. helical scanner
    m. helical scanning
    m. system
multidetector-row
    m.-r. CT (MDCT)

M

NOTES

multidetector-row *(continued)*
    m.-r. CT scan
    m.-r. helical computed tomography
MultiDop P, T, X transcranial Doppler device
multidose vial
multidrug-resistant tuberculosis
multiecho
    m. axial
    m. axial image
    m. coronal image
    m. imaging
    m. multiplane (MEMP)
    m. sequence
    standard m.
multielectrode catheter
multielemental neutron activation analysis
multiexponential relaxation
multifactorial etiologies
multifield beam
multifocal
    m. aggressive infiltrate
    m. anaplastic astrocytoma
    m. area of hyperintensity
    m. autonomic adenoma
    m. brain tumor
    m. breast carcinoma
    m. enhancing brain lesion
    m. glioblastoma multiforme
    m. hemorrhage
    m. infarct
    m. invasive lobular carcinoma
    m. leukoencephalopathy
    m. lymphoma
    m. nephroblastomatosis
    m. osteosarcoma
    m. residual focus
    m. short stenosis
    m. subperitoneal sclerosis
multifollicular ovary
multiformat camera
multiformatted imaging
multiforme
    glioblastoma m. (GBM)
    multifocal glioblastoma m.
multiform ventricular complex
multigated
    m. acquisition (MUGA)
    m. angiography
    m. imaging
    m. pulsed Doppler flow system
    m. spectral Doppler analysis software
    m. spectral Doppler imaging (MSDI)
multigate Doppler

MultiHance
    M. contrast medium
    M. imaging agent
multihole collimator
multiilluminant color correction
multiinfarct dementia
multiinterval
multilamellar periosteal reaction
multilaminar body
multileaf
    m. collimating system
    m. collimator (MLC)
multilevel fusion
multiline scanning technique
Multi-Link
    M.-L. Penta stent
    M.-L. Terra stent
multilobular
    m. cirrhosis
    m. configuration
multilobulated mass
multilocular
    m. cystic lesion
    m. cystic nephroma
    m. renal cyst
multiloculated mass
multilog effect
multimodal image fusion technique
multimodality
    m. imaging
    m. therapy
multimode imaging confocal optical microscope (MIMCOM)
multinodular
    m. goiter
    m. thyroid
multinuclear MRI
Multi-Operatory Dentalaser (MOD)
multiorgan imaging
multiparametric color composite display
multiparticle cyclotron
multipartite
    m. fracture
    m. patella
multipennate muscle
multipharmaceutical chemoembolization solution
multiphase MRA
multiphase-multisection T2-weighted MR imaging
multiphasic
    m. helical CT
    m. multislice MRI technique
    m. multislice spin-echo imaging technique
    m. perfusion computed tomography
    m. renal computerized tomography
multiplanar
    m. compression

m. display (MPD)
m. endorectal ultrasound
m. gradient-echo software
m. gradient recall (MPGR)
m. gradient-recalled echo
m. gradient refocus
m. gradient refocused sequence
m. mode
m. MRI
m. MR imaging
phase-offset m. (POMP)
phase-ordered m. (POMP)
m. reconstruction (MPR)
m. reformation (MPR)
m. reformatted radiographic and digitally reconstructed radiographic imaging
m. reformatting
m. reformatting view
m. scanning
m. transducer
m. transesophageal echocardiography
m. volume reformation (MPVR)
m. volume-reformatted image

multiplane

contiguous slice multiecho m. (CSMEMP)
m. dosage calculation
multiecho m. (MEMP)

multiple

m. accessory spleen
m. aortopulmonary collateral artery (MAPCA)
m. averaging
m. bile duct hamartomas
m. blocks
m. bone myeloma
m. bull's eye lesions bowel wall
m. cartilaginous exostoses
m. chords
m. coil array
m. colon filling defects
m. concentric GI rings
m. congenital anomalies (MCA)
m. congenital fibromatosis
m. cortical infarcts
m. echo single shot (MESS)
m. emboli
m. enchondromatosis
m. endocrine neoplasia (MEN)
m. endocrine neoplasia syndrome
m. epiphysial dysplasia

m. fetuses
m. fibroxanthomata
m. focal lesions of spinal cord
m. foci
m. fractures
m. gated acquisition (MUGA)
m. gated acquisition scan
m. gated blood pool scan
m. gestations
m. gland disease
m. hereditary exostoses
m. idiopathic hemorrhagic sarcoma
m. jointed digitizer
m. jointed digitizer scanner
m. kidney myeloma
m. line scan (MLS)
m. line scan imaging (MLSI)
m. loops of small bowel
m. lucent lung lesions
m. lung nodules
m. lytic bone lesions
m.'s of median
m. mucosal neuroma syndrome
m. mural dilatations
m. organ failure
m. osteochondromatosis
m. osteolysis
m. osteosclerotic lesions
m. overlapping thin-slab acquisition (MOTSA)
m. parotid gland lesions
m. peripheral papillomas
m. planar gradient-recalled image
m. pleural densities
m. polyposis
m. polyps
m. pregnancies
m. projection biplane angiography
m. pterygium syndrome
m. pulmonary calcification
m. pulmonary cysts
m. pulmonary necrobiotic nodules
m. quantum coherence
m. recurrent inversion injuries
m. sclerosis
m. sclerosis plaques
m. sclerotic osteosarcoma
m. sensitive points
m. slice acquisition
m. slice imaging
m. small bowel filling defects
m. small bowel stenosis

NOTES

M

multiple *(continued)*
    m. small bowel ulcers
    m. spin echo
    m. stenotic lesions
    m. stenotic lesions of small bowel
    m. stones
    m. symmetric lipomatosis
    m. system atrophy (MSA)
    m. system atrophy syndrome
    m. thin slab acquisition (MTSA)
    m. thin-walled lung cavity
    m. thyroid cysts
    m. trauma
    m. vascular leiomyomas
multiple-beam interface spacing
multiple-coil arrays
multiple-echo imaging
multiple-electrode probe system
multiple-exposure volumetric holography
multiple-gated blood pool imaging
multiple-headed gamma camera
multiple-injection protocol
multiple-lesion osteosclerosis
multiple-line scanning method
multiple-plane imaging
multiple-sample clearance
multiple-sensitive-point method
multiple-side-hole
    m.-s.-h. infusion catheter
    m.-s.-h. infusion system
multiple-suture synostosis
multiplex
    dysostosis m.
    dysplasia epiphysialis m.
multiplexing
multiplying digital-to-analog converter (MDAC)
multiply tuned coil
Multi-Pro biopsy needle
multipurpose
    m. access port (MPAP)
    m. catheter
multiray fracture
multirod collimator
multiscalar
multiscale image detail contrast amplification (Musica)
multisection
    m. diffuse-weighted magnetic resonance imaging
    m. gradient-echo echo-planar imaging
    m. method
    m. multirepetition acquisition
multisectional dose-volume histogram
multisegment disease
multisensor
    m. structured light range digitizer

    m. structured light-range digitizer scanner
multiseptate appearance
multiseptated gallbladder
multishot
    m. echo-planar imaging (MS-EPI)
    m. spin-echo echo-planar imaging
multi-sideport infusion catheter
multislab magnetic resonance angiography
multislice
    m. acquisition
    m. cardiovolume (MSCV)
    m. computed tomographic angiography (MSCTA)
    m. computed tomography
    m. CT
    m. CT scanner
    2D m.
    ECG-gated m.
    m. first-pass myocardial perfusion imaging
    m. FLASH 2D
    m. flow-related enhancement
    m. full line scan
    m. modality
    m. mode
    m. modified KWE direct Fourier imaging
    m. spin-echo sequence
    m. spin-echo technique
    m. spiral CT (MSCT)
    m. spiral weighting
multislit catheter
multispectral diffuse transillumination
multispin relaxation
Multistar
    M. angiographic unit
    M. Top Plus DSA system
multisweep
    high-resolution m. (HRMS)
multitime point imaging
multitracer
    m. imaging
    m. study
multivane intensity modulation compensator (MIMIC)
multivariant regressional analysis
multiwire proportional chamber
multizone transmit-receive focus
mummy restraint
mural
    m. aneurysm
    m. arch
    m. architecture
    m. change
    m. clot
    m. CNS nodule
    m. defect

m. degeneration
m. dilatation
m. endomyocardial fibrosis
m. fibrosing alveolitis
m. hematoma
m. infiltrate
m. kidney
m. leaflet of mitral valve
m. nodulation
m. pregnancy
m. stratification
m. thickening
m. thrombus
m. thrombus formation
mural-type vein of Galen malformation
muscarinic receptor
muscle

abductor digiti quinti m.
abductor hallucis m.
abductor pollicis brevis m.
accessory m.
adductor magnus m.
Aeby m.
Albinus m.
anconeus m.
anomalous m.
anterior papillary m. (APM)
antigravity m.
m. artifact
auricular m.
axillary m.
BBC m.'s
2-bellied m.
belly of m.
biceps femoris m.
bipennate m.
Bochdalek m.
Bovero m.
Bowman m.
brachioradialis m.
Braune m.
Brücke m.
bulbi m.
bulbocavernosus m.
m. bulk
cardiac m.
Casser m.
casserian m.
cervical m.
Chassaignac m.
circular m.
Coiter m.

conal papillary m.
cone of extraocular m.
m. contracture
Crampton m.
cricopharyngeus m.
m. crushing injury
dartos m.
deep m.
m. of deglutition
detrusor m.
digastric m.
dorsal m.
Dupré m.
Duverney m.
ECRB m.
ECRL m.
ECU m.
EDB m.
EDC m.
EDL m.
EDQ m.
EIP m.
EPB m.
EPL m.
extensor carpi radialis brevis m.
extensor carpi radialis longus m.
extensor carpi ulnaris m.
extensor digiti quinti m.
extensor digitorum brevis m.
extensor digitorum communis m.
extensor digitorum longus m.
extensor hallucis longus m.
extensor indicis proprius m.
extensor pollicis brevis m.
extensor pollicis longus m.
external oblique m.
extraocular m.
extrinsic foot m.
fast-twitch m.
FDL m.
FDQB m.
FDS m.
m. fiber
m. fiber wasting
fibrosed m.
fixator m.
flexor carpi radialis m.
flexor digiti quinti brevis m.
flexor digitorum longus m.
flexor digitorum profundus m.
flexor digitorum superficialis m.
flexor hallucis brevis m.

M

NOTES

muscle *(continued)*

  Folius m.
  frontotemporal m.
  fused papillary m.
  Gantzer m.
  gastrocnemius m.
  Gavard m.
  genioglossus m.
  Guthrie m.
  Hilton m.
  Horner m.
  Houston m.
  hyoglossus m.
  hyperintense m.
  m. hyperintensity
  ileococcygeus m.
  iliocostal m.
  iliopsoas m.
  m. infarct
  infarcted heart m.
  inferior gemellus m.
  infraspinatus m.
  innermost intercostal m.
  intercostal m.
  internal intercostal m.
  interosseous m.
  interspinal m.
  intertransverse m.
  intraauricular m.
  intrinsic foot m.
  m. irritability
  ischiocavernosus m.
  Klein m.
  Lancisi m.
  lateral pterygoid m.
  lateral rectus m.
  latissimus dorsi m.
  left ventricular m.
  lesser m.
  levator m.
  longitudinal m.
  longus colli m.
  Luschka m.
  major m.
  Marcacci m.
  masseter m.
  masticator m.
  medial papillary m.
  medial pterygoid m.
  middle m.
  minimus scalenus m.
  minor m.
  Müller m.
  multipennate m.
  mylohyoid m.
  myocardial m.
  nonstriated m.
  oblique m.
  obturator internus m.

occipitofrontalis m.
Ochsner m.
Oddi m.
ODQ m.
Oehl m.
omohyoid m.
opponens digiti quinti m.
opposing m.
organic m.
m. ossification
palatal m.
papillary m.
paralaryngeal m.
paraspinal m.
Passavant m.
pectineus m.
pectoralis major m.
pectoralis minor m.
peroneal m.
peroneus quartus m.
pharyngeal m.
Phillips m.
piriform m.
piriformis m.
plantaris m.
platysma m.
posterior papillary m. (PPM)
Pozzi m.
psoas m.
pterygoid m.
pubococcygeus m.
pupillary constrictor m.
pyloric m.
quadrate m.
quadriceps m.
reactive disease of smooth m.
m. recruitment pattern
rectus m.
Reisseisen m.
retronuchal m.
rhomboideus major m.
ribbon m.
rider's m.
Riolan m.
rotator cuff m.
Rouget m.
round m.
Ruysch m.
sacrospinalis m.
Santorini m.
sartorius m.
scalenus anterior m.
Sebileau m.
semimembranous m.
semispinal m.
semitendinous m.
septal papillary m.
serratus anterior m.
m. sheath

short m.
shoulder m.
Sibson m.
skeletal m.
slow-twitch m.
smooth m.
Soemmerring m.
soleus m.
somatic m.
m. spasm
sphenomandibularis m.
m. spindle
spindle-shaped m.
sternocleidomastoid m.
sternohyoid m.
sternothyroid m.
m. strain
strap m.
striated m.
styloglossus m.
stylohyoid m.
subaortic m.
subscapularis m.
sucking m.
superficial m.
supraspinatus m.
synergic m.
tailor's m.
temporalis m.
tendinous part of epicranius m.
tensor veli palatini m.
Theile m.
thenar m.
thigh m.
m. tissue
Tod m.
Toynbee m.
transversus abdominis m.
trapezius m.
Treitz m.
triangular m.
trigonal m.
true back m.
unipennate m.
m. uptake
Valsalva m.
vascular smooth m.
vastus medialis m.
ventral m.
vertical m.
visceral m.
vocal m.

vocalis m.
voluntary m.
Wilson m.
wrinkler m.
muscle-eye-brain disease
muscle-fat interface
muscular
    m. atrioventricular septum
    m. branch
    m. bridge
    m. crus
    m. crus of diaphragm
    m. degeneration
    m. dystrophy
    m. hypertrophy
    m. insufficiency
    m. lesion
    m. ring esophagus
    m. slip
    m. subaortic stenosis
    m. tube
    m. twig
    m. ventricular septal defect
muscularis
    mucosa m.
    m. mucosa
    m. propria
musculature
    axial m.
    cervical m.
    longitudinal taenia m.
    paraspinous m.
    paravertebral m.
    scalene m.
musculoaponeurotic
    m. fibroma
    m. fibromatosis
musculocutaneous sarcoidosis
musculofascial pedicle
musculophrenic
    m. artery
    m. branch
    m. vessel
musculoskeletal
    m. imaging
    m. imaging study
    m. lesion
    m. radiography
    m. system
    m. tumor
musculotendinous
    m. cuff

M

NOTES

musculotendinous *(continued)*
    m. junction
    m. retraction
    m. unit
musculotendinous-osseous link
musculotubal canal
musculus, pl. **musculi**
    m. uvula
mushroom
    m. appearance
    m. picker's disease
    m. shape
    m. worker's lung
mushroom-shaped mass
Musica
    multiscale image detail contrast
    amplification
Musset sign
mustard
    L-phenylalanine m. (LPAM)
MUSTPAC
    Medical Ultrasound Three-Dimensional
    Portable Advanced Communications
    MUSTPAC ultrasound imaging
mutant
mutation
    point m.
    reelin m.
mutational dysostosis
mutilans
    arthritis m.
muzzle velocity
MV
    megavolt
    mesenteric vasculitis
MVA
    mitral valve area
MVO
    maximum venous outflow
    mitral valve opening
    mitral valve orifice
MVP
    mitral valve prolapse
MVR
    mitral valve replacement
MVS
    mitral valve stenosis
MVV
    maximal voluntary ventilation
mycalamide A
mycetoma
    m. formation
    kidney m.
mycobacteria
    nontuberculosis m.
mycophenolic acid
mycoplasmal pneumonitis
mycosis, pl. **mycoses**

mycotic
    m. aortic aneurysm
    m. brain aneurysm
    m. intracranial aneurysm
    m. lung infection
    m. plaque
    m. pneumonia
    m. sinusitis
myelencephalon
myelin
    m. ball
    m. ball formation
    m. sheath
myelination
    delayed m.
    nerve fiber m.
    optic pathway m.
myelinolysis
    central pontine m.
    extrapontine m.
    pontine m.
myelitis
    acute transverse m.
    radiation m.
    subacute necrotizing m.
    transverse m.
myeloblastoma
myelocele
myelocisternoencephalography
myelo-CT
myelocystocele
myelocystography
myelodysplasia
myelodysplastic syndrome (MDS)
myelofibrosis
    acute m.
    m. osteosclerosis
myelogenesis
myelogram
myelographic imaging agent
myelography
    air m.
    cervical m.
    complete m.
    computed m.
    computer-assisted m. (CAM)
    CT m.
    extraarachnoid m.
    Hypaque m.
    m. imaging
    lumbar m.
    lumbosacral m.
    magnetic resonance m.
    metrizamide m.
    oil m.
    opaque m.
    oxygen m.
    Pantopaque m.
    positive contrast m.

thoracic m.
water-soluble m.
myeloid
   m. malignancy
   m. metaphysis
myelolipoma
   adrenal m.
myeloma
   amyloidosis of multiple m.
   endothelial m.
   indolent m.
   localized m.
   M-band m.
   multiple bone m.
   multiple kidney m.
   plasmablastic m.
   sclerosing m.
   solitary bone m.
   spinal plasma cell m.
myelomalacia
   cystic m.
myelomatosis
myelopathy
   acute posttraumatic m.
   carcinomatous m.
   cervical spondylotic m. (CSM)
   cystic m.
   delayed posttraumatic m.
   necrotizing m.
   paracarcinomatous m.
   posttraumatic ascending m.
   posttraumatic cystic m.
   progressive posttraumatic m.
   radiation m.
   spondylotic m.
   subacute necrotizing m.
myelophthisic splenomegaly
myeloproliferative disorder
myeloschisis
myelosclerosis
myelotomography
myenteric
   m. plexus
   m. plexus of Auerbach
Myerson sign
mylohyoid
   m. muscle
   m. ridge
myoblastoma
   granular breast-cell m.
   granular lung-cell m.
   granular sella-cell m.

myocardial
   m. band (MB)
   m. blood flow (MBF)
   m. blush
   m. bridge
   m. calcification
   m. cellular degeneration
   m. cellular hypertrophy
   m. centroid
   m. contractile function
   m. contractility
   m. contracture
   m. contrast appearance time (MCAT)
   m. contrast echocardiography (MCE)
   m. contusion
   m. depression
   m. dilatation
   m. disarray
   m. fiber
   m. fibrous degeneration
   m. function assessment
   m. hibernation
   m. I-123 MIBG imaging
   m. incompetence
   m. infarct (MI)
   m. infarct imaging
   m. infarction recovery index
   m. infiltration
   m. inflammation
   m. insufficiency
   m. insult
   m. irritability
   m. ischemia
   m. jeopardy index
   m. mass
   m. metabolism
   m. muscle
   m. necrosis
   m. O_2 demand index
   m. oxygen consumption
   m. perfusion
   m. perfusion echocardiography
   m. perfusion imaging (MPI)
   m. perfusion imaging Q-complex
   m. perfusion reserve (MPR)
   m. perfusion scan
   m. perfusion scintigraphy
   m. perfusion tomography
   m. preservation
   m. protection

NOTES

M

myocardial *(continued)*
>   m. recovery
>   m. reperfusion injury
>   m. revascularization
>   m. rupture
>   m. scar
>   m. stunning
>   m. tagging
>   m. texture analysis
>   m. thallium imaging
>   m. thickening
>   m. tissue viability
>   m. twist
>   m. uptake
>   m. wall
>   m. work

myocardial-specific marker
myocardiopathy
myocarditis
>   fibroid m.
>   fragmentation m.

myocardium
>   asynergic m.
>   calcification of m.
>   dilated m.
>   hibernating m.
>   hypertrophied m.
>   hypokinetic m.
>   infarcted m.
>   inferior apical aspect of m.
>   ischemic reperfused m.
>   ischemic viable m.
>   jeopardized m.
>   necrotic m.
>   noninfarcted m.
>   nonperfused m.
>   perfused m.
>   recovery period of m.
>   refractory period of m.
>   reperfused m.
>   rupture of m.
>   salvage of m.
>   senile m.
>   sparkling appearance of m.
>   stunned m.
>   thinned m.
>   ventricular m.
>   viable m.

myocardium-to-abdomen count ratio
myocutaneous
>   transverse rectus abdominis m.
>   (TRAM)

myocyte
>   cardiac m.
>   m. membrane purinoceptor

myoepithelial sialadenitis
myoepithelioma

myofascial
>   m. disruption
>   m. pain-dysfunction syndrome

myofibrillar disintegration
myofibril volume fraction
myofibroblastoma
>   giant m.
>   intranodal m.

myofibrohistiocytic proliferation
myofibromatosis
>   infantile m.

myogenesis
myoid hamartoma
myoinositol-creatine ratio (Mi-Cr)
myointimal
>   m. hyperplasia
>   m. proliferation

myoma
>   complicated m.
>   intramural m.
>   pedunculated subserous m.
>   serosal m.
>   submucous m.
>   uncomplicated m.
>   uterine m.

myometrial
>   m. contraction
>   m. septum

myometrium
>   uterine m.

myonecrosis
>   calcific m.

myoneural junction
myopathy
>   carcinomatous m.

myosarcoma
Myoscint
>   M. imaging
>   M. imaging agent

MyoSight imaging system
myosin
>   [111]In murine monoclonal antibody
>   Fab to m.

myosis
>   endolymphatic stromal m.

myositis
>   brucellar m.
>   eye m.
>   granulomatous m.
>   m. ossificans circumscripta
>   m. ossificans progressiva
>   m. ossificans traumatica

myostatic contracture
myotendinous
>   m. junction
>   m. junction rupture
>   m. strain

**Myotherm XP cardioplegia delivery
system**

MyoTrac
>M. EMG monitor
>M. 2 EMG monitor

myotube

Myoview imaging agent

myxadenoma

myxedema
>m. of heart
>pretibial m.

myxoglobulosis

myxoid
>m. cyst
>m. degenerative change
>m. extraskeletal chondrosarcoma
>m. malignant fibrous histiocytoma
>m. MFH

myxoma, pl. **myxomata, myxomas**
>atrial m.
>biatrial m.
>cardiac m.

>complex m.
>familial m.
>heart m.
>m. of heart
>left atrial m.
>odontogenic m.
>pedunculated uterine m.
>vascular m.
>ventricular m.

myxomatodes
>fibroma m.

myxomatous
>m. degeneration
>m. liposarcoma
>m. proliferation
>m. valve leaflet

myxomembranous colitis

myxopapillary ependymoma

MZL
>marginal zone lymphoma

NOTES

M

N
nitrogen
N-2
neutron-atomic number ratio
^{13}N
^{13}N ammonia radioactive tracer
^{13}N ammonia uptake
^{14}N
nitrogen 14
^{15}N
nitrogen 15
^{23}Na
sodium 23
^{23}Na magnetic resonance imaging
^{23}Na MR imaging with short echo time
^{24}Na
sodium 24
nabothian
n. cyst
n. follicle
Naclerio
V-sign of N.
nadir
untransformed n.
Naegele obliquity
Naffziger sign
Nägele pelvis
NaI
sodium iodide
NaI detector
nail
n. bed lesion
body of n.
gamma n.
intramedullary n.
Jewett n.
orthopedic n.
n. plate
n. plate avulsion
Smith-Petersen n.
spoon-shaped n.
triflanged n.
Zickel supercondylar n.
nailing
elastic stable intramedullary n. (ESIN)
nail-patella syndrome
nail-plate device
Nakata index
naked-facet sign
naloxone imaging agent
Namaqualand hip dysplasia

nanocolloid
technetium-99m n.
nanocurie (nCi)
nanogram (ng)
nanoparticle
iodinated n.
monocrystalline iron oxide n. (MION)
nanoparticulate imaging agent
naphthalenes
fluorine-18 2-dialkylamino-6-acylmalononitrile substituted n. (FDDNP)
napkin-ring
n.-r. anular lesion
n.-r. anular stenosis
n.-r. anular tumor
n.-r. trachea
Napoleon hat sign
Narcomatic flowmetry
naris, pl. **nares**
NARP
neuropathy, ataxia and retinitis pigmentosa
narrow
n. anteroposterior diameter
n. beam
n. caliber
n. chest
n. collimation
n. gating tolerance
narrow-band spectral-selective radiofrequency pulse
narrow-beam half-thickness
narrowed
n. orifice
n. valve
narrowing
airway n.
antral stomach n.
arterial n.
arteriolar n.
n. of artery
artificial lumen n.
n. asymmetry
atherosclerotic n.
beaklike n.
bile duct n.
bird-beak configuration or n.
bronchiolar n.
n. of bronchiolar passage
carinal angle n.
circumferential n.
colonic n.
concentric n.

N

narrowing *(continued)*
degenerative n.
diffuse n.
discrete n.
disc space n.
duodenal n.
eccentric n.
esophageal n.
n. exchange
focal esophageal n.
n. of forefoot
gastric n.
glottic n.
high-grade n.
intervertebral disc n.
joint space n.
large airway n.
longitudinal n.
long smooth esophageal n.
lower esophageal n.
luminal n.
motional n.
nasopharyngeal n.
neural foraminal n.
oropharyngeal n.
pancompartmental joint space n.
rectal n.
residual luminal n.
retropharyngeal n.
segmental bronchus n.
smooth esophageal n.
n. of spinal canal
stomach n.
subcritical n.
subglottic n.
supraglottic n.
symmetric n.
n. of thecal sac
tracheal n.
vallecular n.

nasal
n. airway resistance
n. bone
n. bridge
n. canal
n. cavity
n. cavity wall
n. concha
n. fracture
n. intubation
n. meatus
n. mucociliary clearance function
n. part of pharynx
n. polyp
n. septum
n. septum hematoma
n. sinus
n. spine
n. suture

n. tip deformity
n. turbinate
n. vault mass
nasal-to-plasma radioactivity ratio
nasi
agger n.
nasion recession
nasobregmatic arc
nasociliary nerve
nasoenteric tube
nasofrontal
n. duct
n. suture
nasogastric
n. intubation
n. (NG) tube
nasojejunal feeding tube
nasolabial
n. cyst
n. lymph node
nasolacrimal
n. canal
n. duct
nasomaxillary
n. fracture
n. suture
nasooccipital arc
nasoorbital fracture
nasopalatal fissure
nasopalatine canal
nasopharyngeal
n. atresia
n. carcinoma (NPC)
n. craniopharyngioma
n. hematoma
n. mass
n. mucous retention cyst
n. narrowing
n. reflux
n. squamous cell carcinoma
nasopharyngography
nasopharynx
nasotracheal
n. intubation
n. tube
nasus
natatory ligament
natiform skull
National Heart, Lung, and Blood Institute (NHLBI)
native
n. aorta
n. aortic valve
n. aortic valve closure
n. atherosclerosis
n. coronary artery
n. image
n. kidney
n. kidney renal artery stenosis

n. kidney renal vein thrombosis
n. lung
n. tissue harmonic imaging (NTIII)
n. ventricle
n. vessel

natural
n. active acquired immunity
n. killer (NK)
n. neon gas
n. radiation
n. radioactivity

Naumoff syndrome

Navarre
N. catheter
N. drainage catheter

navel
n. ring artifact
n. string

Navi Ball guidance system

navicular
n. body
n. body fracture
n. bone
carpal n.
n. to first metatarsal angle
n. hand fracture
ossific nucleus of n.
n. projection
protrusion of n.
target n.
tarsal n.
n. tuberosity
n. view

naviculare
os n.

navicularis
fossa n.

naviculocapitate fracture
naviculocuneiform
n. joint
n. ligament

navigable echo signal
navigated spin-echo diffusion-weighted MR imaging
navigation
computer-assisted intracranial n.

navigator
N. computer workstation
n. echo
n. echo-based real-time respiratory gating and triggering

n. echo motion correction technique
n. pulse
n. shift

navigator-guided motion correction
Navigus cranial electrode system
Navi-Star ablation catheter
Navitrack computer-assisted surgery system
NAWM
normal-appearing white matter
NAWM metabolite concentration

NB
neuroblastoma

NBCA
N-butyl cyanoacrylate

N-butyl-2-cyanoacrylate embolization
N-butyl cyanoacrylate (NBCA)
NB200 vascular access device
N-Cat N-500 tonometric blood pressure monitor
NCCT
noncontrast head CT

nCi
nanocurie

NCP
noncontrast phase
implanted NCP

NCPF
noncirrhotic portal fibrosis

Nd:YAG
neodymium:yttrium-aluminum-garnet
Nd:YAG CTLC
Nd:YAG laser catheter

Nd:YLF
neodymium:yttrium-lithium fluoride
Nd:YLF laser

near
n. field
n. infrared (NIR)
n. infrared spectroscopy (NIRS)

near-anatomic
n.-a. position
n.-a. position of joint

near-infrared optical mammography
near-isotropic reformatted image
near-normal radiotracer uptake
near-resonance spin-lock contrast
near-water
n.-w. attenuation
n.-w. density

N

NOTES

NEC
   noise effective count
necessity
   fracture of n.
neck
   anatomic n.
   n. of aneurysm
   aneurysmal n.
   aneurysm remnant n.
   n. of bladder
   bone n.
   n. coil
   dental n.
   n. emphysema
   femoral n.
   n. of femur
   n. fracture
   n. of gallbladder
   n. germ-cell tumor
   hyperextension of n.
   n. lymphangioma
   Madelung n.
   n. of pancreas
   pancreatic n.
   n. phantom
   posterior triangle of the n.
   potato tumor of n.
   n. of rib
   selective occlusion of
     aneurysmal n.
   n. shaft angle
   surgical n.
   n. of talus
   n. teratoma
   uterine wry n.
   vesical n.
   webbed n.
neck-space anatomy
necleotherapy
necrobiotic nodule
necrolytic
necrosis, pl. **necroses**
   acute cortical n.
   acute native kidney tubular n.
   acute renal transplant tubular n.
   acute sclerosing hyaline n. (ASHN)
   acute tubular n. (ATN)
   alveolar septal n.
   aortic idiopathic n.
   arteriolar n.
   aseptic n.
   asphyxia-related renal n.
   avascular n. (AVN)
   avascular bone n.
   avascular cortical infarction n.
   avascular femoral head n.
   avascular tarsal scaphoid n.
   avascular vertebral body n.
   bilateral cortical n.

biliary piecemeal n.
bloodless zone of n.
bony n.
bowel n.
breast fat n.
bridging n.
caseous n.
central n.
centrilobular n.
coagulation n.
colliquative n.
colonic n.
comedo n.
contraction band n.
cortical kidney n.
cystic medial n.
diffuse n.
dirty n.
embolic n.
encapsulated fat n.
epiphysial ischemic n.
Erdheim cystic medial n.
fascial margin n.
fat n.
fatty n.
fibrinoid n.
fibrosing piecemeal n.
Ficat stage of avascular n.
focal fat n.
focal hepatic n.
frank n.
heart muscle n.
hemorrhagic n.
hepatic n.
hyaline n.
idiopathic avascular n.
indurative n.
intestinal n.
intratumoral n.
ischemic n.
laminar brain n.
liquefaction n.
localized n.
lung n.
margin n.
massive hepatic n.
medial cystic n.
midzonal n.
mucosal n.
myocardial n.
Paget quiet n.
pancreatic n.
papillary n.
peripheral n.
piecemeal n.
postbiopsy fat n.
postpartum pituitary n.
postsurgical fat n.
posttraumatic aseptic n.

posttraumatic fat n.
pressure n.
progressive emphysematous n.
punctate n.
radiation n.
radiation-induced n. (RIN)
radiation-induced cerebral n.
radium n.
renal allograft n.
renal cortical n.
renal papillary n.
renal tubular n.
septal n.
septic n.
soft tissue n.
strangulation n.
stromal n.
subacute hepatic n.
subcapsular hepatic n.
subcutaneous fat n.
subendocardial n.
submassive hepatic n.
superficial n.
total n.
tracheobronchial mucosal n.
transmural n.
traumatic fat n.
tubular n.
tumor n.
vascular n.
ventricular muscle n.
Zenker n.

necrotic
n. bone
n. bone pseudocyst
n. debris
n. flap
n. inflammation
n. lesion
n. metastasis
n. myocardium
n. renal cell carcinoma
n. sequestrum
n. tissue
n. tumor
n. ulcer

necrotizing
n. aspergillosis
n. emphysema
n. enterocolitis
n. external otitis
n. fasciitis

n. gastritis
n. glomerulonephritis
n. myelopathy
n. pancreatitis
n. pneumonia
n. respiratory granulomatosis
n. thrombosis
n. ulcerative gingivitis (NUG)

NECT
nonenhanced computed tomography

NED
no evidence of disease

needle
Abrams biopsy n.
abscission n.
Accucore II biopsy n.
Amplatz angiography n.
Arrow Fischell EVAN N.
aspiration biopsy n.
Bauer-Temno biopsy n.
B-D bone marrow biopsy n.
beveled n.
Bierman n.
BioPince n.
n. biopsy
biopsy n.
Biopty cut n.
blood-containment n.
blunt-end sialogram n.
Brockenbrough n.
BV2 n.
cesium n.
Chiba n.
coaxial sheath cut-biopsy n.
Colapinto n.
Conrad-Crosby bone marrow
   biopsy n.
Cope biopsy n.
core biopsy n.
Core bone biopsy n.
Cournand arteriography n.
Cournand-Grino angiography n.
n. deviation
Dos Santos aortography n.
dumbbell n.
Echo-Coat ultrasound biopsy n.
Echo Tip trocar n.
E-Z-EM cut biopsy n.
flexible biopsy n.
Franseen n.
full-intensity n.
17-gauge coaxial Temno n.

N

NOTES

needle *(continued)*
18-gauge percutaneous access n.
Greene n.
half-intensity n.
Hawkins-Akins n.
Hawkins breast lesion
    localization n.
Hawkins 1-stick n.
Homerlok n.
Homer Mammalok n.
n. hydrophone
iridium n.
Kopans n.
Kormed liver biopsy n.
larger-caliber cutting n.
n. localization
n. localization of breast lesion
n.-localized breast biopsy (NLBB)
Maggi biopsy n.
Majestik shielded angiographic n.
Mammalock n.
n. marker
Mentor prostatic biopsy n.
metallic n.
micropuncture n.
middle-caliber n.
2.1-mm automated biopsy n.
Monoject hypodermic n.
Monopty n.
Multi-Pro biopsy n.
nonferromagnetic n.
Ostycut bone biopsy n.
PercuCut cut-biopsy n.
pronged Franseen-type point n.
n. pyelography
Quick-Core biopsy n.
Quincke spinal n.
^{226}Ra n.
Rosch-Uchida n.
Ross n.
scalp vein n.
Seldinger n.
self-aspirating cut-biopsy n.
sheath n.
sialography n.
single-wall n.
skinny n.
small-caliber n.
Sos Pulse-Vu Bloodless Entry N.
spinal n.
spring-loaded biopsy n.
Temno II cutting n.
T-fastener delivery n.
thin-walled guiding n.
TLA n.
translumbar aortography n.
Tuohy aortography n.
n. visualization
Westcott n.

Whitacre spinal n.
Yueh centesis n.
2-needle biopsy technique
needle-guided excisional biopsy
needle-hookwire localization
needle-localized breast biopsy (NLBB)
needle-shaped breast calcification
Needlestick Safety and Prevention Act
needle-tip bioimpedance
needle-wire system
Neel temperature
Neer
    N. classification of shoulder
        fracture
    N. impingement sign
    N. lateral view
    N. transscapular view
Neer-Horowitz
    N.-H. classification of humeral
        fracture
    N.-H. humerus fracture
        classification
NEFA
    nonesterified fatty acid
    NEFA scintigraphy
Neff percutaneous access set
negative
    n. contrast agent
    n. contrast imaging agent
    n. contrast left atriography
    n. EMA result
    n. image
    n. image pulmonary edema
    n. Mach band
    n. mucin result
    n. predictive value
    pulmonary edema photographic n.
    true n. (TN)
    n. ulnar variance
negative-ion cyclotron
negatron emission
negligible pressure gradient
Nélaton
    N. dislocation
    N. fold
    N. line
Nelson syndrome
NEMD
    nonspecific esophageal motility disorder
neoadjuvant
    n. hormonal therapy
    n. radiotherapy
neoangiogenesis
neoaorta
neoaortic valve
neobladder
    ileal n.
neocerebellum
neocholangiole

neocortex
neodensity
neodymium:YAG laser therapy
neodymium:yttrium-aluminum-garnet
  (Nd:YAG)
    n:y.-a.-g. laser
neodymium:yttrium-lithium fluoride
  (Nd:YLF)
neofissure
neogalactosyl albumin
neointima formation
neointimal
    n. hyperplasia
    n. proliferation
Neo-Iopax
neonatal
    n. adrenal ultrasound
    n. ascites
    n. cardiac failure
    n. choroid plexus hemorrhage
    n. cystic pulmonary emphysema
    n. heart failure
    n. hepatitis
    n. hyperthyroidism
    n. intracerebellar hemorrhage
    n. intracranial hemorrhage
    n. intracranial ischemia
    n. intraventricular hemorrhage
    n. omphalitis
    n. osteomyelitis
    n. pneumonia
    n. radiography
    n. subdural hemorrhage
    n. transfontanellar brain ultrasound
    n. wet lung disease
neonate
    n. encephalomalacia
    n. mediastinal shift
neonatorum
    edema n.
neon particle protocol
neopallium
neoplasia
    exophytic n.
    extrinsic n.
    lobular n.
neoplasm, pl. **neoplasia**
    adrenocortical n.
    benign n.
    bone n.
    breast n.
    bronchopulmonary n.

cavitating n.
cervical intraepithelial n.
choroid plexus n.
colonic n.
connective tissue n.
cranial nerve n.
cystic splenic n.
ductectatic mucinous cystic n.
encapsulated n.
epithelial n.
esophageal n.
external ear n.
firm n.
focally decreased renal n.
functioning n.
gestational trophoblastic n.
gonadal n.
granulosa theca n.
hepatic n.
interdigital n.
intracranial n.
intraductal papillary-mucinous n.
  (IPMN)
intrahepatic biliary n.
intramedullary compartment n.
lethal n.
low-grade n.
macrocystic n.
malignant urethral n.
mesenchymal n.
metastatic renal n.
middle ear n.
mucinous pancreatic cystic n.
multiple endocrine n. (MEN)
neuroepithelial n.
NK-cell n.
osteocartilaginous parasellar n.
ovarian n.
pancreatic n.
papillary epithelial n.
papillary pancreatic cystic n.
pearly n.
pineal gland n.
primary n.
second malignant n. (SMN)
skeletal n.
soft tissue n.
spheric n.
supratentorial n.
T-cell n.
thoracic spinal n.
thymic n.

NOTES

N

neoplasm (continued)
    transitional cell n.
    trochlear nerve n.
    vaginal intraepithelial n.
    vulvar intraepithelial n.
    well-circumscribed n.
neoplastic
    n. aneurysm
    n. calcification
    n. cyst
    n. destruction of spinal element
    n. fracture
    n. hyperplasia
    n. invasion
    n. lesion
    n. process
    n. stenosis
    n. tissue
Neoprobe
    N. 1000, 1500 portable
      radioisotope detector
    N. radioactivity detector
neopterin
neorectum
Neoscan
NeoSpect diagnostic imaging agent
neosphincter
neostigmine methylsulfate
NeoTect imaging agent
neoterminal ileum
neovagina
neovascularity
    tumor n.
neovascularization
    choroidal neovascularization (CNV)
neovasculature
    tumor n.
nepheline pneumoconiosis
nephritic calculus
nephritis, pl. **nephritides**
    acute diffuse bacterial n.
    acute focal bacterial n.
    acute interstitial n. (AIN)
    bacterial n.
    Balkan n.
    chronic hereditary n.
    diffuse bacterial n.
    focal bacterial n.
    glomerular n.
    interstitial n.
    nephrocalcinosis n.
    radiation n.
    salt-losing n.
    tubulointerstitial n.
nephroblastoma
    classical n.
    cystic partially differentiated n.
    polycystic n.

nephroblastomatosis
    panlobar n.
nephroblastomatosis
    multifocal n.
    superficial diffuse n.
nephrocalcinosis
    cortical n.
    medullary n.
    n. nephritis
    renal cortical n.
nephrogenic, nephrogenetic
    n. bladder adenoma
    n. diabetes insipidus
    n. phase
nephrogram
    cortical rim n.
    delayed unilateral n.
    increasingly dense n.
    medullary n.
    obstructive n.
    persistent increasing n.
    rim n.
    n. rim
    segmental n.
    shell n.
    n. shock
    soap-bubble n.
    spotted n.
    striated angiographic n.
    sunburst n.
    Swiss cheese n.
    tubular n.
nephrographic
    generalized n. (GNG)
    n. phase (NP)
nephrography
    isotope n.
nephrolithiasis
nephrolithotomy
    percutaneous n. (PCNL)
nephroma
    congenital mesoblastic n.
    cystic n.
    mesoblastic n.
    multilocular cystic n.
NephroMax balloon catheter
nephronia
    lobar n.
nephronophthisis
    juvenile n.
nephron-sparing surgery
nephropathic cystinosis
nephropathy
    analgesic n.
    Balkan n.
    contrast media–induced n.
    diabetic n.
    HIV n.
    ischemic n.

obstructive n.
radiation n.
radiocontrast-induced n.
radiographic contrast media-
    induced n.
reflux n.
urate n.
uric acid n.
nephroptosis
nephropyelography
nephrosclerosis
    arterial n.
    benign n.
    malignant n.
    senile n.
nephroscope
    Alken-Marberger n.
    flexible n.
    percutaneous n.
    Wickham-Miller n.
nephroscopic fulguration
nephroscopy
nephrosis, pl. **nephroses**
    congenital Finnish n.
nephrosonography
nephrostogram
    n. imaging
    postprocedure n.
nephrostolithotomy
    calyceal n.
    percutaneous n. (PCNL)
nephrostomy
    n. catheter
    circle wire n.
    Cope loop n.
    percutaneous n.
    n. puncture
    n. track
nephrotic
    n. edema
    n. syndrome
nephrotomogram
nephrotomography
    n. imaging
    infusion n.
nephrotoxic contrast medium
nephrotoxicity
    contrast media n.
    cyclosporin n.
    drug-induced n.

nephroureteral
    n. stent
    n. stent system
nephroureterectomy
nephroureterostomy stent
nephrourography
nephrouroradiology
Neptune trident appearance
neptunium
NER
    no evidence of recurrence
NERD
    no evidence of recurrent disease
Nernst equation
nerve
    accessory n.
    acoustic n.
    afferent digital n.
    cluneal n.
    cochlear n.
    cranial n.
    dorsal ramus of spinal n.
    efferent digital n.
    n. entrapment
    excrescentic thickening of optic n.
    facial n.
    femoral n.
    N. Fiber Analyzer GDx
    n. fiber myelination
    fifth cranial n.
    fourth cranial n.
    frontal n.
    fusiform enlargement of optic n.
    glossopharyngeal n.
    greater superficial petrosal n.
    hypoglossal n.
    n. injury
    intercostal n.
    intercostobrachial n.
    interosseous n.
    lacrimal n.
    laryngeal n.
    n. of Latarjct
    left respiratory n.
    lingual n.
    mandibular n.
    median n.
    nasociliary n.
    oculomotor n.
    ophthalmic n.
    optic n.
    peripheral n.

NOTES

N

nerve *(continued)*
    periradicular n.
    peroneal n.
    petrosal n.
    pinched n.
    n. plexus
    posterior interosseous n. (PIN)
    recurrent laryngeal n.
    recurrent meningeal n.
    n. root
    n. root axillary pouch
    n. root compression
    n. root edema
    n. root embarrassment
    n. root impingement
    n. root irritability
    n. roots of cauda equina
    n. root sheath
    n. root sheath effacement
    n. root sleeve
    n. root tumor
    rostral cervical n.
    sacral n.
    saphenous n.
    second cranial n.
    n. sheath tumor
    spinal accessory n.
    subcostal n.
    supraspinatus n.
    sural n.
    trochlear n.
    n. trunk
    vagus n.
    vein, artery, n.
    vestibular division of eighth cranial n.
    vestibulocochlear n.
    vidian n.
    VIII n. complex
nervus intermedius
nesidioblastoma
nesidioblastosis
nest
    junctional n.
nester coil
net
    n. magnetization factor
    n. magnetization vector
    n. shunt
    n. tissue magnetization
    n. transverse magnetization
network
    articular n.
    artificial neural n.
    hypertrophic duct n.
    lymphatic n.
    matching n.
    neural n.

    vascular n.
    venous n.
neural
    n. arch cleft
    n. arch fracture
    n. axis vascular malformation
    n. blockade
    n. canal
    n. crest origin
    n. crest tissue
    n. evaluation algorithm
    n. fibrolipoma
    n. foramen
    n. foramen remodeling
    n. foraminal narrowing
    n. groove
    n. miscommunication
    n. network
    n. origin bone tumor
    n. pathway
    n. placode
    n. sheath
    n. tube
    n. tube defect (NTD)
    n. tuberculosis
    n. vertebral arch
neuralgia
    sphenopalatine n.
neuraxis
    n. radiation therapy
    n. staging
neuraxonal dystrophy
neurenteric canal
neurilemoma, neurilemmoma
    intradermal n.
neurinoma *(var. of* neuroma)
neuritic
    n. plaquing
    n. senile plaque
neuritis, pl. **neuritides**
    axial n.
    brachial plexus n.
    friction n.
    optic n.
neuro
    N. Lobe software
    n. phase-contrast venography
    N. SPGR software
Neuroacryl tissue adhesive
neuroangiography
neuroarthropathy
neuroaugmentation
neuroblastoma (NB)
    adrenal n.
    cerebral n.
    chest wall n.
    dumbbell-type n.
    Hutchinson-type n.
    intracranial n.

intraventricular n.
olfactory n.
stage 4S n.
n. staging
neuroblockage
neurocentral synchondrosis
neurocutaneous syndrome
neurocysticercosis
neurocytoma
central n.
intraventricular n.
neurodegenerative disease
neurodiagnostic
n. imaging
n. scanner
NeuroEcho software
neuroectodermal
n. dysplasia
n. origin
n. tumor
neuroendocrine
n. hepatic metastasis
n. small-cell carcinoma
n. tumor
neuroendoscopy
neuroendovascular interventional
  procedure
neuroenteric cyst
neuroepithelial neoplasm
neurofibrillary tangle
neurofibroma
aryepiglottic fold n.
craniofacial plexiform n.
dumbbell n.
extraspinal n.
paraspinal n.
plexiform n.
neurofibromatosis
abortive n.
central n.
incomplete n.
kidney n.
peripheral n.
segmental n.
n. type 1 (NF1)
type 1, 2 n.
n. type 2 (NF2)
n. with bilateral acoustic neuroma
neurofibrosarcoma
neurofilamentous misalignment
NeuroFOCUS scanner

neurogenic
n. disorder
n. fracture
n. intestinal obstruction
n. lesion
n. pulmonary edema
n. sarcoma
n. shock
n. tumor
neuroglial tumor
neurography
magnetic resonance n. (MRN)
neuroimaging
3D n.
functional n.
n. modality
neurointerventional radiology
NeuroLink II data acquisition system
Neurolite imaging agent
neurologic
n. bladder lesion
n. sequelae
neuroma, neurinoma
acoustic n.
digital n.
interdigital n.
Morton n.
multicystic acoustic n.
neurofibromatosis with bilateral
  acoustic n.
postamputation n.
posttraumatic n.
neuromatosa
elephantiasis n.
neuromeningeal trunk
neuromorphometry
neuromuscular
n. junction
n. system electric induction
neuromyelitis optica
neuromyopathy
carcinomatous n.
neuron
lower motor n.
nigrostriatal dopaminergic n.
pyramidal n.
upper motor n.
neuronal
n. cell origin tumor
n. cytotoxic edema
n. migration

N

NOTES

neuronal (*continued*)
    n. plasticity
    n. proliferation
neuronavigation
neuroorthopedic syndrome
neurootologist
Neuropack 4, 8 EMG
neuropathic
    n. ankle
    n. arthropathy
    n. fracture
    n. midfoot deformity
    n. osteoarthropathy
    n. pain
    n. tarsometatarsal joint
neuropathicum
    papilloma n.
neuropathy
    compression n.
    entrapment n.
    radiation-related optic n. (RON)
neuropathy, ataxia and retinitis pigmentosa (NARP)
neuropore
neuroradiologic
    n. examination
    n. imaging
neuroradiology
    interventional n.
    pediatric n.
neuroreceptor
neuroroentgenography
neurosarcoidosis
neurosarcoma
NeuroScan 3D imager
neurosecretory granule
Neurosector
    N. ultrasound
    N. ultrasound system
Neuroshield
    N. distal protection device
    MedNova N.
neurosonogram
neurosonography
neurosonology
neurospectroscopy
neuroticum
    papilloma n., papilloma
       neuropathicum
neurotomography
neurotoxic effect
neurotransmitter
    excitatory n.
    n. imaging
    inhibitory n.
    n. precursor
neurotrophic
    n. fracture

    n. imaging agent
    n. joint
neurovascular
    n. bundle
    n. compression
    n. lesion
neurulation
neutral
    adduction to n.
    n. amyloid probe
    n. hip position
    n. ulnar variance
neutralization plate
neutrino
    electron n.
neutron
    n. absorption process
    n. activation analysis
    n. beam
    n. bombardment
    epithermal n.
    fast n.
    n. irradiation
    n. number
    n. radiation
    n. radiography
    slow n.
    n. therapy
    n. therapy machine
    thermal n.
neutron-atomic number ratio (N-2, N-Z)
neutron-deficient
    n.-d. nucleus
    n.-d. short-lived isotope
neutron/gamma
    n./g. transmission
    n./g. transmission method
    n./g. transmission therapy
neutron-rich biomedical tracer
neutropenic enterocolitis
neutrophilic leukocyte
Neviaser frozen shoulder classification
nevoid
    n. basal cell carcinoma
    n. basal cell carcinoma syndrome
nevus verrucosus
new bone formation
Newman
    N. classification of radial neck and
      head fracture
    N. radial fracture classification
NewTom CT scanner
Newton guidewire
Newvicon camera tube
NEX
    number of excitation
NexStent
NF1
    neurofibromatosis type 1

NF2
> neurofibromatosis type 2
> Wishart-Lee-Abbott N.

ng
> nanogram

NHLBI
> National Heart, Lung, and Blood Institute

Nicoladoni-Branham sign

Nicolet
> N. Elite Doppler   monitor
> N. Elite Doppler ultrasound
> N. NMR spectrometer

Nicoll bone

nicotinamide
> n. imaging agent
> n. radiosensitizer

Nidek
> N. EC-5000 excimer laser
> N. EC-5000 excimer laser system

nidus
> n. angle
> arteriovenous malformation n.
> n. demarcation
> n. of lesion
> n. patency
> thrombus n.
> tumor n.

Niemann-Pick disease

Niemeier gallbladder perforation

Nievergelt
> N. disease
> N. syndrome

Niewenglowski ray

nightstick fracture

nigra
> substantia n.

nigricans
> acanthosis n.

nigrostriatal dopaminergic neuron

Nihon Kohden Neurofax Electroencephalograph

Nijmegen breakage syndrome

nimodipine
> n. imaging agent
> intraarterial superselective n.

niobium/titanium superconductor

Niopam
> N. contrast medium
> N. imaging agent

NIP
> nonspecific interstitial pneumonia

nipple
> adenoma of n.
> aortic n.
> deep to the n.
> n. marker
> out-of-profile n.
> n. retraction
> n. ring artifact
> n. sector
> n. shadow

nipple-areolar complex

nipplelike
> n. common bile duct
> n. osteophyte formation

NIPS
> noninvasive programmed stimulation

NIR
> near infrared
> NIR contrast agent
> NIR optical mammography
> NIR stent

NIRS
> near infrared spectroscopy

Nishimoto Sangyo scanner

Nissen
> N. antireflux operation
> N. fundoplication
> N. fundoplication procedure

Ni-Ti alloy stent

nitinol
> n. guidewire
> n. inferior vena cava filter
> N. Symphony stent
> n. U-clips
> n. wire core

niton

nitrate
> organic n.

Nitrex
> N. ev3 guidewire
> N. Nitinol guidewire

nitric oxide

nitrocellulose film

nitrogen (N)
> n. 14 (^{14}N)
> n. 15 (^{15}N)
> n. washout

nitrogen-13 ammonia imaging agent

nitroxide-stable free radical

NK
> natural killer
> NK-cell neoplasm

N

NOTES

NLBB
    needle-localized breast biopsy
NMR
    nuclear magnetic resonance
      continuous-wave NMR
      2D NMR
      NMR imaging
      NMR LipoProfile test
      magic angle spinning NMR
      NMR magnetometer probe
      pulse NMR
      pulsed-electron paramagnetic NMR
      NMR quadrature detection array
      NMR scan
      NMR signal
      NMR spectrometer
      surface coil NMR
NMS
    N-methylspiroperidol
NMSP
    N-methylspiperone
no
    no discernible finding
    no evidence of disease (NED)
    no evidence of recurrence (NER)
    no evidence of recurrent disease
      (NERD)
    no frequency wrap
noble
    n. gas
    n. gas in magnetic resonance study
    N. position
***Nocardia* brain abscess**
nocardial osteomyelitis
no-carrier-added
    n.-c.-a. ^{18}F imaging agent
    n.-c.-a. radionuclide
nociceptive pain
nociceptor
    ectopic firing n.
nocturnal polysomnography
nodal
    n. conduction
    n. disease
    n. fibrosis
    n. impulse
    n. metastasis
    n. point
    n. premature contraction
    n. rhythm
    n. rupture
    n. staging
    n. tissue
node
    abdominal lymph n.
    accessory lymph n.
    anorectal lymph n.
    aortic lymph n.
    aortic window n.

apical lymph n.
appendicular lymph n.
Aschoff n.
Aschoff-Tawara n.
atrioventricular n.
auricular lymph n.
AV n.
axillary lymph n. (ALN)
azygos lymph n.
benign n.
bifurcation lymph n.
Bouchard n.
brachial lymph n.
brachiocephalic lymph n.
bronchopulmonary lymph n.
buccinator lymph n.
n. calcification
calcified lymph n.
cardiac n.
cartilaginous n.
caval lymph n.
celiac lymph n.
central lymph n.
cervical paratracheal lymph n.
Cloquet inguinal lymph n.
common iliac lymph n.
companion lymph n.
coronary n.
cubital lymph n.
cystic lymph n.
delphian lymph n.
deltopectoral lymph n.
diaphragmatic lymph n.
Dürck n.
eggshell calcification of lymph n.
epicolic lymph n.
epigastric lymph n.
epitrochlear lymph n.
Ewald n.
external iliac lymph n.
fibular lymph n.
Flack sinuatrial n.
foraminal n.
gastric lymph n.
gastroduodenal lymph n.
gastroepiploic lymph n.
gastrohepatic ligament n.
gastroomental lymph n.
Ghon n.
giant hyperplasia lymph n.
gluteal lymph n.
gouty n.
Haygarth n.
Heberden n.
hemal n.
hemolymph n.
Hensen n.
hepatic lymph n.
hilar lymph n.

ileocolic lymph n.
iliac circumflex lymph n.
ilioinguinal lymph n.
image-intensifier n.
infraclavicular n.
infrahyoid lymph n.
inguinal lymph n.
intercostal lymph n.
interiliac lymph n.
internal mammary lymph n.
interpectoral lymph n.
intramammary n. (IMN)
intramammary lymph n.
intraparenchymal lymph n.
intrapulmonary lymph n.
jugular lymph n.
jugulodigastric n.
juguloomohyoid lymph n.
juxtaintestinal n.
Keith n.
Keith-Flack sinuatrial n.
Koch sinuatrial n.
lacunar n.
lumbar lymph n.
lymph n.
lymphomatous lymph n.
malar lymph n.
mandibular lymph n.
mastoid lymph n.
medial supraclavicular n.
mediastinal n.
mesenteric n.
Meynet n.
multicentric angiofollicular lymph n.
nasolabial lymph n.
obturator lymph n.
occipital lymph n.
Osler n.
pancreatic lymph n.
pancreaticoduodenal lymph n.
pancreaticolienal lymph n.
pancreaticosplenic n.
paraaortic lymph n.
paracardial lymph n.
paracolic lymph n.
paramammary lymph n.
pararectal lymph n.
parasternal lymph n.
paratracheal lymph n.
parauterine lymph n.
paravaginal lymph n.
paravesicular lymph n.

parietal lymph n.
parotid lymph n.
Parrot n.
pectoral lymph n.
pelvic lymph n.
periaortic lymph n.
peribronchial lymph n.
pericardial lymph n.
pericholedochal n.
perisplenic n.
phrenic lymph n.
popliteal n.
porta hepatis n.
postaortic lymph n.
postcaval lymph n.
posterior mediastinal n.
postvesicular lymph n.
potato n.
preaortic lymph n.
precaval lymph n.
prececal lymph n.
prelaryngeal n.
prepericardial lymph n.
pretracheal lymph n.
prevertebral lymph n.
prevesicular lymph n.
pulmonary juxtaesophageal
 lymph n.
pyloric lymph n.
Ranvier n.
rectal lymph n.
regional lymph n.
retroaortic lymph n.
retroauricular lymph n.
retrocecal lymph n.
retrocrural n.
retroperitoneal n.
retropharyngeal lymph n.
retropyloric n.
retrorectal lymph n.
right hilar lymph n.
Rosenmüller n.
Rotter n.
Rouvière n.
SA n.
sacral lymph n.
satellite n.
scalene n.
Schmorl n.
sentinel lymph n. (SLN)
sick sinus n.
sigmoid lymph n.

NOTES

N

node (*continued*)
    signal n.
    singer's n.
    sinoauricular n.
    sinuatrial n. (SAN)
    sinus node
    Sister Mary Joseph n.
    solitary lymph n.
    spinal accessory lymph n.
    splenic lymph n.
    subcarinal lymph n.
    subcentimeter n.
    submandibular lymph n.
    submental lymph n.
    subpyloric n.
    subscapular lymph n.
    superficial inguinal lymph n.
    supraclavicular lymph n.
    suprapyloric n.
    supratrochlear n.
    syphilitic n.
    Tawara atrioventricular n.
    thyroid lymph n.
    tibial n.
    tracheal lymph n.
    tracheobronchial lymph n.
    Troisier n.
    vesicular lymph n.
    vestigial left sinuatrial n.
    Virchow sentinel n.
    Virchow-Troisier n.
    visceral lymph n.
node-negative carcinoma
node-positive carcinoma
nodosa
    periarteritis n.
    polyarteritis n. (PAN)
    salpingitis isthmica n.
nodosum
nodoventricular
    n. bypass fiber
    n. pathway
    n. tachycardia
nodular
    n. adrenal hyperplasia
    n. aneurysm
    n. appearance
    n. density
    n. enhancement
    n. goiter
    n. hyperintense focus
    n. induration of temporal artery
    n. irregularity
    n. lesion
    n. liver
    n. liver regeneration
    n. lung disease
    n. lymphoid hyperplasia
    n. mass

    n. obstruction
    n. proliferation
    n. pulmonary parenchymal opacity
    n. regenerative hyperplasia (NRH)
    n. sclerosis Hodgkin disease
    n. subepidermal fibrosis
    n. synovitis
    n. thyroid disease
nodularity
    calcified n.
    coarse n.
    lung n.
    noncalcified n.
    pulmonary n.
    surface n.
    tendon n.
    vein n.
nodulated
nodulation
    mural n.
nodule
    acinar n.
    airspace n.
    Albini n.
    aortic valve n.
    Arantius n.
    Aschoff n.
    autonomous thyroid n. (ATN)
    Bianchi n.
    calcified lung n.
    Caplan n.
    cartilaginous n.
    cavitating lung n.
    centrilobular n.
    cerebral n.
    circumscribed n.
    cirrhotic n.
    cold thyroid n.
    conglomerate pulmonary n.
    cortical n.
    Cruveilhier n.
    cutaneous n.
    Dalen-Fuchs n.
    discordant thyroid n.
    discrete pulmonary n.
    dysplastic liver n.
    eccentric enhancing n.
    echogenic n.
    enhancing n.
    esophageal mucosal n.
    fibrocartilaginous n.
    fibrous n.
    fluffy pulmonary n.
    Fränkel typhus n.
    functioning n.
    Gamna n.
    Gamna-Gandy n.
    glial n.
    ground-glass n.

n. halo
hemorrhagic lung n.
heterotopic n.
hyperechoic renal n.
hypermetabolic n.
hypointense n.
interstitial n.
Kerckring n.
Koeppe n.
laryngeal n.
lingular n.
Lisch n.
lung n.
meningotheliallike n.
miliary n.
Morgagni n.
mucosal esophageal n.
multiple lung n.'s
multiple pulmonary necrobiotic n.'s
mural CNS n.
necrobiotic n.
noncavitary n.
nondelineated n.
nonenhancing n.
nonfunctioning thyroid n.
ossific n.
peripheral n.
pleura-based lung n.
pleural n.
pneumoconiotic n.
prostatic hyperplastic n.
pulmonary n.
regenerative liver n.
rheumatoid n.
Rokitansky n.
satellite n.
Scheuermann n.
Schmorl n.
semiautonomous n.
shaggy lung n.
silicotic n.
singer's n.
Sister Mary Joseph n.
solitary metastatic lung n.
solitary pulmonary n. (SPN)
solitary pulmonary necrobiotic n.
subcutaneous n.
subpleural n.
surfer's n.
tendon n.
thyroid adenoma n.
thyroid colloid n.

tobacco n.
toxic n.
tuberculous n.
typhoid n.
typhus n.
warm n.
nodule-in-a-nodule appearance
nodule-in-nodule liver
nodulus Arantius
nodus arcus venae azygos
nofetumomab diagnostic imaging agent
noire
atrophie n.
noise
digitalization n.
echogenic n.
n. effective count (NEC)
gaussian n.
gradient switching n.
image n.
lesion-to-cerebrospinal fluid n.
lesion-to-white matter n.
pixel n.
quantum n.
radiographic n.
Rayleigh n.
n. reconstruction kernel
n. spike artifact
statistical n.
structured n.
subtractive n.
systematic n.
thermal n.
total image n.
Nölke position
NOMI
nonocclusive mesenteric ischemia
nomifensine
nominal
n. single dose
n. standard dose
nomogram
nonablative heating
nonaccelerated MRI
nonanaplastic glioma
nonaneurysmal perimesencephalic
subarachnoid hemorrhage
nonarrhythmic myocardial infarct
nonarticular radial head fracture
nonatherosclerotic disease
nonattenuation-corrected
n.-c. image

NOTES

N

nonattenuation-corrected *(continued)*
    n.-c. slice
    n.-c. SPECT imaging
nonavid infarct imaging
nonaxial beam technique
nonbony union
noncalcareous renal calculus
noncalcified
    n. carcinoma
    n. coronary stenosis
    n. fibroadenoma
    n. mitral leaflet
    n. nodularity
    n. nodular mass
    n. ocular process
noncardiac
    n. angiography
    n. pulmonary edema
noncardiogenic pulmonary edema
noncaseating
    n. granuloma
    n. tubercle
noncavitary nodule
nonchromaffin paraganglioma
noncircularity degree
noncirrhotic
    n. liver
    n. portal fibrosis (NCPF)
nonclassifiable interstitial pneumonia
noncleaved cell lymphoma
non-CNS PNET
noncoaxial catheter tip position
noncoiled umbilical cord
noncollagenous pneumonoconiosis
noncollinear directions
noncolonic structure
noncommitted mode
noncommunicating
    n. cyst
    n. hydrocephalus
noncompaction
    left ventricular n.
noncompliant plaque
noncontact imaging technology
noncontiguous
    n. expiratory HRCT
    n. fracture
noncontractile scar tissue
noncontrast
    n. CT scan
    n. head CT (NCCT)
    n. phase (NCP)
noncoplanar
    n. arch technique
    n. arc technique
    n. beam technique
    n. therapy beam

noncoronary
    n. cusp
    n. sinus
noncritical
    n. soft tissue
    n. stenosis
nondeciduate placenta
nondecremental
nondelineated nodule
nondependent lung
nondetachable
    n. balloon
    n. balloon catheter
nondilated system
nondisplaced fracture
nondissociative instability
nondominant
    n. hemisphere lesion
    n. putaminal hemorrhage
    n. vessel
nondynamometric trunk strength measurement
non-ECG-assisted multidetector row CT
nonechogenic tumor
nonembolic infarct
nonenclosed magnet
nonenhanced
    n. computed tomography (NECT)
    n. CT
    n. CT scan
nonenhancing
    n. lesion
    n. nodule
nonesterified
    n. fatty acid (NEFA)
    n. fatty acid scintigraphy
nonexpansile
    n. multilocular bone lesion
    n. osteolysis
    n. unilocular bone lesion
    n. well-demarcated multilocular bone defect
    n. well-demarcated unilocular bone defect
nonfamilial intestinal pseudoobstruction
nonferromagnetic
    n. needle
    n. positioning device
nonfetal
    n. complication
    n. uterine condition
nonfilarial chylocele
nonfilling venous segment
non-flow-compensated sequence
nonforeshortened angiographic view
nonfunctioning
    n. gallbladder
    n. heart valve
    n. islet cell tumor

n. kidney
n. pituitary adenoma
n. thyroid nodule
nonfusion of cranial suture
nongated CT scan
nongranular leukocyte
nonhemorrhagic
n. infarct
n. ischemia
n. mass
nonhomogeneous
n. consolidation
n. enhancement
n. hyperdense mass
nonhyperfunctioning adrenal adenoma
nonidiosyncratic anaphylactoid reaction
nonimmune
n. fetal hydrops
n. hydrops fetalis
noninducible tachycardia
noninfarcted
n. myocardium
n. segment
noninflammatory joint effusion
noninvasive
n. aspergillosis
n. assessment
n. imaging
n. imaging study
n. lesion
n. programmed stimulation (NIPS)
n. technique
n. thermometry
n. thymoma
n. ultrasound
nonionic
n. contrast material
n. dimer contrast medium
n. iodinated contrast agent
n. paramagnetic contrast imaging
agent
n. triiodinated monomer
n. water-soluble contrast medium
nonionizing radiation
nonischemic congestive cardiomyopathy
nonisotropic gradient
nonlethal
n. dwarfism
n. dysplasia
n. myocardial ischemic injury

nonlinear
n. excitation profile
n. sampling
nonlinearity
nonlingular
n. branch
n. branch of upper lobe bronchus
nonlocalized ischemia
nonmagnetization transfer gradient-refocused echo image
nonmagnified
n. image
n. mammography
nonmeningiomatous malignant lesion
nonmetastasizing fibrosarcoma
nonmotile leukocyte
nonmucinous adenocarcinoma
Nonne-Milroy lymphedema
nonneoplastic
n. cyst
n. tumor
nonnephrotoxic contrast agent
nonnipple sector
nonnodular
n. fibrosis
n. silicosis
nonobstructive
n. atelectasis
n. cardiomyopathy
n. hydrocephalus
n. ileus
nonocclusive
n. mesenteric arterial insufficiency
n. mesenteric ischemia (NOMI)
nonodontogenic
nonolfactory cortex
nononcogenic
nonopaque
n. calculus
n. intraluminal mass
n. stone
nonorthogonal plane
nonoscillatory motion
nonossifying fibroma
nonosteogenic fibroma
nonperfused myocardium
nonphysial fracture
nonplanar slice
nonpolar crevice
nonpregnant horn of bicornuate uterus
nonproliferative lesion
nonproton MRI

N

NOTES

nonpulsatile abdominal mass
nonradiopaque
    n. foreign body
    n. stone
nonreplantable amputation
nonresonance Raman spectroscopy
nonrheumatic
    n. aortic insufficiency
    n. valvular aortic stenosis
nonrhizomelic chondrodysplasia punctata
non-rib-bearing vertebra
nonrotational burst fracture
nonrotation of bowel loop
nonsecretor
nonsegmental areas of opacification
nonselective
    n. angiography
    n. pulse
nonseminomatous germ cell tumor
nonseptate
nonseptic embolic brain infarct
non-skin-sparing mastectomy (non-SSM)
non-small cell lung carcinoma (NSCLC)
nonspecific
    n. accumulation
    n. bowel gas pattern
    n. change
    n. conglomerate
    n. esophageal motility disorder
      (NEMD)
    n. finding
    n. interstitial pneumonia (NIP,
      NSIP)
non-SSM
    non-skin-sparing mastectomy
nonstanding lateral oblique view
nonstress
    n. fetal test
    n. test (NST)
nonstriated muscle
nonsubperiosteal cortical defect
nonsubtracted image
nonsubtraction
    n. image
    n. imaging
nonsuppurative
    n. ascending cholangitis
    n. destructive cholangitis
nonsurgical ablative therapy
nonsyndromic
    n. bicoronal synostosis
    n. focal cerebellar dysplasia
    n. unicoronal synostosis
nontarget embolization
nonthromboembolic condition
nonthrombogenic
nontrabeculated atrium

nontransmural
    n. match
    n. myocardial infarct
nontraumatic
    n. DCO
    n. epidural hemorrhage
nontriggered phase-contrast MR
  angiography
nontuberculosis mycobacteria
nontunneled catheter
nonuniform
    n. attenuation
    n. excitation
    n. rotational defect (NURD)
nonuniformity
nonunion
    atrophic n.
    bony n.
    fibrous n.
    fracture n.
    n. of fracture fragment
    hypertrophic n.
    torsion wedge n.
nonunited fracture
nonvalved conduit
nonviable
    n. fetus
    n. gestation
    n. scar
    n. tissue
nonviral vector
nonvisualization
    n. of fetal stomach
    n. of gallbladder
    n. of spleen
nonweightbearing view
Noonan syndrome
noose keyhole pull-away sign
no-reflow phenomenon
Norland
    N. bone densitometry
    N. pQCT XCT2000 scanner
    N. XR26 bone densitometer
normal
    n. anatomic position
    n. anatomic variation
    n. anteroposterior view
    n. axis
    n. bladder caliber
    borderline n.
    n. calcification
    n. caliber bowel
    n. caliber duct
    n. chest film
    n. echogenicity
    n. fold urethrogram
    n. gestation
    n. hemodynamic liver parameter
    high n.

n. lordotic curve
low n.
n. lower esophageal sphincter resting pressure
morphologically n.
n. ossification
n. ovarian surface epithelium (NOSE)
n. perfusion pressure breakthrough
n. planar MR anatomy
n. range
n. renal parenchyma
n. sinus rhythm
n. spleen weight
upper limits of n.
n. variant
n. variant fluorodeoxyglucose uptake distribution
n. variant of Ga-67 uptake
n. whole body fluorodeoxyglucose distribution
normal-appearing
n.-a. bronchus
n.-a. white matter (NAWM)
normalization
interictal n.
spatial n.
normalized
n. average glandular dose
n. cross-section
n. to plasma activity
n. plateau slope
normal-pressure hydrocephalus
normal-region pixel
normochromasia
normochromia
normotensive hydrocephalus
normoxia
Norrie disease
NOS
not otherwise specified
NOSE
normal ovarian surface epithelium
nose
anteater n.
beak-shaped n.
external n.
n. ring artifact
nose-chin position
nose-forehead position
nosocomial infection
notable cerebral insult

notch
anacrotic n.
angular n.
antegonial n.
aortic n.
apical n.
auricular n.
cardiac n.
cerebellar n.
clavicular n.
coracoid n.
costal n.
craniofacial n.
dicrotic n.
digastric n.
ethmoidal n.
fibular n.
Frankfort mandibular n.
n. from gastric sling fiber
frontal n.
greater sciatic n.
greater sigmoid n.
interclavicular n.
intercondylar n.
interpeduncular n.
intervertebral n.
lateral femoral n.
lesser sciatic n.
lucent hilar n.
n. projection
radial sigmoid n.
sacrosciatic n.
scapular n.
sciatic n.
semilunar n.
septal n.
sigmoid n.
spinoglenoid n.
splenic n.
sternal n.
suprasternal n.
trochlear n.
ulnar n.
n. view
notched
n. aortic knob
n. vertebra
notching
cortical n.
pelvic n.
n. of pulmonic valve
rib n.

N

NOTES

notching *(continued)*
    n. ureter
    ureteral n.
Nothnagel syndrome
no-threshold
    n.-t. body
    n.-t. concept
notochordal
    n. canal
    n. process
notochord remnant
not otherwise specified (NOS)
Novacor left ventricular assist system
NovaLine
    N. excimer laser
    N. Litho-S DUV excimer laser
Novalis radiosurgery system
NovaPulse CO_2 laser
novel agent
Novopaque
Novus Medical Image Card
NOX
    number of excitation
nozzle effect
NP
    nephrographic phase
NPC
    nasopharyngeal carcinoma
^{59}NP scintigraphy
NRC
    (U.S.) Nuclear Regulatory Commission
NRH
    nodular regenerative hyperplasia
NSA
    number of signal average
    number of signals averaged
    NSA of femur
NSCLC
    non-small cell lung carcinoma
N-shaped sigmoid loop
NSIP
    nonspecific interstitial pneumonia
NST
    nonstress test
NTD
    neural tube defect
NTHI
    native tissue harmonic imaging
NTP
    nucleoside triphosphate
nuchae
    ligamentum n.
nuchal
    n. cord
    n. cyst
    n. ligament
    n. plane
    n. skin thickening
    n. translucency

nuchofrontal projection
Nuck
    N. canal
    N. diverticulum
nuclear
    n. aggregation
    n. angiography
    n. anular differentiation
    n. atom
    n. bone imaging
    n. cardiovascular imaging
    n. chemistry
    n. decay
    n. disintegration
    n. electric quadripole relaxation
    n. emulsion
    n. enema
    n. energy
    n. fission
    n. force
    n. fusion
    n. gated blood pool imaging
    n. gated blood pool testing
    n. genome
    n. hepatobiliary imaging
    n. herniation
    N. Magnetic Device Lypoo Profile device
    n. magnetic moment
    n. magnetic resonance (NMR)
    n. magnetic resonance Fourier transformation
    n. magnetic resonance image
    n. magnetic resonance imaging
    n. magnetic resonance phantom
    n. magnetic resonance relaxation rate enhancement
    n. magnetic resonance scan
    n. magnetic resonance scanning sequence
    n. magnetic resonance signal intensity
    n. magnetic resonance spectography
    n. magnetic resonance spectral parameter
    n. magnetic resonance spectrometer
    n. magnetic resonance spectroscopy
    n. magnetic resonance spectrum
    n. magnetic resonance tomography
    n. magnetism
    n. matrix
    n. medicine
    n. medicine camera
    n. medicine imaging
    n. medicine information system
    n. Overhauser effect
    n. particle
    n. perfusion imaging
    n. pleomorphism

n. polarization
n. probe
n. pulse amplifier
n. radiationoccupational radiation
n. reaction
n. reactornuclear relaxation
n. renal scintigraphy
n. scanner
n. scanning
n. signal
n. spin
n. spin quantum number
n. structure
(U.S.) N. Regulatory Commission (NRC)

nuclei (*pl. of* nucleus)
nucleide
nucleiform
nucleography
nucleoid
nucleon number
nucleoside
n. phosphonate
n. triphosphate (NTP)

nucleotide scan
Nucletron
N. applicator
N. MicroSelectron/LDR remote afterloader

nucleus, pl. **nuclei**
n. ambiguus lesion
arcuate n.
basal n.
n. basalis lesion
n. of Cajal
caudate n.
cranial n.
n. of Darkschewitsch
dentate nuclei
dorsomedial n.
head of caudate n.
inferior syndrome of red n.
Köllicker n.
lentiform n., lenticular nucleus
magnetic nuclei
motor n.
neutron-deficient n.
oculomotor-trochlear n.
ossific n.
parafascicular n.
pretectal n.

n. pulposus herniation
quadripolar n.
residual n.
sensory n.
sixth n.
n. of solitary tract
ventral cochlear n.

nuclide
n. analysis
daughter n.
n. generator
isobar n.
isomer n.
isotone n.
isotope n.
parent n.
radioactive n.

NUG
necrotizing ulcerative gingivitis

nulled
nulling
gradient moment n. (GMN)

null point
NuLytely bowel preparation
number
average gradient n.
Avogadro n. (Λ)
body atomic n.
clonogen n.
CT n.
effective atomic n.
Euler n.
n. of excitation (NEX, NOX)
Hounsfield n.
Huckman n. (HN)
imaginary n.
mass n.
neutron n.
nuclear spin quantum n.
nucleon n.
n. profile
quantum n.
Reynolds n.
S n.
n. of signal average (NSA)
n. of signals averaged (NSA)
spin quantum n.

numerary renal anomaly
nummular pneumonia
NURD
nonuniform rotational defect

NOTES

N

Nurick
N. classification of spondylosis
N. spondylosis classification
nursemaid's elbow
nutation
n. angle
n. angle measurement
nutcracker
n. esophagus
n. fracture
n. phenomenon
n. syndrome
nutmeg appearance of liver
nutrient
n. artery of femur
n. artery of fibula
n. artery growth
n. foramen

Nutriflex tube
nutritional cirrhosis
Nuvolase 660 laser
NYHA
New York Heart Association
NYHA congestive heart failure classification
nylon
n. catheter
liquid n.
Nyquist
N. criterion
N. frequency
N. limit
N. sampling theorem
N-Z
neutron-atomic number ratio

O₂

oxygen
O₂ consumption index

¹⁵O

oxygen 15

¹⁶O

oxygen 16

¹⁷O

oxygen 17

¹⁸O

oxygen 18

OA

osteoarthritis
ovarian artery

OAF

off-axis factor

OAR

off-axis ratio
OAR malleolar rule

oasis

O. thrombectomy catheter
O. thrombectomy system
O. triple-lumen catheter

oat cell carcinoma

OAV

oculoauriculovertebral

object

o. coordinate system
o. modulation
side-by-side o.
unidentified bright o. (UBO)

object-based

o.-b. interpolation
o.-b. visualization

object-film distance (OFD)

object-plane blur

oblique

o. annihilation photon pair
o. axial MR imaging
o. coronal plane
o. diameter
o. film
o. fissure
o. flow misregistration
o. lateral projection
left anterior o. (LAO)
left posterior o. (LPO)
o. magnetic resonance imaging
mediolateral o. (MLO)
o. muscle
o. pericardial sinus
o. position
o. prescription line
o. radiograph
o. ridge

right anterior o. (RAO)
right posterior o. (RPO)
o. sagittal EKG-gated spin-echo
magnetic resonance imaging
o. sagittal sequence
o. slice
o. spiral fracture
superior o.
trauma o.
T2-weighted fast spin-echo
coronal o.
o. vein
o. vein of left atrium
o. view

oblique-angle reconstruction

obliquely

o. oriented axon
o. oriented fiber

obliquity

degree of neck o.
Litzmann o.
magnitude of o.
Naegele o.
pelvic o.
Roederer o.
varying degrees of o.

obliterans

arteriosclerosis o. (ASO)
atherosclerosis o. (ASO)
bronchiolitis fibrosa o.
endarteritis o.
mastitis o.
postinfectious bronchiolitis o.
thromboangiitis o.

obliterated costophrenic angle

obliteration

balloon-occluded transvenous o.
subdeltoid fat plane o.

obliterative

o. arteriosclerosis
o. bronchiolitis
o. cardiomyopathy
o. inflammation

oblongata

medulla o.

O'Brien

O. classification of radial fracture
O. radial fracture classification

OBS

organic brain syndrome

obscuration arteriosclerosis

observation

fluoroscopic o.

observed maximal uptake

observer variation

O

obstetric, obstetrical
   o. sonography
   o. ultrasound
obstipation
obstructed shunt tube
obstructing embolus arteriosclerosis
obstruction
   acute abdominal o.
   adynamic intestinal o.
   airway o.
   aortic arch o.
   aortic outflow o.
   aortic valve o.
   aortoiliac o.
   aqueductal o.
   arachnoid villi o.
   arterial o.
   ball-valve o.
   benign biliary o. (BBO)
   bilateral o.
   bile flow o.
   biliary tract o.
   biliary tree o.
   bladder outlet o.
   bowel o.
   bronchial o.
   bronchiolar o.
   cardiac o.
   catheter o.
   central venous o.
   cerebrospinal fluid o.
   chronic airway o.
   closed-loop intestinal o.
   colonic o.
   common bile duct o.
   complete bowel o.
   congenital duodenal o.
   congenital left-sided outflow o.
   congenital pelviureteric junction o.
   congenital subpulmonic o.
   congenital ureteric o.
   cystic duct o.
   distal common bile duct o.
   duct o.
   duodenal-gastric outlet o.
   efferent loop o.
   embolic o.
   endobronchial o.
   esophageal o.
   extrahepatic binary o.
   extrathoracic o.
   extrinsic malignant o.
   false colonic o.
   fecal o.
   fetal bowel o.
   fetal renal o.
   fixed airway o.
   fixed coronary o.
   flow-dependent o.

food bolus o.
foreign body upper airway o.
functional ureteral o.
gastric outlet o.
gastrointestinal tract o.
hepatic venous outflow o.
high-grade o.
high small bowel o.
hilar o.
hydrocephalic o.
idiopathic o.
ileal o.
iliac vein o.
incomplete o.
increased pulmonary o.
inferior vena caval o.
infravesical o.
intermittent o.
interposed colon segment o.
intestinal o.
intrapancreatic o.
intrathoracic upper airway o.
intraventricular right ventricular o.
intravesical o.
irreversible airway o.
jejunal o.
large bowel o.
left ventricular inflow tract o.
left ventricular outflow tract o.
  (LVOTO)
low small bowel o.
lymphatic o.
malignant airway o.
mammary duct o.
mechanical biliary o.
mechanical duct o.
mechanical extrahepatic o.
mechanical intestinal o.
mechanical respiratory tract o.
mechanical small bowel o.
neurogenic intestinal o.
nodular o.
otic o.
outflow o.
outlet o.
pancreatic duct o.
paralytic colonic o.
partial small bowel o.
pelvic venous o.
porta hepatis o.
posttransplantation ureteric o.
posttuberculous o.
postural ureteric o.
preocclusive o.
primary acquired nasolacrimal
  duct o. (PANDO)
prostatic o.
pulmonary artery o.
pulmonary outflow o.

pulmonary vascular o.
pulmonary venous o.
pyloric outlet o.
pyloroduodenal o.
rectal o.
renal o.
respiratory tract o.
right ventricular outflow o.
Rigler triad of small bowel o.
secondary o.
segmental biliary o.
sequence o.
simple mechanical o.
small-bowel o. (SBO)
strangulated o.
strangulating o.
subclavian artery o.
subpulmonic o.
subrectus o.
subvalvular aortic o.
subvalvular diffuse muscular o.
superior vena cava o. (SVCO)
suprapancreatic o.
supravesical o.
thrombotic o.
transient shunt o.
tubal o.
UPJ o.
upper airway o.
ureteral renal transplant o.
ureteropelvic junction o.
ureterovesical junction o.
urethral o.
urinary o.
vascular o.
venous o.
ventricular o.
vesical outlet o.

obstructive
o. abnormality
o. airway disease
o. atelectasis
o. biliary cirrhosis
o. calculus
o. component
o. dysfunctional ileitis
o. emphysema
o. hydrocephalus
o. hypertrophic cardiomyopathy
o. hypopnea
o. lesion
o. lung disease

o. nephrogram
o. nephropathy
o. pancreatitis
o. plaque
o. pneumonia
o. pulmonary arterial hypertension
o. pulmonary disease (OPD)
o. pulmonary overinflation
o. renal dysplasia
o. shock
o. thrombus
o. uropathy
o. ventilatory defect

obturating embolus
obturator
o. avulsion fracture
o. externus
o. foramen
o. hernia
o. internus
o. internus fascia
o. internus muscle
o. internus tendon
o. line
o. lymph node
o. membrane
o. nodal chain
o. sign

obtuse
o. marginal (OM)
o. marginal branch (OMB)
o. marginal coronary artery

occipital
o. artery
o. bone
o. bossing
o. cephalocele
o. condyle
o. condyle fracture
o. condyle hypoplasia
o. condyle invasion
o. eminence
o. encephalocele
o. fissure
o. focus
o. fontanelle
o. gyrus
o. horn
o. lesion
o. lobe
o. lobe infarct
o. lymph node

NOTES

O

occipital *(continued)*
- o. meningocele
- o. plane
- o. pole
- o. protuberance
- o. sinus
- o. suture
- o. tip
- o. vessel
- o. view
- o. view of skull

occipitalization
- atlas o.

occipitoanterior

occipitoatlantoaxial
- o. anomaly
- o. fusion
- o. ligament

occipitoaxial
- o. joint
- o. ligament

occipitocervical
- o. angle
- o. articulation
- o. fusion
- o. junction
- o. plate

occipitofrontal
- o. diameter (OFD)
- o. fasciculus

occipitofrontalis muscle

occipitomastoid suture

occipitomental
- o. diameter
- o. projection

occipitoparietal suture

occipitopontine tract

occipitoposterior

occipitosphenoid suture

occipitotemporal
- o. convolution
- o. gyrus
- o. sulcus

occiput

occluded
- o. graft
- o. lumen

occluder
- ameroid o.
- CardioSEAL o.
- clamshell double umbrella o.
- Flo-Rester vessel o.
- radiolucent plastic o.
- Rashkind o.

occluding
- o. agent
- o. spring embolus

occlusal
- o. facet

- o. film
- o. plane
- o. radiograph
- o. segment
- o. surface

occlusion
- angiographic o.
- o. angiography
- o. aorta
- aqueductal o.
- arterial o.
- o. of artery
- atrial septal defect o.
- balloon o.
- balloon test o.
- basilar o.
- bilateral o.
- carotid artery o.
- carotid-cavernous fistula o.
- celiac axis o.
- cerebral sinovenous o.
- complete o.
- coronary o.
- deep venous o.
- diathermic vascular o.
- ductus arteriosus o.
- dural sinus o.
- embolic o.
- fallopian tube o.
- graft o.
- infrapopliteal artery o.
- intermittent o.
- internal carotid artery o.
- intracranial vascular o.
- late graft o.
- o. measurement
- mesenteric artery o.
- mesenteric vascular o.
- middle cerebral artery o.
- parent artery o.
- parent vessel o.
- percutaneous thermal o.
- pulmonary arterial o.
- selective test o.
- side-branch o.
- snowplow o.
- subclavian artery o.
- subclavian vein o.
- subtotal o.
- superficial femoral artery o.
- tandem ICA/MCA o.
- tapering o.
- test balloon o.
- thermal o.
- thrombotic o.
- top of carotid T o.
- total o.
- transrenal ureteric o.
- transvenous o.

traumatogenic o.
tubal o.
unilateral o.
ureteral o.
vascular brain o.
vein graft o.
venous o.
vertebral artery o.
vertebrobasilar o.
vertebrobasilar artery o.
vessel o.

occlusive
    o. arterial thrombus
    o. cerebrovascular disease
    o. cerebrovascular insult
    o. drain
    o. ileus
    o. impedance phlebography
    o. lesion
    o. mesenteric infarct

occult
    o. blood
    o. bone metastasis
    o. cerebral vascular malformation (OCVM)
    o. detection
    o. hydrocephalus
    o. intrasacral meningocele
    o. lesion
    o. osseous fracture
    o. osseous injury
    o. papillary carcinoma
    o. pericardial constriction
    o. phosphaturic mesenchymal tumor
    o. primary tumor of testis
    o. residual herniated disc
    roentgenographically o.
    o. spinal dysraphism
    o. subluxation
    o. thyroid carcinoma
    o. vascular brain malformation

occulta
    spina bifida o. (SBO)

occupational lung disease

OCD
    osteochondral defect

OCG
    oral cholecystogram
    OCG imaging

ochronosis

Ochsner muscle

OCL
    oral colonic lavage
    OCL bowel preparation

O'Connor finger dexterity test

OCR
    off-center ratio

OCT
    optic coherence tomography

octagonal configuration

Octane postprocessing workstation

OctreoScan
    O. 111 radioactive imaging agent
    O. system

octreotide
    o. imaging
    o. imaging agent
    ^{111}In o.
    o. paraganglioma scintigraphy
    ^{99m}Tc-labeled o.
    o. tumor localization scan

ocular
    o. adnexa
    o. globe topography
    o. implant
    o. lesion
    o. magnification system
    o. pneumoplethysmography (OPG)
    o. radiation therapy (ORT)
    o. rhabdomyosarcoma
    o. trauma

OcuLight SL diode laser

oculoauriculovertebral (OAV)

oculomotor
    o. apparatus
    o. nerve

oculomotor-trochlear nucleus

oculopharyngeal dystrophy

oculoplethysmography (OPG)

oculoplethysmography/carotid phonoangiography (OPG/CPA)

oculopneumoplethysmography

oculosubcutaneous syndrome of Yuge

OCVM
    occult cerebral vascular malformation

OD
    optic density

odd-echo dephasing

Oddi
    O. muscle
    sphincter of O.

odds ratio (OR)

Odelca camera unit

O

NOTES

O'Donoghue unhappy triad
odontogenic
- o. cyst
- o. fibromyxoma
- o. keratocyst
- o. myxoma
- o. tumor

odontoid
- o. bone
- o. condyle fracture
- o. dysplasia
- o. erosion
- o. fracture types I–III
- o. ligament
- pannus deformity of o.
- o. process
- o. vertebra
- o. view

odontoma
odontoradiograph
ODQ
- opponens digiti quinti
- ODQ muscle

odynophagia
OEC Series 9600 cardiac system
OEF
- oxygen extraction fraction

Oehl muscle
OER
- oxygen extraction rate

OFD
- object-film distance
- occipitofrontal diameter

off-axis
- o.-a. dose inhomogeneity
- o.-a. factor (OAF)
- o.-a. point localization
- o.-a. ratio (OAR)
- o.-a. rotational acquisition

off-center
- o.-c. cut
- o.-c. modulation
- o.-c. ratio (OCR)

off-lateral projection
off-resonance
- 3D rotating delivery of excitation o.-r.
- rotating delivery of excitation o.-r. (RODEO)
- o.-r. saturation
- o.-r. saturation pulse imaging
- o.-r. spin-locking

off-resonant spin
offset
- chemical shift spatial o.
- E-zero o.
- o. fan-beam
- focal osseous o.
- o. frequency

quarter-detector o.
o. radiofrequency spin echo
resonance o.

Ogden
- O. classification of epiphysial fracture
- O. epiphysial fracture classification

Ogilvie syndrome
Ogston line
Ohio
- O. infuser
- O. Nuclear Delta 50 FS, 2000 scanner

Ohm law
Ohngren line
OHP
- orthogonal-hole test pattern

OI
- osteogenesis imperfecta

OIH
- iodine-123 orthoiodohippurate
- orthoiodohippurate
- ^{123}I OIH
- iodine-131 OIH

oil
- brominated o.
- chloriodized o.
- o. cyst
- o. embolus
- o. emulsion imaging agent
- ethiodized o.
- iodized poppy seed o.
- iophendylate o.
- o. myelography
- silicone o.

oil-aspiration pneumonia
oil-retention enema
oil-soluble contrast medium (OSCM)
oil-water phantom
okadaic acid
Okuda
- O. hepatic compromise stage I–III
- O. transhepatic obliteration of varix

old
- o. hemorrhage
- o. myocardial infarct

olecranon
- o. bursa
- o. bursitis
- o. fossa
- o. process
- o. tip fracture

oleoperitoneography
oleothorax
Olerud and Molander fracture classification
olfactory
- o. area
- o. bulb

o. canal
o. groove meningioma
o. gyrus
o. neuroblastoma
o. sulcus
o. tract
oligemia
mosaic o.
oligemia-related cyanotic CHD
oligoastrocytoma
anaplastic mixed o.
recurrent vermian o.
oligodactylia
oligodendroglia
oligodendroglioma
bifrontal o.
subependymal o.
oligohydramnios
oligomeganephronia
oligonucleotide
antisense o.
o. probe
radiolabeled antisense o.
olisthesis
olivary
o. degeneration
o. hypertrophy
olive
amiculum of o.
inferior o.
posterior o.
Oliver-Cardarelli sign
olivopontocerebellar
o. atrophy
o. degeneration (OPCD)
Ollier disease
OLM
ophthalmic laser microendoscope
Olshevsky tube
Olympus
O. CF-1T100L colonoscope
O. CF-200Z colonoscope
O. CHF-BP30 transduodenal
choledochofiberscope
O. endoscopic ultrasound
O. endoscopic ultrasound scanner
O. ENF-P2 laryngoscope
O. EU-M30 system
O. EVIS Q-200V endoscope
O. Gastrocamera GTF-A
O. GF-UM2, GF-UM3
echoendoscope

O. GIF-1T10 echoendoscope
O. JF1T10 duodenoscope
O. JF1T10 fiberoptic duodenoscope
O. JF-UM20 echoendoscope
O. MH-908 slim ultrasonic probe
O. OSF sigmoidoscope
O. SIF-100 video enteroscope
O. S20-20R transendoscopic
ultrasound probe
O. TJF-100 endoscope
O. VU-M2 echoendoscope
O. XIF-UM3 echoendoscope
O. XQ230 gastroscope
OM
obtuse marginal
orbitomeatal
OM artery
OMB
obtuse marginal branch
omega-sella
Omenn syndrome
omenta (*pl. of* omentum)
omental
o. band
o. bursa
o. cake
o. cyst
o. infarct
o. mass
o. tuberosity
omentoportography
omentum, pl. **omenta**
colic o.
gastric o.
gastrocolic o.
gastrohepatic o.
gastrosplenic o.
greater o.
incarcerated o.
lesser o. (LO)
o. majus
o. minus
pancreaticosplenic o.
sigmoid o.
splenogastric o.
Omni
O. Flex biliary stent
O. Flush 3F, 4F, 5F catheter
O. Selective 0-3 catheter
**Omnilink/Megalink balloon-expanded
stent**

O

NOTES

Omnipaque
    O. 140, 180, 240, 300, 350
      imaging agent
    O. injection
OmniPulse-MAX holmium laser
Omniscan imaging agent
Omniscience valve
Omnisense
    O. multisite QUS device
    O. 7000S bone sonometer
omohyoid muscle
omovertebral bone
omphalic
omphalitis
    neonatal o.
omphalocele
    infraumbilical o.
omphaloma
omphalomesenteric
    o. artery
    o. duct
    o. duct cyst
    o. remnant
omphalopagus twin
onchocerciasis
oncocalyx
oncocytic thyroid adenoma
oncocytoma
    pituitary o.
oncogenesis
    radiation o.
oncogenic osteomalacia
oncology
    PortalVision radiation o. system
on-column preparation
OncoRad OV103
OncoScint
    O. CR103
    O. CR/OV breast imaging agent
    O. OV103
    O. PR
oncosis
OncoTrac
oncotropic
OneStep paracentesis drainage catheter
one-third ejection fraction
onionlike laminar structure
onion peel appearance
onion-shaped dilatation of duodenum
onionskin
    o. appearance
    o. configuration of collagenous
      fiber
    o. lesion
    o. periosteal reaction
onlay graft
OnLine ABG monitor
on-line portal imaging
Onodi cell

on-off phenomenon
onset
on-the-fly random correction
onychoosteodysplasia
    familial o.
Onyx-015 genetically engineered
  adenovirus
oocyte retrieval
oophoroma folliculare
opacification
    arterial o.
    collecting system o.
    contrast o.
    early segmental o.
    extravesical o.
    ground-glass o. (GGO)
    hemithorax o.
    insufficient venous o.
    maxillary sinus o.
    nonsegmental areas of o.
    pedal artery o.
    o. of posterior longitudinal
      ligament
opacified
opacifying
    o. gallstone
    o. injection
opacity
    abnormal lung o.
    airspace o.
    asymmetric lung o.
    basilar reticular o.
    branching centrilobar o.
    bubbly o.
    centrilobar o.
    chronic diffuse confluent lung o.
    chronic multifocal ill-defined
     lung o.
    coarse linear o.
    coarse reticular o.
    conglomerate o.
    dependent o.
    diffuse airspace o.
    generalized hazy o.
    granular o.
    ground-glass o.
    hazy o.
    homogeneous o.
    linear o.
    localized pure ground-glass o.
    lung o.
    Medusa hairlike o.
    nodular pulmonary parenchymal o.
    parenchymal o.
    patchy alveolar o.
    pleura-based area of increased o.
    o. profusion
    pure ground glass o. (pGGO)
    reticular o.

rounded o.
tree-in-bud o.
tubular o.
uterine o.
whole-lung o.

opaque
    o. arthrography
    o. branching structure
    o. calculus
    o. enema
    o. foreign body
    o. material
    o. meal
    o. mediastinography
    o. medium
    o. myelography
    o. powder
    o. stone
    o. synovium
    o. wire suture

OPART MRI
OPCD
    olivopontocerebellar degeneration
OPD
    obstructive pulmonary disease
Opdima digital mammography system
OPD-Scan optical path difference scanning system
open
    o. beam
    o. bronchus sign
    o. dislocation
    o. fontanelle
    o. fracture
    o. magnet
    o. magnetic resonance defecography
    o. MRI
    o. MRI system
    o. neural tube defect
    o. pneumothorax
    o. reduction
    o. reduction and internal fixation (ORIF)
    o. tuberculosis
open-architecture system
open-book fracture
open-break fracture
open-configuration magnetic resonance system
open-cord tendon implant
open-ended guidewire

opening
    aortic o. (AO)
    aortic valve o.
    buttonhole o.
    caval o.
    esophageal o.
    mitral valve o. (MVO)
    peripherally inserted central catheter occlusion line o. (PICCOLO)
    o. slope
    tubal fimbrial o.
    valvular o.
open-mouth
    o.-m. odontoid view
    o.-m. projection
OpenPACS system
opera-glass hand
operating voltage
operation
    3D connect o.
    Fontan o.
    Miles o.
    Nissen antireflux o.
    pulsed-mode o.
    Senning o.
    Whipple o.
operative
    o. arteriography
    o. cholangiogram
operator-dependent positioning
operator exposure
opercular
    o. cortex
    o. segment of middle cerebral artery
operculofrontal artery
operculum, pl. **opercula**
    cerebral o.
    parietal o. (PO)
    sylvian o.
OPES
    oropharyngoesophageal scintigraphy
OPG
    ocular pneumoplethysmography
    oculoplethysmography
    ophthalmoplethysmography
OPG/CPA
    oculoplethysmography/carotid phonoangiography
ophenoxic acid
ophthalmic
    o. artery

O

NOTES

ophthalmic *(continued)*
    o. biometry by ultrasound echography
    o. laser microendoscope (OLM)
    o. nerve
    o. vein
ophthalmopathy
    Mourits criteria (Graves o.)
ophthalmoplegia
ophthalmoplethysmography (OPG)
ophthalmoscope
    Panoramic 200 nonmydriatic o.
ophthalmoscopy
    scanning laser o.
opinion
    in my o. (IMO)
opisthion
opisthotonic position
Opitz thrombophlebitic splenomegaly
OPLL
    ossification of posterior longitudinal ligament
    thoracic OPLL
Opmilas
    O. CO_2 multipurpose laser
    O. 144 Plus laser system
Oppenheim sign
opponens
    o. digiti minimi
    o. digiti quinti muscle
    o. pollicis
opportunistic lung cavity infection
opposed
    o. GRE image
    o. loop-pair quadrature NMR coil
opposed-phase
    o.-p. GRE, MR imaging
    o.-p. MRI
    o.-p. sequence
    o.-p. T1-weighted image
opposing
    o. articular surfaces
    o. muscle
    o. pleural surfaces
opsonized
OPTA
    OPTA 5 angioplasty balloon
    OPTA balloon stent-graft
OptEase permanent vena cava filter
optic
    o. canal
    o. chiasm
    o. chiasm disease
    o. coherence tomography (OCT)
    o. complex tumor
    o. density (OD)
    o. excrescentic thickening
    o. foramen
    o. glioma pathway

    o. globe
    o. glove
    o. isomer
    o. nerve
    o. nerve atrophy
    o. nerve compression
    o. nerve drusen
    o. nerve enlargement
    o. nerve fusiform thickening
    o. nerve glioma
    o. nerve hypoplasia
    o. nerve lesion
    o. nerve sheath meningioma
    o. neuritis
    o. papilla
    o. pathway myelination
    o. radiation
    o. recess
    o. strut
    o. surface imaging (OSI)
optica
    neuromyelitis o.
optical
    O. Biopsy System laser
    O. Path Difference-Scan optical device
Opticath catheter
opticochiasmatic cistern
Opti-Flow dialysis catheter
optimal
    o. angle imaging
    o. imaging plane
    o. modality
    o. visualization
optimally positioned view
OptiMARK contrast agent
optimization
    acquisition o.
    interactive gradient o.
    o. parameter
optimum dose
option
    post reconstruction filtering o.
optional target-to-background ratio
Optiplanimat automated unit
Opti-Plast balloon dilatation catheter
Optiplast Centurion balloon
OptiQue catheter
Optiray 10, 240, 300, 320, 350 imaging agent
Optison sterile injectable sonography contrast agent
Optispike dispensing pin
Optistar MR contrast delivery system
Optistat power injector
OptiVision laser
OR
    odds ratio
OR1 electronic system

ora (*pl. of* os)
Orabilex
oracle
    O. MegaSonics catheter
    O. Micro Plus catheter
    O. PTCA catheter
Oragrafin
    O. calcium imaging agent
    O. sodium imaging agent
oral
    o. cavity tumor
    o. cephalocele
    o. cholecystogram (OCG)
    o. cholecystogram imaging
    o. cholecystography
    o. colonic lavage (OCL)
    o. contrast imaging agent
    o. fissure
    o. intubation
    o. magnetic particle
    o. part of pharynx
    o. radiology
    o. urography
oral-enhanced CT scan
orange
    acridine o.
orbicular
    o. bone
    o. ligament
orbicularis
    zona o.
orbit
    angular process of o.
    o. artifact
    body contour o.
    bony o.
    egg-shaped o.
    electron o.
    floor of o.
    o. measurement
    Rhese view of o.
orbital
    o. abscess
    o. amyloidosis
    o. aneurysm
    o. angiography
    o. apex
    o. apex syndrome
    o. aspect of frontal lobe
    o. base
    o. blood cyst
    o. blowout fracture

    o. bone
    o. canal
    o. capillary hemangioma
    o. cavity
    o. cellulitis
    o. childhood tumor
    o. chocolate cyst
    o. dermoid cyst
    o. edema
    o. electron
    o. emphysema
    o. fissure
    o. floor fracture
    o. granulocytic sarcoma
    o. gyrus
    o. infection
    o. juvenile pilocytic astrocytoma
    o. lymphangioma
    o. lymphoma
    o. mass compression
    o. metastasis
    o. mucocele
    o. plane
    o. plate
    o. pseudotumor
    o. rhabdomyosarcoma
    o. rim
    o. rim stepoff
    o. sarcoidosis
    o. schwannoma
    o. space
    o. superolateral quadrant mass
    o. teratoma
    o. varix
    o. varix ophthalmic vein
    o. wall
orbitofrontal
    o. cortex
    o. dominance
orbitography
orbitomeatal (OM)
    o. line
orbitopathy
    thyroid o.
orbitosphenoidal bone
orbitotomy
    Krönlein o.
Orbix x-ray unit
Orca C-arm fluoroscopy
order
    phase-encoding o.

O

NOTES

ordered
>o. phase encoding
>o. subset expectation maximization (OSEM)

Orfit mask

organ
>accessory o.
>adjacent o.
>anulospiral o.
>o. capsule
>circumventricular o.
>Corti o.
>critical o.
>extraperitoneal o.
>floating o.
>hollow o.
>o. ischemia
>o. piping
>pole of o.
>retroperitoneal o.
>rudimentary o.
>sanctuary o.
>secondary retroperitoneal o.
>target o.
>o. transplant
>Zuckerkandl o.

organelle
>sphere o.

organic
>o. anion transporter polypeptide
>o. brain syndrome (OBS)
>o. free radical
>o. granulomatosis
>o. lesion
>o. muscle
>o. nitrate

organification defect

organization
>World Health O. (WHO)

organized
>o. hematoma
>o. thrombus

organizer
>embryonic o.
>isthmic o.

organizing
>o. focal pneumonia
>o. interstitial pneumonia
>o. pneumonia

organoaxial
>o. rotation
>o. volvulus

organogenesis

organoid structure

organomegaly

organ-sparing treatment approach

organ-specific
>o.-s. concentration
>o.-s. scintigraphic imaging

Oriental
>O. cholangiohepatitis
>O. lung fluke

orientation
>angle of o.
>axial o.
>coronal o.
>cruciate o.
>disc-to-magnetic field o.
>disturbed o.
>sagittal o.
>scan o.
>slice o.
>spatial o.
>temporal o.
>transverse o.

ORIF
>open reduction and internal fixation

orifice
>anal o.
>aortic o.
>atrioventricular nodal o.
>cardiac o.
>coronary o.
>double coronary o.
>esophagogastric o.
>external urethral o.
>gastroduodenal o.
>hypoplastic tricuspid o.
>ileocecal o.
>inferior vena cava o.
>internal urethral o.
>lingular o.
>mitral o. (MO)
>mitral valve o. (MVO)
>narrowed o.
>pharyngeal o.
>pulmonary o.
>pyloric o.
>rectal o.
>regurgitant o.
>segmental bronchus o.
>slitlike o.
>tricuspid o.
>ureteral o.
>urethral o.
>vaginal o.
>valvular o.

orifice-anulus ratio

origin
>aberrant o.
>anomalous o.
>o. of artery
>brown fat o.
>fever of unknown o. (FUO)
>histiocytic bone tumor o.
>neural crest o.
>neuroectodermal o.

spatial o.

o. of vessel

Ormond disease

orodigitofacial syndrome

oroendotracheal tube

orofacial fistula

orogastric tube

oropharyngeal

o. airway

o. dysfunction

o. dysphagia

o. emptying

o. narrowing

oropharyngoesophageal scintigraphy (OPES)

oropharynx

orotracheal intubation

ORT

ocular radiation therapy

Orthicon

O. camera

O. tube

orthocephalic

orthodeoxia

orthodiagram

orthodiagraph

orthodiagraphy

orthodiascopy

orthogonal

o. angiographic projection

o. C-arm fluoroscopy

o. plane

o. projection mammography

o. radiofrequency coil

o. tag line

o. view

o. view on angiography

orthogonal-hole test pattern (OHP)

orthogonally

orthoiodohippurate (OIH)

iodine-123 o. (OIH)

iodine-131 o.

OrthOne 1-tesla extremity MRI

orthonormal diameter

orthopantogram imaging

orthopantograph

orthopantomograph

Orthopantomograph-panoramic digital radiography unit

orthopantomography

orthopedic

o. nail

o. pin

o. plate

o. rod

o. screw

o. staple

orthoroentgenogram imaging

orthoroentgenography

orthostereoscope

orthotic plate

orthotopic

o. liver transplantation

o. total heart replacement

o. ureter

o. ureterocele

orthovoltage

o. radiation therapy

o. radiotherapy

Ortner syndrome

Ortolani

O. sign

O. test

os, pl. **ora, ossa**

bone

os acetabulum

os acromiale

os calcis

os calcis bone

coronary sinus os

os coxae

os cuboides secondarium

external os

os fabella

os infundibulum

internal cervical os

os naviculare

os odontoideum

os peroneum

os peroneum syndrome

os pubis

os styloidium

os supranaviculare

os supratrochleare dorsale

os sustentaculum

os terminale

os tibiale externum

os trigonum

os trigonum syndrome

Osborne ligament

Oscar ultrasonic bone cement removal system

oscillating

o. Bucky

NOTES

O

oscillating (*continued*)
   o. electron
   o. gradient
   o. grid
   o. magnetic field
oscillation
   resonant frequency of o.
oscillatory shear rate
oscillography
oscilloscope tuning station
OSCM
   oil-soluble contrast medium
OSEM
   ordered subsct expectation maximization
Osgood-Schlatter disease
O shell
OSI
   optic surface imaging
Osler
   O. disease
   O. maneuver
   O. node
   O. sign
   O. triad
Osler-Libman-Sacks syndrome
Osler-Weber-Rendu
   O.-W.-R. syndrome
   O.-W.-R. telangiectasia
Osm
   osmole
osmium
osmolality
   low o.
osmole (Osm)
osmotic
   o. edema
   o. effect
   o. gradient
   o. load
ossa (*pl. of* os)
osseocartilaginous
   o. arch
   o. thoracic cage
osseoligamentous arch
osseous, osteal
   o. abnormality
   o. activity
   o. bone contusion
   o. bridge
   o. cervical spine injury
   o. coalition
   o. defect
   o. destructive process
   o. dysplasia
   o. graft
   o. hemangioendothelioma
   o. hemangioma
   o. hydatidosis
   o. instability

o. labyrinth
o. lacuna
o. lesion
o. lymphoma
o. metaplasia
o. metastasis
o. metastatic disease
o. patellar outgrowth
o. pinch mechanism
o. polyp
o. rarefaction
o. remodeling
o. spiral lamina
o. structure
o. survey
o. trauma
o. tumor of soft tissue
o. union
ossicle
   accessory o.
   Kerckring o.
   meniscal o.
   Riolan o.
ossiferous
ossific
   o. nodule
   o. nucleus
   o. nucleus of navicular
ossificans
   fasciitis o.
   labyrinthitis o.
   panniculitis o.
   pseudomalignant myositis o.
   subacute myositis o.
ossification
   abnormal o.
   o. of cartilaginous structure
   o. center
   diaphysial o.
   disc o.
   dural o.
   ectopic o.
   enchondral o.
   extraarticular posterior o.
   flowing anterior vertebra o.
   heterotopic scar o.
   intracartilaginous o.
   intramembranous o.
   irregular enchondral o.
   o. of longitudinal ligament
   muscle o.
   normal o.
   paravertebral o.
   periarticular heterotopic o. (PHO)
   peripheral o.
   o. of posterior longitudinal
     ligament (OPLL)
   primary center of o.
   scar o.

secondary center of o.
soft tissue o.
spine o.
unilateral o.
o. variant
vertebral arch ligament o.
ossified
   o. body
   o. cartilage
   o. posterior longitudinal ligament
   o. scar
ossiform
ossifying
   o. bone fibroma
   o. cochleitis
   o. epiphysis
   o. skull fibroma
ossium
   fibrogenesis imperfecta o.
osteal (*var. of* osseous)
osteite
osteitic lesion of sternum
osteitis
   o. condensans ilii
   o. deformans
   diffuse periapical sclerosing o.
   o. fibrosa
   o. fibrosa cystica
   o. pubis
   radiation o.
   synovitis, acne, pustolosis,
     hyperostosis, o. (SAPHO)
ostemia
ostempyesis
OsteoAnalyzer bone densitometry device
osteoarthritic
   o. cartilage
   o. change
   o. spur
osteoarthritis (OA)
   degenerative o.
   early o.
   erosive o.
   generalized o.
   o. grade
   o. grading classification
   hand o.
   inflammatory o.
   interphalangeal o.
   posttraumatic o.
   premature o.
   traumatic o.

osteoarthropathy
   hypertrophic pulmonary o.
   neuropathic o.
   primary hypertrophic o.
   pulmonary o.
osteoarticular
osteoblastic
   o. activity
   o. bone regeneration
   o. lesion
   o. metastasis
   o. osteosarcoma
   o. presentation
   o. tumor
osteoblastoma
   benign o.
   expansile o.
osteocartilaginous
   o. defect
   o. exostosis
   o. lesion
   o. metaplasia
   o. parasellar neoplasm
   o. tissue
   o. tumor
osteochondral
   o. defect (OCD)
   o. fracture fragment
   o. injury
   o. lesion
   o. loose body
   o. slice fracture
osteochondritis dissecans
osteochondrodysplasia
osteochondrodystrophia deformans
osteochondrodystrophy
osteochondrofibroma
osteochondrolysis
osteochondroma
   benign o.
   coat hanger o.
   epiphysial o.
   soft tissue o.
osteochondromatosis
   bursal o.
   multiple o.
   synovial o.
   tenosynovial o.
osteochondromyxoma
osteochondrophyte
osteochondrosarcoma

O

NOTES

osteochondrosis
    o. deformans juvenilis
    o. dissecans
    intervertebral o.
    spinal o.
    vertebral o.
osteochondrotic
    o. loose body
    o. separation of epiphysis
osteoclasis
osteoclastic
    o. erosion
    o. resorption
osteoclast-mediated bone resorption
osteoclastoma
osteocondensation
osteoconductive polymer
osteocyte
osteocytoma
osteodentin
osteodermia
osteodermopathia hypertrophicans
osteodiastasis
osteodystrophia fibrosa
osteodystrophy
    Albright hereditary o.
    azotemic o.
    congenital renal o.
    fibrous o.
    renal o.
osteoenchondroma
osteofibroma
osteofibromatosis
    cystic o.
osteofibrous dysplasia
osteogenesis
    distraction o.
    o. imperfecta (OI)
    o. imperfecta tarda
osteogenic
    o. bone fibroma
    o. sarcoma
Osteo-Gram bone density test
osteoid
    o. carcinoma
    o. formation
    malignant o.
    o. matrix
    o. osteoma
    o. seam
    tumor o.
osteoid-origin tumor
osteolipochondroma
osteolipoma
osteolucency
osteolysis
    blade-of-grass o.
    candle-flame o.
    carpotarsal o.

    distal clavicle o. (DCO)
    essential o.
    expansile o.
    idiopathic o.
    idiopathic multicentric o.
    lytic o.
    malignant acetabular o.
    mandible o.
    massive o.
    medial end of clavicle o.
    mixed sclerotic o.
    multiple o.
    nonexpansile o.
    o. on both sides of joint
    periprosthetic o.
    sacral o.
    scalloping o.
    skull o.
    temporomandibular joint o.
    trabeculated o.
    o. tuft
    unilocular o.
osteolytic
    o. lesion
    o. metastasis
    o. osseous metastasis
osteoma, pl. **osteomas**
    cancellous osteoid o.
    choroidal o.
    compact o.
    cortical osteoid o.
    costal o.
    o. cutis
    o. durum
    o. eburneum
    fibrous o.
    giant osteoid o.
    intracapsular osteoid o.
    ivory o.
    juxtaarticular osteoid o.
    o. medullare
    osteoid o.
    parosteal o.
    soft tissue o.
    o. spongiosum
    spongy o.
    subperiosteal osteoid o.
    trabecular o.
    tropical ulcer o.
    ulcer o.
osteomalacia
    axial o.
    hematogenous o.
    hypophosphatemic o.
    oncogenic o.
    renal tubular o.
    senile o.
osteomalacic pelvis
osteomatoid

osteomatosis
osteomesopyknosis
osteomyelitic sinus
osteomyelitis
    Ackerman criteria for o.
    active o.
    acute hematogenous o. (AHO)
    bacterial o.
    brucellar o.
    central vertebral o.
    childhood o.
    chronic recurrent multifocal o.
    chronic sclerosing o.
    cystic tuberculous o.
    discovertebral o.
    early o.
    Garré sclerosing o.
    neonatal o.
    nocardial o.
    puncture wound o.
    pyogenic o.
    recurrent multifocal o.
    sacral o.
    o. scintigraphy
    sclerosing nonsuppurative o.
    sneaker o.
    spinal o.
    subligamentous vertebral o.
    tuberculous o.
    vertebral o.
osteomyelofibrosis
osteomyelography
osteonal bone
osteonecrosis
    radiation o.
    spontaneous o.
osteopathia
    o. condensans disseminata
    o. striata
osteopenia
    localized o.
osteopenic bone
osteopetrosis
    autosomal dominant benign form
      of o.
    cranial o.
    malignant o.
osteophyte
    anterior o.
    bony o.
    bridging o.
    cervical o.

    discogenic o.
    floating o.
    o. formation
    fringe of o.
    horseshoe o.
    impinging o.
    jagged o.
    marginal o.
    posterior o.
    spinal o.
osteophytic
    o. bone lip
    o. bridge
    o. defect
    o. lipping
    o. proliferation
    o. spurring
osteophytosis in fluorosis
osteoplastic flap
osteoplasty
    minimally invasive o.
    percutaneous o.
osteopoikilosis
osteoporosis
    o. of bone
    o. circumscripta
    o. circumscripta cranii
    corticosteroid-induced o.
    disuse o.
    ground-glass o.
    juvenile o.
    localized o.
    partial transient o.
    periarticular o.
    picture-framing o.
    postmenopausal o.
    posttraumatic o.
    regional migratory o.
    regional transient o.
    senile o.
    transient regional o.
osteoporotic
    o. bone
    o. compression fracture
osteoradiology
osteoradionecrosis
osteosarcoma
    cardiac o.
    central o.
    chondroblastic o.
    classical o.
    conventional o.

O

NOTES

osteosarcoma *(continued)*
    dedifferentiated parosteal o.
    epithelioid o.
    extraosseous o.
    extraskeletal o.
    extremity o.
    fibroblastic o.
    gnathic o.
    high-grade surface o.
    intracortical o.
    intramedullary o.
    intraosseous o.
    intraosseous low-grade o.
    o. of jaw
    juxtacortical o.
    lytic o.
    metastatic o.
    multicentric o.
    multifocal o.
    multiple sclerotic o.
    osteoblastic o.
    parosteal o.
    periosteal o.
    sacral o.
    sclerosing o.
    secondary o.
    small-cell o.
    surface o.
    telangiectatic o.
osteosarcomatosis
osteosarcomatous
osteosclerosis
    constitutional o.
    diffuse o.
    multiple-lesion o.
    myelofibrosis o.
    solitary o.
    subchondral o.
    o. tuft
    o. vertebral sarcoidosis
osteosclerotic lesion
osteosis
osteospongioma
osteosynthesis
    biologic o.
osteothrombosis
osteotomy
    femoral varus derotational o.
    high tibial o.
    Pemberton o.
    Steele triple innominate o.
OsteoView
    O. desktop hand x-ray system
    O. digital bone densitometer
    O. 2000 digital imaging system
ostial
    o. cannulation
    o. lesion
    o. renal artery stenosis

ostiomeatal
    o. complex
    o. unit
ostitis deformans
ostium, pl. **ostia**
    o. abdominale tubae uterinae
    aneurysmal o.
    aortic o.
    artery o.
    atrioventricular nodal o.
    conus branch ostia
    coronary artery o.
    coronary sinus o.
    fistula o.
    o. primum
    o. primum atrial septal defect
    o. secundum
    o. secundum atrial septal defect
Ostreg spinal marker system
Ostwald solubility coefficient (Λ)
Ostycut bone biopsy needle
2.OT
    Spectro-20000 2.OT
OTD
    organ tolerance dose
otic
    o. capsule
    o. ganglion
    o. obstruction
otitis
    malignant external o.
    necrotizing external o.
OtoLAM laser
otologic implant
otosclerosis
    cochlear o.
    fenestral o.
    retrofenestral o.
    stapedial o.
otospongiosis
Ottawa ankle rule
Otto
    O. disease
    O. pelvis
Otto-Kobak pelvis
OURQ
    outer upper right quadrant
out
    rule o. (R/O)
    silhouetted o.
outcropping of lesion
outer
    o. anular/posterior longitudinal ligament complex
    o. border of uterus
    o. canthus
    o. table of skull
    o. table thickening
    o. upper right quadrant (OURQ)

outer-air
 o.-a. region
 o.-a. segmentation
outflow
 double o.
 o. effect
 hepatic venous o.
 hypoplastic subpulmonic o.
 maximum venous o. (MVO)
 o. obstruction
 subpulmonic o.
 swan-neck shape of ventricular o.
 o. tract
 o. tract gradient
 o. of ventricle
outgrowth
 osseous patellar o.
outlet
 cervical o.
 o. impingement
 o. obstruction
 pelvic o.
 pyloric o.
 thoracic o.
 ventricular o.
 o. view
 o. view radiograph
 widened thoracic o.
outline
 absent kidney o.
 double o.
 gastric o.
 renal o.
 trabeculated o.
out-of-field count
out-of-phase
 o.-o.-p. gradient echo
 o.-o.-p. GRE imaging
out-of-profile nipple
out-of-slice artifact
outpocketing of mucosa
outpouching
 aneurysmal o.
 saccular o.
output
 adequate cardiac o.
 o. amplitude
 augmented cardiac o.
 cardiac o. (CO, Q)
 Dow method for measuring
  cardiac o.

Fick method for measuring
 cardiac o.
Gorlin method for measuring
 cardiac o.
Hamilton-Stewart formula for
 measuring cardiac o.
inadequate cardiac o.
instrument o.
low cardiac o.
o. point
pulmonic o.
reduced systemic cardiac o.
stroke o.
systemic o.
thermodilution cardiac o.
ventricular o.
outrigger arm
outside-to-inside segmentation
OV103
 OncoRad O.
 OncoScint O.
ov, OV
 ovarian
ova (*pl. of* ovum)
Ovadia-Beals tibial plafond fracture classification
oval
 o. aneurysm
 o. aneurysm with bleb
 o. shape
 o. window
ovalbumin
ovale
 centrum o.
 foramen o.
 patent foramen o. (PFO)
 o. skull base of foramen
ovalis
 anulus o.
 fossa o.
ovarian (ov, OV)
 o. abscess
 o. anatomy
 o. artery (OA)
 o. carcinoma
 o. choriocarcinoma
 o. cortex
 o. cystadenofibroma
 o. cystadenoma
 o. dermoid
 o. dermoid cyst
 o. Doppler signal

NOTES

O

ovarian *(continued)*
    o. dysgenesis
    o. dysgerminoma
    o. edema
    o. fibroma
    o. fishnet weave pattern
    o. follicular cyst
    o. fossa
    o. hernia
    o. hyperstimulation syndrome
    o. image signature cyst
    o. mass
    o. medulla
    o. mesonephroid tumor
    o. metastasis
    o. morphology
    o. neoplasm
    o. pregnancy
    o. remnant syndrome
    o. retention cyst
    o. serous cystadenocarcinoma
    o. size
    o. suspensory ligament
    o. systic teratoma
    o. torsion
    o. vein
    o. vein embolization
    o. vein syndrome
    o. vein thrombosis
    o. venography
    o. volume
ovarioabdominal pregnancy
ovary
    atrophied o.
    clear cell neoplasm of o.
    cystic o.
    embryonic o.
    fibroma-thecoma tumor of o.
    o. germ cell tumor
    o. gland
    hilar cell tumor of o.
    hyperstimulation of o.
    ligament of o.
    mulberry o.
    multifollicular o.
    palpable postmenopausal o.
    pearly white o.
    polycystic o.
    postmenopausal o.
    sclerocystic o.
    stromal carcinoid tumor of o.
    suspensory ligament of o.
    teratoblastoma of o.
    teratocarcinoma of o.
    thecoma of o.
    transposition of o.
Ovation falloposcopy system
overaeration
"overcalling" metastasis

overcirculation
    pulmonary vessel o.
    o. vascularity
overcouch
    o. exposure
    o. tube
    o. view
overdamping
overdevelopment
    bone o.
overdiagnostic bias
overdistention
    alveolar o.
    o. of alveolar populations
    pulmonary o.
overdrainage
overdrive suppression
overembolize
overexpansion
    lung o.
    pulmonary o.
overexposure
overframing
    horizontal o.
    mean-diameter o.
    subtotal o.
overgrowth
    bony o.
    cuticular o.
    epiphysial o.
    fibrocartilaginous o.
    vertebral body o.
overhanging
    o. border
    o. margin
Overhauser effect
overhead
    o. film
    o. oblique view
overinflation
    lung o.
    obstructive pulmonary o.
    pulmonary o.
    unilateral o.
overlap
    liver-spleen o.
    o. shadow
overlapping
    o. finger
    o. fracture
    o. image
    o. rib
    o. suture
overlay
    anatomic o.
    o. plate
    venous o.
overlie

overload
    acute hemodynamic o.
    cardiac o.
    chronic hemodynamic o.
    diastolic o.
    fluid o.
    pressure o.
    right ventricular o.
    systolic ventricular o.
    transfusional iron o.
    volume o.
overlying
    o. attenuation artifact
    o. bowel content
    o. bowel gas
    o. bowel shadow
    o. branching pattern
overpenetrated film
overread
overrelaxation factor
override
    aortic o.
overriding
    o. aorta
    o. of fracture fragment
    o. great artery
    o. sutures of fontanelle
    o. toe
oversampled
over-the-wire
    o.-t.-w. design
    o.-t.-w. Greenfield filter
overventilation
    alveolar o.
overview angiogram
overvoltage
oviductal pregnancy
ovoid
    afterloading tandem and o.
    o. heart
    o. high signal intensity
    Manchester o.
    o. ossification center
    o. shape
    tandem and o.
ovulation
    incessant o.
    o. induction

ovulatory
    o. failure
    o. phase
ovum, pl. **ova**
    aspiration of ova
Owen view
owl's eye appearance
oxalosis
    bone o.
    kidney o.
    primary o.
Oxford
    O. magnet
    O. 2-T large-bore imaging system
      scanner
ox heart
oxidase
    cytochrome c o. (COX)
    monoamine o.
oxidation
    Baeyer-Villiger o.
    o. state
oxidative metabolism
oxide
    nitric o.
    superparamagnetic agent iron o.
    superparamagnetic iron o. (SPIO)
    ultrasmall superparamagnetic iron o.
      (USPIO)
oxidized complex
oxidronate
OxiFirst fetal oxygen monitor
Oxilan imaging agent
oxime
    hexamethylpropylencamine o.
    (HMPAO)
    ^{99m}Tc hexamethylpropylene
      amine o.
    technetium-99m hexamethylpropylene
      amine o.
oximetry
    pulse o.
oxine
    ^{111}In o.
oxine-indium
    lipophilic o.-i.
oxycephaly
oxygen (O_2)
    o. 15 (^{15}O)
    o. 16 (^{16}O)
    o. 17 (^{17}O)
    o. 18 (^{18}O)

NOTES

O

oxygen *(continued)*
    activation-induced uncoupling of cerebral o.
    cerebral metabolic rate of o. ($CMRO_2$)
    cistern o.
    o. cisternography
    o. consumption (QO_2)
    o. effect
    o. extraction fraction (OEF)
    o. extraction rate (OER)
    o. imaging agent
    metabolic rate of o.
    o. myelography
    regional cerebral metabolic rate for o. ($rCMRO_2$)
    o. saturation
oxygen-17 NMR spectroscopy
oxygenated perfluorocarbon blood substitute
oxygenation
    extracorporeal membrane o.
    tissue o.

oxygenation-sensitive
    o.-s. functional MR
    o.-s. functional MR imaging
oxygenator
    bubble o.
    disc o.
    extracorporeal membrane o.
    film o.
    membrane o.
    rotating disc o.
    screen o.
oxygen-dependent emphysema
oxygen-enhanced lung MR imaging
oxygen-supersaturated water
Oxyguard endoscopy biteblock
oxyorthosilicate
    cerium-doped lutetium o. (LSO)
    gadolinium o.
oxyphilic adenoma
oyster-pearl breast calcification

P

phosphorus
posterior
  P loop
  P pulmonale pattern
  P sign
  P wave-QRS wave ratio (P-QRS)
P1-P4 segment of posterior cerebral artery
P2 segment aneurysm
³²P, P-32
  phosphorus 32
    sodium phosphate ³²P
PA
  parathyroid adenoma
  pathology
  posteroanterior
  pulmonary artery
    PA and lateral films
    PA position
    PA projection
P-A
  perimeter-area ratio
    P-A ratio
Pa
  protactinium
Paas disease
PABP
  pulmonary artery balloon pump
pacchionian
  p. body
  p. depression
  p. granulation
PACE
  prospective acquisition correction
    PACE technique
pace
  p. mapping
  P. Plus System scanner
pacemaker
  p. artifact
  bipolar p.
  p. effect
  implanted p.
  p. lead
  p. wire
pachydermoperiostosis
pachyfibril
pachygyria
pachymeningitis
pachymeninx, pl. **pachymeninges**
pachymetry
  ultrasonic p.
pachypleuritis

pacing
  p. artifact
  p. lead
Packard Merlin life-monitoring system
packed bead
packing
  edge p.
  endosaccular p.
  p. fraction
packing, extraction, and calculation technique
PACS
  picture archival communication system
    PACS PathSpeed MR imaging
    PACS workstation
PAD
  pressure applied dressing
pad
  antimesenteric fat p.
  decubitus p.
  p. effect
  electrical grounding p.
  epicardial fat p.
  esophagogastric fat p.
  fat p.
  fibrocartilaginous p.
  foveal fat p.
  haversian fat p.
  heel fat p.
  Hoffa fat p.
  ileocecal fat p.
  intracapsular fat p.
  intrapatellar fat p.
  ischiorectal fat p.
  patellar fat p.
  pericardial fat p.
  pre-Achilles fat p.
  Sat P.
  scalene fat p.
  p. sign of aortic insufficiency
  standoff p.
  thickened heel p.
  UltraEase ultrasound p.
  ultrasound p.
  wireless handheld Web p.
padding
  antral p.
  zero p.
paddle
  compression p.
  spot compression p.
  p. wheel method
paddlewheel reformation

P

PADP-PAWP
pulmonary artery diastolic pressure and
pulmonary artery wedge pressure
PAEDP
pulmonary artery end-diastolic pressure
Page kidney
Paget
P. abscess
P. carcinoma
P. disease of bone
P. jaw disease
P. osteitis deformans
P. quiet necrosis
pagetic
pagetoid
p. bone
p. epidermal involvement
Paget-von Schroetter syndrome
PAH
paraaminohippurate
pulmonary arterial hypertension
pain
neuropathic p.
nociceptive p.
periumbilical p.
p. provocation response
painful
p. disc derangement
p. osmotic demyelination syndrome
painless thyroiditis
paint brush striation
pair
electron-positron p.
exon-specific primer p.
line p.
Maxwell p.
oblique annihilation photon p.
p. production
transaxial annihilation photon p.
paired
p. inferior vena cava
p. parietal branch
p. visceral branch
Pais fracture
palatal muscle
palate
palatina
uvula p.
palatine
p. bone
p. canal
p. foramen
p. ridge
p. root
p. shelf
p. suture
palatoethmoidal suture
palatoglossus
palatograph

palatography
palatomaxillary
p. canal
p. suture
palatomyograph
palatopharyngeal fold
palatopharyngeus
palatovaginal canal
paleopathologic and radiologic study
palisade formation
palladium (Pd)
p. 103 (^{103}Pd, Pd-103)
p. imaging agent
p. implant
palliative
p. esophagostomy
p. irradiation
p. radiation therapy
pallidoluysian atrophy
pallidotomy
pallidum
pallidus
globus p.
Pallister-Hall syndrome
palmar
p. angulation
p. aponeurosis
p. arterial arch
p. cutaneous vein
p. displacement
p. fascia
p. fasciitis
p. fibromatosis
p. ganglion
p. interossei
p. metacarpal ligament
p. plate
p. radiocarpal ligament
p. slope
p. surface
p. tilt
p. wrist
palmaris
p. brevis
p. longus
p. longus tendon
Palmaz
P. Genesis balloon-expanded stent
P. Genesis stent
P. large balloon-expanded stent
P. medium balloon-expanded stent
30-mm-long P. stent
P. PS 424 stent
P. P 394 stainless steel balloon-
expandable stent
P. P564 stent
P. stent
P. 424 stent
P. 784 stent

Palmaz-Schatz long medium balloon-expanded stent
palmitate
^{11}C p.
palmitic acid
palmoplantar
Palomar SLP1000 diode
Palomo procedure
palpable
p. aortic ejection sound
p. postmenopausal ovary
p. presystolic bulge
p. pulmonic ejection sound
Palpagraph breast mapping device
palpation-guided approach
palpatory T-stage prostate carcinoma
palpebra, pl. **palpebrae**
levator palpebrae
palpebral
p. fissure
p. raphe
palsy
dyskinetic cerebral p.
progressive supranuclear p.
waiter's tip p.
PAM
pulmonary artery mean pressure
PAM pressure
pamidronate
p. disodium
p. therapy
pampiniform plexus
PAN
polyarteritis nodosa
panacinar emphysema
panaortic
panbronchiolitis
diffuse p.
pancake
p. appearance
p. compression
p. kidney
p. MRI magnet
pancarpal destructive arthritis
panchamber
p. enlargement
p. hypertrophy
Pancoast
P. syndrome
P. tumor
pancolitis

pancompartmental joint space narrowing
pancreas, pl. **pancreata**
aberrant p.
accessory p.
anterior surface of p.
anular p.
Aselli p.
body of the p.
p. cystadenoma
degeneration of p.
p. divisum
dorsal p.
ectopic p.
fat-spared area in p.
p. gland
head of p.
heterotopic p.
interior surface of p.
intraductal papillary mucinous tumor of p.
lesser p.
mature pseudocyst of p.
metastasis to the p.
mucinous ductal ectasia of p.
mucinous ductectatic tumor of p.
neck of p.
posterior surface of p.
tail of p.
p. transplant
p. ultrasonography imaging
uncinate process of p.
ventral p.
pancreatic
p. abscess
p. angiography
p. arteriography
p. ascites
p. atrophy
p. calcification
p. calculus
p. carcinoma
p. cholera syndrome
p. cutaneous fistula
p. cyst
p. cystadenocarcinoma
p. cystic fibrosis
p. cystic lymphangioma
p. degeneration
p. disease
p. divisum
p. dorsal anlage

NOTES

P

pancreatic *(continued)*
  p. duct
  p. ductal adenocarcinoma
  p. duct branch
  p. duct dilatation
  p. duct obstruction
  p. duct sphincter
  p. duct stent
  p. fluid collection
  p. hamartoma
  p. head
  p. hemorrhage
  p. herniation
  p. islet cell tumor
  p. lipomatosis
  p. lymph node
  p. lymphoma
  p. macrocystic adenoma
  p. mass
  p. metastasis
  p. microcystic adenoma
  p. neck
  p. necrosis
  p. neoplasm
  p. phlegmon
  p. pseudocyst
  p. pseudocyst drainage
  p. scan
  p. trauma
  p. vein
pancreatic-enteric continuity
pancreatic herniation
pancreaticobiliary
  p. common channel
  p. disease
  p. ductal junction
  p. function variant
  p. sphincter
  p. tract
  p. ultrasound
pancreaticoblastoma
pancreaticoduodenal
  p. artery
  p. lymph node
pancreaticoduodenectomy
pancreaticohepatic syndrome
pancreaticolienal lymph node
pancreaticopleural fistula
pancreaticosplenic
  p. node
  p. omentum
pancreaticus
  hemosuccus p.
pancreatitis
  acute p.
  chronic calcifying p.
  chronic obstructive p.
  diffuse p.
  edematous p.

focal p.
necrotizing p.
obstructive p.
phlegmonous p.
p. pseudoaneurysm
Santiani-Stone classification of p.
suppurative p.
tropical p.
pancreatocholangiogram
  retrograde p.
pancreatogram
pancreatography
  endoscopic retrograde p.
  p. imaging
  intraoperative p.
  magnetic resonance p. (MRP)
  percutaneous p.
  retrograde p.
pancreatolithiasis
pancytopenia-dysmelia syndrome
panda appearance
Pander island
PANDO
  primary acquired nasolacrimal duct
    obstruction
panduriform placenta
panencephalitis
  progressive rubella p.
  sclerosing p.
  subacute sclerosing p. (SSPE)
panfacial fracture
panhypopituitarism
panlobar nephroblastomatosis
panlobular emphysema
panmyelopathy
panmyelosis
Panner disease
panniculitis
  mediastinal p.
  mesenteric p. (MP)
  p. ossificans
  systemic nodular p.
pannus, pl. panni
  p. deformity
  p. deformity of odontoid
  p. formation
  synovial p.
  p. of synovium
panography
pan-oral radiography
panoramic
  p. CT scan
  p. image
  p. imaging
  P. 200 nonmydriatic
    ophthalmoscope
  p. radiograph
  p. radiography
  p. rotating machine

p. surface projection
p. tomography
p. view
p. x-ray film
Panorex view
pansinusitis
pan synovitis
pansystolic mitral regurgitation
pantalar fusion
pantaloon
   p. embolus
   p. hernia
pantomogram
pantomographic view
pantomography
   concentric p.
   eccentric p.
Pantopaque
   P. cisternography
   P. imaging agent
   P. myelography
PAOD
   peripheral arterial occlusive disease
PAP
   pulmonary alveolar proteinosis
   pulmonary artery pressure
Papavasiliou classification of olecranon
  fracture
paper-doll fetus
Papile classification
papilla, pl. **papillae**
   aberrant p.
   acoustic p.
   bile p.
   circumvallate p.
   p. of columnar epithelium
   duodenal p.
   major duodenal p.
   minor duodenal p.
   optic p.
   renal p.
   Santorini p.
   sloughed p.
   smudged p.
   urethral p.
   p. of Vater
   p. of Vater enlargement
   p. of Vater stenosis
papillary
   p. adenoma of large intestine
   p. apocrine change
   p. bile duct stenosis

p. breast carcinoma
p. cystadenoma lymphomatosum
p. cystic adenoma
p. DCIS
p. duct of Bellini
p. epididymal cystadenoma
p. epithelial neoplasm
p. excrescence
p. fibroelastoma
p. lesion
p. muscle
p. muscle infarct
p. muscle rupture
p. necrosis
p. pancreatic cystic neoplasm
p. projection
p. proliferation
p. renal cell carcinoma
p. serous adenocarcinoma
p. serous carcinoma
p. thyroid carcinoma
p. tumor
papilledema
papillocarcinoma
papillogram
papilloma, pl. **papillomas, papillomata**
   p. acuminata
   basal cell p.
   benign intraductal p.
   p. of bladder
   breast p.
   choroid plexus p.
   cockscomb p.
   p. diffusum
   ductal p.
   p. durum
   fibroepithelial p.
   p. of fourth ventricle
   hard p.
   Hopmann p.
   p. inguinale
   intraductal p.
   inverted p.
   large duct p.
   laryngeal p.
   p. molle
   multiple peripheral papillomas
   p. neuropathicum
   p. neuroticum
   penile squamous p.
   schneiderian p.
   soft p.

NOTES

P

papilloma *(continued)*
    transitional urethral cell p.
    villous p.
papillomatosis
    intraductal breast p.
    invasive p.
    juvenile breast p.
    juvenile laryngeal p.
    laryngeal p.
    pulmonary p.
    recurrent respiratory p.
    tracheobronchial p.
papillomatous growth
papillomavirus
    human p.
Papillon-Lèfevre syndrome (PLS)
Papillon technique
papillotomy
papular lesion
papulonecrotic lesion
PAPVR
    partial anomalous pulmonary venous
    return
papyracea
    lamina p.
papyraceus
    fetus p.
PAR
    plain abdominal radiography
paraaminobenzoic acid
paraaminohippurate (PAH)
paraaminohippuric acid
paraaminosalicylic acid (PAS)
paraanastomotic aneurysmal repair
paraaortic
    p. lymph node
    p. mass
paraarticular
    p. bone remodeling
    p. calcification
parabola
    digital p.
    metatarsal p.
parabolic velocity profile
paracarcinomatous myelopathy
paracardiac
    p. mass
    p. metastasis
    p. tumor
**paracardiac-type total anomalous venous
return**
paracardial lymph node
paracecal appendix
paracentesis
    abdominal p.
    subxiphoid p.
paracentral
    p. artery

    p. gyrus
    p. lobule
paracervical lymphatic
parachute
    p. deformity of mitral valve
    p. mitral valve deformity
paracicatricial emphysema
paracoccidioidal granuloma
paracolic
    p. abscess
    p. gutter
    p. lymph node
paracorporeal heart
paracortical hyperplasia
paracostal
paracystic pouch
paradigm
    block p.
    coregistration p.
    event-related p.
paradiscal lesion
paradoxic, paradoxical
    p. bronchospasm
    p. cerebral embolus
    p. colon dilatation
    p. embolization
    p. enhancement
    p. leaflet motion
    p. middle turbinate
    p. septal motion
    p. suppression
paradoxicum
paradoxus
    pulsus p.
paraduodenal
    p. fold
    p. fossa
    p. hernia
    p. recess
paraesophageal
    p. hernia
    p. varix
paraesophagogastric devascularization
parafascicular
    p. nucleus
    p. thalamotomy
paraffin-embedded tissue
paraffinoma
paraganglioma
    adrenal p.
    chromaffin p.
    extraadrenal p.
    functional p.
    gangliocytic p.
    nonchromaffin p.
    thoracic p.
paragangliomatosis
paraglenoid cyst

paragonimiasis
   brain p.
   lung p.
paragranuloma
parahiatal hernia
parahilar
parahippocampal gyrus
paraileostomal hernia
para-isopropyl-iminodiacetic
   p.-i.-i. acid (PIPIDA)
   p.-i.-i. acid technetium-99m
     hepatobiliary scan
para-isopropyl-iminodiacetic acid
  (PIPIDA)
parakeet fancier's lung
paralabral
   p. cyst
   p. lesion
paralanguage
paralaryngeal
   p. muscle
   p. space
parallax
   p. method
   p. view
parallel
   p. analog mapping
   p. array
   p. cine
   p. data acquisition coil
   p. hole imaging
   p. imaging
   p. mean translation
   p. M line
   p. MRI
   p. opposed unmodified port
   p. pitch line
   p. ray
   p. and spiral flow pattern
   p. tag plane
   p. virtual machine (PVM)
parallel-hole
   p.-h. medium sensitivity collimator
   p.-h. scintigram
parallelism
   p. of articular surface
   p. of facet joint
parallel-line
   p.-l. equal spacing (PLES)
parallel-line-equal-space bar
parallel-opposed beams

parallel-tagged MR image
paralysis, pl. paralyses
   p. of diaphragm
   diaphragmatic p.
   hernia p.
   Klumpke p.
   phrenic nerve p.
   vocal cord p.
paralytic
   p. chest
   p. colonic obstruction
   p. ileus
paralytica
   dysphagia p.
paramagnetic
   p. artifact
   p. cation
   p. contrast agent
   p. contrast-enhanced MR study
   p. contrast enhancement
   p. effect
   p. enhancement accentuation
   p. enhancement accentuation by
     chemical shift imaging
   p. influence
   p. shift
   p. shift relaxation
paramagnetism
   apparent p.
   collective p.
paramalleolar artery
paramammary lymph node
paramedian
   p. infarct
   p. line
   p. pontine reticular formation
     (PPRF)
   p. position
   p. sagittal plane
   p. section
   p. thalamic artery
   p. thalamopeduncular artery
   p. triangle
paramediastinal gland
parameningeal rhabdomyosarcoma
parameniscal cyst
paramesonephric
   p. duct
   p. duct cyst
parameter
   clinical p.
   extrinsic cellular p.

NOTES

P

parameter *(continued)*
    growth p.
    hematologic p.
    intrinsic cellular p.
    kinetic perfusion p.
    normal hemodynamic liver p.
    nuclear magnetic resonance
      spectral p.
    optimization p.
    physiologic p.
    rendering p.
    scan p.
    sonographic p.
    thermal treatment p.
    timing p.
    ventricular function p.
parametrectomy
    radical p.
parametrial fat
parametric image
parametrium, pl. **parametria**
paranasal
    p. sinus
    p. sinus carcinoma
    p. sinusitis
    p. sinus mass
    p. sinus mucocele
paraneoplastic
    p. cerebellar degeneration
    p. process
    p. syndrome
    p. thromboembolism
paraorbital lesion
paraosteoarthropathy
paraovarian
    p. cyst
    p. varicosity
parapatellar plica
parapelvic
    p. cyst
    p. gutter
parapharyngeal
    p. abscess
    p. space
    p. space cyst
paraphysis
parapneumonic effusion
paraprosthetic
    p. leak
    p. leakage
paraprosthetic-enteric fistula
pararectal
    p. abscess
    p. fossa
    p. lymph node
    p. pouch
pararenal
    p. abscess
    p. aortic aneurysm

    p. aortic atherosclerosis
    p. space
parasagittal
    p. depression
    p. image
    p. intracranial mass
    p. lesion
    p. meningioma
    p. plane
parasellar
    p. brain mass
    p. cistern
    p. dermoid tumor
    p. lesion
    p. metastasis
    p. region lesion
paraseptal
    p. emphysema
    p. position
parasinoidal
parasitic
    p. fetus
    p. infiltrate
parasitized collateral
paraspinal
    p. abnormality
    p. abscess
    p. calcification
    p. line
    p. muscle
    p. neurofibroma
    p. pleural stripe
    p. soft tissue mass
    p. soft tissue shadowing
paraspinous musculature
parasternal
    p. bulge
    p. long-axis view
    p. long-axis view echocardiography
    p. lymph node
    p. motion
    p. scanning
    p. short-axis view
    p. short-axis view echocardiography
    p. view of heart
    p. window
parastomal hernia
parastriate cortex
parasympathetic
    p. fiber
    p. ganglia tumor
    p. nervous system
paraterminal gyrus
paratesticular
    p. rhabdomyosarcoma
    p. tumor
parathyroid
    p. adenoma (PA)
    p. carcinoma

p. cyst
ectopic p.
p. hyperplasia
p. insufficiency
p. scintigraphy
technetium-99m sestamibi p.
p. tumor
p. ultrasonography imaging
p. vein

parathyroidectomy
radioguided p.

paratracheal
p. adenopathy
p. convexity
p. lymph node
p. region
p. soft tissue
p. tissue stripe

paratrooper's fracture
paratubal serous cyst
paratumoral injection
paraumbilical
p. anterior abdominal wall
p. vein

paraureteral diverticulum
paraurethral
p. canal
p. cyst
p. duct
p. gland

parauterine lymph node
paravaginal
p. lymph node
p. soft tissue

paravalvular
p. leak
p. regurgitation

paravertebral
p. ganglion
p. groove
p. gutter
p. musculature
p. nerve plexus
p. ossification
p. scanning
p. venous plexus

paravertebrally
p. situated pelvic tumor mass
p. situated thoracic tumor mass

paravesical
p. fossa
p. pouch

paravesicular lymph node
parcellation of structure
parchment
p. heart
p. right ventricle

parenchyma
bleeding into brain p.
brain p.
breast p.
cerebral p.
computerized texture analysis of
lung nodules and lung p.
hepatic p.
liver p.
lung p.
mammary p.
marbling of pancreatic p.
mottling of renal p.
normal renal p.
pulmonary p.
renal p.
spinal cord p.
testicular p.

parenchymal
p. blastoma
p. blood
p. brain metastasis
p. breast pattern
p. change
p. cone
p. consolidation
p. echogenicity
p. enhancement
p. extension
p. fibrous band
p. hematoma
p. infarct
p. laceration
p. lung band
p. opacity
p. peliosis hepatis
p. phase image
p. scarring
p. tissue
p. tracer accumulation
p. transit

parenchymatous
p. atrophy
p. cerebellar degeneration
p. inflammation
p. phase
p. pneumonia

NOTES

P

parenchymography
    endoscopic retrograde p. (ERP)
parenchymous goiter
parent
    p. artery occlusion
    p. element
    p. isotope
    p. nuclide
    p. radionuclide
    p. vein
    p. vessel
    p. vessel occlusion
parentheseslike calcification
Parenti-Fraccaro disease
paresthetica
    meralgia p.
Parham-Martin band
parietal
    p. association area
    p. band
    p. bone
    p. bone thinning
    p. boss
    p. cephalohematoma
    p. convexity
    p. cortex
    p. cortex lesion
    p. diameter
    p. eminence
    p. encephalocele
    p. extension
    p. extension of infundibular septum
    p. eye field (PEF)
    p. fistula
    p. foramen
    p. gyrus
    p. layer
    p. lobe
    p. lobe gray-matter cytosolic
      choline pathogenetic mechanism
      of myocardial fibrosis
    p. lobe lesion
    p. lymph node
    p. middle cerebral artery
    p. operculum (PO)
    p. pelvic fascia
    p. pericardial calcification
    p. pericardium
    p. peritoneum
    p. pleura
    p. pleural scarring
    p. pregnancy
    p. presentation
    p. suture
parietography
    gastric p.
parietomastoid suture
parietooccipital
    p. area

    p. branch of posterior cerebellar
      artery
    p. lesion
    p. region
    p. sulcus
    p. suture
parietoorbital projection
parietotemporal
    p. area
    p. suture
Parinaud syndrome
Paris ultrasound system
park
    p. bench position
    P. Medical Systems scanner
Parkes-Weber syndrome
Parks
    P. bidirectional Doppler flowmeter
    P. 800 bidirectional Doppler
      flowmetry
paroophoron
parosteal
    p. bone lesion
    p. chondrosarcoma
    p. osteogenic sarcoma
    p. osteoma
    p. osteosarcoma
    p. soft tissue angiosarcoma
parotid
    p. abscess
    p. duct
    p. gland
    p. gland sialography
    p. lymph node
    p. pleomorphic adenoma
    p. pneumatocele
    p. tumor
parotitis
    adenoid cystic carcinoma p.
    benign mixed tumor p.
    cylindroma p.
    mucoepidermoid carcinoma p.
    pleomorphic adenoma p.
parovarian cyst
paroxysmal
    p. auricular tachycardia
    p. AV block
    p. change
    p. pulmonary edema
parrot
    frontal bossing of P.
    P. node
parrot-beak
    p.-b. labral tear
    p.-b. meniscus tear
    p.-b. pattern
parry fracture
Parry-Romberg syndrome
pars, pl. **partes**

p. flaccida cholesteatoma
p. infravaginalis gubernaculi
p. interarticularis
p. interarticularis defect
p. interarticularis fracture
pedicles and p.
p. tensa cholesteatoma

Parsons
third intercondylar tubercle of P.
P. tubercle

part
fetal small p.
presenting p.

partes (*pl. of* pars)
1-part fracture
2-part fracture
3-part fracture
4-part fracture
partial
p. anomalous pulmonary venous
connection
p. anomalous pulmonary venous
return (PAPVR)
p. atrioventricular canal defect
p. brain irradiation
p. bursal surface tear
p. collapse of lung
p. complex seizure
p. corpus callosum agenesis
p. dislocation
p. dislodgement
p. flip-angle fast-scan technique
p. Fourier imaging
p. Fourier technique
p. heart block
p. k-space sampling
p. lesion
p. liquid ventilation
p. liquid ventilation with perflubron
p. obliteration of lateral ventricle
p. pericardial abscess
p. pericardial absence
p. placenta previa
p. pulmonary venous connection
p. saturation (PS)
p. saturation pulse sequence
p. saturation spin echo
p. saturation technique
p. small bowel malrotation
p. small bowel obstruction
p. thickening
p. thickness split tear

p. transient osteoporosis
p. transposition of great artery
p. tubular appearance
p. ureter duplication
p. volume averaging
p. volume effect artifact

partial-brain radiation therapy
partially
p. polycystic kidney
p. relaxed Fourier transform
(PRFT)

**partial-ring bismuth germanate-crystal
scanner**
particle
accelerated p.
p. accelerator
alpha p.
p. approach
beta p.
bone p.
calcium/oxyanion-containing p.
charged-p.
embosphere p.
gelatin sponge p.
gold p.
heavy charged p.
p. identification
Ivalon p.
large colloidal p.
magnetic iron oxide p. (MIOP)
p. mask
nuclear p.
oral magnetic p.
polyvinyl alcohol p.
PVA p.
p. size determination
Spongel gelatin sponge p.
submicron magnetic p.'s
superparamagnetic iron oxide p.
viral p.
Zimmermann elementary p.

particle-beam radiation therapy
particulate
p. arterial embolization
p. debris
p. echo
p. embolic agent
magnetic p.
p. matter

partition
atrial p.

NOTES

P

693

partition *(continued)*
    p. coefficient
    gastric p.
partitioning
    recursive p.
parturient canal
parturition
PAS
    paraaminosalicylic acid
    pulmonary artery systolic pressure
pascals of force
PASH
    pseudoangiomatous stromal hyperplasia
PASP-SASP ratio
pass
    p. coaxially
    interleaved imaging p.
passage
    adiabatic fast p. (AFP)
    adiabatic rapid p. (ARP)
    biliary p.
    free air p.
    narrowing of bronchiolar p.
    p. pressure
Passager Nitinol self-expandable stent
Passavant
    P. bar
    P. muscle
    P. ridge
passive
    p. acquired immunity
    p. atelectasis
    p. chest expansion
    p. clot
    p. edema
    p. filling
    p. hepatic congestion
    p. hyperemia
    p. loss of correlation effect
    p. pneumonia
    p. shielding
    p. shimming
    p. track detector
    p. vascular congestion
    p. venous distention
passively
    p. congested lung tissue
    p. shimmed superconducting magnet
PASTA imaging
paste
    ferric ammonium citrate-cellulose p.
pastille, pastil
    p. radiometer
    Sabouraud p.
PASV
    pressure-activated safety valve
    PASV catheter
    PASV valve
    PASV valve technology

Patau syndrome
patch
    ash leaf p.
    blood p.
    p. crinkling
    p. electrode
    epidural blood p.
    p. graft reconstruction
    p. kinking
    p. lesion
    McCallum p.
    Peyer p.
    pigskin p.
    sclerotic calvarial p.
    subcutaneous p.
patch-graft aortoplasty
patchy
    p. alveolar opacity
    p. area of consolidation
    p. area of density
    p. area of pneumonia
    p. atelectasis
    p. atrophy of renal cortex
    p. colonic ulcer
    p. distribution of tracer
    p. edema
    p. migratory infiltrate
    p. zone
patella, pl. **patellae**
    p. alta
    apex of head of p.
    p. baja
    bipartite p.
    chondromalacia p.
    dislocation of p.
    floating p.
    half-moon p.
    high-lying p.
    high-riding p.
    ligamentum patellae
    lower pole of p.
    multipartite p.
    pebble-shaped p.
    skyline view of p.
    squared p.
    subluxation of p. (SLP)
    subluxing p.
    undersurface of p.
patellar
    p. bursa
    p. bursitis
    p. button
    p. cartilage thickness
    p. chondromalacia
    p. contour
    p. dislocation
    p. edge
    p. entrapment
    p. fat pad

p. fossa
p. groove
p. ligament-patellar ratio
p. malalignment
p. pole
p. retinaculum
p. shaving
p. shelf
p. skyline view
p. sleeve fracture
p. subluxation
p. tendinopathy
p. tendinosis
p. tendon
p. tilt
patellectomy
patelliform
patellofemoral
p. angle
p. articular cartilage
p. articulation
p. compartment
p. congruence
p. disorder
p. incongruency
p. index
p. joint
p. joint space
p. realignment
patelloquadriceps tendon
patency
arterial p.
p. of artery
coronary artery bypass graft p.
ductus arteriosus p.
ductus venosus p.
graft p.
long-term p.
modified Blalock-Taussig shunt p.
nidus p.
p. rate
short-term p.
shunt p.
p. trifurcation
p. and valvular reflux of deep
vein
vascular p.
vein p.
p. of vein graft
p. of vessel
patent
p. bifurcation

p. ductus arteriosus (PDA)
p. foramen ovale (PFO)
p. lumen
p. stent
p. urachus
p. vessel
widely p.
Paterson-Parker system
path
p. length
mean free p.
puncture p.
water p.
pathognomonic
p. finding
p. imaging characteristic
pathologic, pathological
p. correlation
p. dislocation
p. fracture
p. intracranial calcification
p. lesion
p. marrow infiltration
pathology (PA)
acute aortic p.
mesenteric lymph node p.
radiographic p.
pathophysiologic change
pathway
amygdalofugal p.
anomalous p.
antegrade fast p.
anterior internodal p.
atrio-His p.
cerebellar p.
cerebropontocerebellar p.
cerebrospinal fluid p.
corticospinal motor p.
dentatoolivary p.
dual atrioventricular node p.
Embden-Meyerhof glycolytic p.
hepatobiliary p.
interhemispheric p.
neural p.
nodoventricular p.
optic glioma p.
reticulocortical p.
retrovestibular neural p.
septal accessory p.
striatal output p.
synaptic p.
Thorel p.

NOTES

P

patient
    p. motion
    p. motion artifact
    p. volume
Patient-Oriented Evidence that Matters (POEM)
Patlak plot
pattern
    abnormal lung p.
    acinar p.
    activation p.
    airway p.
    alveolar p.
    anhaustral colonic gas p.
    anular tear p.
    arborization p.
    architectural p.
    arterial deficiency p.
    atypical vessel colposcopic p.
    ballerina-foot p.
    basket-weave p.
    beam p.
    benign-appearing p.
    bigeminal p.
    blood flow p.
    bony trabecular p.
    bowel gas p.
    branching p.
    broken bough p.
    bronchiectatic p.
    bronchopneumonia p.
    bronchovascular p.
    bubbly p.
    butterfly p.
    cavitating p.
    centrum semiovale p.
    cerebral cortical gyral p.
    circadian p.
    coarse p.
    cobblestone p.
    cobweb p.
    coiled spring p.
    collimator plugging p.
    colonic urticaria p.
    comedo p.
    concertina p.
    contractile p.
    contrast enhancement p.
    convolutional p.
    corduroy cloth p.
    corkscrew p.
    crazy-paving p.
    cribriform p.
    cross-sectional p.
    cystic p.
    degenerative nuclear p.
    p. of destruction
    diffraction p.

    diffuse contrast agent distribution p.
    dissemination p.
    divergent spiculated p.
    dot-and-dash p.
    3D physiologic flow p.
    ductal p.
    early repolarization p.
    echo p.
    echo-dense p.
    echolucent p.
    edema p.
    enhancement p.
    enhancement p. type I–IV
    esophageal achalasia p.
    extended p.
    feathery p.
    fernlike p.
    fibrotic cavitating p.
    fibrous nodular p.
    filigree p.
    fine peripheral reticular p.
    fine reticular p.
    finger-in-glove p.
    fingerprint p.
    fleur-de-lis p.
    flip-flop p.
    focal p.
    fold p.
    folial p.
    follicular p.
    fragmented p.
    gas p.
    gastric mucosal p.
    geographic p.
    ground-glass p.
    gyriform p.
    hairbrush p.
    hanging-fruit p.
    haustral p.
    helical p.
    hemodynamic p.
    hepatic echo p.
    herringbone p.
    heterogeneous internal echo p.
    heterogeneous perfusion p.
    hierarchical scanning p.
    hole p.
    homogeneous echo p.
    homogeneous MR p.
    honeycomb p.
    hourglass p.
    infiltration p.
    inhomogeneous echo p.
    interstitial lung p.
    interstitial tear p.
    intestinal gas p.
    intraaneurysmal inflow p.
    intraaneurysmal outflow p.

inverse follicle p.
juvenile T-wave p.
kidney mass growth p.
lacelike trabecular p.
ladderlike p.
Laue p.
left ventricular contraction p.
left ventricular strain p.
linear interstitial disease p.
liver spoked-wheel p.
lobular alveolar p.
locomotor p.
lymphatic drainage p.
lytic p.
M p.
macronodular p.
magnetic resonance enhancement p.
manometric p.
marrow edema p.
micronodular p.
migrational p.
miliary p.
mimosa p.
mixed lytic and sclerotic p.
moiré p.
mosaic attenuation p.
mosaic duodenal mucosal p.
moth-eaten p.
mottled p.
movement p.
M-shaped mitral valve p.
mucosal fold p.
muscle recruitment p.
nonspecific bowel gas p.
orthogonal-hole test p. (OHP)
ovarian fishnet weave p.
overlying branching p.
parallel and spiral flow p.
parenchymal breast p.
parrot-beak p.
permeative p.
phlebographic p.
pin p.
PLES bar p.
pneumoencephalographic p.
postembolization angiographic p.
P pulmonale p.
proliferative p.
prominent ductal p.
pseudohomogeneous edema p.
pseudoinfarct p.
pseudomantle zone p.

pulmonary flow p.
pulmonary vascular p.
pulsation p.
QR p.
4-quadrant bar p.
quantum mottling p.
railroad track p.
ray p.
recurrence p.
relief p.
restrictive p.
reticular interstitial disease p.
reticular lung p.
reticulogranular p.
reticulonodular p.
reverberating flow p.
rheologic p.
right ventricular strain p.
ringlike p.
rosary bead p.
rugal p.
salt-and-pepper chromatin p.
sawtooth excretory p.
sclerotic p.
segmental alveolar p.
seizure p.
sheetlike growth p.
shish kabob p.
sigmoid hair p.
signet ring p.
sinus p.
slice-of-sausage breast p.
small bowel mucosal p.
snowflake p.
snowstorm breast p.
solid p.
speckled p.
SPECT perfusion p.
spectral p.
spiral flow p.
spoiler gradient p.
spoked wheel p.
p. of spread
star p.
star test p.
start test p.
stellate p.
storiform p.
storiform-pleomorphic p.
strain p.
sulcal p.
sunburst gyral p.

NOTES

P

pattern *(continued)*
    surface convexity p.
    Tabar p.
    tagging p.
    task-rest p.
    temporal sawtooth p.
    thermal convection p.
    tigroid p.
    trabecular p.
    tram-track p.
    transducer beam p.
    tree-in-bud p.
    trigeminal p.
    triple signal p.
    tubular gas p.
    typical cobblestone p.
    V p.
    variegated p.
    ventricular contraction p.
    vesicular p.
    white branching linear p.
    Wolfe DY, NI, P1, P2 p.
    Wolfe mammographic
      parenchymal p.
    zebra stripe p.
patulous
    p. cardia
    p. esophagogastric region
    p. hiatus
PAU
    penetrating atherosclerotic ulcer
pauciarticular
paucilocular
    p. cystic mass
    p. tumor
pauciostotic
paucity
    alveolar p.
    p. of bowel gas
Pauli exclusion principle
Pauly point
pause
    asystolic p.
    compensatory p.
    postextrasystolic p.
    sinus p.
Pauwel
    P. angle
    P. femoral neck fracture
      classification
paving-stone degeneration
PAVM
    pulmonary arteriovenous malformation
Pawlik
    P. triangle
    P. trigone
Pawlow
    P. position
    P. projection

PAWP
    pulmonary artery wedge pressure
Payr sign
Pb
    lead
PBD
    percutaneous biliary drainage
PBF
    pulmonary blood flow
PBI
    protein-bound iodine
PBPI
    penile-brachial pressure index
PBV
    pulmonary blood volume
PBVI
    pulmonary blood volume index
PC
    phase contrast
    posterior commissure
      PC MR angiography
PCA
    posterior cerebral artery
    posterior communicating artery
PCC
    peripheral cholangiocarcinoma
PCD
    percutaneous catheter drainage
    posterior capsular distance
pCi
    picocurie
PCIS
    postcardiac injury syndrome
PCL
    posterior cruciate ligament
    pubococcygeal line
PCLBCL
    primary cutaneous large B-cell
      lymphoma
PC-MRA
    phase contrast MRA
PCNL
    percutaneous nephrolithotomy
    percutaneous nephrostolithotomy
PCoA
    posterior communicating artery
PCOD
    polycystic ovarian disease
PCOS
    polycystic ovary syndrome
PCP
    pulmonary capillary pressure
PCPA
    postcatheterization pseudoaneurysm
PCRA
    percutaneous coronary rotational
      atherectomy
PCS
    proximal coronary

PCWP
pulmonary capillary wedge pressure
Pd
palladium
^{103}**Pd, Pd-103**
palladium 103
^{103}Pd isotope
^{103}Pd prostatic implant
^{103}Pd radioactive material
PDA
patent ductus arteriosus
poorly differentiated adenocarcinoma
posterior descending artery
PDD
percentage depth dose
progressive diaphysial dysplasia
pDEXA
peripheral dual energy x-ray
pDEXA x-ray peripheral bone
densitometer
PDI
power Doppler imaging
PDR
pulsed dose rate
PDS
power Doppler sonography
PDT
photodynamic therapy
PE
pericardial effusion
phase encoding
photographic effect
polyethylene
pulmonary edema
pulmonary embolus
PE catheter
Peacock system
peak
p. airway pressure
p. amplitude
p. aortic flow velocity
p. area
p. arterial frame
backscatter p.
Bragg ionization p.
carotid pulse p.
p. count density
p. diastolic gradient
diffraction p.
p. dP/dt
p. early diastolic filling velocity
early systolic p. (ESP)

p. expiratory flow (PEF)
p. filling
p. filling rate (PFR)
p. fitting
p. flow variability
p. flush flow
frequency-related p.
p. identification
p. inflation pressure
p. instantaneous gradient
juxtaphrenic p.
kilovolt p. (kVp)
p. late diastolic filling velocity
main glow p.
p. of maximum enhancement
(PME)
p. parenchymal activity
photon p.
pressure p.
p. pressure gradient
p. profile
p. pulmonary flow velocity
recirculation p.
p. regurgitant flow velocity
p. regurgitant wave pressure
p. right ventricular-right atrial
systolic gradient
p. scatter factor
p. shape
single p.
p. skin dose (PSD)
p. skin radiation dose
spread Bragg p.
p. systolic aortic pressure
p. systolic and diastolic ratio
p. systolic gradient
p. systolic velocity (PSV)
temporal p. (TP)
time to p. (TTP)
time-to-p.
p. transmitted velocity
p. velocity of blood flow
peak-to-peak pressure gradient
pearl
keratin p.
p. necklace gallbladder
scrotal p.
pearllike breast calcification
pearly
p. body
p. CNS tumor

NOTES

P

pearly (*continued*)
  p. neoplasm
  p. white ovary
pear-shaped
  p.-s. defect
  p.-s. heart
  p.-s. urinary bladder
  p.-s. uterus
Pearson
  P. attachment
  P. correlation coefficient
  P. method
  P. position
  P. syndrome
pea-size
pebble-shaped patella
Pecquet
  cistern of P.
pecten pubis
pectinate
  p. ligament
  p. line
pectineal
pectineus muscle
pectoral
  p. girdle
  p. heart
  p. lymph node
  p. ridge
pectoralis
  p. major muscle
  p. major syndrome
  p. minor muscle
pectus
  p. carinatum deformity
  p. excavatum
  p. excavatum deformity
  p. recurvatum
pedal
  p. artery opacification
  p. bone
  p. lymphangiography
  p. lymphography
  p. pulse
pedal pulse
pedes
pediatric
  p. biplane TEE probe
  p. bronchiolitis
  p. fibroxanthoma
  p. hemangioma
  P. Ingesta Scan metal detector
  p. neuroradiology
  p. nuclear medicine imaging
  p. primary brain tumor
  p. radiology
  p. scintigraphy
  p. solid tumor

pedicle
  p. bone graft
  p. erosion
  p. finger
  p. flap
  p. fracture
  musculofascial p.
  p.'s and pars
  phrenic p.
  p. plate
  pulmonary p.
  p. sclerosis
  p. signal intensity
  spinal p.
  splaying of p.'s
  p. targeting
  vascular p.
  p. of vertebra
pedicolaminar fracture-dislocation
pedis
  malum perforans p.
  calcar p.
  digitus p.
  dorsalis p.
  dorsum p.
  pollex p.
pedobarography
  dynamic p.
PEDRI
  proton-electron double-resonance
    imaging
peduncle
  cerebellar p.
  cerebral p.
  inferior cerebellar p.
peduncular
  p. loop
  p. segment of superior cerebellar
    artery
pedunculated
  p. leiomyoma
  p. lesion
  p. polyp
  p. subserous myoma
  p. thrombus
  p. uterine fibroid
  p. uterine myxoma
  p. vesical tumor
pedunculation
peel
  pleura p.
peel-away
  10F p.-a. sheath
  p.-a. sheath
PEF
  parietal eye field
  peak expiratory flow
PEG
  percutaneous endoscopic gastrostomy

pneumoencephalogram
pneumoencephalography
polyethylene glycol
peg
    cerebellar p.
    rete p.
Pegasus PIV laser
Pegasys workstation
PEHO
    progressive encephalopathy with edema,
      hypsarrhythmia, and optic atrophy
    PEHO syndrome
PEI
    percutaneous ethanol injection
    PEI 1-shot technique
    PEI 2-shot technique
PELA
    peripheral excimer laser angioplasty
peliosis
    spleen p.
Pelizaeus-Merzbacher disease
Pelizzari surface matching method
Pellegrini-Stieda
    P.-S. calcification
    P.-S. disease
pellet
    alanine-silicone p.
    p. artifact
    radiopaque p.
pellucidum
    cavum septum p.
    septum p.
pelves (*pl. of* pelvis)
pelvic
    p. abscess
    p. aneurysm
    p. arteriography
    p. artery
    p. bone
    p. brim
    p. canal
    p. chocolate cyst
    p. collateral vessel
    p. colon
    p. congestion syndrome
    p. cystic mass
    p. diameter
    p. diaphragm
    p. exenteration
    p. exostosis
    p. fascia
    p. femoral angle

p. fibrolipomatosis
p. film for IUD localization
p. floor
p. fluid
p. fracture frame
p. girdle
p. infection
p. inflammatory disease
p. inlet
p. insufficiency fracture
p. lipomatosis
p. lymph node
p. malignancy
p. mass complex
p. mass frequency
p. morphometry
p. notching
p. obliquity
p. organ prolapse
p. outlet
p. peritoneal surface
p. peritoneum
p. phased-array coil
p. plane
p. plexus
p. rim fracture
p. ring
p. ring fracture
p. ring ligament
p. sidewall
p. sonography
p. space
p. spot
p. spur syndrome
p. steal
p. steal test
p. straddle fracture
p. ultrasound
p. ultrasound CT scan
p. unleveling
p. vascular trauma
p. vein thrombosis
p. venous obstruction
p. venous stenosis
p. view
p. viscus
p. wall
pelvicaliceal system
pelvicaliectasis
pelvicalyceal
    p. change
    p. dilatation

NOTES

P

pelvicalyceal *(continued)*
    p. distention
    p. system
pelvicephalography
pelvicephalometry
pelviectasis
pelvimetry
    magnetic resonance p.
    radiographic p.
pelviography
pelvioradiography
pelvioscopy
pelviradiography
pelviroentgenography
pelvis, pl. **pelves**
    aditus p.
    android p.
    anthropoid p.
    assimilation p.
    beaked p.
    bifid p.
    bony p.
    brachypellic p.
    brim of p.
    champagne glass p.
    contracted p.
    cordate p.
    cordiform p.
    Deventer p.
    diameter obliqua p.
    diameter transversa p.
    dolichopellic p.
    dwarf p.
    elephant ears p.
    extrarenal renal p.
    false p.
    female p.
    flat p.
    frozen p.
    funnel-shaped p.
    goblet-shaped p.
    greater p.
    gynecoid p.
    hardened p.
    heart-shaped p.
    intrarenal p.
    inverted p.
    juvenile p.
    p. of kidney
    Kilian p.
    kyphoscoliotic p.
    kyphotic p.
    lesser p.
    longitudinal oval p.
    lordotic p.
    male p.
    masculine p.
    mesatipellic p.

    Mickey Mouse ears p.
    Nägele p.
    osteomalacic p.
    Otto p.
    Otto-Kobak p.
    platypelloid p.
    postmenarchal female p.
    pseudoosteomalacic p.
    rachitic p.
    renal p.
    reniform p.
    Rokitansky p.
    scoliotic p.
    small p.
    spider p.
    spondylolisthetic p.
    tombstone p.
    transverse oval p.
    trident p.
    true p.
    windswept p.
    wine glass p.
pelviureteric junction (PUJ)
pelviureterography
pelvocaliectasis
pelvocalyceal effacement
pelvocephalography
PEM
    positron emission mammography
Pemberton osteotomy
Pena-Shokeir syndrome
pencil
    p. dosimeter
    p. electron beam
pencil-beam
    p.-b. approach
    p.-b. navigator echo
pencil-in-cup
    p.-i.-c. appearance
    p.-i.-c. deformity
penciling
    p. deformity
    p. of the distal clavicle
    p. of rib
    p. of terminal tuft
pencillike deformity
pencil-point metatarsal deformity
pendent positioning
pendetide
    [111]In satumomab p.
Pendred syndrome
PenduLaser
    Kaplan P. 115
pendulous
    p. heart
    p. pouch
    p. reference axis (PRA)
    p. urethra

pendulum
>cor p.
>p. movement

penes (*pl. of* penis)
penetrability
penetrating
>p. aortic ulcer
>p. atherosclerotic ulcer (PAU)
>p. fracture
>p. lung injury
>p. trauma
>p. TRD
>p. wound

penetration
>acoustic p.
>bowel wall p.
>p. fraction
>insufficient acoustic p.
>lack of acoustic p.
>radiographic p.
>rectal p.

penetrometer
>Benoist p.

penile
>p. artery
>p. fibromatosis
>p. implant
>p. plaque
>p. raphe
>p. sonography
>p. squamous papilloma
>p. urethra
>p. vein
>p. vessel

penile-brachial pressure index (PBPI)
penis, pl. **penes**
>bulb of p.
>bulbospongiosus muscle of p.
>clubbed p.
>concealed p.
>corpora cavernosa p.
>corpus spongiosum p.
>crus of p.
>deep fascia of p.
>dorsal artery of p.
>dorsal nerve of p.
>dorsum of p.
>double p.
>glans p.
>hypoplastic p.
>ischiospongiosus muscle of p.
>root of p.

>suspensory ligament of p.
>webbed p.

penlscopy
penoscrotal
PenRad mammography clinical reporting system
Penta balloon
pentacene
pentagastrin imaging agent
pentalogy
>Cantrell p.
>p. of Fallot

pentavalent DMSA imaging agent
Pentax ELLB 6000, 6500 ultrasound gastroscope
Pentax-Hitachi FG32UA endosonographic system
pentetate
>^{111}In imciromab p.

pentetic acid imaging agent
pentetide
>satumomab p.

pentetreotide
>p. imaging agent
>^{111}In p.
>p. tumor localization scan

pentose cycle
penultimate section
penumbra, pl. **penumbrae**
>dosimetric p.
>hemodynamic p.
>ischemic p.
>p. zone

PEP
>preejection period

pepper
>P. syndrome
>P. tumor

peppermint oil imaging agent
pepper-pot pitting
peptic
>p. esophagitis
>p. stricture
>p. ulcer
>p. ulcer disease (PUD)

peptide imaging agent
percentage
>p. classification
>p. depth dose (PDD)
>p. signal intensity loss

Perception scanner
perceptual linearization

NOTES

P

perched facet joint
Percheron
    artery of P.
perchlorate
    potassium p.
    p. washout test
Perclose
    P. arterial closure device
    P. diagnostic device
    P. 6F Closer
    P. PVS suture system
    P. therapeutic device
percreta
    placenta p.
PercuCut cut-biopsy needle
Percuflex stent
percussion sensitivity
Percusurg distal protection device
percutaneous
    p. abscess drainage
    p. antegrade biliary drainage
    p. antegrade pyelography
    p. antegrade urography
    p. arterial closure device
    p. atherectomy
    p. automated discectomy
    p. biliary drainage (PBD)
    p. catheter drainage (PCD)
    p. cavity drainage catheter
    p. cecostomy
    p. cementoplasty
    p. chemical ablation
    p. cholecystocholedochostomy
    p. cholecystotomy catheter
    p. choledochoscopy
    p. coronary rotational atherectomy
     (PCRA)
    p. dilatation of biliary duct
    p. dissolution of thrombus
    p. drainage
    p. electrical nerve stimulation
    p. embolectomy
    p. embolotherapy
    p. endofluoroscopy
    p. endoluminal placement
    p. endometrial drug delivery
    p. endopyelotomy
    p. endoscopic gastrostomy (PEG)
    p. endoscopy
    p. ethanol injection (PEI)
    p. ethanol injection therapy
    p. ethanol instillation
    p. ethanol sclerotherapy
    p. femoral arteriography
    p. gastroenterostomy
    18-gauge p. access needle
    p. hepaticojejunostomy
    p. hepatobiliary cholangiography
    p. interventional radiology

    p. intraaortic balloon
    p. intracoronary angioscopy imaging
    p. mechanical thrombectomy (PMT)
    p. microwave coagulation therapy
    7 × 40-mm p. transluminal
     angioplasty balloon
    p. nephrolithotomy (PCNL)
    p. nephroscope
    p. nephrostolithotomy (PCNL)
    p. nephrostomy
    p. nonvascular abdominal
     intervention
    p. osteoplasty
    p. pancreatography
    p. pericardioscopy
    p. peritoneovenous shunt creation
    p. pin insertion
    p. radiofrequency catheter ablation
    p. retrograde transfemoral technique
    p. splenoportography
    p. stent
    p. suture-mediated arteriotomy
     closure device
    p. suture-mediated closure device
    p. thermal occlusion
    p. thrombin injection
    p. transcatheter therapy
    p. transhepatic biliary drainage
     (PTBD)
    p. transhepatic cholangial drainage
     (PTCD)
    p. transhepatic cholangiogram (PTC,
     PTCA, PTHC)
    p. transhepatic cholangiography
     (PTHC)
    p. transhepatic cholecystostomy
    p. transhepatic decompression
    p. transhepatic endoluminal biliary
     biopsy
    p. transhepatic liver biopsy
    p. transhepatic lymphography (PTL)
    p. transhepatic portography
    p. transluminal angioplasty (PTA)
    p. transluminal balloon dilatation
    p. transluminal coronary angioplasty
     (PTCA)
    p. transluminal coronary
     recanalization technique
    p. transluminal renal angioplasty
     (PTRA)
    p. transperineal seed implantation
    p. transthoracic needle biopsy
     (PTNB)
    p. transtracheal bronchography
    p. tube insertion
    p. tumor treatment
    p. ultrasound-guided thrombin
     injection

p. vascular surgical device
p. vertebroplasty
percutaneously cannulated
Perez sign
Perflex stainless steel balloon-expandable stent
perflubron
p. imaging agent
partial liquid ventilation with p.
perfluorocarbon-exposed sonicated dextrose albumin (PESDA)
perfluorocarbon imaging agent
perfluorochemical
perfluorooctyl bromide (PFOB)
perflutren lipid microsphere injectable suspension
perforans
perforated
p. aortic cusp
p. cholecystitis
p. diverticulum
p. gangrenous appendix
p. hollow viscus
p. ulcer
perforating
p. aneurysm
p. artery
p. branch
p. colorectal carcinoma
p. fracture
p. vein
p. wound
perforation
bladder p.
bowel p.
cardiac p.
colonic p.
common bile duct spontaneous p.
duodenal ulcer p.
esophageal p.
gallbladder p.
iatrogenic esophageal p.
idiopathic gastric p.
intestinal p.
Niemeier gallbladder p.
renal transplant GI tract p.
septal p.
spontaneous p.
transseptal p.
ulcer p.
ureteral p.

vascular p.
ventricular p.
perforative lesion
perforator
incompetent p.
septal p.
p. vessel
Performa mammography system
perfusate vessel
perfused
p. myocardium
p. needle applicator
p. twin
perfusion
p. abnormality
adequate coronary p.
p. agent
antegrade p.
blood p.
brain p.
capillary p.
continuous hyperthermic peritoneal p.
p. CT
decreased distal p.
diminished airway p.
diminished systemic p.
first-pass cardiac p.
gated stress myocardial p. (GMP)
p. gradient
homogeneous p.
hypothermic p.
impaired renal p.
increment of p.
p. index
inhomogeneous p.
intraperitoneal hyperthermic p. (IPHP)
isolation p.
limb p.
lung p.
p. lung scan
luxury p.
maldistribution of ventilation and p.
p. measurement technique
misery p.
mosaic p.
p. MRI
p. MR imaging
myocardial p.
peripheral p.

NOTES

perfusion *(continued)*
poor p.
p. pressure
pulsatile p.
quantitative cardiac p.
regional cerebral p.
regional pulmonary p.
regional vascular p.
renal p.
resting p.
retrograde cardiac p.
p. scintigraphy
p. study
p. time
tissue p.
unilateral lung p.
p. and ventilation lung imaging
perfusion-metabolism mismatch
perfusion-weighted
p.-w. imaging (PWI)
p.-w. MRI
periadventitial fibrosis
perialveolar fibrosis
periampullary
p. carcinoma
p. diverticulum
p. duodenal tumor
perianal
p. abscess
p. hematoma
periaortic
p. area
p. fibrosis
p. lymph node
p. mediastinal hematoma
periaortitis
chronic p.
periapical
p. cemental dysplasia
p. granuloma
p. lesion
p. radiograph
periappendiceal
p. abscess
p. structure
periaqueductal
p. gray matter
p. hemorrhage
periareolar fistula
periarteriolar lymphoid sheath
periarteritis nodosa
periarthritis
adhesive p.
periarticular
p. calcification
p. fluid collection
p. fracture
p. heterotopic ossification (PHO)
p. margin

p. osteoporosis
p. tissue
periauricular region
peribiliary cyst
peribronchial
p. alveolar space
p. connective tissue
p. cuffing
p. distribution
p. fibrosis
p. hemorrhage
p. infiltrate
p. lymph node
p. marking
p. micronodule
p. thickening
peribronchovascular interstitial compartment
peribursal fat
pericaliceal cyst
pericallosal
p. artery
p. lipoma
p. vein
p. vessel
pericapsular fat infiltrate
pericardia (*pl. of* pericardium)
pericardiacophrenic vein
pericardiac pleura
pericardial
p. aorta
p. calcification
p. cavity
p. chyle with tamponade
p. defect
p. diaphragmatic adhesion
p. disease
p. duplication cyst
p. effusion (PE)
p. empyema
p. fat pad
p. flap
p. fluid
p. fold
p. halo
p. hematoma
p. infusion
p. knock sound
p. lymph node
p. reserve volume
p. sac
p. silhouette
p. sinus
p. sleeve recess
p. space
p. tamponade
p. vein
p. window
pericardiectomy

pericardiocentesis
    hand-carried ultrasound-guided p.
pericardioperitoneal canal
pericardioscopy
    percutaneous p.
pericarditis
    bread-and-butter p.
    constrictive p.
    diffuse p.
    hemorrhagic p.
    postmeningococcal p.
    radiation-induced p.
pericardium, pl. **pericardia**
    adherent p.
    autologous p.
    p. calcareous deposit
    calcified p.
    congenitally absent p.
    crus p.
    diaphragmatic p.
    p. fibrosum
    fibrous p.
    inelastic p.
    parietal p.
    rheumatic adherent p.
    roughened state of p.
    serous p.
    shaggy p.
    soldier's patches of p.
    visceral p.
pericarinal injury
pericatheter
    p. thrombosis
    p. thrombus
pericaval
pericavernous
pericecal abscess
pericentral fibrosis
pericerebral fluid
pericholecystic
    p. abscess
    p. edema
    p. fluid
    p. fluid collection
pericholedochal
    p. node
    p. varix
perichondral
    p. bone
    p. cell seeding
    p. ring
perichondrium

pericicatricial emphysema
pericolic abscess
pericolonic
    p. abscess
    p. fat
    p. fluid
pericranii
    sinus p.
pericyst
pericystic edema
peridental space
peridiaphragmatic hematoma
peridiploid
peridiverticulitis
periductal
    p. calcification
    p. fibrosis
peridural fibrosis
periesophageal fluid
perifascial fluidlike collection
perifocal
    p. edema
    p. emphysema
perigastric
    p. deformity
    p. fat
perigestational hemorrhage
perigraft
    p. fluid
    p. hematoma
    p. seroma
perihepatic
    p. abscess
    p. space
perihepatitis
    focal p.
perihilar
    p. area
    p. batwing infiltrate
    p. density
    p. edema
    p. fat
    p. fibrosis
    p. lung disease
    p. marking
    p. region
periileal
periinfarction
    p. block
    p. ischemia
perilabral sulcus
perilesional white matter

NOTES

P

perilobular
- p. connective tissue
- p. duct

perilunar
- p. dislocation
- p. instability

perilunate
- p. dislocation
- p. fracture-dislocation
- p. instability

perimedial
- p. dysplasia
- p. fibroplasia
- p. renal fibroplasia artery

perimedullary

perimembranous ventricular septal defect

perimeniscal capsular plexus

perimesencephalic
- p. cistern
- p. nonaneurysmal subarachnoid hemorrhage

perimeter-area ratio (P-A)

perimetry testing

perimuscular
- p. fibrosis
- p. plexus

perimylolysis

perinatal
- p. anoxia
- p. asphyxia
- p. injury

perineal
- p. descent
- p. fascia
- p. sinus
- p. space

perineogram imaging

perineoplastic edema

perineovaginal fistula

perinephric
- p. abscess
- p. air injection
- p. fat
- p. fluid collection
- p. hematoma
- p. space
- p. space hemorrhage

perinephritic abscess

perineum, pl. **perinea**

perineural
- p. arachnoid cyst
- p. fat
- p. fibroblastoma
- p. fibroblastoma tumor
- p. fibrosis
- p. glial proliferation
- p. invasion

- p. sacral cyst
- p. tumor spread

perinuclear halo

period
- antegrade refractory p.
- diastasis heart p.
- diastolic filling p.
- effective refractory p. (ERP)
- embryonic p.
- fetal p.
- functional refractory p. (FRP)
- immediate postictal p.
- isoelectric p.
- isovolumetric p.
- phase-encoding p.
- postbiopsy p.
- preejection p. (PEP)
- radiofrequency p.
- rapid filling p.
- raster p.
- reduced ventricular filling p.
- relative refractory p. (RRP)
- retrograde refractory p.
- roentgen equivalent man p. (REMP)
- systolic ejection p. (SEP)
- total atrial refractory p. (TARP)
- ventricular effective refractory p. (VERP)
- window p.

periodic
- p. acid-Schiff
- p. synchronous discharge (PSD)

periodically rotated overlapping parallel lines with enhanced reconstruction (PROPELLER)

periodicity
- circadian p.

periodontal
- p. disease
- p. ligament

perioptic meningioma

periorbital
- p. bidirectional Doppler
- p. directional Doppler ultrasonography
- p. edema

periosseous soft tissue mass

periosteal
- p. artery
- p. bone
- p. bone collar
- p. cloaking
- p. creep
- p. desmoid
- p. dysplasia
- p. elevation
- p. fibroma
- p. fibrosarcoma

p. ganglion
p. new bone formation
p. osteosarcoma
p. reaction
p. resorption
p. sarcoma
periosteum, pl. **periostea**
p. of rib
periostitis
florid reactive p.
medial malleolus p.
periotic bone
peripancreatic
p. artery
p. fluid collection
p. lymphadenopathy
peripartum dilated cardiomyopathy
peripelvic
p. collateral vessel
p. cyst
p. fat proliferation
p. lipomatosis
peripheral
p. airspace disease
p. arterial disease
p. arterial occlusive disease
(PAOD)
p. arteriography
p. arteriosclerosis
p. blood
p. blood flow
p. bolus chase
p. border
p. bronchogenic carcinoma
p. cholangiocarcinoma (PCC)
p. chondrosarcoma
p. circulation
p. circulatory vasoconstriction
p. consolidation
p. cutaneous vasoconstriction
p. directional atherectomy
p. dual energy x-ray (pDEXA)
p. embolus
p. excimer laser angioplasty
(PELA)
p. expansion
p. fracture
p. hematopoietic intermediate signal
intensity marrow
p. hypoperfusion
p. infiltrate
p. intravenous infusion line

p. laser angioplasty
p. lesion enhancement
p. loading
p. lung disease
p. lymphoma
p. meniscocapsular tear
p. MR angiography
p. necrosis
p. nerve
p. nerve decompression
p. nerve injury
p. nerve lesion
p. nervous system
p. neuroectodermal tumor
p. neurofibromatosis
p. nodule
p. ossification
p. ossifying fibroma
p. parenchymal atelectasis
p. perfusion
p. perimeniscal capillary ingrowth
p. pneumonia
p. pseudoaneurysm
p. puddling
p. pulmonary artery stenosis
(PPAS)
p. pulse gating
p. quantitative computed
tomography (pQCT)
p. runoff
p. skeleton
p. small airway study
p. synovitis
p. texture
p. vascular disease (PVD)
p. vascular imaging
p. vascular occlusive disease
p. vascular resistance (PVR)
p. vasculature
p. vasogenic edema
p. venography
p. vessel
peripherally
p. inserted central catheter (PICC)
p. inserted central catheter line
p. inserted central catheter
occlusion line opening
(PICCOLO)
periphery
p. of anulus
echogenic p.
lung p.

NOTES

P

periportal
    p. area
    p. cirrhosis
    p. collar
    p. fibrosis
    p. sinusoidal dilatation
    p. tracking
    p. tracking of blood
periprocedural monitoring
periprosthetic
    p. bone resorption
    p. fluid collection
    p. fracture
    p. leak
    p. osteolysis
periprosthetic fluid collection
periradicular
    p. nerve
    p. sheath
perirectal
    p. abscess
    p. fat
perirenal
    p. abscess
    p. air study
    p. bleeding
    p. compartment
    p. fat
    p. hematoma
    p. hemorrhage
    p. insufflation
    p. lymphoma
    p. mass
    p. septum
    p. space
perirolandic parietal cortex
perisellar vascular lesion
perisigmoid colon
perisinusoidal space
perisplenic node
peristalsis
    abnormal esophageal p.
    absence of primary p.
    absent p.
    accelerated p.
    anterograde p.
    bowel p.
    decreased p.
    esophageal p.
    hyperactive p.
    increased p.
    meconium p.
    primary esophageal p.
    retrograde p.
    reversed p.
    secondary p.
    small bowel p.
    ureteral seesaw p.
    visible p.

    yo-yo esophageal p.
    yo-yo ureteral p.
peristaltic
    p. activity
    p. contraction
    p. rush
    p. sequence
    p. wave
peristriate cortex
perisylvian cortex
peritendinitis
peritendinous
    p. adhesion
    p. calcification
perithyroid vein
peritoneal
    p. abscess
    p. attachment
    p. band
    p. carcinomatosis
    p. cavity
    p. cavity fluid
    p. dialysis catheter
    p. effusion
    p. enhancement
    p. fold
    p. gutter
    p. hernia
    p. inclusion cyst
    p. lymphopneumatosis
    p. mass
    p. mesothelioma
    p. metastasis
    p. metastatic implant
    p. mouse
    p. part of inguinal ligament
    p. recess
    p. sac
    p. scintigraphy
    p. seeding
    p. shunting
    p. sign
    p. space
peritoneal-venous shunt patency test
peritonei
    carcinomatosis p.
    gliomatosis p.
    pseudomyxoma p.
peritoneocele
peritoneogram imaging
peritoneography
    CT, MR p.
peritoneopericardial diaphragmatic hernia
peritoneopleural communication
peritoneoscintigraphy
peritoneovenous shunt (PVS)
peritoneum
    p. desmoid tumor

parietal p.
pelvic p.
visceral p.
peritonitis
bile p.
chemical p.
meconium p.
tuberculous p.
peritrigonal white matter
peritrochanteric fracture
peritubular vascular bed
peritumoral
p. cyst
p. edema
p. enhancement
p. tissue
periumbilical
p. pain
p. swelling
periungual fibroma
periureteral fibrosis
periurethral gland
perivalvular
p. leak
p. pseudoaneurysm
perivascular
p. cloaking
p. cuffing
p. distribution
p. edema
p. fibrosis
p. infiltrate
p. mass
p. pseudorosette
p. space
periventricular
p. blush
p. bright signal
p. calcification
p. echogenicity (PVE)
p. gray (PVG)
p. gray matter
p. halo
p. hemorrhagic infarct
p. hypodensity
p. lesion
p. leukoencephalopathy
p. leukomalacia (PVL)
p. plaque
p. white matter
perivenular fibrosis
perivesical

Perkin line
Perkins-Ombrdanne line
permanent
p. brachytherapy
p. callus
p. interstitial implant
p. magnet
p. stoma
PermCath
Quinton P.
permeability
capillary p.
p. constant
constant p.
Crone-Renkin index of p.
magnetic p.
membrane p.
pulmonary capillary p.
p. pulmonary edema
tumor capillary p.
permeation
permeative
p. bone destruction
p. lesion
p. pattern
permutation
pernio lupus
peroneal
p. artery
p. bone
p. brevis tendon
p. longus tendon
p. muscle
p. nerve
p. retinaculum
p. sign
p. tendon injury
p. tendon subluxation
p. tenosynovitis
p. thrombus
p. trochlea
p. tubercle
p. vein
p. vessel
peroneal-to-anterior compartment ratio
peroneum
os p.
peroneus
p. brevis tendon
p. longus
p. longus muscle avulsion
p. longus tendon

NOTES

P

peroneus *(continued)*
    p. quartus muscle
    p. tertius
    p. tertius tendon
peroral
    p. cone radiation therapy
    p. implantation
    p. retrograde pancreaticobiliary
        ductography
peroxidase
    tracer horseradish p.
peroxyl
perpendicular
    p. mean translation
    method of p.'s
Persantine
    P. imaging agent
    P. thallium imaging
persistent
    p. bronchopleural fistula
    p. common atrioventricular canal
    p. cortical kidney lobation
    p. ductus arteriosus
    p. fetal circulation
    p. generalized lymphadenopathy
    p. hyperparathyroidism
    p. increasing nephrogram
    p. left inferior vena cava
    p. left superior vena cava
    p. metopic suture
    p. ossiculum terminale
    p. ostium atrioventriculare commune
    p. primitive trigeminal artery
    p. pulmonary hypertension
    p. pylorospasm
    p. renal lobation
    p. sciatic artery
    p. splenomegaly
    p. truncus arteriosus (PTA)
personal
    p. ionization chamber
    p. space
personal space
perspective volume rendering (PVR)
Pertechnegas
pertechnetate
    p. scintigraphy
    sodium p.
    technetium-99m p. (TcO$_4$)
Perthes
    P. disease
    P. epiphysis
    P. lesion
Perthes-Bankart lesion
pertrochanteric fracture
perturbation
    cytoskeletal p.
    magnetic field p.
    radiation dose p.

perturbing magnetic field
pertussoid eosinophilic pneumonia
perversus
    situs p.
pervious duct of Botallo
pes
    p. abductus
    p. adductus
    p. anserine bursa
    p. anserinus
    p. anserinus bursitis
    p. arcuatus
    p. arcuatus clawfoot deformity
    p. calcaneocavus
    p. calcaneovalgus
    p. calcaneus
    p. calvaneovalgus
    p. cavovalgus
    p. cavovarus
    p. cavus
    p. cavus clawfoot deformity
    p. contortus
    p. equinovalgus
    p. equinovarus
    p. equinus
    p. malleus valgus
    p. planovalgus
    p. planovalgus deformity
    p. plantigrade planus
    p. planus deformity
    p. pronation
    p. pronatus
    p. varus
PESDA
    perfluorocarbon-exposed sonicated
        dextrose albumin
PET
    positron emission tomography
    PET balloon
    cardiac PET
    PET compound
    PET full-ring scanner
    PET lung imaging
    PET measurement of dopamine
        receptor availability
    PET metabolic imaging
    PET myocardial fatty acid imaging
    PET perfusion metabolism imaging
    PET radioligand
    PET radiopharmaceutical
    PET scan
    PET target material
    tyrphostin radiotracer for PET
petal-fugal flow
PET/CT scanner
petiole
petit
    P. ligament

p. mal seizure
P. sinus
Pétrequin ligament
petrobasilar suture
petroclinoid ligament
petromastoid
petrosal
    p. bone
    p. cerebellum
    p. foramen
    p. ganglion
    greater p.
    lesser p.
    p. nerve
    p. sinus
    p. vein
petrositis
    apical p.
petrosphenobasilar suture
petrosphenoid
petrosphenooccipital
    p. suture
    p. suture of Gruber
petrosquamosal suture
petrosquamous suture
petrous
    p. apex
    p. apex dumbbell mass
    p. carotid canal
    p. carotid canal stenosis
    p. ICA
    p. pyramid
    p. pyramid scalloping
    p. ridge
    p. segment of internal carotid
    artery
    p. temporal bone
    p. tip
PETT
    positron emission transaxial tomography
    positron emission transverse tomography
    PETT imaging
    PETT VI PET scanner
Peutz-Jeghers
    P.-J. gastrointestinal polyposis
    P.-J. polyp
    P.-J. syndrome
Peyer patch
Peyronie disease
PFA
    platelet function analyzer
PFA-100 system

Pfaundler-Hurler
    P.-H. disease
    P.-H. syndrome
Pfeiffer
    P. acrocephalosyndactyly
    P. disease
    P. syndrome
Pfeiffer-Comberg method
PFFD
    proximal focal femoral deficiency
PFI
    private finance initiative
Pfizer 200 FS, 400 scanner
PFO
    patent foramen ovale
PFOB
    perfluorooctyl bromide
PFR
    peak filling rate
pGGO
    pure ground glass opacity
PGSE
    pulsed-gradient spin echo
PHA
    proper hepatic artery
    pulse-height analyzer
PHACES
    posterior fossa malformations, facial
    hemangiomas, arterial anomalies,
    cardiac anomalies and aortic
    coarctation, eye anomalies, and sternal
    clefting and/or supraumbilical raphe
    PHACES syndrome
phagedenic ulcer
phakomatosis, pl. **phakomatoses**
phalangeal
    p. bone
    p. branch
    p. diaphysial fracture
    p. glenoidal ligament
    p. herniation
    p. preponderance
    p. shortening
phalanx, pl. **phalanges**
    base of p.
    drumstick p.
    hourglass p.
    ivory p.
    rectangular p.
Phalen
    P. maneuver
    P. position

NOTES

P

phantogeusia
global p.
phantom
Alderson anthropomorphic p.
p. bone
p. breast tumor
chest p.
p. dosimetry
flood p.
gelatin p.
Hine-Duley p.
p. image
p. limb syndrome
p. lung tumor
mammographic p.
metal line-pair p.
neck p.
nuclear magnetic resonance p.
oil-water p.
p. pregnancy
p. radiograph
reference p.
p. simulating cardiac motion
p. study
velocity-evaluation p.
wax p.
phantosmia
birhinal p.
unirhinal p.
pharmacoangiography
pharmacodynamics
pharmacologic
p. dilatation
p. stress
p. stress dual-isotope myocardial
perfusion SPECT
p. stress echocardiography
pharmacomechanical thrombolysis
pharmacoradiologic disimpaction of
esophageal foreign body
pharmacoradiology
PharmaSeed palladium-103 seeds
pharyngeal
p. abscess
p. area
p. artery
p. canal
p. muscle
p. orifice
p. plexus
p. pouch
p. recess
p. space mass
p. tonsil
p. wall carcinoma
pharynges (*pl. of* pharynx)
pharyngobasilar fascia
pharyngoesophageal
p. diverticulum

p. function
p. sphincter
pharyngoesophagogram
pharyngoesophagography
pharyngography
pharyngotonsillitis
pharyngotympanic tube
pharynx, pl. **pharynges**
p. cross-section
laryngeal part of p.
nasal part of p.
oral part of p.
postcricoid p.
phase
accelerated p.
accumulation p.
p. analysis
p. angle
arterial p.
blastic p.
blood pool p.
p. cancellation
cardiac p.
chronic p.
p. coherence
p. contrast (PC)
p. contrast MRA (PC-MRA)
p. contrast sequence
p. correction
corticomedullary p.
p. cycling
p. delay
delayed p.
diastolic depolarization p.
p. difference mapping
p. discontinuity artifact
p. effect
p. encoding (PE)
equilibrium p.
excretory p. (EP)
expiratory p.
fat-water out of p.
p. filtering
follicular p.
p. gain
hepatic arterial p. (HAP)
p. identification
p. image
inspiratory p.
p. instability
interictal p.
p. inversion harmonic imaging
late p.
luteal p.
midarterial p.
p. mismapping
nephrogenic p.
nephrographic p. (NP)
noncontrast p. (NCP)

ovulatory p.
parenchymatous p.
plateau p.
portal venous p. (PVP)
portal venous-dominant p. (PVP)
prolonged expiratory p.
prolonged inspiratory p.
rapid early repolarization p.
rapid ventricular filling p.
p. relation
p. sampling ratio (PSR)
p. shift
spent p.
static bone p.
thallium redistribution p.
vascular p.
p. velocity imaging
venous p.
ventilation scintigraphy
  equilibrium p.
wash-in p.
washout p.
zero p.
2-phase
2-p. computed tomographic imaging
2-p. CT imaging
2-p. helical computed tomography
2-p. helical CT
3-phase
3-p. bone scan
3-p. bone scintigraphy (TPBS)
3-p. current
3-p. generator
3-p. imaging
3-p. system
3-p. technetium study
3-p. voltage supply
3-p. whole-body bone imaging
  (TPWBBI)
phase-angle display redundancy
4-phase bone scintigraphy
phase-contrast
p.-c. angiography
p.-c. cine MRI
phase-corrected GRE image
phased-array
p.-a. body coil MR imaging
2.0-MHz p.-a. probe
p.-a. MRI
p.-a. multicoil imaging
p.-a. multicoils
p.-a. scanner

p.-a. surface coil
p.-a. surface coil MR imaging
p.-a. torso coil
p.-a. transducer
phased array coil
phase-dependent spectroscopic imaging
phase-encode
p.-e. pulse
p.-e. time-reduced acquisition
  sequence
p.-e. time-reduced acquisition
  sequence imaging
phase-encoding
p.-e. direction
p.-e. gradient
p.-e. motion artifact
p.-e. order
p.-e. period
p.-e. step
phase-inversion method
phase-offset multiplanar (POMP)
phase-ordered multiplanar (POMP)
phase-preserving reconstruction
phase-sensitive
p.-s. detector
p.-s. flow measurement
p.-s. gradient-echo MR imaging
phase-shift
p.-s. artifact
p.-s. effect
p.-s. velocity mapping
phase-shifting interferometry
phase-specific action
phase-unwrapping method
phase-velocity image
phasic
p. contraction
p. pressure
phasicity
phasing-in time
Phemister triad
phenazopyridine
phenobarbital
p. biliary atresia
p. imaging agent
phenoltetrachlorophthalein
**phenomenological effective surface
  potential**
phenomenon, pl. **phenomena** (*See* disease,
  syndrome)
Ashman p.
Austin Flint p.

NOTES

P

phenomenon *(continued)*
   autoimmune p.
   Bancaud p.
   Bell p.
   common cavity p.
   crankshaft p.
   Cushing p.
   dip p.
   embolic p.
   extinction p.
   flare p.
   flow p.
   fogging p.
   Friedreich p.
   Gärtner p.
   glove p.
   Hurst p.
   interference p.
   irradiation p.
   Jod-Basedow p.
   Katz-Wachtel p.
   kindling p.
   magic angle p.
   no-reflow p.
   nutcracker p.
   on-off p.
   pivot shift p.
   Raynaud p.
   resonance p.
   R-on-T p.
   Schiff-Sherrington p.
   seizure p.
   spin-phase p.
   staircase p.
   steal p.
   treppe p.
   truncation p.
   unilateral Raynaud p.
   vacuum disc p.
   vertebral steal p.
   Wenckebach p.
phenotype
phenoxyacetic acid
phentetiothalein
phenyloxazolyl
pheochromocytoma
   adrenal p.
   bladder p.
   p. rule of 10
Philips
   P. DVI 1 system
   P. Gyroscan ACS, NT, NT5,
   NT15, S5, T5 scanner
   P. Gyroscan ACS NT
   superconducting magnet
   P. Integris 5000 digital subtraction
   angiography system
   P. linear accelerator
   P. 1.5 NT-Intera scanner

   P. 1.5-T NT MR scanner
   P. Tomoscan 350, SR 6000 CT
   scanner
   P. 4.7-T small-bore system scanner
Phillips muscle
phlebectasia
   malformed p.
phlebectatic peliosis hepatis
phlebitis
   postvenography p.
phlebogram
   ascending contrast MR p.
   direct puncture MR p.
   impedance MR p.
phlebograph
phlebographic pattern
phlebography
   ascending contrast p.
   cervical magnetic resonance p.
   (CMRP)
   direct puncture p.
   impedance p.
   magnetic resonance p.
   occlusive impedance p.
phlebolith
phlebolithlike calcification
phleborheography (PRG)
phlebosclerosis
phlebostasis
phlebostenosis
phlebothrombosis
phlegmasia cerulea dolens
phlegmon
   Holz p.
   mesenteric p.
   pancreatic p.
phlegmonous
   p. abscess
   p. gastritis
   p. mass
   p. pancreatitis
phlyctenule lesion
PHO
   periarticular heterotopic ossification
phocomely, phocomelia
phonation study
phonoangiography
   carotid p.
   oculoplethysmography/carotid p.
   (OPG/CPA)
phonocardiography
phonophotography
PhorMax CR desktop workstation
   system
phosphate
   chromium p.
   p. enema
   linear p.
   membrane p.

phosphorus-32 sodium p.
  sodium p. (P-32)
  ^{99m}Tc p.
phosphaturic
  p. intraosseous lesion
  p. mass
  p. material
  p. tumor
phosphaturic-inducing tumor
phosphomonoester (PME)
  p. signal
phosphonate
  nucleoside p.
phosphor
  cesium iodide input p.
  fluorescent p.
  photostimulable p. (PSP)
  p. plate
phosphorated
phosphorescence
phosphoric acid imaging agent
phosphorus (P)
  p. 31
  p. 32 (^{32}P, P-32)
  colloidal chromic p.
  p. imaging agent
  inorganic p.
  p. isotope
  labeled p.
  p. magnetic resonance spectroscopy
   (P-MRS)
  p. metabolism
  radioactive p.
phosphorus-32
  p.-32 intracavitary irradiation
  p.-32 sodium phosphate
phosphorus-31 magnetic resonance spectroscopy
phosphorylase
  thymidine p. (TP)
Phospho-Soda
phosphosoda enema
Phosphotec
Phosphotope oral solution
photic
photo
  analog p.
  p. plotter film
  p. transformation
photoacoustic ultrasound
photoactinic

photoaffinity
photoaging
photoangioplasty
photocathode
photocell plethysmography
photochemotherapy
  extracorporeal p.
photochromogen
photocoagulation
  interstitial laser p.
  intraoperative laser p.
  krypton laser p.
photocoagulator
  xenon arch p.
photodeficient region
photodensitometry
photodetector
  CCD p.
photodiode
photodisintegration
photodisplay unit
photodisruption
photodynamic therapy (PDT)
photoechoic effect
photoelasticity
photoelectric
  p. absorption
  p. effect
  p. emission
  p. interaction
  p. system
photoelectron
photoexcitation
photoflow
photofluorogram
photofluorographic
photofluorography
photofluoroscope
PhotoGenica V-Star laser
photographic
  p. effect (PE)
  p. radiometer
photography
  CT bone window p.
  moiré p.
  Raster stereo p.
photolysis
  flash p.
photometer
  HemoCue p.

NOTES

P

photomicrograph
    cystic hyperplasia p.
photomultiplier (PM)
    p. tube (PMT)
photon (hv)
    annihilation p.
    p. attenuation
    p. attenuation measurement
    p. cataract removal system
    Compton scattering p.
    p. correlation spectroscopy
    p. deficiency
    degraded p.
    p. dcnsitometry
    p. density
    dual p.
    p. energy
    p. fluence
    p. flux
    gamma p.
    p. interaction depth
    linear p.
    p. mottle
    p. peak
    p. radiosurgery system (PRS)
    soft p.
    p. starvation
    p. theory of radiation
    p. therapy beam line
photon-deficient
    p.-d. area
    p.-d. bone lesion
    p.-d. lesion bone scintigraphy
photoneutron
photonic medicine
photon-neutron mixed-beam radiation therapy
photonuclear
    p. effect
    p. reaction
photooptical detection
photopeak
    p. breadth
    p. fraction
photopenia
photopenic
    p. area
    p. defect
    p. region
Photopic Imaging ultrasound system
photoplethysmographic
    p. digit
    p. monitoring
photoplethysmography (PPG)
PhotoPoint
    P. laser
    P. photodynamic therapy
photoprotein
photoradiation

photoradiometer
photoreceptor
    p. fractional velocity error
    p. motion
photorecording
photoroentgenography
photoscan
photoscanner
photostimulable
    p. luminescence intensity
    p. phosphor (PSP)
    p. phosphor computed radiography
    p. phosphor dental radiography
    p. phosphor digital imaging
    p. phosphor plate
phototherapeutic keratectomy (PTK)
photothermal sclerosis
phototimer
phototoxic
phototoxicity
phototube output circuit
photovolt pH meter
PHP
    pseudohypoparathyroidism
phrenic
    p. ampulla
    p. artery
    p. lymph node
    p. nerve injury
    p. nerve paralysis
    p. pedicle
    right inferior p.
phrenicocolic ligament
phrenicolienal ligament
phrenicosplenic ligament
phrenoesophageal, phrenicoesophageal
    p. ligament
phrenogastric ligament
phrenopericardial angle
phrenosplenic ligament
phrenovertebral junction
phrygian
    p. cap
    p. cap deformity
phrynoderma
phthalocyanine
phthinoid chest
phthisis
    p. bulbi
phyllode
    cystosarcoma p.
    p. tumor
physes (*pl. of* physis)
physial, physeal
    p. bar
    p. bony bridging
    p. cartilage
    p. closure
    p. damage

p. distraction
p. injury
p. plate fracture
physician
Fellow of the American College of Nuclear P.'s
physics
radiation p.
physiologic
p. atrophy
p. herniation
p. high activity
p. hyperplasia
p. hypertrophy
p. imaging
p. ovarian cyst
p. parameter
p. regurgitation
p. shunt flow
p. sphincter
p. uterine blush
physiologically immature lung
physis, pl. **physes**
distal tibial p.
fibular p.
fused p.
medial p.
unfused p.
phytobezoar
PI
pulmonic insufficiency
pia arachnoid
pial
p. AVM
p. vessel
piano key sign
PICA
posterior-inferior cerebellar artery
pica artifact
PICC
peripherally inserted central catheter
Groshong NXT PICC
PICC line
Vaxcel PICC
PICCOLO
peripherally inserted central catheter occlusion line opening
PICCOLO study
PICD
Projecto de Intervenção do Chafariz de Dentro (Lisbon)

pick
P. body
P. bundle
P. disease
P. tubular adenoma
Picker
P. camera
P. Eclipse MR unit
P. Magnascanner
P. MR scanner
P. PQ 5000 helical CT scanner
P. PQ 2000 spiral CT scanner
P. PRISM 3000 PET scanner
P. SPECT attenuation correction
P. Synerview 600 scanner
P. system
picket
p. fence appearance
P. Fence stereotactic localizer
pick-off artifact
pickup tube
picocurie (pCi)
picometer (pm)
picomole (pmol)
picosecond pulse
picture
p. archival communication system (PACS)
p. archiving and communication system
p. element
p. frame appearance
p. frame pattern of vertebral body
p. frame vertebra
picture-frame-like
picture-framing osteoporosis
PIE
postinfectious encephalomyelitis
pulmonary interstitial emphysema
piece
chin-occiput p.
pole p.
piecemeal necrosis
Piedmont fracture
Pierre Robin syndrome
piezoelectric
p. effect
p. transducer
pigeon
p. chest
p. fancier's lung
pigeon-breast deformity

NOTES

P

719

Pigg-O-Stat
  P.-O-S. mechanical immobilizer
  P.-O-S. pediatric positioning device
pigmented
  p. basal cell carcinoma
  p. iris hamartoma
  p. villonodular synovitis
pigmentosa
  neuropathy, ataxia and retinitis p.
    (NARP)
pigment stone
pigskin patch
pigtail
  p. catheter
  p. stent
PIHI
  pulse-inversion harmonic imaging
pilar
  p. sheath
  p. tumor
pilaris
pile
  sentinel p.
pile-up
  pulse p.-u.
pill
  barium p.
  p. esophagitis
pillar
  faucial p.
  p. fracture
  p. projection
  tonsillar p.
  P. view
pill-induced inflammation
pillion fracture
pillow
  cervical skull p.
  foam vacuum p.
  p. fracture
pilocytic
  p. astrocytoma
  p. tumor
piloid astrocytoma
pilomatricoma
pilon ankle fracture
pilonidal
  p. cyst
  p. fistula
  p. sinus
  p. tract
pilorum
  vortices p.
pilosebaceous unit
pilosity
PIN
  positive-intrinsic-negative
  posterior interosseous nerve
  PIN diode

pin
  Hagie p.
  lead p.
  Optispike dispensing p.
  orthopedic p.
  p. pattern
  resorbable p.
  revolving Ge-68 p.
  track of p.
pinchcock
  p. effect
  p. mechanism
pinched nerve
pinch-off syndrome
pincushion distortion
Pindborg tumor
pineal
  p. apoplexy
  p. body
  p. cyst
  p. dysgerminoma
  p. germ-cell tumor
  p. germinoma
  p. gland
  p. gland calcification
  p. gland neoplasm
  p. gland shift
  p. gland teratocarcinoma
  p. gland tumor
  p. gland tumor classification
  p. mass
  p. parenchymal tumor
  p. region
  p. region tumor
  p. teratoma
  p. ventricle
pinealcytoma
pinealoblastoma, pineoblastoma
pinealoma
  ectopic p.
pineocytoma
ping-pong
  p.-p. ball deformity
  p.-p. fracture
  p.-p. heart volume
pinguecula lesion
pinhole
  bone p.
  p. camera
  p. collimator
  p. image
  p. scintigram
  p. technique
pink tetralogy
Pinnacle
  P. Destination renal guiding sheath
Pinnacle₃ radiotherapy planning system
PINNACLE R/O II radiopaque marker

pinning
> hip p.
> in situ p.

PinPoint stereotactic arm

Pins sign

pion
> p. beam
> p. dosimetry

PIOPED
> prospective investigation of pulmonary
> embolus diagnosis
> > PIOPED criteria

Piotrowski sign

PIP
> proximal interphalangeal
> > PIP articulation
> > PIP joint

pipe
> endoscopic washing p.

pipestem
> p. artery
> p. cirrhosis
> p. fibrosis
> p. ureter

pipe-stemming of ankle-brachial index

PIPIDA
> para-isopropyl-iminodiacetic acid
> > PIPIDA hepatobiliary imaging
> > PIPIDA scan
> > technetium-99m PIPIDA

piping
> organ p.

PIPJ
> proximal interphalangeal joint

Pipkin femoral fracture classification

Pirie
> P. bone
> P. method
> P. transoral projection

piriform, pyriform
> p. muscle
> p. recess
> p. sinus
> p. sinus carcinoma

piriformis, pyriformis
> apertura p.
> p. muscle

Pirogoff
> P. amputation
> P. angle

PISA
> proximal isovelocity surface area

pisiform
> p. bone
> p. fracture

pisohamate ligament

pisometacarpal ligament

pisoscaphoid distance

pisotriquetral
> p. articulation
> p. joint

pisounciform ligament

pisouncinate ligament

pistol-grip
> p.-g. appearance
> p.-g. femur deformity

pistoning

pistonlike reflux

pit
> anal p.
> articular p.
> auditory p.
> central p.
> colonic p.
> costal p.
> cutaneous p.
> gastric p.
> herniation p.
> pitch ratio p.
> postanal p.
> primitive p.
> scan pitch p.
> spiral CT pitch p.
> p. of stomach
> synovial herniation p.

pitch
> beam p.
> calcaneal p.
> data p.
> high p.
> high-quality p.
> high-speech p.
> low p.
> p. ratio
> p. ratio pit
> recon p.
> scan p.
> spiral CT p.

pitchblende

pitted cartilage

pitting
> pepper-pot p.

Pittsburgh pneumonia

pituicytoma

NOTES

P

pituilith
pituitary
    p. adenoma
    p. adenoma chromophobe
    p. apoplexy
    p. bright spot
    p. cyst
    p. dwarfism
    p. failure
    p. fossa
    p. gland
    p. gland anatomy
    p. gland enlargement
    p. hyperplasia
    p. infarct
    p. infundibulum
    p. macroadenoma
    p. microadenoma
    p. oncocytoma
    p. stalk
    p. stone
    p. tumor
pivot
    p. of calcar
    p. joint
    p. shift
    p. shift phenomenon
pivoting table
pivot-shift sign
pixel
    aliased p.
    8x8 p. block
    p. count method
    edge-region p.
    maximum intensity p. (MIP)
    p. noise
    normal-region p.
    p. shift program
    p. value
pixel-oriented algorithm
pixel-wise
Pixsys FlashPoint camera
pizoelectric generator
PLA
    polylactic acid
placement
    anular p.
    catheter p.
    double-J stent p.
    extragastric p.
    iliac artery stent p.
    intracoronary stent p.
    intragastric p.
    intrapericardial patch lead p.
    line p.
    minimally invasive endovascular
      stent p.
    percutaneous endoluminal p.
    radiotherapy field p.

shim p.
shunt p.
subanular p.
subject p.
superselective microcatheter p.
transcatheter filter p.
transjugular portosystemic stent
    shunt p.
transluminal endovascular stent-
    graft p.
transpapillary p.
placenta, pl. **placentae**
    abnormal adherence of p.
    abruptio placentae
    accessory p.
    p. accreta
    adherent p.
    anterofundal p.
    anular p.
    battledore p.
    bilobate p.
    p. biopsy
    chorioallantoic p.
    circummarginate p.
    cirsoid p.
    deciduate p.
    Duncan p.
    p. enlargement
    extrachorial p.
    fetal p.
    first-trimester p.
    fundal p.
    horseshoe p.
    incarcerated p.
    p. increta
    kidney-shaped p.
    low-lying p.
    marginal p.
    maternal p.
    p. membranacea
    p. migration
    nondeciduate p.
    panduriform p.
    p. percreta
    premature senescence p.
    p. previa
    retained p.
    p. rotation
    Schultze p.
    second-trimester p.
    third-trimester p.
    p. tumor
    vascular space of p.
    velamentous p.
    villous p.
placental
    p. abruption
    p. circulation
    p. disc

p. edema
p. grade
p. hemorrhage
p. infarct
p. localization
p. metastasis
p. polyp
p. septal cyst
p. septum
p. souffle
p. villus
placentation abnormality
placentogram
displacement p. (DPG)
placentography
indirect p.
placode
neural p.
unneurulated neural p.
plafond
p. fracture
tibial p.
plagiocephaly
deformation posterior p.
posterior p.
synostotic posterior p.
plain
p. abdominal radiography (PAR)
p. film
p. film imaging
p. radiograph
p. tomogram
p. view
plain-paper image
plan
isodose p.
posterior transaxial scan p.
plana
coxa p.
vertebra p.
planar
p. circular coil
p. detector
p. diagnostic 1231 scintigraphy
p. exercise thallium-201
scintigraphy
p. left anterior oblique image
p. plate
p. radionuclide imaging
p. spin imaging
p. thallium imaging
p. thallium scan

p. thallium with quantitative
analysis
p. view
Planck
P. constant
P. quantum theory
plane
AC-PC p.
Aeby p.
anatomic p.
areolar p.
axial p.
axiolabiolingual p.
axiomesiodistal p.
Baer p.
biparietal p.
bite p.
Blumenbach p.
Bolton p.
Bolton-nasion p.
Broadbent-Bolton p.
buccolingual p.
Calvé vertebra p.
capsular p.
4-chamber p.
circular p.
p. of cleavage
clip-editing p.
coronal p.
count per p.
cross-sectional p.
Daubenton p.
E p.
eye-ear p.
facial p.
fascial p.
fat p.
first parallel pelvic p.
flexion-extension p.
fourth parallel pelvic p.
Frankfort horizontal p.
frontal biauricular p.
frontoparallel p.
German horizontal p.
gonion-gnathion p.
Hensen p.
Hodge p.
horizontal p.
imaging p.
interiliac p.
internervous p.
intersphincteric p.

NOTES

P

723

plane *(continued)*
interspinal p.
interspinous p.
intertubercular p.
ischiorectal fossa p.
kx-ky p.
limited-cut p.
Ludwig p.
magnetic focal p.
Meckel p.
medial sagittal p.
median raphe p.
median sagittal p.
mesiodistal p.
midclavicular p.
midcoronal p.
midfrontal p.
midsagittal p.
midthalamic p.
Morton p.
nonorthogonal p.
nuchal p.
oblique coronal p.
occipital p.
occlusal p.
optimal imaging p.
orbital p.
orthogonal p.
parallel tag p.
paramedian sagittal p.
parasagittal p.
pelvic p.
Poschl p.
principal p.
radial p.
p. of reference
reverse Waters p.
sagittal p.
scan p.
sella-nasion p.
semicoronal p.
sensitive p.
p. sensitivity
short axis p.
slicing p.
spinous p.
sternoxiphoid p.
subadventitial p.
subcostal p.
subintimal cleavage p.
supracristal p. (SCP)
suprasternal notch p.
p. suture
tag p.
temporal p.
thalamic p.
thoracic p.
transaxial scan p.
transmedial p.

transpyloric p.
transtubercular p. (TTP)
transumbilical p. (TUP)
transverse p.
tumor cleavage p.
umbilical p.
valve p.
varus-valgus p.
vertical p.
Virchow p.
XY p.
ZY p.
2-plane
2-p. fluorometry
2-p. view
planigram
planigraphic principle
planigraphy
planimeter
planimetry
planing
planithorax
planning
3D radiation treatment p.
radiation therapy p. (RTP)
radiation treatment p. (RTP)
p. target volume (PTV)
planogram
planography
planovalgus
p. foot
p. foot deformity
pes p.
plantar
p. aponeurosis
p. arterial arch
p. aspect
p. axial view
p. bursa
p. calcaneal enthesophyte
p. calcaneal spur
p. capsule
p. compartment
p. compartmental anatomy
p. fasciitis
p. fibromatosis
p. flexion-inversion deformity
p. flexion stress view
p. hyperplasia
p. interossei
p. ligament
p. metatarsal angle
p. metatarsal artery
p. plate
p. shift
p. surface
p. vault
plantarward
plantodorsal projection

planum sphenoidale
planus
    pes plantigrade p.
plaque
    arterial p.
    arteriosclerotic p.
    asbestos pleural p.
    atheromatous p.
    beta amyloid senile p.
    calcified p.
    carotid artery p.
    p. cleaving
    p. compression
    concentric atherosclerotic p.
    p. constituent
    p. cracker
    discrete p.
    disrupted p.
    eccentric atherosclerotic p.
    echogenic p.
    echolucent p.
    endocardial p.
    p. erosion
    esophageal p.
    fatty p.
    fibrofatty p.
    fibrotic p.
    fibrous intima p.
    fissured atheromatous p.
    florid p.
    focal pleural p.
    p. fracture
    fungal p.
    gastrointestinal p.
    p. hemorrhage
    heterogeneous carotid p.
    p. histomorphometry
    homogeneous carotid p.
    Hutchinson p.
    hypoechoic p.
    iliac p.
    infiltrating p.
    intraluminal p.
    lipid-laden p.
    luminal p.
    meningioma en p.
    multiple sclerosis p.'s
    mycotic p.
    neuritic senile p.
    noncompliant p.
    obstructive p.
    penile p.

    periventricular p.
    pleural p.
    pleuroparenchymal p.
    pulverized p.
    Randall p.
    p. regression
    p. remodeling
    residual p.
    p. rupture
    sclerotic p.
    senile p.
    sequential paired opposed p.
    (SPOP)
    sessile p.
    p. splitting
    stenotic p.
    talc p.
    p. tearing
    ulcerated atheromatous p.
    ulcerated carotid artery p.
    uncalcified pleural p.
    p. vaporization
plaque-containing artery
plaquelike
    p. lesion
    p. linear defect
plaquing
    p. calcification
    neuritic p.
plasma
    p. cell granuloma
    p. cell pneumonia
    p. emission spectroscopy
    P. 1000 ICP-AES unit
    p. iron turnover
    p. radioiron disappearance rate
    p. radioiron turnover rate
    p. volume
plasmablast
plasmablastic
    p. lymphoma
    p. myeloma
plasmacytoma
    anaplastic p.
    extramedullary p. (EMP)
    primary pulmonary p.
    solitary p.
    solitary bone p. (SBP)
plasmodium embolus
plaster
    x-ray in p. (XIP)
    x-ray out of p. (XOP)

NOTES

P

plastic
>p. bowing fracture
carbon fiber-reinforced p.
p. clot
p. pleurisy
p. Vortex Port system

plastica
>linitis p.

plasticity
>brain p.
neuronal p.

plate
>acetabular reconstruction p.
alar p.
amorphous selenium p.
anal p.
anchor p.
auditory p.
axial p.
basal p.
blade p.
bone fixation p.
bony p.
buttress p.
cap p.
cardiogenic p.
cartilaginous growth p.
cloacal p.
cloverleaf p.
compression p.
condylar p.
connecting p.
cortical p.
cranial fixation p.
cribriform p.
3D p.
dorsal p.
dual p.
end p.
epiphysial cartilage p.
epiphysial growth p.
ethmovomerine p.
femoral p.
fenestrated compression p.
fibrocartilaginous volar p.
flat p.
flexor p.
foot p.
Fresnel zone p.
frontal p.
fusion p.
ground p.
growth p.
hilar p.
hyaline cartilage p.
interfragmentary p.
intertrochanteric p.
localization-compression grid p.

>low-contact dynamic compression p.
(LC-DCP)
meningioma of cribriform p.
microfixation p.
nail p.
neutralization p.
occipitocervical p.
orbital p.
orthopedic p.
orthotic p.
overlay p.
palmar p.
pedicle p.
phosphor p.
photostimulable phosphor p.
planar p.
plantar p.
Plexiglas p.
prochordal p.
PSP imaging p.
pterygoid p.
quadrigeminal p.
quadrilateral p.
p. reader
resorbable p.
p. and screw fixation
selenium p.
septal cartilage p.
sinodural p.
skull p.
Spli-Prest p.
stabilization p.
stainless steel p.
stem base p.
subchondral bone p.
supracondylar p.
tarsal p.
tectal p.
tendon p.
tissue p.
titanium p.
vertebral body p.
volar p.
xeroradiographic selenium p.
Y bone p.

plateau
>p. phase
p. tibia fracture
tibial p.

platelet-fibrin embolus
platelet function analyzer (PFA)
platelet-rich thrombus
platelike atelectasis
platform
>positioning p.
transcatheter intravascular ring p.
(TIRP)

platinocyanoide
    barium p.
platinum (Pt)
    p. coil
    p. coil embolization
    0.0015-inch p. wire
    0.00175-inch p. wire
    p. microcoil
    P. Plus guidewire
    p. tip guidewire
platinum-marked stent
platinum-resistant ovarian carcinoma
platybasia
platycephaly
platypelloid, platypellic
    p. pelvis
platypodia
platysma muscle
platyspondylia
platyspondylosis
platyspondyly generalisata
play
    joint p.
pleat
    accordion-shaped p.
pleating
    p. of ligamentum flavum
    p. of small bowel
pledget
    gelatin sponge p.
pleomorphic
    p. adenoma parotitis
    p. calcification
    p. liposarcoma
    p. lung adenoma
    p. microcalcification
    p. rhabdomyosarcoma
    p. sarcoma
    p. T-cell lymphoma
    p. type
    p. xanthoastrocytoma (PXA)
pleomorphism
    nuclear p.
pleonosteosis
    Leri p.
PLES
    parallel-line equal spacing
    PLES bar
    PLES bar pattern
plesiocurie therapy
plesiography
plesiosectional tomography

plesiotherapy
Pletal
plethora-related cyanotic CHD
plethysmograph
    Medgraphics body p.
plethysmography
    air p.
    body box p.
    computer strain-gauge p. (CSGP)
    digital p.
    Doppler ultrasonic velocity detector
      segmental p.
    exercise strain gauge venous p.
    impedance p. (IPG)
    Medsonic p.
    photocell p.
    segmental bronchus p.
    strain-gauge p.
    thermistor p.
    venous p.
pleura, pl. **pleurae**
    cervical p.
    congested p.
    costal p.
    costodiaphragmatic recess of p.
    crus p.
    diaphragmatic p.
    edematous p.
    fibrous tumor p.
    hyaloserositis p.
    inflamed p.
    localized fibrous tumor of p.
    mediastinal p.
    p. metastasis
    parietal p.
    p. peel
    pericardiac p.
    p. pseudotumor
    pulmonary p.
    scarification of p.
    silicotic visceral p.
    solitary fibrous tumor of p.
      (SFTP)
    visceral p.
    wrinkled p.
pleura-based
    p.-b. area of increased opacity
    p.-b. lung nodule
pleural
    p. apical hematoma cap
    p. calcification
    p. canal

NOTES

P

pleural (*continued*)
    p. cavity
    p. change
    p. cupula
    p. cyst
    p. density
    p. disease
    p. effusion
    p. empyema
    p. fibromyxoma
    p. fistula
    p. flap
    p. fluid
    p. fluid aspiration
    p. fluid collection
    p. line
    p. margin
    p. mass
    p. mesothelioma
    p. nodule
    p. plaque
    p. reaction
    p. recess
    p. rind
    p. sac
    p. scarring
    p. shunting
    p. space
    p. stripe
    p. thickening
    p. tube
pleurisy
    acute p.
    Bends asbestos p.
    blocked p.
    chronic p.
    circumscribed p.
    costal p.
    diaphragmatic p.
    diffuse p.
    double p.
    dry p.
    encysted p.
    exudative p.
    fibrinopurulent p.
    fibrinous p.
    hemorrhagic p.
    ichorous p.
    indurative p.
    interlobar p.
    latent p.
    mediastinal p.
    metapneumonic p.
    plastic p.
    primary p.
    proliferation p.
    pulmonary p.
    pulsating p.
    purulent p.

    sacculated p.
    secondary p.
    septic p.
    serofibrous p.
    serous p.
    single p.
    suppurative p.
    typhoid p.
    visceral p.
    wet p.
pleuritic pneumonia
pleuritis
    viral p.
pleurocutaneous fistula
pleurodesis
    chemical p.
pleuroesophageal
    p. line
    p. stripe
pleurography
pleuroparenchymal
    p. plaque
    p. reflection
pleuropericardial
    p. adhesion
    p. canal
    p. cyst
    p. effusion
pleuroperitoneal
    p. canal
    p. communication
    p. fold
pleuropulmonary
    p. adhesion
    p. blastoma
    p. complication
pleuropulmonary complication
pleuroscopy
plexiform neurofibroma
Plexiglas plate
plexogenic pulmonary arteriopathy
plexus, pl. **plexus, plexuses**
    abdominal aortic p.
    anterior coronary p.
    anterior pulmonary p.
    aortic p.
    autonomic p.
    axillary p.
    basilar p.
    Batson p.
    biliary p.
    brachial p.
    cardiac p.
    carotid p.
    cavernous p.
    celiac p.
    cervical p.
    choroid p.
    ciliary ganglionic p.

coccygeal p.
colic p.
colonic myenteric p.
common carotid p.
coronary p.
cystic p.
dangling choroid p.
deep cardiac p.
deferential p.
enteric p.
epidural venous p.
esophageal p.
Exner p.
extradural vertebral p.
facial p.
femoral p.
gastric p.
gastroesophageal variceal p.
glomus of choroid p.
great cardiac p.
hemorrhoidal p.
hepatic nerve p.
hypogastric p.
ileocolic p.
inferior mesenteric p.
p. injury
intermesenteric p.
left coronary p.
lumbar p.
lumbosacral p.
lymph p.
Meissner p.
myenteric p.
nerve p.
pampiniform p.
paravertebral nerve p.
paravertebral venous p.
pelvic p.
perimeniscal capsular p.
perimuscular p.
pharyngeal p.
posterior coronary p.
posterior pulmonary p.
presacral p.
prostatic venous p.
pterygoid p.
pulmonary p.
rectal p.
retrovertebral p.
right coronary p.
sacral p.
sciatic p.

solar p.
spinal nerve p.
subareolar p.
submucosal venous p.
superficial p.
superior hypogastric p.
superior mesenteric p.
tympanic p.
uterovaginal p.
vaginal p.
vascular p.
venous p.
vertebral venous p.
vesical venous p.
plica, pl. **plicae**
infrapatellar p.
medial p.
parapatellar p.
p. resection
suprapatellar p.
symptomatic lateral synovial p.
p. syndrome
synovial p.
plicated dural sheath
plication
p. defect
disc p.
transmesenteric p.
PLIF
posterior lumbar interbody fusion
P-Link software
PLL
posterior longitudinal ligament
plot
box-and-whisker p.
Patlak p.
PLS
Papillon-Lèfevre syndrome
plug
bile p.
biodegradable collagen p.
bone p.
collagen p.
dermoid p.
echogenic p.
fingerlike mucous p.
p. flow
gamma-irradiated p.
hydrogel p.
interbody bone p.
Ivalon p.
keratin p.

NOTES

P

plug *(continued)*
    luminal p.
    meconium p.
    mucous p.
    P. n View 3D medical imaging
      software
    Porstmann Ivalon p.
plugging
    mucous p.
pluglike appearance
Plumbicon
plumbline view
Plummer
    P. disease
    P. sign
Plummer-Vinson syndrome
plump vessel
plurality of slices
plural pregnancy
**pluripotential bronchial epithelial stem
  cell**
plus
    GuardWire P.
    4096 P. PET scanner
plus-density artifact
plutonism
plutonium
    environmental p.
PM
    photomultiplier
    posterior mitral
Pm
    promethium
pm
    picometer
PMC
    primary motor cortex
    PMC activation
PME
    peak of maximum enhancement
    phosphomonoester
    time to PME (tPME)
PMF
    progressive massive fibrosis
PML
    progressive multifocal
      leukoencephalopathy
pML
    posterior mitral leaflet
PMMA
    polymethylmethacrylate
pmol
    picomole
PMRA
    pulmonary magnetic resonance
      angiography
P-MRS
    phosphorus magnetic resonance
      spectroscopy

PMT
    percutaneous mechanical thrombectomy
    photomultiplier tube
      PMT imaging agent
      PMT robotic fulcrumless
        tomographic system
PMV
    prolapsed mitral valve
PMVL
    posterior mitral valve leaflet
PNC
    premature nodal contraction
PNET
    primitive neuroectodermal tumor
    non-CNS PNET
pneumarthrogram
pneumarthrography
pneumatic
    p. bone
    p. reduction of intussusception
pneumatization
pneumatocele
    p. cranii
    extracranial p.
    intracranial p.
    parotid p.
    postinfectious p.
    traumatic p.
pneumatocyst
pneumatogram
pneumatograph
pneumatosis
    p. coli
    cystic p.
    p. cystoides intestinalis
    epidural p.
    gastric p.
    p. sphenoidale
    stomach p.
pneumencephalography
    lumbar p.
pneumoalveolography
pneumoangiogram
pneumoangiography
pneumoarthrogram
pneumoarthrography
pneumobilia
pneumocardiograph
pneumocardiography
pneumocele
pneumocephalus
    intracranial p.
pneumocolon
pneumoconiosis, pl. **pneumoconioses**
    aluminum p.
    barium p.
    bauxite p.
    p. classification
    coal worker's p. (CWP)

complicated p.
fiberglass p.
fibrogenic p.
Fuller earth p.
inert p.
inert dust p.
kaolin p.
mica p.
nepheline p.
rheumatoid p.
sericite p.
silicate p.
sillimanite p.
talc p.
tungsten carbide p.
zeolite p.
pneumoconiotic nodule
pneumoconstriction
pneumocystic infection
pneumocystography
breast p.
pneumocystosis
cutaneous p.
pneumocystotomography
pneumoencephalogram (PEG)
pneumoencephalographic pattern
pneumoencephalography (PEG)
cerebral p.
fractional p.
pneumoencephalomyelogram
pneumoencephalomyelography
pneumoenteric
p. canal
p. defect
pneumofasciogram
pneumogastrography
pneumogram
pneumography
cerebral p.
retroperitoneal p.
pneumogynogram
pneumohemothorax
pneumohydrothorax
pneumointestinalis
pneumolith
pneumomediastinogram
pneumomediastinography
pneumomediastinum
postoperative p.
radiolucent p.
spontaneous p.
traumatic p.

pneumomyelography
pneumonectomy chest
pneumonia
acute eosinophilic p.
acute interstitial p. (AIP)
adenovirus p.
alcoholic p.
allergic p.
alveolar p.
anthrax p.
apical p.
aspiration p.
asthmatic p.
atypical bronchial p.
atypical interstitial p.
atypical measles p.
atypical primary p.
bilateral lower lobe p.
bilious bronchial p.
bronchiolitis obliterans with
organizing p. (BOOP)
Buhl desquamative p.
capillary p.
caseous p.
catarrhal p.
cavitating p.
central p.
cerebral p.
cheesy p.
chelonian p.
chemical p.
chronic interstitial p.
community-acquired p.
concomitant p.
consolidative p.
contusion p.
cryptogenic organizing p.
deglutition p.
delayed resolution of p.
desquamative interstitial p. (DIP)
diffuse p.
double p.
Eaton agent p.
embolic p.
endogenous lipid p.
eosinophilic p.
ephemeral p.
exogenous lipoid p.
extensive bilateral p.
fibrinous p.
fibrous p.
focal organizing p.

NOTES

P

731

pneumonia *(continued)*
    Friedländer p.
    fungal p.
    gangrenous p.
    giant cell interstitial p. (GIP)
    granulomatous p.
    Hecht p.
    hemorrhagic p.
    herpesvirus p.
    hypersensitivity p.
    hypostatic p.
    idiopathic interstitial p.
    incomplete resolution of p.
    indurative p.
    infantile p.
    inhalation p.
    interstitial organizing p.
    interstitial plasma cell p.
    irradiation p.
    lingular p.
    lipoid endogenous p.
    lobar p.
    lobular p.
    Löffler p.
    lower lobe p.
    lymphocytic interstitial p. (LIP)
    lymphoid interstitial p. (LIP)
    massive p.
    measles p.
    migratory p.
    mycotic p.
    necrotizing p.
    neonatal p.
    nonclassifiable interstitial p.
    nonspecific interstitial p. (NIP, NSIP)
    nummular p.
    obstructive p.
    oil-aspiration p.
    organizing p.
    organizing focal p.
    organizing interstitial p.
    parenchymatous p.
    passive p.
    patchy area of p.
    peripheral p.
    pertussoid eosinophilic p.
    Pittsburgh p.
    plasma cell p.
    pleuritic p.
    postobstructive p.
    posttraumatic p.
    purulent p.
    pyogenic p.
    radiation p.
    recurrent p.
    resolving p.
    right-sided p.
    round p.

    SARS-associated coronavirus p.
    secondary p.
    segmental p.
    septic p.
    superficial p.
    suppurative p.
    terminal p.
    toxic p.
    traumatic p.
    tuberculous p.
    tularemic p.
    unresolved p.
    usual interstitial p. (UIP)
    walking p.
    white p.
pneumonic infiltrate
pneumonitis
    acute interstitial p.
    acute radiation p.
    aspiration p.
    bacterial p.
    basilar p.
    chemical p.
    chronic p.
    diffuse p.
    drug-induced p.
    early p.
    giant cell p.
    granulomatous p.
    hypersensitivity p.
    idiopathic interstitial p.
    interstitial p.
    lipoid p.
    lymphocytic interstitial p.
    lymphoid interstitial p.
    mycoplasmal p.
    radiation p.
    unusual interstitial p.
    usual interstitial p.
    ventilation p.
pneumonocirrhosis
pneumonoconiosis
    noncollagenous p.
pneumonograph
pneumonography
pneumoorbitography
pneumopathy
    cobalt p.
pneumopericardium
pneumoperitoneal
pneumoperitoneography
pneumoperitoneum
    balanced p.
    diagnostic p.
    drop test for p.
    transabdominal p.
pneumoplethysmography
    ocular p. (OPG)
pneumopreperitoneum

pneumopyelogram
pneumopyelography
pneumorachicentesis
pneumorachis
pneumoradiography
    retroperitoneal p.
pneumoretroperitoneum
pneumoroentgenogram
pneumoroentgenography
pneumoscrotum
pneumothorax, pl. pneumothoraces (PT)
    artificial p.
    basilar p.
    blowing p.
    catamenial p.
    closed p.
    congenital p.
    diagnostic p.
    extrapleural p.
    induced p.
    life-threatening p.
    open p.
    positive-pressure p.
    pressure p.
    recurrent p.
    simultaneous bilateral
      spontaneous p. (SBSP)
    spontaneous tension p.
    sucking p.
    tension p.
    therapeutic p.
    traumatic p.
    tuberculous p.
    uncomplicated p.
    valvular p.
pneumotomography
pneumoventriculogram
pneumoventriculography
PNL
    posterior nipple line
PO
    parietal operculum
Po
    polonium
pocket
    air p.
    p. chamber
    p. Doppler
    p. dosimeter
    infraclavicular p.
    rectus sheath p.
    regurgitant p.

    p. shot
    subcutaneous p.
    subpectoral p.
    valve p.
    p. of Zahn
pocketed calculus
pocketing of barium
POEM
    Patient-Oriented Evidence that Matters
POEMS
    polyneuropathy, organomegaly,
      endocrinopathy, monoclonal
      gammopathy, skin changes
    POEMS syndrome
point
    A p.
    Addison p.
    alveolar p.
    apophysial p.
    auricular p.
    p. Ba
    bleeding p.
    Bolton p. (craniometric) (Bo)
    branch p.
    breast trigger p.
    Cannon p.
    Cannon-Boehm p.
    cardinal p.
    Chauffard p.
    choroid p.
    Clado p.
    coaptation p.
    commissural p.
    congruent p.
    Cope p.
    coplanar contour p.
    craniometric p.
    Crowe pilot p.
    D p.
    dorsal p.
    end p.
    entry p.
    equilibrium p.
    Erb p.
    frontopolar p.
    glenoid p.
    Griffith p.
    Hartmann p.
    ICRU reference p.
    p. imaging
    interventional reference p. (IRP)
    J p.

NOTES

P

point (*continued*)
    Kienböck-Adamson p.
    Lanz p.
    lead p.
    p. localization
    Mackenzie p.
    McBurney p.
    midinguinal p.
    Morris p.
    multiple sensitive p.'s
    p. mutation
    nodal p.
    null p.
    output p.
    Pauly p.
    preauricular p.
    pressure p.
    random p.
    reentry p.
    p. resolved spectroscopy (PRESS)
    Rolando p.
    sacrococcygeal inferior pubic p.
    (SCIPP)
    saddle p.
    scanned focal p. (SFP)
    p. scanning
    seed p.
    sensitive p.
    p. sensitivity
    Sudeck p.
    sylvian p.
    target p.
    time p.
    white p.
3-point
    3-p. Dixon technique
    3-p. Dixon water-fat separation
    sequence
pointer
    hip p.
    metallic p.
    shoulder p.
point-in-space stereotactic biopsy
point-resolved
    p.-r. spectroscopy localization
    technique
    p.-r. spectroscopy sequence
    (PRESS)
4-point-restraint
point-spread function (PSF)
point-to-point protocol (PPP)
Poiseuille
    P. flow
    P. law
poisoning
    radiation p.
Poisson
    P. distributed activity concentration
    P. distribution

    P. noise fluctuation
    P. ratio
Poisson-Pearson formula
poker spine
Poland
    P. epiphysial fracture classification
    P. syndrome
polar
    p. coordinate system
    P. Vantage XL heart rate monitor
polar-bound water
polarimetry
    scanning laser p.
Polaris
    P. 1.32 Nd:YAG laser
    P. X steerable diagnostic catheter
Polaris-Dx steerable diagnostic catheter
polarity-altered
    p.-a. spectral-selective acquisition
    p.-a. spectral-selective acquisition
    imaging
polarization
    cell p.
    chemically-induced dynamic
    nuclear p.
    dynamic nuclear p. (DNP)
    linear p.
    nuclear p.
polarized light microscopy
polarographic
    p. needle electrode
    p. needle electrode measurement
Polaroid film
pole
    abapical p.
    cephalic p.
    fetal p.
    p. figure texture analysis
    frontal p.
    germinal p.
    inferior p.
    kidney p.
    lower p.
    magnetic p.
    middle p.
    occipital p.
    p. of organ
    patellar p.
    p. piece
    scaphoid p.
    p. of scaphoid bone
    superior p.
    temporal p.
    p. tip
    upper p.
    p. of vessel
pole-to-pole length of kidney
Polhemus 3D digitizer
polidocanol sclerosing agent

polka-dot appearance
pollex pedis
pollicis
adductor p.
p. longus tendon
opponens p.
pollicization
Riordan finger p.
pollicized ray
polonium (Po)
POLPSA
posterior labroscapular periosteal
avulsion
POLPSA lesion
polyadenopathy
angiofollicular and plasmacytic p.
polyalveolar lobe
polyangiitis
microscopic p.
Pólya procedure
polyarcuate diaphragm
polyarteritis nodosa (PAN)
polyarthritis
juvenile chronic p.
polyarthropathy
**polyarticular symmetric tophaceous joint
inflammation**
polychondritis
relapsing p.
polychromatic radiation
polycycloidal tomography
polycystic
p. kidney
p. kidney disease
p. liver
p. liver disease
p. lung
p. nephroblastoma
p. ovarian disease (PCOD)
p. ovary
p. ovary syndrome (PCOS)
polydactyly
Wassel classification of thumb p.
polydirectional tomography
polyethylene (PE)
p. catheter
p. glycol (PEG)
p. stent
p. tube
Polyflex stent
polyglycolide
self-reinforced p.

polygonal elongate cell
polygon mirror
polygyria
polyhydramnios
polylactic acid (PLA)
polylobar liver
polymastia
polymer
p. dosimetry
osteoconductive p.
polymerization
fibrin p.
polymerizing agent
polymethylmethacrylate (PMMA)
polymethyl methacrylate implant
polymicrogyria
polymorphism
single-strand conformational p.
(SSCP)
polymorphonuclear leukocyte
polymyalgia rheumatica
Polynesian bronchiectasis
**polyneuropathy, organomegaly,
endocrinopathy, monoclonal
gammopathy, skin changes (POEMS)**
**polynomial stepwise multilinear
regression**
polynuclear neutrophilic leukocyte
polyostotic
p. bone lesion
p. fibrous dysplasia
polyp
adenomatous p. (AP)
angiomatous nasal p.
antral p.
antrochoanal p.
bleeding p.
broad-based p.
bronchial p.
cardiac p.
carpet p.
cervical p.
choanal p.
cholesterol gallbladder p.
colonic adenomatous p.
colonic hamartomatous p.
colorectal p.
cyst or p.
cystic p.
dental p.
duodenal p.
endometrial p.

NOTES

P

735

polyp (*continued*)
    epithelial colonic p.
    fibrinous p.
    fibroepithelial urethral p.
    fibroid p.
    fibrous urinary tract p.
    fibrovascular p.
    filiform p.
    gallbladder p.
    gastric p.
    hamartomatous gastric p.
    Hopmann p.
    hydatid p.
    hyperplastic adenomatous p.
    hyperplastic colon p.
    hyperplastic gastric p.
    hyperplastic stomach p.
    inflammatory colonic p.
    inflammatory esophagogastric p.
    inflammatory fibroid p.
    inflammatory stomach p.
    intraluminal p.
    juvenile p.
    laryngeal p.
    lipomatous p.
    lymphoid p.
    metaplastic p.
    metastatic p.
    mucous p.
    multiple p.'s
    nasal p.
    osseous p.
    pedunculated p.
    Peutz-Jeghers p.
    placental p.
    postinflammatory p.
    rectal p.
    regenerative gastric p.
    retention colon p.
    retention stomach p.
    sessile p.
    sigmoid p.
    single p.
    p. stalk
    tubular p.
    tubulovillous p.
    uterine fibroid p.
    vascular fibrous p.
    villoglandular p.
    villous stomach p.
polypeptide
    organic anion transporter p.
polypharmacy
polyphase generator
polyphebus
polyphosphate
polyphosphonate
    technetium p.

polypoid
    p. adenoma
    p. calcified irregular mass
    p. carcinoma
    p. dysplasia
    p. fibroma
    p. fibroma collecting system
    p. filling defect
    p. lesion
    p. lesion of lower esophagus
    p. lymphoid hyperplasia
    p. lymphoma
    p. mucosa
polyposa
    colitis p.
polyposis
    diffuse mucosal p.
    familial adenomatous p. (FAP)
    familial colorectal p.
    familial gastrointestinal p.
    familial intestinal p.
    familial juvenile p.
    familial multiple p.
    filiform p.
    gastric hamartomatous p.
    intestinal p.
    juvenile p.
    lymphomatous p. (LP)
    multiple p.
    Peutz-Jeghers gastrointestinal p.
    postinflammatory p.
    sinonasal p.
polypropylene catheter
polyradiculomyelitis
polyradiculoneuropathy
polyradiculopathy
polysomnogram
polysomnography
    nocturnal p.
polysplenia syndrome
polystotic
polytetrafluoroethylene (PTFE)
    p. graft
polythelia
polytomogram
polytomographic radiology
polytomography
    mastoid p.
polytrauma
Polytron DSA equipment
polyurethane
    p. foam embolus
    p. stent
polyvinyl
    p. alcohol (PVA)
    p. alcohol particle
    p. alcohol particle embolization

p. butyral (PVB)
p. chloride (PVC)
polyvinylpyrrolidone (PVP)
POMP
phase-offset multiplanar
phase-ordered multiplanar
POMP imaging
Pompe disease
Ponderal Index
pond fracture
pons
basilar p.
bifid p.
caudal p.
infarct of p.
rostral p.
tegmentum of p.
ponticulus posticus
pontine, pontile
p. angle
p. angle tumor
p. artery
central p.
p. cistern
p. contusion
p. glioma
p. hemorrhage
p. hydatid cyst
p. infarct
p. isthmus
p. lesion
p. myelinolysis
p. reticular formation
p. tegmentum
pontine-medullary level
pontis
basis p.
brachium p.
pontocerebellar
p. fiber
p. glioma
p. hypoplasia
pontomedullary
p. junction
p. sulcus
pontomesencephalic
p. junction
p. vein
pool
blood p.
focal p.

gastric p.
miscible p.
vascular blood p.
pooling
genital blood p.
venous p.
poor
p. perfusion
p. screen/film contact
p. sensitivity
p. shimming of MRI magnet
p. vascular reserve
p. visualization
poorly
p. circumscribed tumor
p. concentrated isotope
p. differentiated adenocarcinoma (PDA)
p. differentiated tumor
popcorn calcification
popcornlike
p. appearance
p. calcification
p. reticulated lesion
popliteal
p. artery
p. artery aneurysm
p. artery entrapment syndrome
p. artery occlusive disease
p. artery pulsation artifact
p. artery trifurcation
p. cavity
p. cyst
p. fossa
p. hiatus
p. ligament
p. line
p. node
p. pulse
p. recess
p. space
p. tendinitis
p. tendon
p. vein
popliteus
p. bursa
p. tendon
poppet
barium-impregnated p.
disc p.
poppy seedlike calcification

NOTES

P

737

population
  overdistention of alveolar p.
  uneven recruitment of alveolar p.
porcelain
  p. aorta
  p. gallbladder
Porcher method
porcine
  p. gallbladder
  p. heart xenograft
porencephalic cyst
porencephaly
  acquired p.
  agenetic p.
  encephaloclastic p.
  true p.
porokeratosis plantaris discreta
porosis
  cerebral p.
porous
  p. bone
  p. ingrowth
  p. kidney
  p. metallic stent
Porstmann Ivalon plug
PORT
  postoperative radiotherapy
  PORT radiofrequency electrode
    design
port
  BardPort low-profile p.
  BardPort MRI full size p.
  Cordis multipurpose access p.
  p. film
  implantable infusion p.
  injection p.
  multipurpose access p. (MPAP)
  parallel opposed unmodified p.
  radiation p.
  radiotherapy p.
  simulation of converging p.
  single p.
  subcutaneous implanted injection p.
  tangential p.
  treatment p.
porta
  p. cirrhosis
  p. hepatis
  p. hepatis defect
  p. hepatis low-density mass
  p. hepatis node
  p. hepatis obstruction
portable
  p. C-arm image intensifier
    fluoroscopy
  p. C-arm intensifier
  p. chest film
  p. imaging procedure
  p. radiography

  p. view
  p. x-ray
portacamera
Port-A-Cath
portacaval
  p. shunt
  p. space
portal
  p. canal
  p. decompression
  p. fibrosis
  p. fissure
  p. flow
  p. hypertension
  p. portography
  radiation p.
  radiocarpal p.
  simulation of tangential p.
  p. space
  superomedial p.
  p. triad
  p. vascular bed
  p. vein
  p. vein aneurysm
  p. vein anomaly type I–V
  p. vein cavernoma
  p. vein congestion index
  p. vein enhancement
  p. vein lesion
  p. vein system
  p. vein thrombosis (PVT)
  p. vein velocity
  p. venography
  p. venous anastomosis
  p. venous dominant
  p. venous-dominant phase (PVP)
  p. venous gas
  p. venous phase (PVP)
  p. venous phase imaging
  p. venous pressure (PVP)
portal-phased spiral CT scan
portal-to-portal
  p.-t.-p. bridge
  p.-t.-p. fibrosis
port-catheter system
portion
  cavernous p.
  intrapericardial p.
  supraclinoid p.
portio vaginalis
portogram
portography
  arterial p.
  computed tomography during
    arterial p. (CTAP)
  double-spiral CT arterial p.
  percutaneous transhepatic p.
  portal p.
  splenic p.

transhepatic p.
transjugular p.
umbilical p.

portohepatic
portomesenteric venous thrombosis
portophlebography
portopulmonary shunt
portosplenic thrombosis
portosplenography
portosystemic

p. anastomosis
p. collateral
p. collateral circulation
p. collateral vessel
p. gradient
p. shunt

portovenography
portovenous
Posada fracture
Posadas-Wernicke coccidioidomycosis
Poschl plane
Posicam HZ PET scanner
position

abduction p.
abduction-external rotation p.
ABER p.
adduction p.
Albers-Schönberg p.
Albert p.
anatomic p.
anterior oblique p.
anteroposterior p.
barber-chair p.
bayonet fracture p.
beach-chair p.
Beclere p.
Benassi p.
Bertel p.
bladder neck p.
Broden p.
brow-down p.
brow-up p.
Caldwell p.
cardiac p.
catheter tip p.
central venous line p.
Chassard-Lapiné p.
Cleaves p.
Clements-Nakayama p.
cock-robin p.
conus medullaris p.
cross-table lateral p.

decubitus p.
dorsal decubitus p.
dorsal recumbent p.
dorsosacral p.
dwell p.
p. encoding
erect p.
eversion p.
extension p.
Feist-Mankin p.
fetal p.
Fick p.
figure-4 p.
Fleischner p.
flexion p.
Fowler p.
Friedman p.
frogleg p.
Fuchs p.
full lateral p.
Grashey p.
Haas p.
heart p.
Hickey p.
high Fowler p.
horizontal p.
infragenicular p.
infrapulmonary p.
inlet p.
inversion p.
jackknife p.
Johnson p.
LAO p.
Larkin p.
lateral decubitus p.
lateral left anterior oblique p.
lateral recumbent p.
Law p.
Lawrence p.
left anterior oblique p.
left posterior oblique p.
left-side-down decubitus p.
Lewis p.
Lilienfelds p.
lithotomy p.
lordotic p.
Lorenz p.
lotus p.
Low-Beers p.
LPO p.
Mayer p.
Miller p.

NOTES

P

739

position *(continued)*
    near-anatomic p.
    neutral hip p.
    Noble p.
    Nölke p.
    noncoaxial catheter tip p.
    normal anatomic p.
    nose-chin p.
    nose-forehead p.
    oblique p.
    opisthotonic p.
    PA p.
    paramedian p.
    paraseptal p.
    park bench p.
    Pawlow p.
    Pearson p.
    Phalen p.
    prone p.
    pulmonary capillary wedge p.
    3-quarters prone p.
    reclining p.
    rectus p.
    recumbent p.
    reverse Trendelenburg p.
    reverse Waters p.
    right anterior oblique p.
    right posterior oblique p.
    right-side-down decubitus p.
    Schüller p.
    semiaxial p.
    semierect p.
    semi-Fowler p.
    semilateral p.
    semirecumbent p.
    semisupine p.
    semiupright p.
    Settegast p.
    side-lying p.
    Sims p.
    spatial p.
    squatting p.
    Staunig p.
    Stecher p.
    steep Trendelenburg p.
    Stenver p.
    stepping-source p.
    submentovertex p.
    supine p.
    supine head-first p.
    swimmer's p.
    Tarrant p.
    Taylor p.
    tibial sesamoid p.
    Titterington p.
    Towne p.
    Trendelenburg p.
    tripod p.
    Twining p.

    upright p.
    ventral decubitus p.
    verticosubmental p.
    Walcher p.
    Waters p.
    Wigby-Taylor p.
    Zanelli p.
positional
    p. dysfunction
    p. variation
positioner
    basilar block skull p.
    dual lateral hand p.
    dual oblique hand p.
    Waters p.
positioning
    arms-up p.
    automatic endoscopic system for
      optimal p. (AESOP)
    p. error
    flap p.
    motion-free p.
    operator-dependent p.
    pendent p.
    p. platform
positive
    p. cephalopelvic disproportion index
    p. contrast agent
    p. contrast encephalography
    p. contrast myelography
    p. electron
    p. end-expiratory pressure
    ER p.
    estrogen-receptor p.
    p. node basin
    p. predictive value (PPV)
    p. ray
    true p. (TP)
    p. ulnar variance
    p. washout test
positive-intrinsic-negative (PIN)
    positive-intrinsic-negative diode
positive-ion cyclotron
positive-pressure pneumothorax
positrocephalogram
positron *(See* PET, PETT)
    p. decay
    p. emission mammography (PEM)
    p. emission tomography (PET)
    p. emission tomography with
      fluorodeoxyglucose (FDG-PET)
    p. emission transaxial tomography
      (PETT)
    p. emission transverse tomography
      (PETT)
    energetic p.
    labeled p.
    p. matter-antimatter annihilation
      reaction

p. range
p. scanning
p. scintillation camera
positron-coincidence
positron-emitting radionucleotide
positronium half-life
Possis AngioJet Xpeedior catheter
post
p. Diamox state
p. ECT sequelae
p. fatty meal cholecystography
p. fire image
p. PTCA residual stenosis
p. reconstruction filtering option
postablation
postamputation neuroma
postanal pit
postangioplasty
p. angiography
p. aortography
p. intimal flap
p. mural thrombosis
p. restenosis
p. stenosis
postaortic lymph node
postaugmentation
postbeat filtration
postbiopsy
p. change
p. eggshell calcification
p. fat necrosis
p. period
p. renal AV fistula
p. scarring
postbulbar
p. duodenum
p. ulcer
postbypass spasm
postcapillary venule
postcaptopril radioisotope study
postcardiac injury syndrome (PCIS)
**postcardiotomy lymphocytic
    splenomegaly**
**postcatheterization pseudoaneurysm
    (PCPA)**
postcaval
p. lymph node
p. ureter
postcentral
p. gyrus
p. sulcus
postchemoembolization liver abscess

postcontrast
p. echocardiography
p. MR imaging
postcricoid
p. area
p. carcinoma
p. defect
p. pharynx
p. soft tissue
p. web
postcubital
postdilatation arteriography
postdrainage
p. cystogram
p. imaging
p. projection
postductal
p. aortic coarctation
p. coarctation of aorta
Postel destructive coxarthrosis
postembolization
p. angiographic pattern
p. angiography
p. syndrome
postenhancement sequence
posterior (P)
p. abdominal wall
p. acoustic enhancement
p. acoustic shadowing
ampulla ossea p.
p. anulus
p. aorta transposition of great
    artery
p. apical segment
p. arch fracture
p. aspect
p. auricular vein
p. axillary line
p. basal segmental bronchus
p. border
p. border of heart
p. calcaneal bursitis
p. capsular distance (PCD)
p. cardinal vein
p. central gyrus
p. central indentation
p. cerebral artery (PCA)
p. cerebral territory infarct
p. cervical line
p. cervical space
p. cervical triangle
p. choroidal artery

NOTES

P

posterior *(continued)*

p. cingulate functional impairment
p. circulation territory
p. circumflex humeral artery
p. cistern
p. colliculus
p. column deficit
p. column demyelination
p. column lesion
p. column of spine
p. column syndrome
p. commissure (PC)
p. communicating artery (PCA, PCoA)
p. communicating artery aneurysm
p. compartment
p. compartment lesion
p. concavity
p. coronary groove
p. coronary plexus
p. cranial fossa
p. cruciate ligament (PCL)
p. cruciate ligament injury
p. cusp
p. descending artery (PDA)
p. descending branch
p. disc margin
p. element fracture
p. embryotoxon
p. epidural fat
p. fascicular block
p. fontanelle
p. fossa circulation
p. fossa cyst
p. fossa-foramen magnum lesion
p. fossa hematoma
p. fossa lesion
p. fossa malformations, facial hemangiomas, arterial anomalies, cardiac anomalies and aortic coarctation, eye anomalies, and sternal clefting and/or supraumbilical raphe (PHACES)
p. fossa meningioma
p. fossa tumor
p. fracture-dislocation
p. free wall
p. ghosting artifact
p. gray column of cord
p. gray horn
p. iliac crest
p. impingement
p. impingement syndrome
p. inferior iliac spine
p. inferior spine
p. inferior tibiofibular ligament
p. intercostal artery
p. intercostal branch
p. interosseous nerve (PIN)

p. interosseous nerve entrapment
p. interventricular groove
p. interventricular sulcus
p. interventricular vein
p. intraoccipital synchondrosis
p. joint syndrome
p. junction line
p. labroscapular periosteal avulsion (POLPSA)
p. language area lesion
p. lateral talar process
p. leaflet prolapse
p. lie
p. lip
p. longitudinal ligament (PLL)
p. longitudinal ligament tear
p. lumbar interbody fusion (PLIF)
p. lumbar vessel
p. median septum
p. mediastinal mass
p. mediastinal node
p. mediastinum
p. membrane articulation
p. metatarsal arch
p. midbody of corpus callosum
p. mitral (PM)
p. mitral leaflet (pML)
p. mitral valve leaflet (PMVL)
p. neck surface coil
p. neural arch
p. nipple line (PNL)
p. oblique ligament
p. olive
p. osteophyte
p. palatine suture
p. papillary muscle (PPM)
p. parietal artery
p. patch aortoplasty
p. pharyngeal wall carcinoma
p. pituitary fossa
p. pituitary gland ectopia
p. plagiocephaly
p. pleural recess
p. predominance
p. probability
p. projection
p. pulmonary plexus
p. rectus sheath
p. retrocrural approach
p. reversible encephalopathy syndrome (PRES)
p. ring fracture
p. root entry zone
p. root ganglion
p. scalloping of vertebra
p. semicircular canal
p. septal space
p. skull view
p. spinal artery

p. spinal cord horn
p. spine fusion (PSF)
p. spinocerebellar tract
p. spur
p. subluxation
superior labral anterior to p. (SLAP)
superior labral anterior p.
p. surface
p. surface of pancreas
p. surface of prostate
p. talofibular (PTF)
p. talofibular ligament
p. temporal artery
p. temporal vertical (PTV)
p. thalamic arteries of Lazorthes
p. tibial artery
tibialis p.
p. tibial pulse
p. tibial tendon (PTT)
p. tibial vein
p. tibiotalar ligament
p. tracheal band
p. transaxial scan plan
p. transcaval approach
p. triangle of the neck
p. turn of the aortic arch
p. urethra
p. urethral injury
p. urethral valve (PUV)
p. urethrovesical angle (PUVA)
p. vagal trunk
p. ventricular branch
p. vertebral element blowout lesion
p. vertebral scalloping
p. wall (PW)
p. wall fracture
p. wall motion
p. wall myocardial infarct
p. wall thickness (PWT)
posterior-inferior cerebellar artery (PICA)
posteroanterior (PA)
p. chest film
p. lordotic projection
p. view
posteroapical defect
posterobasal
p. segment
p. wall myocardial infarct
posteroexternal
posteroinferior myocardial infarct

posterointernal
posterolateral
p. aspect
p. capsule
p. compartment
p. corner injury
p. disc herniation
p. fontanelle
p. rotatory instability
p. rotatory subluxation
p. sclerosis
p. segment
p. spinal artery
p. wall
p. wall motion
p. wall myocardial infarct
posteromedial
p. compartment
p. tibia
posteromedian
posterooblique view
posteroparietal
posterosuperior glenoid impingement
posterotransverse diameter
postevacuation
p. film
p. view
postexercise
p. echocardiography
p. film
p. image
p. imaging
p. index
p. stunning
postextrasystolic
p. pause
p. potentiation
postfiltering
low-pass three-dimensional p.
postgadolinium scan
postganglionic
p. gray fiber
p. sympathetic fiber
postglomerular arteriolar constriction
postglucose loading examination
posthemorrhagic hydrocephalus
posthepatic cirrhosis
postictal cerebral blood flow scan
postimplant radiation survey
postinfarction
p. ventricular aneurysm
p. ventriculoseptal defect

NOTES

P

743

postinfectious
- p. bronchiectasis
- p. bronchiolitis obliterans
- p. demyelination
- p. encephalitis
- p. encephalomyelitis (PIE)
- p. hydrocephalus
- p. pneumatocele

postinflammatory
- p. adenopathy
- p. polyp
- p. polyposis
- p. pulmonary fibrosis
- p. renal atrophy
- p. scarring

postinjection
- p. attenuation scan
- p. echocardiography
- p. imaging
- p. scan delay

postintraarticular paramagnetic contrast injection T1-weighted image

postirradiation
- p. fracture
- p. MFH
- p. osteogenic sarcoma
- p. vascular insufficiency

postischemic
- p. atrophy
- p. recovery

postlaminectomy
- p. instability
- p. kyphosis

postlumpectomy skin thickening
postlymphangiography
postmastectomy lymphedema
postmaturity syndrome
postmediastinal
postmediastinum
postmenarchal female pelvis
postmeningococcal pericarditis
postmenopausal
- p. adnexal cyst
- p. endometrial thickness
- p. endometrium
- p. estrogen therapy
- p. osteoporosis
- p. ovary
- p. uterine atrophy

postmetrizamide
- p. CT imaging
- p. CT scan

postmyelography CT
postmyocardial
- p. infarct
- p. infarction echocardiography
- p. infarction syndrome

postmyocardiotomy infarct
postmyocarditis dilated cardiomyopathy

postnatal injury
postnecrotic
- p. cirrhosis
- p. scarring

postobstructive
- p. atelectasis
- p. pneumonia
- p. renal atrophy

postoperative
- p. angiography
- p. breast hematoma
- p. cholangiography
- p. cholangiography imaging
- p. chylothorax
- p. emphysema
- p. ileus
- p. mediastinal hemorrhage
- p. pneumomediastinum
- p. radiotherapy (PORT)
- p. resorption atelectasis
- p. scar tissue
- p. seroma
- p. skull defect
- p. stenosis
- p. thoracic deformity
- p. view

postorchiectomy paraaortic radiation therapy
postpartum
- p. cardiomyopathy
- p. pituitary apoplexy
- p. pituitary necrosis

postperfusion lung
postpericardiotomy syndrome
postpharyngeal soft tissue
postphlebitic
- p. leg
- p. valvular incompetence

postpolio syndrome
postprimary pulmonary tuberculosis
postprocedure nephrostogram
postprocessing
- image p.
- p. procedure
- p. workstation

postprocessor
postpyelonephritis cortical scarring
postradiation
- p. calcification
- p. fibrosis

postradiotherapy implant survey reading
postreduction
- p. film
- p. mammoplasty
- p. view
- p. x-ray

postrelease radiography
postrheumatic cusp retraction
postrolandic parietal cortex

postsphenoid bone
poststenotic dilatation
poststress
    p. ankle/arm Doppler index
    p. image
    p. stunning
postsurgical
    p. change
    p. emphysema
    p. fat necrosis
    p. pseudoaneurysm
    p. recurrent ulcer
posttemporal middle cerebral artery
postterm
    p. fetus
    p. pregnancy
posttherapy change
postthoracotomy change
postthrombolytic coronary reocclusion
posttourniquet occlusion angiography
posttransplant
    p. acute renal failure
    p. coronary artery disease
    p. lymphoproliferative disorder
posttransplantation ureteric obstruction
posttraumatic
    p. angulation
    p. arthritis
    p. ascending myelopathy
    p. aseptic necrosis
    p. atrophy of bone
    p. cavus
    p. central spinal cord syrinx
    p. chondrolysis
    p. cystic myelopathy
    p. fat necrosis
    p. fibrosis
    p. hemorrhage
    p. hydrocephalus
    p. intradiploic pseudomeningocele
    p. neuroma
    p. oil cyst
    p. osteoarthritis
    p. osteoporosis
    p. pneumonia
    p. pulmonary insufficiency
    p. spinal cord cyst
    p. subcapsular hepatic fluid
      collection
    p. syringomyclia
posttuberculous obstruction

postulate
    Avogadro p.
postulnar bone
postural
    p. reduction
    p. ureteric obstruction
posture
    benediction p.
posturography
    moving platform p.
postvagotomy
    p. dysphagia
    p. effect
    p. small-bowel distention
postvasectomy change in epididymis
postvenography phlebitis
postvesicular lymph node
postviral leukoencephalopathy
postvoid
    p. radiography
    p. residual urine
    p. residual urine volume
    p. view
postvoiding film
Potain sign
potassium (K)
    p. 38 (^{38}K)
    p. 39 (^{39}K)
    p. 40 (^{40}K)
    p. 42 (^{42}K)
    p. 43 (^{43}K)
    p. bromide contrast medium
    p. imaging agent
    p. iodide
    ionic p.
    p. perchlorate
    total exchangeable p. (TEK)
potassium-titanyl-phosphate (KTP)
potato
    p. node
    p. tumor of neck
potential
    p. difference
    electrostatic p.
    p. energy
    p. gradient
    ionization p.
    low metastatic p.
    movement-related cortical p.
    phenomenological effective
      surface p.
    recruitment p.

NOTES

P

potential (*continued*)
    resting phase of cardiac action p.
    sorption p.
    upstroke phase of cardiac action p.
    variable tube p.
potentiation
    postextrasystolic p.
potentiator
potentiometer
Pott
    P. abscess
    P. aneurysm
    P. ankle fracture
    P. disease
    P. puffy tumor
Potter
    P. classification
    P. dysplasia
    P. facies
    P. sequence
    P. syndrome
    P. type IV kidney
Potter-Bucky
    P.-B. diaphragm
    P.-B. grid
Potts shunt
pouce flottant
pouch
    antral p.
    apophysial p.
    arachnoid retrocerebellar p.
    axillary p.
    Blake p.
    blind upper esophageal p.
    branchial p.
    Broca pudendal p.
    celomic p.
    collecting venous p.
    deep perineal p.
    Douglas rectouterine p.
    dural root p.
    endodermal p.
    endorectal ileal p.
    fourth branchial cleft p.
    gastric p.
    Hartmann p.
    haustral p.
    Heidenhain p.
    hepatorenal p.
    hernia p.
    hypophysial p.
    ileal S p.
    ileoanal p.
    ileocecal p.
    Indiana p.
    jejunal p.
    Kock p.
    lateral hypopharyngeal p. (LHP)
    2-loop ileal J p.

    Mainz p.
    mature p.
    Morison p.
    nerve root axillary p.
    paracystic p.
    pararectal p.
    paravesical p.
    pendulous p.
    pharyngeal p.
    Prussak p.
    Rathke p.
    rectal p.
    rectouterine p.
    rectovaginal p.
    rectovaginouterine p.
    rectovesical p.
    renal p.
    Seessel p.
    S-shaped p.
    Studer p.
    superficial inguinal p.
    superficial perineal p.
    suprapatellar p.
    UCLA p.
    ultimobranchial p.
    uterovesical p.
    venous p.
    vesicouterine p.
    Willis p.
    W-shaped ileal p.
    Zenker p.
pouchogram
pouchography
    evacuation p.
poudrage
    thoracoscopic p.
Poupart inguinal ligament
Pourcelot index
powder
    barium p.
    bone p.
    E-Z-EM barium p.
    gelatin sponge p.
    licorice p.
    opaque p.
    p. pseudocalcification
    tantalum p.
    tungsten p.
Powell method
power
    backscattered p.
    p. Doppler
    p. Doppler imaging (PDI)
    p. Doppler signal
    p. Doppler sonography (PDS)
    p. Doppler ultrasound
    p. gain
    p. injection
    p. injector

mass collision stopping p.
p. ratio
resolving p.
scanning p.
p. spectral analysis (PSA)
stopping p.
stroke p.
P. Trak 6000 gradient
POWERstation LNX workstation
PowerVision ultrasound
Pozzi muscle
PPAS
peripheral pulmonary artery stenosis
PPG
photoplethysmography
PPH
primary pulmonary hypertension
PPM
posterior papillary muscle
PPP
point-to-point protocol
PPRF
paramedian pontine reticular formation
PPV
positive predictive value
pQCT
peripheral quantitative computed
tomography
pQCT measurement
pQCT scanner
PQ 5000 CT scanner
P-QRS
P wave-QRS wave ratio
PR
pulmonic regurgitation
OncoScint PR
Pr
praseodymium
PRA
pendulous reference axis
practicable
as low as readily p. (ALARP)
praecox
praseodymium (Pr)
PRE
proton relaxation enhancement
T2 PRE
T2 proton relaxation enhancement
preablation
pre-Achilles fat pad
preacinar arterial wall thickness
preamplifier

preampullary portion of bile duct
preangioplasty stenosis
preaortic lymph node
preauricular point
precancer
precancerous change
precapillary lung hypertension
precaptopril radioisotope study
precarcinomatous
precatheterization
precautions
airborne p.
contact p.
standard p.
transmission-based p.
precaval lymph node
prececal lymph node
precentral
p. artery
p. cerebellar vein
p. gyrus
p. sulcus
precentroblast
precessing proton
precession
p. angle
fast imaging with steady-state p.
(FISP)
free p.
Larmor p.
reverse fast imaging with steady-
state free p. (PSIF)
steady-state free p. (SSFP)
true fast imaging with steady-
state p. (TrueFISP)
precessional
p. frequency
p. motion
precharred fiber
prechiasmal optic nerve lesion
precipitate evacuation
precipitating event
precipitation
contrast p.
Precise self-expanding stent
precision
test-retest p.
precocity
isosexual p.
precommunicating
p. segment of anterior cerebral
artery

NOTES

precommunicating *(continued)*
　　p. segment of posterior cerebral
　　　artery
precontrast
　　p. echocardiography
　　p. imaging
　　p. scan
precordial
　　p. bulge
　　p. lead
　　p. mapping
precordium, pl. **precordia**
　　active p.
　　anterior p.
　　bulging p.
　　lateral p.
precoronal sagittal sinus
precuneus
precursor
　　BH4 p.
　　bone marrow myeloid p.
　　neurotransmitter p.
　　p. sign to rupture of aneurysm
predental space
predetector
predicted
　　p. cardiac index
　　p. maximal uptake
　　p. target heart rate
prediction
　　linear p. (LP)
predictor
predisposition
　　hereditary p.
prediverticular
　　p. change
　　p. disease
predominance
　　anterior p.
　　basilar p.
　　posterior p.
　　temporal p.
predominant flow load
preductal aortic coarctation
preejection
　　p. interval
　　p. period (PEP)
preembolization aortography
preemphasis
preenhancement sequence
preepiglottic
　　p. soft tissue
　　p. space
preesophageal dysphagia
preexcitation
　　ventricular p.
preexposure prophylaxis
preferential flow
prefilled syringe

pre-filtering
　　3D p.-f.
prefire image
preformed clot
prefragmentation
prefrontal
　　p. artery
　　p. bone of von Bardeleben
pregnancy
　　abdominal ectopic p.
　　ampullar p.
　　anembryonic p.
　　bigeminal p.
　　broad ligament p.
　　cervical p.
　　combined p.
　　compound p.
　　compromised p.
　　cornual ectopic p.
　　diamniotic p.
　　dichorionic diamniotic twin p.
　　ectopic p. (EP)
　　extrauterine p.
　　failed p.
　　fallopian p.
　　false p.
　　gemellary p.
　　heterotopic p.
　　hydatid p.
　　hypervolemia of p.
　　interstitial ectopic p.
　　intraligamentary p.
　　intraperitoneal p.
　　intrauterine p. (IUP)
　　membranous p.
　　mesenteric p.
　　molar p.
　　monochorionic diamniotic twin p.
　　monochorionic monoamniotic
　　　twin p.
　　multiple pregnancies
　　mural p.
　　ovarian p.
　　ovarioabdominal p.
　　oviductal p.
　　parietal p.
　　phantom p.
　　plural p.
　　postterm p.
　　prevalence ectopic p.
　　prolonged p.
　　pseudointraligamentary p.
　　ruptured ectopic p.
　　sarcofetal p.
　　sarcohysteric p.
　　selective reduction of p.
　　sextuplet p.
　　spurious p.
　　stump p.

tubal p.
tuboabdominal p.
tuboligamentary p.
tuboovarian p.
tubouterine p.
p. tumor
twin ectopic p.
uteroabdominal p.
uterotubal p.
p. wastage
pregnancy-induced uterine blush
pregnant
p. uterus
p. uterus rupture
preinjection echocardiography
preinsular gyrus
preintegration complex
preinterparietal bone
preinvasive
p. carcinoma
p. disease of cervix, vagina, and vulva
Preiser disease
prelaryngeal node
preliminary
p. film
p. view
preload
left ventricular p.
p. reserve
preloading radiation survey
premalleolar bursa
premammillary
p. artery
p. branch
premasseteric
p. space
p. space abscess
premature
p. atherosclerosis
p. calcification
p. closure of ductus arteriosus
p. mid diastolic closure of mitral valve
p. nodal contraction (PNC)
p. osteoarthritis
p. placental senescence
p. senescence placenta
p. suture synostosis
p. uterine membrane rupture
p. valve closure
p. ventricular contraction (PVC)

prematurely closed suture
premaxillary
p. bone
p. suture
premedication
premedullary arteriovenous fistula
premolar teeth
premonitory sign
premotor
p. area
p. coret activation
p. cortex
premyocardial infarction echocardiography
prenatal
p. diagnosis
p. injury
p. radiation
preocclusive obstruction
preoperative
p. angiography
p. imaging
p. localization
p. radiotherapy
p. resting MUGA scan
p. view
preosteonecrosis marrow edema
prep
preparation
LoSo Prep
Tagitol prep
touch prep
prepapillary bile duct
preparation (prep)
bowel p.
Colyte bowel p.
crush p.
dry bowel p.
Dulcolax bowel p.
Emulsoil bowel p.
p. error
Evac-Q-Kwik bowel p.
Fleet Phospho-Soda bowel p.
flow cytometry sample p.
GoLYTELY bowel p.
inadequate bowel p.
international reference p.
kit p.
NuLytely bowel p.
OCL bowel p.
on-column p.
Tridrate bowel p.

NOTES

P

preparation *(continued)*
 wet bowel p.
 X-Prep bowel p.
prepared
 magnetization p. (MP)
prepatellar
 p. bursa
 p. bursitis
prepectoral fascia
prepectorally
prepericardial lymph node
preperitoneal fat
preplacental hemorrhage
preponderance
 phalangeal p.
prepontine
 p. cistern
 p. white epidermoidoma
prepubertal
 p. female breast
 p. testicular mass
prepulse
 shared p. (SHARP)
 spin-lock p.
prepyloric
 p. antrum
 p. atresia
 p. fold
 p. sphincter
 p. ulcer
 p. vein
prereduction
 p. view
 p. x-ray
prerenal
 p. aortic aneurysm
 p. failure
 p. fat
prerupture of aneurysm
PRES
 posterior reversible encephalopathy
 syndrome
presacral
 p. anomaly
 p. cystic lesion
 p. mass
 p. plexus
 p. space
presaturation
 p. bolus tracking
 fat-selective p.
 p. projection
 p. pulse
 spatial p.
 p. technique
presbyesophagus
presbyophrenia
prescan
 MRI p.

prescapula
presence
 inferred p.
presenile arteriosclerosis
presentation
 breech p.
 brow p.
 cephalic p.
 compound p.
 cord p.
 face p.
 footling p.
 frank breech p.
 midline incense p.
 osteoblastic p.
 parietal p.
 shoulder p.
 transverse p.
 vertex p.
presenting part
preservation
 myocardial p.
 p. of native aortic valve
 sphincter p.
 zone of partial p. (ZPP)
presinusoidal
preslip
 p. change
 p. staging
presphenoid bone
PRESS
 point resolved spectroscopy
 point-resolved spectroscopy sequence
pressor unit
pressure
 acoustic p.
 airway p.
 alveolar p.
 p. amplitude
 ankle-arm p.
 ankle systolic p.
 aortic root p.
 p. applied dressing (PAD)
 arterial peak systolic p.
 atmospheric p.
 atrial p.
 A-wave p.
 bile duct p.
 blood p.
 bone marrow p. (BMP)
 brachial artery cuff p.
 brachial artery end-diastolic p.
 brachial artery peak systolic p.
 brachial artery pulse p.
 bursting p.
 capillary hydrostatic p.
 capillary wedge p.
 cardiac filling p.
 cardiovascular p.

catheter bursting p.
central aortic p.
central venous p. (CVP)
cerebral perfusion p. (CPP)
colloid oncotic p. (COP)
coronary perfusion p.
coronary wedge p.
CT-estimated superimposed
  hydrostatic p.
p. cuff
C-wave p.
damping of catheter tip p.
diastolic filling p. (DFP)
diastolic perfusion p.
distal coronary perfusion p.
Doppler ankle systolic p.
Doppler blood p.
draining with venous p.
drifting wedge p.
elevated lower esophageal sphincter
  resting p.
endocardial p.
end-systolic p. (ESP)
p. epiphysis
p. equalization
equalized diastolic p.
esophageal peristaltic p.
extravascular p.
feeding mean arterial p. (FMAP)
filling p.
p. fracture
p. half-time
p. half-time technique
hepatic wedge p. (HWP)
high filling p.
high interstitial p.
high wedge p.
increased central venous p.
increased intracranial p.
increased intrapericardial p.
increased pulmonary arterial p.
p. injector
inspiratory increase in venous p.
interstitial fluid hydrostatic p.
intracardiac p.
intracranial p. (ICP)
intracranial pulse p.
intraductal p.
intraluminal esophageal p.
intramuscular fluid p.
intrapericardial p.
intrapleural p.

intrapulmonary p.
intrathoracic p.
jugular venous p.
labile blood p.
left atrial p. (LAP)
left atrial end-diastolic p.
left-sided heart p.
left subclavian central venous p.
  (LSCVP)
left ventricular p. (LVP)
left ventricular cavity p.
left ventricular end-diastolic p.
  (LVEDP)
left ventricular filling p.
left ventricular peak systolic p.
left ventricular systolic p.
lower esophageal sphincter p.
  (LESP)
low urethral p. (LUP)
maximum inflation p.
mean aortic p.
mean arterial p. (MAP)
mean blood p.
mean brachial artery p.
mean circulatory filling p.
mean left atrial p.
mean pulmonary artery p. (MPAP)
mean pulmonary artery wedge p.
mean pulmonary capillary p.
  (MPCP)
mean right atrial p.
p. measurement
minimum blood p.
p. necrosis
normal lower esophageal sphincter
  resting p.
p. overload
PAM p.
passage p.
p. peak
peak airway p.
peak inflation p.
peak regurgitant wave p.
peak systolic aortic p.
perfusion p.
p. perfusion imaging
p. perfusion study
phasic p.
p. pneumothorax
p. point
portal venous p. (PVP)
positive end-expiratory p.

NOTES

751

pressure *(continued)*

pulmonary arterial systolic pressure to systemic arterial systolic p.

pulmonary arterial wedge p.

pulmonary artery p. (PAP)

pulmonary artery diastolic pressure and pulmonary artery wedge p. (PADP-PAWP)

pulmonary artery end-diastolic p. (PAEDP)

pulmonary artery mean p. (PAM)

pulmonary artery peak systolic p.

pulmonary artery systolic p. (PAS)

pulmonary artery wedge p. (PAWP)

pulmonary capillary p. (PCP)

pulmonary capillary wedge p. (PCWP)

pulmonary venous wedge p.

pulmonary wedge p. (PWP)

pulse p.

p. reading

recoil p.

regional cerebral perfusion p. (rCPP)

right atrial p. (RAP)

right-sided heart p.

right ventricular p. (RVP)

right ventricular diastolic p.

right ventricular end-diastolic p.

right ventricular peak systolic p.

right ventricular volume p.

segmental bronchus lower extremity Doppler p.

shockwave p.

stump p.

subatmospheric p.

superior vena cava p.

supersystemic pulmonary artery p.

systemic diastolic blood p.

systemic mean arterial p. (SMAP)

systolic-diastolic blood p.

torr p.

transmyocardial perfusion p.

transpulmonary p. (Ptp)

venous p.

ventricular p.

ventricularization of p.

in vivo balloon p.

V-wave p.

p. wave

p. waveform

wedge p.

wedge hepatic venous p. (WHVP)

withdrawal p.

X-wave p.

Y-wave p.

Z-point p.

pressure-activated safety valve (PASV)

pressure-controlled intermittent coronary occlusion technique

pressure-detachable silicone balloon

pressure-flow gradient

pressure-gradient wire system

pressure-volume loop

PressureWire sensor

pressurized fluid jet

prestenotic dilatation

prestomal ileitis

prestyloid recess

pretectal

p. lesion

p. nucleus

pretendinous

p. band

p. cord

pretherapy imaging

pretibial

p. dimple

p. myxedema

pre-TIPS gradient

pretracheal lymph node

Preussmann algorithm

prevalence ectopic pregnancy

prevertebral

p. fascia

p. ganglion

p. lymph node

p. soft tissue (PVST)

p. soft tissue swelling

p. space

p. space mass

p. width

prevesicular lymph node

previa

central placenta p.

complete placenta p.

incomplete placenta p.

lateral placenta p.

marginal placenta p.

partial placenta p.

placenta p.

total placenta p.

vasa p.

previable fetus

PRFT

partially relaxed Fourier transform

PRG

phleborheography

prickle cell carcinoma

Prima laser

primary

p. achalasia

p. acquired cholesteatoma

p. acquired nasolacrimal duct obstruction (PANDO)

p. adrenal insufficiency

p. adrenal lymphoma

p. amyloidosis
p. aspergillosis
p. atelectasis
p. auditory cortex
p. beam
p. benign liver tumor
p. biliary cirrhosis
p. bone lymphoma
p. brain lymphoma
cancer of unknown p. (CUP)
p. cartilage joint
p. center of ossification
p. CNS cholesteatoma
p. CNS lymphoma
p. CNS tumor classification
p. coccidioidomycosis
p. complex
p. congenital megaureter
p. cutaneous large B-cell
  lymphoma (PCLBCL)
p. cyst of spleen
p. digital acquisition
p. esophageal peristalsis
p. familial xanthomatosis
p. gastric non-Hodgkin lymphoma
p. hepatocellular carcinoma
p. HIV encephalitis
p. hydrocele
p. hydrocephalus
p. hyperparathyroidism
p. hypertrophic osteoarthropathy
p. hypothyroidism
p. implanted tumor
p. intracerebral hematoma
p. intracranial germ cell tumor
p. intraosseous carcinoma
p. irritant
p. left bronchus
p. lesion
p. malignant liver tumor
p. megaureter
p. motor cortex (PMC)
p. motor strip
p. myeloid metaphysis
p. neoplasm
p. neuroendocrine small-cell
  carcinoma
p. optic atrophy
p. ovarian choriocarcinoma
p. oxalosis
p. peristaltic wave

p. pigmented nodular adrenocortical
  disease
p. pleurisy
p. progressive cerebellar
  degeneration
p. pulmonary hemangiopericytoma
p. pulmonary hypertension (PPH)
p. pulmonary lobule
p. pulmonary lymphangiectasis
p. pulmonary malignancy
p. pulmonary malignant fibrous
  histiocytoma
p. pulmonary plasmacytoma
p. pulmonary tuberculosis
p. radiation
p. ray
p. refractory Burkitt lymphoma
p. renal tumor
p. retroperitoneal fibrosis
p. rhabdomyosarcoma
p. right bronchus
p. sarcoma
p. sclerosing cholangitis
p. sequestrum
p. subclavian-axillary vein
  thrombosis
p. teeth
p. temporal bone cholesteatoma
p. thrombus
p. tumor bed
unknown p.
p. vasospasm
p. vesical calculus
p. visual cortex
p. vitreous
p. yolk sac

PRIME
  Projects in Medical Education
priming effect
primitive
  p. acoustic artery
  p. bone
  p. dislocation
  p. gut
  p. hindgut
  p. hypoglossal artery
  p. neuroectodermal tumor (PNET)
  p. neuroepithelial tumor
  p. pit
  p. streak
  p. trigeminal artery (PTA)
  p. ventricle

NOTES

P

primitive *(continued)*
    p. vertebra
    p. yolk sac
primordial
    p. follicle
    p. tooth cyst
primum
    ostium p.
    septum p.
primus
    digitus p.
PrinceStar electrophysiologic imaging
    study system
principal
    p. artery of pterygoid canal
    p. bronchus
    p. eigenvector
    p. plane
principle
    Dodge p.
    Doppler shift p.
    Fick p.
    Fuchs p.
    Grossman p.
    Huygens p.
    indicator fractionation p.
    line focus p.
    Pauli exclusion p.
    planigraphic p.
    tracer p.
    uncertainty p.
print reflectance modulation
prion protein (PrP)
prior probability
prism
    P. 3-head system
    p. interpolation
    p. method for ventricular volume
private finance initiative (PFI)
PROACT
    Prolyse in acute cerebral
       thromboembolism
       PROACT I, II trial
proactinium
probability
    absolute emission p.
    emission p.
    posterior p.
    prior p.
PROBE
    proton brain examination
probe
    Aloka SSD ultrasound system
       and p.
    AngeLase combined mapping-
       laser p.
    P. balloon dilatation system
    biplane sector p.
    bipolar circumactive p. (BICAP)

Bowman p.
Bruel-Kjaer transvaginal
    ultrasound p.
Cardiac View p.
p. dilatation
Doppler flow echocardiographic p.
electrohydraulic p.
electromagnetic flow p.
fiberoptic p.
freehand p.
gamma p.
gamma-detection p.
GE proton head coil p.
hand-held exploring electrode p.
hand-held mapping p.
hand-held 8-MHz Doppler p.
high-frequency miniature p.
hot-tipped laser p.
hybrid p.
hybridization p.
hyperthermia p.
interstitial p.
intraoperative gamma p.
laparoscopic p.
laparoscopic ultrasound p.
laser-Doppler flowmetry p.
LeVeen RF p.
linear array transrectal
    ultrasound p.
localizing p.
magnetometer p.
MH-908 slim ultrasonic p.
2.0-MHz phased-array p.
neutral amyloid p.
NMR magnetometer p.
nuclear p.
oligonucleotide p.
Olympus MH-908 slim
    ultrasonic p.
Olympus S20-20R transendoscopic
    ultrasound p.
pediatric biplane TEE p.
relaxation p.
scintillation p.
shift p.
side-firing p.
side-hole cannulated p.
Teflon p.
transesophageal echocardiography p.
Transonics flow p.
truncated NMR p.
ultrasonic p.
ultrasound p.
USCI p.
Versadopp ultrasonic Doppler p.
probehead
    MRI p.
probe-surface distance

PROBE-SV
proton brain exam-single voxel
PROBE-SV spectrometry
problematic abdominal activity
problem-focused history
proboscis lateralis
Probst callosal bundle
probucol
halofuginone p.
procedure
artificial pleural effusion p.
button p.
Cabrol composite graft p.
Carson p.
catheter-directed interventional p.
Chamberlain p.
diagnostic p.
DKS p.
edge-detection p.
Eloesser p.
endoscopic p.
gastric pull-through p.
Glenn p.
Guidant Ancure endograft p.
Hofmeister p.
interventional p.
intestinal bypass p.
invasive radiological vascular p.
Kasai p.
limb-lengthening p.
magnetic resonance angiography-
directed bypass p.
mobile imaging p.
neuroendovascular interventional p.
Nissen fundoplication p.
Palomo p.
Pólya p.
portable imaging p.
postprocessing p.
provocative p.
psoas hitch p.
revascularization p.
Roux-en-Y p.
segmentation p.
Senning p.
spatial localization p.
2-step p.
stereotactic p.
STING p.
Swenson pull-through p.
uroradiologic p.
Whipple p.

Proceed vascular interventional CT process
accessory p.
acromion p.
alar p.
alveolar consolidative p.
apical p.
articular p.
ascending p.
auditory p.
basilar p.
bony p.
bremsstrahlung p.
calcaneal p.
capitular p.
carrier-free separation p.
caudate p.
clinoid p.
cochleariform p.
condyloid p.
conoid p.
consolidative p.
coracoacromial p.
coracoid p.
coronoid p.
costal p.
cribriform p.
cystic p.
destructive p.
2D filtering p.
energy transfer p.
ensiform p.
ethmoidal p.
falciform p.
fanning of the spinous p.
fibroplastic p.
frontal p.
frontonasal p.
frontosphenoidal p.
glenoid p.
inflammatory synovial p.
intercondylar p.
interspinous p.
intravascular clotting p.
jugular p.
knobby p.
lateral talar p.
left ventricular posterior superior p.
leptomeningeal p.
lumbar transverse p.
mastoid p.
maxillary p.

NOTES

P

755

process *(continued)*
    monarticular p.
    neoplastic p.
    neutron absorption p.
    noncalcified ocular p.
    notochordal p.
    odontoid p.
    olecranon p.
    osseous destructive p.
    paraneoplastic p.
    posterior lateral talar p.
    prominent xiphoid p.
    pterygoid p.
    radial styloid p.
    radiostyloid p.
    sacral p.
    sacralized transverse p.
    Sand p.
    space-occupying p.
    spinous p.
    SSFP p.
    Stieda p.
    styloid p.
    superior articulating p.
    supracondylar p.
    supracondyloid p.
    temporal p.
    p. tomography (PT)
    transverse p.
    trigonal p.
    trochlear p.
    ulnar styloid p.
    uncinate p.
    vermiform p.
    vertebral p.
    vertebrospinous p.
    within-slice filtering p.
    xiphoid p.
    zygomatic p.
processing
    digital imaging p. (DIP)
    enterocytic p.
    intrapixel sequential p. (IPSP)
    maximum entropy p.
    MIP image p.
    signal p.
processor
    array p.
    conventional p.
    daylight p.
    fast-array p.
    Kodak RP X-OMAT p.
    ML 700 daylight p.
    RP X-OMAT p.
    p. sensitometry
    sequence p.
processor-related artifact
processus vaginalis
prochordal plate

procoagulant
ProCol vascular bioprosthesis
proctogram
    balloon p.
    defecating p.
    video p.
proctographic feature
proctography
    evacuation p.
proctopathy
    radiation p.
proctostat
procurvature deformity
Prodigy bone densitometer
product
    brightness area p. (BAP)
    decay p.
    dose area p. (DAP)
    dose-length p. (DLP)
    fibrin-split p.
    fission p.
    iodine-labeled p.
    respiratory burst p.
    spallation p.
production
    Cerenkov radiation p.
    fast routine p.
    lactoferrin p.
    mitochondrial ATP p.
    pair p.
    radionuclide p.
    radiopharmaceutical p.
    remote-controlled p.
    secondary electron p.
    1-step p.
Profasi HP
profile
    autocalibration k-space p.
    CH20 Kernal and slim 2 p.
    3D dose p.
    excitation p.
    flat time-intensity p.
    flow velocity p.
    fluence p.
    P. mammography system
    nonlinear excitation p.
    number p.
    parabolic velocity p.
    peak p.
    projection p.
    p. ray view
    rectangular section p.
    section-sensitivity p.
    slice sensitivity p. (SSP)
    ultra-low p. (ULP)
    velocity p.
profilogram
profluens
Proforma catheter

profundal popliteal collateral index
profundus
  flexor digitorum p.
  p. tendon
profusion
  opacity p.
progeny
  radon p.
progeria
  adult p.
prognathic dilatation
prognathism
programmable
  p. stepper motor
  p. ventricular shunt valve
programmer
  pulse p.
  p. wand
progression
  inexorable p.
  inflow disease p.
  interval p.
  true fast imaging and steady p.
    (FISP)
progressive
  p. coccidioidomycosis
  p. degeneration
  p. diaphysial dysplasia (PDD)
  p. dysphagia
  p. emphysematous necrosis
  p. encephalopathy with edema,
    hypsarrhythmia, and optic atrophy
    (PEHO)
  p. familial cirrhosis
  p. hydrocephalus
  p. interstitial pulmonary fibrosis
  p. massive fibrosis (PMF)
  p. multifocal leukoencephalopathy
    (PML)
  p. nodular pulmonary fibrosis
  p. posttraumatic myelopathy
  p. primary tuberculosis
  p. rubella panencephalitis
  p. spin saturation
  p. stroke
  p. subcortical gliosis
  p. suppurative cholangitis
  p. supranuclear palsy
  p. systemic sclerosis
  p. uptake

ProHance
  P. contrast medium
  P. imaging agent
projectile horn
projection
  p. angiogram
  anterior p.
  anteroposterior lordotic p.
  AP p.
  apical lordotic p.
  average pixel p. (APP)
  axial p.
  axillary p.
  back p.
  ball-catcher p.
  base p.
  basilar p.
  basovertical p.
  p. binning
  biplane p.
  blowout view p.
  bony vertebra p.
  brow-down p.
  brow-up p.
  Caldwell p.
  carpal tunnel p.
  cartographic p.
  caudad p., caudal p.
  caudocranial p.
  centroid-based maximum
    intensity p.
  Chassard-Lapiné p.
  Chausse III p.
  Chaussier p.
  coronal maximum-intensity p.
  craniocaudal p.
  cross-sectional transverse p.
  cross-table lateral p.
  cylindrical map p.
  divergent ray p.
  dorsoplantar p.
  3D stereotactic surface p.
  erect fluoro spot p.
  fan-beam p.
  fast Fourier p. (FFP)
  FI p.
  p. fiber damage
  filtered back p. (FBP)
  fingerlike p.
  Fletcher p.
  flexion-extension p.
  p. formula

NOTES

P

projection *(continued)*
    frogleg lateral p.
    full-scan p.
    full scan with interpolation p.
    Granger p.
    half-axial anteroposterior p.
    half-scan with extrapolation p.
    Hermodsson tangential p.
    intraoral p.
    Lambert p.
    LAO p.
    lateral oblique axial p.
    lateral transcranial p.
    lateral transfacial p.
    lateromedial oblique p.
    left anterior oblique p.
    left lateral p.
    left posterior oblique p.
    Low-Beers p.
    L5-S1 p.
    lumbosacral p.
    maximum intensity p. (MIP)
    maximum-intensity sliding thin
      slab p.
    medial oblique axial p.
    mediolateral oblique p.
    Mercator p.
    minimal intensity p. (minIP)
    minimum-intensity sliding thin
      slab p.
    modified p.
    mortise p.
    navicular p.
    notch p.
    nuchofrontal p.
    oblique lateral p.
    occipitomental p.
    off-lateral p.
    open-mouth p.
    orthogonal angiographic p.
    PA p.
    panoramic surface p.
    papillary p.
    parietoorbital p.
    Pawlow p.
    pillar p.
    Pirie transoral p.
    plantodorsal p.
    postdrainage p.
    posterior p.
    posteroanterior lordotic p.
    presaturation p.
    p. profile
    radiographic p.
    ramp-filtered back p.
    ray-sum p.
    p. reconstruction imaging
    recumbent lateral p.
    reversed Stenvers p.

    Rhese p.
    right anterior oblique p.
    right posterior oblique p.
    rotating tomographic p.
    Runström p.
    saturation inversion p. (SIP)
    scaphoid p.
    Schüller p.
    semiaxial anteroposterior p.
    semiaxial transcranial p.
    Settegast p.
    simulated annealing method p.
    skyline p.
    sliding thin-slab maximum
      intensity p. (STS-MIP)
    steep left anterior oblique p.
    steep Towne p.
    Stenver p.
    stereographic p.
    stereo right lateral p.
    stereotactic surface p. (SSP)
    straight lateral p.
    stress p.
    Stryker notch p.
    submentovertex p.
    sunrise p.
    superoinferior p.
    surface p.
    swimmer's p.
    tangential p.
    thin-slab minimum intensity p.
    Towne p.
    p. tract imaging
    transaxial maximum-intensity p.
    transthoracic p.
    tunnel p.
    under-filled submentovertical p.
    under-scan method p.
    variable p. (VARPRO)
    verticosubmental p.
    Vogt bone-free p.
    Waters p.
    p. x-ray microscope
projectional image
projection-reconstruction technique
Projecto de Intervenção do Chafariz de
    Dentro (Lisbon) (PICD)
projector
    cine p.
    liquid crystal display p.
    white light pattern p.
Projects in Medical Education (PRIME)
prolactin-secreting pituitary
    macroadenoma
prolapse
    anterior leaflet p.
    p. of aortic valve
    billowing mitral valve p.
    cord p.

gastroduodenal mucosal p.
gastrojejunal mucosal p.
holosystolic mitral valve p.
intestinal p.
intracranial fat p.
mitral valve p. (MVP)
mitral valve leaflet systolic p.
pelvic organ p.
posterior leaflet p.
rectal p.
p. of right aortic valve cusp
p. of spleen
systolic p.
tricuspid valve p.
p. of umbilical cord
valve p.

prolapsed
p. antral mucosa
p. gastric mucosa
p. mitral valve (PMV)
p. stoma
p. tumor

proliferation
angiofibroblastic p.
p. area
astrocytic p.
benign sclerosing ductal p.
bile duct p.
bizarre parosteal
    osteochondromatous p.
bizarre subparosteal
    osteochondromatous p.
p. of bone
bony p.
collagen tissue p.
connective tissue p.
extranodal p.
fibroplastic p.
p. of fibrous tissue
glandular p.
intimal p.
myofibrohistiocytic p.
myointimal p.
myxomatous p.
neointimal p.
neuronal p.
nodular p.
osteophytic p.
papillary p.
perineural glial p.
peripelvic fat p.
p. pleurisy

p. rate
reactive fibrovascular arachnoid p.
synovial p.
villous p.
proliferative
p. bronchiolitis
p. change
p. glomerulonephritis
p. index
p. inflammation
p. lesion
p. pattern
p. phase endometrium
prolonged
p. ejection time
p. expiratory phase
p. inspiratory phase
p. interval
p. left ventricular impulse
p. pregnancy
**Prolyse in acute cerebral
    thromboembolism (PROACT)**
promethium (Pm)
prominence
aortic p.
p. of bone
bony p.
hilar p.
interstitial p.
mediastinal p.
styloid p.
tibial tubercle p.
upper lobe vein p.
prominent
p. ductal pattern
p. ductal vascular structure
p. liver
p. pyramidal thyroid lobe
p. rim of radiolucency
p. septal lymphatic
p. spur
p. tubercle
p. uptake
p. vertebra
p. xiphoid process
promontory
p. mass
sacral p.
pronate
pronation
hallucal p.
pes p.

NOTES

P

759

pronation-abduction
    p.-a. fracture
    p.-a. injury
pronation-eversion fracture
pronation-external
    p.-e. rotation
    p.-e. rotation injury
pronator
    p. quadratus
    p. quadratus line
    round p.
    p. teres (PT)
    p. teres tendon
pronatus
    pes p.
prone
    p. angled view
    p. film
    p. lateral view
    p. position
pronephron
    rudimentary p.
pronephros, pl. **pronephroi**
pronged Franseen-type point needle
pronunciation
    artifact p.
propagation speed artifact
Propaq Encore vital signs monitor
PROPELLER
    periodically rotated overlapping parallel
    lines with enhanced reconstruction
        PROPELLER FSE technique
        PROPELLER MRI
        PROPELLER technique
proper
    p. digital nerve branch
    p. hepatic artery (PHA)
properitoneal
    p. fat
    p. fat line
    p. flank stripe
    p. hernia
prophylactic IVC filter
prophylaxis
    preexposure p.
propidium iodide
proportion
    aneurysmal p.
proportional
    p. counter
    p. ratio
proportionality
    cephalofacial p.
propria
    lamina p.
    muscularis p.
    substantia p.
    tunica p.

propulsive
    p. mechanism
    p. movement
propyliodone imaging agent
prosencephalon
ProSound SSD-5500 ultrasound
prospective
    p. acquisition correction (PACE)
    p. analysis
    p. investigation of pulmonary
      embolus diagnosis (PIOPED)
    p. synchronization
ProSpeed CT scanner
prostaglandin
    p. E_1
    p. E_1 injection
    p. infusion
Prostalase laser system
Prostar-Techstar suture-mediated closure device
Prostar XL 8, 10 suture mediated closure device
ProstaScint
    P. monoclonal antibody imaging
      agent
    P. scan
prostate
    p. abscess
    p. anatomy
    apex of p.
    p. capsule
    p. carcinoma
    floating p.
    p. gland
    p. hypoechoic lesion
    p. implant
    inferolateral surface of p.
    lateral lobe of p.
    lymph vessel of p.
    median lobe of p.
    posterior surface of p.
    p. seeding
    transrectal ultrasound-guided biopsy
      of the p.
    transurethral incision of p.
    transurethral resection of p.
      (TURP)
    visual laser ablation of p. (VLAP)
prostatectomy
    transurethral ultrasound-guided laser-
      induced p. (TULIP)
prostatic
    p. adenoma
    p. bed
    p. calculus
    p. carcinoma
    p. cyst
    p. duct
    p. fluid

p. hyperplasia
p. hyperplastic nodule
p. obstruction
p. sinus
p. stent
p. transition zone
p. urethra (PU)
p. urethroplasty
p. uterus
p. venous plexus
prostaticovesical junction
prostatitis
cavitary p.
diverticular p.
prostatography
prosthesis
Angelchik reflux p.
Medtronic Talent p.
prosthetic
p. cup
p. femoral distal graft
p. heart valve
p. implant
p. mitral valve
p. replacement
p. valve embolus
prostrema
area p.
Protg
P. GPS self-expanding Nitinol
stent-biliary system
P. GPS stent
P. self-expanding stent
protactinium (Pa)
protect
Cardiac P.
protection
p. factor
myocardial p.
radiation p.
region of p.
protective
p. cold saline infusion
p. isolation
6F Protégé self-expanding stent
protein
carrier p.
CSF 14-3-3 p.
macrophage inflammatory p. (MIP)
prion p. (PrP)
proteinase
protein-bound iodine (PBI)

protein-fat fluid level
protein-losing enteropathy
**protein-nucleic acid synthesis in tumor
cell**
proteinosis
alveolar p.
pulmonary alveolar p. (PAP)
proteoglycan matrix
Proteus syndrome
protium
protocol
axial BMD center with agreed
joint p.
axial T1-SE p.
biphasic injection p.
Cornell p.
CT scan with renal stone p.
default display p.
2D GRE dynamic p.
Ellestad p.
experimental p.
Heidelberg p.
helical CT scanning p.
low-dose/high-dose p.
MP-RAGE p.
multiple-injection p.
neon particle p.
point-to-point p. (PPP)
proton relaxometric p.
single-injection p.
telomere repeat amplification p.
transmission control
protocol/Internet p. (TCP/IP)
UCLA imaging p.
Protoco$_2$l automated CO$_2$ insufflator
protodensity MR imaging
protodiastolic reversal of blood flow
proton
p. beam
p. brain examination (PROBE)
p. brain exam-single voxel
(PROBE-SV)
p. chemical shift imaging
p. dipole-dipole interaction
p. electron dipole-dipole
excited p.
high-energy p.
interstitial water p.
p. irradiation
lactate p.
p. magnetic resonance
methyl p.

NOTES

P

761

proton *(continued)*
    p. MR spectroscopic imaging
    p. MR spectroscopy
    p. nuclear magnetic resonance
      spectroscopy
    p. nuclear magnetic resonance
      spectrum
    precessing p.
    p. relaxation
    p. relaxation enhancement (PRE)
    p. relaxometric protocol
    p. spin-lattice relaxation time
    p. therapy
proton-density
    p.-d. axial image
    p.-d. axial MR scan
proton-density-weighted
    p.-d.-w. fast spin-echo image
    p.-d.-w. imaging
    p.-d.-w. MRI
proton-electron double-resonance imaging (PEDRI)
proton-proton magnetization exchange
protoplasmic astrocytoma
protopulmonary bilharziasis
protracted
    p. exposure sensitization
    p. radiation
    p. venous infusion (PVI)
protruded disc
protruding
    p. atheroma
    p. fat
protrusio acetabuli
protrusion
    acetabular p.
    anal p.
    broad-based disc p.
    coil p.
    p. of cystocele
    disc p.
    hip p.
    p. of navicular
    spicular p.
    spoonlike p.
    vascular p.
protuberance
    bony p.
    occipital p.
protuberans
    dermatofibrosarcoma p.
provisional callus
provocable ischemia
provocative procedure
proximal
    p. acinar emphysema
    p. anterior descending artery
    p. anterior tibial artery
    p. aorta

    p. articular set angle
    p. aspect
    p. brain shift
    p. carpal row
    p. circumflex artery
    p. coil
    p. colon
    p. convoluted tubule
    p. coronary (PCS)
    p. digital artery
    p. dilation
    p. and distal portion of vessel
    p. esophagitis dilatation
    p. femoral fracture
    p. femur
    p. fibula
    p. focal femoral deficiency (PFFD)
    p. humeral fracture
    p. interphalangeal (PIP)
    p. interphalangeal joint (PIPJ)
    p. interphalangeal joint articulation
    p. isovelocity surface area (PISA)
    p. jejunum
    p. left anterior descending artery
    p. loop syndrome
    p. part of dorsal duct
    p. popliteal artery
    p. radioulnar joint
    p. segment
    p. small bowel
    p. third shaft
    p. tibia
    p. tibial metaphysial fracture
    p. trochlear groove
    p. tubular adenoma
proximally
proximity
    p. arteriography
    p. injury
    stent p.
PrP
    prion protein
PRS
    photon radiosurgery system
prune belly syndrome
pruned
    p. appearance of pulmonary
      vasculature
    p. hilum
    p. tree appearance
pruned-tree appearance
pruned-tree-appearance bile duct
pruning
    p. of pancreatic duct branch
    pulmonary artery p.
Prussak
    P. pouch
    P. space

PS
>   partial saturation
>   pulmonary sequestration

PSA
>   power spectral analysis

psammoma
>   p. body
>   p. body meningioma
>   Virchow p.

psammomatoid ossifying fibroma

psammomatous
>   p. calcification
>   p. meningioma
>   p. microcalcification

psathyrosis

PSC
>   public sector comparator

PSD
>   peak skin dose
>   periodic synchronous discharge

pseudarthrosis (*var. of* pseudoarthrosis)

pseudoacardia

pseudoachondroplasia

pseudoaneurysm
>   anastomotic p.
>   aortic p.
>   arterial p.
>   chronic posttraumatic aortic p.
>   extrahepatic p.
>   femoral artery p.
>   p. formation
>   heart p.
>   hepatic artery p.
>   iatrogenic p.
>   inguinal p.
>   p. of mitral-aortic fibrosa
>   pancreatitis p.
>   peripheral p.
>   perivalvular p.
>   postcatheterization p. (PCPA)
>   postsurgical p.
>   renal transplant p.
>   saccular p.
>   splenic artery p.
>   traumatic aortic p.
>   uterine artery p.

pseudoangiomatous stromal hyperplasia (PASH)

pseudoangiosarcoma

pseudoarthritis

pseudoarthrosis, pseudarthrosis
>   long bone p.
>   tibial p.

pseudoarticulation

pseudoascites

pseudo-AV block

pseudobulbar affect

pseudocalcification
>   powder p.

pseudocalculus bile duct

pseudocapsule
>   radiopaque p.

pseudocarcinoma

pseudocarcinomatous

pseudocavitation
>   lung p.

pseudochylous effusion

pseudocirrhosis
>   cholangiodysplastic p.

pseudocoarctation of aorta

pseudocolor B-mode

pseudocryptorchidism

pseudocyst
>   adrenal p.
>   gelatinous brain p.
>   mature pancreatic p.
>   meconium p.
>   necrotic bone p.
>   pancreatic p.
>   pulmonary p.
>   splenic p.
>   subarticular p.
>   umbilical cord p.

pseudocystic hygroma

pseudo-Dandy-Walker malformation

pseudodefect

pseudodextrocardia

pseudodiffusion

pseudodisease

pseudodislocation

pseudodissection

pseudodiverticula
>   small bowel p.

pseudodiverticulosis
>   intramural esophageal p.

pseudodiverticulum
>   retrograde ureteral p.

pseudodynamic MR imaging

pseudoepiphysis

pseudoexstrophy

pseudofollicle

pseudofollicular salpingitis

NOTES

P

pseudofracture
  p. artifact
  milkman's p.
pseudogating
  diastolic p.
pseudogestational sac
pseudogland formation
pseudoglioma
pseudogout
pseudogynecomastia
pseudohaustration
pseudohermaphroditism
  female p.
pseudohomogeneous edema pattern
pseudo-Hurler deformity
pseudohypertrophy
pseudohypoparathyroidism (PHP)
pseudoinfarct pattern
pseudointimal
  p. formation
  p. hyperplasia
pseudointraligamentary pregnancy
pseudointussusception
pseudo-Jefferson fracture
pseudojoint
pseudokidney sign
pseudolesion
pseudoluxation
pseudolymphoma
  breast p.
  gastric p.
  lung p.
pseudomalignant
  p. myositis ossificans
  p. tumor
pseudomantle zone pattern
pseudomass
  mediastinal p.
  mucous p.
pseudomembrane
  fetal neck p.
pseudomembranous
  p. colitis
  p. inflammation
  p. radiation gastritis
pseudomeningocele
  posttraumatic intradiploic p.
pseudomitral leaflet
pseudomucinous cystadenocarcinoma
pseudomyxoma peritonei
pseudoneoplasm
pseudonephritis
  athlete's p.
pseudoneuroma
pseudoneuropathic joint
pseudoobstruction
  bowel p.
  chronic idiopathic intestinal p.
    (CIIP)

colonic p.
familial intestinal p.
idiopathic intestinal p.
nonfamilial intestinal p.
pseudoomphalocele
pseudoorbital tumor
pseudoosteomalacic pelvis
pseudopancreatitis
pseudoperiostitis
pseudoplaque
pseudopneumoperitoneum
pseudopod formation
pseudopodia
pseudopolyp definition
pseudopolyposis lymphatica
pseudoporencephaly
pseudopost Billroth I appearance
pseudopregnancy
pseudopseudohypoparathyroidism
pseudopyogenic granuloma
pseudorosette
  perivascular p.
pseudosac
pseudosacculation
pseudosarcoma
  esophageal p.
pseudosarcomatous fasciitis
pseudosclerosis
  spastic p.
pseudosheath
pseudospondylolisthesis
  Junghans p.
pseudostenosis
  sigmoid p.
pseudostone
pseudostricture
  colon p.
pseudosubluxation
  C-spine p.
pseudotear
pseudothickening
pseudothrombophlebitis syndrome
pseudothrombosis
pseudotrabecula
pseudotrochanteric bursitis
pseudotruncus arteriosus
pseudotumor
  abdominal p.
  p. appearance
  atelectatic asbestos p.
  p. cerebri (PTC)
  fibrosing inflammatory p.
  hemophilic p.
  inflammatory carotid p.
  inflammatory idiopathic orbital p.
  inflammatory intestinal p.
  intraosseous hemophilic p.
  kidney p.
  orbital p.

pleura p.
renal p.
small bowel p.
vermian p.
xanthomatous p.

pseudotumoral lesion
pseudo-Turner syndrome
pseudoulceration
pseudoureterocele
pseudovagina
pseudo-Whipple disease
pseudowidening
joint space p.
pseudoxanthoma elasticum
pseudo-Zollinger-Ellison syndrome
PSF
point-spread function
posterior spine fusion
PSH-25GT transcranial imaging transducer
PSIF
reverse fast imaging with steady-state free precession
P sign
psoas
p. abscess
p. fascia
p. hitch procedure
p. line
p. major
p. margin
p. muscle
p. shadow
p. shadow angle
p. sign
p. stripe
psoralen and ultraviolet A (PUVA)
PSP
photostimulable phosphor
PSP imaging plate
^{31}P spectroscopy
PSR
phase sampling ratio
PSV
peak systolic velocity
psychotherapeutic drug
PT
pneumothorax
process tomography
pronator teres
Pt
platinum
PTA
percutaneous transluminal angioplasty
persistent truncus arteriosus
primitive trigeminal artery
suprainguinal PTA
PTBD
percutaneous transhepatic biliary drainage
PTC
percutaneous transhepatic cholangiogram
pseudotumor cerebri
PTCA
percutaneous transhepatic cholangiogram
percutaneous transluminal coronary angioplasty
PTCA Registry
PTCD
percutaneous transhepatic cholangial drainage
pterion
pterional transsylvian approach
p-terphenyl
pterygium colli
pterygoid
p. artery
p. bone
p. canal
p. chest
p. fossa
p. muscle
p. plate
p. plexus
p. process
pterygoideus hamulus
pterygomandibular
p. ligament
p. raphe
pterygopalatine
p. canal
p. fossa
p. ganglion
pterygospinous ligament
PTF
posterior talofibular
PTF ligament
PTFE
polytetrafluoroethylene
PTFE stent
PTHC
percutaneous transhepatic cholangiogram
percutaneous transhepatic cholangiography

NOTES

P

PTK
phototherapeutic keratectomy
PTL
percutaneous transhepatic lymphography
PTNB
percutaneous transthoracic needle biopsy
ptosis, pl. **ptoses**
ptotic kidney
Ptp
transpulmonary pressure
PTRA
percutaneous transluminal renal
angioplasty
PTT
posterior tibial tendon
pulse transit time
PTV
planning target volume
posterior temporal vertical
ptyalography
PU
prostatic urethra
PU catheter
pubescent uterus
pubic
p. arch
p. bone
p. bone maldevelopment
p. crest
p. ramus
p. symphysis
p. tubercle
pubica
symphysis p.
pubis
mons p.
os p.
osteitis p.
pecten p.
symphysis ossium p.
widened symphysis p.
public sector comparator (PSC)
pubocapsular ligament
pubocervical ligament
pubococcygeal line (PCL)
pubococcygeus muscle
pubofemoral ligament
puboischial area
puboprostatic ligament
puborectalis loop
pubovesical ligament
Puck film changer
PUD
peptic ulcer disease
puddle sign
puddling
p. of contrast
peripheral p.

pudenda
ulcerating granuloma of p.
pudendal
p. blood supply
p. branch
p. canal
p. cleft
p. vein
p. vein reflux
PUJ
pelviureteric junction
pullback
p. across aortic valve
aortic p.
p. arterial marking
p. esophagram
p. imaging
p. pressure gradient
p. pressure recording
p. study
pulley
bone p.
p. of finger
pull maneuver
pull-type gastrostomy tube
pull-up
gastric p.-u.
pulmoaortic canal
pulmogram
pulmolith
pulmolithiasis
pulmonale
atrium p.
cor p.
pulmonary
p. abscess
p. adenopathy
p. alveolar microlithiasis
p. alveolar proteinosis (PAP)
p. alveolus
p. amyloidosis
p. angioma
p. aplasia
p. arborization
p. arc
p. arterial circulation
p. arterial flow insufficiency
p. arterial hypertension (PAH)
p. arterial input impedance
p. arterial malformation
p. arterial marking
p. arterial occlusion
p. arterial resistance index
p. arterial systolic pressure to
systemic arterial systolic pressure
p. arterial vent
p. arterial wedge pressure
p. arteriography
p. arteriolar resistance

p. arteriolar vasoconstriction
p. arteriosclerosis
p. arteriovenous aneurysm
p. arteriovenous fistula
p. arteriovenous malformation (PAVM)
p. artery (PA)
p. artery agenesis
p. artery apoplexy
p. artery atresia
p. artery balloon pump (PABP)
p. artery bifurcation
p. artery blockage
p. artery-bronchus ratio
p. artery compression ascending aortic aneurysm
p. artery diastolic pressure and pulmonary artery wedge pressure (PADP-PAWP)
p. artery dilatation
p. artery embolization
p. artery end-diastolic pressure (PAEDP)
p. artery hemorrhage
p. artery interruption
p. artery intima
p. artery mean pressure (PAM)
p. artery obstruction
p. artery peak systolic pressure
p. artery pressure (PAP)
p. artery pruning
p. artery to right ventricle diastolic gradient
p. artery sarcoma
p. artery stenosis
p. artery stenting
p. artery systolic pressure (PAS)
p. artery wedge angiography
p. artery wedge pressure (PAWP)
p. asbestosis
p. aspergillosis
p. aspiration
p. atrium
p. barotrauma
p. blood flow (PBF)
p. blood flow redistribution
p. blood flow study
p. blood volume (PBV)
p. blood volume index (PBVI)
p. calcification
p. capillary endothelium
p. capillary hemangiomatosis

p. capillary permeability
p. capillary pressure (PCP)
p. capillary wedge position
p. capillary wedge pressure (PCWP)
p. capillary wedge tracing
p. and cardiac sclerosis
p. cartilage
p. cavitation
p. cavity
p. cirrhosis
p. confluence
p. consolidation
p. contusion
p. cyst
p. cystic lymphangiectasis
p. density
p. dysmaturity
p. edema (PE)
p. edema photographic negative
p. embolic septic disease
p. embolus (PE)
p. failure
p. flow pattern
p. function test
p. gas
p. gas exchange
p. hamartoma
p. heart
p. hilum
p. histoplasmosis
p. hyalinizing granuloma
p. hyperinflation
p. hypertension
p. hypoperfusion
p. hypoplasia
p. idiopathic fibrosis
p. incompetence
p. infarct
p. interstitial abnormality
p. interstitial disease
p. interstitial emphysema (PIE)
p. interstitial idiopathic fibrosis
p. interstitial thinning
p. interstitium
p. juxtaesophageal lymph node
p. Kaposi sarcoma
p. lesion
p. ligament
p. linearity
p. lobe
p. lymphangiomatosis

NOTES

P

pulmonary *(continued)*
p. lymphoid disorder
p. lymphoma
p. magnetic resonance angiography (PMRA)
p. mainline granulomatosis
p. mass
p. meningioma
p. metastasis
p. microcirculation
p. microvasculature
p. neuroendocrine cell hyperplasia
p. nodularity
p. nodule
p. nodule enhancement
p. orifice
p. osteoarthropathy
p. outflow gradient
p. outflow obstruction
p. overdistention
p. overexpansion
p. overinflation
p. papillomatosis
p. parenchyma
p. parenchymal change
p. parenchymal infection
p. parenchymal infiltrate
p. parenchymal injury
p. parenchymal window
p. pedicle
p. perfusion imaging
p. perfusion MRI contrast agent
p. perfusion and ventilation
p. pleura
p. pleurisy
p. plexus
p. pseudocyst
p. quantitative differential function study
p. resection
p. sarcoidosis
p. scar
p. scintigraphy
p. sclerosing hemangioma
p. segment
p. sequestration (PS)
p. sequestration spectrum
p. sinus
p. sling
p. sling complex
p. squamous cell carcinoma
p. stable echo-enhancer
p. stenosis
p. structural maturation
p. subcutaneous encephalitis emphysema
p. sulcus
p. talcosis
p. telangiectasia

p. thromboembolic disease
p. thromboembolism
p. thromboembolization
p. thrombosis
p. time activity curve
p. trunk
p. trunk bifurcation
p. trunk idiopathic dilatation
p. tuberculosis
p. tumor
p. valve
p. valve anulus
p. valve area
p. valve atresia
p. valve cusp
p. valve deformity
p. valve dysplasia
p. valve insufficiency
p. valve stenosis
p. valve stenosis dilatation
p. varix
p. vascular bed
p. vascular bed impedance
p. vascular congestion
p. vascularity
p. vascular marking
p. vascular obstruction
p. vascular pattern
p. vascular redistribution
p. vascular reserve
p. vascular resistance (PVR)
p. vascular resistance index (PVRI)
p. vasculature
p. vasoreactivity
p. vein
p. vein apoplexy
p. vein atresia
p. vein fibrosis
p. vein stenosis
p. vein wedge angiography
p. venous congestion (PVC)
p. venous drainage
p. venous hypertension
p. venous obstruction
p. venous recess
p. venous return
p. venous system
p. venous-systemic air embolus
p. venous wedge pressure
p. ventilation imaging
p. vesicle
p. vessel
p. vessel overcirculation
p. wedge pressure (PWP)

pulmonic
p. area
p. atresia
p. infiltrate
p. insufficiency (PI)

p. output
p. output flow
p. output index
p. regurgitation (PR)
p. stenosis
p. valve (PV)
p. valve gradient
p. valve regurgitation
p. valvular stenosis
p. versus systemic flow
pulmonic-systemic flow ratio
pulmonis
crista p.
lingula p.
pulp
p. abscess
p. canal
p. of finger
p. space
p. stone
pulpal abscess
pulposus
herniated nucleus p. (HNP)
pulsatile perfusion
pulsatility
arterial p.
p. indices
p. measurement
pulsating
p. current
p. empyema
p. mass
p. metastasis
p. pleurisy
p. vein
pulsation
p. artifact
capillary p.
mean venous p.
p. pattern
pulse
adiabatic slice-selective
radiofrequency p.
p. amplifier
apical p.
balanced fast-field-echo p.
brachial p.
carotid p.
compensated composite spin-lock p.
composite p.
dampened obstructive p.
DANTE-selective p.

depth p.
p. design
diastolic depolarization p.
Doppler p.
p. Doppler interrogation
dorsalis pedis p.
2D spatially selective
radiofrequency p.
E point of cardiac apex p.
p. fashion pulse spray
fat suppression p.
femoral p.
p. flip angle
flow respiratory artifact obliteration
with directed orthogonal p.'s
(FRODO)
frequency-selective p.
globally optimized alternating-phase
rectangular p. (GARP)
gradient p.
p. height spectral analysis
2010 P. Holter system
inversion p.
p. labeling
p. length
motion compensation gradient p.
MP inversion p.
narrow-band spectral-selective
radiofrequency p.
navigator p.
p. NMR
nonselective p.
p. oximetry
pedal p.
phase-encode p.
picosecond p.
p. pile-up
popliteal p.
posterior tibial p.
presaturation p.
p. pressure
p. programmer
P. Pro heart rate monitor
radial p.
radiofrequency p.
radiofrequency excitation p.
p. reappearance time
p. repetition frequency
p. repetition time
resting p.
RF p.
saturation p.

NOTES

P

pulse *(continued)*
    section-select p.
    selective p.
    p. sequence
    p. sequence echo-planar imaging
    p. shape
    small water-hammer p.
    spatially selective inversion p.
    p. spray infusion
    synchronous carotid arterial p.
    tailored p.
    temporal p.
    tidal wave of carotid arterial p.
    time following inversion p. (TI)
    p. transit time (PTT)
    trough of venous p.
    twin-peaked p.
    velocity-compensating gradient p.
    vertical synchronization p.
    p. voltage
    p. volume recording (PVR)
    p. volume waveform
    V peak of jugular venous p.
    p. width (PW)
    p. width variation

PULSEcdc
    P. compact gamma camera
    P. gamma camera

pulsed
    p. arterial spin labeling
    p. arterial spin labeling sequence
    p. Doppler flowmeter
    p. Doppler transesophageal
      echocardiography
    p. Doppler ultrasound
    p. Doppler waveform
    p. dose rate (PDR)
    p. dye laser therapy
    p. electron paramagnetic imaging
    p. infrared laser
    p. L-band ESR spectrometry
    p. magnetization transfer MR
      imaging
    p. metal vapor laser
    p. mode
    p. nuclear magnetic resonance
    p. pump
    p. therapeutic low-intensity
      ultrasound
    p. wave
    p. wave Doppler ultrasonography

pulsed-dye
    p.-d. laser
    p.-d. laser lithotripsy

pulsed-electron paramagnetic NMR
pulsed-gradient
    p.-g. spin echo (PGSE)

    p.-g. spin-echo echo-planar pulse
      sequence
    p.-g. spin-echo technique

pulsed-mode operation
pulsed-wave
    p.-w. Doppler
    p.-w. Doppler echocardiography
    p.-w. Doppler recording
    p.-w. spectral color Doppler signal

pulse-echo
    p.-e. distance measurement
    p.-e. image
    p.-e. imaging
    p.-e. method
    p.-e. technique

pulse-height analyzer (PHA)
pulse-inversion
    p.-i. harmonic imaging (PIHI)
    p.-i. harmonic ultrasound
    p.-i. imaging

PulseMaster laser
12-pulse, 3-phase generator
6-pulse, 3-phase generator
Pulse-Spray
    P.-S. injector
    P.-S. pulsed infusion system

Pulse-Spray/PRO infusion catheter
pulse-spray technique
pulsing current
pulsion
    p. diverticulum
    P. FS laser

Pulsolith
    P. laser
    P. laser lithotripter

pulsus
    p. alternans
    p. paradoxus
    p. tardus et parvus

pulverized
    p. plaque
    p. plaque particulate matter

pulvinar
    p. hip joint
    p. hyperintensity
    p. sign
    p. sign of vCJD
    p. of thalamus

pump
    AutoCAT intraaortic balloon p.
    balloon p.
    efflux p.
    gradient p.
    implantable infusion p.
    intraaortic balloon p. (IABP)
    intraarterial chemotherapy p.
    ion p.
    p. lung

pulmonary artery balloon p.
(PABP)
pulsed p.
punch
Sweet sternal p.
punched-out
p.-o. appearance
p.-o. area
p.-o. bony defect
p.-o. lytic bone lesion
p.-o. ulcer
punch-through
puncta (*pl. of* punctum)
punctata
chondrodysplasia p.
dysplasia epiphysialis p.
nonrhizomelic chondrodysplasia p.
rhizomelic chondrodysplasia p.
punctate
p. calcification
p. enhancement
p. hyperintense focus
p. infiltrate
p. lesion
p. necrosis
p. ulcer
p. white matter hyperintensity
punctation
PunctSURE vascular access imaging
punctum, pl. **puncta**
puncture
antegrade p.
cisternal p.
CT-directed p.
diagnostic p.
direct needle p.
fine-needle p.
p. fracture
p. guidance
lumbar p. (LP)
maxillary sinus p.
nephrostomy p.
p. path
retrograde nephrostomy p.
stereotactic p.
p. transducer
p. ulcer
ultrasound-guided nephrostomy p.
p. wound osteomyelitis
pupillary
p. constrictor muscle
p. sign

pupillometer
Pupilscan II p.
Pupilscan II pupillometer
pure
p. ground glass opacity (pGGO)
p. word alexia
purging
bone marrow p.
immunomagnetic p.
purinoceptor
myocyte membrane p.
purity
radiochemical p.
radioisotopic p.
radionuclide p.
radiopharmaceutical p.
Purkinje fiber
purpose
Low Energy All P. (LEAP)
purse-stringing effect
purulent
p. lesion
p. pleurisy
p. pneumonia
p. salpingitis
p. synovitis
pushability
stent p.
pushable coil
push maneuver
push-pull
p.-p. ankle stress view
p.-p. hip view
pustulotic arthroosteitis
putamen, pl. **putamina**
putaminal hemorrhage
putty kidney
PUV
posterior urethral valve
PUVA
posterior urethrovesical angle
psoralen and ultraviolet A
PUVA radiation
PUVA therapy
PV
pulmonic valve
PVA
polyvinyl alcohol
PVA particle
PVB
polyvinyl butyral

NOTES

P

PVC
> polyvinyl chloride
> premature ventricular contraction
> pulmonary venous congestion
>> PVC catheter

PVD
> peripheral vascular disease

PVE
> periventricular echogenicity

PVG
> periventricular gray
>> PVG matter

PVI
> protracted venous infusion

PVL
> periventricular leukomalacia

PVM
> parallel virtual machine

PVP
> polyvinylpyrrolidone
> portal venous-dominant phase
> portal venous phase
> portal venous pressure
>> PVP image

PVR
> peripheral vascular resistance
> perspective volume rendering
> pulmonary vascular resistance
> pulse volume recording
>> PVR fly-through viewing

PVRI
> pulmonary vascular resistance index

PVS
> peritoneovenous shunt

PVST
> prevertebral soft tissue
>> PVST shadow

PVT
> portal vein thrombosis

PW
> posterior wall
> pulse width

P wave-QRS wave ratio (P-QRS ratio)

PWI
> perfusion-weighted imaging

PWP
> pulmonary wedge pressure

PWT
> posterior wall thickness

PXA
> pleomorphic xanthoastrocytoma

pyarthrosis, pl. pyarthroses
pycnodysostosis
pyelectasia
pyelectasis
> fetal p.

pyelitis
> p. cystica
> emphysematous p.

pyelocaliceal, pyelocalyceal
pyelocaliectasis
pyelofluoroscopy
pyelogenic cyst
pyelogram
> dragon p.
> hydrated p.
> infusion p.

pyelographic appearance time
pyelography
> air p.
> antegrade p.
> ascending p.
> drip infusion p.
> p. by elimination
> excretion p.
> excretory intravenous p.
> p. imaging
> infusion p.
> intravenous p. (IVP)
> lateral p.
> needle p.
> percutaneous antegrade p.
> rapid-sequence intravenous p.
> respiration p.
> retrograde p.
> washout p.

pyelolymphatic backflow
pyelolysis
pyelonephritis
> acute focal bacterial p.
> acute suppurative p.
> atrophic p.
> chronic atrophic p.
> emphysematous p. (EPN)
> suppurative p.
> xanthogranulomatous p.

pyeloplasty
pyelorenal backflow
pyeloscopy
pyelostogram
pyelotomy
> Davis intubated p.

pyelotubular backflow
pyeloureteritis cystica
pyeloureterography
pyeloureterostomy
pyelovenous backflow
pyemic embolus
pygopagus twin
Pyle
> P. disease
> P. dysplasia

pyloric
> p. antrum
> p. canal
> p. cap
> p. channel
> p. channel length

p. channel ulcer
p. diameter
p. hypertrophy
p. index
p. insufficiency
p. lymph node
p. muscle
p. orifice
p. outlet
p. outlet obstruction
p. ring
p. sphincter
p. stenosis
p. stricture
p. teat
p. valve
p. volume

pyloroduodenal
p. junction
p. obstruction

pyloroplasty
pylorospasm
infantile p.
persistent p.

pylorus
hypertrophic p.
torus p.

pyocele
pyocephalus
pyoderma granulosa
pyogenic
p. brain abscess
p. cholangitis
p. liver
p. liver abscess
p. osteomyelitis
p. pneumonia

pyometra
pyomyositis
pyonephrosis
pyopneumothorax
pyosalpinx
pyothorax

pyothorax-associated pleural lymphoma
pyoureter ectopic ureterocele
PYP
pyrophosphate
PYP imaging
PYP technetium myocardial scan

pyramid
medullary p.
p. method for ventricular volume
petrous p.
renal medullary p.

pyramidal
p. bone
p. eminence
p. fracture
p. hemorrhagic zone
p. layer of cerebral cortex
p. lobe
p. neuron
p. sign
p. system
p. tract

pyridine
ACS-grade p.

pyridone derivative
pyriform (*var. of* piriform)
pyriformis (*var. of* piriformis)
pyrimidine
p. analog
halogenated p.

pyrogen testing
Pyrolite kit
pyrophosphate (PYP)
p. arthropathy
p. crystal
p. imaging
p. scintigraphy
stannous p.
^{99m}Tc p.
technetium-99m p. (^{99m}Tc-PYP)
p. technetium myocardial scan
tetrasodium p. (TSPP)

NOTES

P

Q
> cardiac output
> quotient
>> Q angle
>> Q space

QCA
> quantitative coronary angiography
> quantitative coronary arteriography

Q-catheter catheterization recording system

Q-complex
> myocardial perfusion imaging Q-c.

QCSI
> quantitative chemical shift imaging

QCT
> quantitative computed tomography
>> QCT bone densitometry system
>> QCT imaging
>> QCT 3000 system for bone densitometry

QDA
> quadratic discriminant analysis

QDE
> quantum detection efficiency

QDR-1500 bone densitometer

QDR-2000 bone densitometer

QECT
> quantitative contrast-enhanced computed tomography

QEEG
> quantitative electroencephalography

QF
> quality factor

QGS
> quantitative gated SPECT

QHS
> quantitative hepatobiliary scintigraphy

QM
> quantization matrix

qMRI, QMRI
> quantitative magnetic resonance imaging

QO₂
> oxygen consumption

QPD
> quadrature phase detector

QR pattern

QRS
> QRS interval
> QRS score
> QRS synchronized shock
> QRS vector

QRST angle

Q-switched
> Q-s. Nd:YAG laser
> Q-s. ruby laser

Q-switching

QuaDDS-QP2 stent

QuaDDS stent

Quad 7000, 12000 high-field open MRI scanner

quadrangle cartilage

quadrangulation of Frouin

quadrant
> q. of death
> q. energy
> left lower q. (LLQ)
> left upper q. (LUQ)
> lower inner q. (LIQ)
> lower outer q. (LOQ)
> lower right q. (LRQ)
> outer upper right q. (OURQ)
> right lower q. (RLQ)
> right upper q. (RUQ)
> upper inner q. (UIQ)
> upper left q. (ULQ)
> upper outer q. (UOQ)
> upper right q. (URQ)

quadrantal

4-quadrant bar pattern

quadrate
> q. gyrus
> q. ligament
> q. lobe of liver
> q. muscle

quadratic
> q. dependence
> q. discriminant analysis (QDA)
> q. phase gain

quadrature
> q. body coil
> q. cervical spine coil
> q. detection
> q. excitation
> q. head coil
> q. phase detector (QPD)
> q. phase detector artifact
> q. radiofrequency receiver coil
> q. setting
> q. surface coil MRI system
> q. terminal latency surface coil
> q. transmit/receive head coil

quadratus
> q. femoris
> q. femoris fascia
> q. lumborum
> q. plantae
> pronator q.

quad resonance NMR probe circuit

quadriceps
> q. apron

quadriceps *(continued)*
  q. femoris
  q. femoris tendon reflex test
  q. muscle
  q. tendon
  q. tendon tear
quadricuspid
  q. aortic valve
  q. pulmonary valve
quadrigeminal
  q. plate
  q. plate cistern
  q. segment of posterior cerebral artery
  q. vein
quadrigeminy
quadrilateral
  q. bone
  q. brim
  q. plate
  q. retinoblastoma
  q. space syndrome
quadrilocular
quadripartite
quadriplegia
quadriplegic
quadripolar
  q. nucleus
  q. signal broadening
quadripole
quadrisect
quadrisection
quadritubercular
quadrupole moment
QuaDS drug-eluting stent
Quain fatty degeneration of heart
qualitative
  q. analysis
  q. assessment
  q. index
  q. study
quality
  q. factor (QF)
  image q.
quanta *(pl. of* quantum)
quantification
  acoustic q.
  automated q.
  flow q.
  rapid fluid q.
  shunt q.
quantimeter
quantitative
  q. amniotic fluid volume
  q. analysis
  q. brain imaging
  q. cardiac perfusion
  q. chemical shift imaging (QCSI)
  q. computed tomography (QCT)

  q. contrast-enhanced computed tomography (QECT)
  q. coronary angiography (QCA)
  q. coronary arteriography (QCA)
  q. CT densitometry
  q. CT during expiration
  q. digital radiography
  q. Doppler assessment
  q. electroencephalography (QEEG)
  q. exercise thallium-201 variable
  q. fluorescence imaging
  q. gated SPECT (QGS)
  q. hepatobiliary scintigraphy (QHS)
  q. image processing system (QUIPS)
  q. imaging of perfusion using a single subtraction
  q. imaging technique
  q. index
  q. Levovist myocardial contrast echocardiography
  q. lung perfusion imaging
  q. magnetic resonance imaging (qMRI, QMRI)
  q. magnetization transfer
  q. multilevel mapping
  q. regional myocardial flow measurement
  q. region lung function study
  q. scan
  q. spirometrically controlled CT
  q. spirometrically controlled CT imaging
  q. track etch autoradiography
quantitization
  vector q.
quantity
  spectrophotometric q.
quantization
  q. error
  q. matrix (QM)
  q. matrix scaling
  sequential scalar q. (SSQ)
  wavelet scalar q. (WSQ)
quantizer-design algorithm
quantum, pl. **quanta**
  q. detection efficiency (QDE)
  q. energy
  q. limit
  q. Monorail balloon catheter
  q. mottle
  q. mottle index
  q. mottling pattern
  q. noise
  q. number
  q. sink
  q. theory
  q. unit

Q

Quant-X color quantification imaging tool
quarter-detector offset
3-quarters prone position
quartisect
quartz
>   q. glass
>   q. lamp

quasiaccelerated fractionation
quasiradiographic image
Queckenstedt sign
quellung reaction
Quénu-Muret sign
questionable lesion
QueST stent
quick
>   Q. CT9800 scanner
>   Q. Spin Sephadex G-50 column

Quick-Core
>   Q.-C. biopsy needle
>   Q.-C. biopsy system

QuickSeal femoral arterial closure system
quiescence

Quik-Prep
>   Quinton Q.-P.

Quimby implant system
Quinby classification of pelvic fracture
Quincke
>   Q. sign
>   Q. spinal needle

Quintero umbilical artery blood flow stage 1–4
quinti
>   abductor digiti q. (ADQ)
>   extensor digiti q. (EDQ)

Quinton
>   Q. PermCath
>   Q. Quik-Prep

QUIPS
>   quantitative image processing system

Quotane
quotient (Q)
>   amnionic head q. (AHQ)
>   Rayleigh q.

QUS-2 calcaneal ultrasonometer
Q-wave myocardial infarct
QX/I CT scanner

NOTES

R

radius
resistance
roentgen
root

R1

longitudinal relaxivity

R2

transverse relaxivity

r

roentgen

RA

right atrium
rotational angiography
rotational atherectomy
Integris 3D RA

Ra

radium

^{226}Ra

radium 226
^{226}Ra needle

RAA

right atrial appendage

RAB

remote afterloading brachytherapy

rabbit ear strand

racemose

r. aneurysm
r. cyst

racetrack microtron accelerator

rachioscoliosis

rachischisis of atlas

rachitic

r. pelvis
r. rosary

RAD

radiation-absorbed dose
reactive airway disease
right axis deviation

rad

radian
radiation adsorbed dose
rad surface dose

radarkymography

radiability

radiable

radiad

radial

r. anular tear
r. aplasia
r. artery to cephalic vein fistula
r. blurring
r. bone
r. breast scar
r. bursa

r. collateral ligament
r. deviation
r. digital artery
r. drift
r. epiphysial displacement
r. facing of metacarpal head
r. fossa
r. glial fiber
r. head
r. head fracture
r. head subluxation
r. height
r. inclination
r. length
r. metacarpal ligament
r. neck fracture
r. neck groove
r. plane
r. pulse
r. ray anomaly
r. ray defect
r. resistive force
r. ridge
r. scar
r. scarlike mammographic
    appearance
r. sclerosing lesion
r. shift
r. sigmoid notch
r. split tear
r. styloid fracture
r. styloid process
r. technique
r. tuberosity
r. vascular thermal injury
r. width

radialis

flexor carpi r.
r. sign

radialized

radian (rad)

radiant energy

radiate sternocostal ligament

radiation

adjuvant r.
r. adsorbed dose (rad)
afterloading r.
alpha r.
annihilation r.
background r.
backscattered r.
r. barrier
r. beam
r. beam monitor
beta r.

radiation *(continued)*
r. biology
bone injury r.
braking r.
bremsstrahlung r.
r. burn
r. carcinogenesis
r. cataract
Cerenkov r.
characteristic r.
r. chemistry
r. chimera
corpuscular r.
cosmic r.
r. counter
cyclotron r.
r. cystitis
r. detector
diagnostic r.
direct r.
dose equivalent r.
R. Dose in Interventional
  Radiology (RAD-IR)
r. dose perturbation
r. dosimetry
r. dosimetry calculation
r. dosimetry of 18F-fluorocholine
r. effect
electromagnetic r.
r. energy
r. enhancement
r. enteritis
r. enteropathy
r. erythema
r. exposure
external beam r.
fatal dose of r.
r. fistula
fractionated r.
gamma r.
r. gastritis
r. of Gratiolet
r. hepatitis
heterogeneous r.
high linear energy transfer r.
homogeneous r.
r. hormesis
Huldshinsky r.
hyperfractionated r.
hysterectomy and r. (H&R)
infrared r.
r. injury
r. intensity
r. interrogation
interstitial r.
intracoronary artery r.
ionization r.
ionizing r.
K r.

r. leakage
man-made environmental r.
Maxwell theory of r.
megavoltage r.
monochromatic synchrotron r.
monoenergetic r.
r. myelitis
r. myelopathy
natural r.
r. necrosis
r. nephritis
r. nephropathy
neutron r.
nonionizing r.
nuclear radiationoccupational r.
r. oncogenesis
r. oncology
optic r.
r. osteitis
r. osteonecrosis
photon theory of r.
r. physics
r. pneumonia
r. pneumonitis
r. poisoning
polychromatic r.
r. port
r. portal
prenatal r.
primary r.
r. proctopathy
r. protection
protracted r.
PUVA r.
radiofrequency r.
recoil r.
rectum r.
remnant r.
r. response (RR)
r. risk
Rollier r.
scatter r.
scattered r.
secondary r.
r. seed
r. sensitivity testing
r. sensitizer
r. sickness
solar r.
specific r.
spontaneous r.
r. stenosis
stray r.
superficial r.
supervoltage r.
synchrotron r.
r. synovectomy
terrestrial r.
therapeutic external r.

R

r. therapy (RT)
r. therapy planning (RTP)
r. therapy planning system
r. therapy sequela
r. therapy system (RTS)
thermal r.
thorny bone r.
tissue tolerance to r.
r. treatment planning (RTP)
ultraviolet r.
useful-beam r.
r. warning symbol
r. weighting factor
white r.
whole-body r. (WBR)
r. window
radiation-associated papillary tumor
radiation-attenuating surgical glove
radiation-induced
　　r.-i. cancer
　　r.-i. carcinoma
　　r.-i. cerebral atrophy
　　r.-i. cerebral necrosis
　　r.-i. change
　　r.-i. colitis
　　r.-i. fibrosis (RIF)
　　r.-i. ischemia
　　r.-i. leukoencephalopathy
　　r.-i. liver disease (RILD)
　　r.-i. necrosis (RIN)
　　r.-i. pericarditis
　　r.-i. peripheral nerve tumor
　　r.-i. pulmonary toxicity
　　r.-i. sarcoma
　　r.-i. sclerosing adenosis
　　r.-i. skin injury
　　r.-i. ulcer
　　r.-i. upregulation
radiation-related
　　r.-r. ischemia
　　r.-r. ischemic change
　　r.-r. optic neuropathy (RON)
radiation-treated astrocytoma
radical
　　free r.
　　heterocyclic free r.
　　r. irradiation
　　leucine r.
　　nitroxide-stable free r.
　　organic free r.
　　r. parametrectomy

stable free r.
r. vulvectomy
radices (*pl. of* radix)
radiciform
radicular
　　r. artery
　　r. compression
　　r. cyst
　　r. vessel
radiculomedullary artery
radiculomeningeal fistula
radiculomyelitis
radiculopathy
　　cervical spondylotic r.
radiculospinal artery
radiferous
Radifocus
　　R. Glidecath
　　R. Glidewire
　　R. hydrophilic coated guidewire
radii (*pl. of* radius)
Radinyl
radioactive
　　r. aerosol
　　r. atom
　　r. bolus
　　r. brain scan
　　r. cancer-specific targeting agent
　　r. cobalt
　　r. colloid
　　r. constant (Λ)
　　^{11}C palmitic acid r.
　　r. cyanocobalamin
　　r. decay
　　r. disintegration
　　r. effluents
　　r. element
　　r. emission
　　r. equilibrium
　　r. fallout
　　r. fibrinogen imaging
　　r. fibrinogen scan
　　r. gallium
　　r. gas
　　r. half-life
　　r. iodide conversion ratio
　　r. iodinated serum albumin (RISA)
　　r. iodinated serum albumin scan
　　r. iodine
　　r. iodine ablation
　　r. iodine scan
　　r. iodine uptake (RAIU)

NOTES

radioactive *(continued)*
  r. iron
  r. isotope
  r. isotope imaging agent
  r. label
  r. labeling
  r. lead
  r. material
  r. metal
  r. nuclide
  r. phosphorus
  r. radon
  r. renogram test
  r. seeding
  r. series
  r. sodium
  r. source
  r. stent
  r. string marker
  r. strontium
  r. sulfur
  r. tag
  r. thorium
  r. tracer
  r. xenon clearance
  r. xenon gas inhalation
radioactively tagged
radioactivity
  artificial r.
  r. detection
  r. distribution
  induced r.
  natural r.
  r. per volume
  unit of r.
radioactor
radioaerosol
  r. clearance
  r. imaging study
radioanaphylaxis
radioassay
radioautogram
radioautograph
radioautography
radiobe
radiobioassay
radiobiologic, radiobiological
radiobiologist
radiobiology
radiocalcium
radiocapitellar
  r. articulation
  r. joint
  r. joint ganglion
  r. line
radiocarbon
radiocarcinogenesis
radiocardiogram
radiocardiography

radiocarpal
  r. angle
  r. articulation
  r. compartment
  r. dislocation
  r. joint
  r. ligament
  r. portal
radioccipital
radiocephalic
radiocephalpelvimetry
radiocesium
radiochemical
  r. purity
  r. study
radiochemistry
radiochemotherapy
radiochemy
radiochlorine
radiocholangiography
radiocholecystography
radiocholesterol scanning
radiochroism
radiochromatography
radiochromic
  r. dosimetry medium
  r. film
radiocineangiocardiography
radiocineangiography
radiocinematograph
radiocinematography
radiocobalt
radiocolloid
  r. lymphoscintigraphy
  r. mapping
radiocontaminant
radiocontrast
radiocontrast-associated
radiocontrast-induced
  r.-i. injury
  r.-i. nephropathy
radiocurability
radiocurable
radiode
radiodense lesion
radiodensity area
radiodermatitis
radiodermatography
radiodiagnosis
radiodiagnostics
radiodiaphane
radiodigital
radioelectrocardiogram
radioelectrocardiograph
radioelectrocardiography
radioelement
  r. solution
  surface application of r.
radioencephalogram

R

radioencephalography
radioenzyme
radioepidermitis
radioepithelitis
radiofibrinogen uptake scan
radiofluorinated
radiofluorine
radiofrequency (RF, rf)
   r. ablation (RFA)
   r. ablation therapy
   r. absorption
   r. balloon
   r. catheter ablation (RFCA)
   r. coil
   r. electromagnetic field
   r. energy
   r. excitation pulse
   r. gangliolysis
   gaussian r.
   r. generator
   r. hyperthermia
   r. lesion
   r. magnetic shield
   r. modification transcatheter
   r. overflow artifact
   r. percutaneous myocardial
     revascularization (RF-PMR)
   r. period
   r. pulse
   r. radiation
   r. radiogenic leukopenia
   r. radiogold
   r. radiographic control
   r. radiographic hallmark
   r. saturation band
   r. screen
   sinc-Hanning r.
   r. spatial distribution problem
     reconstruction artifact
   r. spin-echo
   r. spoiled 3D GRE sequence
   r. spoiled Fourier-acquired steady
     state (RF-FAST)
   r. spoiling
   r. subsystem
   r. thermal ablation
   r. tongue base reduction
   r. transmitter-receiver coil
   r. wave
radiogallium
radiogenesis
radiogenic leukopenia

radiogold
   r. colloid
   radiofrequency r.
radiogram
radiogrammetry
radiograph (See radiography)
   axial r.
   biplane r.
   bitewing r.
   cephalometric r.
   Code and Carlson r.
   coned-down r.
   contact r.
   conventional r.
   decubitus r.
   digital abdominal r.
   digital chest r.
   digitally reconstructed r. (DRR)
   double-contrast r.
   dual-energy r. (DER)
   erect lateral flexion/extension r.
   extraoral r.
   frontal cephalometric r.
   internal oblique r.
   intraoral r.
   lateral cephalometric r.
   lateral decubitus r.
   lateral flexion/extension r.
   lateral oblique jaw r.
   lateral ramus r.
   lateral skull r.
   maxillary sinus r.
   mortise r.
   oblique r.
   occlusal r.
   outlet view r.
   panoramic r.
   periapical r.
   phantom r.
   plain r.
   scout r.
   scout digital r.
   soft tissue r.
   spot r.
   submentovertex r.
   supine r.
   survey r.
   tangent r.
   Trendelenburg r.
   tunnel r.
   Waters view r.
radiographer

NOTES

radiographic
- r. baseline
- r. blurring
- r. cephalometry
- r. contrast
- r. contrast media-induced nephropathy
- r. control
- r. criterion
- r. density
- r. distention
- r. effect
- r. and fluoroscopic (R&F)
- r. image
- r. interpretation
- r. mottle
- r. noise
- r. parallel line shadow
- r. pathology
- r. pelvimetry
- r. penetration
- r. pincushion distortion
- r. projection
- r. spiculation
- r. stability of lesion

radiographically
- r. firm synostosis
- r. normal imaging
- r. occult fracture

radiographic-dense breast

radiography
- advanced multiple-beam equalization r. (AMBER)
- air-gap r.
- barium r.
- bedside r.
- biomedical r.
- body section r.
- cardiac r.
- computed r. (CR)
- computed dental r. (CDR)
- computerized r.
- contrast r.
- dental r.
- diagrammatic r.
- digital r. (DR)
- digital video gastrointestinal r.
- direct digital r.
- double-contrast r.
- electron r.
- filmless r.
- film-screen r.
- flexion-extension r.
- gamma r.
- high-resolution, low-speed r.
- horizontal-beam r.
- interventional r.
- intraoperative r.
- intraoral periapical r.

- magnification r.
- mobile r.
- moving slot r.
- mucosal relief r.
- musculoskeletal r.
- neonatal r.
- neutron r.
- pan-oral r.
- panoramic r.
- photostimulable phosphor computed r.
- photostimulable phosphor dental r.
- plain abdominal r. (PAR)
- portable r.
- postrelease r.
- postvoid r.
- quantitative digital r.
- rapid serial r.
- scanned projection r. (SPR)
- scanning equalization r.
- sectional r.
- selective r.
- selenium r.
- serial r.
- slit r.
- soft-copy computed r.
- specimen r.
- spot film r.
- stereoscopic r.
- stress r.
- video digital gastrointestinal r.

radioguided
- r. laparotomy
- r. parathyroidectomy
- r. surgery

radiohepatographic

radiohumeral
- r. articulation
- r. bursitis
- r. meniscus

radioimmunity

radioimmunoassay (RIA)
- r. method
- scintillation proximity r.

radioimmunoconjugate

radioimmunodetection (RAID)

radioimmunodiffusion

radioimmunoguided surgery (RIGS)

radioimmunoimaging

radioimmunolocalization

radioimmunoluminography

radioimmunoprecipitation test

radioimmunoscintigraphy

radioimmunosorbent

radioimmunotherapy

radioinduced sarcoma

radioinduction

radioiodide

radioiodinated serum albumin (RISA)

radioiodination
  direct r.
  electrophilic r.
radioiodine
  r. test
  r. uptake
radioiron
  r. oral absorption
  r. red cell utilization
radioisotope
  r. calibrator
  r. camera
  carrier-free r.
  cistern r.
  r. cisternography
  r. cisternography imaging
  r. delivery system (RDS)
  r. gallium imaging
  Gd-DTPA r.
  r. indium-labeled white blood cell
    imaging
  r. labeling
  r. lung scan
  r. renogram test
  r. scanner
  r. scanning
  r. scintigraphy
  r. stent
  r. synovectomy
  r. technetium imaging
  transplutonium r.
  trapping of r.
  r. uptake
  r. voiding cystogram
radioisotopic purity
radiokymography
radiolabel
radiolabeled
  r. antibody
  r. antibody imaging
  r. anti-CEA
  r. antisense oligonucleotide
  r. compound
  r. estrogen analog
  r. fibrinogen
  r. marker substrate
  r. MoAb
  r. MoAb imaging agent
  r. peptide alpha-M^2
  r. platelet
  r. water study
  r. WBCs

radiolabeling
  area of increased r.
radiolead
radiolesion
radioligand
  PET r.
radiologic
  r. anatomy
  r. diagnosis
  r. guidance
  r. percutaneous gastrostomy
  r. stigmata
  r. technology
radiological contrast medium
radiologic-anatomic correlation
radiologic-histopathologic study
radiologic-pathologic
  r.-p. concordance
  r.-p. correlation
  r.-p. discordance
radiology
  American College of R. (ACR)
  cardiovascular r.
  chest r.
  computed r. (CR)
  dental r.
  diagnostic r.
  intraoral r.
  neurointerventional r.
  oral r.
  r. outcomes data
  pediatric r.
  percutaneous interventional r.
  polytomographic r.
  Radiation Dose in Interventional R.
    (RAD-IR)
  radionuclide r.
  skeletal r.
  Society of Interventional R.
  storage phosphor r.
  r. telephone access system
  therapeutic r.
radiolucency
  linear band of maximal r.
  prominent rim of r.
  relative r.
  soap-bubble r.
radiolucent
  r. area
  r. cleft
  r. crescent line
  r. density

NOTES

radiolucent *(continued)*
    r. fat
    r. fat halo
    r. focus
    r. gallstone
    r. joint space
    r. lesion
    r. linear filling defect
    r. medium
    r. operating room table extension
    r. plastic occluder
    r. pneumomediastinum
    r. roll
    r. spine frame
    r. stone
radiolunate articulation
radiolunotriquetral ligament
radiolymphoscintigraphy
    intraoperative r.
radiolysis
radiomedullary artery
radiometallography
radiometer
    pastille r.
    photographic r.
radiometric
    r. analysis
    r. assay
radiomicrometer
radiomimetic
radiomuscular
radiomutation
radion
radionecrosis
    cerebral r.
radioneuritis
Radionics CRW stereotactic head frame
radionitrogen
radionuclear venography
radionucleotide
    positron-emitting r.
radionuclide
    absorption of r.
    r. angiocardiography
    r. angiogram (RNA)
    r. angiography
    r. blood flow study
    r. bone scan
    r. bone scintigraphy
    r. camera
    r. cardiography
    r. carrier
    carrier added r.
    carrier free r.
    r. carrier system
    r. cerebral angiogram
    r. cholescintigraphy
    r. cineangiography
    r. cisternography

    concentration of r.
    r. contamination
    r. cystogram
    r. cystography
    r. ejection fraction
    r. emission tomography
    r. esophageal dead time
    r. esophagram
    r. flow scan
    r. generator
    gold-195m r.
    r. inflammation
    inhaled r.
    r. injection
    r. label
    r. liver scan
    lung perfusion r.
    r. mammography
    metastable r.
    r. milk imaging
    r. milk scan
    no-carrier-added r.
    parent r.
    r. production
    r. purity
    r. radiology
    renal r.
    r. renal imaging
    r. renography imaging
    r. scanning
    r. shuntogram
    r. signal
    r. stenosis
    r. stroke volume
    r. synovectomy
    r. table
    r. testicular scintigraphy
    r. therapy
    r. thyroid imaging
    r. thyroid scan
    uptake of r.
    r. venography
    ventilation r.
    r. ventriculogram (RNV, RVG)
    r. voiding cystourethrography
    r. voiding study
radionuclide-gated
    r.-g. blood pool imaging
    r.-g. blood pool scan
radiopacity
    linear r.
radiopaque
    r. bone cement
    r. contrast media (ROCM)
    r. density
    r. distal tip
    r. drain
    r. fluid extravasation
    r. foreign body

r. gold marker
r. imaging agent
r. lesion
r. marker
r. medium
r. medium thorium dioxide
r. pellet
r. pseudocapsule
r. urine
r. vesical calculus
r. wire of counteroccluder buttonhole
r. xenon gas
radioparency
radioparent
radiopathology
radiopelvimetry
radiopharmaceutical
r. ablation
r. agent
brain imaging r.
r. chemistry
r. dacryocystography
diagnostic r.
r. dose
r. dosimetry
r. localization
PET r.
r. production
r. purity
r. quality control
r. synovectomy
^{99m}Tc-ECD r.
^{99m}Tc-HMPAO r.
^{99m}Tc-iminodiacetic acid derivative r.
^{99m}Tc-MAG3 r.
^{99m}Tc-MIBI r.
^{99m}Tc polyphosphate compound r.
technetium-99m isonitriles r.
r. therapy
trace amount of r.
r. tracer
r. uptake
r. voiding cystogram
r. volume-dilution technique
radiopharmacy
radiophobia
radiophosphate
radiophosphorus
radiophotography
radiophylaxis

radiopotassium
radiopotentiation
radioprotectant
radioprotective agent
radioprotector
radiopulmonography
radioreaction
radioreceptor
radioresistance
radioresistant
radioresponsiveness
radioscaphocapitate ligament
radioscaphoid
r. articulation
r. joint
r. ligament
radioscapholunate ligament
radioscintigraphy
radioscopy
radiosensibility
radiosensitiveness
radiosensitive tumor
radiosensitivity
fibroblast r.
radiosensitization
radiosensitizer
carbogen r.
halogenated thymidine analog r.
nicotinamide r.
radiosodium
radiospirometry
radiostereoscopy
radiostrontium
radiostyloid process
radiosulfur
radiosurgery
Bragg peak r.
charged-particle r.
dynamic stereotactic r.
gamma knife r.
heavy-charged particle Bragg peak r.
image-guided r.
interstitial r.
LINAC r.
modified linear accelerator r.
multiarc LINAC r.
stereotactic r. (SRS)
Winston-Lutz for LINAC-based r.
radiotellurium
radiotherapeutic agent

NOTES

radiotherapist
radiotherapy, radiation therapy (RT)
   arc r.
   AVM r.
   computerized r.
   contact r.
   continuous hyperfractionated
     accelerated r.
   3-dimensional conformal r.
   dynamic r.
   electron-beam intraoperative r.
     (EBIORT)
   extended-field r.
   external beam r.
   fast neutron r.
   r. field placement
   fractionated stereotactic r. (FSR)
   hemibody r.
   high-dose r.
   high-voltage r.
   hyperfractionated r.
   iceberg r.
   interstitial r.
   intracavitary r.
   intraoperative r.
   inverted Y field r.
   large-field r.
   r. localization
   locoregional field r.
   mantle r.
   megavoltage r.
   neoadjuvant r.
   orthovoltage r.
   r. port
   postoperative r. (PORT)
   preoperative r.
   rotational r.
   salvage r.
   short-distance r.
   skeletal targeted r. (STR)
   split-course accelerated r.
   stereotactic r.
   supervoltage r.
   teletherapy r.
   whole-body r.
   whole-brain r. (WBRT)
   r. with hyperthermia
   r. without hyperthermia
radiothermy
radiothorium
radiothyroidectomy
radiothyroxin
radiotomy
radiotoxemia
radiotoxicity
radiotracer
   r. accumulation
   r. activity
   decreased uptake of r.

   r. deposition
   r. foil method
   increased uptake of r.
   ^{99m}Tc-HMPAO r.
   r. technique
   r. uptake
radiotransparency
radiotransparent
radiotropic
radioulnar
   r. articulation
   r. joint
   r. proximodistal translation
   r. subluxation
   r. surface
RAD-IR
   Radiation Dose in Interventional
   Radiology
   RAD-IR study
radium (Ra)
   r. beam therapy
   r. emanation
   intracavitary r.
   r. necrosis
   r. radioactive source
radium 226 (^{226}Ra)
radius, pl. radii (R)
   Bohr r.
   r. of curvature
   r. hypoplasia
   sigmoid cavity of r.
radix, pl. radices
radix-2 algorithm
RadNet radiology information system
radon (Rn)
   r. 222 (^{222}Rn, Rn-222)
   r. progeny
   radioactive r.
   r. seed implantation
RadPICC catheter
RadStat hemostasis device
RADstation radiology workstation
radwaste radioactivity detection
RAE
   right atrial enlargement
Raeder paratrigeminal syndrome
Rael cell
RAGE
   rapid gradient echo
ragged urethra
ragpicker's disease
RAID
   radioimmunodetection
Raider triangle
RAILL test
railroad
   r. track appearance
   r. track calcification
   r. track ductus arteriosus

r. track pattern
r. track sign
railway spine
ralser
stress r.
RAIU
radioactive iodine uptake
rake ulcer
RAM
reduced-acquisition matrix
Raman spectroscopy
Ramesh and Pramod algorithm
rami (*pl. of* ramus)
ramification
ramify
ramp
r. down
r. filter
folded step r.
maximum slew rate r.
r. reconstruction
r. time
r. up
ramp-filtered back projection
ramping
Ramsay
R. Hunt cerebellar myoclonic
dyssynergia
R. Hunt syndrome
ramus, pl. **rami**
dorsal primary r.
inferior pubic r.
r. intermedius artery
r. intermedius artery branch
ischiopubic r.
r. of ischium
r. of lateral sulcus
mandibular r.
r. medialis artery
r. medialis artery branch
pubic r.
superior r.
superior pubic r.
ventral primary r.
Ranawat method
Randall plaque
Rand microballoon
random
r. coincidence event
r. count
r. error

r. motion
r point
randomized clinical trial (RCT)
Ranfac cholangiographic catheter
range
absorbed dose r.
r. ambiguity artifact
dynamic r.
emission r.
frequency r.
gray-scale r.
normal r.
positron r.
reference r.
r. resolution
slew r.
therapeutic r.
water r.
range-gated
r.-g. Doppler spectral flow analysis
r.-g. pulsed Doppler
ranging
echo r.
ranine vein
rank
Spearman r.
Ranke
R. angle
R. complex
ranula
Ranvier
R. groove
R. node
RAO
right anterior oblique
RAP
right atrial pressure
Rapamune
Rapamycin
rapamycin
raphe
abdominal r.
amnionic r.
anococcygeal r.
anogenital r.
longitudinal r.
median r.
palpebral r.
penile r.
posterior fossa malformations, facial
hemangiomas, arterial anomalies,
cardiac anomalies and aortic

NOTES

R

raphe *(continued)*
    coarctation, eye anomalies, and
    sternal clefting and/or
    supraumbilical r. (PHACES)
    pterygomandibular r.
    scrotal r.
    tendinous r.
    unicusp with central r.
RAPI
    resting ankle pressure index
rapid
    r. acquisition computed tomography
    r. acquisition spin echo (RASE)
    r. acquisition with relaxation
    enhancement (RARE)
    r. axial MR imaging
    r. biplane angiocardiography
    r. computed tomography
    r. deceleration injury
    r. dephasing
    r. dissolution formula
    r. distribution
    r. early repolarization phase
    r. exchange (RX)
    r. filling (RF, rf)
    r. filling period
    r. filling wave (RFW)
    r. film changer
    r. fluid expansion
    r. fluid quantification
    r. gantry rotation
    r. gradient echo (RAGE)
    r. gradient reversal
    r. half-Fourier T2-weighted image
    r. image transfer
    r. inspiratory flow rate
    r. oscillatory motion
    r. pull-through technique (RPT)
    r. scan technique
    r. screen
    r. sequential CT scan
    r. serial radiography
    r. telephone access system (RTAS)
    r. thoracic compression technique
    r. tracer washout
    R. Transit catheter
    R. Transit microcatheter
    r. ventricular filling phase
    r. ventricular rate
    r. ventricular response
rapid computed tomography
rapid-excitation MR imaging
Rapid-Scan Spectrometery
RapidScreen
    R. RS-2000 CAD
    R. RS-2000 x-ray equipment
rapid-sequence
    r.-s. imaging

    r.-s. intravenous pyelography
    r.-s. IVP
Rapidtransit microcatheter
Rappaport classification
RAR
    renal-aortic ratio
RARE
    rapid acquisition with relaxation
    enhancement
    RARE sequence
    single-shot thick-slab RARE
    RARE technique
RARE-derived pulse sequence
rare-earth
    r.-e. scintillator
    r.-e. screen
rarefaction
    bony r.
    r. of cortex
    fluffy r.
    osseous r.
rarefied area
RAS
    renal artery stenosis
RASE
    rapid acquisition spin echo
Rashkind
    R. double umbrella device
    R. occluder
Rasmussen
    R. encephalitis
    R. mycotic aneurysm
raster
    r. frequency
    r. line
    r. period
    r. spacing error
    R. stereo photography
rat-bite erosion
ratchet
rate
    ACR r.
    r. analysis
    atrial r. (AR)
    count r.
    digital sampling r.
    dipole-dipole relaxation r.
    disintegration r.
    exogenous glucose r.
    flow r.
    glomerular filtration r. (GFR)
    gradient slew r.
    high-dose r. (HDR)
    high frame r.
    inspiratory flow r.
    instantaneous enhancement r.
    intraoperative high dose r.
    (IOHDR)
    lipid fraction relaxation r.

low frame r.
LVOT flow r.
magnet r.
maximum midexpiratory flow r. (MMFR)
maximum predicted heart r. (MPHR)
mean circumferential fiber shortening r. (MCFSR)
r. meter (R-meter)
oscillatory shear r.
oxygen extraction r. (OER)
patency r.
peak filling r. (PFR)
plasma radioiron disappearance r.
plasma radioiron turnover r.
predicted target heart r.
proliferation r.
pulsed dose r. (PDR)
rapid inspiratory flow r.
rapid ventricular r.
relaxation r.
shear strain r.
Solomon-Bloembergen theory of dipole-dipole relaxation r.
specific absorption r. (SAR)
spirometer flow r.
standby r.
stone-free r.
stroke ejection r.
time-to-peak filling r. (TPFR)
transverse relaxation r.
ultra-low dose r. (ULDR)
valley-to-peak dose r.
variable response r.
ventricular r.

ratemeter
Rathke

R. cleft cyst
R. duct
R. pouch
R. pouch tumor

ratio

adenoidal-nasopharyngeal r. (AN)
adrenal-spleen r. (ASR)
ankle-brachial pressure r.
aortic root r.
aortic valve opening to aortic valve closing r. (AO/AC)
apnea-bradycardia r.
artery-aortic velocity r.
artery bronchus r. (ABR)

bicaudate r.
blank-to-trues r.
blood-to-fat contrast r.
blood-to-myocardium contrast r.
bone age r.
bone and limb growth velocity r.
brain Glx/Cr r.
brain-to-background r.
branching r.
bronchus-to-pulmonary artery r.
cardiothoracic r. (CT, CTR)
carpal content r.
carpal height r.
r. of caudate to right hepatic lobe
cerebral blood volume to cerebral blood flow r. (CBV-CBF)
chemical shift r.
compression r.
conduction r.
contrast-to-noise r. (CNR, C/N)
conversion r.
cord subarachnoid space r.
CT r.
diaphysial bone length r.
diastolic velocity r.
differential uptake r.
distention r.
dome-to-neck r.
dose nonuniformity r. (DNR)
E-A wave r.
end-systolic pressure-end-systolic volume r. (ESP-ESV)
end-systolic wall index:end-systolic volume r.
escape-peak r.
Evans r.
false-negative r.
false-positive r.
flattening r. (FR)
gray-to-white matter activity r.
gray-to-white matter contrast r.
gray-to-white matter utilization r.
grid r.
gyromagnetic r.
head circumference-to-abdominal circumference r. (HC-AC)
heart count-mediastinum count r. (H-M)
heart-lung r. (HLR)
heart-to-background r.
hilar height r.
Holdaway r.

NOTES

791

ratio *(continued)*
>   inferior-anterior count r.
>   infundibular-bulb r.
>   infundibular systolic/diastolic r.
>   Insall r.
>   Insall-Salvati r.
>   inspiratory to expiratory r. (I-E)
>   inverse inspiratory-expiratory time r.
>   iodine-particle r.
>   isotopic r.
>   kidney length to body height r.
>   (KBR)
>   kidney-to-background r.
>   L-A peak r.
>   L-B r.
>   left atrium-aortic root r. (LA-AR)
>   left ventricular systolic time
>   interval r.
>   lesion-background r.
>   lesion-brain r. (L-B)
>   lesion-countersite r. (L-C)
>   lesion-muscle r.
>   lesion-nonlesion count r.
>   lesion-normal tissue r.
>   likelihood r. (LR)
>   limb bone length r.
>   Lindegaard r.
>   liver-to-aorta peak r.
>   liver-to-liver peak r.
>   liver-to-muscle contrast r.
>   L-LP r.
>   LQ r.
>   magnetization transfer r. (MTR)
>   magnetogyric r.
>   maximum diameter to minimum
>   diameter r.
>   metatarsal length r.
>   myocardium-to-abdomen count r.
>   myoinositol-creatine r. (Mi-Cr)
>   nasal-to-plasma radioactivity r.
>   neutron-atomic number r. (N-2, N-
>   Z)
>   odds r. (OR)
>   off-axis r. (OAR)
>   off-center r. (OCR)
>   optional target-to-background r.
>   orifice-anulus r.
>   P-A r.
>   PASP-SASP r.
>   patellar ligament-patellar r.
>   peak systolic and diastolic r.
>   perimeter-area r. (P-A)
>   peroneal-to-anterior compartment r.
>   phase sampling r. (PSR)
>   r. of photoelectric to Compton
>   absorption
>   pitch r.
>   Poisson r.
>   power r.

>   proportional r.
>   pulmonary artery-bronchus r.
>   pulmonic-systemic flow r.
>   P wave-QRS wave r. (P-QRS)
>   radioactive iodide conversion r.
>   renal-aortic r. (RAR)
>   repetition time to echo time r.
>   (TR-TE)
>   right ventricular to left ventricular
>   systolic pressure r. (RVP-VP)
>   scatter-air r. (SAR)
>   scatter-maximum r. (SMR)
>   scatter-primary r.
>   sensitizer enhancement r.
>   septal-to-free wall r.
>   signal intensity r.
>   signal-to-clutter r.
>   signal-to-noise r. (SNR, S-N, S:N)
>   SI joint-sacrum r.
>   spleen-to-liver r.
>   standardized uptake r. (SUR)
>   stroke count r.
>   stroke volume r.
>   systolic-diastolic r. (S-D)
>   systolic velocity r.
>   target-to-background r.
>   target-to-nontarget r.
>   thallium-to-scalp r.
>   thermal enhancement r. (TER)
>   thickness-diameter of ventricle r.
>   tissue-air r. (TAR)
>   tissue-maximum r. (TMR)
>   tissue-phantom r. (TPR)
>   TME r.
>   r. transformer
>   trapezium-metacarpal eburnation r.
>   tumor-to-gray matter r.
>   tumor-to-normal brain r.
>   tumor-to-white matter r.
>   unfavorable neutron-to-proton r.
>   uptake r. (UR)
>   ventilation-perfusion r.
>   ventricle-brain r. (VBR)

**RatioVision digital fluorescent imaging
system**
Ratliff avascular necrosis classification
rat-tail
>   r.-t. common bile duct
>   r.-t. esophagus

rature
>   r. detector
>   r. surface coil system

Rau
>   apophysis of R.

Rauchfuss triangle
rave
>   fracture en r.

Raw
>   airway resistance

ray

actinic r.
alpha r.
r. amputation
anode r.
beta r.
Bucky r.
r. casting technique
cathode r.
central r. (CR)
chemical r.
corresponding r.
delta r.
digital r.
direct r.
fluorescent r.
gamma r.
glass r.
grenz r.
H r.
hard r.
hypermobile first r.
incident r.
indirect r.
infrared r.
infraroentgen r.
intermediate r.
keV gamma r.
long axis r.
Niewenglowski r.
parallel r.
r. pattern
pollicized r.
positive r.
primary r.
reflected r.
roentgen r.
scattered r.'s
secondary r.
soft r.
r. sum
terahertz r.
r. therapeutic
r. tracing
ultraviolet r.
vertical r.
W r.

ray-casting method

Rayleigh

R. noise
R. quotient

R. scattering
R. scattering law

Rayleigh-Tyndall scattering

Raymond-Cestan syndrome

Raynaud

R. phenomenon
R. syndrome

ray-sum

r.-s. projection
r.-s. view

Ray-Tec x-ray detectable surgical sponge

Rb

rubidium

^{82}Rb, Rb-82

rubidium 82

^{82}Rb-based cardiac imaging

RBBB

right bundle-branch block

RBC

red blood cell
labeled RBC
^{99m}Tc-labeled RBC
^{99m}Tc-tagged RBC
UltraTag RBC

RBE

relative biologic effectiveness

RB-ILD

respiratory bronchiolitis-associated interstitial lung disease

RBL

Reid baseline

RC

retrograde cystogram

RCA

retained cortical activity
right coronary angiography
right coronary artery
rotational coronary atherectomy

rCBF

regional cerebral blood flow
rCBF PET scan

rCBV

regional cerebral blood volume
relative cerebral blood volume

RCM

red cell mass

rCMRO$_2$

regional cerebral metabolic rate for oxygen

rCPP

regional cerebral perfusion pressure

R

NOTES

793

RCT
  randomized clinical trial
Rd
  rutherford
RDF
  rotary door flap
RDPA
  right descending pulmonary artery
RDS
  radioisotope delivery system
  respiratory distress syndrome
RDS-like deficiency
RDX coronary radiation catheter delivery system
RE
  reflux esophagitis
    Biafine RE
Re
  rhenium
^{186}Re
  rhenium 186
^{188}Re
  rhenium 188
    generator-produced ^{188}Re
reabsorption
  r. atelectasis
  bony r.
  sodium r.
reaccumulation
reactance
  capacitive r.
  inductive r. (XL)
reaction
  allergic r.
  anaphylactic r.
  anaphylactoid r.
  annihilation r.
  arrest r.
  biomolecular r.
  chemotoxic r.
  choriodecidual r.
  complex periosteal r.
  Crohn-like lymphoid r.
  dependency r.
  desmoplastic r.
  dystonic r.
  Eisenmenger r.
  endoergic r.
  exoergic r.
  extrapyramidal r.
  first-order r.
  flare r.
  fluffy periosteal r.
  hair-on-end periosteal r.
  hexokinase r.
  hilar r.
  hypersensitivity r.
  idiosyncratic anaphylactoid r.
  inflammatory r.

  interrupted periosteal r.
  Jones-Mote r.
  lamellar periosteal r.
  multilamellar periosteal r.
  nonidiosyncratic anaphylactoid r.
  nuclear r.
  onionskin periosteal r.
  periosteal r.
  photonuclear r.
  pleural r.
  positron matter-antimatter annihilation r.
  quellung r.
  r. recovery time
  sarcoidlike r.
  scar tissue r.
  Schultz r.
  shell-type of periosteal r.
  soft tissue r.
  solid periosteal r.
  sunburst periosteal r.
  symmetric periosteal r.
  thermonuclear r.
  vasomotor r.
  vasovagal r.
  r. vial
reactivation tuberculosis
reactive
  r. airway disease (RAD)
  r. airway dysfunction syndrome
  r. arteriole
  r. arthritis
  r. bone sclerosis
  r. cyst cord
  r. disease of smooth muscle
  r. fibrosis
  r. fibrous lesion
  r. fibrovascular arachnoid proliferation
  r. follicular hyperplasia
  r. gliosis
  r. hyperemia
  r. interface
  r. lymphadenopathy
  r. lymphoid hyperplasia
  r. lymphoid lesion
  r. marrow edema
  r. remodeling
  r. spinal cyst
reactivity
  bronchial r.
reactor
  breeder r.
  fast-breeder r.
reader
  AC 3 plate r.
  first r.
  Immuno-mini NJ-2300 microplate r.
  microplate r.

R

R. paratrigeminal syndrome
plate r.

reading
postradiotherapy implant survey r.
pressure r.
wet r.

readout
r. delay
echo planar r.
r. gradient
steady-state projection imaging with
dynamic echo-train r. (SPIDER)
r. wavelength

ReadyPET support services

reagent
lanthanide shift r. (LSR)
shift r.
splenic r.

REAL
Revised European American Lymphoma
REAL classification

realignment
intrarun r.
patellofemoral r.

Reality Engine graphics

real signal

real-time
r.-t. assessment
r.-t. biplanar needle tracking
r.-t. chirp Z transformer
r.-t. color Doppler imaging
r.-t. compression
r.-t. CT fluoroscopy
r.-t. 2D blood flow imaging
r.-t. 2-dimensional Doppler flow-
imaging system
r.-t. display
r.-t. Doppler
r.-t. 4D ultrasound imaging system
r.-t. echocardiography
r.-t. echo-planar image
r.-t. enhancement
r.-t. format converter
r.-t. magnetic resonance imaging
tracking
r.-t. phase-contrast flow
r.-t. position management (RPM)
r.-t. quantitative flow
r.-t. respiratory feedback
r.-t. scan
r.-t. scan ultrasound
r.-t. sector scanning

r.-t. sonogram
r.-t. sonography
r.-t. ultrasonography
r.-t. volume rendering

rear
r. endoluminal view
r. projection screen

rearfoot varus

rebleeding of aneurysm

rebound
r. excitation
r. sign

rebreathing ventilation scan

recalcitrant

recall
multiplanar gradient r. (MPGR)

recanalization
endovascular r.
endovascular photo acoustic r.
(EPAR)
fallopian tube r.
r. technique
transcervical fallopian tube r.

recanalized
r. artery
r. ductus

recapture
mobile with r.
mobile without r.
stuck with r.
stuck without r.

receive-only circular surface coil

receiver
r. coil
r. dead time
Medtronic radiofrequency r.
r. operating characteristic (ROC)
r. operating characteristic curve
r. operating characteristic method

recent dislocation

receptor
r. binding
r. expression
r. imaging
muscarinic r.

recess
attic r.
azygoesophageal r.
Baumgarten r.
cecal r.
cerebellopontine r.
cochlear r.

NOTES

recess *(continued)*
   costodiaphragmatic r.
   costomediastinal r.
   costophrenic r.
   duodenojejunal r.
   epitympanic r. (EPR)
   hepatorenal r.
   ileocecal r.
   inferior duodenal r.
   infraglenoid r.
   intersigmoid r.
   lacrimal r.
   lateral r.
   lumbosacral lateral r.
   mild r.
   optic r.
   paraduodenal r.
   pericardial sleeve r.
   peritoneal r.
   pharyngeal r.
   piriform r.
   pleural r.
   popliteal r.
   posterior pleural r.
   prestyloid r.
   pulmonary venous r.
   rectouterine r.
   rectovesical r.
   retrocecal r.
   retroduodenal r.
   sacciform r.
   sphenoethmoidal r.
   splenorenal r.
   step-like r.
   sublabral r.
   subphrenic r.
   subscapularis r.
   superior azygoesophageal r.
   superior duodenal r.
   twining r.

recession
   nasion r.
   rib r.

reciprocal
   r. agonist-antagonist relaxation
   r. change
   r. depression
   r. rhythm

reciprocating conduction
reciprocity theorem dose
recirculation peak
RECIST
   Response Evaluation Criteria in Solid
   Tumors

Recklinghausen
   R. disease of bone
   R. tumor

reclining position
recoarctation of aorta

recognizer
   exposure data r. (EDR)

recoil
   r. atom
   r. electron
   r. energy
   r. pressure
   r. radiation

recombinant
   r. thyrotropin contrast agent (rTSH)
   r. tissue plasminogen activator

recon pitch
reconstitution
   artery r.
   r. of blood flow in artery
   r. via profunda artery

reconstructed
   3D acquired/2D r.
   r. image
   r. radiographic imaging

reconstruction
   ACV r.
   adaptive cardiac volume r.
   r. algorithm
   analytic r.
   r. of aorta
   aortic r.
   aortobifemoral r.
   r. artifact
   coronal r.
   curved r.
   curvilinear r.
   3D r.
   3D image r.
   Dor r.
   external gamma dose r.
   fan-beam r.
   Fourier 2-dimensional projection r.
   Fourier transformation r.
   r. from projections imaging
   gated 3D r.
   image r.
   r. interval
   iterative r.
   magnitude r.
   MIP r.
   multiplanar r. (MPR)
   oblique-angle r.
   patch graft r.
   periodically rotated overlapping
    parallel lines with enhanced r.
    (PROPELLER)
   phase-preserving r.
   ramp r.
   renovascular r.
   respiration gated 3D r.
   sagittal r.
   segmental correction using spine r.
   1-sided image r.

single pixel r.
spatial r.
r. study
transanular patch r.
r. view
zygomaticomalar r.

reconstructive imaging
reconstructor
dynamic planar r. (DPR)
dynamic spatial r. (DSR)

recording
color Doppler r.
continuous-wave Doppler r.
pullback pressure r.
pulsed-wave Doppler r.
pulse volume r. (PVR)
segmental limb pressure r.
simultaneous r.
split-screen r.

recovery
arrhythmia-insensitive flow-sensitive
alternating inversion r. (A-FAIR)
cardiac r.
3D turbo fluid-attentuated
inversion r.
fast short tau inversion r.
R. filter
flow-sensitive alternating
inversion r. (FAIR)
fluid-attenuated inversion r.
(FLAIR)
inversion r. (IR)
myocardial r.
R. Nitinol filter
r. period of myocardium
postischemic r.
saturation r. (SR)
selective saturation r.
shape r.
short-inversion-time inversion r.
(STIR)
short tau inversion r. (STIR)
short TI inversion r.
short T1 inversion r. (STIR)
silver r.
spectral presaturation with
inversion r. (SPIR)
r. time (RT)
r. time image
total saturation r. (TSR)
turbo short tau inversion r.
turbo short tau/TI inversion r.

recrudescence
recrudescent tuberculosis
recruitment potential
recta
vasa r.

rectal
r. ampulla
r. balloon
r. carcinoma
r. contrast medium
r. dilatation
r. distention
r. duplication cyst
r. endoscopic ultrasonography
r. endosonography
r. fascia
r. fisting
r. fistula
r. fold
r. intussusception
r. lesion
r. lymph node
r. multiplane transducer
r. muscle cuff
r. narrowing
r. obstruction
r. orifice
r. penetration
r. plexus
r. polyp
r. pouch
r. prolapse
r. radiation injury
r. sheath hematoma
r. shelf
r. stenosis
r. stump
r. tear
r. tip
r. valve
r. vault

rectangular
r. disc
r. field of view
r. phalanx
r. section profile

recti (*gen. and pl. of* rectus)
rectification
full-wave r.
4-valve-tube r.

rectifier
full-wave r.

R

NOTES

rectifier *(continued)*
    silicon-controlled r. (SCR)
    r. subblock
    r. tube
rectilinear
    r. biphasic waveform for external
       defibrillation
    r. bone scan
    r. bone scan imaging
    r. scanner
    r. thyroid scan
    r. tomography
rectocele
rectogenital septum
rectorectal intussusception
rectosigmoid
    r. carcinoma
    r. function
    r. index
    r. junction
    r. manometry
    r. polypoid lesion
rectouterine
    r. fold
    r. fossa
    r. pouch
    r. recess
rectovaginal
    r. fistula
    r. pouch
    r. septum
rectovaginouterine pouch
rectovesical
    r. fistula
    r. pouch
    r. recess
    r. septum
rectum
    benign lymphoma of r.
    Hartmann closure of r.
    r. radiation
rectus, gen. and pl. **recti**
    ampulla recti
    r. femoris
    r. femoris tendon
    gyrus recti
    r. muscle
    r. position
    r. sheath
    r. sheath pocket
recumbency
recumbent
    r. lateral projection
    r. position
    r. view
recurrence
    ipsilateral breast tumor r. (IBTR)
    local r. (LR)
    no evidence of r. (NER)

    r. pattern
    tumor r.
recurrent
    r. artery of Heubner
    r. bronchiectasis
    r. canal
    r. digital fibroma
    r. dislocation
    r. embolus
    r. fleeting infiltrate
    r. high-grade malignant glioma
    r. hyperparathyroidism
    r. laryngeal nerve
    r. lateral patellar subluxation
    r. lesion
    r. lymphoma
    r. meningeal nerve
    r. multifocal osteomyelitis
    r. pneumonia
    r. pneumothorax
    r. pyogenic cholangitis
    r. pyogenic hepatitis
    r. respiratory papillomatosis
    r. sialadenitis
    r. stricture
    r. ulcer
    r. vermian oligoastrocytoma
recursive
    r. partitioning
    r. partitioning analysis
recurvatum
    r. deformity
    genu r.
    pectus r.
red
    r. blood cell (RBC)
    r. blood cell iron turnover
    r. cell ghost
    r. cell mass (RCM)
    r. infarct
Reddick cystic duct cholangiogram
    catheter
redirection of inferior vena cava
redistributed thallium scan
redistribution
    blood flow r.
    flow r.
    pulmonary blood flow r.
    pulmonary vascular r.
    r. study
    r. thallium-201 imaging
    vascular r.
Redi-Vu teleradiology system
red-out
REDS
    remote endoscopic digital spectroscopy
reduced
    r. acquisition
    r. alveolar ventilation

R

r. circulation
r. compliance of chamber
r. filling
r. lung volume
r. plasma volume
r. prominence of pulmonary vessel
r. pulmonary compliance
r. signal intensity
r. stroke volume
r. subluxation
r. systemic cardiac output
r. ventricular filling period

reduced-acquisition
r.-a. matrix (RAM)
r.-a. matrix FAST

reducing stent

reduction
anatomic r.
blood viscosity r.
closed r.
concentric r.
congruent r.
r. deformity
3D field echo acquisition with short repetition time and echo r. (3D FASTER)
electrolytic r.
field echo acquisition with short repetition time and echo r. (FASTER)
fracture r.
gradient moment r. (GMR)
limb r.
open r.
postural r.
radiofrequency tongue base r.
stable r.

redundancy
r. of interposed colon segment
phase-angle display r.

redundant
r. aortic valve leaflet
r. capsule
r. carotid artery
r. mitral valve leaflet
r. scallop of posterior anulus
r. ureter

reefing
capsular r.
r. of medial retinaculum of knee

reelin mutation

reentrant
r. loop
r. well chamber

reentry
bundle-branch r. (BBR)
r. circuit
functional r.
intraatrial r.
r. point
sinus nodal r.

reexpansion
lung r.
r. pulmonary edema

reexploration

reference
chemical shift r.
r. compound
r. coordinate system
distal line of r. (DLR)
r. dose
r. image
r. line
r. phantom
plane of r.
r. range
rotating frame of r.
r. site
r. standard
sternospinal r.
r. wave

referral teleradiology

refill
capillary r.

Refinity Coblation System

reflectance-guided laser selection

reflected
r. edge of Poupart ligament
r. inguinal ligament
r. ray

reflection
r. coefficient
pleuroparenchymal r.
second-order r.
vascular r.

reflectivity
echo r.
high r.

reflectometer tuning unit

reflector
diffuse r.
specular r.

NOTES

reflex
    r. arc
    cat's eye r.
    conditioned r. (CR)
    genitourinary r.
    r. ileus
    stapedius r.
    r. sympathetic dystrophy
    r. sympathetic dystrophy syndrome
refluoromyelography
reflux
    acid r.
    r. activity
    r. atrophy
    r. of barium
    bile r.
    congenital vesicoureteral r.
    cortical venous r.
    duodenobiliary r.
    duodenogastric r. (DGR)
    duodenogastroesophageal r.
    duodenopancreatic r.
    esophageal r.
    r. esophagitis (RE)
    free r.
    r. gastritis
    gastroesophageal r. (GER)
    gonadal vein r.
    r. grade (I–V)
    hepatojugular r.
    r. ileitis
    intrarenal r.
    nasopharyngeal r.
    r. nephropathy
    pistonlike r.
    pudendal vein r.
    r. regurgitation
    vesicoureteral r. (VUR)
    vesicoureteric r.
refluxing spastic neurogenic bladder
refocus
    multiplanar gradient r.
refocusing
reformat
reformation
    coronal r.
    curved multiplanar r. (CPR)
    curved planar r.
    DentaScan multiplanar r.
    image r.
    multiplanar r. (MPR)
    multiplanar volume r. (MPVR)
    paddlewheel r.
reformatted
    r. computed tomography
    r. T1 magnetic resonance image
reformatting
    cardiac oblique r.

    3D r.
    multiplanar r.
refraction
refractive shadowing
refractory
    r. congestive heart failure
    r. hepatic hydrothorax
    r. hypertension
    r. period of myocardium
    r. TLE
    r. to treatment
    r. tumor
refractured bone
regeneration
    imperfect r.
    nodular liver r.
    osteoblastic bone r.
    r. of tissue
regenerative
    r. chondrocyte
    r. gastric polyp
    r. liver nodule
regimen
    lifetime r.
region
    r. of activation
    Broca r.
    dark r.
    distention of esophagogastric r.
    esophagogastric r.
    hyperechoic r.
    hypermetabolic r.
    hypervariable r.
    insular r.
    r. of interest (ROI)
    r. of interest fluoroscopy
    r. of interest imaging technique
    intersphincteric r.
    isthmic r.
    laterocervical r.
    limbic r.
    outer-air r.
    paratracheal r.
    parietooccipital r.
    patulous esophagogastric r.
    periauricular r.
    perihilar r.
    photodeficient r.
    photopenic r.
    pineal r.
    r. of protection
    subpial r.
regional
    r. asynergy
    r. cerebral blood flow (rCBF)
    r. cerebral blood flow response
    r. cerebral blood volume (rCBV)
    r. cerebral metabolic rate for
      oxygen (rCMRO$_2$)

r. cerebral oxygen saturation
r. cerebral perfusion
r. cerebral perfusion pressure
(rCPP)
r. colitis
r. contractile reserve
r. differences in aeration
r. dyskinesia
r. dyssynergia
r. ejection fraction
r. enteritis
r. granulomatous lymphadenitis
r. hypokinesis
r. hypokinetic wall motion
r. ileitis
r. infusion
r. intraarterial infusion
r. left ventricular function
r. lymph node
r. mean transit time (rMTT)
r. migratory osteoporosis
r. myocardial blood flow
r. myocardial dysfunction
r. myocardial function
r. myocardial ischemia
r. myocardial mass distribution
r. oxygen extraction fraction
(rOEF)
r. perfusion abnormality
r. pulmonary perfusion
r. spread
r. tracer uptake
r. transient osteoporosis
r. transmural ischemia
r. tumor confinement
r. vascular perfusion
r. ventilation
r. wall motion assessment
r. washout measurement

registration
r. and alignment of 3D image
automatic image r. (AIR)
combined anatomic r.
2D portal image r.
feasibility of image r.
image r.
intermodality image r.
landmark r.
robust r.
spastic r.
spatial r.
surface r.

registry
PTCA R.
Regnauld degeneration of MTP joint
Regnauld-type great toe degeneration
regressed cyst
regression
r. analysis
caudal r.
plaque r.
polynomial stepwise multilinear r.
spontaneous r.
stepwise r.
regressive remodeling
regridding algorithm
regrowth delay
regular
r. connective tissue
r. wedge delay
regularization
Tikhonov r.
regulation
volume r.
regurgitant
r. flow delay
r. fraction
r. jet
r. lesion
r. lesion delay
r. orifice
r. orifice area (ROA)
r. pandiastolic flow
r. pocket
r. stream
r. stroke volume (RSV)
r. systolic flow
r. valve
r. velocity
regurgitation
aortic r. (AR)
congenital aortic r.
congenital mitral r. (CMR)
Dexter-Grossman classification of
mitral r.
Doppler tricuspid r.
factitious r.
Grossman scale for r.
ischemically mediated mitral r.
massive aortic r.
mitral r. (MR)
mitral valve r.
pansystolic mitral r.
paravalvular r.

NOTES

regurgitation *(continued)*
 physiologic r.
 pulmonic r. (PR)
 pulmonic valve r.
 reflux r.
 semilunar aortic valve r.
 semilunar pulmonic valve r.
 silent r.
 syphilitic aortic r.
 transient tricuspid r.
 tricuspid orifice r.
 tricuspid valve r.
 valvular r. (VR)
Reichert
 R. canal
 R. flexible sigmoidoscope
Reichert-Mundinger-Fischer stereotactic frame
Reid
 R. baseline (RBL)
 R. line
 R. lobule
Reil
 R. band
 R. island
reimplantation
 r. lung response
 r. technique
reinfarction
reinjection thallium stress examination
Reinke space
reinnervation
 motor r.
reintimalization
reirradiation
Reisseisen muscle
Reiter
 R. syndrome
 R. syndrome arthritis
[188]**Re-labeled self-expanding Nitinol stent**
relapse
 bone marrow r.
 solitary r.
 testicular r.
relapsing
 r. course
 r. polychondritis
relation
 end-diastolic pressure-volume r.
 end-systolic pressure-volume r.
 force-frequency r.
 force-length r.
 force-velocity r.
 Frank-Starling r.
 phase r.
relationship
 atlantoaxial r.
 complex anatomic r.
 dentoskeletal r.

 dose-time r.
 dose-volume r.
 globe-orbit r.
 Karplus r.
 Reynolds r.
 tumor cell-host bone r.
relative
 r. biologic effectiveness (RBE)
 r. cerebral blood flow
 r. cerebral blood volume (rCBV)
 r. conversion factor
 r. error
 r. hypoxia
 r. mitral stenosis
 r. peak height
 r. radiolucency
 r. refractory period (RRP)
 r. regional blood flow (rrBF)
 r. shunt flow
 r. value scale
relativistic mass
relaxation
 absent lower esophageal sphincter r.
 r. atelectasis
 r. enhancement technique
 esophageal sphincter r.
 ferromagnetic r.
 incomplete lower esophageal sphincter r.
 isovolumetric r.
 longitudinal r.
 molecular weight dependence of r.
 multiexponential r.
 multispin r.
 nuclear electric quadripole r.
 nuclear reactornuclear r.
 paramagnetic shift r.
 r. probe
 proton r.
 r. rate
 r. rate frequency dependence
 reciprocal agonist-antagonist r.
 sinusoidal r.
 spin-lattice r.
 spin-spin r.
 r. time
 tissue-based T2 r.
 transverse r.
 T2 star r.
relaxed lower esophageal sphincter
relaxivity
 r. data
 longitudinal r. (R1)
 transverse r. (R2)
relaxometer
 Bruker PC-10 r.
 Bruker TC-10 r.
 IBM field-cycling research r.

relaxometry
> time-efficient T2 r.
> tissue r.

relaxor
> ferroelectric r.

releasing factor

relief pattern

reloading
> anode tube r.

REM
> roentgen equivalent man

remasking

remineralization

remitting course

remnant
> cystic duct r.
> ductal r.
> gastric r.
> heart r.
> notochord r.
> omphalomesenteric r.
> r. radiation
> thyroglossal duct r.

remodeling
> balloon r.
> bone r.
> bony r.
> cord r.
> coronary r.
> craniofacial r.
> intimal r.
> neural foramen r.
> osseous r.
> paraarticular bone r.
> plaque r.
> reactive r.
> regressive r.
> stress-induced r.
> r. technique
> thrombus r.

remote
> r. afterloading brachytherapy (RAB)
> r. afterloading system
> r. endoscopic digital spectroscopy (REDS)
> r. ischemia
> r. lower motor neuron lesion

remote-controlled
> r.-c. implantation of radioactive source
> r.-c. production

removal
> brachytherapy implant r.

REMP
> roentgen equivalent man period

remyelinization

Renaissance 3D workstation

renal
> r. abscess
> r. adenocarcinoma
> r. agenesis
> r. allograft
> r. allograft necrosis
> r. amyloidosis
> r. angiography
> r. angiography imaging
> r. angiomyolipoma
> r. anomaly
> r. anticoagulant-related bleeding
> r. aortography
> r. arteriography
> r. arteriosclerosis
> r. artery
> r. artery aneurysm
> r. artery dissection
> r. artery fibromuscular dysplasia
> r. artery hypertension
> r. artery revascularization
> r. artery stenosis (RAS)
> r. artery stenosis screening MR
> r. artery transplant thrombosis
> r. axis
> r. calcification
> r. calculus
> r. calyx
> r. capsule
> r. carbuncle
> r. carcinoma
> r. carcinosarcoma
> r. cell carcinoma stage I, II, IIIA, IIIB, IIIC, IVA, IVB
> r. cholesterol embolus
> r. choristoma
> r. clearance
> r. cocktail
> r. colic
> r. collecting structure
> r. collecting system
> r. collecting system atony
> r. column
> r. cortex
> r. cortical adenoma
> r. cortical isotope scanning agent

NOTES

renal (*continued*)
r. cortical necrosis
r. cortical nephrocalcinosis
r. CT imaging
r. cystic disease
r. cyst imaging
r. cyst study
r. Doppler
r. duplex imaging
r. duplex scan
r. duplication
r. dwarfism
r. dysfunction
r. edema
r. failure
r. fascia
r. flow curve
r. function differential
r. function impairment
r. function study
r. fungal infection
r. fungus ball
r. gallium scintigraphy
r. glomerulus
r. hamartoma
r. helical CT
r. hemangiopericytoma
r. hilar vessel
r. hilum
r. image
r. impression
r. infarct
r. inflammation
r. injury
r. insufficiency
r. interstitium
r. isthmus
r. labyrinth
r. leiomyoma
r. length measurement
r. lithiasis
r. lymphoma
r. malrotation
r. mass lesion
r. medulla
r. medullary pyramid
r. metastasis
r. obstruction
r. osteodystrophy
r. outline
r. papilla
r. papillary necrosis
r. parenchyma
r. parenchymal blush
r. parenchymal disease
r. parenchymal malakoplakia
r. pelvic fibrolipomatosis
r. pelvis
r. perfusion

r. pouch
r. pseudotumor
r. radionuclide
r. reflux atrophy
r. resistive index
r. scarring
r. sclerosis
r. shadow
r. shutdown
r. sinus
r. sinus complex
r. sinus cyst
r. sinus echo
r. sinus fat
r. sinus lipomatosis
r. sinus mass
r. size
r. stone
r. stone mineral composition
r. surface
r. transplant
r. transplant GI tract perforation
r. transplant hypertension
r. transplant lymphocele
r. transplant pseudoaneurysm
r. transplant urine extravasation
r. trauma
r. tuberculosis
r. tubular degeneration
r. tubular dysgenesis
r. tubular ectasia
r. tubular necrosis
r. tubular osteomalacia
r. tubule
r. tumor
r. ultrasonography imaging
r. ultrasound
r. vascular anatomy
r. vascular damage
r. vascular hypertension (RVH)
r. vein
r. vein renin assay
r. vein thrombosis (RVT)
r. vein transplant thrombosis
r. venogram
r. venography
vertebral, anal, tracheal,
  esophageal, r. (VATER)
renal-aortic ratio (RAR)
rendering
3D surface r.
interactive volume r.
r. parameter
perspective volume r. (PVR)
real-time volume r.
shaded surface r. (SSR)
transparent r.
volume r. (VR)

renegade
R. Hi-Flo microcatheter
R. microcatheter
reniform
r. contour
r. mass
r. pelvis
renin-angiotensin-dependent outer cortex
reninculus
reninoma
renin-secreting tumor
ren lobatus
RenoCal-76
renocystogram
Renografin-76
Renografin-60 imaging agent
renogram
captopril r.
r. curve
diuresis r.
F-15 r.
r. imaging
isotope r.
renography
ACE inhibition r.
acetazolamide r.
diuretic r.
DTPA r.
emission r.
enalaprilat-enhanced r.
exercise r.
Lasix r.
technetium-99m MAG3 r.
Reno-M-30
Reno-M-60
renovascular
r. disease
r. hypertension
r. reconstruction
r. stent
Renovist
R. II imaging agent
R. II injector
Renovue-65 imaging agent
Renovue-Dip imaging agent
rent
fascial r.
reocclusion
postthrombolytic coronary r.
reordering
MRA using 3D k-space r.
r. of phase encoding

REP
roentgen equivalent-physical
repair
endovascular r.
endovascular aneurysm r. (EVAR)
paraanastomotic aneurysmal r.
reparative giant cell granuloma
repeated free-induction decay
reperfused
r. artery
r. myocardium
reperfusion
r. injury of postischemic lung
r. lung edema
r. therapy
repetition
r. time (RT)
r. time to echo time ratio (TR-TE)
time-to-r. (TR)
repetitive
r. anterior subluxation of the tibia
r. microtrauma
r. pulse sequence
r. seizures
r. strain injury (RSI)
r. stress injury (RSI)
rephased transverse magnetization
rephasing
echo r.
even-echo r.
field-echo sequence with even-echo r. (FEER)
field-even echo r. (FEER)
r. gradient
gradient moment r. (GMR)
gradient motion r. (GMR)
replacement
aortic root r.
aortic valve r. (AVR)
bipolar hip r.
r. bone
r. fibrosis
hip r.
low-signal-intensity r.
mitral valve r. (MVR)
orthotopic total heart r.
prosthetic r.
spongiosa r.
valve r.
replacing oblique view
replantable amputation

NOTES

replantation of finger
replanted digit
repolarization
    ventricular r.
report
    unusual occurrence r. (UOR)
reporting
    structured r. (SR)
    structured platform-independent data
      entry and r. (SPIDER)
reproducibility index
reproducible baseline
reproduction
    colorimetric color r.
reproductive tract embryology
reprogramming therapy
requirement
    increased myocardial oxygen r.
rerotation
    varus r.
reroute
resampling
    volumetric r.
rescue
    autologous bone marrow r.
    bone marrow r.
resectability
resectable
    r. colorectal carcinoma
    r. lesion
resecting fracture
resection
    absolute curative r.
    absolute noncurative r.
    atrial septal r.
    r. cavity
    colosigmoid r.
    computer-assisted stereotactic r.
    en bloc r.
    extraarticular r.
    r. of mobile aortic arch atheroma
    plica r.
    pulmonary r.
    rim r.
    subtotal gastric r.
    transurethral r. (TUR)
    wedge r.
resectoscope
    Iglesias fiberoptic r.
reserve
    blood flow r.
    brain perfusion r.
    cardiac r.
    r. cardiac function
    contractile r.
    coronary flow r. (CFR)
    diastolic r.
    r. force
    left ventricular systolic functional r.

    myocardial perfusion r. (MPR)
    poor vascular r.
    preload r.
    pulmonary vascular r.
    regional contractile r.
    stenotic flow r. (SFR)
    systolic r.
    vascular r.
    ventricular r.
reservoir
    r. effect
    ICV r.
    shunt r.
residual
    r. aneurysmal sac
    r. barium
    r. cement
    r. ductal tissue
    fibrocalcific r.
    fibrocystic r.
    fibrotic r.
    r. focus
    gastric r.
    r. gradient
    r. imaging agent
    r. interstitial change
    r. limb-shaped change
    r. luminal narrowing
    r. magnetization
    r. metal fragment shaving
    r. nucleus
    r. plaque
    r. stone
    r. stress analysis
    r. urine
    r. urine accumulation
    r. volume (RV)
    r. volume/total lung capacity
      (RV/TLC)
residue
    fecal r.
residuum morphology
resilient artery
resin
    IRA-400 r.
    r. sphere
resistance (R)
    acquired radiation r.
    airway r. (Raw)
    arteriolar r.
    r. blood flow
    calculated r.
    coronary vascular r.
    decreased peripheral vascular r.
    decreased systemic r.
    drug-induced drug r.
    efferent arteriolar r.
    end organ r.
    expiratory r.

R

fixed pulmonary valvular r.
increased cerebrovascular r.
increased outflow r.
increased peripheral r.
increased pulmonary vascular r.
index of runoff r.
nasal airway r.
peripheral vascular r. (PVR)
pulmonary arteriolar r.
pulmonary vascular r. (PVR)
systemic vascular r. (SVR)
total peripheral r. (TPR)
total pulmonary r. (TPR)
vascular systemic r.
r. wire heater
Wood units index of r.

resistive
r. exercise table
r. index (RI)
r. index angiography
r. magnet

resistivity
conductor r.

resistor

resolution
anatomic r.
angle variation r.
anisotropic r.
axial r.
contrast r.
depth r.
r. element
energy r.
fibrotic r.
high temporal r.
image spatial r.
in-plane spatial r.
interval r.
intrinsic energy r.
isotropic r.
lateral r.
low-energy ultra-high r. (LEUHR)
range r.
spatial r.
r. stage
temporal r.
R. ultrasonic catheter
wide aperture kinematic table with
  isotropic r. (WakiTrak)

Resolve non-locking draining catheter

resolving
r. ischemic neurologic defect

r. pneumonia
r. power
r. time

resonance
bandbox r.
biphasic magnetic r.
r. capture
computerized
  tomography/magnetic r. (CT/MR)
cough r.
cracked-pot r.
electron paramagnetic r. (EPR)
electron spin r. (ESR)
fast-scan magnetic r.
focused nuclear magnetic r.
r. frequency
functional magnetic r. (fMR)
gated inflow magnetic r.
r. generator
high-resolution magnetic r. (HR-
  MR)
lactate r.
r. line
localized magnetic r. (LMR)
low-field magnetic r.
magnetic r. (MR)
mobile magnetic r.
nuclear magnetic r. (NMR)
r. offset
r. phenomenon
proton magnetic r.
pulsed nuclear magnetic r.
skodaic r.
split water r.
tagging cine magnetic r.
topical magnetic r. (TMR)
T1-weighted magnetic r.
velocity-encoded cine magnetic r.
  (VEC-MR)

resonant
r. frequency
r. frequency of oscillation

resonator
bird-cage r.
bridged loop-gap r.
detunable elliptic transmission
  line r.
Faraday shielded r.
flexible surface-coil-type r. (FSCR)
250 MHz crossed-loop r.
multicoupled loop-gap r.

NOTES

resorbable
  r. pin
  r. plate
  r. rod
  r. screw
resorcinol spray
resorption
  r. atelectasis
  bone r.
  cortical bone r.
  dependent edema fluid r.
  fluid r.
  r. lacuna
  osteoclastic r.
  osteoclast-mediated bone r.
  periosteal r.
  periprosthetic bone r.
  r. phase of healing
  subarticular bone r.
  subchondral bone r.
  subperiosteal bone r.
  terminal tuft r.
  total r.
  trabecular bone r.
resorptive atelectasis
Resovist MR contrast medium
respiration
  cardiac-gated r.
  r. gated 3D reconstruction
  r. pyelography
respiratory
  r. atrium
  r. bronchiolar dilatation
  r. bronchiole
  r. bronchiolitis
  r. bronchiolitis-associated interstitial
    lung disease (RB-ILD)
  r. burst
  r. burst product
  r. capacity
  r. chain complex I–VI
  r. compensation
  r. compromise
  r. decompensation
  r. diaphragm
  r. distress syndrome (RDS)
  r. disturbance of acid base
  r. effort
  r. embarrassment
  r. failure
  r. frequency
  r. gated imaging
  r. gating
  r. insufficiency
  r. modulation of vascular
    impedance
  r. motion
  r. motion artifact
  r. muscle weakness

  r. ordered phase encoding (ROPE)
  r. sorted phase encoding
  r. spasm
  r. system
  r. tract
  r. tract infection
  r. tract obstruction
  r. trigger
  r. triggered
  r. triggered fast SE technique
  r. triggered fat-saturated axial
    image
  r. triggering
  r. volume
  r. zoonosis
respiratory-esophageal fistula
response
  abnormal ejection fraction r.
  autoimmune r.
  blood flow r.
  blood oxygenation level-
    dependent r.
  blood pressure r.
  BOLD r.
  cardioinhibitory r.
  clinical complete r.
  clinical partial r.
  controlled ventricular r.
  deconditioned exercise r.
  desmoplastic r.
  end-organ r.
  R. Evaluation Criteria in Solid
    Tumors (RECIST)
  graft-versus-tumor r.
  healing flare r.
  hemodynamic r.
  high-rate ventricular r.
  immune r.
  line of r. (LOR)
  magnet r.
  metabolic r.
  pain provocation r.
  radiation r. (RR)
  rapid ventricular r.
  regional cerebral blood flow r.
  reimplantation lung r.
  slow ventricular r.
  synovial inflammatory r.
  therapeutic r.
  vasoactive r.
  vasoconstrictor r.
  vasodepressor r.
  vasodilatory r.
  ventricular r.
  whole-body inflammatory r.
responsiveness
  airway r.
rest
  cervical r.

glial r.
r. injection
knee r.
r. left ventricular function
r. magnetization
r. myocardial perfusion imaging
r. redistribution examination
r. redistribution imaging
r. right ventricular function
r. thallium-201 myocardial imaging

rest-and-exercise-gated nuclear angiography

restenosis
in-stent r.
postangioplasty r.

restiform body

restiformia
corpora r.

resting
r. ankle pressure index (RAPI)
r. echocardiography
r. electrocardiogram
r. end-systolic wall stress
r. energy expenditure
r. forefoot supination angle
r. heart
r. left ventricular ejection fraction
r. lower esophageal sphincter
r. MUGA imaging
r. myocardial echocardiography
r. perfusion
r. phase of cardiac action potential
r. pulse
r. regional myocardial blood flow
r. regional myocardial hypoperfusion

resting-redistribution thallium-201 scintigraphy

restoration
r. algorithm
r. of flow

restraint
r. caliper
foam-padded Velcro r.
mummy r.

restricted
r. diffusion
r. water diffusion

restriction
cortical diffusion r.
intrauterine growth r.
unilateral flow r.

restrictive
r. abnormality
r. bulboventricular foramen
r. cardiomyopathy
r. hemodynamic syndrome
r. lung disease
r. myocardial disease
r. pattern
r. pulmonary emphysema
r. ventilatory defect

restrictor
beam r.

restructuring

result
concordant r.
false-negative r.
false-positive r.
negative EMA r.
negative mucin r.
suboptimal r.
true-positive r.

resurfacing
Silk Touch laser skin r.

retained
r. barium
r. common bile duct stone
r. cortical activity (RCA)
r. dead fetus
r. fetal lung fluid
r. foreign body
r. gallstone
r. gastric antrum
r. placenta
r. root
r. secretion
r. urine

retardation (*See* IUGR)
asymmetric intrauterine growth r.
fetal growth r.
growth r.
intrauterine growth r. (IUGR)

Retavase

rete, pl. **retia**
r. mirabile
r. peg
r. ridge
r. testis

retention
r. of barium
CO_2 r.
r. colon polyp
r. cyst

NOTES

retention (*continued*)
  r. enema
  fluid r.
  r. of food
  r. meal
  r. of secretion
  r. stomach polyp
  r. of stool
  uptake and r.
  water r.
retentivity
  magnetic r.
Reteplase
rethrombosis
retia (*pl. of* rete)
reticula (*pl. of* reticulum)
reticular
  r. abnormality
  r. activating formation
  r. activating substance
  r. connective tissue
  r. formation (RF, rf)
  r. formation of brainstem
  gray r.
  r. infiltrate
  r. interstitial disease pattern
  r. lung pattern
  r. opacity
  r. type
  r. varicosities
reticularis
  livedo r.
  zona r.
reticulated bone
reticulation
  r. artifact
  chronic diffuse r.
  coarse lung r.
  diffuse fine lung r.
  lower lobe r.
  r. with hilar adenopathy
reticule
reticulocortical pathway
reticuloendothelial
  r. imaging
  r. imaging agent
  r. system
  r. tumor
reticuloendotheliosis
reticulogranular
  r. appearance
  r. pattern
  r. pulmonary density
reticulohistiocytic granuloma
reticulohistiocytosis
  multicentric r.
reticuloid
  actinic r.

reticulonodular
  r. infiltrate
  r. lung disease
  r. pattern
reticulosis
  mast cell r.
  midline malignant r.
reticulospinal tract
reticulum, pl. **reticula**
  r. bone cell sarcoma
  r. brain cell sarcoma
  hematopoietic r.
retina
  angiomatosis of r.
retinacular
  r. disruption
  r. ligament
retinaculum, pl. **retinacula**
  avulsed r.
  cubital tunnel r.
  retinacula cutis
  extensor r.
  flexor r.
  free-floating r.
  inferior extensor r.
  inferior peroneal r.
  inferior quadriceps r.
  patellar r.
  peroneal r.
  superior extensor r.
  superior peroneal r. (SPR)
retinal
  r. angiomatosis
  r. anlage tumor
  r. artery
  r. astrocytoma
  r. degeneration
  r. dysplasia
  r. embolus
  r. hemangioblastoma
  r. microaneurysm
retinalis
retinoblastoma
  r. hereditary human carcinoma
  quadrilateral r.
  trilateral r.
retinocerebellar angiomatosis
retinochoroiditis
retinocortical time
retinocytoma
retinoma
retinopathy
retracted
  r. rib
  r. stoma
retractile
  r. mesenteritis
  r. testis

retraction
    chest wall r.
    clot r.
    costa r.
    fiber r.
    inspiratory r.
    intercostal r.
    late systolic r.
    leaflet r.
    mediastinal r.
    midsystolic r.
    mild subcostal r.
    musculotendinous r.
    nipple r.
    postrheumatic cusp r.
    sternocleidomastoid r.
    sternum r.
    substernal r.
    superior r.
    suprasternal r.
    systolic r.
    upward r.

retractor
    external r.

retrievable IVC filter

retrieval
    microvascular r.
    oocyte r.
    transvaginal oocyte r.
    transvesical oocyte r.

retroaortic
    r. lymph node
    r. renal vein

retroappendiceal fossa

retroareolar
    r. density
    r. dysplasia

retroauricular lymph node

retrobulbar
    r. fat
    r. hemorrhage
    r. mass

retrocalcaneal
    r. bursa
    r. bursitis
    r. exostosis
    r. spur

retrocardiac
    r. area
    r. density
    r. infiltrate

    r. mass
    r. space

retrocaval ureter

retrocecal
    r. appendix
    r. lymph node
    r. recess

retrocerebellar
    r. arachnoid cyst
    r. CSF collection

retrochiasmal lesion

retroclavicular

retrococcygeal air study

retrocrural
    r. adenopathy
    r. air
    r. lymphadenopathy
    r. node
    r. space

retrodiscal
    r. temporomandibular joint pad
      inflammation
    r. tissue

retrodisplaced fracture

retroduodenal recess

retroesophageal
    r. aorta
    r. arch
    r. right subclavian artery
    r. vessel

retrofenestral otosclerosis

retroflexed
    r. uterus
    r. view

retroflexion
    uterine r.

retrogasserian target

retrogastric space

retroglandular lesion

retrograde
    r. angiocardiography
    r. arteriography
    r. atherectomy
    r. atrial activation mapping
    r. block
    r. blood flow across valve
    r. blood velocity
    r. cannulation
    r. cardiac perfusion
    r. cardioangiography
    r. cholangiogram
    r. coronary sinus infusion

R

NOTES

retrograde *(continued)*
  r. cystogram (RC)
  r. cystography
  r. cystourethrography
  r. degeneration
  r. embolus
  r. femoral aortography
  r. femoral arterial approach
  r. femoral artery catheterization
  r. filling
  r. flow of gastric content
  r. injection
  r. jejunoduodenogastric
    intussusception
  r. left ventriculogram
  r. nephrostomy puncture
  r. pancreatocholangiogram
  r. pancreatography
  r. peristalsis
  r. pyelography
  r. refractory period
  r. systolic flow
  r. transaxillary aortography
  r. transfemoral aortography
  r. translumbar aortography
  r. transurethral prostatic
    urethroplasty
  r. ureteral pseudodiverticulum
  r. ureterogram
  r. ureterography
  r. ureteropyelogram
  r. urethrocystography
  r. urethrogram (RUG)
  r. urogram (RU)
  r. urography
  r. venous route
  r. ventriculoatrial conduction
retrohepatic vena cava
retroileal appendix
retroiliac ureter
retrolental fibroplasia
retrolisthesis
  vertebral body r.
retromalleolar
  r. groove
  r. sulcus
retromammary
  r. fascia
  r. fat
  r. fluid collection
  r. space
  r. space view
retromandibular
retromedullary arteriovenous
  malformation
retromembranous hematoma
retromolar trigone carcinoma
retronuchal muscle
retroorbital space

retropancreatic tunnel
retroparotid space
retropectoral mammary implant
retroperfusion
  coronary sinus r.
  synchronized r.
retroperitoneal
  r. actinomycosis
  r. adenopathy
  r. air
  r. air study
  r. area
  r. calcification
  r. cavity
  r. cyst
  r. drain
  r. fat stripe displacement
  r. fibrosis (RPF)
  r. fistula
  r. gas insufflation
  r. hematoma
  r. hemorrhage
  r. infection
  r. leiomyosarcoma
  r. liposarcoma
  r. lymphadenopathy
  r. lymphangioma
  r. lymphatic vessel
  r. lymphoma
  r. mass
  r. node
  r. organ
  r. pneumography
  r. pneumoradiography
  r. space
  r. tumor
  r. tunnel
  r. viscus
retroperitoneum
retropharyngeal
  r. abscess
  r. hematoma
  r. hemorrhage
  r. lymph node
  r. narrowing
  r. soft tissue
  r. space
  r. space mass
retroplacental
  r. hematoma
  r. hemorrhage
retropneumoperitoneum
retropulsed fracture fragment
retropulsion
  vertebral body r.
retropyloric node
retrorectal
  r. cystic hamartoma
  r. lymph node

retrosomatic cleft
retrospective
    r. respiratory gating
    r. review
    r. synchronization
retrosphenoidal space
retrosternal
    r. airspace
    r. area
    r. mass
    r. soft tissue
    r. space
    r. thyroid
retrotorsion
    femoral r.
retrotracheal
    r. adenoma
    r. goiter
    r. soft tissue
    r. vessel
retrovascular goiter
retroversion
    r. of acetabular cup
    femoral r.
retrovertebral plexus
retroverted uterus
retrovesical
    r. septum
    r. space
retrovestibular neural pathway
retrusion
    midface r.
Rett syndrome
return
    anomalous pulmonary venous r.
    arterial r.
    r. to baseline
    impaired venous r.
    infracardiac-type total anomalous
      venous r.
    interatrial transposition of venous r.
    paracardiac-type total anomalous
      venous r.
    partial anomalous pulmonary
      venous r. (PAPVR)
    pulmonary venous r.
    supracardiac total anomalous
      venous r.
    systemic venous r.
    total anomalous pulmonary
      venous r. (TAPVR)
    venous r.

Retzius
    R. foramen
    R. ligament
    line of R.
    space of R.
    R. system
    R. vein
REV
    room's eye view
revalidation
revascularization
    cerebral r.
    coronary ostial r.
    endosteal r.
    foot r.
    graft r.
    infragenicular r.
    infrainguinal r.
    myocardial r.
    r. procedure
    radiofrequency percutaneous
      myocardial r. (RF-PMR)
    renal artery r.
    robotic coronary r.
    transmyocardial r. (TMR)
revascularized tissue
Reveal XVI PET/CT imaging system
reverberating flow pattern
reverberation
    r. artifact
    r. echo
reversal
    r. of cervical lordosis
    end-systolic r.
    gradient r.
    mirror image r.
    rapid gradient r.
    shunt r.
    r. sign
reverse
    r. Barton fracture
    r. Colles fracture
    r. 3 configuration
    r. distribution
    r. fast imaging with steady-state
      free precession (PSIF)
    r. Hill-Sachs lesion
    r. isolation
    r. Monteggia fracture
    r. pattern of signal intensity
    r. peripheral bat-wing infiltrate
    r. pivot shift (RPS)

R

NOTES

reverse *(continued)*
  r. Segond fracture
  r. S sign
  r. tennis elbow
  r. transport
  r. Trendelenburg position
  r. Waters plane
  r. Waters position
reversed
  r. coarctation
  r. coarctation of aorta
  r. ductus arteriosus
  r. greater saphenous vein
  r. peristalsis
  r. shunt
  r. Stenvers projection
  r. vein graft
  r. vertebral blood flow
reverse isolation
reversible
  r. airway disease
  r. bronchiectasis
  r. ischemic defect
  r. ischemic neurologic deficit
  r. myocardial ischemia
  r. posterior leukoencephalopathy
    syndrome (RPLS)
  r. temporary myocardial dysfunction
  r. vasogenic edema
review
  retrospective r.
Revised European American Lymphoma
  (REAL)
Revitalase erbium cosmetic laser
revolving Ge-68 pin
Reynolds
  R. number
  R. relationship
REZ
  root exit zone
RF, rf
  radiofrequency
  rapid filling
  reticular formation
    RF coil
    RF pulse
    RF shielding
    RF spin echo
    RF spoiling
R&F
  radiographic and fluoroscopic
    R&F camera
RFA
  radiofrequency ablation
    minimally invasive saline enhanced
      RFA
    RFA with perfused needle
      applicator

RFCA
  radiofrequency catheter ablation
RF-FAST
  radiofrequency spoiled Fourier-acquired
    steady state
RF-PMR
  radiofrequency percutaneous myocardial
    revascularization
RF-shielded cupboard
RF-spoiled FAST
RFW
  rapid filling wave
Rh
  rhodium
rhabdoid
  r. suture
  r. tumor
rhabdomyoblast
rhabdomyolysis
  exertional r.
rhabdomyoma
  cardiac r.
  r. of heart
rhabdomyosarcoma (RMS)
  alveolar r.
  bladder-prostate r.
  botryoid r.
  cardiac r.
  chest wall r.
  childhood r.
  embryonal r.
  extremity r.
  female genital tract r.
  genitourinary r.
  metastatic r.
  ocular r.
  orbital r.
  parameningeal r.
  paratesticular r.
  pleomorphic r.
  primary r.
  truncal r.
rhabdosarcoma
rhebosis
rhenium (Re)
  r. 186 (^{186}Re)
  r. 188 (^{188}Re)
  r. imaging agent
  r. isotope
rhenium-186 etidronate
rheography
  light reflection r.
rheologic pattern
rheolytic mechanical thrombectomy
  device
Rhese
  R. projection
  R. view
  R. view of orbit

rheumatic
  r. adherent pericardium
  r. aortic insufficiency
  r. aortic valvular stenosis
  r. granuloma
  r. heart disease
  r. heart valve
  r. lesion
  r. mitral stenosis
  r. tricuspid stenosis
  r. valvular disease
rheumatica
  polymyalgia r.
  synovitis in active polymyalgia r.
rheumatism
  articular r.
  desert r.
  hydroxyapatite r.
rheumatoid
  r. arthritis
  r. factor
  r. lung disease
  r. nodule
  r. pneumoconiosis
  r. spondylitis
rheumatologist
rhinencephalic mamillary body
rhinitis gangrenosa progressiva
rhinoplasty
rhinoscintigraphy
  ^{99m}Tc MAA r.
rhinoscleroma
rhinosinusitis
rhizolysis
rhizomelia
rhizomelic
  r. chondrodysplasia punctata
  r. dysplasia
rhizotomy
  trigeminal r.
rhm, Rhm
  roentgen(s) (per) hour (at one) meter
rhodium (Rh)
  r. anode
  r. filter
  r. isoimmunization
rhodium-rhodium target filter combination (Rh-Rh)
rhombencephalitis
rhombencephalon
rhombencephalosynapsis
rhombic lip

rhomboid
  r. fossa
  r. ligament
  r. major
  r. of Michaelis
  r. minor
rhomboideus major muscle
rho° transformation
Rh-Rh
  rhodium-rhodium target filter combination
RHV
  right hepatic vein
rhythm
  atrial bigeminal r.
  atrioventricular nodal r.
  bisferious pulse r.
  escape-capture r.
  idioventricular r. (IVR)
  mu r.
  nodal r.
  normal sinus r.
  reciprocal r.
  sinus r.
  transitional r.
  ventricular r.
rhythmeur
rhythmic
  r. paradoxic eruption
  r. segmentation
RI
  resistive index
RIA
  radioimmunoassay
  CA15-3 RIA
rib
  angle of r.
  beaded r.
  bed of r.
  bicipital r.
  bifid r.
  bone lesion of r.
  cervical r.
  r. contusion
  cough fracture of r.
  dense r.
  r. detail
  double-exposed r.
  false r.
  fifth r.
  first r.
  floating r.

NOTES

rib *(continued)*
    r. fracture
    fused r.
    guillotine r.
    gumma of r.
    head of r.
    hyperlucent r.
    hypoplastic horizontal r.
    inferior margin of superior r.
    jail-bar r.
    r. lesion
    lumbar r.
    minced r.
    neck of r.
    r. notching
    overlapping r.
    penciling of r.
    periosteum of r.
    r. recession
    retracted r.
    rudimentary r.
    r. shadowing
    shaft of r.
    short r.
    slipping r.
    sternal r.
    Stiller r.
    superior border of r.
    superior margin of inferior r.
    true r.
    r. tubercle
    twisted ribbonlike r.
    vertebral r.
    vertebrocostal r.
    vertebrosternal r.
    r. view
    wide r.
rib-bearing vertebra
Ribbing disease
ribbon
    r. application
    r. bowel
    hollow r.
    ^{192}Ir r.
    r. muscle
    seed r.
    r. uterus
ribonucleic acid (RNA)
D-ribose
ribosyl
ribothymidine
ribulose
rib-vertebral angle difference
rice joint body
ricelike muscle calcification
Richter
    R. hernia
    R. syndrome
Richter-Monroe line

rickets classification
rickettsial lung infection
rider's
    r. bone
    r. muscle
    r. tendon
ridge
    alveodental r.
    alveolar r.
    apical ectodermal r. (AER)
    basal r.
    bisagittal r.
    bony r.
    broad maxillary r.
    buccogingival r.
    bulbar r.
    cerebral r.
    cranial r.
    cutaneous r.
    dental r.
    dorsal r.
    epicondylar r.
    epidermal r.
    epipericardial r.
    fibrocartilaginous r.
    fibromuscular r.
    ganglion r.
    gastrocnemial r.
    genital r.
    gluteal r.
    humeral r.
    interarticular r.
    interosseous r.
    intertrochanteric r.
    interureteric r.
    longitudinal r.
    marginal r.
    mylohyoid r.
    oblique r.
    palatine r.
    Passavant r.
    pectoral r.
    petrous r.
    radial r.
    rete r.
    sagittal r.
    semicircular r.
    septal r.
    sphenoid r.
    supraaortic r.
    supracondylar r.
    supracoronary r.
    supraorbital r.
    tentorial r.
    transverse r.
    triangular r.
    ulnar r.
    urethral r.
ridged-convoluted villus

riding
- r. embolus
- r. stomach

Ridley sinus

Riedel
- R. lobe
- R. struma
- R. thyroiditis

Rieder
- R. cell
- R. cell leukemia

Riemann classification

Rieux hernia

RIF
- radiation-induced fibrosis

right
- r. anterior oblique (RAO)
- r. anterior oblique position
- r. anterior oblique position ventriculogram
- r. anterior oblique projection
- r. anterior oblique view
- r. aortic arch
- r. aortic arch with mirror image branching
- r. atrial appendage (RAA)
- r. atrial chamber
- r. atrial cuff
- r. atrial enlargement (RAE)
- r. atrial extension of uterine leiomyosarcoma
- r. atrial hypertrophy
- r. atrial pressure (RAP)
- r. atrial sarcoma
- r. atrium (RA)
- r. atrium oxygen saturation
- r. auricle
- r. axis deviation (RAD)
- r. border of heart
- r. brain
- r. bundle branch
- r. bundle-branch block (RBBB)
- r. cardiophrenic angle mass
- r. colon
- r. colonic flexure
- r. coronary angiography (RCA)
- r. coronary artery (RCA)
- r. coronary cusp
- r. coronary plexus
- r. crus
- r. descending pulmonary artery (RDPA)
- r. dominant coronary anatomy
- r. femoral artery
- r. gutter
- r. heart catheterization
- r. hemisphere
- r. hepatic duct
- r. hepatic vein (RHV)
- r. hilar lymph node
- r. ileocolic artery
- r. inferior epigastric artery
- r. inferior phrenic
- r. internal iliac artery
- r. internal jugular artery
- r. lateral decubitus view
- r. and left ankle index
- r. and left atrial phasic volumetric function
- r. or left lateral decubitus film
- r. lobe bronchus
- r. lobe of liver
- r. lower lobe (RLL)
- r. lower lobe lesion
- r. lower quadrant (RLQ)
- r. lung
- r. mainstem bronchus
- r. mediastinum
- r. middle lobe (RML)
- r. middle lobe lingula
- r. middle lobe syndrome
- r. ovarian artery
- r. paratracheal stripe
- r. posterior oblique (RPO)
- r. posterior oblique position
- r. posterior oblique projection
- r. primary bronchus
- r. pulmonary artery (RPA)
- r. pulmonary vein (RPV)
- r. subclavian central venous (RSCVP)
- r. triangular ligament
- r. upper lobe (RUL)
- r. upper lobe lesion
- r. upper quadrant (RUQ)
- r. ventricle
- r. ventricle of heart
- r. ventricle-pulmonary artery conduit
- r. ventricle-to-ear time
- r. ventricular apex (RVA)
- r. ventricular apical electrogram
- r. ventricular assist device (RVAD)

NOTES

right *(continued)*

r. ventricular branch of right
coronary artery
r. ventricular cardiomyopathy
r. ventricular chamber
r. ventricular coil
r. ventricular conduction defect
r. ventricular diastolic pressure
r. ventricular dilatation
r. ventricular dimension (RVD)
r. ventricular dysfunction (RVD)
r. ventricular dysplasia
r. ventricular ejection fraction
(RVEF)
r. ventricular electrogram
r. ventricular end-diastolic pressure
r. ventricular end-diastolic volume
(RVEDV)
r. ventricular end-systolic volume
(RVESV)
r. ventricular enlargement (RVE)
r. ventricular failure
r. ventricular hypertrophy (RVH)
r. ventricular infarct
r. ventricular inflow view
r. ventricular infundibulum
r. ventricular internal diameter
(RVID)
r. ventricular to left ventricular
systolic pressure ratio (RVP-VP)
r. ventricular to main pulmonary
artery pressure gradient
r. ventricular mass (RVM)
r. ventricular outflow obstruction
r. ventricular outflow tract (RVOT)
r. ventricular overload
r. ventricular peak systolic pressure
r. ventricular pressure (RVP)
r. ventricular strain
r. ventricular strain pattern
r. ventricular stroke volume
r. ventricular stroke work (RVSW)
r. ventricular stroke work index
(RVSWI)
r. ventricular systolic/diastolic
function
r. ventricular volume pressure

right-angle chest tube
right-angled
r.-a. isosceles triangle board
r.-a. telescopic lens
right-handedness
ventricular r.-h.
right inferior phrenic
right-sided
r.-s. angiocardiography
r.-s. arch
r.-s. cardiomyopathy
r.-s. empyema

r.-s. heart failure
r.-s. heart pressure
r.-s. pneumonia
right-sidedness
bilateral r.-s.
right-side-down decubitus position
right-to-left
r.-t.-l. shift
r.-t.-l. shunting of blood
rightward
rigid
r. endofluoroscopy
r. manipulation
r. ureter
rigidity
lead-pipe r.
rigidus
hallux r.
**RigiScan Plus rigidity assessment
system**
Rigler
R. sign
R. triad
R. triad of small bowel obstruction
RIGS
radioimmunoguided surgery
RIGS system
RIGScan CR49 imaging agent
RILD
radiation-induced liver disease
Riley-Day syndrome
rim
r. apophysis
bony glenoid r.
r. of capsule
r. of cartilage
dark signal intensity r.
r. degeneration
dorsal r.
r. enhancement
r. of fascia
glenoid r.
high-density r.
hypoechoic r.
intercartilaginous r.
low-density r.
r. nephrogram
nephrogram r.
orbital r.
r. resection
sclerotic r.
r. sign
signal intensity r.
volar r.
rim-enhancing lesion
rimlike calcium distribution
RIN
radiation-induced necrosis

rind
    pleural r.
rindlike thickening
ring
    abdominal r.
    amnion r.
    anorectal r.
    r. apophysis
    r. apophysis calcification
    arc r.
    r. badge
    R. biliary drainage catheter
    r. blush on cerebral arteriography
    Carpentier r.
    Carpentier-Edwards r.
    cartilaginous r.
    ciliary r.
    common tendinous r.
    congenital r.
    constriction r.
    r. detector
    distal esophageal r.
    double-populated detector r.
    drop-lock r.
    Duran r.
    echogenic r.
    r. enhancement
    r. epiphysis
    esophageal mucosal r.
    esophageal muscular r.
    external inguinal r.
    felt enforcing r.
    femoral r.
    fibrous r.
    r. finger
    r. fracture
    R. guidewire
    half-r.
    halo r.
    Ilizarov r.
    inguinal r.
    internal abdominal r.
    internal inguinal r.
    Kayser-Fleischer r.
    r. lesion
    r. ligament
    low-density r.
    lower esophageal mucosal r.
    r. man shoulder
    mitral valve r.
    mucosal r.
    multiple concentric GI r.'s

    pelvic r.
    perichondral r.
    pyloric r.
    r. scanner
    Schatzki r.
    r. shadow
    r. sign
    silastic r.
    silicone elastomer r.
    sodium iodide r.
    stereotactic r.
    sugar r.
    superficial inguinal r.
    supravalvular r.
    symptomatic vascular r.
    tracheal r.
    R. transjugular intrahepatic access set
    trophoblastic r.
    tubal r.
    umbilical r.
    valve r.
    vascular r.
    r. of Vieussens
    Waldeyer r.
    Wimberger r.
ring-and-arc calcification
ring-disrupting fracture
ring-down
    r.-d. artifact
    r.-d. echo
ring-enhancing
    r.-e. brain lesion
    r.-e. mass
ringing
    edge r.
    Gibbs r.
ringlike
    r. appearance
    r. configuration
    r. contraction
    r. lesion
    r. pattern
    r. structure
Ring-McLean sump drainage set
ring-of-bone concept
ring-shaped form
ring-type
    r.-t. imaging
    r.-t. imaging system
ring-wall lesion

NOTES

Riolan
- R. arch
- R. artery
- R. muscle
- R. ossicle

Riordan
- R. club hand classification
- R. finger pollicization

ripple voltage

RISA
- radioactive iodinated serum albumin
- radioiodinated serum albumin

Riseborough-Radin intercondylar fracture classification

rise time

risk
- radiation r.

risk-adapted CSI

Risser
- R. sign
- R. stage

Ritchie index

Rivero-Carvallo maneuver

Rivinus
- R. canal
- R. duct

RLL
- right lower lobe

RLQ
- right lower quadrant

R-meter
- rate meter

RML
- right middle lobe

RMS
- rhabdomyosarcoma

rMTT
- regional mean transit time

Rn
- radon

²²²Rn, Rn-222
- radon 222

RNA
- radionuclide angiogram
- ribonucleic acid
- gated RNA

RNV
- radionuclide ventriculogram

R/O
- rule out

ROA
- regurgitant orifice area

roadmap

road-mapping
- r.-m. mode
- r.-m. technique

Roadrunner NaviGuide guidewire

Robert ligament

robertsonian translocation

Roberts syndrome

Robin
- R. anomalad
- R. sequence

Robinow syndrome

robotic
- r. coronary revascularization
- r. mitral valve surgery

robotics-controlled stereotactic frame

Robson
- R. modification of Flocks-Kadesky system
- R. staging classification

robust
- r. registration
- r. registration technique

ROC
- receiver operating characteristic
- ROC curve
- ROC method

rocker-bottom
- r.-b. foot
- r.-b. foot deformity

rocker deformity

rocking
- r. curve measurement
- r. precordial motion

Rockwood acromioclavicular injury classification

ROCM
- radiopaque contrast media

rod
- Alta reconstruction r.
- Alta tibial/humeral r.
- r. eyelet
- Harrington r.
- Hopkins r.
- IM r.
- Isolar r.
- Luque r.
- medullary r.
- orthopedic r.
- resorbable r.
- r. source
- thermoluminescent dosimeter r.
- TLD r.

rodding
- IM r.
- intramedullary r.

rodent ulcer

RODEO
- rotating delivery of excitation off-resonance
- 3D RODEO
- RODEO imaging technical

rod-shaped calcification

Roederer obliquity

rOEF
    regional oxygen extraction fraction
roentgen (R, r)
    r. equivalent man (REM)
    r. equivalent man period (REMP)
    r. equivalent-physical (REP)
    r. knife
    r. kymography
    r. meter
    r.'s per second (R/s)
    r. ray
    r. stereophotogrammetric
    r. stereophotogrammetric analysis
      (RSA)
    r. tube
    r. unit (RU)
roentgen-equivalent-physical
roentgenkymogram
roentgenkymograph
roentgenkymography
roentgenogram
roentgenographic
    r. change
    r. control
    r. diagnosis
    r. finding
    r. silhouette
roentgenographically occult
roentgenography
    abdominal r.
    double-contrast r.
    magnification r.
    mucosal relief r.
    sectional r.
    selective r.
roentgenologic
roentgenological
roentgenologist
roentgenology
roentgenometer
roentgenoscope
roentgenotherapy
roentgen(s) (per) hour (at one) meter
    (rhm, Rhm)
roentgentherapy
    intraoral r.
    intravaginal r.
Rogan teleradiology system
Roger
    R. disease
    maladie de R.

    R. system
    R. ventricular septal defect
ROI
    region of interest
Rokitansky
    R. diverticulum
    R. lobe
    R. nodule
    R. pelvis
Rokitansky-Aschoff sinus
Rokitansky-Cushing ulcer
Rokitansky-Mayer-Küster-Hauser
    syndrome
Rokus view
rolandic
    r. artery
    r. cortex
    r. fissure
    r. sulcus
Rolando
    R. angle
    R. area
    fissure of R.
    R. fracture
    R. line
    R. point
    R. tubercle
    R. zone
rolandoparietal glioma
roll
    log r.
    radiolucent r.
rolled
    r. edge deformity
    r. view
roller mark artifact
Rollet stroma
Rollier radiation
rolling
    r. hiatal hernia
    r. membrane
    r. membrane Wallstent cobalt-based
      alloy balloon-expandable stent
roll-off
Romano-Ward syndrome
Romberg sign
Romberg-Wood syndrome
Romhilt-Estes score for left ventricular
    hypertrophy
ROMI
    rule out myocardial infarct

NOTES

RON
radiation-related optic neuropathy
R-on-T phenomenon
roof
acetabular r.
r. of fourth ventricle
r. of insula
intercondylar r.
roofless fourth ventricle diverticulum
room
r. shielding
room's eye view (REV)
root (R)
anatomic r.
aortic r.
cervical nerve r.
cochlear r.
r. compression
coronary sinus r.
cranial r.
dental r.
dilacerated tooth r.
dilated aortic r.
r. end granuloma
r. entry zone
r. entry-zone lesion
r. exit zone (REZ)
extrathecal nerve r.
facial r.
insula r.
intradural nerve r.
intrathecal r.
lateral r.
lingual r.
lumbar nerve r.
lung r.
r. of mesentery
motor r.
nerve r.
palatine r.
r. of penis
retained r.
sensory r.
spinal r.
ventral r.
ventricle r.
rootlet
intradural r.
root-mean-squared gradient measurement
ROPE
respiratory ordered phase encoding
ropelike cord
ropy
Rosai-Dorfman disease
rosary
r. bead configuration
r. beading
r. beading bone scintigraphy
r. beading esophagus

r. bead pattern
rachitic r.
Rosch hepatic catheter
Rosch-Uchida
R.-U. liver access set
R.-U. needle
rose
r. bengal dye
r. bengal ^{131}I radioactive agent
r. bengal sodium I-131 biliary
imaging
R. criteria
r. thorn sign
Rose-Bradford kidney
Rosen
R. curved guidewire
R. wire
Rosenbach sign
Rosenmüller
R. fossa
R. node
R. valve
Rosenthal
basal vein of R. (BVR)
R. canal
rosette shape
Ross needle
rostral
r. body of corpus callosum
r. brainstem ischemia
r. cervical nerve
r. connection
r. hypothalamus
r. medulla
r. pons
r. spinal cord
r. terminus
rostrocaudal extent signal abnormality
rostrum
r. of corpus callosum
r. sphenoidale
Rotablator thrombectomy system
rotary
r. ankle instability
r. deviation
r. door flap (RDF)
r. subluxation of scaphoid
r. thoracolumbar scoliosis
rotatable pigtail catheter
rotated
abducted and externally r. (ABER)
r. craniocaudal view
rotate-rotate scan
rotate-stationary scan
rotating
r. anode
r. anode tube
r. delivery of excitation off-
resonance (RODEO)

r. delivery of excitation off-resonance MR imaging
r. disc oxygenator
r. endoprobe
r. frame
r. frame imaging
r. frame of reference
r. gamma camera
r. Ge-68 rod source
r. hemostatic valve
r. raw cine data
r. tomographic projection
r. ultra-fast imaging sequence (RUFIS)

rotating-frame zeugmatography

rotation
360° r.
r. angle
anisotropic r.
r. anomaly
axial r.
degree of head r.
gantry r.
instantaneous axis of r. (IAR)
internal femoral r.
medial r.
organoaxial r.
r.'s per minute (rpm)
placenta r.
pronation-external r.
rapid gantry r.
SPECT center of r.
r. therapy
tibiotalar r.
tube position r.

rotational
r. alignment
r. angiography (RA)
r. atherectomy (RA)
r. atherectomy system
r. burst fracture
r. contact lithotripsy
r. coronary atherectomy (RCA)
r. correlation time
r. deformity
r. dislocation
r. displacement
r. field
r. force
r. frequency
r. instability
r. malalignment

r. method
r. motion
r. radiotherapy
r. scanography
r. therapy technique
r. tomography

rotationally invariant imaging
rotation-shearing injury
rotator
r. cuff
r. cuff arthropathy
r. cuff lesion
r. cuff muscle
r. cuff tear
r. interval

rotatory
r. instability
r. load
r. load on spine

Rotch sign
Roth spot
Rotograph
R. Plus imaging system
R. Plus panoramic dental tomography imaging system

rotography
Rotor syndrome
rotoscoliosis
rotoscoliotic deformity
Rotter node
rotundum
foramen r.

Rouget muscle
roughened
r. articular surface
r. cartilage
r. state of pericardium

rough zone
round
r. bone cell tumor
r. cancer of breast
r. cell sarcoma
r. heart
r. ligament
r. ligament artery
r. ligament of uterus
r. lucent lesion
r. muscle
r. pneumonia
r. pronator
r. shift

NOTES

R

round *(continued)*
  r. shoulder deformity
  r. ulcer
roundback deformity
round-cell tumor
rounded
  r. appearance
  r. atelectasis
  r. border of lung
  r. convex border
  r. lesion
  r. opacity
Rous
  R. sarcoma
  R. tumor
route
  hematogenous r.
  retrograde venous r.
  thoracic duct r.
  translumbar aortic r.
  urinary excretory r.
routine magnification view
Rouvière
  R. ligament
  R. node
Roux-en-Y
  R.-e.-Y. limb
  R.-e.-Y. procedure
Roux loop
Rovighi sign
Rovsing sign
row
  carpal r.
  distal carpal r.
  first carpal r.
  proximal carpal r.
Rowasa enema
Rowe calcaneal fracture classification
Rowe-Lowell fracture-dislocation classification
row-mode sinogram imaging
Royal Flush 4F pigtail catheter
RPA
  right pulmonary artery
RPF
  retroperitoneal fibrosis
RPLS
  reversible posterior leukoencephalopathy syndrome
RPM
  real-time position management
  RPM tracking system
rpm
  rotations per minute
RPO
  right posterior oblique
RPS
  reverse pivot shift

RPT
  rapid pull-through technique
RPV
  right pulmonary vein
RP X-OMAT processor
RR
  radiation response
rrBF
  relative regional blood flow
RRP
  relative refractory period
R/s
  roentgens per second
RSA
  roentgen stereophotogrammetric analysis
RSCVP
  right subclavian central venous
RSI
  repetitive strain injury
  repetitive stress injury
RSV
  regurgitant stroke volume
RT
  radiation therapy
  radiotherapy
  recovery time
  repetition time
    RT 3200 Advantage ultrasound
    RT 3200 Advantage ultrasound scanner
    RT 6800 ultrasound
    RT 6800 ultrasound scanner
RTAS
  rapid telephone access system
R-to-R imaging
RTP
  radiation therapy planning
  radiation treatment planning
    3D RTP
    RTP system
RTS
  radiation therapy system
    MammoSite RTS
rTSH
  recombinant thyrotropin contrast agent
RU
  retrograde urogram
  roentgen unit
Ru
  ruthenium
rubber
  r. drain
  r. vessel loop
rubidium (Rb)
  r. 82 (^{82}Rb, Rb-82)
  r. chloride imaging agent
Rubratope
Rubratope-57 imaging agent
Rudick red flag

rudimentary
　　r. bone
　　r. lung
　　r. organ
　　r. outlet chamber
　　r. pronephron
　　r. rib
　　r. sinus
　　r. ventricle
　　r. ventricular chamber
Ruedi-Allgower
　　R.-A. tibial plafond fracture
　　R.-A. tibial plafond fracture
　　　classification
ruffled border formation
RUFIS
　　rotating ultra-fast imaging sequence
RUG
　　retrograde urethrogram
ruga, pl. **rugae**
　　gastric rugae
rugal
　　r. fold
　　r. pattern
rugger
　　r. jersey appearance
　　r. jersey sign
　　r. jersey spine
　　r. jersey vertebra
rugose, rugous
RUL
　　right upper lobe
rule
　　Buffalo malleolar r.
　　modified Simpson r.
　　OAR malleolar r.
　　r. of 3
　　Ottawa ankle r.
　　r. out (R/O)
　　r. out myocardial infarct (ROMI)
rule-based scheme
ruler
　　endocatheter r.
Rumstrom view
run
　　high-frame-rate r.
　　low-frame-rate r.
Rundles-Falls syndrome
runner's
　　r. bump
　　r. knee

runoff
　　absent r.
　　aortic r.
　　aortofemoral r.
　　arterial r.
　　r. arteriography
　　digital r.
　　distal r.
　　r. film
　　inadequate r.
　　peripheral r.
　　r. resistance index
　　single-vessel r.
　　suboptimal r.
　　vessel r.
　　2-vessel r.
　　3-vessel r.
Runström projection
Runyon classification
RUPS-100 liver access set
rupture
　　Achilles tendon r.
　　amnion r.
　　aneurysmal r.
　　aortic r.
　　appendix r.
　　arch r.
　　arterial dilatation and r.
　　Berry aneurysm r.
　　bladder r.
　　breast prosthesis r.
　　bronchial r.
　　bulbomembranous urethral r.
　　buttonhole r.
　　cardiac r.
　　chordae tendineae r.
　　chordal r.
　　complex extraperitoneal r.
　　contained aneurysmal r.
　　contained aortic r.
　　delayed splenic r.
　　diaphragmatic r.
　　esophageal r.
　　extraperitoneal bladder r.
　　forniceal r.
　　frank r.
　　hemidiaphragm r.
　　hepatic capsular r.
　　hernia r.
　　interventricular septal r.
　　intramural esophageal r.
　　intraperitoneal r.

R

NOTES

rupture *(continued)*
  intratendinous r.
  mesenteric r.
  myocardial r.
  r. of myocardium
  myotendinous junction r.
  nodal r.
  papillary muscle r.
  plantaris r.
  plaque r.
  pregnant uterus r.
  premature uterine membrane r.
  silicone implant r.
  simple extraperitoneal r.
  splenic r.
  subbursal r.
  tendon r.
  testicular r.
  tracheobronchial r.
  traumatic aortic r.
  urinary bladder r.
  ventricular free wall r.
  ventricular septal r.
  vessel r.
ruptured
  r. aneurysm
  r. aortic cusp
  r. capillary
  r. chordae tendineae
  r. disc
  r. ectopic pregnancy
  r. emphysematous bleb
  r. follicle
  r. hollow viscus
  r. pelvic varix
  r. spleen
  r. thoracic duct
  r. ulcer
RUQ
  right upper quadrant
Rusch catheter
rush
  peristaltic r.
Russell
  R. body
  R. effect
Russell-Rubinstein cerebrovascular malformation classification
Russell-Silver
  R.-S. dwarfism
  R.-S. syndrome
ruthenium (Ru)
rutherford (Rd)
  R. clinical stage (peripheral vascular disease)
  r. unit

Rutherford-Becker
  R.-B. claudication category 1–5
Rutner balloon dilatation helical stone extractor set
Ruvalcaba-Myhre-Smith syndrome
Ruysch
  R. disease
  R. muscle
RV
  residual volume
RVA
  right ventricular apex
  RVA electrogram
RVAD
  right ventricular assist device
RVD
  right ventricular dimension
  right ventricular dysfunction
RVE
  right ventricular enlargement
RVEDV
  right ventricular end-diastolic volume
RVEF
  right ventricular ejection fraction
RVESV
  right ventricular end-systolic volume
RVG
  radionuclide ventriculogram
RVH
  renal vascular hypertension
  right ventricular hypertrophy
RVID
  right ventricular internal diameter
RVM
  right ventricular mass
RVOT
  right ventricular outflow tract
RVP
  right ventricular pressure
RVP-VP
  right ventricular to left ventricular systolic pressure ratio
RVSW
  right ventricular stroke work
RVSWI
  right ventricular stroke work index
RVT
  renal vein thrombosis
RV/TLC
  residual volume/total lung capacity
RX
  rapid exchange
  RX stent delivery system

S
sulfur
S contour
S distortion
S number
S shape
S sign of Golden
S value
S670
S670 over-the-wire coronary stent
S670 stent
^{35}S, S-35
sulfur 35
S7 AVE stent
SA
sarcoma
serratus anterior
sinoatrial
splenic artery
subcarinal angle
SA node
SAAV
simultaneous acquisition of artery and
vein
SAB
sinuatrial block
saber-sheath trachea
saber-shin
s.-s. appearance
s.-s. deformity
sabot
coeur en s.
s. heart
Sabouraud-Noire instrument
Sabouraud pastille
sac
abdominal s.
air s.
alveolar s.
amnionic s.
s. of aneurysm
aneurysmal s.
aortic s.
bursal s.
chorionic s.
common dural s.
cystic s.
decidual s.
dental s.
double decidual s.
dural s.
embryonic s.
empty gestational s.
endolymphatic s.
enterocele s.

false s.
fluid-filled s.
gestational s. (GS)
greater peritoneal s.
heart s.
hernia s.
hydronephrotic s.
indirect hernia s.
intrauterine s.
lacrimal s.
lesser peritoneal s.
lymphatic s.
narrowing of thecal s.
pericardial s.
peritoneal s.
pleural s.
primary yolk s.
primitive yolk s.
pseudogestational s.
residual aneurysmal s.
sacral s.
secondary yolk s.
spinal s.
terminal air s.
thecal s.
tight dural s.
wide-mouth s.
wrapped aneurysmal s.
yolk s. (YS)
sacciform
s. aneurysm
s. kidney
s. recess
saccular
s. bronchiectasis
s. cerebral aneurysm
s. collection
s. dilatation
s. ectasia
s. formation
s. malformation
s. mass
s. outpouching
s. pseudoaneurysm
sacculated pleurisy
sacculation
saccule
sacculocochlear canal
sacculoutricular canal
sacculus ventricularis
Sack-Barabas syndrome
saclike
s. cavity
s. space

S

827

sacral
 s. agenesis
 s. ala
 s. aneurysm
 s. bone
 s. bone tumor
 s. canal
 s. chordoma
 s. crest
 s. cyst
 s. dysgenesis
 s. foramen
 s. gutter
 s. hyperintensity
 s. insufficiency fracture (SIF)
 s. lymph node
 s. meningocele
 s. nerve
 s. osteolysis
 s. osteomyelitis
 s. osteosarcoma
 s. plexus
 s. process
 s. promontory
 s. sac
 s. spine
 s. vertebra
sacralization
sacralized transverse process
sacrococcygeal
 s. chordoma
 s. inferior pubic point (SCIPP)
 s. inferior pubic point line
 s. joint
 s. remnant tumor
sacrococcyx
sacrodural ligament
sacrogenital fold
sacrohorizontal angle
sacroiliac (SI)
 s. articulation
 s. disease
 s. fracture
 s. infection
 s. joint
 s. joint fusion
 s. joint widening
 s. sprain
 s. subluxation
sacrolumbar dysgenesis
sacropubic diameter
sacrosciatic
 s. foramen
 s. notch
sacrospinalis muscle
sacrospinous ligament
sacrotuberous ligament
sacrouterine
sacrovertebral angle

sacrum
 cornu of s.
 tilted s.
SACT
 sinuatrial conduction time
saddle
 s. clot
 s. coil
 s. embolus
 s. joint
 s. lesion
 s. peristalsis ureter
 s. point
saddle-shaped
 s.-s. uterine fundus
 s.-s. uterus
Sadowsky breast marking system
SAE
 stimulated acoustic emission
SAECG, SaECG
 signal-averaged electrocardiogram
Saemisch ulcer
Saethre-Chotzen acrocephalosyndactyly
SafeFlo IVC filter
SAFHS
 sonic-accelerated fracture-healing system
 Exogen 2000 SAFHS
 SAFHS 2000 sonic accelerated
  fracture healing system
Saf-T-Intima integrated IV catheter
Sage-Salvatore classification of
 acromioclavicular joint injury
sagging brain
sagittal
 s. canal diameter (SCD)
 s. celloidin section
 s. and coronal reconstruction view
 s. cranial suture
 s. fast spin-echo T2-weighted MR
  imaging
 s. fat-suppressed T1-weighted 3D
  spoiled gradient-echo image
 s. fontanelle
 s. gradient-echo imaging
 s. groove
 s. HR-MR
 s. localization
 s. magnetization transfer view
 s. oblique imaging
 s. orientation
 s. paraffin section
 s. plane
 s. plane fault
 s. plane loop
 s. plane vectorcardiography
 s. porta hepatis
 s. reconstruction
 s. ridge
 s. roll spondylolisthesis

s. scan
s. scout image
s. sinus
s. slice
s. synostosis
s. thrombosis
s. tomogram
s. transabdominal imaging
s. T1-weighted MR image
s. ultrasound

SAH
subarachnoid hemorrhage

Sahara
S. clinical bone sonometer
S. portable bone densitometer

saillike tricuspid valve
sail sign
Saint triad
Sakellarides classification of calcaneal fracture
Saldino-Noonan syndrome
Salem sump tube
saline
s. chaser
s. enema
s. implant
s. infusion sonohysterography (SIS)
s. solution
s. solution flush
s. torch

saline-enhanced
s.-e. MR arthrography
s.-e. MR imaging
s.-e. radiofrequency tissue ablation

salivary
s. calculus
s. gland
s. gland carcinoma
s. gland dysfunction
s. gland function study
s. gland infection
s. gland lymphoepithelioma
s. gland scan
s. gland scintigraphy
s. stone

Salla disease
salmon-patch hemorrhage
salpinges (*pl. of* salpinx)
salpingitis
chronic interstitial s.
follicular s.
hemorrhagic s.

interstitial s.
s. isthmica nodosa
pseudofollicular s.
purulent s.
tuberculous s.

salpingogram
salpingography
selective osteal s.

salpingopharyngeus
salpinx, pl. **salpinges**
salt-and-pepper
s.-a.-p. chromatin pattern
s.-a.-p. duodenal erosion

saltans
coxa s.
hallux s.

Salter-Harris
S.-H. classification of epiphysial fracture groups 1–5
S.-H. growth plate injury classification

Salter-Harris-Rang epiphysial fracture classification
salt-losing nephritis
Saltzman anatomy
salvage
s. of myocardium
s. radiotherapy
s. therapy

salvo of echoes
SAM
scanning acoustic microscope
systolic anterior motion

samarium (Sm)
s. imaging agent
s. scintigraphy

samarium 153 (^{153}Sm, Sm-153)
samarium-153 ethyl-enediaminetetramethylenephosphonic acid therapy
SAMBA imaging system
same-day
s.-d. exercise-rest Tc-99m tetrofosmin myocardial perfusion scintigraphy
s.-d. microsurgical arthroscopic lateral-approach laser-assisted fluoroscopic discectomy

sampling
angular s.
asymmetric data s.
s. error

NOTES

S

sampling *(continued)*
Gibbs s.
length-biased s.
nonlinear s.
partial k-space s.
s. window
zonal s.
SAN
sinuatrial node
Sanchez-Perez cassette changer
sanctuary
s. organ
s. site
sand
S. process
s. tumor
sandal-gap deformity
sandbagging fracture
sandbag hazard
Sanders sign
sandlike lucency
sandwich
s. appearance
s. configuration
s. configuration adenopathy
s. patch closure
s. sign
s. technique
s. vertebra
sandwiched gadolinium
Sanfilippo syndrome
sanguifacient
sanguiferous
sanguification
sanguineous, sanguinous
Sansom sign
Sansregret method
Santavuori-Haltia disease
Santiani-Stone classification of pancreatitis
Santorini
S. canal
S. duct
S. ligament
S. muscle
S. papilla
SAPA
spatial average-pulse average
saphenofemoral junction
saphenous
s. nerve
s. system
s. varix
s. vein
s. vein bypass graft
s. vein incompetence
s. vein mapping
s. vein stenosis

SAPHO
synovitis, acne, pustolosis, hyperostosis, osteitis
SAPHO syndrome
SAP-MS
sodium acrylate and vinyl alcohol copolymer microsphere
superabsorbent polymer microsphere
SAP-MS transarterial embolization
saponated cresol solution
Sappey
S. inferior vein
S. ligament
S. line
saprophytic
s. aspergillosis
s. colonization
SAR
scatter-air ratio
specific absorption rate
sarcocarcinoma
sarcofetal pregnancy
sarcohysteric pregnancy
sarcoid
s. granuloma
lung s.
sarcoidlike reaction
sarcoidosis
acinar s.
alveolar s.
bone s.
cardiac s.
endobronchial s.
hepatic s.
musculocutaneous s.
orbital s.
osteosclerosis vertebral s.
pulmonary s.
spinal cord s.
spleen s.
sarcoma (SA)
African Kaposi s.
alveolar soft-part s. (ASPS)
ameloblastic s.
angiolithic s.
bone-forming s.
botryoid s.
breast s.
cardiac s.
cerebellar s.
cervical s.
chloroma granulocytic s.
clear cell s.
diaphragmatic s.
embryonal liver s.
endobronchial Kaposi s.
endometrial stromal s.
epithelioid s.
Ewing s.

extraosseous Ewing s.
fascicular s.
giant cell s.
granulocytic s.
hemangioendothelial bone s.
hemangioendothelial liver s.
hepatic anaplastic s.
high-grade surface osteogenic s.
intracortical osteogenic s.
intrathoracic Kaposi s.
juxtacortical osteogenic s.
Kaposi s. (KS)
Kupffer cell s.
low-grade central osteogenic s.
lymphatic s.
malignant myeloid s.
meningeal s.
mesenterial s.
mesodermal s.
mixed cell s.
multicentric osteogenic s.
multiple idiopathic hemorrhagic s.
neurogenic s.
orbital granulocytic s.
osteogenic s.
parosteal osteogenic s.
periosteal s.
pleomorphic s.
postirradiation osteogenic s.
primary s.
pulmonary artery s.
pulmonary Kaposi s.
radiation-induced s.
radioinduced s.
reticulum bone cell s.
reticulum brain cell s.
right atrial s.
round cell s.
Rous s.
sclerotic osteogenic s.
soft tissue s.
synovial s.
telangiectatic osteogenic s.
tendosynovial s.
undifferentiated liver s.
vascular s.
vasoablative endothelial s. (VABES)
sarcomatode
sarcomatoid
sarcomatosis
diffuse s.
sclerosing osteogenic s.

sarcomatous
sarcomere
SARS
severe acute respiratory syndrome
SARS-associated coronavirus pneumonia
sartorius
s. insertion
s. muscle
s. tendon
SAS
supravalvular aortic stenosis
SA-SD
subacromial-subdeltoid
SA-SD bursitis
Sassouni analysis
SATA
spatial average-temporal average
satellite
s. cartilaginous focus
s. lesion
s. metastasis
s. node
s. nodule
s. structure
satellite-borne phased array (SBPA)
satellitosis
Sat Pad
satumomab
s. pendetide imaging agent
s. pentetide
saturated potassium iodide solution (SSKI)
saturation
s. analysis
aortic oxygen s.
arterial oxygen s.
s. band
s. current
fat s.
frequency-selective fat s.
gaussian line s.
s. index (SI)
s. inversion projection (SIP)
jugular venous oxygen s.
line s.
lorentzian line s.
mixed venous s.
MT s.
off-resonance s.
oxygen s.
partial s. (PS)
progressive spin s.

S

NOTES

saturation *(continued)*
> s. pulse
> s. recovery (SR)
> s. recovery image
> s. recovery sequence
> s. recovery technique
> regional cerebral oxygen s.
> right atrium oxygen s.
> selective s.
> spatial-spectral prepulses for fat s.
> spectral s.
> s. stripe
> systemic oxygen s.
> s. transfer
> T1-weighted axial image with fat s.

saucerization of vertebra
saucer-shaped excavation
sausage
> s. digit
> s. finger
> s. segment effect

sausage-shaped appearance
sausaging of vein
Sauvage filamentous velour graft
SAVANT
> surgical anatomy visualization and navigation tools
> SAVANT imaging system

sawtooth
> s. appearance
> s. configuration
> s. edge
> s. excretory pattern
> s. irregularity of bowel contour
> s. sign
> s. ureter

sawtoothlike thickening
SBDX
> scanning-beam digital x-ray

SBE
> small bowel enteroscopy

SBF
> systemic blood flow

SBFT
> small-bowel follow-through

SBO
> small-bowel obstruction
> spina bifida occulta

SBP
> solitary bone plasmacytoma

SBPA
> satellite-borne phased array

SBS
> shaken baby syndrome

SBSP
> simultaneous bilateral spontaneous pneumothorax

Sc
> scandium

⁴⁷Sc, Sc-47
> scandium 47

SCA
> single-channel analyzer
> superior cerebellar artery

scabbard trachea
SCAD
> spontaneous coronary artery dissection

scalar
> s. coupling
> s. effect

scalariform
scale
> abbreviated injury s. (AIS)
> Bloch s.
> color-flame s.
> digital gray s.
> expanded-disability status s. (EDSS)
> false color s.
> Flint colon injury s.
> Glasgow outcome s.
> gray s.
> Hunt and Hess subarachnoid hemorrhage s.
> injury severity s. (ISS)
> relative value s.
> Scandinavian Stroke s.

scalene
> s. anticus syndrome
> s. fat pad
> s. maneuver
> s. musculature
> s. node
> s. triangle
> s. tubercle

scalenus
> s. anterior
> s. anterior muscle
> s. anticus muscle hypertrophy
> s. anticus syndrome
> s. medius
> s. minimus

scaler
> s. counter
> decade s.

scaling
> s. device
> quantization matrix s.

scalloped
> s. appearance
> s. appearance of white matter
> s. border
> s. bowel lumen
> s. commissure
> s. luminal configuration

scalloping
> bone tumor s.

s. contour
cortical s.
endosteal s.
s. of margin of vertebral body
s. osteolysis
petrous pyramid s.
posterior vertebral s.
vertebral s.

scalp

s. branch of external carotid artery
s. hematoma
s. hypothermia
s. vein needle

scalpcl

s. cut
interactive electronic s.
ultrasonically activated s.

scan (*See* scanning)

A s.
abdominal CT s.
adrenal s.
aerosol ventilation s.
A-mode amplitude modulation s.
attenuation s.
axial s.
axial unenhanced CT s.
B s.
Becton-Dickinson FAC s.
bile duct s.
biphasic helical CT s.
blank s.
blood pool radionuclide s.
B-mode brightness modulation s.
bone marrow s.
brain s.
bremsstrahlung s.
brightness modulation s.
C s.
capillary blockade perfusion C-
mode s.
cardiac s.
CardioTec s.
CE-FAST s.
cerebral perfusion SPECT s.
cine CT s.
cine view in MUGA s.
clearance phase ventilation s.
^{11}C-methionine PET s.
coincidence detection s.
colloid shift on s.
color-flow duplex s.
computed tomography s.

contiguous s.
s. converter
coregistered s.
coronal s.
coronary artery s. (CAS)
CT s.
s. decrement
s. defect
dental s.
DEXA s.
diffusion s.
diuretic renal s.
dot s.
double helical CT s.
2D sector s.
dual-phase s.
dynamic CT s.
dynamic emission s.
elbow coronal s.
electromagnetic interference s.
enhanced CT s.
equilibrium MUGA s.
FDG-PET s.
^{18}FDG-PET s.
flow portion of bone s.
fluorescent s.
full-body CT s.
^{67}Ga bone s.
gadolinium s.
gallium s.
gamma s.
gastric emptying s.
gated blood pool s.
3-head s.
Heart CT s.
helical thin-section CT s.
hepatobiliary s.
hepatoiminodiacetic acid s.
HIDA s.
ictal PET s.
^{125}I fibrinogen s.
indium-111-labeled white blood
cell s.
infarct s.
In-111 pentetreotide s.
Insight Millennium s.
interictal SPECT s.
intravenously enhanced CT s.
iodine-131 whole-body s.
isotope bone s.
isotopic lung s.
kidney s.

NOTES

scan *(continued)*
- krypton s.
- labeled leukocyte s.
- lacrimal s.
- left-side-down decubitus s.
- left ventricular gated blood pool s.
- liver s.
- liverlung s.
- liver-spleen s.
- longitudinal s.
- lung s.
- MAG3 Lasix renal s.
- mechanical compound s.
- Meckel s.
- medronate s.
- MET-PET s.
- MIBG SPECT s.
- Miraluma s.
- M-mode time motion s.
- MUGA s.
- multidetector-row CT s.
- multiple gated acquisition s.
- multiple gated blood pool s.
- multiple line s. (MLS)
- multislice full line s.
- myocardial perfusion s.
- NMR s.
- noncontrast CT s.
- nonenhanced CT s.
- nongated CT s.
- nuclear magnetic resonance s.
- nucleotide s.
- octreotide tumor localization s.
- oral-enhanced CT s.
- s. orientation
- pancreatic s.
- panoramic CT s.
- para-isopropyl-iminodiacetic acid technetium-99m hepatobiliary s.
- s. parameter
- pelvic ultrasound CT s.
- pentetreotide tumor localization s.
- perfusion lung s.
- PET s.
- 3-phase bone s.
- PIPIDA s.
- s. pitch
- s. pitch pit
- planar thallium s.
- s. plane
- portal-phased spiral CT s.
- postgadolinium s.
- postictal cerebral blood flow s.
- postinjection attenuation s.
- postmetrizamide CT s.
- precontrast s.
- preoperative resting MUGA s.
- ProstaScint s.
- proton-density axial MR s.

- PYP technetium myocardial s.
- pyrophosphate technetium myocardial s.
- quantitative s.
- radioactive brain s.
- radioactive fibrinogen s.
- radioactive iodinated serum albumin s.
- radioactive iodine s.
- radiofibrinogen uptake s.
- radioisotope lung s.
- radionuclide bone s.
- radionuclide flow s.
- radionuclide-gated blood pool s.
- radionuclide liver s.
- radionuclide milk s.
- radionuclide thyroid s.
- rapid sequential CT s.
- rCBF PET s.
- real-time s.
- rebreathing ventilation s.
- rectilinear bone s.
- rectilinear thyroid s.
- redistributed thallium s.
- renal duplex s.
- rotate-rotate s.
- rotate-stationary s.
- sagittal s.
- salivary gland s.
- scintillation s.
- sector s.
- segmental lung defect s.
- segmenting dual-echo MR head s.
- selective excitation line s.
- s. sequence
- Seratec s.
- serial duplex s.
- single-pass s.
- single-photon emission-computed tomography technetium sestamibi s.
- single sweep s.
- spatially normalized PET and SPECT s.
- spin-echo s.
- spiral CT s.
- spleen s.
- splenic perfusion measurement by dynamic CT s.
- s. spot
- stacked s.
- static emission s.
- stereotactic CT s.
- stimulation s.
- stress thallium s.
- strip s.
- sulfur colloid s.
- suppression s.
- survey s.

^{99m}Tc HMPAO-labeled leukocyte total-body s.
^{99m}Tc-labeled macroaggregated albumin s.
TcO₄ thyroid s.
^{99m}Tc WBC s.
teboroxime cardiac s.
TechneLite s.
technetium-99m hepatoiminodiacetic acid s.
technetium-99m phytate s.
thallium-201 s.
thallium myocardial s.
thallium single-photon emission computed tomography s.
thorium-201 SPECT s.
thyroid stimulation s.
thyroid suppression s.
thyroid whole-body s.
s. time
transabdominal ultrasound s.
transaxial CT s.
transaxial joint s.
transaxial PET s.
transmission s.
transverse s.
triple-phase bone s.
T2-weighted s.
unenhanced magnetic resonance imaging s.
uniform phantom s.
venous s.
ventilation lung s.
ventilation-perfusion lung s.
s. volume
volumetric s.
V/Q lung segment s.
washout phase ventilation s.
water path s.
water signal on magnetic resonance imaging s.
whole-body bone s.
whole-body PET s.
whole-body transmission s.
s. with contrast enhancement
ZeroRad MRI s.
Scandinavian Stroke scale
Scanditronix
S. 1024-7B camera

S. MLC system
S. PET scanner
scandium (Sc)
scandium 47 (⁴⁷Sc, Sc-47)
Scanmaster DX x-ray film digitizer scanner
scannable tumor
scanned
s. focal point (SFP)
s. projection radiography (SPR)
scanned-slot detector system
scanner
Acuson 128EP s.
Acuson Sequoia 512 s.
Acuson XP 10 s.
Advanced NMR Systems s.
Agfa Medical s.
All-Tronics s.
Aloka ultrasound linear s.
Aloka ultrasound sector s.
American Shared-CuraCare s.
ANMR Insta-scan MR s.
Aquilion combined CT-fluoroscopy s.
Aquilion plus V-detector CT s.
Artoscan MRI s.
ATL Mark 600 real-time sector s.
ATL Neurosector real-time s.
Aura Laser helical s.
Aurora MR breast imaging system s.
BioSpec MR imaging system s.
biplane sector s.
Bruel-Kjaer ultrasound s.
Bruker s.
Canon s.
Cardio Data MK3 Holter s.
cardiovascular computed tomographic s. (CVCT)
Cencit surface s.
charge-coupled device s.
cine CT s.
C-150 LXP EBT s.
coincidence imaging s.
combined CT-fluoroscopy s.
C-PET s.
CT9000, 9800 s.
CT body s.
CTI 933/04 ECAT s.
CTI 931 PET s.
CT Max 640 s.
dedicated head s.

NOTES

scanner *(continued)*
dedicated PET s.
Delarnette s.
Diasonics ultrasound s.
Discovery LS, ST⁴ PET/CT s.
Dornier s.
DSR s.
3D surface digitizer s.
dual-probe rectilinear s.
duplex s.
DuPont s.
Eastman Kodak s.
EBT s.
Echospeed Signa LX 1.5 T s.
electron beam CT s.
8000-element linear array CCD s.
Elscint Excel 905 s.
Elscint MR s.
Elscint Twin CT s.
EMED s.
EMI 7070 s.
EMI brain s.
EMI CT 500 s.
Esaote extremity s.
Evolution CT s.
Evolution XP s.
Flexart MRI s.
FONAR-360 MRI s.
full ring s.
Galen Scan s.
gamma ray s.
Gammex RMI s.
gated CT s.
GE Advance PET s.
GE CT Advantage s.
GE CTI 9800 s.
GE CTI single detector s.
GE CT Max s.
GE CT Pace s.
GE 8800 CT/T s.
GE CT/T7 s.
GE CT/T 8800 s.
GE Genesis CT s.
GE GN 500-MHz s.
GE 9800 high-resolution CT s.
GE HiSpeed Advantage helical
  CT s.
GE HiSpeed single detector s.
GE Lightspeed CT s.
GE MR Max s.
GE MR Signa s.
GE MR Vectra s.
GE Omega 500-MHz s.
GE Pace CT s.
GE QE 300-MHz s.
GE Signa 4.7 MRI s.
GE Signa 1.5-T s.
GE Signa 5.2 with SR-230 3-axis
  EPI gradient upgrade s.

GE Spiral CT s.
GE Vectra MR s.
Gyroscan ACS-NT MRI s.
Gyroscan ACS-NT 1.5 T MR s.
Gyroscan Interna s.
Gyroscan S15 s.
Harvard multidetector s.
helical CT s.
Hewlett-Packard s.
high-field open MRI s.
high-field-strength s.
HighSpeed CT s.
HiLight Advantage System CT s.
HiSpeed Advantage helical s.
HiSpeed Advantage System CT s.
Hitachi CT s.
Hitachi MR s.
Hitachi Open MRI system s.
Hitachi 0.3-T unit s.
Hologic 2000 s.
Hologic QDR 1000W dual-energy
  x-ray absorptiometry s.
Horizon LX s.
Howtek Scanmaster DX s.
IDSI s.
Imatron C-100 EBT s.
Imatron C-150L EBCT s.
Imatron C-1000 UFCT s.
Imatron C-100 Ultrafast CT s.
Imatron C-150XL CT s.
Imatron C-100XP CT s.
Imatron Fastrac C-100 cine x-ray
  CT s.
Imatron Ultrafast CT s.
Indomitable s.
Innervision MR s.
InstaScan s.
Integris 3000 s.
Irex Exemplar ultrasound s.
IRIS s.
Konica s.
large-bore 0.6-T, 1,5-T imaging
  system s.
LightSpeed   CT s.
LightSpeed multidetector CT s.
LightSpeed QX/i s.
LightSpeed QXi CT s.
low-field MR s.
Lumiscan LS 85 s.
Lumisys 20 digital x-ray s.
Lunar s.
lutetium oxyorthosilicate-based
  PET s.
LymphoScan nuclear imaging
  system s.
3M s.
Magna-SL s.
Magnes 2500 whole-blood s.
MAGNETOM SP63 s.

MAGNETOM Symphony MR s.
MAGNETOM 1.5-T s.
MAGNETUM Vision s.
Magnex MR s.
Mallinckrodt s.
Malvern 2600 Sizer laser
  diffraction s.
Max Plus MR s.
mechanical sector s.
MedImage s.
Medison s.
Medspec MR imaging system s.
Medspec 30/80 tesla MR s.
MedX s.
microCT-20 s.
Microtek ScanMaker 9600XL s.
midget MRI s.
mobile spiral computed
  tomography s.
modified electron-beam CT s.
mPower PET s.
MR catheter imaging and
  spectroscopy system s.
multidetector CT s.
multidetector helical s.
multiple jointed digitizer s.
multisensor structured light-range
  digitizer s.
multislice CT s.
neurodiagnostic s.
NeuroFOCUS s.
NewTom CT s.
Nishimoto Sangyo s.
Norland pQCT XCT2000 s.
nuclear s.
Ohio Nuclear Delta 50 FS,
  2000 s.
Olympus endoscopic ultrasound s.
Oxford 2-T large-bore imaging
  system s.
Pace Plus System s.
Park Medical Systems s.
partial-ring bismuth germanate-
  crystal s.
Perception s.
PET/CT s.
PET full-ring s.
PETT VI PET s.
Pfizer 200 FS, 400 s.
phased-array s.
Philips Gyroscan ACS, NT, NT5,
  NT15, S5, T5 s.

Philips 1.5 NT-Intera s.
Philips 1.5-T NT MR s.
Philips Tomoscan 350, SR 6000
  CT s.
Philips 4.7-T small-bore system s.
Picker MR s.
Picker PQ 5000 helical CT s.
Picker PQ 2000 spiral CT s.
Picker PRISM 3000 PET s.
Picker Synerview 600 s.
4096 Plus PET s.
Posicam HZ PET s.
PQ 5000 CT s.
pQCT s.
ProSpecd CT s.
Quad 7000, 12000 high-field open
  MRI s.
Quick CT9800 s.
QX/I CT s.
radioisotope s.
rectilinear s.
ring s.
RT 3200 Advantage ultrasound s.
RT 6800 ultrasound s.
Scanditronix PET s.
Scanmaster DX x-ray film
  digitizer s.
scintillation s.
SCU-1200, SCU-2200 digital color
  ultrasound s.
SDCT s.
sector s.
SFP s.
Shimadzu CT s.
Shimadzu MR s.
Siemens DRH CT s.
Siemens Ecat EXACT HR+ CTI
  PET s.
Siemens Magnetom GBS II s.
Siemens Magnetom SP 4000 s.
Siemens Magnetom 1.5-T s.
Siemens Magnetom Vision s.
Siemens One Tesla s.
Siemens Plus 4 Volume Zoom
  multidetector s.
Siemens Somaform 512 CT s.
Siemens SOMATOM DR2, DR3
  whole-body s.
Siemens SOMATOM Plus CT s.
Siemens Sonoline Elegra
  ultrasound s.

NOTES

scanner *(continued)*

Signa Horizon LX SR 77 gradients 1.5-T MR s.
Signa MRI s.
Signa 1.5T s.
Signa VH/i3.0-T MR s.
single-detector helical s.
single-detector row s.
small-bore s.
SmartPrep s.
SOMATOM DR CT s.
SOMATOM Plus-S CT s.
spiral CT, XCT s.
supercam scintillation s.
Swissray s.
TCT900S helical CT s.
Technicare Delta 2020 s.
Tecmag Libra-S16 system s.
1.5 T Magnetom Symphony whole-body s.
tomographic multiplane s.
Tomoscan AVEU spiral CT s.
Tomoscan SR 7000 s.
Toshiba MR s.
Toshiba 900S helical CT s.
Toshiba 900S/XII s.
Toshiba TCT-80 CT s.
Toshiba Xpress SX helical CT s.
Toshiba X-Vigor s.
Toshiba Xvision s.
Trionix s.
4T whole-body GI Signa MRI s.
ultrafast computed tomography s.
Ultramark 9 s.
UM 4 real-time sector s.
Varian CT s.
Vidar s.
Vision Ten V-scan s.
Vision 1.5 T Siemens MRI s.
whole-body 1.5 Tesla s.
whole-body 3T MRI system s.
whole-body 1.5-T Siemens Vision s.
Xpress/SW helical CT s.
Xpress/SX helical CT s.
X-Vigor s.
X-Vigor CT s.

scanning *(See* scan)

s. acoustic microscope (SAM)
s. arm
s. beam digital system
body s.
breath-hold s.
close-space thin-section s.
collimation s.
combined ^{99m}Tc-DMSA and ^{99m}Tc-DTPA s.
continuous s.

contrast material-enhanced s.
delayed phase s.
diagnostic radioiodine s. (DxRaI)
diffusion-weighted s.
discontinuous s.
dual isotope s.
electrical impedance s. (EIS)
s. electron microscope (SEM)
s. equalization radiography
external s.
full-line s.
gamma s.
gated equilibrium blood pool s.
high-resolution ultrasound s.
IDA s.
interleaved BOLD-fMRI s.
intraoperative MIBG s.
laser diffraction s.
s. laser ophthalmoscopy
s. laser polarimetry
light s.
line s. (LS)
linear s.
s. locus
M-mode s.
multidetector helical s.
multiplanar s.
nuclear s.
parasternal s.
paravertebral s.
point s.
positron s.
s. power
radiocholesterol s.
radioisotope s.
radionuclide s.
real-time sector s.
sector s.
sensitive point s.
spiral CT s.
spot s.
subsecond s.
suprasternal s.
^{99m}Tc (V) DMSA s.
s. technique
total body s.
transabdominal s.
triplex s.
whole-body ^{29}FDG s.
wide-beam s.
xenon CT s.

scanning-beam digital x-ray (SBDX)

scanogram imaging

scanography

rotational s.
slit s.
spot s.

3-Scape real-time 3D imaging

scaphocapitate
- s. joint
- s. syndrome

scaphocephalic head shape

scaphocephaly

scaphoid
- s. bone
- congenital bipartite s.
- s. facet
- s. fat stripe
- s. hand fracture
- s. pole
- s. projection
- rotary subluxation of s.
- s. shape
- s. stomach

scapholunate (SL)
- s. advanced collapse (SLAC)
- s. arthritic collapse
- s. dislocation
- s. dissociation
- s. joint
- s. ligament
- s. space
- s. widening

scaphotrapeziotrapezoid (STT)
- t. joint

scaphotriquetral ligament

scapula, pl. **scapulae**
- body of s.
- high-riding s.
- inferior tip of s.
- margin of s.
- swallowtail malformation of s.
- winged s.

scapulae
- incisura s.
- levator s.

scapular
- s. angle
- s. body
- s. bone
- dorsal s.
- s. flap
- s. margin
- s. notch
- s. snapping
- s. winging

scapuloclavicular articulation

scapulocostal syndrome

scapulothoracic
- s. joint
- s. motion

scapulovertebral border

scar (*See* scarring)
- s. band
- s. carcinoma
- central pancreatic lesion s.
- s. contracture
- dense s.
- s. emphysema
- femoral physial s.
- fibrocartilaginous s.
- s. formation
- infarcted s.
- s. lesion
- lung starfish s.
- myocardial s.
- nonviable s.
- s. ossification
- ossified s.
- pulmonary s.
- radial s.
- radial breast s.
- s. tissue
- s. tissue entrapment
- s. tissue reaction
- tumor of liver s.
- well-demarcated s.

scarification of pleura

scarified duodenum

Scarpa
- canal of S.
- S. fascia
- S. ganglion
- ligament of S.
- method of S.
- S. triangle

scarred
- s. duodenum
- s. kidney

scarring (*See* scar)
- apical s.
- basilar pleural s.
- fibrotic s.
- glial s.
- interstitial s.
- parenchymal s.
- parietal pleural s.
- pleural s.
- postbiopsy s.
- postinflammatory s.

S

NOTES

scarring *(continued)*
   postnecrotic s.
   postpyelonephritis cortical s.
   renal s.
   selective s.
   valvular s.
scatter
   s. activity
   s. compensation
   s. correction
   s. degradation factor
   s. dose
   s. fraction
   s. graph
   s. grid
   low-frequency s.
   s. radiation
   s. and veiling glare (SVG)
scatter-air ratio (SAR)
scattered
   s. air bronchogram
   s. coincidence event
   s. count
   s. radiation
   s. rays
scatterer
   s. depth
   echogenicity s.
scattergram
scattering
   broad-beam s.
   classical s.
   coherent s.
   collimator s.
   Compton s.
   s. foil
   s. foil compensator
   forward-angle light s.
   image-degrading s.
   low-angle s.
   Rayleigh s.
   Rayleigh-Tyndall s.
   side s.
   small-angle multiple s.
   s. system
   Thomson s.
scatter-maximum ratio (SMR)
scatterplot
scatter-primary ratio
scavenging system
SCD
   sagittal canal diameter
scene
   s. coordinate system
   s. domain
   s. intensity
scene-based
   s.-b. interpolation
   s.-b. visualization

Sceratti goniometer
SCFE
   slipped capital femoral epiphysis
Scharff-Bloom-Richardson
   S.-B.-R. grade
   S.-B.-R. histologic grade system
Schatzker fracture classification
Schatzki
   S. ring
   S. view
Schaumann body
Scheibe dysplasia
Scheie syndrome
scheme
   6-ablation, 14-ablation s.
   computer-aided diagnosis s.
   cylindrical-ablation s.
   decay s.
   gradient s.
   rule-based s.
   single-ablation s.
   zero-filling interpolation s.
Schepelmann sign
Scheuermann
   S. disease
   S. juvenile kyphosis
   S. nodule
Schick sign of tuberculosis
Schiff-Sherrington phenomenon
Schilder disease
Schiller-Duval body
schistosomal bladder carcinoma
schistosomiasis
schizencephaly
Schlemm
   S. canal
   S. ligament
Schlesinger
   S. sign
   S. vein
Schmid disease
Schmid-like metaphysial
   chondrodysplasia
Schmidt optics system
Schmid-type metaphysial dysplasia
Schmincke tumor
Schmorl
   S. disease
   S. node
   S. nodule
Schneider
   S. enteral stent
   S. Guider catheter
schneiderian
   s. carcinoma
   s. papilloma
Schoemaker line
Schonander film changer
Schönlein-Henoch syndrome

Schroedinger equation
Schüller
    S. position
    S. projection
    S. view
Schultze
    S. bundle
    S. placenta
Schultz reaction
Schumacher criterion
Schwann
    S. cell
    S. cell of myelin sheath
    S. tumor
schwannoma
    acoustic s.
    facial s.
    geniculate ganglion s.
    jugular foramen s.
    orbital s.
    trigeminal s.
    vestibular s.
Schwartz
    S. criterion
    S. test for patency of deep
      saphenous veins
Schwartze sign
Schwartz-Jampel syndrome (SJS)
SCl
    spinal cord injury
sciatic
    s. endometriosis
    s. notch
    s. plexus
scimitar
    s. deformity
    shadow s.
    s. sign
    s. syndrome
    s. vein
scimitar-shaped
    s.-s. flap
    s.-s. shadow
scintiangiography
scinticisternography
Scinticore multicrystal scintillation
   camera
scintigram
    parallel-hole s.
    pinhole s.
    spatial resolution s.
    ^{99m}Tc MDP skeletal s.

scintigraphic
    s. angiography
    s. balloon
    s. balloon topography
    s. evidence
    s. perfusion defect
    s. scan imaging
    s. study
scintigraphy
    ACE inhibition s.
    adrenal s.
    antifibrin s.
    s. artifact
    bleeding s.
    blood pool s.
    bone marrow s.
    brain perfusion s.
    captopril-enhanced renal s.
    cardiac s.
    cerebral s.
    cholesterol-based s.
    cold defect renal s.
    combined ventilation-perfusion s.
    cortical s.
    dipyridamole thallium-201 s.
    dual intracoronary s.
    dynamic antral s.
    dynamic radionuclide renal s.
    early bone s.
    exercise myocardial perfusion s.
    exercise stress-redistribution s.
    exercise thallium s.
    functional radioiodine s.
    ^{67}Ga citrate s.
    gallium bone s.
    gallium lung s.
    gallium tumor s.
    gastrointestinal s.
    gated blood pool s.
    GI tract s.
    heart s.
    hepatobiliary s.
    ^{123}I metaiodobenzylguanidine s.
    ^{111}In antimyosin s.
    In-pentetreotide s.
    iodine s.
    iodine-131 whole-body s.
    iodomethyl-norcholesterol-59 s.
    isotope s.
    labeled free fatty acid s.
    lacrimal s.
    liver s.

S

NOTES

scintigraphy *(continued)*
long segmental diaphysial uptake bone s.
lung s.
lymphoma gallium s.
marrow agent bone s.
MIBG s.
microsphere perfusion s.
morphine sulfate s.
myocardial perfusion s.
NEFA s.
^{59}NP s.
nuclear renal s.
octreotide paraganglioma s.
oropharyngoesophageal s. (OPES)
osteomyelitis s.
parathyroid s.
pediatric s.
perfusion s.
peritoneal s.
pertechnetate s.
3-phase bone s. (TPBS)
4-phase bone s.
photon-deficient lesion bone s.
planar diagnostic 123I s.
planar exercise thallium-201 s.
pulmonary s.
pyrophosphate s.
s. quality control
quantitative hepatobiliary s. (QHS)
radioisotope s.
radionuclide bone s.
radionuclide testicular s.
renal gallium s.
resting-redistribution thallium-201 s.
rosary beading bone s.
salivary gland s.
samarium s.
same-day exercise-rest Tc-99m tetrofosmin myocardial perfusion s.
sestamibi parathyroid s. (SPS)
single-photon planar s. (SPPS)
soft tissue uptake bone s.
somatostatin receptor s. (SRS)
source of artifact s.
SPECT brain perfusion s.
SPECT thallium s.
splenic s.
split-function s.
stress perfusion s.
sulfur colloid s.
^{99m}Tc depreotide s.
^{99m}Tc-DMSA s.
^{99m}Tc HIG s.
^{99m}Tc human polyclonal immunoglobulin G s.
^{99m}Tc human serum albumin s.
Tc-labeled red blood cell s.

^{99m}Tc-labeled white blood cell s.
^{99m}Tc-methoxyisobutylisonitrile s.
TcO$_4$ MIBI subtraction s.
^{99m}Tc-PYP s.
technetium-99m heat-denatured RBC splenic s.
technetium-99m (V) DMSA s.
thallium-201 myocardial s.
thallium perfusion s.
thyroid s.
thyroidal lymph node s.
time course fracture s.
transit s.
ventilation s.
ventilation-perfusion pulmonary s.
vesicoureteral s.
white blood cell with indium-111 s.

scintillascope

scintillation
s. camera
s. camera field uniformity
s. camera geometry
s. camera linearity
s. camera linearity differential
s. camera uniformity differential
s. counter
s. counting technique
s. crystal
s. detector
s. imaging
migrainous s.
s. probe
s. proximity radioimmunoassay
s. scan
s. scanner
s. spectrometer
s. spectrometry

scintillator
caesium iodide s.
cesium iodide s.
rare-earth s.

scintillometer

scintimammography (SMM)
^{99m}Tc glucoheptanoate s.
technetium-99m methoxyisobutylisonitrile s.

scintiphoto
combined transmission-emission s.

scintiphotograph

scintiphotography
liver s.

scintirenography

scintiscan

Scintiview nuclear computer system

Scintron IV nuclear computer system

SCIPP
sacrococcygeal inferior pubic point

scirrhous
>s. breast carcinoma
>s. infiltrating adenocarcinoma
>s. lesion
>s. tumor

scission
>double-strand s.
>single-strand s.

scissoring of legs
SCIWORA
>spinal cord injury without radiographic
>abnormality

SCL
>sinus cycle length

SCLBCL
>secondary cutaneous large B-cell
>lymphoma

SCLC
>small-cell lung carcinoma

scleral canal
sclerocystic ovary
scleroderma
>complicated s.
>diffuse s.
>s. of esophagus

ScleroLaser laser system
scleroma
ScleroPLUS
>S. HP
>S. HP laser system

sclerosant
sclerosed temporal bone
sclerosing
>s. adenitis
>s. adenosis
>s. agent
>s. basal cell carcinoma
>s. cholangitis
>s. duct hyperplasia
>s. hemangioma
>s. hepatic carcinoma (SHC)
>s. inflammation
>s. injection
>s. lesion
>s. lipogranuloma
>s. mediastinitis
>s. mesenteritis
>s. myeloma
>s. nonsuppurative osteomyelitis
>s. osteogenic sarcomatosis

>s. osteosarcoma
>s. panencephalitis

sclerosis, pl. **scleroses**
>aortic s.
>arterial s.
>arteriocapillary s.
>arteriolar s.
>Baló concentric s.
>bony s.
>calcified s.
>chronic subperitoneal s.
>congenital hippocampal s.
>coronary s.
>cyst s.
>diaphysial s.
>diffuse CNS s.
>diffuse myeloclastic s.
>disseminated s.
>endocardial s.
>endplate s.
>esophageal variceal s.
>focal bone s.
>gastric s.
>hepatic s.
>hepatoportal s.
>hippocampal s.
>idiopathic hypertrophic subaortic s.
> (IHSS)
>incisural s.
>Krabbe diffuse s.
>laser s.
>lobar s.
>marginal s.
>marked s.
>medial calcific s.
>mesenteric s.
>mesial temporal s.
>multifocal subperitoneal s.
>multiple s.
>pedicle s.
>photothermal s.
>posterolateral s.
>progressive systemic s.
>pulmonary and cardiac s.
>reactive bone s.
>renal s.
>segmental vein s.
>subchondral low-signal-intensity s.
>subendocardial s.
>systemic s.
>temporal bone s.
>thick rind s.

NOTES

sclerosis *(continued)*
    tuberous s. (TS)
    tumefactive multiple s.
    unilateral mesial temporal s.
    valvular s.
    variceal s.
    vascular s.
    venous s.

sclerostenosis

sclerotherapy
    percutaneous ethanol s.
    talc s.

sclerotic
    s. area
    s. border
    s. calvarial patch
    s. calvarium bone island
    s. coronary artery
    s. degeneration
    s. kidney
    s. lesion
    s. margin
    s. osteogenic sarcoma
    s. pattern
    s. plaque
    s. rim
    s. stomach

sclerotomy
    ab externo laser s.
    ab interno laser s.

SCM
    spinal cord malformation

SCNB
    stereotactic core needle biopsy

scoliosis
    adolescent idiopathic s. (AIS)
    Aussies-Isseis unstable s.
    Cobb measurement of s.
    congenital s.
    dextrorotary s.
    Dwyer correction of s.
    Ferguson method for measuring s.
    fixation of s.
    functional s.
    idiopathic s.
    s. index
    juvenile idiopathic s.
    King classification of thoracic s.
    King-Moe s.
    levorotary s.
    lumbar s.
    S. Research Society
    rotary thoracolumbar s.
    S-shaped s.
    thoracic s.
    thoracolumbar s.
    uncompensated rotary s.
    Winter-King-Moe s.

scoliotic
    s. pelvis
    s. spine

SCOOP model polyurethane intratracheal catheter

ScopeGuide
    S. magnetic resonance imaging device
    S. MRI device

Scopix Laser film

scorbutic white line

score
    Agatston s.
    aortic valve calcium s.
    biophysical profile s. (BPS)
    coronary artery calcium s. (CACS)
    densitometry z s.
    electron-beam CT-derived CAC s.
    fetal biophysical profile s.
    injury severity s. (ISS)
    late effect toxicity s.
    LENT s.
    Mallampati s.
    mean wall motion s.
    MRI Severity Scale s.
    QRS s.
    stroke scale s.
    thallium SPECT s.
    total calcium s. (TCS)
    volume s.
    wall motion s.

scored cartilage

scoring
    calcium s.

scotograph

scotometry

scottie, scotty
    s. dog appearance
    s. dog fracture
    s. dog view

scout
    s. digital radiograph
    s. film
    s. image
    s. imaging
    s. radiograph
    s. sequence
    s. view

SCP
    supracristal plane

SCR
    silicon-controlled rectifier

scrambled image

screen
    s. craze artifact
    fluorescent s.
    guilt s.
    intensifying s.
    Kodak Min-R s.

Lanex medium s.
s. oxygenator
radiofrequency s.
rapid s.
rare-earth s.
rear projection s.
s. type film
Ultra Vision Rapid s.

screener
AutoPAP 300 QC automatic
Pap s.

screen-film
s.-f. contact
s.-f. mammography

screening
biplane s.
breast cancer s.
s. mammography
s. technique

screening-detected abnormality
screen-intensifying factor (IF)
screenless mammography film
screw
bicortical s.
bone s.
cancellous s.
compression plate and s.
DHS s.
s. fixation
interference s.
lag s.
metallic s.
orthopedic s.
resorbable s.
transfixing s.
unicortical s.

scroll bone
scrotal
s. abscess
s. anatomy
s. area
s. calcification
s. fasciitis
s. fibroma
s. gas
s. hematocele
s. hernia
s. histiocytoma
s. mass
s. pearl
s. raphe

s. vein
s. wall thickening

scrotum, pl. scrota, scrotums
acutely symptomatic s.

SCT
Sertoli cell tumor
spiral computed tomography
star-cancellation test

SCTA
spiral computed tomography
arteriography

SCU-1200, SCU-2200 digital color ultrasound scanner
Scully tumor
scyphoid
SD
septal defect

S-D
systolic-diastolic ratio

SDCT
single-detector computed tomography
SDCT scanner

SDD
surfactant deficiency disorder

SDH
subdural hemorrhage
succinate dehydrogenase

SDRI
small, deep, recent infarct

SE
ischemic injury
spin-echo
SE proton-density weighted image

Se
selenium

⁷⁵Se, Se-75
selenium 75
⁷⁵Se selenomethionine radioactive
agent

SEA
spinal epidural abscess

seagull
s. joint
s. sign

seal
water s.

sealed
mechanically s.

seal-fin deformity
seam
osteoid s.

NOTES

S

seatbelt
>   s. fracture
>   s. injury

sea urchin granuloma

sebaceous
>   s. adenoma
>   s. carcinoma
>   s. cyst
>   s. gland calcification

sebaceum
>   adenoma s.

SEBI
>   stereotactic external-beam irradiation

Sebileau muscle

second
>   s. branchial arch
>   s. branchial cleft cyst
>   s. cranial nerve
>   s. cuneiform bone
>   cycle per s. (cps)
>   s. diagonal branch
>   S. Look breast imaging device
>   S. Look CAD system
>   s. malignant neoplasm (SMN)
>   meters per s. (MPS, mps, m/sec)
>   s. order subtraction
>   s. portion of duodenum
>   roentgens per s. (R/s)
>   s. ventricle of cerebrum

secondary
>   s. achalasia
>   s. acquired cholesteatoma
>   s. amyloidosis
>   s. archnoid cyst
>   s. atelectasis
>   s. axillary adenopathy
>   s. axillary lymphadenopathy
>   s. biliary cirrhosis
>   s. brain lymphoma
>   s. bronchus
>   s. calcification
>   s. cartilaginous joint
>   s. center of ossification
>   s. central venous thrombosis
>   s. chondromatosis
>   s. coccidioidomycosis
>   s. collimation
>   s. contracture
>   s. cutaneous large B-cell lymphoma
>   (SCLBCL)
>   s. degeneration
>   s. electron
>   s. electron production
>   s. extravasation
>   s. fracture
>   s. gliosis
>   s. hydrocele
>   s. hydrocephalus
>   s. hyperparathyroidism

>   s. hypoparathyroidism
>   s. hypothyroidism
>   s. intracranial hypertension (SIH)
>   s. lesion
>   s. lymphangiectasis
>   s. malignancy
>   s. myeloid metaphysis
>   s. obstruction
>   s. osteosarcoma
>   s. ovarian tumor
>   s. peristalsis
>   s. pleurisy
>   s. pneumonia
>   s. pulmonary lobule
>   s. radiation
>   s. ray
>   s. retroperitoneal fibrosis
>   s. retroperitoneal organ
>   s. sclerosing cholangitis
>   s. sequestrum
>   s. sonographic finding
>   s. teeth
>   s. ulcer
>   s. union
>   s. venous insufficiency
>   s. wave
>   s. yolk sac

second-degree
>   s.-d. AV block
>   s.-d. heart block

second-echo image

second-harmonic imaging

second-look arthroscopy

second-order
>   s.-o. chorda
>   s.-o. compensation
>   s.-o. correction
>   s.-o. reflection

second-trimester
>   s.-t. gestational dating
>   s.-t. placenta

secretin-enhanced dynamic MRCP

secretion
>   adrenocortical s.
>   bowel s.
>   gastric s.
>   hyperdense sinus s.
>   inspissated s.
>   mineralocorticoid s.
>   retained s.
>   retention of s.
>   sinonasal s.
>   tubular kidney s.

secretion-filled bronchus

secretory
>   s. adenocarcinoma
>   s. calcification
>   s. capacity
>   s. carcinoma

s. component
s. phase endometrium

section

axial celloidin s.
celloidin s.
contiguous interleaved axial s.
coronal s.
cross s.
distal leg cross s.
flood s.
frontal s.
hip muscle cross s.
midfrontal plane coronal s.
paramedian s.
penultimate s.
sagittal celloidin s.
sagittal paraffin s.
serial s.
serpiginous s.
step s.
thin s.
s. timing correction
tomographic s.
transverse s.

sectional

s. radiography
s. roentgenography
s. segmental anatomy

section-select

s.-s. flow compensation
s.-s. pulse

section-sensitivity profile

sector

lower field visual s.
2.5-, 5-MHz s. transducer
nipple s.
nonnipple s.
s. scan
s. scanner
s. scanning
Sommer s.
s. transducer

sector-scan echocardiography imaging

secular equilibrium

secundum

s. atrial septal defect
ostium s.
septum s.

sedation

conscious s.
deep s.

light s.
moderate s.

sedimented calcium

seed

encapsulated radioactive s.
gold s.
I-Plant brachytherapy s.'s
PharmaSeed palladium-103 s.'s
s. point
radiation s.
s. ribbon
Symmetra I-125 brachytherapy s.'s
s. voxel

seeding

intracranial s.
metastatic s.
perichondral cell s.
peritoneal s.
prostate s.
radioactive s.
subarachnoid s.
subependymal s.
TheraSeed s.
tumor s.

seeker

bone s.

seen on end

seesaw peristalsis ureter

Seessel pouch

see-through image

segment

aganglionic s.
akinetic s.
angulated s.
anterobasal s.
anterolateral s.
aortic s.
aperistaltic distal ureteral s.
apical s.
apicoposterior s.
arterial s.
atretic s.
atretic aortic s.
blind s.
bronchopulmonary s.
cardiac s.
coarcted s.
contiguous s.
Couinaud liver s. 1–8
diaphragmatic s.
distal s.
s. distraction

S

NOTES

segment *(continued)*
    diversity s.
    duodenal s.
    expansile aortic s.
    hypokinetic s.
    infarcted lung s.
    inferoapical s.
    inferobasal s.
    inferoposterior s.
    intercalated s.
    interleaved inversion-readout s.
    interposed colon s.
    intradiaphragmatic aortic s.
    intramuscular aortic s.
    ischemic s.
    Jackson and Huber classification of
      bronchial s.'s
    joint s.
    liver s.
    meatal s.
    nonfilling venous s.
    noninfarcted s.
    occlusal s.
    posterior apical s.
    posterobasal s.
    posterolateral s.
    proximal s.
    pulmonary s.
    redundancy of interposed colon s.
    septal wall s.
    superior s.
    taillike s.
    variable s.
    vaterian s.
    venous s.
    view per s. (VPS)
segmental
    s. alveolar pattern
    s. asynergy
    s. biliary obstruction
    s. bone defect
    s. bone loss
    s. bowel infarct
    s. branch of artery
    s. bronchus
    s. bronchus consolidation
    s. bronchus defect
    s. bronchus fracture
    s. bronchus ischemia
    s. bronchus lesion
    s. bronchus lower extremity
      Doppler pressure
    s. bronchus narrowing
    s. bronchus orifice
    s. bronchus perfusion abnormality
    s. bronchus plethysmography
    s. bronchus renal artery waveform
    s. bronchus symptom

    s. correction using spine
      reconstruction
    s. correction using x-ray
      measurement
    s. demyelination
    s. dyssynergia
    s. k-space turbo gradient-echo
      breath-hold sequence imaging
    s. limb pressure recording
    s. liver anatomy
    s. lung defect scan
    s. lung density
    s. necrotizing glomerulonephritis
    s. nephrogram
    s. neurofibromatosis
    s. omental infarct
    s. pneumonia
    s. portal hypertension
    s. pressure measurement
    s. renal artery branch
    s. resorption atelectasis
    s. spinal dysgenesis (SSD)
    s. stenosis
    s. transcatheter arterial
      chemoembolization
    s. vein
    s. vein sclerosis
    s. wall motion
segmentation
    anatomy-oriented colon s. (AOCS)
    s. anomaly
    automatic lumen edge s.
    automatic lung nodule s.
    barium s.
    GM s.
    inside-to-outside s.
    lung s.
    s. method
    s. method for real-time display
    MRI s.
    outer-air s.
    outside-to-inside s.
    s. procedure
    rhythmic s.
    semiautomated cerebrospinal fluid s.
    time-resolved imaging by automatic
      data s. (TRIADS)
    vascular s.
segmented
    s. cine
    s. echo-planar imaging (SEPI)
    s. k-space cardiac tagging
    s. k-space data acquisition
    s. k-space time-of-flight MR
      angiography
segmenting
    s. dual-echo MR head scan
    s. dual-echo MR imaging
Segond fracture

Segre chart
SEH
    spinal epidural hemorrhage
SEI
    subendocardial infarct
Seidelin body
Seidlitz powder test
Seinsheimer classification of femoral fracture
seizure
    absence s.
    generalized s.
    grand mal s.
    s. localization
    partial complex s.
    s. pattern
    petit mal s.
    s. phenomenon
    repetitive s.'s
    s. threshold
SELCA
    smooth excimer laser coronary angioplasty
Seldinger
    S. angiography
    S. catheterization
    S. needle
    S. percutaneous technique
select
    BimOdal Slice S. (BOSS)
Selecta 7000 laser
selection
    s. bias
    coil s.
    delay time s.
    gradient s.
    guidance system s.
    reflectance-guided laser s.
    slice s.
selective
    s. angiocardiography
    s. arterial injection
    s. arterial magnetic resonance angiography
    s. cannulation
    s. cerebral arteriography
    s. coronary arteriography
    s. coronary arteriography view
    s. coronary cineangiography
    s. excitation
    s. excitation line scan
    s. excitation method

    s. excitation projection reconstruction imaging
    s. hole burning
    s. internal radiation therapy (SIRT)
    s. irradiation
    s. laser sintering (SLS)
    s. occlusion of aneurysmal neck
    s. osteal salpingography
    s. partial inversion-recovery (SPIR)
    s. partial inversion-recovery MRI (SPIR)
    s. population inversion (SPI)
    s. population transfer (SPT)
    s. presaturation MR angiography
    s. pulse
    s. radiography
    s. reduction of pregnancy
    s. roentgenography
    s. saturation
    s. saturation method
    s. saturation recovery
    s. scarring
    s. separation
    s. test occlusion
    s. venography
    s. venous magnetic resonance angiography
    s. visceral aortography
    s. visceral arteriography
    s. visualization
selectivity
    spatial s.
Selectron system
Selenia imaging system
selenium (Se)
    s. 75 (^{75}Se, Se-75)
    amorphous s.
    s. imaging agent
    s. plate
    s. radiography
selenium-based digital chest system
selenium-drum-detector system
selenium-labeled bile acid imaging
selenomethylcholesterol
self-administered cleansing enema
self-aspirating cut-biopsy needle
self-expandable metal stent
self-expanding
    s.-e. covered stent
    s.-e. metallic endoprosthesis
    s.-e. open mesh stent
    s.-e. stent

S

NOTES

self-expanding *(continued)*
    s.-e. stent graft
    s.-e. tulip sheath
8 × 50-mm self-expanding Easy Wallstent
self-injury
self-quenched counter tube
self-reinforced polyglycolide
self-retaining Cope loop pigtail catheter
self-reversed parallel wire balloon technique
self-scattering
self-sealing latex balloon
self-selection bias
self-shielding
sella, pl. **sellae**
    ballooned s.
    decalcified dorsum s.
    diaphragma s.
    dorsum s.
    empty s.
    s. enlargement
    J-shaped s.
    tuberculum s.
    s. turcica
    s. turcica calcification
    s. turcica diaphragm
sella-nasion plane
sellar
    s. destruction
    s. floor
    s. tomography
Selvester QRS scoring system
SEM
    scanning electron microscope
semialdehyde
    succinic s.
semiautomated
    s. cerebrospinal fluid segmentation
    s. computed tomography angiography
semiautonomous nodule
semiaxial
    s. anteroposterior projection
    s. position
    s. transcranial projection
semicircular
    s. canal
    s. canal hydrops
    s. ridge
semicommitted mode
semiconductor
    complementary metal oxide s. (CMOS)
    s. detector
    metal oxide s. (MOS)
semicoronal plane
semidynamic splint

semierect
    s. film
    s. position
semiflexed MTP
semi-Fowler position
semihorizontal heart
semiinvasive aspergillosis
semilateral position
semiliquid feces
semilobar holoprosencephaly
semilunar
    s. aortic valve regurgitation
    s. bone
    s. bone formation
    s. calcification
    s. cartilage
    s. fold
    s. indentation
    s. line
    s. notch
    s. pulmonic valve regurgitation
    s. valve
    s. valve cusp
semilunaris
    hiatus s.
    linea s.
semimembranosus
    s. bursa
    s. tendon
semimembranosus-tibial collateral ligament bursa
semimembranous muscle
seminal
    s. colliculus
    s. tract
    s. vesicle
    s. vesicle atrophy
    s. vesicle cyst
    s. vesicle hypoplasia
    s. vesicle invasion (SVI)
    s. vesiculography
seminiferous
    s. tubular damage
    s. tubular ectasia
    s. tubule
seminoma
    extragonadal s.
    mediastinal s.
    s. mediastinum
    testicular s.
seminomatous tumor
semiopaque
semiovale
    centrum s.
semiquantitative
    s. measurement
    s. technique
semirecumbent position
semispinal muscle

semisupine position
semitendinosus tendon
semitendinous muscle
semiupright
    s. position
    s. view
semivertical heart
^{77}Se MRI spectroscopy
send-receive phased-array extremity coil
senescence
    premature placental s.
senescent
    s. aortic stenosis
    s. change
Sengstaken-Blakemore tube
senile
    s. amyloidosis
    s. ankylosing hyperostosis
    s. arteriosclerosis
    s. change
    s. degeneration
    s. emphysema
    s. fibroma
    s. myocardium
    s. nephrosclerosis
    s. osteomalacia
    s. osteoporosis
    s. plaque
    s. subcapital fracture
senilis
    coxa s.
Senning
    S. operation
    S. procedure
senograph
Senographe
    S. 2000D digital mammography
    imaging
    S. 2000D digital mammography
    system
    S. DMRt mammography system
    S. 500T, 600T, 700T, 800T
    mammography
senography
SenoScan
    S. full-field digital imaging system
    S. full field digital mammography
    system
    S. full field mammography system
Sens-A-Ray
    S.-A.-R. dental imaging system

S.-A.-R. 2000 dental imaging
    system
sensation
    Siemens SOMATOM S. 64
SENSE
    sensitivity encoded
    sensitivity encoding
    generalized SENSE (GSENSE)
    SENSE method
    modified SENSE (mSENSE)
    SENSE MRI
    time-adaptive SENSE (TSENSE)
    SENSE with half-Fourier single-
    shot turbo spin echo (SShTSE)
sensing
    s. coil
    s. error
sensitive
    s. plane
    s. plane projection reconstruction
    imaging
    s. point
    s. point scanning
    s. volume
sensitivity
    s. analysis
    contrast s.
    C sign s.
    s. encoded (SENSE)
    s. encoding (SENSE)
    s. encoding method
    index of s.
    line-shape s.
    percussion s.
    plane s.
    point s.
    poor s.
    spectral s.
    uniform s.
sensitization
    protracted exposure s.
sensitizer
    s. enhancement ratio
    radiation s.
sensitizing gradient
sensitometer
    electroluminescent s.
sensitometric
    s. curve
    s. strip
sensitometry
    processor s.

S

NOTES

sensor
  Bispectral Index S. (BIS)
  PressureWire s.
  temperature s.
sensorimotor
  s. cortex
  s. gyrus
sensory
  s. ganglion
  s. impairment
  s. nucleus
  s. paralytic bladder
  s. root
  s. strip
  s. tract
sentinel
  s. clot sign
  s. fold
  s. fracture
  s. loop
  s. loop sign
  s. lymph node (SLN)
  s. node dissection
  s. node localization and biopsy
  s. pile
  s. transoral hemorrhage
SEP
  systolic ejection period
separation
  acromioclavicular joint s.
  aortic cusp s.
  atlantoaxial s.
  atlantooccipital s.
  s. of bowel loop
  carrier-free s.
  chorioamnionic s.
  chromatographic s.
  collagen fiber s.
  costochondral junction s.
  E point to septal s. (EPSS)
  fat-water signal s.
  fracture fragment s.
  frequency s.
  s. of ghosts
  leaflet s.
  meniscocapsular s.
  meniscotibial s.
  mitral valve septal s.
  selective s.
  septal s.
  shoulder s.
  small bowel s.
separator tube
Sephadex bead
SEPI
  segmented echo-planar imaging
  spiral EPI
septa (*pl. of* septum)
  enhancing s.

septal
  s. accessory pathway
  s. amplitude
  s. arcade
  s. area
  s. asymmetry
  s. band
  s. bone
  s. cartilage plate
  s. cirrhosis
  s. cusp
  s. cusp of Calvé
  s. defect (SD)
  s. deviation
  s. dip
  s. hyperperfusion
  s. hypertrophy
  s. hypokinesis
  s. hypoperfusion
  s. leaflet
  s. line
  s. malformation
  s. myocardial infarct
  s. necrosis
  s. notch
  s. papillary muscle
  s. perforating branch
  s. perforation
  s. perforator
  s. perforator artery
  s. placenta cyst
  s. ridge
  s. separation
  s. thickening
  s. tricuspid anulus
  s. vein
  s. wall
  s. wall motion
  s. wall segment
  s. wall thickness
septal-to-free wall ratio
septate
  s. appearance
  s. hypertrophy
septation
  gallbladder s.
  s. septal defect
septic
  s. arthritis
  s. bursitis
  s. cholangitis
  s. discitis
  s. lung
  s. necrosis
  s. pleurisy
  s. pneumonia
  s. pulmonary embolus
  s. pulmonary infarct

s. shock
s. thrombosis
septomarginal
s. band
s. trabecula
septooptic dysplasia
septostomy
atrial s.
balloon atrial s.
septum, pl. **septa**
alveolar s.
anal intermuscular s.
anteroapical trabecular s.
aortic s.
aortopulmonary s.
atrial s.
atrioventricular nodal s.
s. band
s. of Bertin
bronchial s.
bulbar s.
canal s.
cartilaginous s.
s. cavum vergae
conal s.
connective tissue s.
conus s.
crural s.
distal bulbar s.
dyskinetic s.
epirenal s.
femoral s.
fibrous s.
gingival s.
infundibular s.
intact ventricular s.
interatrial s. (IAS)
interhaustral s.
interlobar s.
interlobular lung s.
intermuscular s.
internal intermuscular s.
interventricular s.
intraventricular s.
Kürner s.
lipomatous hypertrophy of
  interatrial s.
low-signal-intensity fibrous s.
median s.
mediastinal s.
membranous s.
muscular atrioventricular s.

myometrial s.
nasal s.
parietal extension of infundibular s.
s. pellucidum
s. pellucidum cavity
perirenal s.
placental s.
posterior median s.
s. primum
rectogenital s.
rectovaginal s.
rectovesical s.
retrovesical s.
s. secundum
sinus s.
subarachnoid s.
thickened s.
s. transversum
s. transversum defect
ventricular s. (VS)
sequela, pl. **sequelae**
late normal tissue s.
post ECT sequelae
radiation therapy s.
significant s.
tissue s.
sequence
amnion rupture s.
black blood s.
breath-hold fast-recovery fast SE
  pulse s.
breath-hold gradient-recalled echo s.
s. bypass graft
cardiac-gated PGSE s.
Carr-Purcell s.
Carr-Purcell-Meiboom-Gill s.
cine-FFE breath-hold s.
cine gradient-echo s.
conventional pulse s.
CP s.
CPMG s.
DANTE s.
3DFT-CISS s.
3D gadolinium s.
diffusion pulse s.
diffusion-sensitive s.
diffusion-weighted pulse s.
double inversion recovery s.
3D spoiled gradient-recalled
  echo s.
3D time-of-flight magnetic
  resonance angiographic s.

S

NOTES

sequence *(continued)*
3D transesophageal echocardiographic s.
dual-echo s.
dual gradient-recalled echo pulse s.
dysplasia-carcinoma s.
ECG-triggered phase contrast cine-gradient-echo s.
s. echo-planar imaging
echo-planar pulse s.
fast FLAIR s.
fast gradient-echo s.
FAST pulse s.
fat-suppressed T2-weighted fast spin-echo s.
fat-suppression pulse s.
field-echo pulse s.
FISP pulse s.
flow-compensated gradient-echo s.
gradient-echo imaging s.
gradient-echo pulse s.
GRASS pulse s.
Hahn spin-echo s.
high-resolution volumetric s.
hypervariable s.
in-phase s.
interleaved GRE s.
inversion recovery s.
IRSE s.
Klippel-Feil s.
long-echo-train fast spin-echo s.
long TR-TE s.
magnetization-prepared rapid acquisition gradient-echo s.
Meiboom-Gill s.
missing pulse steady-state free precession s.
s. monophasic shock
multiecho s.
multiplanar gradient refocused s.
multislice spin-echo s.
non-flow-compensated s.
nuclear magnetic resonance scanning s.
oblique sagittal s.
s. obstruction
opposed-phase s.
partial saturation pulse s.
peristaltic s.
phase contrast s.
phase-encode time-reduced acquisition s.
3-point Dixon water-fat separation s.
point-resolved spectroscopy s. (PRESS)
postenhancement s.
Potter s.
preenhancement s.

s. processor
pulse s.
pulsed arterial spin labeling s.
pulsed-gradient spin-echo echo-planar pulse s.
s. quantitative MR imaging
radiofrequency spoiled 3D GRE s.
RARE s.
RARE-derived pulse s.
repetitive pulse s.
Robin s.
rotating ultra-fast imaging s. (RUFIS)
saturation recovery s.
scan s.
scout s.
Shine-Dalgamo s.
short repetition time s.
short TI inversion recovery pulse s.
single breath-hold s.
single-echo versus multiple-echo s.
SL-GRE s.
spin-echo imaging s.
spin-echo pulse s.
spin-warp pulse s.
spiral-pulse s.
SPIR-FLAIR s.
spoiled gradient echo pulse s.
spoiled gradient-recalled echo s. (SPGR)
steady-state free precession s.
STEAM s.
STIR s.
susceptibility-sensitive s.
s. time
TONE s.
turboFLASH s.
turbo inversion recovery s.
turbo IR s.
turbo pulse s.
turbo SE s.
turbo spin-echo T2-weighted s.
T2-weighted combination s.
T1-weighted coronal fat-suppressed fast spin-echo s.
T2-weighted fat-saturated s.
T2-weighted pulse s.
T2-weighted spin-echo s.
twin-reversed arterial perfusion s.
ultrafast FLASH 2D s.
velocity-encoded s.
VIBE s.
voiding s.
water suppression pulse s.

sequencing
2D TOF pulse s.

sequential
s. balloon inflation

s. circulator
s. determinant
s. extraction-radiotracer technique
s. films
s. first pass imaging
s. image acquisition
s. line imaging
s. mode
s. paired opposed plaque (SPOP)
s. plane imaging
s. point imaging
s. postcontrast MR image
s. quantitative MR imaging
s. scalar quantization (SSQ)
sequestered
s. disc
s. lobe
s. lobe of lung
sequestra (*pl. of* sequestrum)
sequestral
sequestration
bronchopulmonary s.
disc s.
extralobar s.
extrapulmonary s.
fluid s.
intralobar s.
labeled red blood cell s.
pulmonary s. (PS)
s. system
third-space s.
sequestrum, pl. **sequestra**
associated s.
bony s.
kissing s.
necrotic s.
primary s.
secondary s.
tertiary s.
Sequoia ultrasound system
sequoiosis
Seratec scan
serendipity view
serial
s. change
s. cholangiogram
s. contrast MR imaging
s. CT slice
s. cut film technique
s. diffusion-weighted MR imaging
and proton MR spectroscopy
s. duplex imaging

s. duplex scan
s. dynamic imaging
s. film changer
s. injection
s. lesion
s. radiographic survey
s. radiography
s. section
s. splinting
s. subtraction film
serialoangiocardiography
serialogram
serialograph
serialography imaging
sericite pneumoconiosis
series, pl. **series**
abdominal s.
acute abdominal s. (AAS)
basophilic s.
cardiac s.
decay s.
diagnostic skull s.
dynamic s.
factor analysis of dynamic s.
(FADS)
FCS s.
full cervical spine s.
gallbladder s. (GBS)
gallbladder-gastrointestinal s.
gastrointestinal s.
GB-GI s.
intubated small bowel s.
Kempe s.
lumbosacral s.
metabolic bone s.
motor meal barium GI s.
radioactive s.
sinus s.
small bowel s.
upper gastrointestinal s.
seriograph
seriography
serioscopy
SER-IV
supination-external rotation IV
SER-IV fracture
serofibrinous pericardial effusion
serofibrous pleurisy
serohemorrhagic fluid
seroma
mediastinal s.

NOTES

seroma *(continued)*
    perigraft s.
    postoperative s.
seromuscular layer
seronegative rheumatoid arthritis
serosa
    cecal s.
serosal
    s. endometrial implant
    s. myoma
    s. surface
    s. tear
serosanguineous fluid
serous
    s. adenocarcinoma
    s. carcinoma
    s. cystadenocarcinoma
    s. cystadenoma
    s. effusion
    s. intraparenchymatous cyst
    s. ligament
    s. membrane
    s. ovarian tumor
    s. pericardium
    s. pleurisy
    s. tumor
serpentine
    s. aneurysm
    s. appearance
    s. asbestos
    s. enhancement
    s. signal void
    s. structure
serpiginosum
    angioma s.
serpiginous
    s. band
    s. low signal intensity border
    s. luminal filling defect
    s. section
    s. ulcer
serrated
    s. appearance
    s. suture
serration
    esophageal margin s.
    marginal s.
serratus
    s. anterior (SA)
    s. anterior muscle
Sertoli cell tumor (SCT)
Sertoli-Leydig cell tumor
Servelle vein
server
    AquariusNET 2D/3D medical
      imaging s.
services
    ReadyPET support s.

servomotor
    magnetic s.
servo power amplifier
Servox amplifier
sesamoid
    s. bone
    s. complex
    fibular hallux s.
    s. injury
    s. ligament
    s. migration
    tibial hallux s.
sesamoidometatarsal joint
sesamophalangeal ligament
sessile
    s. adenoma
    s. filling defect
    s. hydatid
    s. lesion
    s. nodular carcinoma
    s. plaque
    s. polyp
    s. tumor
sestamibi
    s. imaging agent
    s. parathyroid scintigraphy (SPS)
    s. polar map
    s. stress scan imaging
    ^{99m}Tc s.
    s. ^{99m}Tc with dipyridamole stress
      test
    s. technetium-99m
set

    access s.
    Amplatz dilator s.
    s. angle
    coaxial micropuncture needle s.
    Codman Cranioplastic Type 1
      Slow S.
    Curry intravascular retriever s.
    3D anatomic data s.
    data s.
    3D MRI data s.
    foreshortened image data s.
    Greene biopsy s.
    Hawkins accordion catheter
      drainage s.
    Hawkins inside-out nephrostomy s.
    Huisman percutaneous drainage s.
    image s.
    McNamara coaxial catheter
      infusion s.
    minimally invasive access s.
    Neff percutaneous access s.
    Ring-McLean sump drainage s.
    Ring transjugular intrahepatic
      access s.
    Rosch-Uchida liver access s.
    RUPS-100 liver access s.

Rutner balloon dilatation helical stone extractor s.
telescopic bougie s.
Van Sonnenberg chest drain s.
volumetric data s.

Sethotope radioactive imaging agent
seton
Settegast
S. method
S. position
S. projection

setting
discriminator s.
quadrature s.
simulation-aided field s.
soft tissue window s.
wide window s.
window/level s.

setting-sun sign
Sever disease
severe acute respiratory syndrome (SARS)
Severin
S. classification
S. grade

SEW
slice excitation wave

sextuplet pregnancy
Seze
angle of Lequesne and de S.

SF$_6$
sulfur hexafluoride

SFA
superficial femoral artery

SFD
source-film distance

SFP
scanned focal point
SFP scanner

S-F Precise stent
SFR
stenotic flow reserve

SFTP
solitary fibrous tumor of pleura

SGE
spoiled gradient echo

shaded
s. surface display
s. surface display imaging
s. surface rendering (SSR)

shading
s. appearance
image s.

shadow (*See* shadowing)
acoustic s.
bandlike s.
batwing s.
bony s.
s. box
breast s.
butterfly breast s.
calcific s.
cardiac s.
cardiomediastinal s.
cardiothymic s.
cardiovascular s.
centrilobular s.
clean s.
companion s.
concatenation of s.'s
cortical signet ring s.
discoid s.
double-arc gallbladder s.
double-bubble s.
dumbbell-shaped s.
edge s.
effusion s.
fusiform s.
gloved-finger s.
heart s.
hilar s.
iliopsoas muscle s.
kidney s.
large thymus s.
line s.
linear s.
mitral configuration of cardiac s.
nipple s.
overlap s.
overlying bowel s.
psoas s.
PVST s.
radiographic parallel line s.
renal s.
ring s.
s. scimitar
scimitar-shaped s.
s. shield
snowstorm s.
soft tissue s.
sound s.
spindle-shaped s.

S

NOTES

shadow *(continued)*
    summation of s.'s
    superimposition of bowel s.
    thymic s.
    toothpaste s.
    tramline s.
    tumorlike s.
    vascular s.
    wall-echo s. (WES)
    widened heart s.
shadowgram
shadowgraph
shadowgraphy
shadowing
    dirty acoustic s.
    hyperechoic structure with s.
    hypointense signal s.
    interstitial s.
    lateral wall refractive s.
    marked hypoechogenicity s.
    paraspinal soft tissue s.
    posterior acoustic s.
    refractive s.
    rib s.
    s. stone
shaft
    bone s.
    femoral s.
    s. flange
    s. fracture
    middle third s.
    proximal third s.
    s. of rib
shag
    aortic s.
shagging of cardiac border
shaggy
    s. contour to bowel
    s. esophagus
    s. heart border
    s. lung nodule
    s. pericardium
shagreen lesion
shaken baby syndrome (SBS)
shallow
    s. inspiration
    s. inspiratory effort
shank bone
shape
    aneurysm with simple s.
    baseball bat s.
    brachycephalic head s.
    cardiac s.
    cricket bat s.
    dumbbell s.
    exponential s.
    gaussian line s.
    gooseneck s.
    half-moon s.

    head s.
    heat s.
    horseshoe s.
    hourglass s.
    ice cream cone s.
    irregular s.
    line s.
    lobulated s.
    S. Maker system
    mesocephalic head s.
    mushroom s.
    oval s.
    ovoid s.
    peak s.
    pulse s.
    s. recovery
    rosette s.
    S s.
    scaphocephalic head s.
    scaphoid s.
    sickle s.
    spheric s.
    spheroid s.
    vertebral body s.
    wine glass s.
shaper
    beam s.
shaping
    heat s.
shared
    s. coronary artery
    s. prepulse (SHARP)
SHARP
    shared prepulse
    SHARP fat saturation technique
sharp
    S. angle
    s. border of lung
    s. carina
    s. dissection
    s. lateral margin
Sharpey fiber
**Sharplan SilkTouch Flashscan surgical
    laser**
**sharply demarcated circumferential
    lesion**
sharpness
    image s.
Sharp-Purser test
shattered
    s. kidney
    s. spleen
Shaver disease
shaving
    femoral condylar s.
    patellar s.
    residual metal fragment s.
SHC
    sclerosing hepatic carcinoma

shear
s. fracture
s. interface
s. strain
s. strain rate
s. stress
shearing
axonal s.
s. force
s. of white matter
s. white matter injury
shear-strain deformation
sheath
Amplatz Teflon s.
angioplasty s.
anterior rectus s.
ArrowFlex s.
arterial s.
axillary s.
bicipital synovial s.
bicipital tendon s.
carotid s.
catheter s.
caudal s.
Check-Flo s.
check-valve s.
Colapinto s.
common synovial flexor s.
Cordis s.
crural s.
dentinal s.
dural s.
extensor carpi ulnaris s.
fascial s.
femoral s.
fenestrated s.
fibrous s.
flexor tendon s.
5F minipuncture s.
10F peel-away s.
5F Pinnacle s.
giant cell tumor of the tendon s.
guiding s.
Henle s.
hockey-stick guiding s.
intratendon s.
s. ligament
muscle s.
myelin s.
s. needle
nerve root s.
neural s.

peel-away s.
periarteriolar lymphoid s.
periradicular s.
pilar s.
Pinnacle Destination renal
    guiding s.
plicated dural s.
posterior rectus s.
rectus s.
Schwann cell of myelin s.
self-expanding tulip s.
s. and side-arm
Spectranetics laser s. (SLS)
straight guiding s.
synovial s.
tendon s.
Terumo Pinnacle R/OII radiopaque
    marker introducer s.
transseptal s.
tulip s.
unplicated s.
vascular s.
venous s.
working s.
sheathing canal
Shebele physician reporting workstation
Sheehan syndrome
sheet
amnionic s.
s. immobilizer
sheetlike
s. dysplasia
s. growth pattern
Sheffield gamma unit
shelf, pl. **shelves**
Blumer rectal s.
buccal s.
dental s.
lateral s.
medial s.
mesocolic s.
palatine s.
patellar s.
rectal s.
synovial s.
shell
acetabular s.
K s.
L s.
M s.
s. nephrogram
O s.

S

NOTES

shelling off of cartilage
shelllike demarcation
shell-of-bone appearance
shell-type of periosteal reaction
Shelton femur fracture classification
shelving edge of Poupart ligament
Shenton line
shepherd
Shepherd fracture
shepherd's
    s. crook configuration
    s. crook deformity
Shepp-Logan filter function
SHG
    sonohysterography
Shibley sign
shibuol
shield
    acrylic syringe s.
    AME PinSite s.
    apron s.
    Faraday s.
    lead apron s.
    lead eye s.
    lead gonad s.
    radiofrequency magnetic s.
    shadow s.
    thyroid s.
    Tungsten eye s.
    Tungsten syringe s.
shielded gradient coil
shielding
    active s.
    faulty radiofrequency s.
    gonadal s.
    magnetic s.
    passive s.
    RF s.
    room s.
shift
    anterior capsular s.
    aromatic solvent-induced s. (ASIS)
    chemical s.
    colloid s.
    diamagnetic s.
    distal s.
    Doppler frequency s.
    flow-related phase s.
    s. of heart
    intracranial s.
    lanthanide-induced s.
    left-to-right s.
    mediastinal s.
    midline s.
    motion-induced phase s.
    navigator s.
    neonate mediastinal s.
    paramagnetic s.
    phase s.

pineal gland s.
pivot s.
plantar s.
s. probe
proximal brain s.
radial s.
s. reagents
reverse pivot s. (RPS)
right-to-left s.
round s.
simple s.
square brain s.
ST-segment s.
superior frontal axis s.
tracheal s.
velocity-induced phase s.
s. of ventricle
ventricular s.
shim
    s. coil
    s. inhomogeneities
    s. placement
Shimadzu
    S. CT scanner
    S. HeadTome Set-031 camera
    S. HeadTome system
    S. MR scanner
shimmed magnet
shimmering
    visual s.
shimming
    active s.
    localized s.
    passive s.
shin bone
Shine-Dalgamo sequence
Shiner radiopaque tube
Shinnar-LeRoux algorithm
Shirmer test
shish
    s. kabob esophagus
    s. kabob pattern
shiver
    esophageal s.
shock
    anaphylactic s.
    bowel s.
    cardiac s.
    cardiogenic s.
    circulation s.
    distributive s.
    hypovolemic s.
    Joule s.
    lung s.
    nephrogram s.
    neurogenic s.
    obstructive s.
    QRS synchronized s.
    septic s.

sequence monophasic s.
vasogenic s.

shockwave pressure
shoemaker's breast
Shone
    S. anomaly
    S. syndrome
shoot-through lateral x-ray film
Shope fibroma
short
    s. acquisition window
    s. axis acquisition
    s. axis image
    s. axis parasternal view
    s. axis plane
    s. axis slice
    s. axis view echocardiography
    s. bone
    s. echo point resolved
      spectroscopic sequence spectrum
    s. esophagus–type hiatal hernia
    s. gut syndrome
    s. half-life
    s. head
    s. head of biceps
    s. insular gyrus
    s. inversion recovery imaging
    s. limb dysplasia
    s. muscle
    s. oblique fracture
    s. radiolunate ligament
    s. repetition time sequence
    s. rib
    s. rib-polydactyly syndrome
    s. scale contrast
    s. tau inversion recovery (STIR)
    s. tau inversion recovery image
    s. TE proton MR spectroscopy
    s. TI inversion recovery
    s. TI inversion recovery imaging
    s. TI inversion recovery pulse
      sequence
    s. T1 inversion recovery (STIR)
    s. T1 relaxation time
    s. TR-TE
short-bore magnet
short-cannula coaxial method
short-distance
    s.-d. radiation therapy
    s.-d. radiotherapy

short-echo-time
    s.-e. t. chemical shift imaging
    s.-e.-t. proton spectroscopy
shortened
    fat-suppressed acquisition with TE
      and TR times s.
shortening
    Achilles tendon s.
    circumferential s.
    s. fraction
    fractional s. (FS)
    fractional myocardial s.
    left ventricular functional s.
      (LVFS)
    leg s.
    phalangeal s.
    skeleton s.
    suboccipital s.
    systolic fractional s.
    T1 s.
    T2 s.
    tendon s.
    T2-weighted s.
short-increment sensitivity index
short-inversion-time inversion recovery
    (STIR)
short-range isotope
short-segment Barrett esophagus (SSBE)
short-term patency
shot
    cusp s.
    fast low-angle s. (FLASH)
    fluid-attenuated inversion recovery-
      fast low-angle s.
    guiding s.
    multiple echo single s. (MESS)
    pocket s.
    turbo fast low-angle s.
      (turboFLASH)
1-shot echo-planar imaging
shoulder
    s. ankylosis
    arthrotomography of s.
    baseball s.
    curvilinear threshold s.
    s. dislocation
    s. dome
    double-contrast arthrotomography
      of s.
    drooping s.
    drop s.
    dynamic ultrasound of s. (DUS)

NOTES

shoulder *(continued)*
    s. dystocia
    flail s.
    football player s.
    frozen s.
    s. girdle
    s. of heart
    s. immobilizer
    s. impingement
    s. impingement syndrome
    intrathoracic dislocation of s.
    s. isocenter
    s. joint
    s. joint instability
    knocked-down s.
    s. labral capsular complex
    Little Leaguer s.
    loose s.
    s. muscle
    s. pointer
    s. presentation
    ring man s.
    s. separation
    subcoracoid dislocation of s.
    subglenoid dislocation of s.
    s. surface coil
    swimmer's s.
    tennis s.
shoulder-hand syndrome
shower
    s. of echoes
    embolic s.
    s.'s of microemboli
Shprintzen velocardiofacial syndrome
shrapnel
Shrapnell membrane
shrinkage
    aneurysm sac s.
    brain s.
    graft s.
    tumor s.
shriveled kidney
shrunken
    s. bladder
    s. folia
    s. gallbladder
    s. liver
    s. lung
SH U 508A contrast agent
shudder
    carotid s.
shunt
    barium-sulfate impregnated s.
    bidirectional s.
    biliopancreatic s.
    Blalock s.
    Blalock-Taussig s.
    cardiac atrial s.

    cardiovascular s.
    cerebral s.
    Cimino AV s.
    Cimino dialysis s.
    cystoatrial s.
    Davidson s.
    Denver s.
    dialysis s.
    direct intrahepatic portacaval s.
     (DIPS)
    distal splenorenal s.
    esophageal s.
    s. evaluation
    s. fraction
    gastrorenal s.
    Glenn s.
    indwelling nonvascular s.
    IVC to portal vein s.
    jejunoileal s.
    JI s.
    mesocaval s.
    net s.
    s. patency
    peritoneovenous s. (PVS)
    s. placement
    portacaval s.
    portopulmonary s.
    portosystemic s.
    Potts s.
    s. quantification
    s. reservoir
    s. reversal
    reversed s.
    small bowel s.
    splenorenal s.
    s. thrombosis
    transjugular intrahepatic
     portosystemic s. (TIPS)
    s. tube
    VA s.
    s. valve
    ventriculoatrial s.
    ventriculoperitoneal s.
    VP s.
    Waterston s.
    Waterston-Cooley s.
    s. with normal left atrium
shunted
    s. blood
    s. hydrocephalus
    s. tracer
shunting
    s. circuit
    lumboperitoneal s.
    peritoneal s.
    pleural s.
    syringosubarachnoid s.
    s. of tracer to bone marrow

shuntogram
s. imaging
radionuclide s.
shuntography
shutdown
renal s.
shuttering
white s.
Shwachman syndrome
SI
sacroiliac
saturation index
signal intensity
sinus irregularity
stroke index
SI joint
SI joint-sacrum ratio
S/I
superior/inferior
Si
silicon
Si (Li) detector
sialadenitis
acute suppurative s.
autoimmune s.
chronic recurrent s.
myoepithelial s.
recurrent s.
sialadenitis (*var. of* sialoadenitis)
sialadenography
sialangiography
sialectasis
sialoadenitis, sialadenitis
sialogram
sialography
CT s.
s. imaging
magnetic resonance s.
s. needle
parotid gland s.
submaxillary s.
sialolithiasis
sialometaplasia
sialometry
sialosis
siboroxime
technetium-99m s.
Sibson
S. fascia
S. groove
S. muscle

sick
s. sinus node
s. sinus syndrome
sickle shape
sickle-shaped fold
sickling
intravascular s.
sickness
decompression s.
radiation s.
SID
source-to-image receptor distance
side
s. branch
s. effect
s. fire
s. lobe artifact
s. scattering
side-arm
sheath and s.-a.
sideband
total suppression of s. (TOSS)
side-branch occlusion
side-by-side
s.-b.-s. object
s.-b.-s. transposition of great artery
1-sided image reconstruction
side-exiting
s.-e. coaxial needle system
s.-e. coaxial system
s.-e. guide
side-firing probe
side-hole cannulated probe
side-lying position
sideplate
Sideris buttoned double-disc device
sideropenic dysphagia
siderotic
s. nodule in spleen
s. splenomegaly
sideswipe fracture
sidewall
s. impingement
pelvic s.
Sidewinder
S. catheter
S. diagnostic catheter
SIE
stroke in evolution
Siemens
S. AG system
S. DRH CT scanner

S

NOTES

Siemens *(continued)*

S. Ecat EXACT HR+ CTI PET scanner

S. gamma camera

S. HICOR/BICOR x-ray system

S. ICON

S. Lithostar lithotripter

S. Magnetom GBS II scanner

S. Magnetom SP 4000 scanner

S. Magnetom 1.5-T scanner

S. Magnetom Vision scanner

S. Magnetom Vision whole-body MR device

S. Mammomat Novation DM full field digital mammography system

S. Mevatron 74 linear accelerator

S. One Tesla scanner

S. Orbiter large-field-of-view camera

S. Plus 4 Volume Zoom multidetector scanner

S. Satellite CT evaluation console

S. Somaform 512 CT scanner

S. SOMATOM DR2, DR3 whole-body scanner

S. SOMATOM nonhelical unit

S. SOMATOM Plus CT scanner

S. SOMATOM Plus-4 CT system

S. SOMATOM Sensation 64

S. Sonoline Elegra ultrasound scanner

S. 1.5-T system

SieScape

S. imaging technology

S. ultrasound

sieve bone

sievert (Sv)

SIF

sacral insufficiency fracture

sigma filter

sigmoid

s. carcinoma

s. cavity

s. cavity of radius

s. cavity of ulna

s. colon

s. colon volvulus

s. density curve

s. diverticulitis

s. diverticulum

s. flexure

s. fold

s. hair pattern

s. kidney

s. loop

s. lymph node

s. mesocolon

s. notch

s. omentum

s. polyp

s. pseudostenosis

s. sinus

s. sulcus

s. valve

sigmoidoscope

Olympus OSF s.

Reichert flexible s.

sigmoidoscopy

sigmoid-shaped configuration

sign

Aaron s.

Abrahams s.

absent bow-tie s.

absent diaphragm s.

accordion s.

air-crescent s.

air-meniscus s.

Allis s.

Amoss s.

angel-wing s.

antecedent s.

anterior drawer s.

aortic nipple s.

apical cap s.

arrowhead s.

Aunt Minnie s.

banana s.

Battle s.

B6 bronchus s.

beaded septum s.

beak s.

Beevor s.

Bergman s.

big rib s.

blade of grass s.

Blumberg s.

bowler hat s.

bowstring s.

bow-tie s.

Bozzolo s.

Bragard s.

Braunwald s.

brim s.

bronchial cuff s.

bronchus s.

Brudzinski s.

Bryant s.

bubble s.

C s.

calcium s.

Cantelli s.

cardinal s.

cardiorespiratory s.

Carman s.

Carnett s.

carotid string s.

Carvallo s.

catheter coiling s.

Chaddock s.
Chilaiditi s.
Claybrook s.
clockwise whirlpool s.
cobblestone s.
cobra-eye s.
Codman s.
Cogan lid twitch s.
cogwheel s.
coiled spring s.
collapsing cord s.
collar s.
Collier s.
colon cutoff s.
comb s.
comet-tail s.
commemorative s.
Comolli s.
continuous diaphragm s.
contralateral s.
Coopernail s.
cord s.
Corrigan s.
cortical rim s.
cortical vein s.
Courvoisier s.
cranial nerve s.
crescent s.
crescent-in-doughnut s.
Cullen s.
cupola s.
cutoff s.
dagger s.
Dance s.
David Letterman s.
Dawbarn s.
deep sulcus s.
Dejerine s.
Delbet s.
delta s.
Demianoff s.
de Musset s.
dense MCA s.
d'Espine s.
Dorendorf s.
double-bleb s.
double-bubble s.
double decidual sac s.
double density s.
double diaphragm s.
double duct s.
double-halo s.

double lesion s.
double line s.
double-ring esophageal s.
double track s.
double wall s.
doughnut s.
drooping lily s.
Drummond s.
Duchenne s.
duct-penetrating s.
Dupuytren s.
Duroziez s.
Ebstein s.
echogenic star burst s.
empty delta s.
Erichsen s.
Ewart s.
extrapleural s.
falciform ligament s.
fallen-fragment s.
fallen lung s.
false localizing s.
fan s.
fat-blood interface s.
fat pad s.
FBI s.
feeding vessel s.
figure-3 s.
Finkelstein s.
Fischer s.
fissure s.
fleck s.
Fleischner s.
flipped meniscus s.
floating viscera s.
floppy-thumb s.
flush-tank s.
focal neurologic s.
football s.
Friedreich s.
Froment s.
frontal lobe s.
Frostberg s.
Gaenslen s.
Galeazzi s.
garland s.
Gerhardt s.
geyser s.
Glasgow s.
gloved-finger s.
Goldthwait s.
Gordon s.

NOTES

sign (*continued*)

Gottron s.
Gowers s.
Grey Turner s.
Griesinger s.
Grocco s.
Gunn crossing s.
half-moon s.
halo s.
Hamman s.
harlequin s.
hatchet s.
Hawkins s.
hay-fork s.
Heim-Kreysig s.
hilar s.
Hildreth s.
Hill s.
Hirschberg s.
Hoffmann s.
Hoover s.
Horner s.
hot nose s.
Howship-Romberg s.
hyperdense middle cerebral
  artery s.
iliopsoas s.
insular ribbon s.
interface s.
interrupted duct s.
intradecidual s.
inverted teardrop s.
inverted-V s.
Jaccoud s.
Jackson s.
Kanavel s.
Kantor string s.
Karplus s.
Kehr s.
Kellock s.
Kernig s.
Klemm s.
Kussmaul s.
Lachman s.
Lancisi s.
Landolfi s.
Lasègue s.
lateralizing s.
Lazarus s.
Leichtenstern s.
lemon s.
leptomeningeal ivy s.
Leri s.
Livierato s.
localizing s.
long tract s.
luftsichel s.
Macewen s.
Maisonneuve s.

Mannkopf s.
Martorell s.
McGinn-White s.
melting s.
Meltzer s.
meniscus s.
Mennell s.
metacarpal s.
Minor s.
Morquio s.
Mulder s.
Müller s.
Musset s.
Myerson s.
Naffziger s.
naked-facet s.
Napoleon hat s.
Neer impingement s.
Nicoladoni-Branham s.
noose keyhole pull-away s.
obturator s.
Oliver-Cardarelli s.
open bronchus s.
Oppenheim s.
Ortolani s.
Osler s.
P s.
Payr s.
Perez s.
peritoneal s.
peroneal s.
piano key s.
Pins s.
Piotrowski s.
pivot-shift s.
Plummer s.
Potain s.
premonitory s.
pseudokidney s.
psoas s.
puddle s.
pulvinar s.
pupillary s.
pyramidal s.
Queckenstedt s.
Quénu-Muret s.
Quincke s.
radialis s.
railroad track s.
rebound s.
reversal s.
reverse S s.
Rigler s.
rim s.
ring s.
Risser s.
Romberg s.
Rosenbach s.
Rose thorn s.

rose thorn s.
Rotch s.
Rovighi s.
Rovsing s.
rugger jersey s.
sail s.
Sanders s.
sandwich s.
Sansom s.
sawtooth s.
Schepelmann s.
Schlesinger s.
Schwartze s.
scimitar s.
seagull s.
sentinel clot s.
sentinel loop s.
setting-sun s.
Shibley s.
signet ring s.
silhouette s.
Sister Mary Joseph s.
Skoda s.
slim carotid artery s.
sonographic Murphy s.
Spalding s.
spinal s.
spine s.
Spurling s.
squeeze s.
steeple s.
Steinberg s.
stepladder s.
Sternberg s.
Stewart-Holmes s.
Stierlin s.
string s.
string-of-beads s.
string-of-pearls s.
stripe s.
Strümpell s.
Strunsky s.
Sumner s.
superior triangle s.
tail s.
target s.
Terry Thomas s.
thread-and-streaks s.
Thurston Holland s.
thymic sail s.
tibialis s.
Tinel s.

Traube s.
tree-in-bud s.
triple-bubble s.
triple track s.
Troisier s.
trolley-track s.
trough s.
Trousseau s.
Turyn s.
twin peak s.
Uhthoff s.
Vanzetti s.
Waddell s.
Wartenberg s.
Wegner s.
Weill s.
Weiss s.
Westermark s.
whirl s.
whirlpool s.
white cerebellum s.
Wimberger s.
windsock s.
yin-yang s.

Signa
S. Advantage system
S. EXCITE 3.0T MRI system
S. Horizon LX MRI system
S. Horizon LX SR 77 gradients
 1.5-T MR scanner
S. Horizon X-Echo-Speed
S. MR imaging system
S. MRI scanner
S. 1.5T scanner
S. VH/i3.0-T MR scanner

signal
abnormal bright s.
s. acquisition
s. attenuation
s. average
s. blooming
BOLD s.
bright s.
s. change
s. characteristic
color Doppler s.
composite s.
D s.
s. dephasing
s. depth
differential s.
Doppler blood flow velocity s.

NOTES

signal *(continued)*
    Doppler ovary s.
    s. drop-out artifact
    s. enhancement
    s. fallout
    flow velocity s.
    fluid s.
    free induction decay s.
    gamma s.
    GE-Amersham merger s.
    s. halo
    high-intensity s.
    high-intensity transient s. (HITS)
    high-pitched s.
    hyperintense s.
    hypointense s.
    hypointense marrow s.
    imaginary s.
    increased echo s.
    s. intensity (SI)
    s. intensity inhomogeneity
    s. intensity measurement
    s. intensity ratio
    s. intensity rim
    s. intensity time curve
    isointense s.
    s. joint
    linear low s.
    lipid s.
    s. loss
    magnetic resonance s.
    s. magnification
    mosaic jet s.
    navigable echo s.
    NMR s.
    s. node
    nuclear s.
    ovarian Doppler s.
    periventricular bright s.
    phosphomonoester s.
    power Doppler s.
    s. processing
    pulsed-wave spectral color
     Doppler s.
    radionuclide s.
    real s.
    s. sonographic feature analysis
    s. source
    SSFP s.
    stimulus-correlated water s.
    superimposition of s.
    s. suppression
    symmetric abnormal increased s.
    s. time course
    s. transducer
    s. transduction
    turbulent s.
    T2-weighted s.
    unsuppressed water s.

    velocity-encoded color Doppler s.
    s. void
    weak s.
signal-averaged electrocardiogram
    (SAECG, SaECG)
signaling molecule
signal-to-clutter ratio
signal-to-noise
    s.-t.-n. calculation
    s.-t.-n. ratio (SNR, S-N, S:N)
    s.-t.-n. threshold
signature
    echo s.
    gut s.
    tissue s.
    tumor s.
signet
    s. ring cell carcinoma
    s. ring pattern
    s. ring sign
significance level
significant
    s. axis deviation
    s. residual deficit
    s. sequela
SIH
    secondary intracranial hypertension
SIL
    squamous intraepithelial lesion
silastic
    s. collar-reinforced stoma
    s. finger joint
    s. ring
silence
    electrocerebral s. (ECS)
silent
    s. area of brain
    s. cerebral embolus
    s. gallstone
    s. ischemic episode
    s. mitral stenosis
    s. myocardial infarct (SMI)
    s. myocardial ischemia
    s. patent ductus arteriosus
    s. regurgitation
    s. sinus syndrome
silhouette
    cardiac s.
    cardiothymic s.
    cardiovascular s.
    enlarged cardiac s.
    heart s.
    s. imaging
    S. laser system
    luminal s.
    pericardial s.
    roentgenographic s.
    s. sign
    s. sign of Felson

s. technique
widened cardiac s.
silhouetted out
silhouetting
silicate pneumoconiosis
silicon (Si)
amorphous s.
s. diode array
s. diode dosimeter
silicon-controlled rectifier (SCR)
silicone
s. caoutchouc
s. elastomer band
s. elastomer ring
s. elastomer rubber ball implant
s. fluid
s. granuloma
s. implant leakage
s. implant rupture
s. injection
s. microsphere
s. oil
s. stent
s. wrist implant
Silicon Graphics Reality Engine system
silicoproteinosis
acute s.
silicosis
accelerated s.
chronic simple s.
complicated s.
Liverpool s.
nonnodular s.
simple s.
silicotic
s. fibrosis of lung
s. nodule
s. visceral pleura
silicotuberculosis
silk
s. suture
S. Touch laser skin resurfacing
s. tuft
SilkLaser
S. aesthetic carbon dioxide laser
S. aesthetic laser system
2040 erbium S.
Sillence classification of osteogenesis imperfecta
sillimanite pneumoconiosis

silo-filler's
s.-f. disease
s.-f. lung
silver
s. finisher's lung
s. fork fracture
Grocott methenamine s.
s. halide film
s. iodide
s. polisher's lung
s. recovery
S. Speed 0.010-inch guidewire
s. wire effect
Silverhawk catheter
simian griffe
Simmond disease
Simmons catheter
Simon
S. focus
S. Nitinol filter
S. Nitinol IVC filter
S. Nitinol vena cava filter
Simonart
S. band
S. ligament
SIM/Plant
simple
s. block
s. bolus
s. bone cyst
s. breast cyst
s. capillary lymphangioma
s. cortical renal cyst
s. dislocation
s. extraperitoneal rupture
s. goiter
s. mechanical obstruction
s. meningocele
s. shift
s. silicosis
s. skull fracture
s. ureterocele
simplex
carcinoma s.
xanthoma tuberosum s.
SimpliCT interventional guidance system
Simpson
S. atherectomy
S. Coronary AtheroCath (SCA) system
S. directional atherectomy catheter

NOTES

S

Simpson *(continued)*
    S. rule method for ventricular volume
    S. white line
Sims position
simulated
    s. annealing
    s. annealing method
    s. annealing method projection
    s. echo
    s. equilibrium factor study
simulation
    s. of converging port
    s. film
    MCPT s.
    Monte Carlo photon transport s.
    s. of tangential portal
simulation-aided field setting
simulator
    AcQsim CT s.
    magnetic resonance s.
    Maxwell 3D field s.
    virtual reality s.
    Ximatron s.
simultaneous
    s. acquisition of artery and vein (SAAV)
    s. acquisition of spatial harmonics (SMASH)
    s. balloon inflation
    s. bilateral spontaneous pneumothorax (SBSP)
    s. fluoroscopy
    s. MSDI
    s. multifilm tomography
    s. multislice acquisition
    s. recording
    s. slice
    s. volume imaging
sincalide
    s. cholescintigraphy
    s. imaging agent
sinc-Hanning radiofrequency
sinc interpolation
sincipital cephalocele
Sinding-Larsen-Johansson disease (SLJD)
sine wave
singer's
    s. node
    s. nodule
Singh osteoporosis index
single
    s. atrium
    s. axis
    s. breath-hold
    s. breath-hold dynamic subtraction CT with multidetector row helical technology
    s. breath-hold sequence

    s. collision energy loss
    s. colonic filling defect
    s. fill/void technique
    s. functioning kidney
    s. isocenter
    s. label
    s. peak
    s. photon/maximum intensity
    s. pixel reconstruction
    s. pleurisy
    s. polyp
    s. popliteal vein
    s. port
    s. section 2D image
    s. shot TSE (SShTSE)
    s. suture synostosis
    s. sweep scan
    s. umbilical artery
    s. umbilical artery spectrum
    s. ventricle
    s. voxel proton brain spectroscopy imaging
    s. voxel proton MR spectroscopy (1H-MRS)
    s. voxel stimulated echo acquisition mode MR spectroscopy
    s. voxel in vivo proton spectrum
    s. x-ray dosimetry
single-ablation scheme
single-bevel stylet
single-breath view
single-cannula atrial cannulation
single-cavity cochlea
single-channel analyzer (SCA)
single-contrast
    s.-c. arthrography
    s.-c. barium enema
    s.-c. study
single-crystal endoprobe
single-curved Cobra catheter
single-detector
    s.-d. computed tomography (SDCT)
    s.-d. CTA
    s.-d. helical CT
    s.-d. helical scanner
    s.-d. row scanner
single-dose gadolinium imaging
single-echo
    s.-e. diffusion imaging
    s.-e. versus multiple-echo sequence
single-energy x-ray absorptiometer (SXA)
single-field hyperthermia technique
single-headed instrument
single-head rotating gamma camera
single-hole collimator
single-injection protocol
single-lumen silicone breast implant
single-needle biopsy technique

single-outlet heart
single-pass scan
single-phase current
single-photon
    s.-p. absorptiometry (SPA)
    s.-p. counting system
    s.-p. densitometer
    s.-p. emission-computed tomography (SPECT)
    s.-p. emission-computed tomography technetium sestamibi scan
    s.-p. emission CT
    s.-p. emission tomography (SPET)
    s.-p. planar scintigraphy (SPPS)
single-plane angiography
single-pole double-throw (SPDT)
single-power injector
single-sample
    s.-s. clearance
    s.-s. technique
single-shot
    s.-s. embolization of micro-AVM
    s.-s. fast spin echo (SSFSE)
    s.-s. gradient echo-planar imaging
    s.-s. imaging technique
    s.-s. MR cholangiogram
    s.-s. thick-slab RARE
single-slice
    s.-s. CTA
    s.-s. eight-echo technique
    s.-s. gradient-echo image
    s.-s. helical CT
    s.-s. long-axis tomogram
single-stick
    s.-s. catheter introduction
    s.-s. system
single-strand
    s.-s. conformational polymorphism (SSCP)
    s.-s. scission
single-stripe colitis (SSC)
single-vessel
    s.-v. disease
    s.-v. runoff
single-view oblique mammography
single-voxel proton brain examination
single-wall needle
singular valve decompensation (SVD)
sinistral portal hypertension
sinistrum
    atrium s.

sink
    s. effect
    quantum s.
sink-trap malformation
sinoatrial (*var. of* sinuatrial) **(SA)**
sinoauricular node
sinodural plate
Sinografin imaging agent
sinogram
sinography
sinonasal
    s. carcinoma
    s. cavity
    s. lesion
    s. lymphoma
    s. polyposis
    s. psammomatoid ossifying fibroma
    s. secretion
    s. tumor
sinotubular junction
sinovaginal bulb
sintering
    selective laser s. (SLS)
sinuatrial, sinoatrial
    s. block (SAB)
    s. branch
    s. bundle
    s. conduction time (SACT)
    s. exit block
    s. nodal reentry tachycardia
    s. node (SAN)
    s. node artery
    s. node dysfunction
    s. node infarct
sinus
    accessory s.
    alternating s.
    aortic valve s.
    s. arrest
    artery of inferior cavernous s. (AICS)
    basilar s.
    branchial s.
    bronchial s.
    carotid s.
    cavernous s.
    s. cavity
    cerebral venous s.
    cervical s.
    circular s.
    cloudy s.
    coccygeal s.

NOTES

S

sinus (continued)
    coronary s. (CS)
    costomediastinal s.
    costophrenic s.
    cranial s.
    s. cycle length (SCL)
    dilated intercavernous s.
    distal coronary s. (DCS)
    dorsal dermal s.
    dorsal enteric s.
    draining s.
    dural venous s.
    dura mater venous s.
    endodermal s.
    s. of epididymis
    ethmoid s.
    frontal s.
    frontalis s.
    granulomatous lesion of s.
    Guérin s.
    s. histiocytosis
    s. hyperplasia
    hypoechoic renal s.
    s. hypoplasia
    inferior sagittal s. (ISS)
    intercavernous s.
    s. irregularity (SI)
    lactiferous s.
    lateral s.
    s. lateralis
    left coronary s.
    s. lipomatosis
    lumbosacral dermal s.
    lymph node s.
    manual pressure over carotid s.
    marginal s.
    mastoid s.
    maxillary s.
    s. mechanism
    medullary s.
    middle coronary s. (MCS)
    s. of Morgagni
    nasal s.
    s. nodal artery
    s. nodal reentry
    s. node
    s. node automaticity
    s. node depression
    s. node dysfunction
    s. node electrogram
    s. node exit block
    s. node recovery time (SNRT)
    noncoronary s.
    oblique pericardial s.
    occipital s.
    osteomyelitic s.
    paranasal s.
    s. pattern
    s. pause

    pericardial s.
    s. pericranii
    perineal s.
    Petit s.
    petrosal s.
    pilonidal s.
    piriform s.
    precoronal sagittal s.
    prostatic s.
    pulmonary s.
    s. of pulmonary trunk
    renal s.
    s. rhythm
    s. rhythm mapping
    Ridley s.
    Rokitansky-Aschoff s.
    rudimentary s.
    sagittal s.
    s. septum
    s. series
    sick s. syndrome
    sigmoid s.
    s. slowing
    sphenoid s.
    sphenoparietal s.
    straight s.
    subeustachian s.
    superior petrous s. (SPS)
    superior sagittal s. (SSS)
    tarsal s.
    s. tarsi syndrome
    thickened s.
    s. thrombosis
    s. tract
    s. tract imaging
    s. tract study
    transverse pericardial s.
    urachal s.
    urogenital s.
    s. of Valsalva
    s. of Valsalva aneurysm
    s. of vena cava
    s. venosus
    s. venosus atrial septal defect
    venous s.
    vertebral articular s.
sinusitis
    acute s.
    allergic s.
    bacterial s.
    bronchiectasis-ethmoid s.
    s. cerebritis
    chronic s.
    mycotic s.
    paranasal s.
    sphenoidal s.
sinusography
    cerebral s.

sinusoid
> hepatic s.
> s. reference function

sinusoidal
> s. capillary
> s. histiocyte
> s. lesion
> s. relaxation
> s. vascular space
> s. waveform

sinusoidalization
sinuvertebral nerve of Luschka
SIP
> saturation inversion projection

siphon
> carotid s.

Sipple syndrome
SIR
> Sirtex Medical Limited

Siremobil Iso-C3d isocentric C-arm
sirenomelia
sirolimus
sirolimus-eluting SMART Nitinol stent
SIR-Spheres radioactive sphere
SIRT
> selective internal radiation therapy

Sirtex Medical Limited (SIR)
SIS
> saline infusion sonohysterography

SISCOM
> Subtraction ictal SPECT coregistered to MRI

SISCO spectrometer
Sister
> S. Mary Joseph node
> S. Mary Joseph nodule
> S. Mary Joseph sign

site
> anastomotic s.
> binding s.
> bleeding s.
> cellular binding s.
> donor s.
> extraadrenal s.
> extranodal s.
> fracture s.
> implantation s.
> ipsilateral antegrade s.
> s. of maximal intensity
> metastatic s.
> reference s.
> sanctuary s.

> termination s.
> unknown primary s.

Site-Rite
> S.-R. II ultrasound system
> S.-R. ultrasound system

site-specific labeling
sitting-up
> s.-u. view
> s.-u. view angiography

situ
> adenocarcinoma in s.
> carcinoma in s.
> ductal carcinoma in s. (DCIS)
> in s.
> intracystic breast papillary carcinoma in s.
> lobular carcinoma in s. (LCIS)

situs
> atrial s.
> s. atrialis solitus
> s. concordance
> D-loop ventricular s.
> s. inversus
> s. inversus totalis
> s. inversus viscerum
> L-loop ventricular s.
> s. perversus
> s. transversus
> s. viscerum inversus

Sitzmarks
> S. capsule
> S. radiopaque marker

sixth
> s. compartment
> s. nucleus
> s. ventricle

size
> abnormal placental s.
> borderline heart s.
> decreased placenta s.
> effective focal spot s.
> embryo s.
> s. estimation error
> gallbladder s.
> kernel s.
> kidney s.
> matrix s.
> ovarian s.
> renal s.
> s. of spinal cord
> top normal limits of s.
> uterine s.

NOTES

size *(continued)*
    ventricular s.
    vertebral body s.
    voxel s.
    x-ray beam s.
Sjögren-Larsson syndrome
Sjögren syndrome
SJS
    Schwartz-Jampel syndrome
    Swyer-James syndrome
skeletal
    s. amyloidosis
    s. bed
    s. biopsy
    s. disruption
    s. dysplasia
    s. emphysema
    s. hyperostosis
    s. hypoplasia
    s. lesion
    s. lymphoma
    s. maturation
    s. maturity
    s. metastasis
    s. muscle
    s. muscle fiber
    s. neoplasm
    s. radiology
    s. survey
    s. system
    s. targeted radiotherapy (STR)
    s. tuberculosis
skeletally
    s. immature
    s. mature
skeletography
skeletology
skeleton
    appendicular s.
    s. appendiculare
    articulated s.
    axial s.
    s. axiale
    bony s.
    cardiac s.
    fibrous s.
    gill arch s.
    laryngeal s.
    peripheral s.
    s. shortening
    spidering s.
    spiky s.
    sulcal s.
    s. thoracis
    visceral s.
skeletonizing
skeletopia
skeletopy
skiagram

skiagraph
skiagraphy
skier's
    s. fracture
    s. injury
    s. thumb
ski jump view
Skillern fracture
skimming of magnetic field
skin
    s. bridge
    s. calcification
    s. carcinoma
    s. crease artifact
    s. depth
    s. dose
    s. effect
    s. fold
    s. fold artifact
    s. lesion artifact
    s. line
    s. staple
    s. thickening
Skinlight erbium YAG laser
Skinner line
skinny needle
skin-rolling scapular tenderness
skin-sparing effect
skip
    s. aganglionosis
    s. area
    s. lesion
    s. metastasis
    s. tomography
skodaic resonance
Skoda sign
skull
    abnormally thin s.
    anterior cerebral artery crawling
      under s.
    s. asymmetry
    base of s. (BOS)
    beaten brass s.
    beaten silver appearance of s.
    button sequestrum s.
    cloverleaf s.
    dentate suture of s.
    s. film
    s. fracture
    geographic s.
    hair-on-end of s.
    hammered-silver s.
    hammer-marked s.
    hot-cross bun s.
    s. hyperostosis
    indented fracture of s.
    inner table of s.
    lacunar s.
    lytic lesion of s.

maplike s.
molding of s.
natiform s.
occipital view of s.
s. osteolysis
outer table of s.
s. plate
sonolucent s.
suture of s.
synchondrosis of s.
thin s.
West-Engstler s.
West lacuna s.

skull-base

s.-b. approach
s.-b. foramen
s.-b. tumor

SKYLight gantry-free nuclear medicine gamma camera

skyline

s. projection
s. view
s. view of patella

SL

scapholunate
spin-lock
SL joint
SL ligament
SL technique

slab

coronal s.
3D MRA s.
interleaved axial s.
s. thickness

slab-MIP

SLAC

scapholunate advanced collapse
SLAC wrist

slant hole collimator

SLAP

superior labral anterior to posterior
SLAP lesion
SLAP tear

slat collimator

sleeve

conjoined root s.
s. fracture
s. lobectomy
nerve root s.
Smitt s.
thoracic root s.

SLE 2000 ventilator

slew range

SL-GRE

spin lock gradient-echo
SL-GRE sequence

slice

angled s.
apical short-axis s.
axial s.
basal short-axis s.
contiguous s.
coronal s.
cross s.
digitized CT s.
direct s.
2D sequential s.
s. excitation wave (SEW)
s. format
s. fracture
gated stress myocardial perfusion s.
s. geometry
horizontal long axis s.
s. interference
intermediate CT s.
long-axis s.
midventricular short-axis s.
nonattenuation-corrected s.
nonplanar s.
oblique s.
s. orientation
s. overlap artifact
plurality of s.'s
s. profile artifact
sagittal s.
s. select gradient (SS)
s. selection
s. sensitivity profile (SSP)
serial CT s.
short axis s.
simultaneous s.
STIR s.
texture s.
s. thickness
tissue s.
tomographic s.
transaxial s.
transverse s.
vertical long-axis s.
s. volume

4-slice acquisition

slice-of-sausage breast pattern

slice-point MRS

slice-selective excitation

S

NOTES

slicing plane
slider crank theory
sliding

s. board transfer
s. hiatal hernia
s. interleaved Ky (SLINKY)
s. thin-slab maximum intensity projection (STS-MIP)
s. thin-slab maximum intensity projection image
s. thin-slab minimum intensity projection technique

slim carotid artery sign
sling

cardiac s.
s. muscle fiber
pulmonary s.
s. ring complex
tendon s.
vascular s.

SLINKY

sliding interleaved Ky

slip

s. angle
diaphragmatic s.
muscular s.
s. of tendon

slip-angle spondylolisthesis
slip-in connection
slippage

epiphysial s.
film s.

slipped

s. capital femoral epiphysis (SCFE)
s. tendon
s. upper femoral epiphysis (SUFE)

slipping

s. rib
s. rib syndrome

slip-ring

s.-r. camera
s.-r. CT
s.-r. gantry system
s.-r. imaging
s.-r. technology

slit

s. collimator
s. hemorrhage
s. radiography
s. scanography
s. ventricle
s. ventricle syndrome

slit-lamp biomicroscopy
slitlike

s. lumen
s. orafice
s. residual lucency

slit-shaped vessel lumen

sliver

bone s.

SLJD

Sinding-Larsen-Johansson disease

SLL

spinolaminar line

SLN

sentinel lymph node

slope

acromial s.
s. blot analysis
closing s.
decreased E-to-F s.
disappearance s.
downward s.
D-to-E s.
E-to-F s.
flat diastolic s.
flattened E-to-F s.
mitral deceleration s.
normalized plateau s.
opening s.
palmar s.
ST/HR s.
ST segment/heart rate slope
triquetrohamate helicoid s.
valve opening s.

slot-scanning detector
slotted tube stent
sloughed

s. mucosa
s. papilla
s. urethra syndrome

sloughing ulcer
slow

s. exchange soft tissue
s. filling wave
s. neutron
s. stroke
s. ventricular response

slow-channel blocking drug
slow-flow

s.-f. lesion
s.-f. vascular anomaly
s.-f. vascular malformation

slow-flowing giant saccular aneurysm
slowing

background s.
sinus s.

slowly

s. developing atelectasis
s. developing lesion

slow-twitch muscle
slow-wave activity
SLP

subluxation of patella

SLS

selective laser sintering

Spectranetics laser sheath
SLS laser
sludge
aggregated s.
s. ball
biliary s.
blood s.
gallbladder s.
tumefactive s.
tumefactive biliary s.
sludgelike intraluminal echo
sludging of retinal vein
sluggish flow
slurry
Sm
samarium
^{153}**Sm, Sm-153**
samarium 153
SMA
spinal muscular atrophy
superior mesenteric artery
Doppler sonography of the SMA
SMAI
superior-medial acetabular index
small
s. adrenal tumor
s. airway
s. airway dysfunction
s. aorta syndrome
s. B-cell lymphoma
s. bowel
s. bowel adenocarcinoma
s. bowel adenoma
s. bowel atresia
s. bowel benign tumor
s. bowel carcinoma
s. bowel cavitary lesion
s. bowel content
s. bowel delayed transit
s. bowel disease
s. bowel diverticulum
s. bowel duplication cyst
s. bowel enema
s. bowel enteroscopy (SBE)
s. bowel filling defect
s. bowel fold anatomy
s. bowel fold atrophy
s. bowel gas
s. bowel hemangioma
s. bowel hemorrhage
s. bowel infarct
s. bowel leiomyoma

s. bowel leiomyosarcoma
s. bowel loop
s. bowel malignant tumor
s. bowel malrotation
s. bowel meal
s. bowel metastasis
s. bowel motility
s. bowel mucosal pattern
s. bowel multiple ulcer
s. bowel peristalsis
s. bowel pseudodiverticula
s. bowel pseudotumor
s. bowel separation
s. bowel series
s. bowel shunt
s. bowel transit time
s. bowel volvulus
s. bowel wall thickening
s. cardiac vein
s. colonic J-pouch
s., deep, recent infarct (SDRI)
s. feminine aorta
s. field-of-view MR imaging
s. gallbladder
s. for gestational age fetus
s. gut
s. internal auditory canal
s. intestine
s. intestine carcinoma
s. intestine mesentery
s. left colon syndrome
s. LITT applicator
s. lymphocytic T-cell lymphoma
s. part of fetus
s. particle iron oxide contrast
s. pelvis
s. round cell carcinoma
s. saphenous vein
s. spleen
s. vertebral body
s. water-hammer pulse
small-angle multiple scattering
small-bore scanner
small-bowel
s.-b. follow-through (SBFT)
s.-b. obstruction (SBO)
small-caliber needle
small-cell
s.-c. cribriform carcinoma
s.-c. lung carcinoma (SCLC)
s.-c. osteosarcoma
s.-c. undifferentiated carcinoma

NOTES

small-droplet fatty liver
small-lunged emphysema
small-step distraction
small-vessel stroke
small-volume tissue ablation
small-voxel acquisition
SMAP
    systemic mean arterial pressure
SMART
    S. Control self-expanding stent
    S. Nitinol self-expandable stent
    S. self-expanding stent
    S. stent
SmartBeam IMRT
SmartNeedle
SmartPrep
    S. imaging agent
    MR S.
    S. scanner
SmartScore CT imaging
SmartSPOT high-resolution digital imaging system
Smartstent
SMAS
    superior mesenteric artery syndrome
SMASH
    simultaneous acquisition of spatial harmonics
        variable density SMASH (VD-auto-SMASH)
smear fragment
Smelloff-Cutter valve
SMI
    silent myocardial infarct
Smith
    S. dislocation
    S. fracture
    S. orthogonal hole test
    S. sesamoid position classification
Smith-Lemli-Opitz syndrome
Smith-Petersen nail
Smith-Robinson bone graft
Smitt sleeve
SMM
    scintimammography
SMN
    second malignant neoplasm
smoked glass image
smokelike echo
smoker's
    s. bronchiolitis
    s. lung
smooth
    s. border
    s. brain
    s. contour
    s. esophageal narrowing
    s. excimer laser coronary angioplasty (SELCA)

    s. hyperplasia
    s. mover
    s. muscle
    s. muscle hypertrophy
    s. muscle tumor
    s. tapered appearance
    s. thickened mucosal fold
Smoothbeam laser
smooth-bordered
smoothed curve fit
smoothie
smoothing
    gaussian s.
    spatial s.
    temporal s.
smooth-walled bladder
SMR
    scatter-maximum ratio
smudged papilla
SMV
    superior mesenteric vein
S-N (*var. of* SNR)
S:N (*var. of* SNR)
Sn
    stannum
    tin
^{113}Sn
    tin 113
snake graft
snake's head appearance
snapping
    s. fascia lata
    s. hip
    s. hip syndrome
    scapular s.
    s. triceps syndrome
snapshot
    contrast-enhanced dynamic s.
    dynamic s.
    s. fashion
snare
    Amplatz Goose Neck s.
sneaker osteomyelitis
Sneddon syndrome
Sneppen fracture of talus
sniff test
Sniper
    S. Elite hydrophilic guidewire
    S. Elite hydrophilic Ni-Ti alloy guidewire
snowboarder fracture
snowflakelike calcification
snowflake pattern
snowman
    s. abnormality
    s. appearance of heart
    s. configuration
    s. deformity

snowplow
    s. effect
    s. occlusion
snowstorm
    s. breast pattern
    s. shadow
SNR, S-N, S:N
    signal-to-noise ratio
SNRT
    sinus node recovery time
snuffbox
    anatomic s.
Snyder classification
soap
    calcium bile s.
    s. suds enema
soap-bubble
    s.-b. appearance
    s.-b. nephrogram
    s.-b. radiolucency
SOC
    sum of cylinder
society
    American Cancer S. (ACS)
    S. of Interventional Radiology
    Scoliosis Research S.
socket-stump interface
Socrates telementoring system
sodium
    s. 23 (^{23}Na)
    s. 24 (^{24}Na)
    acetrizoate s.
    s. acrylate and vinyl alcohol
      copolymer microsphere (SAP-MS)
    s. and/or methylglucamine
      diatrizoate contrast agent
    s. bicarbonate imaging agent
    s. chloride imaging agent
    s. diatrizoate imaging agent
    ^{18}F s. fluoride imaging agent
    fluorescein s.
    s. imaging
    s. iodide (NaI)
    s. iodide detector
    s. iodide iodine-131
    s. iodide ring
    s. iodide ring imaging agent
    iodohippurate s.
    s. iodohippurate imaging agent
    iothalamate s.
    s. iothalamate imaging agent
    ioxaglate s.

ipodate s.
    s. ipodate imaging agent
liothyronine s.
    s. meglumine ioxaglate contrast
      agent
    s. metrizoate acid contrast agent
    s. morrhuate
    s. pertechnetate
    s. pertechnetate imaging agent
    s. phosphate (P-32)
    s. phosphate ^{32}P
radioactive s.
    s. reabsorption
technetium-99m pertechnetate s.
tetrabromophenolphthalein s.
    s. tetradecyl sulfate
tetraiodophenolphthalein s.
total exchangeable s. (TENa)
tyropanoate s.
    s. tyropanoate imaging agent
warfarin s.
ytterbium pentetate s.
sodium-2-mercaptoethane sulfonate
sodium-potassium ATPase-dependent
  exchange mechanism
Soemmerring
    S. ligament
    S. muscle
soft
    s. disc herniation
    s. food dysphagia
    s. infiltrate
    s. palate carcinoma
    s. papilloma
    s. photon
    s. pigment stone
    s. ray
    s. tissue
    s. tissue ablation
    s. tissue abnormality
    s. tissue abscess
    s. tissue attenuation value
    s. tissue canal encroachment
    s. tissue chondroma
    s. tissue contracture
    s. tissue contrast
    s. tissue contusion
    s. tissue convexity
    s. tissue defect
    s. tissue density
    s. tissue density mass
    s. tissue density structure

S

NOTES

soft (*continued*)
  s. tissue derangement
  s. tissue distraction
  s. tissue entrapment
  s. tissue envelope
  s. tissue fibroma
  s. tissue ganglion
  s. tissue gas
  s. tissue hemangioma
  s. tissue injury
  s. tissue interposition
  s. tissue kernel
  s. tissue lesion classification
  s. tissue lipoma
  s. tissue lipomatosis
  s. tissue necrosis
  s. tissue neoplasm
  s. tissue ossification
  s. tissue osteochondroma
  s. tissue osteoma
  s. tissue pathoanatomy in
    melorheostosis
  s. tissue radiograph
  s. tissue reaction
  s. tissue sarcoma
  s. tissue shadow
  s. tissue stranding
  s. tissue stroma
  s. tissue swelling
  s. tissue uptake bone scintigraphy
  s. tissue window
  s. tissue window setting
  S. Torque uterine catheter
softball sliding injury
soft-copy computed radiography
softening
  s. of brain
  s. of cartilage
SoftLight laser
Softouch catheter
Softscan
  S. laser
  S. laser mammography system
Soft-Tip catheter
Soft-Vu angiographic catheter
software
  autotriggering s.
  BrainVoyager interactive s.
  calcium scoring s.
  CareGraph skin dose mapping s.
  CT Perfusion 2 s.
  DecThreads s.
  3-Dimensional Perfusion/Motion
    Map s.
  FuncTool s.
  GammaPlan s.
  GE Viewer s.
  HeartView cardiac reconstruction s.
  image-processing s.

  IP-plus image processing s.
  Kodak s.
  linear combination model s.
  LX 8.3 s.
  magnetic resonance user
    interface s.
  modified vessel image processor s.
  MRUI s.
  multigated spectral Doppler
    analysis s.
  multiplanar gradient-echo s.
  NeuroEcho s.
  Neuro Lobe s.
  Neuro SPGR s.
  P-Link s.
  Plug n View 3D medical
    imaging s.
  SPARC s.
  SPOT mobile 3D ultrasound
    system and s.
  Starlink s.
  StereoPlan stereotactic planning
    software
  TeraRecon s.
  VERT s.
  ViewMax s.
  Vitrea 2 3D CT angiographic s.
  Voxel-Man s.
  VoxelView s.
software-controlled internal hardware
  filter
SOG
  supraorbital groove
sojourn time
solar
  s. plexus
  s. radiation
solarization
soldier's
  s. heart
  s. patches of pericardium
  s. spot
soleal
  s. line
  s. vein
sole cluster of microcalcification
solenoid surface coil
soleus
  s. muscle
  s. syndrome
solid
  s. bolus challenge
  s. bone
  s. bony union
  s. circumscribed breast carcinoma
  s. component
  s. consolidation
  s. and cystic pancreatic tumor
  s. DCIS

s. echo
s. edema
s. edema of lung
s. food dysphagia
s. lesion spleen
s. lesion thymus
s. mass
s. matrix
s. organ transplant (SOT)
s. ovarian teratoma
s. ovarian tumor
s. and papillary pancreatic carcinoma
s. pattern
s. periosteal reaction
s. pilocytic astrocytoma
s. primary tumor
s. pseudopapillary tumor
s. splenic lesion
s. thymic lesion
s. viscus
s. viscus injury

solidifying agent
solid-phase extraction tube
solid-rod ureteroscope
solid-state
s.-s. manometry catheter
s.-s. nuclear track detector

solitary
s. adenoma
s. bone cyst
s. bone myeloma
s. bone plasmacytoma (SBP)
s. cold lesion
s. collapsed vertebra
s. dilated duct
s. fibrous tumor of pleura (SFTP)
s. gallstone
s. left IVC
s. lymph node
s. mass
s. metastatic lung nodule
s. osteosclerosis
s. osteosclerotic lesion
s. plasmacytoma
s. pleura tumor
s. pulmonary necrobiotic nodule
s. pulmonary nodule (SPN)
s. rectal ulcer
s. rectal ulcer syndrome
s. relapse
s. rib hot spot

s. rib lesion
s. small bowel filling defect
s. sternal lesion
s. sternal metastasis

solitus
abdominal situs s.
atrial situs s.
cardiac situs s.
situs atrialis s.
visceral situs s.

Solomon-Bloembergen
S.-B. equation
S.-B. theory of dipole-dipole relaxation rate

Solomon syndrome
solubilize
solution
aqueous s.
Blancophor FFG, SV s.
Bracco A-C-D s.
Carnoy s.
chemoembolization s.
Hartmann s.
hundredth-normal s.
hyperosmotic s.
hypertonic s.
isosmotic water s.
lidocaine-adrenaline s.
MACRO-P s.
Melrose s.
molal s.
multipharmaceutical chemoembolization s.
Phosphotope oral s.
radioelement s.
saline s.
saponated cresol s.
saturated potassium iodide s. (SSKI)

Solutrast 200, 250, 300, 370 contrast medium
solvent
s. suppression
s. water TI frequency dependence
SOM
supraorbital margin
somatic muscle
SOMATOM
S. DR CT scanner
S. Plus 4 CT
S. Plus-S CT scanner

S

NOTES

SOMATOM (*continued*)
    S. Sensation 64
    S. Volume Zoom CT system
somatosensory cortex
somatostatin
    s. imaging agent
    s. receptor scintigraphy (SRS)
    ^{99m}Tc-labeled s.
somatostatinoma
Sommer sector
Sonablate 200 ultrasound system
sonar
sonarography
Sonata imager
Sonazoid contrast agent
Sones
    S. cineangiography technique
    S. selective coronary arteriography
Song covered duodenal stent
SONIA
    Strokes Outcome and Neuroimaging of
      Intracranial Atherosclerosis
    SONIA trial
**sonic-accelerated fracture-healing system
(SAFHS)**
sonicated
    s. albumin microbubbles
    s. dextrose albumin imaging agent
    s. saline contrast medium
Sonicath Ultra imaging catheter
sonication
Sonicator portable ultrasound
sonic effect
SonicWAVE phacoemulsification system
Sonifer sonicating system
SONK
    spontaneous osteonecrosis of knee
**Sonnenberg classification of erosive
esophagitis**
SonoAce 6000 II ultrasound system
sonoangiogram
SonoCT real-time compound imaging
Sonocut ultrasonic aspirator
sonodynamic therapy
sonofluoroscopy
sonogram
    dual transverse linear-array s.
    fatty meal s. (FMS)
    real-time s.
    transabdominal s.
sonographer
sonographic
    s. assessment
    s. detection
    s. diagnosis
    s. echo
    s. feature analysis
    s. guidance

    s. hip type
    s. measurement of subtalar joint
      instability
    s. Murphy sign
    s. parameter
    S. Planning of Oncology Treatment
      (SPOT)
sonography
    abdominal s.
    Acuson computed s.
    Acuson transvaginal s.
    breast s.
    carotid s.
    color-coded duplex s. (CCDS)
    color-coded real-time s.
    color Doppler s. (CDS)
    color-flow Doppler s.
    color power transcranial Doppler s.
    compression s.
    contrast-enhanced transrectal s.
    Doppler s.
    duplex s. (DS)
    duplex-pulsed Doppler s.
    dynamic s.
    endoanal s.
    endoluminal s.
    endoscopic s.
    endovaginal s.
    fatty meal s.
    fetal s.
    follow-up duplex Doppler s.
    freehand interventional s.
    graded compression s.
    gray-scale s.
    hysterosalpingo-contrast s.
    intraaortic endovascular s.
    intraoperative s. (IOS)
    obstetric s.
    pelvic s.
    penile s.
    power Doppler s. (PDS)
    real-time s.
    TCD s.
    thoracic s.
    tissue harmonic s.
    transabdominal color Doppler s.
    transcranial color-coded s.
    transcranial color-coded Doppler s.
    transcranial color-coded duplex s.
      (TCCS)
    transcranial real-time color-flow
      Doppler s.
    transrectal s.
    transvaginal s. (TVS)
    triplex mode Doppler s.
    s. unit
    velocity-encoded color Doppler s.
    whole-breast s.

SonoHeart ELITE personal hand-carried ultrasound system
sonohysterography (SHG)
    saline infusion s. (SIS)
Sonolayer model SSA-270A ultrasound
Sonoline
    S. Antares 4-D ultrasound imaging
    S. Elegra ultrasound system
    S. Sierra ultrasound imaging device
Sonolith Praktis lithotripter
sonolucent
    s. area
    s. cystic lesion
    s. cystic mass
    s. doughnut
    s. halo
    s. layer
    s. skull
    s. zone
sonometer
    Omnisense 7000S bone s.
    Sahara clinical bone s.
    SoundScan 2000 bone s.
    SoundScan Compact bone s.
    UBIS 5000 ultrasound bone s.
SonoRx oral ultrasound contrast agent
SonoSite
    S. digital ultrasound
    S. hand-carried ultrasound
    S. 180 hand-carried ultrasound device
    S. iLook 24 ultrasound
    S. MicroMaxx laptop ultrasound
    S. 180Plus ultrasound
    S. pulsed wave Doppler
    S. Titan ultrasound
    S. 180 ultrasound system
Sonos 2000 ultrasound unit
Sonotron electronic therapeutic device
SonoVue
Sopha DSX1 camera
Sophy
    S. camera
    S. programmable valve
Sorbie calcaneal fracture classification
sorbitol 70% imaging agent
Sorbol heel
sorption
    s. kinetics
    s. potential
sorter
    FACSVantage cell s.

fluorescence-activated cell s. (FACScan)
Sos Pulse-Vu Bloodless Entry Needle
SOT
    solid organ transplant
Sotos syndrome
souffle
    funic s.
    placental s.
    systolic mammary s.
sound
    s. beam
    bowel s.
    heart s.
    palpable aortic ejection s.
    palpable pulmonic ejection s.
    pericardial knock s.
    s. shadow
    speed of s.
    s. transmission
    s. wave
SoundScan
    S. 2000 bone sonometer
    S. Compact bone sonometer
source
    americium radioactive s.
    s. of artifact scintigraphy
    cobalt radioactive s.
    Cornell high energy synchrotron s. (CHESS)
    ^{137}Cs point s.
    diagnostic x-ray camera and imaging s.
    discrete bleeding s.
    dummy s.
    s. of emission
    external heat generating s.
    fiberoptic light s.
    flood s.
    gold radioactive s.
    heat-generating s.
    s. imaging
    interstitial heat-generating s.
    intracavitary radiation s.
    intrastitial radiation s.
    iodine radioactive s.
    radioactive s.
    radium radioactive s.
    remote-controlled implantation of radioactive s.
    rod s.
    rotating Ge-68 rod s.

S

NOTES

source (*continued*)
    signal s.
    yttrium radioactive s.
source-film distance (SFD)
source-skin distance (SSD)
source-surface distance (SSD)
source-to-image receptor distance (SID)
source-tray distance (STD)
SP6 camera
SPA
    single-photon absorptiometry
SPACE
    spatial and chemical-shift encoded
      excitation
space (*See* spacing)
    abdominal s.
    acromioclavicular s.
    action s.
    alveolar dead s.
    anatomic dead s.
    antecubital s.
    anterior clear s.
    anterior pararenal s. (APS)
    arachnoid s.
    axillary s.
    Bogros s.
    Bowman s.
    buccal s.
    capsular s.
    carotid s.
    cartilage joint s.
    cavitary s.
    cisternal s.
    coracoclavicular s.
    cortical liquoral s.
    Crookes s.
    CY color s.
    dead s.
    s. deficit
    disc s.
    Disse s.
    dorsal subaponeurotic s.
    dorsal subcutaneous s.
    echo s.
    echo-free s.
    enlarged presacral s.
    enlargement of subarachnoidal s.
    epicardial s.
    epidural s.
    episcleral s.
    epitympanic s.
    extraaxial s.
    extracellular s.
    extradural s.
    extrapleural s.
    fifth intercostal s.
    fluid s.
    foraminal s.
    fourth intercostal s.

free pericardial s.
gingival s.
hip joint s.
Holzknecht s.
hyperintense marrow s.
increased lateral joint s.
infraglottic s.
inframesocolic s.
intercellular s.
intercondylar joint s.
intercostal s.
interlobar s.
intermetatarsal s.
interosseous s.
interpeduncular s.
interpleural s.
interstitial fluid s.
intervertebral disc s.
intrathecal s.
intravascular s.
joint s.
lateral joint s.
left intercostal s. (LICS)
masticator s.
medial joint s.
midpalmar s.
orbital s.
paralaryngeal s.
parapharyngeal s.
pararenal s.
patellofemoral joint s.
pelvic s.
peribronchial alveolar s.
pericardial s.
peridental s.
perihepatic s.
perineal s.
perinephric s.
perirenal s.
perisinusoidal s.
peritoneal s.
perivascular s.
personal s.
pleural s.
popliteal s.
portacaval s.
portal s.
posterior cervical s.
posterior septal s.
predental s.
preepiglottic s.
premasseteric s.
presacral s.
prevertebral s.
Prussak s.
pulp s.
Q s.
radiolucent joint s.
Reinke s.

retrocardiac s.
retrocrural s.
retrogastric s.
retromammary s.
retroorbital s.
retroparotid s.
retroperitoneal s.
retropharyngeal s.
retrosphenoidal s.
retrosternal s.
retrovesical s.
s. of Retzius
s. of Retzius abscess
saclike s.
scapholunate s.
sinusoidal vascular s.
spatial frequency s.
subacromial s.
subarachnoid s.
subdural s.
subhepatic s.
subperitoneal s.
subphrenic s.
subpulmonic pleural s.
subumbilical s.
supralevator s.
supratentorial s.
Talairach stereotaxic s.
thenar s.
tissue s.
ventricular s.
Virchow-Robin perivascular s.
visceral s.
widened joint s.

space-occupying
s.-o. intracranial lesion
s.-o. mass
s.-o. process

spacing
gray-level s.
interecho s.
multiple-beam interface s.
parallel-line equal s. (PLES)

spade
s. field
s. finger

spadelike
s. appearance
s. hand

spade-shaped valvotome
Spalding sign
spall

spallation product
SPAMM
spatial modulation of magnetization
SPAMM technique

span
levator s.
liver s.
ventricular s.

SPARC software
sparing
arytenoid s.
fatty s.

spark
s. chamber
s. gap generator

sparkling appearance of myocardium
SPARS
spatially resolved spectroscopy

sparsity of bone formation
spasm
arterial s.
bowel s.
bronchial smooth muscle s.
catheter-induced coronary artery s.
colonic s.
coronary artery s. (CAS)
diffuse arteriolar s.
diffuse esophageal s. (DES)
esophageal s.
hemifacial s.
inspiratory s.
intermittent diffuse esophageal s.
muscle s.
postbypass s.
respiratory s.
vascular s.
venous s.

spasmodic stricture
spastic
s. bowel syndrome
s. colon
s. electron paramagnetic resonance
imaging
s. equinovarus deformity
s. esophagus
s. heart
s. hindfoot valgus deformity
s. ileus
s. mapping
s. pseudosclerosis
s. registration

S

NOTES

spastica
    dysphagia s.
spatial
    s. average-pulse average (SAPA)
    s. average-pulse average intensity
    s. average-temporal average (SATA)
    s. average-temporal average
       intensity
    s. and chemical-shift encoded
       excitation (SPACE)
    s. distribution
    s. dose distribution
    s. encoding
    s. filter
    s. frequency
    s. frequency domain
    s. frequency error
    s. frequency space
    s. harmonics
    s. localization procedure
    s. mapping
    s. misregistration artifact
    s. modulation of magnetization
       (SPAMM)
    s. modulation of magnetization
       image
    s. normalization
    s. offset image artifact
    s. orientation
    s. origin
    s. peak-temporal average (SPTA)
    s. peak-temporal average intensity
    s. position
    s. presaturation
    s. presaturation band
    s. reconstruction
    s. registration
    s. resolution
    s. resolution scintigram
    s. selectivity
    s. smoothing
    s. vectorcardiography
spatially
    s. localized spectroscopy
    s. normalized PET and SPECT
       scan
    s. resolved spectroscopy (SPARS)
    s. selective inversion pulse
spatial-spectral prepulses for fat
    saturation
SPDT
    single-pole double-throw
Spearman
    S. correlation coefficient
    S. rank
    S. rank test
spear tackler's spine
special bolus

specific
    s. absorption rate (SAR)
    s. activity
    s. modulation
    s. radiation
specified
    not otherwise s. (NOS)
specimen radiography
specious finding
speck finger
speckled pattern
speckling
    heterogeneous color s.
SPECT
    single-photon emission-computed
       tomography
       acetazolamide-enhanced SPECT
       brain perfusion SPECT
       SPECT brain perfusion scintigraphy
       SPECT center of rotation
       cerebral SPECT
       dual-head SPECT
       dual-isotope SPECT
       dynamic volumetric SPECT
       electrocardiogram-gated SPECT
       FDG SPECT
       ^{67}Ga SPECT
       GE SPECT
       ictal ^{99m}Tc HMPAO brain SPECT
       SPECT imaging
       interictal brain SPECT
       methoxyisobutyl isonitrile SPECT
       SPECT perfusion pattern
       pharmacologic stress dual-isotope
          myocardial perfusion SPECT
       SPECT quality control
       quantitative gated SPECT (QGS)
       stress-rest SPECT
       ^{99m}Tc-HMPAO SPECT
       ^{99m}Tc red blood cell SPECT
       technetium-99m somatostatin analog
          SPECT
       SPECT thallium scintigraphy
       Trionix SPECT
       SPECT uniformity
spectamine
    s. brain imaging
    ^{123}I brain imaging s.
SPECT-CT
    Symbia TruePoint SPECT-CT
spectography
    nuclear magnetic resonance s.
spectra (*pl. of* spectrum)
spectral
    s. analysis
    s. broadening
    s. diffusion
    s. Doppler
    s. Doppler imaging

s. editing
s. emission
s. line
s. noise distribution
s. pattern
s. presaturation with inversion recovery (SPIR)
s. saturation
s. sensitivity
s. ultrasound
s. waveform
s. width
s. window

spectral-spatial
s.-s. fat suppression
s.-s. image

Spectranetics
S. excimer laser
S. laser sheath (SLS)

spectrin

Spectris
S. MR-compatible injector
S. power injector

spectrofluorometry

spectrometer
beta-ray s.
Bragg s.
Bruker AMX 300 NMR s.
Compton suppression s.
EDXRF s.
gamma ray s.
GE GN300 7.05-T/89-mm bore multinuclear s.
GE NMR s.
IBM NMR s.
liquid scintillation s.
mass s.
Mossbauer s.
Nicolet NMR s.
NMR s.
nuclear magnetic resonance s.
Rapid-Scan S.
scintillation s.
SISCO s.
Varian Associates 11.7-T, 51-mm bore s.
Varian NMR s.
VT multinuclear s.
x-ray s.

spectrometry
accelerator mass s. (AMS)
Fourier transform NMR s.

inductively coupled plasma atomic emission s. (ICP-AES)
liquid scintillation s.
PROBE-SV s.
pulsed L-band ESR s.
scintillation s.

Spectro-20000 2.OT
spectrophotofluorometer
spectrophotometer
absorption s.
F-1200, 2000, 4500 fluorescence s.
U-1100 UV-Vis s.

spectrophotometric
s. calculation
s. quantity

spectrophotometry
atomic absorption s.
ultraviolet s.

spectroscope
direct vision s.

spectroscopic voxel
spectroscopy
atomic absorption s.
brain proton magnetic resonance s.
carbon 13 s.
circular dichroism s.
COSY H-1 MR s.
CSI s.
depth-resolved surface s. (DRESS)
diffusion s.
2D J-resolved 1H MR s.
double-spin echo proton s.
3D proton MR s.
elastic scattering s.
electrospray ionization mass s.
flame emission s. (FES)
fluorescence s.
fluorine-19 s.
Fourier transform infrared s.
Fourier transform Raman s.
glutamate s.
H-1 MR s.
hydrogen-1, -2, -3 MR s.
image-selected in vivo s. (ISIS)
INVOS 2100 optical s.
laser correlational s. (LCS)
light-induced autofluorescence s.
localized H1 s.
localized proton magnetic resonance s.
long TE MR s.
magnetic resonance s. (MRS)

S

NOTES

spectroscopy *(continued)*
    MR proton s.
    near infrared s. (NIRS)
    nonresonance Raman s.
    nuclear magnetic resonance s.
    oxygen-17 NMR s.
    ^{31}P s.
    phosphorus magnetic resonance s.
      (P-MRS)
    phosphorus-31 magnetic
      resonance s.
    photon correlation s.
    plasma emission s.
    point resolved s. (PRESS)
    proton MR s.
    proton nuclear magnetic
      resonance s.
    Raman s.
    remote endoscopic digital s.
      (REDS)
    ^{77}Se MRI s.
    serial diffusion-weighted MR
      imaging and proton MR s.
    short-echo-time proton s.
    short TE proton MR s.
    single voxel proton MR s. (1H-
      MRS)
    single voxel stimulated echo
      acquisition mode MR s.
    spatially localized s.
    spatially resolved s. (SPARS)
    surface coil rotating-frame s.
    in vivo MR s.
    in vivo optical s. (INVOS)
    in vivo 31P MR s.
    in vivo 31-P MR s.
    in vivo proton MR s.
spectrum, pl. **spectra, spectrums**
    absorption x-ray s.
    artery s.
    chromatic s.
    color s.
    continuous x-ray s.
    Dandy-Walker s.
    S. DG-P pediatric cradle
    Doppler frequency s.
    electromagnetic s.
    energy s.
    excitation s.
    frequency s.
    gamma ray s.
    infinitesimal Z s.
    infrared s.
    invisible s.
    localized single-voxel proton s.
    midsystolic notching of velocity s.
    nuclear magnetic resonance s.
    proton nuclear magnetic
      resonance s.

    pulmonary sequestration s.
    short echo point resolved
      spectroscopic sequence s.
    single umbilical artery s.
    single voxel in vivo proton s.
    thermal s.
    ultraviolet s.
    VACTERL s.
    velocity s.
    water-suppressed proton s.
    Wiener s.
    x-ray s.
specular
    s. echo
    s. reflector
speech area
speed
    film s.
    s. of sound
Spence
    axillary tail of S.
    tail of S.
Spengler fragment
Spens syndrome
spent phase
spermatic
    s. artery
    s. calculus
    s. cord
    s. cord torsion
    s. vein
    s. venography
spermatocele
spermatogonia
sperm granuloma
SPET
    single-photon emission tomography
SPGR
    spoiled gradient-recalled echo sequence
    spoiled GRASS
S-phase
    S-p. analysis
    S-p. fraction
    S-p. fractionation
sphenocephaly
sphenoethmoidal
    s. encephalocele
    s. recess
    s. suture
sphenofrontal suture
sphenoid
    s. angle
    s. bone
    s. bone fracture
    s. dysplasia
    s. fontanelle
    s. ridge
    s. ridge meningioma
    s. ridge tumor

s. sinus
s. sinus metastasis
s. wing
s. wing meningioma
sphenoidal
s. encephalocele
s. fossa
s. sinusitis
s. turbinated bone
sphenoidale
planum s.
pneumatosis s.
rostrum s.
sphenomalar suture
sphenomandibularis muscle
sphenomandibular ligament
sphenomaxillary
s. encephalocele
s. suture
sphenooccipital
s. chordoma
s. suture
s. synchondrosis
sphenoorbital
s. encephalocele
s. meningioma
s. suture
sphenopalatine
s. canal
s. foramen
s. ganglion
s. neuralgia
sphenoparietal
s. sinus
s. sulcus
s. suture
sphenopetrosal suture
sphenopharyngeal
s. canal
s. encephalocele
s. meningoencephalocele
sphenosquamous suture
sphenotemporal suture
sphenovomerine suture
sphenozygomatic suture
sphere
s. organelle
resin s.
SIR-Spheres radioactive s.
spheric
s. disc
s. kernel

s. lesion
s. map
s. mass
s. neoplasm
s. shape
s. structure
spheroid
s. shape
tumor s.
spherule
sphincter
anal s.
antral s.
s. atony
basal s.
bicanalicular s.
s. of bile duct
Boyden s.
canalicular s.
cecal s.
choledochal s.
colic s.
cricopharyngeal s.
duodenal s.
duodenojejunal s.
s. dysfunction
external anal s.
external urethral s.
extrinsic s.
first duodenal s.
functional s.
hypertensive lower esophageal s.
s. incompetence
inferior esophageal s. (IES)
lower esophageal s. (LES)
s. of Oddi
s. of Oddi manometry
pancreatic duct s.
pancreaticobiliary s.
pharyngoesophageal s.
physiologic s.
prepyloric s.
s. preservation
pyloric s.
relaxed lower esophageal s.
resting lower esophageal s.
tonically contracted s.
upper esophageal s. (UES)
sphincteric mechanism
sphingomyelinase deficiency
sphingomyelin lipidosis
sphygmography

NOTES

sphygmomanometer
SPI
 selective population inversion
spicular
 s. density
 s. protrusion
spiculated
 s. border
 s. carcinoma
 s. distortion
 s. margin
 s. mass
 s. scirrhous lesion
spiculation
 radiographic s.
spicule
 bony s.
SPIDER
 steady-state projection imaging with
  dynamic echo-train readout
 structured platform-independent data
  entry and reporting
spider
 s. angioma
 s. finger
 s. pelvis
 stainless steel s.
 s. x-ray view
spidering skeleton
spiderlike
 s. calyx
 s. pelvocaliceal system
spiderweb
 s. appearance
 s. circulation
Spielmeyer-Vogt disease
spigelian
 s. fascia
 s. hernia
 s. lobe
spike
 s. averaging
 s. loading
 s. staple
 sterile vent s.
spike-related functional MR imaging
spiking
 interictal s.
spiky skeleton
spill
 ileal s.
spin
 s. coupling
 s. density
 s. density weighted
 s. dephasing
 s. diffusion
 s. echo
 electron s.

 s. exchange
 s. flip
 flowing s.
 high s.
 incoherent s.
 s. lock gradient-echo (SL-GRE)
 nuclear s.
 off-resonant s.
 s. quantum number
 stationary s.
 s. tagging
 transverse relaxation of proton s.
 uncoupled s.
 unsaturated s.
 s. vector
spina, pl. **spinae**
 s. bifida
 s. bifida aperta
 s. bifida occulta (SBO)
 erector spinae
 s. ventosa
spinal
 s. accessory lymph node
 s. accessory nerve
 s. angiogram
 s. angulation
 s. anomaly
 s. arteriography
 s. artery
 s. axis
 s. axis tumor
 s. capillary hemangioblastoma
 s. chordoma
 s. column stabilization
 s. concussion
 s. cord
 s. cord angiography
 s. cord atrophy
 s. cord caliber
 s. cord canal
 s. cord cleft
 s. cord compression
 s. cord decompression
 s. cord depression
 s. cord diameter
 s. cord ependymoma
 s. cord glioma
 s. cord hemisection
 s. cord infarct
 s. cord injury (SCI)
 s. cord injury without radiographic
  abnormality (SCIWORA)
 s. cord laceration
 s. cord lesion
 s. cord malformation (SCM)
 s. cord metastasis
 s. cord parenchyma
 s. cord sarcoidosis
 s. cord stroke

s. cord syrinx
s. cord transsection
s. cord tumor
s. degeneration
s. dermoid
s. diastematomyelia
s. dorsal horn
s. dural arteriovenous fistula
s. dural AVF
s. empyema
s. endplate change
s. epidural abscess (SEA)
s. epidural hemorrhage (SEH)
s. epidural lymphoma
s. fixation
s. fixation device
s. fluid
s. fracture
s. fusion
s. ganglion
s. growth
s. hemiplegia
s. hydatid cyst
s. infection
s. inflammation
s. instability
s. integrity
s. lordosis
s. medulla
s. meningioma
s. muscular atrophy (SMA)
s. needle
s. nerve plexus
s. nerve root avulsion
s. osteochondrosis
s. osteomyelitis
s. osteophyte
s. pedicle
s. plasma cell myeloma
s. root
s. sac
s. sign
s. stenosis
s. subarachnoid hemorrhage
s. subdural hemorrhage (SSH)
s. syndesmophyte
s. teratoma
s. tophaceous gout
s. tuberculosis
s. vascular malformation
ventral derotating s. (VDS)
s. videofluoroscopy

spindle
aortic s.
s. colonic groove
His s.
muscle s.
ureteral s.
spindle-shaped
s.-s. aneurysm
s.-s. muscle
s.-s. shadow
spindling
spine
alar s.
s. angioreticuloma
angulation of s.
anterior column of s.
anterior-inferior iliac s.
anterior maxillary s.
anterior-superior iliac s. (ASIS)
anteroposterior iliac s.
arachnoid loculation of the s.
bamboo s.
basilar s.
biomechanically normal s.
caroticojugular s.
cervical fusion of s.
Charcot s.
cleft s.
coccygeal s.
dendritic s.
dens view of cervical s.
dorsal s.
dysraphic s.
epidermoid s.
extension injury of s.
fetal s.
functional units of s.
s. hyperflexion
iliac s.
intermaxillary s.
ischial s.
kinetic cervical s.
kissing s.
s. lipoma
lumbar s.
lumbarized s.
lumbosacral s. (LS)
maxillary s.
mental s.
microcystic lumbar s.
midthoracic s.
s. morphology

S

NOTES

spine *(continued)*
nasal s.
s. ossification
poker s.
posterior column of s.
posterior inferior s.
posterior inferior iliac s.
railway s.
rotatory load on s.
rugger jersey s.
sacral s.
scoliotic s.
s. sign
spear tackler's s.
static cervical s.
thin-plate s.
thoracic s.
thoracolumbar s.
tibial s.
trochanteric s.
vertebral s.
wedge fracture of s.
spin-echo (SE)
axial single shot fast s.-e.
breath-hold turbo s.-e.
s.-e. cardiac imaging
dual-echo turbo s.-e.
fast s.-e. (FSE)
half-Fourier acquisition single-shot
turbo s.-e. (HASTE)
s.-e. imaging sequence
inversion recovery s.-e. (IRSE)
s.-e. magnetic resonance imaging
s.-e. pilot image
s.-e. pulse sequence
radiofrequency s.-e.
s.-e. scan
s.-e. technique
s.-e. train
turbo s.-e. (TSE)
T1-weighted conventional s.-e.
s.-e. T1-weighted image
s.-e. T1-weighted transaxial MR
imaging
s.-e. using repeated gradient echoes
spinescope
Clarus s.
spin-label
s.-l. method
s.-l. technique
spin-lattice
s.-l. relaxation
s.-l. relaxation time
spin-lock (SL)
s.-l. imaging technique
s.-l. and magnetization transfer
imaging
s.-l. prepulse

spin-lock-induced T1-rho weighted
image
spin-locking
off-resonance s.-l.
spinning
variable-angle s. (VAS)
spinning-top
s.-t. test
s.-t. urethra
spinocerebellar
s. degeneration
s. tract
spinoglenoid
s. ligament
s. notch
spinogram
spinographic
s. angle
s. line
spinography
digitized s.
spinolaminar line (SLL)
spinoreticular tract
spinosum
foramen s.
spinothalamic tract
spinous
s. foramen
s. plane
s. process
s. process avulsion
s. process fracture
s. tarsus ligament
spin-phase
s.-p. graph
s.-p. phenomenon
spin-spin
s.-s. coupling
s.-s. relaxation
s.-s. relaxation time
spintharicon
spinthariscope
spin-warp
s.-w. imaging
s.-w. method
s.-w. pulse sequence
SPIO
superparamagnetic iron oxide
SPIO-enhanced MR imaging
spiperone
SPIR
selective partial inversion-recovery
selective partial inversion-recovery MRI
spectral presaturation with inversion
recovery
spiral
s. appearance
s. arthrosis
s. band of Gosset

s. computed tomography (SCT)
s. computed tomography
  arteriography (SCTA)
s. CT pitch
s. CT pitch pit
s. CT scan
s. CT scanning
s. CT, XCT scanner
s. dissection
s. echo-planar technique
s. EPI (SEPI)
s. flow pattern
s. fold
s. imaging method
s. k-space coverage
s. ligament
s. multidetector CT
s. oblique fracture
s. scanning technique
s. valve
s. volumetric CT
s. x-ray computed tomography
  (SVCT, SXCT)
spiral-pulse sequence
SPIR-FLAIR
SPIR-FLAIR image
SPIR-FLAIR sequence
spirometer flow rate
spirometric
s. acquisition
s. gating
**spirometrically controlled CT lung
  densitometry**
spirometry
full-volume loop s.
splanchnapophysis
splanchnic
s. aneurysm
s. AV fistula
s. blood
s. vascular imaging
s. vasculature
s. venous system
s. vessel
splanchnography
splanchnoskeleton
SPLATT
split anterior tibial tendon
splayed cranial suture
splayfoot deformity

splaying
s. of frontal horn
s. of pedicles
spleen
aberrant s.
absence of s.
accessory s.
s. angiosarcoma
delayed rupture s.
s. density
s. diameter
s. dimension
ectopic s.
epithelial s.
floating s.
hamartoma s.
hyperdense s.
increased density s.
s. inflammation
inflammatory s.
s. laceration
large s.
s. lesion
liver, kidneys, and s. (LKS)
long axis of s.
malpighian body of s.
microabscess of s.
multiple accessory s.
nonvisualization of s.
s. peliosis
primary cyst of s.
prolapse of s.
ruptured s.
s. sarcoidosis
s. scan
shattered s.
siderotic nodule in s.
small s.
solid lesion s.
tail of the s.
tip of s.
s. ultrasonography imaging
wandering s.
spleen-to-liver ratio
splenatrophy
splenauxe
splenculus
splenectasis
splenectopia
splenelcosis
spleneolus
splenia (*pl. of* splenium)

S

NOTES

splenial branch of posterior cerebral artery
splenic
  s. abscess
  s. amyloidosis
  s. angle
  s. arteriography
  s. artery (SA)
  s. artery aneurysm
  s. artery pseudoaneurysm
  s. AV fistula
  s. B-cell lymphoma
  s. bleeding
  s. bump
  s. calcification
  s. capsule
  s. cleft
  s. congestion
  s. epidermoid cyst
  s. flexure
  s. flexure carcinoma
  s. hamartoma
  s. hemangioma
  s. hilum
  s. hyperplasia
  s. infarct
  s. lesion
  s. lobule
  s. lymph node
  s. metastasis
  s. microabscess
  s. notch
  s. perfusion measurement by dynamic CT scan
  s. portal venography
  s. portography
  s. pseudocyst
  s. reagent
  s. rupture
  s. scintigraphy
  s. torsion
  s. trauma
  s. vein
  s. vein thrombosis
  s. vessel
spleniculus, pl. **spleniculi**
splenium, pl. **splenia**
  s. of corpus callosum
splenization
splenobronchial fistula
splenocaval
splenocolic ligament
splenogastric omentum
splenogonadal fusion
splenography
splenoma
splenomalacia
splenomedullary

splenomegaly
  congenital s.
  congestive s.
  Egyptian s.
  fibrocongestive s.
  Gaucher s.
  hemolytic s.
  infectious s.
  myelophthisic s.
  Opitz thrombophlebitic s.
  persistent s.
  postcardiotomy lymphocytic s.
  siderotic s.
splenomyelomalacia
splenoncus
splenonephric
splenopancreatic
splenophrenic
splenoportal
  s. junction
  s. venography
splenoportogram
splenoportography
  direct s.
  s. imaging
  percutaneous s.
splenorenal
  s. anastomosis
  s. angle
  s. arterial bypass graft
  s. ligament
  s. recess
  s. shunt
splenosis
  abdominal s.
  thoracic s.
splenunculus, pl. **splenunculi**
spline curve
splint
  bird-cage s.
  semidynamic s.
  thigh s.
splintered
  s. bone
  s. fracture
splinting
  serial s.
Spli-Prest
  S.-P. latex
  S.-P. negative control
  S.-P. plate
  S.-P. positive control
split
  s. anterior tibial tendon (SPLATT)
  s. atlas
  s. brain
  s. compression fracture
  s. cranium
  s. foot deformity

s. image artifact
s. notochord syndrome
s. peroneus brevis
s. renal function decrease
s. spinal cord
s. spinal cord malformation
(SSCM)
s. water resonance

split-brain
s.-b. imaging
s.-b. study

split-cord syndrome
split-course
s.-c. accelerated radiotherapy
s.-c. hyperfractionated radiation
therapy
s.-c. technique

split-function scintigraphy
split-heel fracture
split-liver transplantation
split-screen recording
splitter
beam s.

splitting
s. fracture
plaque s.
sternal s.
zero-field s.

SPN
solitary pulmonary nodule

SPOCS
Surgical Planning and Orientation
Computer System

spoiled
s. gradient echo (SGE)
s. gradient echo pulse sequence
s. gradient-recalled
s. gradient-recalled echo sequence
(SPGR)
s. GRASS (SPGR)

spoiler
s. gradient pattern
Lucite beam s.

spoiling
radiofrequency s.
RF s.
surface s.

spoke bone
spoked wheel pattern
spondylarthritis

spondylitic
s. change
s. deformity

spondylitis
ankylosing s.
cryptococcal s.
s. deformans
discovertebral s.
juvenile ankylosing s.
lung ankylosis s.
rheumatoid s.
staphylococcal discovertebral s.
tuberculous s.

spondyloarthritis, pl. **spondyloarthritides**
spondyloarthropathy
destructive s.
juvenile s.

spondylocostal dysplasia
spondylodiskitis drainage
spondyloepiphysial dysplasia
spondylolisthesis
degenerative s.
isthmic s.
sagittal roll s.
slip-angle s.
spondylolytic s.
traumatic s.

spondylolisthetic pelvis
spondylolysis
traumatic s.

spondylolytic spondylolisthesis
spondylomalacia
spondylosis
cervical spine s.
s. deformans
degenerative s.
diffuse s.
Nurick classification of s.

spondylosyndesis
spondylothoracic dysplasia
spondylotic myelopathy
sponge
blood-filled bone s.
gelatin s.
Ivalon s.
s. kidney
medullary s.
Ray-Tec x-ray detectable
surgical s.
surgical s.
Vistec x-ray detectable s.

Spongel gelatin sponge particle

NOTES

spongiform
>   s. change
>   s. degeneration
>   s. leukoencephalopathy

spongioblastoma

spongiocytoma

spongiosa
>   s. of mitral valve
>   s. replacement

spongiosis

spongiosum
>   corpus s.
>   osteoma s.

spongy
>   s. appearance
>   s. bone
>   s. osteoma
>   s. white matter degeneration

spontaneous
>   s. carotid dissection
>   s. closure of defect
>   s. conversion
>   s. coronary artery dissection (SCAD)
>   s. detorsion
>   s. disintegration
>   s. drainage
>   s. echo contrast
>   s. fetal movement
>   s. fracture
>   s. hematoma
>   s. hemodialysis catheter fracture and embolization
>   s. infantile ductal aneurysm
>   s. intracranial hypotension
>   s. involution
>   s. lesion
>   s. osteonecrosis
>   s. osteonecrosis of knee (SONK)
>   s. perforation
>   s. perforation of common bile duct
>   s. pneumomediastinum
>   s. radiation
>   s. regression
>   s. renal hemorrhage
>   s. tension pneumothorax
>   s. transient vasoconstriction
>   s. urinary extravasation

spoonlike
>   s. protrusion
>   s. protrusion of leaflet

spoon-shaped nail

SPOP
>   sequential paired opposed plaque
>   SPOP technique

sporadic
>   s. Burkitt lymphoma
>   s. colorectal carcinoma
>   s. tumor

SPOT
>   Sonographic Planning of Oncology Treatment
>   SPOT mobile 3D ultrasound system and software

spot
>   blooming focal s.
>   capitate soft s.
>   Carleton s.
>   cold s.
>   s. compression
>   s. compression image
>   s. compression magnification mammography
>   s. compression paddle
>   s. compression view
>   cotton-wool s.
>   EIS s.
>   s. film
>   s. film device
>   s. film fluorography
>   s. film radiography
>   flying focal s.
>   focal s. (FS)
>   focal liver hot s.
>   hematocystic s. (HCS)
>   hot-s.
>   hyperechoic splenic s.
>   s. magnification
>   pelvic s.
>   pituitary bright s.
>   s. radiograph
>   Roth s.
>   scan s.
>   s. scanning
>   s. scanography
>   soldier's s.
>   solitary rib hot s.
>   thermal hot s.
>   tree-shaped s.
>   z-flying focal s.

spot-magnification image

spotted nephrogram

SPPS
>   single-photon planar scintigraphy

SPR
>   scanned projection radiography
>   superior peroneal retinaculum

sprain
>   acute s.
>   chronic s.
>   eversion s.
>   s. fracture
>   inversion s.
>   sacroiliac s.
>   syndesmosis s.

spray
>   pulse fashion pulse s.
>   resorcinol s.

spread
    s. Bragg peak
    distant s.
    hematogenous s.
    intraocular s.
    lymphatic tumor s.
    pattern of s.
    perineural tumor s.
    regional s.
    subependymal s.
    s. suture
    transfascial s.
    s. of tumor
Sprengel deformity
spring
    s. ligament
    s. onion ureter
spring-driven system
Springer fracture
spring-loaded biopsy needle
sprinter's fracture
Sprint fixed-detector research system
sprodiamide imaging agent
SPS
    sestamibi parathyroid scintigraphy
    superior petrous sinus
SPT
    selective population transfer
SPTA
    spatial peak-temporal average
SPTL-1b vascular lesion laser
spur
    acromial s.
    anterior s.
    bone s.
    bronchial s.
    calcaneal s.
    calcific s.
    degenerative s.
    drum s.
    s. formation
    heel s.
    impingement s.
    inferior s.
    marginal s.
    medial traction s.
    osteoarthritic s.
    plantar calcaneal s.
    posterior s.
    prominent s.
    retrocalcaneal s.

    traction s.
    uncovertebral s.
spuriae
    costae s.
    vertebra s.
spurious
    s. aneurysm
    s. ankylosis
    s. finding
    s. pregnancy
Spurling sign
spurring
    bony s.
    degenerative s.
    hypertrophic marginal s.
    marginal s.
    osteophytic s.
    ulnar traction s.
Spyglass angiography catheter
SPY intraoperative imaging system
SQFT
    subcutaneous quadriceps fat thickness
squamosal suture
squamosomastoid suture
squamosoparietal suture
squamososphenoid suture
squamous
    s. intraepithelial lesion (SIL)
    s. metaphysis
    s. metaplasia
    s. metaplasia white epithelium
    s. odontogenic tumor
    s. part of frontal bone
    s. part of occipital bone
    s. part of temporal bone
    s. suture
square
    s. brain shift
    least s. (LS)
    s. wave
squared
    s. patella
    s. vertebral body
squared-off
    s.-o. heart
    s.-o. thorax
squatting
    s. facet
    s. maneuver
    s. position
squeeze sign
Squibb system

NOTES

S

SQUID
superconducting quantum interference
device
SR
saturation recovery
structured reporting
Sr
strontium
Sr 87m
⁸⁹Sr
strontium 89
⁸⁹Sr bracelet
⁹⁰Sr
strontium 90
⁹⁰Sr-loaded eye applicator
SRO 2550 x-ray tube
SRS
somatostatin receptor scintigraphy
stereotactic radiosurgery
SS
slice select gradient
SSBE
short-segment Barrett esophagus
SSC
single-stripe colitis
SSCM
split spinal cord malformation
SSCP
single-strand conformational
polymorphism
SSD
segmental spinal dysgenesis
source-skin distance
source-surface distance
surface shaded display
SSD algorithm
SSD imaging
SSFP
steady-state free precession
SSFP magnetization
SSFP process
SSFP signal
SSFSE
single-shot fast spin echo
SSH
spinal subdural hemorrhage
S-shaped
S-s. gallbladder
S-s. pouch
S-s. scoliosis
SShTSE
SENSE with half-Fourier single-shot
turbo spin echo
single shot TSE
SSKI
saturated potassium iodide solution
SSP
slice sensitivity profile
stereotactic surface projection

SSPE
subacute sclerosing panencephalitis
SSQ
sequential scalar quantization
SSR
shaded surface rendering
SSS
superior sagittal sinus
SSS thrombosis
ST
ST segment/heart rate (ST/HR)
ST segment/heart rate slope
(ST/HR slope)
stability
bony s.
s. of fracture
magnet s.
stabilization
electronic s.
s. plate
spinal column s.
stabilizer
dynamic s.
static s.
stabilizing bullet
stable
s. cavitation
s. fracture
s. free radical
s. isotope
s. reduction
s. Xenon CT
stable-state tuberculosis
stacked
s. ovoid lesion
s. scan
s. tomogram
stacked-coin appearance
stacked-foil technique
stacked-metaphor workstation
stacked-scan imaging
stack mode display
stack-of-coins mucosal fold
stack-of-spirals trajectory
Stafne idiopathic bone cavity
stage
Okuda hepatic compromise s. I–III
Quintero umbilical artery blood
flow s. 1–4
resolution s.
Risser s.
s. 4S neuroblastoma
2-stage
2-s. amputation
2-s. fusion
2-s. venous cannulation
1-stage amputation
2-staged stent implantation

stage-matched
    s.-m. intervention
    s.-m. intervention on repeat
        mammography
staghorn
    s. calculus
    s. stone
staging
    distraction-flexion s. (DFS)
    Ficat s.
    invasive surgical s. (ISS)
    Kadish s.
    lymphoma s.
    malignant melanoma s.
    neuraxis s.
    neuroblastoma s.
    nodal s.
    preslip s.
stagnant-loop syndrome
stag wound
stain
    Bielschowsky s.
    hematoxylin and eosin s.
    mucicarmine s.
stained-glass appearance
staining
    alloxan-Schiff s.
    immunocytochemical s.
    tumor s.
stainless
    s. steel coil
    s. steel mesh stent
    s. steel microsphere
    s. steel plate
    s. steel spider
stainless-steel Greenfield filter
staircase phenomenon
stairstep
    s. air-fluid level
    s. artifact
    s. fracture
stalk
    body s.
    fibrovascular s.
    infundibular s.
    pituitary s.
    polyp s.
    tumor s.
    yolk s.
standard
    ACR teleradiology s.
    s. atlas

criterion s.
    s. deviation
    s. exchange wire
    s. fixed core guidewire
    international s. (IS)
    s. LITT applicator
    s. multiecho
    s. precautions
    reference s.
    s. single echo
    s. uptake value (SUV)
**standard-dose enhanced conventional T1
    weighted image**
standardized uptake ratio (SUR)
standby rate
standing
    s. dorsoplantar view
    s. false profile view
    s. lateral view
    s. postvoid view
    s. wave
    s. weight-bearing view
standoff
    acoustic s.
    s. pad
standstill
    atrial s.
    cardiac s.
    ventricular s.
Stanford
    S. aortic dissection classification
    S. type B aortic dissection
    S. type B dissection closure
    S. and Wheatstone stereoscope
Stanley cervical ligament
stannosis
stannous
    s. chloride
    s. pyrophosphate
stannum (Sn)
stapedial
    s. artery
    s. nerve anatomy
    s. otosclerosis
stapedius reflex
stapes, pl. **stapedes**
staphylococcal discovertebral spondylitis
staphyloma
staple
    metallic s.
    orthopedic s.
    skin s.

S

NOTES

staple *(continued)*
   spike s.
   stone s.
   surgical s.
star
   s. artifact
   s. effect
   s. pattern
   s. test pattern
Starcam camera
star-cancellation test (SCT)
Starling curve
Starlink software
STARRT falloposcopy system
star-shaped vessel lumen
start test pattern
starvation
   photon s.
stasis, pl. **stases**
   antral s.
   bile s.
   bladder s.
   s. of blood flow
   chronic venous s.
   circulation s.
   s. cirrhosis
   complete vascular s.
   s. edema
   s. esophagitis
   s. gallbladder
   intrahepatic biliary s.
   s. liver
   s. ulcer
   ureteral s.
   urinary s.
   vascular s.
   venous s.
state
   cardiac steady s.
   chronic constrictive s.
   contrast-enhanced Fourier-acquired
     steady s. (CE-FAST)
   double-mode steady s.
   s. equilibrium
   fast adiabatic trajectory in
     steady s. (FATS)
   Fourier-acquired steady s. (FAST)
   free precession sequence steady s.
   gradient-recalled acquisition in
     steady s. (GRASS)
   ground s.
   high-output s.
   hypoperfused s.
   inducibility basal s.
   metastable s.
   oxidation s.
   post Diamox s.
   radiofrequency spoiled Fourier-
     acquired steady s. (RF-FAST)

Statham electromagnetic flowmetry
static
   s. bone phase
   s. cervical spine
   s. coupling
   s. 3D FLASH imaging
   s. emission scan
   s. foot deformity
   s. image
   s. image display
   s. liver imaging
   s. lung
   s. magnetic field
   s. rCBF tracer
   s. stabilizer
   s. view
station
   American Thoracic Society node s.
   calf-foot s.
   lower s.
   oscilloscope tuning s.
stationary
   s. anode
   s. field
   s. focus
   s. spin
   s. zero-order motion
statistical noise
STATLase-SDL diode laser
STATus
   Cardiac S.
Stauffer syndrome
Staunig position
STD
   source-tray distance
STE
   stimulated echo
steady-state
   s.-s. coherent
   s.-s. free precession (SSFP)
   s.-s. free precession imaging
   s.-s. free precession magnetization
   s.-s. free precession sequence
   s.-s. gradient-echo imaging
   s.-s. projection imaging with
     dynamic echo-train readout
     (SPIDER)
steal
   arterial s.
   s. effect
   false s.
   pelvic s.
   s. phenomenon
   subclavian s.
   s. syndrome
   transmural s.
STEAM
   stimulated echo acquisition mode
   STEAM sequence

steatosis
    hepatic s.
    liver s.
    macrovesicular s.
Stecher position
steel coil
Steele triple innominate osteotomy
steep
    s. left anterior oblique projection
    s. left anterior oblique view
    s. Towne projection
    s. Trendelenburg position
steeple sign
steerable guide wire system
steering
    beam s.
    coaxial s.
    electronic independent beam s.
Steerocath-Dx octapolar and valve mapping catheter
steganography
Steinberg
    S. classification
    S. sign
Steinbrocker rheumatoid arthritis classification
Steinert epiphysial fracture classification
Stein-Leventhal syndrome
Steinstrasse calculus
Stejskal-Tanner gradient
stellate
    s. abnormality
    s. border breast lesion
    s. configuration
    s. confluence
    s. crease
    s. defect
    s. ganglion block
    s. granuloma
    s. ligament
    s. mass
    s. pattern
    s. skull fracture
    s. tear
    s. undepressed fracture
stem
    s. base plate
    brain s.
    bronchus s.
    straight s.
stem-loop structure
Stener lesion

stenion
stenocardia
stenogyria
stenoobstructive lesion
stenosed aortic valve
stenosing
    s. ring of left atrium
    s. tenosynovitis
stenosis, pl. stenoses
    acquired aortic valve s.
    acquired mitral s.
    acquired spinal s.
    ampullary s.
    anal s.
    anastomotic s.
    antral s.
    s. of aorta
    aortic s. (AS)
    aortoiliac s.
    aqueduct s.
    aqueductal s.
    s. area
    arterial s.
    atheromatous s.
    atherosclerotic s.
    atypical aortic valve s.
    benign papillary s.
    benign tracheobronchial s.
    bicuspid valvular aortic s.
    bilateral carotid s.
    bowel s.
    branch pulmonary artery s.
    bronchial s.
    buttonhole mitral s.
    calcific bicuspid valvular s.
    calcific senile aortic valvular s.
    canal s.
    candy-wrapper s.
    carotid artery s.
    central canal s.
    central spinal s.
    cephalic arch s.
    cerebral artery s.
    cervical s.
    choledochoduodenal junctional s.
    circumferential venous s.
    common pulmonary vein s.
    concentric hourglass s.
    coronary artery s.
    coronary luminal s.
    coronary ostial s.
    critical coronary s.

NOTES

stenosis *(continued)*
  critical valvular s.
  cross-sectional area s.
  culprit s.
  s. diameter
  diffuse s.
  discrete focal s.
  discrete subaortic s.
  discrete subvalvular aortic s.
   (DSAS)
  duodenal hourglass s.
  dynamic subaortic s.
  eccentric s.
  edge s.
  s. encroachment
  esophageal s.
  external iliac s.
  femoropopliteal atheromatous s.
  fibromuscular renal artery s.
  fibromuscular subaortic s.
  fishmouth mitral s.
  fixed-orifice aortic s.
  flow-limiting s.
  focal eccentric s.
  foraminal s.
  graft s.
  granulation s.
  hemodialysis-related venous s.
  hemodynamically significant s.
  hepatic artery s.
  high-grade proximal s.
  hourglass s.
  hypercalcemic supravalvular
   aortic s.
  hypertrophic infundibular
   subpulmonic s.
  hypertrophic pyloric s. (HPS)
  hypertrophic pyloric string sign s.
  hypertrophic pyloric target sign s.
  hypertrophic subaortic s.
  idiopathic hypertrophic subaortic s.
  ileal s.
  iliac artery s.
  iliofemoral venous s.
  infrainguinal bypass s.
  infrarenal s.
  infundibular pulmonary s.
  infundibular subpulmonic s.
  innominate artery s.
  in-stent s.
  intragraft s.
  intrarenal s.
  intrinsic vein graft s.
  irislike s.
  juxtaanastomotic s.
  lateral recess s.
  linear s.
  lumbar spinal s.
  luminal s.

  membranous subaortic s.
  membranous subvalvular aortic s.
  midgraft s.
  mitral s. (MS)
  mitral valve s. (MVS)
  multifocal short s.
  multiple small bowel s.
  muscular subaortic s.
  napkin-ring anular s.
  native kidney renal artery s.
  neoplastic s.
  noncalcified coronary s.
  noncritical s.
  nonrheumatic valvular aortic s.
  ostial renal artery s.
  papillary bile duct s.
  papilla of Vater s.
  pelvic venous s.
  peripheral pulmonary artery s.
   (PPAS)
  petrous carotid canal s.
  postangioplasty s.
  postoperative s.
  post PTCA residual s.
  preangioplasty s.
  pulmonary s.
  pulmonary artery s.
  pulmonary valve s.
  pulmonary vein s.
  pulmonic s.
  pulmonic valvular s.
  pyloric s.
  radiation s.
  radionuclide s.
  rectal s.
  relative mitral s.
  renal artery s. (RAS)
  rheumatic aortic valvular s.
  rheumatic mitral s.
  rheumatic tricuspid s.
  saphenous vein s.
  segmental s.
  senescent aortic s.
  silent mitral s.
  spinal s.
  stomal s.
  string-sign s.
  subaortic s.
  subclavian artery s.
  subglottic s.
  subinfundibular s.
  subsonic s.
  subvalvular aortic s.
  subvalvular pulmonary s.
  supraaortic s.
  supraclavicular aortic s.
  suprarenal s.
  supravalvular aortic s. (SAS,
   SVAS)

supravalvular mitral s.
supravalvular pulmonary s.
tapering s.
tendon sheath s.
thoracic outlet s. (TOS)
TOCU for internal carotid artery s.
tracheal s.
tricuspid s.
true mitral s.
truncal renal artery s.
tubular s.
tunnel subaortic s.
tunnel subvalvular aortic s.
uncomplicated supraclavicular s.
unicuspid aortic valve s.
unilateral carotid s.
ureteral s.
valvular aortic s.
valvular pulmonic s.
vein graft s.
vertebral artery s.

stenotic

s. change
s. coronary artery
s. esophagogastric anastomosis
s. flow reserve (SFR)
s. gradient
s. isthmus
s. lesion
s. plaque
s. tricuspid valve

Stensen

S. canal
S. duct
S. foramen
S. gland

stent

Acculink s.
active MRI s. (AMRIS)
AneuRx s.
aSpire covered s.
Assurant balloon-expanded s.
AVE s.
AVE Bridge Flexible balloon-
  expanded s.
AVE Bridge SE self-expanding s.
AVE bridge stainless steel balloon-
  expandable s.
balloon-expandable s.
Bard Saxx S.
biliary s.
biodegradable s.

BiodivYsio s.
brachiocephalic s.
Bx Velocity s.
CardioCoil coronary s.
Cary-Coon biliary s.
C-flex s.
cobalt alloy s.
coil vascular s.
compliance matching s. (CMS)
Conformexx biliary s.
Cordis Palmaz Corinthian s.
Cordis Palmaz Schatz long
  medium s.
Cordis Smart Nitinol s.
Corinthian stainless steel balloon-
  expandable s.
covered s.
Cragg s.
Cragg Endopro system I
  covered s.
Cypher s.
Dacron s.
deployed s.
s. deployment
detachable balloon-modified
  reducing s.
double-helix prostatic s.
double-J ureteral s.
Dynalink 0.018 sclf-cxpanding s.
Dynalink 0.035 self-expanding s.
Easy Wallstent s.
electropolished s.
Endeavor drug-eluting s.
EsophaCoil s.
esophageal s.
ev3 premounted balloon
  expandable s.
ev3 self-expanding s.
ev3 unmounted balloon
  expandablc s.
expandable Gianturco metallic s.
s. expansion
Express balloon-expanded s.
Express biliary LD s.
Fabian s.
Flamingo s.
6F Protégé self-expanding s.
FreeFlo proximal Nitinol s.
Genesis s.
Gianturco s.
Gianturco-Rosch biliary s.
gold-marked s.

NOTES

S

stent *(continued)*

Guidant Megalink peripheral s.
Hemobahn s.
indwelling s.
internal biliary s.
internal ureteral s.
IntraCoil s.
IntraCoil self-expanding s.
IntraCoil self-expanding
  peripheral s.
IntraStent balloon-expanded s.
IntraStent biliary s.
IntraStent DoubleStrut biliary s.
IntraStent DS balloon-expanded s.
IntraStent LD balloon-expanded s.
IntraStent LP balloon-expanded s.
intravascular s.
^{192}Ir-loaded s.
Jomed Flexmaster s.
Jomed peripheral s.
Jostent covered s.
Jostent SelfX Nitinol s.
kissing s.
Luminexx biliary s.
Luminexx self-expanding s.
MedNova s.
MEGALINK s.
Memotherm Nitinol self-
  expandable s.
s. mesh
metallic s.
s. migration
Miller double mushroom biliary s.
ML-Ultra balloon s.
30-mm-long Palmaz s.
Monorail Wallstent self-
  expanding s.
Multi-Link Penta s.
Multi-Link Terra s.
nephroureteral s.
nephroureterostomy s.
NIR s.
Ni-Ti alloy s.
Nitinol Symphony s.
Omni Flex biliary s.
Omnilink/Megalink balloon-
  expanded s.
Palmaz s.
Palmaz 424 s.
Palmaz 784 s.
Palmaz Genesis s.
Palmaz Genesis balloon-expanded s.
Palmaz large balloon-expanded s.
Palmaz medium balloon-expanded s.
Palmaz P564 s.
Palmaz PS 424 s.
Palmaz P 394 stainless steel
  balloon-expandable s.

Palmaz-Schatz long medium
  balloon-expanded s.
pancreatic duct s.
Passager Nitinol self-expandable s.
patent s.
Percuflex s.
percutaneous s.
Perflex stainless steel balloon-
  expandable s.
pigtail s.
platinum-marked s.
polyethylene s.
Polyflex s.
polyurethane s.
porous metallic s.
Precise self-expanding s.
prostatic s.
Protg GPS s.
Protg self-expanding s.
s. proximity
PTFE s.
s. pushability
QuaDDS s.
QuaDDS-QP2 s.
QuaDS drug-eluting s.
QueST s.
radioactive s.
radioisotope s.
reducing s.
^{188}Re-labeled self-expanding
  Nitinol s.
renovascular s.
rolling membrane Wallstent cobalt-
  based alloy balloon-expandable s.
S670 s.
S7 AVE s.
Schneider enteral s.
self-expandable metal s.
self-expanding s.
self-expanding covered s.
self-expanding open mesh s.
S-F Precise s.
silicone s.
sirolimus-eluting SMART Nitinol s.
slotted tube s.
SMART s.
SMART Control self-expanding s.
SMART Nitinol self-expandable s.
SMART self-expanding s.
Song covered duodenal s.
S670 over-the-wire coronary s.
stainless steel mesh s.
straight s.
Strecker balloon-expanded s.
Strecker Nitinol self-expandable s.
Strecker tantalum balloon-
  expandable s.
s. strut
Supra G s.

Symphony Nitinol self-expandable s.
Symphony self-expanding s.
TAG Excluder s.
tandem s.
tantalum s.
Taxus Express s.
Temp Tip ureteral s.
s. thrombosis
transhepatic biliary s.
T-tube s.
Ultraflex s.
Ultrathane Amplatz ureteral s.
urethral metallic s.
urinary s.
U-tube s.
vascular s.
V-Flex Plus s.
Viabahn covered s.
Viabil s.
Vistaflex balloon-expanded s.
Wallgraft cobalt-based alloy balloon-expandable s.
Wallgraft covered s.
Wallstent s.
Wallstent Iliac RP self-expanding s.
Wallstent RP self-expanding s.
XT radiopaque coronary s.
ZA-stent Nitinol self-expandable s.
Zenith stainless steel self-expandable s.
zigzag s.
Zilver s.
Zilver self-expanding s.

stent-graft
AneuRx s.-g.
Cragg EndoPro s.-g.
endovascular s.-g.
Excluder s.-g.
FreeFlo s.-g.
Gore covered biliary s.-g.
Hemobahn PTFE-covered s.-g.
Jomed peripheral s.-g.
OPTA balloon s.-g.
Wallgraft endoprosthesis s.-g.

stenting
antegrade ureteral s.
brachiocephalic artery s.
bronchial s.
carotid artery s.
colon s.

endobiliary s.
iliac artery s.
innominate artery s.
intracoronary s.
intravascular s.
pulmonary artery s.
subclavian artery s.
tracheobronchial s.
ureteral s.
venous s.
stentless porcine aortic valve
stent-mounted
s.-m. allograft valve
s.-m. heterograft valve
stent-related artifact
stent-vessel wall contact
Stenver
S. position
S. projection
S. view
step
modality performed procedure s. (MPPS)
phase-encoding s.
s. section
s. wedge
2-step
2-s. procedure
2-s. technique
step-and-shoot
s.-a.-s. mode
s.-a.-s. technique
step-down transformer
stepladder
s. appearance
s. sign
step-like recess
step-oblique mammography
stepoff
s. of fracture
orbital rim s.
stepping-source position
stepping-table MRA
1-step production
step-up transformer
stepwise
s. infusion
s. regression
s. regression analysis
stercora
stercoraceous
stercoral ulcer

NOTES

stercoroma
stercorous
stercus
stereo
    s. mammography
    s. right lateral projection
stereocinefluorography
stereoencephalotomy
stereofluoroscopy
stereogram
stereograph
stereographic projection
stereography
StereoGuide
    LORAD S.
    S. prone breast biopsy system
    S. stereotactic needle core biopsy
stereolithography
StereoLoc upright biopsy system
stereologic method of volume estimation
stereomammography
stereometry
stereomicroradiography
stereophotogrammetric
    roentgen s.
StereoPlan stereotactic planning
  software
stereoradiogram
stereoradiography
stereoroentgenogram
stereoroentgenography
stereoroentgenometry
stereosalpingography
stereoscope
    binocular s.
    Stanford and Wheatstone s.
stereoscopic
    s. radiography
    s. view
    s. vision
    s. zonography
stereoscopy
stereoskiagraphy
stereotactic, stereotaxic
    s. ablation
    s. apparatus
    s. automated technique
    s. breast biopsy
    s. breast biopsy system
    s. cerebral angiography
    s. core needle biopsy (SCNB)
    s. CT scan
    s. data
    s. device
    s. external-beam irradiation (SEBI)
    s. head frame
    s. localization
    s. localization frame
    s. mammography

    s. percutaneous lumbar discectomy
    s. percutaneous needle biopsy
    s. procedure
    s. proton irradiation
    s. puncture
    s. radiation therapy
    s. radiosurgery (SRS)
    s. radiotherapy
    s. ring
    s. surface projection (SSP)
    s. surgery
    s. tractotomy
    s. vacuum-assisted biopsy
    s. vacuum-assisted breast biopsy
      (SVABB)
stereotaxically guided interstitial laser
  therapy
stereotaxis
    computer-assisted volumetric s.
    imaging-based s.
    volumetric minimally invasive s.
stereotaxy
    frameless s.
sterile
    s. barium
    s. vent spike
sterna (*pl. of* sternum)
sternal
    s. abscess
    s. angle
    s. angle of Louis
    s. apex
    s. border
    s. cartilage
    s. clip
    s. edge
    s. joint
    s. lesion
    s. lift
    s. marrow
    s. notch
    s. part of diaphragm
    s. rib
    s. splitting
    s. suture
    s. vertebra
    s. view
Sternberg
    S. myocardial insufficiency
    S. sign
Sterner lesion
sterni
    corpus s.
sternochondral junction
sternoclavicular
    s. angle
    s. dislocation
    s. hyperostosis
    s. joint

s. joint disc
s. ligament
sternocleidomastoid
clavicular head of s.
s. muscle
s. muscle border
s. retraction
s. tumor
sternocostal
s. joint
s. part of diaphragm
s. surface of heart
sternohyoid muscle
sternomanubrial joint
sternopericardial ligament
sternospinal reference
sternothyroid muscle
sternotomy wire
sternoxiphoid plane
sternum, pl. **sterna**
anterior bowing of s.
osteitic lesion of s.
s. retraction
tie s.
stethoscope
ultrasound s.
Steward-Milford fracture classification
Stewart-Hamilton equation
Stewart-Holmes sign
Stewart-Treves syndrome
ST/HR
ST segment/heart rate
ST/HR slope
Stickler syndrome
1-stick system
Stieda
S. fracture
S. process
Stierlin sign
stiff
s. guidewire
s. lung syndrome
s. man syndrome
s. noncompliant lung
stiffness
aortic s.
s. coefficient
lung s.
ventricular s.
stigmata
radiologic s.
Still disease

Stiller rib
Stilling canal
Stimucath continuous nerve block catheter
stimulated
s. acoustic emission (SAE)
s. echo (STE)
s. echo acquisition mode (STEAM)
s. echo artifact
s. echo-tagging technique
stimulation
alternating hemifield s.
cardiosynchronous s.
electric s.
high-voltage s. (HVS)
high-voltage pulsed galvanic s. (HVPGS)
intraoperative electrocortical s.
magnetic s.
s. mode
noninvasive programmed s. (NIPS)
percutaneous electrical nerve s.
s. scan
vagus nerve s. (VNS)
stimulator
AME bone growth s.
bone growth s.
DTU-215 cardiac digital s.
transcutaneous electrical nerve s.
stimulus-correlated water signal
STING
subureteric Teflon injection
STING procedure
stippled
s. appearance
s. calcification
s. mineralization
s. soft tissue
stippling of lung field
STIR
short-inversion-time inversion recovery
short tau inversion recovery
short T1 inversion recovery
fast STIR
STIR imaging
STIR sequence
STIR slice
STIR technique
stirrup bone
stochastic effect
Stoerck loop

S

NOTES

Stokes theorem
stoma, pl. **stomata**
    abdominal s.
    anastomotic s.
    bowel s.
    diverting s.
    gastroenterostomy s.
    gastrointestinal s.
    permanent s.
    prolapsed s.
    retracted s.
    silastic collar-reinforced s.
stomach
    aberrant umbilical s.
    s. adenocarcinoma
    air contrast view of the s.
    angulus of s.
    antrum of s.
    s. atony
    s. bed
    bilocular s.
    body of the s.
    s. bubble
    s. calculus
    canal of s.
    cardiac s.
    cascade s.
    cobblestone appearance s.
    contrast-filled s.
    convex border of s.
    coronary artery of s.
    cup-and-spill s.
    s. curvature
    s. defect incisura
    distal blind s.
    distended s.
    s. diverticulum
    dumping s.
    s. filling defect
    s. fundus
    greater curvature of s.
    hourglass s.
    intrathoracic s.
    J-shaped s.
    leather bottle s.
    s. leiomyoma
    s. leiomyosarcoma
    lesser curvature of s.
    s. margin
    miniature s.
    mucous lake of s.
    s. narrowing
    nonvisualization of fetal s.
    pit of s.
    s. pneumatosis
    riding s.
    scaphoid s.
    sclerotic s.
    thoracic s.

    trifid s.
    s. tube
    s. ulcer
    upside-down s.
    s. varioliform erosion
    s. varix
    s. volvulus
    s. wall
    waterfall s.
    water-trap s.
    wet s.
stomal
    s. edema
    s. intussusception
    s. stenosis
stone
    barrel-shaped s.
    bile duct s.
    biliary tract s.
    bilirubinate s.
    black faceted s.
    bladder s.
    bosselated s.
    common bile duct s.
    cystic duct remnant s.
    cystine s.
    dropped s.
    s. extraction
    extrahepatic s.
    fecal s.
    gallbladder s.
    gas-containing s.
    s. heart
    high-attenuation s.
    impacted urethral s.
    s. impaction
    intrahepatic s.
    intraluminal s.
    intravesical s.
    kidney s.
    lung s.
    matrix s.
    metabolic s.
    multiple s.'s
    nonopaque s.
    nonradiopaque s.
    opaque s.
    pigment s.
    pituitary s.
    pulp s.
    radiolucent s.
    renal s.
    residual s.
    retained common bile duct s.
    salivary s.
    shadowing s.
    soft pigment s.
    staghorn s.
    s. staple

ureteral s.
urinary bladder s.
vein s.
womb s.

stone-free rate
stonelike calculus
stony mass
stool
retention of s.
s. tagging

stool-tagging agent
stop
crimp s.
s. test

stop-action
s.-a. image
s.-a. imaging

stopcock
Accel s.
3-way s.

3-stopcock manifold
stopping power
1-stop-shop examination
storage
digital s.
magnetic tape s.
s. phosphor-based technique
s. phosphor imaging
s. phosphor radiology
s. phosphor system

storiform pattern
storiform-pleomorphic
s.-p. malignant fibrous histiocytoma
s.-p. MFH
s.-p. pattern

storm
thyroid s.

Storz
S. infant bronchoscope
S. thoracoscope

stoved finger
STR
skeletal targeted radiotherapy

strabismus convergens alternans
straddle
s. fracture
s. injury

straddling
chondroblastoma s.
s. embolus

straight
s. anterior vertebral border

s. AP pelvic injection
s. chest tube
s. cord
s. end-hole catheter
s. guidewire
s. guiding sheath
s. interposition graft
s. lateral projection
s. side-hole catheter
s. sinus
s. stem
s. stent
s. tubule
s. ureter

straight-line flow
strain
adductor muscle s.
s. fracture
left ventricular hypertrophy with s.
ligamentous s.
lumbosacral spine s.
muscle s.
myotendinous s.
s. pattern
right ventricular s.
shear s.

strain-gauge plethysmography
strain-rate MR imaging
strand
s.'s of increased density
rabbit ear s.

stranding
fascial s.
fat s.
glial s.
mesenteric fat s.
soft tissue s.

strangulated
s. bowel
s. inguinal hernia
s. obstruction
s. viscus

strangulating obstruction
strangulation necrosis
strap muscle
strata (*pl. of* stratum)
stratification
mural s.

stratified
stratiform
stratigraphy

S

NOTES

Stratis II MRI system
stratum, pl. **strata**
strawberry gallbladder
strawberry-shaped head
stray
    s. neutron field
    s. radiation
streak
    s. artifact
    s. of atelectasis
    atherosclerotic fatty s.
    fatty intima s.
    s. of increased density
    primitive s.
streaklike
    s. artifact
    s. configuration
stream
    electron s.
    regurgitant s.
streaming
    tram-track s.
Strecker
    S. balloon-expanded stent
    S. Nitinol self-expandable stent
    S. tantalum balloon-expandable
      stent
Streeter dysplasia
strength
    air-kerma s.
    diffusion encoding s.
    field s.
    high gradient field s.
    hoop s.
    magnetic field s.
streptavidin peroxidase technique
streptokinase
stress
    adduction s.
    biomechanical s.
    s. Broden view
    s. cystogram
    s. echocardiography
    s. endpoint
    s. eversion view
    s. film
    s. fracture
    hoop s.
    s. incontinence
    s. injury
    s. inversion view
    mediolateral s.
    s. perfusion and rest function
    s. perfusion scintigraphy
    pharmacologic s.
    s. projection
    s. radiography
    s. raiser
    resting end-systolic wall s.

    shear s.
    s. thallium image
    s. thallium-201 myocardial imaging
    s. thallium scan
    torque s.
    torsion s.
    s. ulcer
    valgus s.
    varus s.
    wall shear s.
stress-and-rest image
stress-gated blood pool cardiac
  examination
stress-induced
    s.-i. ischemia
    s.-i. left ventricular dilatation
    s.-i. remodeling
stress-injected
stress-only perfusion imaging
stress-redistribution
    s.-r. examination
    s.-r. imaging
stress-rest
    s.-r. reinjection examination
    s.-r. SPECT
stress-strain curve
stretched
    s. lung
    s. out ligament
stria, pl. **striae**
    s. diagonalis
    s. laminae granularis externae
    s. laminae granularis internae
    s. laminae molecularis
    s. laminae pyramidalis internae
    s. longitudinalis lateralis corporis
      callosi
    s. mallearis membranae tympani
    s. malleolaris membranae tympani
    s. medullaris thalami
    s. olfactoria lateralis
    s. olfactoria medialis
    s. terminalis
    s. vascularis ductus cochlearis
striatal
    s. lesion
    s. output pathway
striate
    s. cortex
    s. hemorrhage
    s. vein
striated
    s. angiographic nephrogram
    s. muscle
striation
    s. across image
    fiber-bundle s.
    intermediate signal s.

paint brush s.
urothelial s.
striatonigral degeneration
striatothalamic groove
striatum
corpus s.
Strichman SME-810 camera
Strickler method
strict isolation
stricture
anal s.
anastomotic s.
antral s.
anular esophageal s.
benign biliary s.
benign peptic s.
bile duct s.
biliary s.
bronchial s.
choledochojejunostomy s.
cicatricial s.
colonic s.
common bile duct s.
congenital urethral s.
contractile s.
duodenal s.
enteric s.
esophageal peptic s.
gastroesophageal junction s.
irritable s.
longitudinal esophageal s.
peptic s.
pyloric s.
recurrent s.
spasmodic s.
tracheal s.
ureteral s.
ureteroenteral anastomotic s.
urethral s.
string
s. cell carcinoma
s. guideline
navel s.
s. sign
stringlike bands of fibrous tissue
string-of-beads
s.-o.-b. appearance
s.-o.-b. sign
string-of-pearls
s.-o.-p. appearance
s.-o.-p. nuclear arrangement
s.-o.-p. sign

string-sign stenosis
strip
primary motor s.
s. scan
sensitometric s.
sensory s.
stripe
aortopulmonary mediastinal s.
central high-signal intensity s.
central intraluminal saturation s.
endometrial s.
esophageal-pleural s.
fat s.
flank s.
Gennari s.
paraspinal pleural s.
paratracheal tissue s.
pleural s.
pleuroesophageal s.
properitoneal flank s.
psoas s.
right paratracheal s.
saturation s.
scaphoid fat s.
s. sign
tracheal s.
tracheal wall s.
vertebral s.
striping
horizontal s.
stripped atom
stripping
fibrin sleeve s.
stroke
anterior spinal artery s.
cardiogenic embolic s.
cerebrovascular s.
completed s.
s. count image
s. count ratio
s. ejection rate
embolic s.
s. in evolution (SIE)
s. force
hemisphere s.
hemorrhagic s.
hyperacute s.
hypertensive s.
incomplete s.
s. index (SI)
lacunar s.

NOTES

S

stroke *(continued)*
    S.'s Outcome and Neuroimaging of
      Intracranial Atherosclerosis
      (SONIA)
    S.'s Outcome and Neuroimaging of
      Intracranial Atherosclerosis trial
    s. output
    s. power
    progressive s.
    s. scale score
    slow s.
    small-vessel s.
    spinal cord s.
    thromboembolic s.
    vertebrobasilar distribution s.
    s. volume (SV)
    s. volume image
    s. volume index (SVI)
    s. volume ratio
stroke-work index (SWI)
stroma, pl. **stromata**
    bone marrow s.
    cartilage s.
    cervical s.
    extralobular s.
    fibrocollagenous s.
    gonadal s.
    Rollet s.
    soft tissue s.
    vascular s.
stromal
    s. carcinoid tumor of ovary
    s. cell tumor
    s. matrix
    s. necrosis
    s. pattern of breast
strongyloidiasis
strontium (Sr)
    s. 89 (^{89}Sr)
    s. 90 (^{90}Sr)
    s. isotope
    radioactive s.
    s. with yttrium 90
strontium-89
    s.-89 chloride
    s.-89 imaging agent
structural
    s. abnormality
    s. anomaly
    s. epilepsy
    s. lesion
    s. pulmonary immaturity
    s. weakness
structurally immature lung
structure
    biliary s.
    bony s.
    brain s.
    branching linear s.

    branching tubular s.
    calcified density s.
    central hilar s.
    cervical s.
    collagenous s.
    cord s.
    cystic s.
    demineralized bony s.
    denture-supporting s.
    3D shape of neuroanatomic s.
    elongated s.
    extracolonic s.
    high-density s.
    hilar s.
    hollow s.
    hypoechoic s.
    intracranial s.
    intratumoral s.
    labyrinthine s.
    linear s.
    low-contrast s.
    low-density s.
    mediastinal s.
    midline cystic s.
    noncolonic s.
    nuclear s.
    onionlike laminar s.
    opaque branching s.
    organoid s.
    osseous s.
    ossification of cartilaginous s.
    parcellation of s.
    periappendiceal s.
    prominent ductal vascular s.
    renal collecting s.
    ringlike s.
    satellite s.
    serpentine s.
    soft tissue density s.
    spheric s.
    stem-loop s.
    superior mediastinal s.
    supraglottic s.
    target parenchymal s.
    test tube s.
    thin linear s.
    treelike airway s.
    tuboreticular s.
    tubular s.
    vascular s.
structured
    s. coil electromagnet
    s. light
    s. noise
    s. platform-independent data entry
      and reporting (SPIDER)
    s. reporting (SR)
    s. water
struma, pl. **strumae**

s. ovarii
Riedel s.
Strümpell sign
Strunsky sign
strut
    bone s.
    s. chorda
    corticocancellous s.
    s. fracture
    optic s.
    stent s.
    s. thickness
    tricuspid valve s.
    valve outflow s.
Struthers
    S. arcade
    S. ligament
struvite calculus
Stryker
    S. frame
    S. notch projection
    S. notch view
ST-segment shift
STS-MIP
    sliding thin-slab maximum intensity
    projection
STT
    scaphotrapeziotrapezoid
    STT joint
stuck
    s. without recapture
    s. with recapture
studded fissure
Studer pouch
study
    air contrast s.
    anatomopathologic s.
    anisotropic volume s.
    antegrade pressure s.
    barium meal s.
    biplane pelvic oblique s.
    bladder contractility s.
    blood flow s.
    bone density s.
    bone length s.
    bone mineral content s.
    brain activation s.
    cardiac-gated s.
    carotid duplex s.
    cerebral blood flow s.
    cerebral perfusion s.
    cine s.

complete stress/rest s.
compressibility and phasicity s.
conventional s.
cornflake esophageal motility s.
correlative Doppler s.
Doppler flow probe s.
double-contrast barium s.
double-probe pH s.
DPTA CSF flow s.
dual-contrast s.
dynamic contrast-enhanced
    subtraction s.
dynamic supine s.
efficacy s.
electromagnetic blood flow s.
endovascular flow wire s.
factor analysis of dynamic s.
first-pass s.
fistula tract s.
flow s.
gallbladder s.
gas ventilation s.
gated imaging s.
gated planar s.
Gd-DOTA-enhanced subtraction
    dynamic s.
horizontal beam s.
ictal phase s.
imaging s.
inhalation s.
interictal PET FDG s.
interictal SPECT s.
intervention s.
iodized oil s.
isotopic 3D s.
isotopic volume s.
kidney function s.
kinematic MRI s.
lumbar flexion and extension s.
MAA s.
marker transit s.
minute-sequence s.
morphine-augmented s.
motility s.
MR flow quantification s.
MRI CSF flow s.
multibreath washout s.
multitracer s.
musculoskeletal imaging s.
noble gas in magnetic resonance s.
noninvasive imaging s.
paleopathologic and radiologic s.

S

NOTES

study *(continued)*
    paramagnetic contrast-enhanced MR s.
    perfusion s.
    peripheral small airway s.
    perirenal air s.
    phantom s.
    3-phase technetium s.
    phonation s.
    PICCOLO s.
    postcaptopril radioisotope s.
    precaptopril radioisotope s.
    pressure perfusion s.
    pullback s.
    pulmonary blood flow s.
    pulmonary quantitative differential function s.
    qualitative s.
    quantitative region lung function s.
    radioaerosol imaging s.
    radiochemical s.
    radiolabeled water s.
    radiologic-histopathologic s.
    radionuclide blood flow s.
    radionuclide voiding s.
    RAD-IR s.
    reconstruction s.
    redistribution s.
    renal cyst s.
    renal function s.
    retrococcygeal air s.
    retroperitoneal air s.
    salivary gland function s.
    scintigraphic s.
    simulated equilibrium factor s.
    single-contrast s.
    sinus tract s.
    split-brain s.
    technetium albumin s.
    thymidine suicide s.
    tracer s.
    transmission electron microscopic s.
    T1-weighted s.
    ureteral reflux s.
    urodynamic pressure-flow s.
    ventilation s.
    videotape s.
    in vivo disposition s.
    voiding s.
    wall motion s.
    wash-in/wash-out s.
    washout s.
    xenon washout s.

stump
    appendiceal s.
    bulbous s.
    s. carcinoma
    cystic duct s.
    duodenal s.

    gastric s.
    s. pregnancy
    s. pressure
    rectal s.

stumped off appearance
stunned myocardium
stunning
    myocardial s.
    postexercise s.
    poststress s.
    thyroid s.

stunted fetus
Sturge-Weber
    S.-W. syndrome
    S.-W. telangiectasia

Sturge-Weber-Dimitri syndrome
stylet
    S. esophageal MRI coil
    single-bevel s.

styloglossus muscle
stylohyoid
    s. ligament
    s. muscle

styloid
    s. process
    s. prominence
    ulnar s.

styloideum
    os s.

stylomandibular ligament
stylomastoid foramen
stylomaxillary ligament
stylopharyngeus
subacromial
    s. bursa
    s. bursal adhesion
    s. bursitis
    s. enthesophyte
    s. space

subacromial-subdeltoid (SA-SD)
    s.-s. bursa
    s.-s. septic bursitis

subacute
    s. bacterial endocarditis
    s. bronchopneumonia
    s. cardiac tamponade
    s. combined spinal cord degeneration
    s. denervation atrophy
    s. encephalitis
    s. extrinsic allergic alveolitis
    s. granulomatous
    s. hemorrhage
    s. hepatic necrosis
    s. inflammation
    s. ischemic brain infarct
    s. myocardial infarct
    s. myositis ossificans
    s. necrotizing encephalomyelopathy

s. necrotizing myelitis
s. necrotizing myelopathy
s. renal vein thrombosis
s. sclerosing panencephalitis (SSPE)
s. subdural hematoma
s. testicular torsion
s. thyroiditis
subadditivity
subadventitial
s. fibrosis
s. hyperplasia
s. plane
s. tissue
subanular
s. calcification
s. placement
subaortic
s. curtain
s. gland
s. muscle
s. stenosis
subapical bronchus
subaponeurotic abscess
subarachnoid
s. cavity
s. cistern
s. clot
s. cyst
s. hemorrhage (SAH)
s. hemorrhage Fisher grade 1–4
s. injection
s. instillation
s. metastatic disease
s. nerve block
s. phenol block
s. seeding
s. septum
s. space
s. space disease
subareolar
s. breast density
s. carcinoma
s. duct
s. lesion
s. mass
s. plexus
subarticular
s. bone resorption
s. cyst
s. pseudocyst
subastragalar dislocation
subastrocytic tumor

subatheromatous ulcer
subatmospheric pressure
subband
wavelet s.
subblock
rectifier s.
subbursal rupture
subcallosal gyrus
subcapital fracture
subcapsular
s. bleed
s. hepatic necrosis
s. renal hematoma
subcardinal vein
subcarina
subcarinal
s. angle (SA)
s. lymph node
subcecal appendix
subcentimeter node
subchondral
s. bone
s. bone plate
s. bone resorption
s. collapse
s. cyst
s. cystic cavity
s. fracture
s. fracture line
s. insufficiency
s. lesion
s. low-signal-intensity sclerosis
s. marrow edema
s. marrow hyperemia
s. microfracture
s. osteosclerosis
s. trabecular compression
subchorionic
s. hematoma
s. hemorrhage
subclavian
s. aneurysm
s. arteriography
s. artery
s. artery obstruction
s. artery occlusion
s. artery stenosis
s. artery stenting
s. flap
s. flap aortoplasty
s. line
s. loop

S

NOTES

subclavian *(continued)*
   s. steal
   s. turndown technique
   s. vein
   s. vein occlusion
   s. vein thrombosis
   s. vessel
   s. vessel thrombosis
subclavian-innominate vein
subclavicular
subclavius
subcollateral gyrus
subcoracoid
   s. bursitis
   s. dislocation of shoulder
subcortical
   s. arteriosclerotic encephalopathy
   s. atherosclerotic encephalopathy
   s. CNS hamartoma
   s. cyst
   s. defect
   s. infarct
   s. intracerebral hemorrhage
   s. intracranial lesion
   s. ischemic vascular dementia
   s. low-intensity lesion
   s. Sudeck osteoporotic atrophy
   s. tumor
subcostal
   s. artery
   s. branch
   s. 4-chamber view
   s. long-axis view
   s. margin
   s. nerve
   s. plane
   s. short-axis view
   s. short-axis view echocardiography
   s. window
subcritical narrowing
subcutaneous
   s. air
   s. array electrode
   s. arterial bypass graft
   s. connective tissue
   s. edema
   s. emphysema
   s. fascia
   s. fat
   s. fat line
   s. fat necrosis
   s. fibroma
   s. fracture
   s. hemangioma
   s. implanted injection port
   s. infiltrate
   s. infusion
   s. injection
   s. injection of contrast artifact

   s. nodule
   s. patch
   s. pocket
   s. quadriceps fat thickness (SQFT)
   s. sacrococcygeal myxopapillary
    ependymoma
   s. tissue gas
   s. tumor
   s. tunnel
   s. vein
subdeltoid
   s. bursa
   s. bursal adhesion
   s. bursal effusion
   s. bursitis
   s. fat plane obliteration
subdiaphragmatic
   s. abscess
   s. fat
subdural
   s. abscess
   s. blood
   s. button
   s. cavity
   s. clot
   s. contrast injection
   s. effusion
   s. empyema
   s. hemorrhage (SDH)
   s. hygroma
   s. interhemispheric hematoma
   s. space
   s. window
subendocardial
   s. infarct (SEI)
   s. injury
   s. ischemia
   s. myocardial infarct
   s. necrosis
   s. sclerosis
subendometrial halo
subependymal
   s. cyst
   s. germinolysis
   s. giant cell astrocytoma
   s. hamartoma
   s. hemorrhage
   s. heterotopia
   s. oligodendroglioma
   s. seeding
   s. spread
   s. vein
subependymal/subpial focus
subependymoma
subepicardial fat
suberosis
subeustachian sinus
subfalcine herniation

subfascial
    s. hematoma
    s. transposition
subfascially
subfrontal meningioma
subgaleal
    s. abscess
    s. cerebrospinal fluid
    s. hematoma
    s. hemorrhage
subglandular implant
subglenoid dislocation of shoulder
subglottic
    s. area
    s. carcinoma
    s. edema
    s. hemangioma
    s. narrowing
    s. stenosis
subglottis
subgluteus
    s. maximus bursa
    s. medius bursa
subhepatic
    s. abscess
    s. area
    s. cecum
    s. space
subinfundibular stenosis
subinsular mass
subintimal
    s. cleavage plane
    s. dissection
    s. fibrosis
    s. filling
subject
    s. contrast
    s. placement
sublabral
    s. foramen
    s. recess
subligamentous
    s. disc herniation
    s. extension
    s. vertebral osteomyelitis
sublimis
    flexor digitorum s. (FDS)
    s. tendon
sublingual
    s. gland
    s. varix
sublux

subluxation
    anterior tibial s.
    s. articulation
    atlantoaxial s.
    s. complex
    distal radioulnar s.
    element s.
    forward s.
    lateral s.
    occult s.
    s. of patella (SLP)
    patellar s.
    peroneal tendon s.
    posterior s.
    posterolateral rotatory s.
    radial head s.
    radioulnar s.
    recurrent lateral patellar s.
    reduced s.
    sacroiliac s.
    tendon s.
    unilateral facet s.
subluxed
    s. facet joint
    s. vertebra
subluxing patella
submandibular
    s. duct
    s. duct calculus
    s. ganglion
    s. gland
    s. lymph node
    s. triangle
submassive
    s. hemorrhage
    s. hepatic necrosis
    s. pulmonary embolus
submaxillary
    s. gland
    s. sialography
    s. view
submembranous placental hematoma
submental
    s. lymph node
    s. vertex view
submentovertex
    s. position
    s. projection
    s. radiograph
submentovertical view
submerged segment of esophagus
submetatarsal bursa

S

NOTES

submicron magnetic particles
submillimeter collimation
submucosal
   s. circular fold
   s. colon tumor
   s. esophageal tumor
   s. fibroid
   s. hemorrhage
   s. lesion
   s. lymphangiectasis
   s. thickening
   s. venous plexus
submucous myoma
suboccipital shortening
suboccipitobregmatic diameter
suboptimal
   s. detail
   s. effort
   s. examination
   s. film
   s. result
   s. runoff
   s. visualization
suboptimally visualized
subpectoral
   s. implant
   s. pocket
subperiosteal
   s. abscess
   s. bone resorption
   s. cortical abrasion
   s. cortical defect
   s. desmoid
   s. fracture
   s. hematoma
   s. hemorrhage
   s. infection
   s. new bone
   s. osteoid osteoma
subperitoneal space
subphrenic
   s. abscess
   s. biloma
   s. fluid
   s. recess
   s. space
subpial
   s. arteriovenous malformation
   s. lipoma
   s. region
subpleural
   s. air cyst
   s. bleb
   s. curvilinear line
   s. dot
   s. effusion
   s. honeycombing
   s. lymphatic
   s. micronodule

   s. nodule
   s. pulmonary arcade
subpubic arch
subpulmonic
   s. effusion
   s. fluid
   s. obstruction
   s. outflow
   s. pleural space
subpyloric node
subrectus obstruction
subsartorial
   s. canal
   s. tunnel
subscapular
   s. artery
   s. bursa
   s. echocardiographic view
   s. fossa
   s. lymph node
subscapularis
   s. muscle
   s. recess
   s. tendon
subsecond
   s. FLASH imaging
   s. scanning
subsegmental
   s. bibasilar atelectasis
   s. bronchus
   s. lower lobe atelectasis
   s. perfusion abnormality
   s. perfusion defect
   s. renal artery branch
subsegment of lung
subselective cannulation
subseptus
   uterus s.
subserosal
   s. fibroid
   s. fibrosis
   s. hemorrhage
   s. layer
   s. lymphangiectasis
   s. tumor
subsite
subsonic stenosis
subspinous dislocation
substance
   bone s.
   brain s.
   diamagnetic s.
   reticular activating s.
substantia
   s. nigra
   s. propria
substernal
   s. angle
   s. goiter

s. retraction
s. thyroid
s. thyroid gland
substitute
bone s.
oxygenated perfluorocarbon blood s.
substrate
main energy s.
radiolabeled marker s.
subsystem
radiofrequency s.
subtalar
s. angle
s. articulation
s. axis
s. instability
s. joint
s. varus
s. view
subtendinous bursa
subtentorial lesion
subthalamus
subtle
s. gradation
s. haziness
s. malalignment
s. microcalcification
subtotal
s. gastric exclusion
s. gastric resection
s. lesion
s. occlusion
s. overframing
subtracted image
subtraction
s. angiography
background s.
s. cloning
complex s.
computer-assisted blood
background s. (CABBS)
digital s.
dual-energy s.
energy s.
s. film
S. ictal SPECT coregistered to
MRI (SISCOM)
s. image
s. imaging
second order s.
s. technique

vector s.
s. venography
subtractive noise
subtrochanteric
s. fracture
s. varus deformity
subumbilical space
subungual
s. abscess
s. fibroma
s. glomus tumor
subunit
functional s. (FSU)
subureteric Teflon injection (STING)
subvalvular
s. aneurysm
s. aortic obstruction
s. aortic stenosis
s. diffuse muscular obstruction
s. gradient
s. pulmonary stenosis
subvesical duct
subxiphoid
s. implantation
s. paracentesis
s. view
succenturiate placental lobe
succimer
succinate dehydrogenase (SDH)
succinic semialdehyde
sucking
s. muscle
s. pneumothorax
Sucquet-Hoyer
S.-H. anastomosis
S.-H. canal
sucralfate
gadolinium s.
sucrose
s. dosimeter
s. polyester imaging agent
suction
s. polyp trap
s. tube
sudden
s. blockage of coronary artery
s. cardiac death
Sudeck
S. atrophy
S. dystrophy
S. point

NOTES

SUFE
   slipped upper femoral epiphysis
suffocative goiter
sugar
   s. ring
   s. tumor
suit
   MAST s.
suite
   Avantx LC angiography s.
sulcal
   s. atrophy
   s. dilatation
   s. enhancement
   s. enlargement
   s. marking
   s. pattern
   s. skeleton
sulcation
sulci
   too few s.
sulcocommissural
   s. artery
   s. branch
sulcus, pl. **sulci**
   s. angle
   angularis s.
   atrioventricular s.
   basilar s.
   blunted posterior s.
   s. calcanei
   calcarine s.
   callosal s.
   carotid s.
   central s.
   cerebral s.
   s. chiasmaticus
   cingulate s.
   collateral s.
   coronary s.
   cortical s.
   costal s.
   costophrenic s.
   s. dilatation
   dilatation of s.
   s. effacement
   frontal s.
   Harrison s.
   hippocampal s.
   hypothalamic s.
   lateral femoral s.
   lateral occipital s.
   lip of lateral s.
   mapping of cerebral s.
   occipitotemporal s.
   olfactory s.
   parietooccipital s.
   perilabral s.
   pontomedullary s.

   postcentral s.
   posterior interventricular s.
   precentral s.
   pulmonary s.
   ramus of lateral s.
   retromalleolar s.
   rolandic s.
   sigmoid s.
   sphenoparietal s.
   superior frontal s.
   superior pulmonary s.
   superior temporal s.
   supracallosal s.
   s. talus
   temporal s.
   ulnar s.
   widened s.
sulfasalazine-induced pulmonary
   infiltrate
sulfate
   barium s. (BaSO$_4$)
   barium lead s.
   barium strontium s.
   E-Z-CAT Dry barium s.
   manganese s.
   sodium tetradecyl s.
   tetradecyl s.
   Varibar honey barium s.
   Varibar nectar barium s.
   Varibar pudding barium s.
   Varibar thin honey barium s.
   Varibar thin liquid barium s.
sulfide
   tin s.
sulfobromophthalein imaging agent
sulfonate
   sodium-2-mercaptoethane s.
sulfur (S)
   s. 35 (^{35}S, S-35)
   s. colloid
   colloidal s.
   s. colloid imaging agent
   s. colloid scan
   s. colloid scintigraphy
   s. hexafluoride (SF$_6$)
   radioactive s.
sum
   s. of cylinder (SOC)
   field-echo s.
   s. peak coincidence
   ray s.
summation
   s. shadow artifact
   s. of shadows
summing correction
summit
   ventricular septal s.
Sumner sign

sump

s. drain
s. drainage catheter
s. tube

sum-peak method

sun

Brett s.
s. lamp
S. SPARCstation system
S. workstation

sunburst

s. appearance
s. brain vascularity
s. gyral pattern
s. nephrogram
s. periosteal reaction

sun-ray appearance

sunrise

s. projection
s. view

sunset view

super

S. Angiorex model G DSA system
S. 50 CP high-voltage generator

superabsorbent

s. polymer embolic material
s. polymer microsphere (SAP-MS)

superacute

supercam scintillation scanner

superciliary arch

superconducting

s. magnet
s. open-magnet system
s. quantum interference device
(SQUID)
1.0T, 1.5T s. magnet

superconductive

s. magnet
s. MR system

superconductor

niobium/titanium s.

superdominant left anterior descending artery

Superdup'r SD6891 left heart system

superfecundation

superfetation

superficial

s. angioma
s. basal cell carcinoma
s. depressed carcinoma
s. diffuse nephroblastomatosis
s. dorsal sacrococcygeal ligament

s. external pudendal artery
s. femoral artery (SFA)
s. femoral artery occlusion
s. femoral vein
s. hyperthermia treatment
s. inguinal lymph node
s. inguinal pouch
s. inguinal ring
s. lesion
s. lymphadenopathy
s. lymphatic vessel
s. muscle
s. necrosis
s. palmar arterial arch
s. palmaris longus tendon
s. pedal vein
s. perineal pouch
s. plexus
s. pneumonia
s. posterior compartment
s. posterior sacrococcygeal ligament
s. radiation
s. spreading esophageal carcinoma
s. spreading stomach carcinoma
s. temporal artery
s. temporalis fascia
s. temporoparietal fascia
s. tendo-Achilles bursa
s. transverse metacarpal ligament
s. transverse metatarsal ligament

superficialis

s. arcade
flexor digitorum s. (FDS)
s. tendon

superimage

superimposed

s. acute partial tear
s. bowel gas
s. fungal infection

superimposition

s. artifact
s. of bowel shadow
s. of signal

superincumbent spinal curve

superior

apertura pelvis s.
s. articular facet
s. articulating process
s. aspect
s. azygoesophageal recess
s. bilateral vena cava
s. border

NOTES

superior (*continued*)
    s. border of heart
    s. border of rib
    s. bronchial artery
    s. caval defect
    s. cerebellar artery (SCA)
    s. cervical ganglion
    s. colliculus
    s. costal facet
    s. costotransverse ligament
    s. duodenal fold
    s. duodenal recess
    s. epigastric artery
    s. extensor retinaculum
    s. frontal axis shift
    s. frontal gyrus
    s. frontal sulcus
    s. genicular artery
    s. gluteal vessel
    s. hypogastric plexus
    s. hypogastric plexus block
    s. intercostal artery
    s. intercostal vein
    s. jugular vein bulb
    s. labral anterior to posterior (SLAP)
    s. labral anterior posterior
    s. labral anterior-posterior injury
    s. labral anterior-posterior lesion
    s. labral anterior to posterior tear
    s. lobe
    s. lobe bronchus
    s. lobe of lung
    s. longitudinal fasciculus
    s. marginal defect
    s. margin of inferior rib
    s. maxillary foramen
    s. mediastinal structure
    s. mediastinum
    s. mesenteric
    s. mesenteric arteriography
    s. mesenteric artery (SMA)
    s. mesenteric artery syndrome (SMAS)
    s. mesenteric ganglion
    s. mesenteric plexus
    s. mesenteric vein (SMV)
    s. oblique
    s. occipitofrontal fasciculus
    s. olivary complex
    s. ophthalmic vein
    s. ophthalmic vein thrombosis
    s. orbital fissure
    s. orbital fissure anatomy
    s. parietal lobule gyrus
    s. peroneal retinaculum (SPR)
    s. peroneal retinaculum disruption
    s. petrosal sinus catheterization
    s. petrous sinus (SPS)

    s. phrenic branch
    s. pole
    s. pubic ligament
    s. pubic ramus
    s. pulmonary artery
    s. pulmonary sulcus
    s. pulmonary sulcus tumor
    s. pulmonary vein
    s. ramus
    s. rectal vein
    s. retraction
    s. sagittal sinus (SSS)
    s. sagittal sinus thrombosis
    s. segment
    s. segmental bronchus
    s. temporal gyrus
    s. temporal sulcus
    s. thoracic aperture
    s. thyroid artery
    s. transverse rectal fold
    s. transverse scapular ligament
    s. triangle sign
    s. turbinated bone
    s. vena cava (SVC)
    s. vena cava obstruction (SVCO)
    s. vena cava pressure
    s. vena cava syndrome
    zygapophysis s.
superior/inferior (S/I)
superior-inferior flow direction
superioris
superior-medial acetabular index (SMAI)
supernormal
    s. artery
    s. excitation
supernumerary
    s. digit
    s. kidney
    s. parathyroid gland
    s. sesamoid bone
    s. teeth
superoinferior
    s. heart
    s. projection
    s. view
superolateral
    s. aspect
    s. displacement
superolaterally
superomedial
    s. margin
    s. portal
    s. surface
superoxide dismutase
superparamagnetic
    s. agent iron oxide
    s. iron oxide (SPIO)
    s. iron oxide blood pool agent

s. iron oxide imaging agent
s. iron oxide MR imaging
s. iron oxide particle
s. microsphere
Superpump System SPS3891
Superscan
superselective
s. angio-CT
s. angiography
s. infusion
s. mesenteric artery catheterization
s. microcatheter placement
super-stiff
s.-s. glide wire
s.-s. guidewire
SuperStitch
S. closure device
Sutura 8F S.
supersystemic pulmonary artery pressure
supervoltage
s. generator
s. radiation
s. radiotherapy
s. technique
supinate
supination
s. deformity
s., external rotation type IV fracture
supination-adduction
s.-a. fracture
s.-a. injury
supination-eversion fracture
supination-external
s.-e. rotation injury
s.-e. rotation IV (SER-IV)
supination-outward rotation injury
supinator
supine
s. bicycle stress echocardiography
s. film
s. full view
s. head-first position
s. position
s. radiograph
supplemental beam filtration
supply
accessory blood s.
arterial scrotum s.
collateral blood s.
dual blood s.

indirect blood s.
lenticulostriate s.
longitudinal blood s.
3-phase voltage s.
pudendal blood s.
tumor blood s.
vascular s.
support
basic life s. (BLS)
biventricular s. (BVS)
elevated leg s.
lateral lumbar s.
ligamentous s.
wedge-shaped s.
suppressed tissue
suppression
chemsat fat s.
Cytomel s.
DIET method of fat s.
drug-induced bone marrow s.
fat s.
fat signal s.
FSE-T2 with fat s.
s. of heart pulsation artifact
overdrive s.
paradoxic s.
s. scan
signal s.
solvent s.
spectral-spatial fat s.
suppuration
suppurative
s. ascending cholangitis
s. inflammation
s. pancreatitis
s. pleurisy
s. pneumonia
s. pyelonephritis
s. thyroiditis
supraanal fascia
supraanular constriction
supraaortic
s. lesion
s. ridge
s. stenosis
supracallosal
s. gyrus
s. sulcus
supracardiac total anomalous venous return
supracardinal vein
supraceliac aorta

S

NOTES

923

supracervical hysterectomy
supraclavicular
    s. aortic stenosis
    s. fossa
    s. lymph node
    s. node involvement
    s. triangle
supraclinoid
    s. carotid aneurysm
    s. ICA
    s. portion
    s. segment of internal carotid
      artery
supracolic compartment
supracollicular spike of cortical bone
supracondylar
    s. femoral fracture
    s. humeral fracture
    s. plate
    s. process
    s. ridge
    s. Y-shaped fracture
supracondyloid process
supracoronary ridge
supracricoid interval
supracristal
    s. plane (SCP)
    s. ventricular septal defect
supradditivity
supradiaphragmatic
    s. aorta
    s. extension
supraepicondylar
supraepitrochlear
supraglenoid tubercle
supraglottic
    s. carcinoma
    s. edema
    s. laryngectomy
    s. larynx
    s. narrowing
    s. structure
supraglottis
Supra G stent
suprahepatic
    s. caval cuff
    s. hypertension
    s. inferior vena cava anastomosis
    s. vena cava
suprahisian block
suprahyoid
suprailiac aortic mesenteric graft
suprainguinal PTA
suprainterparietal bone
supralevator
    s. fistula
    s. space
supraligamentous disc herniation
supramalleolar open amputation

supramarginal gyrus
supramesocolic compartment
supranaviculare
    os s.
supranuclear lesion
supraoccipital bone
supraorbital
    s. artery
    s. canal
    s. fissure
    s. foramen
    s. groove (SOG)
    s. margin (SOM)
    s. ridge
suprapancreatic obstruction
suprapatellar
    s. bursa
    s. plica
    s. pouch
suprapharyngeal bone
suprapubic
    s. area
    s. transabdominal ultrasound
suprapyloric node
suprarenal
    s. aortic aneurysm
    s. extension of aneurysm
    s. gland
    s. impression
    s. stenosis
suprascapular
    s. ligament
    s. nerve entrapment
    s. notch syndrome
suprasellar
    s. adenoma
    s. aneurysm
    s. atypical teratoma
    s. capsule
    s. extension
    s. extension of tumor
    s. hemorrhagic germinoma
    s. low-density lesion
    s. mass
    s. mass calcification
    s. meningioma
    s. subarachnoid cistern
suprasphincteric fistula
supraspinatus
    s. muscle
    s. musculotendinous junction
    s. nerve
    s. tendinosis
    s. tendon
supraspinous
    s. ligament
    s. ligament disruption
suprasternal
    s. bone

s. bulge
s. notch
s. notch plane
s. notch view
s. retraction
s. scanning
s. window
suprasyndesmotic fixation
supratentorial
s. astrocytoma
s. brain tumor
s. cerebral blood flow
s. flow compensation
s. glioma
s. gray matter
s. lesion
s. neoplasm
s. primitive neuroectodermal tumor
s. space
s. volume
s. white matter
suprathreshold
supratip nasal tip deformity
supratrochlear
s. artery
s. node
supratubercular ridge of Meyer
supravalvular
s. aortic stenosis (SAS, SVAS)
s. aortography
s. mitral stenosis
s. pulmonary stenosis
s. ring
supravaterian duodenum
supraventricular
s. crest (SVC)
s. level
s. tachyarrhythmia
s. tachycardia
s. venous echo
supraventricularis
crista s.
supravesical obstruction
supreme turbinate bone
SUR
standardized uptake ratio
sural nerve
SureStart contrast tracking
surface
acromial articular s.
anterolateral s.
anteromedial s.

s. application of radioelement
apposing articular s.
articular s.
articulating s.
arytenoidal articular s.
attenuated cortical s.
auricular s.
axial s.
basal s.
bone s.
bosselated s.
buccal s.
calcaneal articular s.
carpal articular s.
cartilaginous joint s.
cerebral s.
s. coil
s. coil localization
s. coil method
s. coil NMR
s. coil rotating-frame spectroscopy
colic s.
s. configuration
contiguous articular s.
s. convexity pattern
corrugated fat pad s.
costal s.
cuboidal articular s.
diaphragmatic s.
distal s.
s. distance
s. dose variation
endosteal s.
endothelial s.
epicardial s.
s. epithelium
erosion of articular s.
fibular articular s.
gastric s.
glenoid s.
grooving of articular s.
immunostained s.
joint articular s.
s. matching technique
mediastinal lung s.
s. nodularity
s. normal overlap method
occlusal s.
opposing articular s.'s
opposing pleural s.'s
s. osteosarcoma
s. ovarian epithelium tumor

S

NOTES

925

surface *(continued)*
  palmar s.
  parallelism of articular s.
  pelvic peritoneal s.
  plantar s.
  posterior s.
  s. projection
  s. radioelement application
  radioulnar s.
  s. registration
  renal s.
  roughened articular s.
  serosal s.
  s. shaded display (SSD)
  s. spoiling
  superomedial s.
  synovial s.
  s. tension of lung
  s. variable-attenuation correction
  ventral s.
  weightbearing s.
surfactant
  s. deficiency
  s. deficiency disorder (SDD)
surfer's
  s. knot
  s. nodule
surgeon
  American Academy of
    Orthopaedic S.'s (AAOS)
surgery
  coronary artery bypass s. (CABS)
  CT-guided stereotactic s.
  gastric bypass s. (GBS)
  image-guided s.
  nephron-sparing s.
  radioguided s.
  radioimmunoguided s. (RIGS)
  robotic mitral valve s.
  stereotactic s.
  telecollaboration s.
surgical
  s. anatomy visualization and
    navigation tools (SAVANT)
  s. angle
  s. artifact
  s. asepsis
  s. decompression
  s. emphysema
  s. endarterectomy
  s. inspection
  s. neck
  s. neck fracture
  s. neck of humerus
  S. Planning and Orientation
    Computer System (SPOCS)
  s. simulation CT
  s. sponge
  s. staple

  s. venous interruption
  s. wound
surgically
  s. corrected transposition of the
    great artery
  s. created resection cavity
Surgilase
  S. 150 high-powered CO_2 laser
  S. Nd:YAG laser
SurgiScope
Surgitron portable radiosurgical unit
Surgiview laparoscope
Surgi-Vision MRI coil
surveillance
  endoscopic s.
  imaging s.
survey
  bone s.
  s. film
  isotopic skeletal s.
  joint s.
  long bone s.
  metabolic bone s.
  metastatic bone s.
  osseous s.
  postimplant radiation s.
  preloading radiation s.
  s. radiograph
  s. scan
  serial radiographic s.
  skeletal s.
  traumatic bone s.
  4-view wrist s.
survival
  failure-free s.
susceptibility
  s. artifact
  bulk magnetic s. (BMS)
  s. contrast-weighted MRI
  diamagnetic s.
  s. effect
  magnetic s.
  s. mapping
susceptibility-sensitive sequence
susceptibility-weighted MR imaging
suspended
  s. heart
  s. inspiration
suspension
  barium s.
  s. characteristic
  chromic phosphate s.
  colloidal s.
  Definity injectable s.
  Enecat CT concentrated rectal s.
  E-Z-Paque barium s.
  fast exchange-cellular s.
  galactose-based s.
  s. of kidney

S

liquid barium s.
perflutren lipid microsphere
  injectable s.
suspensory
  s. ligament
  s. ligament of ovary
  s. ligament of penis
  s. muscle of duodenum
suspicious
  s. lesion
  s. mass
sustained
  s. anterior parasternal motion
  s. apical impulse
  s. left ventricular heave
sustentacular trauma
sustentaculi
sustentaculum
  s. lienis
  os s.
  s. tali
Sutura 8F SuperStitch
sutural
  s. bone
  s. calcification
  s. ligament
  s. marking
suture
  anterior palatine s.
  apical s.
  basilar s.
  bioabsorbable Dexon s.
  biparietal s.
  bony s.
  bregmatomastoid s.
  s. calcification
  coronal s.
  cranial s.
  delayed closure of s.
  dentate s.
  denticulate s.
  diastasis of s.
  diastatic lambdoid s.
  ethmoidolacrimal s.
  ethmoidomaxillary s.
  false s.
  flat s.
  frontal s.
  frontoethmoidal s.
  frontolacrimal s.
  frontomalar s.
  frontomaxillary s.

frontonasal s.
frontoparietal s.
frontosphenoid s.
frontozygomatic s.
Gillies s.
Gruber s.
incisive s.
infiltration s.
infraorbital s.
intermaxillary s.
internasal s.
interpalatine s.
interparietal s.
jugal s.
lacrimoconchal s.
lacrimoethmoidal s.
lacrimomaxillary s.
lacrimoturbinal s.
lambdoid s.
lambdoidal cranial s.
limbus s.
s. line
s. line carcinoma
s. lock
longitudinal s.
malomaxillary s.
mamillary s.
mastoid s.
median palatine s.
metallic s.
metopic s.
middle palatine s.
nasal s.
nasofrontal s.
nasomaxillary s.
nonfusion of cranial s.
occipital s.
occipitomastoid s.
occipitoparietal s.
occipitosphenoid s.
opaque wire s.
overlapping s.
palatine s.
palatoethmoidal s.
palatomaxillary s.
parietal s.
parietomastoid s.
parietooccipital s.
parietotemporal s.
persistent metopic s.
petrobasilar s.
petrosphenobasilar s.

NOTES

927

suture (*continued*)
 petrosphenooccipital s.
 petrosquamosal s.
 petrosquamous s.
 plane s.
 posterior palatine s.
 prematurely closed s.
 premaxillary s.
 rhabdoid s.
 sagittal cranial s.
 serrated s.
 silk s.
 s. of skull
 sphenoethmoidal s.
 sphenofrontal s.
 sphenomalar s.
 sphenomaxillary s.
 sphenooccipital s.
 sphenoorbital s.
 sphenoparietal s.
 sphenopetrosal s.
 sphenosquamous s.
 sphenotemporal s.
 sphenovomerine s.
 sphenozygomatic s.
 splayed cranial s.
 spread s.
 squamosal s.
 squamosomastoid s.
 squamosoparietal s.
 squamososphenoid s.
 squamous s.
 sternal s.
 temporal s.
 temporomalar s.
 temporozygomatic s.
 true s.
 wide s.
 zygomaticofrontal s.
 zygomaticotemporal s.

SUV
 standard uptake value

SV
 stroke volume

Sv
 sievert

SV-5 guidewire

SVABB
 stereotactic vacuum-assisted breast
  biopsy

SVAS
 supravalvular aortic stenosis

SVC
 superior vena cava
 supraventricular crest
  SVC syndrome

SVCO
 superior vena cava obstruction

SVCT
 spiral x-ray computed tomography

SVD
 singular valve decompensation

SVG
 scatter and veiling glare

SVI
 seminal vesicle invasion
 stroke volume index

SvO$_2$
 systemic vascular resistance index

SVR
 systemic vascular resistance

SVRI
 systemic vascular resistance index

swallow
 barium s.
 dry s.
 Gastrografin s.
 Hypaque s.
 ice-water s.
 video barium s.
 water-soluble contrast esophageal s.
 wet s.

swallowing
 s. artifact
 s. center
 s. dysfunction
 fetal s.
 s. function
 s. mechanism

swallowtail
 s. configuration
 s. malformation of scapula

swamp-static artifact

Swan-Ganz balloon catheter

swan-neck
 s.-n. finger deformity
 s.-n. shape of ventricular outflow
 s.-n. tubular lesion

Swanson finger joint

sweat
 s. duct adenoma
 s. gland carcinoma

sweep
 duodenal s.
 finger s.
 iterative s.
 whole-body s.
 widened duodenal s.

sweet
 S. method
 S. sternal punch

swelling
 ankle s.
 blennorrhagic s.
 brain s.
 bulbar s.
 s. of cartilage

congestive brain s.
fusiform s.
joint s.
periumbilical s.
prevertebral soft tissue s.
soft tissue s.
Swenson pull-through procedure
SWI
stroke-work index
swimmer's
s. position
s. projection
s. shoulder
s. view
swimming pool granuloma
swinging heart
swirling
s. motion
s. smokelike echoes
Swiss
S. Alps appearance
S. cheese air bronchogram
S. cheese appearance
S. cheese nephrogram
S. cheese ventricular septal defect
S. lithoclast intracorporeal
lithotripter
S. roll technique
Swissray scanner
switchable coil
swollen
s. brain hemisphere
s. tissue
Swyer-James-Macleod syndrome
Swyer-James syndrome (SJS)
Swyer syndrome
SXA
single-energy x-ray absorptiometer
SXCT
spiral x-ray computed tomography
Syed-Neblett template
Syed-Puthawala-Hedger esophageal
applicator
Syed template
sylvian
s. aqueduct
s. aqueduct syndrome
s. candelabra
s. cistern
s. fissure
s. operculum

s. point
s. triangle
sylvian-rolandic junction
Sylvius
aqueduct of S.
cistern of S.
S. fossa
hereditary stenosis of the aqueduct
of S. (HSAS)
S. ventricle
Symbia TruePoint SPECT-CT
symbol
radiation warning s.
Syme ankle disarticulation amputation
Symington body
Symmers fibrosis
Symmetra I-125 brachytherapy seeds
symmetric
s. abnormal increased signal
bilaterally s.
s. chest
s. confluent high signal intensity
s. consolidation
s. distribution
s. echo
s. heart hypertrophy
s. IUGR
s. loss of DAT
s. narrowing
s. pattern of radiotracer uptake
s. periosteal reaction
s. phased array
s. pulmonary congestion
s. thorax
symmetry
architectural s.
bilateral s.
inverse s.
sympathetic
s. block
s. blockade
s. chain
s. denervation
s. discharge
s. dystrophy
s. ganglia tumor
s. ganglion
s. innervation
s. nervous tissue
s. vascular instability
sympathicoblastoma
sympathicogonioma

NOTES

sympathicolysis
 MR-guided lumbar s.
sympathoblastoma
sympathogonia
sympathogonioma
symphony
 S. MR imaging system
 S. MR unit
 S. Nitinol self-expandable stent
 S. self-expanding stent
symphyseal
symphysis, pl. **symphyses**
 s. cartilage joint
 s. intervertebralis
 s. of mandible
 s. manubriosternalis
 s. ossium pubis
 pubic s.
 s. pubica
symptom
 constellation of s.'s
 constitutional s.
 segmental bronchus s.
 vasomotor s.
symptomatic
 s. coarctation of aorta
 s. gallstone
 s. lateral synovial plica
 s. metastatic spinal cord
  compression
 s. obstructive hydrocephalus
 s. vascular ring
synaptic
 s. cleft
 s. dopamine concentration
 s. pathway
 s. vesicle
sync
 V sync
syncephalus
synchondrosis, pl. **synchondroses**
 cartilaginous s.
 disruption of cartilaginous s.
 low signal intensity s.
 s. manubriosternalis
 neurocentral s.
 posterior intraoccipital s.
 s. of skull
 s. sphenoethmoidalis
 sphenooccipital s.
 s. sphenopetrosa
 s. sternalis
 s. sternocostalis costae primae
 s. xiphosternalis
synchronicity
synchronization
 s. device
 prospective s.
 retrospective s.

synchronized retroperfusion
synchronous
 s. carotid arterial pulse
 s. disease
 s. lesion
 s. transitional cell carcinoma
synchrony
 ventricular s.
synchrotron
 monochromatic s.
 s. radiation
synclitic
syncliticism
synclitism
syncytium
 circular s.
syndactylization of digit
syndactyly in fetus
syndesmophyte
 marginal s.
 spinal s.
syndesmosis, pl. **syndesmoses**
 distal tibiofibular s.
 s. radioulnaris
 s. sprain
 tibiofibular s.
 s. tibiofibularis
 s. tympanostapedialis
syndesmotic
 s. diastasis
 s. impingement
 s. ligament
 s. ligament complex
syndrome (*See* disease, phenomenon)
 abdominal muscle deficiency s.
 acquired adult Fanconi s.
 acquired immunodeficiency s.
  (AIDS)
 acute central cord s.
 acute chest s.
 acute compartment s.
 acute radiation s. (ARS)
 acute respiratory distress s.
  (ARDS)
 acute retroviral s.
 Adams-Stokes s.
 adductor canal s.
 adductor insertion avulsion s.
 adrenogenital s.
 adult respiratory distress s. (ARDS)
 afferent loop s.
 Aicardi s.
 Aicardi-Goutières s.
 Alagille s.
 Albright s.
 Albright-McCune-Sternberg s.
 Alibert-Bazin s.
 Alpers-Huttenlocher s. (AHS)
 amnionic band s.

angiomatous s.
angioosteohypertrophy s.
anterior compartment s.
anterior cord s.
anterior impingement s.
anterior spinal artery s.
anterior tarsal tunnel s.
anterolateral impingement s.
aortitis s.
apallic s.
apple-peel s.
Arnold-Chiari s.
Asherson s.
atherosclerotic occlusive s.
autoerythrocyte sensitization s.
Avellis s.
axonopathic neurogenic thoracic
  outlet s.
Ayerza s.
Bäfverstedt s.
Balint s.
Bannayan-Riley-Ruvalcaba s.
Banti s.
Barlow s.
Barré-Lieou s.
Bartter s.
basal cell nevus s.
basilar artery s.
Bazex s.
beat-knee s.
Beckwith-Wiedemann s.
Behr s.
Berdon s.
Bernard-Horner s.
Bernard-Soulier s.
Bertolotti s.
Beuren s.
biliary obstruction s.
Bing-Horton s.
Blackfan-Diamond s.
Bland-Garland-White s.
Blesovsky s.
blind loop s.
blind pouch s.
blueberry muffin s.
blue-digit s.
blue rubber-bleb nevus s.
blue-toe s.
Boerhaave s.
bone marrow edema s.
Bouveret s.
Brissaud s.

Brown-Séquard s.
Brugada s.
Budd-Chiari s.
Caffey s.
Caffey-Kempe s.
capillary leak s.
Caplan s.
carcinoid s.
cardiac disturbance s.
cardiocutaneous s.
cardiosplenic s.
Carney s.
carotid blowout s.
carotid sinus s. (CSS)
carpal tunnel s.
cat's cry s.
cauda equina s. (CES)
caudal regression s.
cavernous sinus s.
Cayler s.
Ceelen-Gellerstedt s.
celiac artery compression s.
celiac axis s.
central cervical cord s.
cerebellar s.
cerebral steal s.
cerebrohepatorenal s. (CHRS)
cervical disc s.
cervical pain s.
cervical rib s.
Cestan-Chenais s.
Chédiak-Steinbrinck-Higashi s.
Chilaiditi s.
CHILD s.
chronic overuse s.
Churg-Strauss s.
Clarke-Hadefield s.
Claude s.
cleft face s.
Clerc-Levy-Cristico s.
clinically isolated s.
COACH s.
coarctation s.
Cobb s.
Cockayne s.
Collet-Sicard s.
compartment s.
compression s.
congenital adrenogenital s.
congenital pulmonary venolobar s.
congenital vascular-bone s. (CVBS)
Conn s.

NOTES

syndrome *(continued)*

Conradi-Hünermann s.
constriction band s.
coronary artery steal s.
coronary-subclavian steal s.
costoclavicular s.
Courvoisier-Terrier s.
Cowden s.
craniofacial pain s.
craniomandibular s.
craniosynostosis s.
CRASH s.
CREST s.
cri-du-chat s.
Cronkhite-Canada s.
Crouzon s.
Crow-Fukase s.
crush s.
cubital tunnel s.
Cushing s.
Cyriax s.
Dandy-Walker s.
Davies-Colley s.
defibrination s.
Degos s.
de Lange s.
Demons-Meigs s.
de Morsier s.
Denys s.
Diamond-Blackfan s.
DiFerrante s.
DiGeorge s.
Di Guglielmo s.
disconnected duct s.
disconnected pancreatic duct s.
disseminated intravascular
    coagulation s.
distal intestinal obstruction s.
Down s.
Drash s.
Dressler s.
Dubin-Johnson s.
dumping s.
Dyke-Davidoff-Masson s.
dysarthria clumsy hand s.
Eagle-Barrett s.
ectopic ACTH s.
ectrodactyly-ectodermal dysplasia-
    clefting s.
Edwards s.
Ehlers-Danlos s.
Eisenmenger s.
Ellis-van Creveld s.
empty sella s.
encephalotrigeminal s.
enlarged vestibular vascular
    aqueduct s.
excessive lateral pressure s. (ELPS)
facet s.

facioauriculovertebral s.
failed back s. (FBS)
failed back surgery s. (FBSS)
Fallot s.
familial adenomatous polyposis s.
Fanconi s.
Fanconi-Hegglin s.
fat embolism s. (FES)
Felty s.
feminizing testes s.
fetal alcohol s. (FAS)
fetal cardiosplenic s.
Feuerstein-Mims s.
fibrocystic breast s.
Fiessinger-Leroy s.
Fiessinger-Leroy-Reiter s.
Fitz-Hugh and Curtis s.
floppy valve s.
Foix-Alajouanine s.
Foix-Chavany-Marie s.
Forney s.
functional bowel s.
Gaisböck s.
Gardner bone s.
gas-bloat s.
Gasser s.
gastrocardiac s.
generalized lymphadenopathy s.
Gerstmann s.
Gianotti-Crosti s.
Goldenhar s.
Goodpasture s.
Gorlin s.
Gorlin-Goltz s.
Graham-Burford-Mayer s.
Grisel s.
Gsell-Erdheim s.
Haglund s.
Hajdu-Cheney s.
Hallermann-Streiff-François s.
Hamman-Rich s.
Hare s.
Hegglin s.
hemisensory s.
hemolyticuremic s.
Hennekam s.
Henoch-Schönlein s.
hepatorenal s. (HRS)
hereditary flat adenoma s.
Hermansky-Pudlak s.
heterotaxy s.
holiday heart s.
Holmes s.
Holt-Oram s.
Horner s.
Howell-Evans s.
Hoyeraal-Hreidarsson s.
Hughes-Stovin s.
Hurler s. (HS)

Hurler-Scheie s.
Hutchinson s.
Hutchinson-Gilford s.
Hutinel-Pick s.
hyperabduction s.
hypoplastic left heart s. (HLHS)
hypoplastic left parietal s.
hypoplastic right heart s.
ileocecal s.
iliac vein compression s.
iliotibial band friction s.
immature lung s.
s. of impending thrombosis
impingement s.
inferior vena cava s.
infrapatellar contracture s. (IPCS)
inguinal ligament s.
inhibitory s.
innominate artery compression s.
intermediate coronary s.
intestinal Behçet s.
intestinal hypoperistalsis s.
irritable bowel s.
Ivemark CHD s.
Jadassohn-Lewandowsky s.
Jaffe-Campanacci s.
Jarcho-Levin s.
Jeune s.
Joubert s.
jugular foramen s.
juvenile polyposis s. (JPS)
Kallmann s.
Kartagener s.
Kasabach-Merritt s.
Kast s.
Katayama s.
Kearns-Sayre s.
Kimmelstiel-Wilson s.
Kinsbourne s.
Kleffner-Landau s.
Klippel-Feil s.
Klippel-Trenaunay s.
Klippel-Trenaunay-Weber s.
Lady Windermere s.
Lambert-Eaton myasthenic s.
Landau-Kleffner s.
Larsen s.
lateral recess s.
Laubry-Pezzi s.
leaky lung s. (LLS)
left heart s.
Leigh s.

Lemierre s.
Lennox-Gastaut s.
Leriche s.
Leri-Weill s.
Lesch-Nyhan s.
Lhermitte-Duclos s.
Lhermitte-Duclos-Cowden s.
Lightwood s.
linear sebaceous nevus s.
locked-in s.
Löffler s.
Löfgren s.
Louis-Bar s.
low back s.
low-flow s.
Lown-Ganong-Levine s. (LGL)
luteinized unruptured follicle s.
Lutembacher s.
luxury perfusion s.
lymphadenopathy s.
lymph node s.
Macleod s.
Maffucci s.
male Turner s.
Mallory-Weiss s.
malperfusion s.
Marchiafava-Micheli s.
Marcus Gunn s.
Marfan s.
Marine-Lenhart s.
Marinesco-Sjögren s.
Maroteaux-Lamy s.
Martin-Bell s.
Martorell aortic arch s.
Mayer-Rokitansky-Küster-Hauser s.
May-Thurner s.
Mazabraud s.
McCune-Albright s.
McKusick-Kaufman s.
Meadows s.
Meckel s.
Meckel-Gruber s.
meconium aspiration s.
meconium plug s.
medial tibial stress s.
megacystis-microcolon-intestinal
  hypoperistalsis s.
Meigs s.
Meigs-Cass s.
Meigs-Salmon s.
Melnick-Needles s.
Mendelson s.

S

NOTES

syndrome *(continued)*

Ménière s.
Menkes s.
mermaid s.
metastatic carcinoid s.
midaortic s. (MAS)
middle aortic s.
middle fossa s.
middle lobe s.
Mikity-Wilson s.
Mikulicz s.
milk-alkali s.
milk leg s.
Milkman s.
Miller-Dieker s.
Milwaukee shoulder s.
Minot-von Willebrand s.
Mirizzi s.
Mohr s.
Morgagni s.
Morgagni-Adams-Stokes s.
Morquio s.
Morquio-Brailsford s.
Mosse s.
Mounier-Kuhn s.
moyamoya s.
Moynahan s.
MSA s.
mucocutaneous lymph node s.
  (MCLS)
mucosal prolapse s.
Muir-Torre s.
multiple endocrine neoplasia s.
multiple mucosal neuroma s.
multiple pterygium s.
multiple system atrophy s.
myelodysplastic s. (MDS)
myofascial pain-dysfunction s.
nail-patella s.
Naumoff s.
Nelson s.
nephrotic s.
neurocutaneous s.
neuroorthopedic s.
nevoid basal cell carcinoma s.
Nievergelt s.
Nijmegen breakage s.
Noonan s.
Nothnagel s.
nutcracker s.
Ogilvie s.
Omenn s.
orbital apex s.
organic brain s. (OBS)
orodigitofacial s.
Ortner s.
Osler-Libman-Sacks s.
Osler-Weber-Rendu s.
os peroneum s.

os trigonum s.
ovarian hyperstimulation s.
ovarian remnant s.
ovarian vein s.
Paget-von Schroetter s.
painful osmotic demyelination s.
Pallister-Hall s.
Pancoast s.
pancreatic cholera s.
pancreaticohepatic s.
pancytopenia-dysmelia s.
Papillon-Lèfevre s. (PLS)
paraneoplastic s.
Parinaud s.
Parkes-Weber s.
Parry-Romberg s.
Patau s.
Pearson s.
pectoralis major s.
PEHO s.
pelvic congestion s.
pelvic spur s.
Pena-Shokeir s.
Pendred s.
Pepper s.
Peutz-Jeghers s.
Pfaundler-Hurler s.
Pfeiffer s.
PHACES s.
phantom limb s.
Pierre Robin s.
pinch-off s.
plica s.
Plummer-Vinson s.
POEMS s.
Poland s.
polycystic ovary s. (PCOS)
polysplenia s.
popliteal artery entrapment s.
postcardiac injury s. (PCIS)
postembolization s.
posterior column s.
posterior impingement s.
posterior joint s.
posterior reversible
  encephalopathy s. (PRES)
postmaturity s.
postmyocardial infarction s.
postpericardiotomy s.
postpolio s.
Potter s.
Proteus s.
proximal loop s.
prune belly s.
pseudothrombophlebitis s.
pseudo-Turner s.
pseudo-Zollinger-Ellison s.
quadrilateral space s.
Raeder paratrigeminal s.

Ramsay Hunt s.
Raymond-Cestan s.
Raynaud s.
reactive airway dysfunction s.
Reader paratrigeminal s.
reflex sympathetic dystrophy s.
Reiter s.
respiratory distress s. (RDS)
restrictive hemodynamic s.
Rett s.
reversible posterior
  leukoencephalopathy s. (RPLS)
Richter s.
right middle lobe s.
Riley-Day s.
Roberts s.
Robinow s.
Rokitansky-Mayer-Küster Hauser s.
Romano-Ward s.
Romberg-Wood s.
Rotor s.
Rundles-Falls s.
Russell-Silver s.
Ruvalcaba-Myhre-Smith s.
Sack-Barabas s.
Saldino-Noonan s.
Sanfilippo s.
SAPHO s.
scalene anticus s.
scalenus anticus s.
scaphocapitate s.
scapulocostal s.
Scheie s.
Schönlein-Henoch s.
Schwartz-Jampel s. (SJS)
scimitar s.
severe acute respiratory s. (SARS)
shaken baby s. (SBS)
Sheehan s.
Shone s.
short gut s.
short rib-polydactyly s.
shoulder-hand s.
shoulder impingement s.
Shprintzen velocardiofacial s.
Shwachman s.
sick sinus s.
silent sinus s.
sinus tarsi s.
Sipple s.
Sjögren s.
Sjögren-Larsson s.

slipping rib s.
slit ventricle s.
sloughed urethra s.
small aorta s.
small left colon s.
Smith-Lemli-Opitz s.
snapping hip s.
snapping triceps s.
Sneddon s.
soleus s.
solitary rectal ulcer s.
Solomon s.
Sotos s.
spastic bowel s.
Spens s.
split-cord s.
split notochord s.
stagnant-loop s.
Stauffer s.
steal s.
Stein-Leventhal s.
Stewart-Treves s.
Stickler s.
stiff lung s.
stiff man s.
Sturge-Weber s.
Sturge-Weber-Dimitri s.
superior mesenteric artery s.
  (SMAS)
superior vena cava s.
suprascapular notch s.
SVC s.
Swyer s.
Swyer-James s. (SJS)
Swyer-James-Macleod s.
sylvian aqueduct s.
synovitis, acne, pustulosis,
  hyperostosis, osteitis s.
systemic inflammatory response s.
TAR s.
tarsal tunnel s.
Taussig-Bing s.
Taussig-Snellen-Alberts s.
terminal reservoir s.
tethered cord s. (TCS)
thoracic inlet s.
thoracic outlet s. (TOS)
thrombocytopenia-absent radius s.
Tietze s.
tight filum terminale s.
Tolosa-Hunt s.
Torre s.

NOTES

syndrome *(continued)*
    Touraine-Solente-Golé s.
    transient bone marrow edema s.
    Treacher Collins s.
    trisomy 8 s.
    trisomy D, E s.
    Trousseau s.
    Turcot s.
    Turner s.
    twiddler's s.
    twin embolization s.
    twin-to-twin transfusion s. (TTTS)
    ulnar impaction s.
    ulnar tunnel s.
    ulnolunate impaction s.
    uncal herniation s.
    unroofed coronary sinus s.
    urethral s.
    VACTERL s.
    van Buchem s.
    Van der Hoeve s.
    vanishing lung s.
    vanishing testes s.
    vascular leak s.
    venolobar s.
    venous statis s.
    Verner-Morrison s.
    vertebral artery s.
    vertebrobasilar artery s.
    vestibular aqueduct s. (VAS)
    Villaret-Mackenzie s.
    von Hippel-Lindau s.
    Waardenburg s.
    Walker-Walburg s.
    Wallenberg lateral medullary s.
    Weil s.
    Weill-Marchesani s.
    Wermer s.
    Werner s.
    Wernicke-Korsakoff s.
    West s.
    wet lung s.
    Widal s.
    Wiedemann-Beckwith s.
    Wilkie s.
    Williams s.
    Williams-Beuren s.
    Williams-Campbell s.
    Wilson-Mikity s.
    s. with multiple cortical renal cyst
    Wolff-Parkinson-White s.
    Wolf-Hirschhorn s.
    Wolfram s.
    Wyburn-Mason s.
    s. X
    XY s.
    Young s.
    Yunis-Varon s.
    Zellweger s.

    Zieve s.
    Zollinger-Ellison s. (ZES)
synechia, pl. **synechiae**
    uterine s.
    s. vulvae
synergic muscle
Synergy ultrasound system
syngeneic
    s. bone marrow transplant
    s. tissue
syngraft
synkinesis
synophridia
synophrys
synostosis, synosteosis, pl. **synostoses**
    bicoronal s.
    cervical s.
    congenital radioulnar s.
    coronal suture s.
    cranial s.
    craniofacial s.
    lambdoid s.
    metatarsal s.
    multiple-suture s.
    nonsyndromic bicoronal s.
    nonsyndromic unicoronal s.
    premature suture s.
    radiographically firm s.
    sagittal s.
    single suture s.
    terminal s.
    tibiofibular s.
    unicoronal s.
synostotic posterior plagiocephaly
synovectomy
    radiation s.
    radioisotope s.
    radionuclide s.
    radiopharmaceutical s.
synovial
    s. bursa
    s. cavity
    s. chondromatosis
    s. cyst
    s. diarthroidal joint
    s. diffuse lipoma
    s. envelope
    s. fluid
    s. fringe
    s. gutter
    s. hemangioma
    s. herniation pit
    s. inflammatory response
    s. ligament
    s. membrane
    s. osteochondromatosis
    s. pannus
    s. plica
    s. proliferation

s. sarcoma
s. sheath
s. shelf
s. surface
s. thickening
s. tissue
synoviogram
synovioma
synoviorthesis
synovitis
s., acne, pustolosis, hyperostosis, osteitis (SAPHO)
s. in active polymyalgia rheumatica
boggy s.
brucellar s.
intraarticular localized nodular s.
nodular s.
pan s.
peripheral s.
pigmented villonodular s.
purulent s.
toxic s.
transient s.
s. tumor
synovium
boggy s.
exuberant s.
hyperplastic s.
opaque s.
pannus of s.
synovium-filled degenerative cyst
synovium-lined fascicle
synpneumonic empyema
synspondylism
cervical s.
synthesizer
frequency s.
synthetic
s. bone implant
s. graft bypass to ankle
s. valve
s. vascular bypass graft
syntropy
syphilis
bone s.
tertiary s.
syphilitic
s. aortic aneurysm
s. aortic regurgitation
s. node
syringe
electric s.

Isovue prefilled s.
Isovue-370 prefilled s.
prefilled s.
tuberculin s.
Ultraject prefilled s.
syringes (*pl. of* syrinx)
syringobulbia
syringocarcinoma
syringocele
syringoencephalia
syringoencephalomyelia
syringohydromyelia
holocord s.
syringohydromyelic cavity
syringoma
chondroid s.
syringomeningocele
syringomyelia
ape hand of s.
cervical s.
Chiari-associated s.
communicating s.
posttraumatic s.
syringopontia
syringosubarachnoid shunting
syrinx, pl. **syringes**
s. cavity
central spinal cord s.
fusiform s.
posttraumatic central spinal cord s.
spinal cord s.
traumatic s.
syrup
diet cola and metoclopramide s.
syssarcosic
syssarcosis
syssarcotic
system (*See also* device, machine, scanner, unit)
ABBI s.
Ablatherm HIFU s.
AbMap electrophysiologic imaging s.
accuDEXA bone mineral density assessment s.
AccuLength arthroplasty measuring s.
ACIST contrast delivery injection s.
Acuson 128XP ultrasound s.
Add-On Bucky image acquisition s.

S

NOTES

system *(continued)*

Advanced Cardiovascular S.'s (ACS)
Advantx-E Legacy s.
Advantx LC+ cardiovascular imaging s.
Aegis sonography management s.
AESOP Hermes-Ready s.
Agfa ADC 70 storage phosphor s.
Agfa CR, PACS s.
air-filtration s.
AIRIS II MR s.
Alexa 1000 s.
Aloka SSD ultrasound s.
American Medical Association Ligament Injury Classification S.
Amplatz Anchor S.
AneuRx bifurcated stent-graft s.
Angioflow meter s.
Angiomat 3000, 6000 contrast delivery s.
Angiomat ILLUMENA injector s.
AngioRad radiation s.
Angio-Seal s.
AngioSURF s.
anterolateral s.
aortoiliac inflow s.
Apogee CX100, CX200 echocardiography s.
Apogee RX400 diagnostic ultrasound s.
Apollo DXA bone densitometry s.
AquaSens FMS 1000 fluid monitoring s.
archival s.
arrhythmia mapping s.
arterial port catheter s.
ArthroCare Coblation-based cosmetic surgery s.
ArthroProbe laser s.
Artoscan MRI s.
Ashhurst fracture classification s.
Aspen digital ultrasound s.
Aspen ultrasound s.
Aspire continuous imaging s.
Atlas 2.0 diagnostic ultrasound s.
ATL HDI 3000, 3500, 4000, 5000 ultrasound s.
ATL ultrasound s.
Aurora dedicated breast MRI s.
Aurora diode-based dental laser s.
automated angle-encoder s.
automated biopsy s.
automated cellular imaging s. (ACIS)
automated infusion s.
autonomic nervous s.
Avera breast imaging s.
Aviva mammography s.

BAK interbody fusion s.
Bard CPS s.
Bard percutaneous cardiopulmonary support s.
BAT s.
Batson vertebral brain s.
Beta-Cath s.
Biad SPECT imaging s.
biliary s.
BiliBed phototherapy s.
biograph molecular imaging s.
Biosound AU3, AU4, AU5 s.
BioSpec MR imaging s.
BioZ s.
biplane s.
biplane image intensifier s.
Bonopty needle s.
BrainLAB VectorVision neuronavigation s.
Brasfield scoring s.
Breast cancer s. 2100
Breast Imaging Reporting and Data S. (BI-RADS)
BreastScan IR s.
Bremer Halo Crown s.
Broselow-Luten Pediatric S.
Brown-Roberts-Wells stereotactic s.
Bruker CSI Omega MR s.
BRW stereotactic s.
CAAS QCA s.
CADx SecondLook s.
calyceal s.
cardiopulmonary support s.
cardiovascular s.
cardiovascular angiography analysis s. (CAAS)
C-arm DSA s.
carrier-mediated transport s.
cartesian reference coordinate s.
CARTO EP navigation s.
cascade s.
catenary s.
CathScanner ultrasound imaging s.
CathTrack catheter locator s.
CDRPan digital x-ray s.
Cemax/Icon PACS s.
Centauri Er:YAG dental laser s.
central nervous s. (CNS)
CerASPECT s.
CGR biplane angiographic s.
2-channel phased-array RF receiver coil s.
Checkmate s.
Chemo-Port vascular access s.
circumflex s.
collateral s.
collecting s.
collimating s.
ColonoSight s.

2-compartment s.
3-compartment s.
COMPASS stereotactic s.
Compton suppression s.
computer information s.
Computerized Thermal Imaging s.
continuous-wave Doppler
  ultrasound s.
continuous-wave laser s.
Cordis endovascular s.
Coroskop Plus cardiac
  angiography s.
Cotrel-Dubousset s.
CRYOguide ultrasound guidance s.
CryoHit tumor ablation s.
CrystalEyes endoscopic video s.
Curix Capacity Plus film
  processing s.
CVIS information s.
CyberKnife stereotactic
  radiosurgery s.
Cyberware 3D scanning s.
data-acquisition s. (DAS)
data collection s.
da Vinci surgical s.
dedicated mammography s.
Delta 32 digital stereotactic s.
DELTAmanager MedImage s.
Delta 32 TACT 3-dimensional
  breast imaging s.
detector s.
16-detector PET s.
digestive s.
digital Add-On Bucky image
  acquisition imaging s.
Digital Add-On Bucky radiographic
  detector image acquisition s.
digital chest imaging s.
Digital Equipment s.
digital flat-panel amorphous silicon
  detector-radiography s.
digital holography s.
digital mammographic s.
Digital Medical s.
digital selenium-based chest
  imaging s.
Digital Traumex s.
Digitron digital subtraction
  imaging s.
DirectView CR 900 imaging s.
Discovery LS imaging s.
display s.

display coordinate s.
DOBI s.
Dodick Laser Photolysis S.
dryer s.
DryView laser imaging s.
DTU-one UltraSure imaging s.
dual-head coincidence detection s.
duplicated renal collecting s.
3D-VIEWNIX software s.
dye laser s.
dynamic optical breast imaging s.
  (DOBI)
DynaRad portable x-ray s.
E.CAM dual-head emission
  imaging s.
ECAT Reveal PET/CT imaging s.
Eccocee CS ultrasound s.
EchoEyc 3-D ultrasound imaging s.
EchoEye ultrasound imaging s.
Eclipse MR S.
Edwards Thrombex PMT s.
electrostatic imaging s.
Elscint Prestige MRI s.
endovascular s.
EndoVasix EPAR laser s.
EnSite 3000 imaging s.
EPAR laser s.
EP2000 electrophysiology
  imaging s.
EPISTAR Diode Laser S.
Evans-D'Angio staging s.
ExAblate 2000 ultrasound s.
excimer laser s.
Exogen 2000+ low-intensity,
  ultrasound fracture healing s.
Explorer X70 intraoral
  radiography s.
Express biliary LD premounted
  stent s.
extracranial carotid s.
extrapyramidal s.
femoropopliteal s.
femtosecond laser s.
fetal musculoskeletal s.
Ficat and Axlet staging s.
fiducial alignment s.
FilmFax teleradiology s.
flexible over-wire s.
Flocks and Kadesky s.
FluoroPlus Cardiac digital
  imaging s.

S

NOTES

system *(continued)*

FluoroPlus real-time digital imaging s.
fluoroptic thermometry s.
FluoroTrak fluoroscopy-based surgical navigation s.
flying spot excimer laser s.
FONAR Standing Ovation MRI s.
Fuji AC2 storage phosphor computed radiology s.
Fuji FCR9000 computed radiology s.
full-field digital mammography s.
Galen teleradiology s.
Galileo intravascular radiotherapy s.
gasless laparoscopic s.
gated s.
GE CT HiSpeed Advantage CT s.
generation 6 integrated radiotherapy s.
generator s.
GentleLASE Plus laser s.
GE Senographe 2000D digital mammography s.
GE Voluson 730 4D ultrasound s.
Given Diagnostic imaging s.
GliaSite radiotherapy s.
gradient s.
GRASS s.
greater saphenous s.
Gyrus endourology s.
HDI 1000, 3000, 3500, 4000, 5000 ultrasound imaging s.
3-head gamma camera-based SPECT s.
Helios laser s.
hepatic artery s.
hepatic ductal s.
hepatic venous s.
HERMES s.
Hewlett-Packard phased-array ultrasound imaging s.
high-field s.
Hi-Star MRI s.
Hitachi Altaire Open MRI s.
Hitachi EUB-555 diagnostic ultrasound s.
Hitachi four-head s.
Hitachi rotating detector array s.
homonuclear spin s.
House grading s.
HP SONOS 5500 ultrasound echocardiography s.
HP SONOS 5500 ultrasound imaging s.
Hunt and Hess aneurysm grading s.
Hydra Vision Plus DR, ES, HP urological imaging s.

HydroCoil Embolic S.
hydrodynamic thrombectomy s.
Hyperion LTK s.
HyperPACS teleradiology s.
IDIS angiography s.
IDXrad radiology information s.
image analysis s.
Imagecast imaging s.
ImageChecker CT CAD software s.
image-forming s.
image intensifier s.
image recording s.
IMPAX PACS s.
implantable drug delivery s.
Indigo LaserOptic treatment s.
infrared navigational s.
InnerVasc vascular access s.
integrated clinical information s. (ICIS)
Integris III-V DSA s.
Integris V 3000 digital subtraction s.
intensified radiographic imaging s. (IRIS)
internal carotid s.
Interspec Apogee RX400 Diagnostic Ultrasound s.
Intrabeam intraoperative radiotherapy s.
intramedullary skeletal kinetic distractor s.
Intra-Op autotransfusion s.
intrarenal collecting s.
IntraStent DoubleStrut ParaMount premounted stent-biliary s.
IntraStent DoubleStrut ParaMount XS premounted stent-biliary s.
INVOS 3100, 3100A cerebral oximeter monitoring s.
iON IntraOperative Navigation S.
ISKD s.
Isocam scintillation imaging s.
Isocam SPECT imaging s.
Jackson staging s.
Kadish staging s.
Kaplan PenduLaser 115 laser s.
Kelly-Goerss Compass stereotactic s.
Kretztechnik ultrasound s.
Krigel staging s.
Lagios classification s.
Laitinen CT guidance s.
laser s.
LaTIS endovascular laser s.
left iliac s.
left ventricular support s.
Leksell stereotactic s.
LENT scoring s.
lesser saphenous s.

Liebel-Flarsheim CT 9000 contrast delivery s.
LIFE-Lung fluorescence endoscopy s.
LightSpeed Ultra CT s.
limbic s.
linear compartmental s.
lipophilic sequestration s.
LocaLisa cardiac navigation s.
LORAD full-field digital mammography s.
lower pole collecting s.
low-field MRI s.
LPI laser s.
LP^2 stainless steel delivery s.
LTX3000 lumbar rehabilitation s.
Luma cervical imaging s.
Luxtec fiberoptic s.
LVs s.
LX EchoSpeed 1.5T CV/i, NVi MR s.
LymphoScan nuclear imaging s.
Magnes biomagnetometer s.
Magnetic Surgery S.
MAGNETOM Open s.
MAGNETOM Sonata 1.5T MR s.
MAGNETOM Trio 3T unlimited MRI s.
MAGNETOM Vision 1.5T MR imaging s.
Magnex Alpha MR s.
mamillary s.
MAMMEX TR computer-aided mammography diagnosis s.
Mammo Plus mammography s.
MammoReader computer-aided dectection s.
MammoReader mammography s.
Mammotest breast biopsy s.
Mammotome ultrasound s.
Manchester LDR implant s.
Marex MRI s.
Massachusetts (General Hospital) Utility Multiprogramming S.
Meddars cardiac catheterization analysis s.
Medilase angioscope-laser delivery s.
Medi-tech ureteral stent s.
Medspec MR imaging s.
Med Tec Vac Loc immobilization s.

Medweb clinical reporting s.
microSelectron rapid delivery s.
microwave cardiac ablation s.
Millennium VG SPECT s.
Mini-Balloon s.
MIR s.
Mitsuyasu staging s.
Mobetron electron beam s.
Mobetron intraoperative radiation therapy treatment s.
mobile artery and vein imaging s. (MAVIS)
mucosal mass collecting s.
multicrystal BGO ring s.
multidetector s.
multigated pulsed Doppler flow s.
multileaf collimating s.
multiple-electrode probe s.
multiple-side-hole infusion s.
Multistar Top Plus DSA s.
musculoskeletal s.
MyoSight imaging s.
Myotherm XP cardioplegia delivery s.
Navi Ball guidance s.
Navigus cranial electrode s.
Navitrack computer-assisted surgery s.
needle-wire s.
nephroureteral stent s.
NeuroLink II data acquisition s.
Neurosector ultrasound s.
Nidek EC-5000 excimer laser s.
nondilated s.
Novacor left ventricular assist s.
Novalis radiosurgery s.
nuclear medicine information s.
Oasis thrombectomy s.
object coordinate s.
OctreoScan s.
ocular magnification s.
OEC Series 9600 cardiac s.
Olympus EU-M30 s.
Opdima digital mammography s.
OPD-Scan optical path difference scanning s.
open-architecture s.
open-configuration magnetic resonance s.
open MRI s.
OpenPACS s.
Opmilas 144 Plus laser s.

S

NOTES

system *(continued)*

Optistar MR contrast delivery s.
OR1 electronic s.
Oscar ultrasonic bone cement
  removal s.
OsteoView desktop hand x-ray s.
OsteoView 2000 digital imaging s.
Ostreg spinal marker s.
Ovation falloposcopy s.
Packard Merlin life-monitoring s.
parasympathetic nervous s.
Paris ultrasound s.
Paterson-Parker s.
Peacock s.
pelvicaliceal s.
pelvicalyceal s.
PenRad mammography clinical
  reporting s.
Pentax-Hitachi FG32UA
  endosonographic s.
Perclose PVS suture s.
Performa mammography s.
peripheral nervous s.
PFA-100 s.
3-phase s.
Philips DVI 1 s.
Philips Integris 5000 digital
  subtraction angiography s.
PhorMax CR desktop
  workstation s.
photoelectric s.
photon cataract removal s.
photon radiosurgery s. (PRS)
Photopic Imaging ultrasound s.
Picker s.
picture archival communication s.
  (PACS)
picture archiving and
  communication s.
Pinnacle$_3$ radiotherapy planning s.
plastic Vortex Port s.
PMT robotic fulcrumless
  tomographic s.
polar coordinate s.
polypoid fibroma collecting s.
portal vein s.
PortalVision radiation oncology s.
port-catheter s.
pressure-gradient wire s.
PrinceStar electrophysiologic
  imaging study s.
Prism 3-head s.
Probe balloon dilatation s.
Profile mammography s.
Prostalase laser s.
Protg GPS self-expanding Nitinol
  stent-biliary s.
pulmonary venous s.
2010 Pulse Holter s.

Pulse-Spray pulsed infusion s.
pyelocalyceal s.
pyramidal s.
Q-catheter catheterization
  recording s.
QCT bone densitometry s.
quadrature surface coil MRI s.
quantitative image processing s.
  (QUIPS)
Quick-Core biopsy s.
QuickSeal femoral arterial
  closure s.
Quimby implant s.
radiation therapy s. (RTS)
radiation therapy planning s.
radioisotope delivery s. (RDS)
radiology telephone access s.
radionuclide carrier s.
RadNet radiology information s.
rapid telephone access s. (RTAS)
RatioVision digital fluorescent
  imaging s.
rature surface coil s.
RDX coronary radiation catheter
  delivery s.
real-time 2-dimensional Doppler
  flow-imaging s.
real-time 4D ultrasound imaging s.
Redi-Vu teleradiology s.
reference coordinate s.
Refinity Coblation S.
remote afterloading s.
renal collecting s.
respiratory s.
reticuloendothelial s.
Retzius s.
Reveal XVI PET/CT imaging s.
RigiScan Plus rigidity
  assessment s.
RIGS s.
ring-type imaging s.
Robson modification of Flocks-
  Kadesky s.
Rogan teleradiology s.
Roger s.
Rotablator thrombectomy s.
rotational atherectomy s.
Rotograph Plus imaging s.
Rotograph Plus panoramic dental
  tomography imaging s.
RPM tracking s.
RTP s.
RX stent delivery s.
Sadowsky breast marking s.
SAFHS 2000 sonic accelerated
  fracture healing s.
SAMBA imaging s.
saphenous s.
SAVANT imaging s.

Scanditronix MLC s.
scanned-slot detector s.
scanning beam digital s.
scattering s.
scavenging s.
scene coordinate s.
Scharff-Bloom-Richardson histologic
  grade s.
Schmidt optics s.
Scintiview nuclear computer s.
Scintron IV nuclear computer s.
ScleroLaser laser s.
ScleroPLUS HP laser s.
Second Look CAD s.
Selectron s.
Selenia imaging s.
selenium-based digital chest s.
selenium-drum-detector s.
Selvester QRS scoring s.
Senographe 2000D digital
  mammography s.
Senographe DMRt mammography s.
SenoScan full-field digital
  imaging s.
SenoScan full field digital
  mammography s.
SenoScan full field
  mammography s.
Sens-A-Ray dental imaging s.
Sens-A-Ray 2000 dental imaging s.
sequestration s.
Sequoia ultrasound s.
Shape Maker s.
Shimadzu HeadTome s.
side-exiting coaxial s.
side-exiting coaxial needle s.
Siemens AG s.
Siemens HICOR/BICOR x-ray s.
Siemens Mammomat Novation DM
  full field digital mammography s.
Siemens SOMATOM Plus-4 CT s.
Siemens 1.5-T s.
Signa Advantage s.
Signa EXCITE 3.0T MRI s.
Signa Horizon LX MRI s.
Signa MR imaging s.
Silhouette laser s.
Silicon Graphics Reality Engine s.
SilkLaser aesthetic laser s.
SimpliCT interventional guidance s.
Simpson Coronary AtheroCath
  (SCA) s.

single-photon counting s.
single-stick s.
Site-Rite II ultrasound s.
Site-Rite ultrasound s.
skeletal s.
slip-ring gantry s.
SmartSPOT high-resolution digital
  imaging s.
Socrates telementoring s.
Softscan laser mammography s.
SOMATOM Volume Zoom CT s.
Sonablate 200 ultrasound s.
sonic-accelerated fracture-healing s.
  (SAFHS)
SonicWAVE phacoemulsification s.
Sonifer sonicating s.
SonoAce 6000 II ultrasound s.
SonoHeart ELITE personal hand-
  carried ultrasound s.
Sonoline Elegra ultrasound s.
SonoSite 180 ultrasound s.
spiderlike pelvocaliceal s.
splanchnic venous s.
spring-driven s.
Sprint fixed-detector research s.
SPY intraoperative imaging s.
Squibb s.
STARRT falloposcopy s.
steerable guide wire s.
StereoGuide prone breast biopsy s.
StereoLoc upright biopsy s.
stereotactic breast biopsy s.
1-stick s.
storage phosphor s.
Stratis II MRI s.
Sun SPARCstation s.
Super Angiorex model G DSA s.
superconducting open-magnet s.
superconductive MR s.
Superdup'r SD6891 left heart s.
Surgical Planning and Orientation
  Computer S. (SPOCS)
Symphony MR imaging s.
Synergy ultrasound s.
systemic venous s.
TCD100M digital transcranial
  Doppler s.
Tecmag Libra-S16 s.
TEGwire ST s.
Telocin diagnostic ultrasound s.
Tesla s.
thermal dosimetry s.

S

NOTES

system *(continued)*
ThinPRep Imaging s.
Thrombex PMT s.
tibioperoneal runoff s.
time-of-flight PET imaging s.
titanium Vortex Port s.
Tmx-2000 BPH thermotherapt
thermotherapy s.
Tomolex tomographic s.
Tomomatic five-slice SPECT
imaging s.
Tomomatic three-slice SPECT
imaging s.
Tomomatic two-slice SPECT
imaging s.
TomoTherapy Hi-ART s.
Total Recall digital imaging s.
Transonics s.
TransScan TS2000 electrical
impedance breast scanning s.
treatment planning s.
Trex digital mammography s.
(TDMS)
Triad SPECT imaging s.
TRON 3 VACI cardiac imaging s.
trumpet-like pelvocaliceal s.
1.5T whole-body MR imaging s.
UltraFine Erbium laser s.
UltraPACS diagnostic imaging s.
ultrasound s.
UltraSTAR computer-based
ultrasound reporting s.
UltraSure DTR-one imaging
ultrasound s.
UMC-I microwave delivery s.
University of Florida staging s.
Univision echocardiographic s.
s. unsharpness
uPACS picture archiving s.
upper pole collecting s.
USCI Probe balloon-on-a-wire
dilatation s.
Vac-Lok patient immobilization s.
vacuum cassette s.
Varian brachytherapy s.
Varian MLC s.
VasoView balloon dissection s.
VAX 4100 s.
Vbeam pulsed dye laser s.
ventricular s.
VentTrak monitoring s.
Versatome D8 Perioperative
Doppler S.
vertebral artery s.
vertebrobasilar s.
VEST s.
Viatronix Virtual Colonoscopy s.
view shadow projection
microtomographic s.

Vingmed CFM ultrasound s.
virtual retinal display s.
Virtuoso imaging s.
Virtuoso portable 3D imaging s.
Vision high-performance gradient s.
Vision MR imaging s.
VISX Star S2 excimer laser s.
VISX WaveScan Wavefront S.
Vitrea 3D s.
VNUS closure s.
Voluson ultrasound s.
Vortex port s.
VoxelView s.
whole-body compact MR s.
widened collecting s.
xenon trap s.
Xillix LIFE-GI fluorescence
endoscopy s.
Xillix LIFE-Lung fluorescence
endoscopy s.
XKnife stereotactic radiosurgery s.
Xplorer 1000 digital imaging s.
Xplorer imaging s.
x-ray shadow projection
microtomographic s.
Yaglazr s.
Zeus s.
Zlatkin grading s.

systematic
s. error
s. noise
s. relaxation effect
s. ultrasound-guided biopsy

systemic
s. adjuvant therapy
s. arterial circulation
s. arterial hypertension
s. arterial vasoconstriction
s. arteriolar resistance index
s. blood flow (SBF)
s. brain lymphoma
s. diastolic blood pressure
s. disorder
s. erythematosus lupus
s. granulomatous disease
s. heart
s. hypoperfusion
s. inflammatory response syndrome
s. intravenous infusion
s. juvenile rheumatoid arthritis
s. lesion
s. mastocytosis
s. mean arterial pressure (SMAP)
s. micrometastasis
s. nodular panniculitis
s. output
s. output flow
s. output index
s. oxygen saturation

s. sclerosis
s. vascular resistance (SVR)
s. vascular resistance index (SvO$_2$, SVRI)
s. vein
s. venous
s. venous hypertension
s. venous return
s. venous system

systole
atrial s.
cervical CSF s.
CSF ventricular s.
end s. (ES)
end of atrial s.
left ventricular internal dimension at end s. (LVIDs)
left ventricular internal end s.
ventricular s.

systolic
s. acceleration time
s. anterior motion (SAM)
s. anterior motion of mitral valve
s. anterior movement
s. atrial volume
s. ejection fraction

s. ejection period (SEP)
s. fractional shortening
s. function
s. gating
s. gradient
s. heart failure
s. hypertension
s. impulse
left ventricular s. (LVs)
s. mammary souffle
s. pressure-time index
s. prolapse
s. prolapse of mitral valve leaflet
s. reserve
s. retraction
s. retraction of apex
s. S wave
s. toe/brachial index
s. upstroke time
s. velocity ratio
s. velocity-time integral
s. ventricular overload
systolic-diastolic blood pressure
systolic-diastolic ratio (S-D)
Syvek Patch closure device

NOTES

S

γ-T
  gamma tocopherol
T
  temperature
  temporal
  thoracic
  tocopherol
  torque
    T artifact
    T axis
    T condylar fracture
    T configuration
    T fracture
    T loop
    T tubogram
    T vector
T1
    T1 shortening
    T1, T2 relaxation time
    T1, T2 value
1.5T
    1.5T Signa MR unit
    1.5T Signa whole body
      imager/spectrometer
    1.5T whole-body MR imaging
      system
T2
    T2 dephasing effect
    T2 image
    T2 PRE
    T2 proton relaxation enhancement
      (T2 PRE)
    T2 quantitative MRI
    T2 shortening
    T2 star relaxation
    T2 time constant
T₄
  thyroxine
T$_E$
  echo train echo time
t
  transformer
T1-contamination artifact
T2-gradient refocused image
T4 uptake
TA
  true apex
Ta
  tantalum
¹⁷⁸Ta
  tantalum 178
¹⁸²Ta
  tantalum 182
Tabar pattern

tabes
  burned-out t.
  t. dorsalis
table
  asymmetric "look-up" t.
  binary opacity t.
  critical dose t.
  dual lookup t.
  Hydradjust IV t.
  inner t.
  MobiTrak automated t.
  MobiTrak moving t.
  t. movement
  pivoting t.
  t. of radiation dose
  radionuclide t.
  resistive exercise t.
  tilt t.
tabletop
  auxiliary CT t.
TACE
  transarterial chemoembolization
  transcatheter arterial chemoembolization
tachyarrhythmia
  supraventricular t.
tachycardia
  atrial ectopic automatic t.
  atrioventricular nodal reentry t.
  nodoventricular t.
  noninducible t.
  paroxysmal auricular t.
  sinuatrial nodal reentry t.
  supraventricular t.
  ventricular paroxysmal t.
tachycardia-induced cardiomyopathy
tachyphylaxis
tachypnea
  transient t.
tackler's exostosis
tacrolimus
TACT
  tuned aperture computed tomography
tactile disc
TAD steerable guidewire
TAE
  transcatheter arterial embolization
taenia tissue
TAFI
  thrombin-activatable fibrinolysis inhibitor
TAG
  T. Excluder stent
tag
  t. of cartilage
  t. image file format (TIFF)

T

tag *(continued)*
> t. plane
> radioactive t.

Tagarno 3SD cine projector for angiography

tagged
> t. atom
> radioactively t.
> t. red cell

tagging
> barium-based fecal t.
> bolus t.
> cine magnetic resonance t.
> t. cine magnetic resonance
> myocardial t.
> t. pattern
> segmented k-space cardiac t.
> spin t.
> stool t.

Tagitol prep

Tagitol V

TAGM
> tris-acryl gelatin microsphere

TAI
> traumatic aortic injury

tail
> t. bone
> t. of breast
> dural t.
> t. of epididymis
> hippocampal head, body, and t.
> long dural t.
> t. of pancreas
> t. sign
> t. of Spence
> t. of the spleen
> t. vertebra
> wool t.

tailgut cyst

taillike segment

tailored
> t. excitation
> t. pulse

tailor's
> t. ankle
> t. muscle

Takayasu
> T. aortitis
> T. arteritis
> T. disease

takeoff
> t. of artery
> t. of vessel

Talairach
> T. coordinate
> T. stereotaxic space

talar
> t. avulsion fracture
> t. beaking

> t. body fusion
> t. dome
> t. dome articular cartilage
> t. dome cyst
> t. dome fracture
> t. dome ischemia
> t. dome osteochondral injury
> t. impingement
> t. neck fracture
> t. osteochondral fracture
> t. tilt angle

talc
> t. plaque
> t. pneumoconiosis
> t. sclerotherapy

talcosis
> lung t.
> pulmonary t.

talent
> T. bifurcated abdominal aortic stent graft
> T. stent graft

tali (*pl. of* talus)

talipes
> t. arcuatus
> t. calcaneus
> t. calcaneus calcaneocavus
> t. cavovalgus
> t. cavus
> t. cavus calcaneocavus
> t. equinovarus
> t. valgus
> t. varus

talocalcaneal
> t. angle
> anteroposterior t. (APTC)
> t. articulation
> t. coalition
> t. index
> t. index classification
> t. joint
> lateral t. (LATC)
> t. ligament

talocalcaneonavicular
> t. articulation
> t. joint

talocrural
> t. angle
> t. fusion
> t. joint

talofibular
> t. impingement
> t. joint
> t. ligament
> t. ligament injury
> posterior t. (PTF)

talohorizontal angle

talometatarsal angle

talonavicular
- t. angle
- t. articulation
- t. beaking
- t. capsule
- t. coalition
- t. joint
- t. ligament

talus, pl. **tali**
- beaking of head of t.
- t. bone
- Cedell fracture of t.
- congenital vertical t.
- flat-top t.
- t. foot deformity
- lateral process of the t.
- neck of t.
- Sneppen fracture of t.
- sulcus t.
- sustentaculum tali
- vertical t.

tam-o-shanter appearance

Tamp catheter

tamponade
- balloon t.
- cardiac t.
- chronic t.
- esophagogastric t.
- ferromagnetic t.
- florid cardiac t.
- full-blown cardiac t.
- heart t.
- low-pressure cardiac t.
- pericardial t.
- pericardial chyle with t.
- subacute cardiac t.

tandem
- t. applicator
- external beam with t.
- Fletcher-Suit-Delclos t.
- t. ICA/MCA occlusion
- t. lesion
- MIR intrauterine t.
- t. and ovoid
- t. stent
- t. technique
- t. transplant

tangential
- t. breast field
- t. constriction
- t. cut
- t. layer of hand

- t. port
- t. projection
- t. scapular view

tangentially

tangent radiograph

tangle
- intraneuronal neurofibrillary t.
- neurofibrillary t.

tanned red cell (TRC)

tannex
- bisacodyl t.

tantalate
- lutetium t.

tantalum (Ta)
- t. 178 (^{178}Ta)
- t. 182 (^{182}Ta)
- t. bronchogram
- t. imaging agent
- t. mesh
- t. powder
- t. stent
- t. tracer

tantalum-178 contrast medium

taper
- fiberoptic t.

tapered
- t. core guidewire
- t. finger

tapered-tip guidewire

tapering
- t. border
- t. dose
- t. occlusion
- t. stenosis

tapetal

tapetoretinal dysplasia

tapetum corporis callosi

tapeworm

tapir mouth

tapiroid

TAPVD
- total anomalous pulmonary venous drainage

TAPVR
- total anomalous pulmonary venous return

tap water enema

TAR
- tissue-air ratio
  - TAR syndrome

tar
- coal t.

T

NOTES

tarda
  osteogenesis imperfecta t.
tardive dyskinesia
tardus-parvus
  t.-p. technique
  t.-p. waveform
target
  angiographic t.
  t. appearance
  t. arch
  t. bone
  t. calcification
  t. canal
  t. coalition
  t. depth
  3D reconstructed t.
  gas t.
  internal cyclotron t.
  t. lung lesion
  t. material
  metal technetium t.
  minimal deformation t. (MDT)
  molybdenum t.
  t. navicular
  t. organ
  t. parenchymal structure
  t. point
  retrogasserian t.
  t. sign
  t. tissue
  tungsten t.
targeted
  t. contrast agent
  t. EIS
target-film distance (TFD)
target-filter combination
targeting
  angiographic t.
  t. bead
  B-mode acquisition and t. (BAT)
  pedicle t.
targetoid growth
target-skin distance (TSD)
target-to-background ratio
target-to-nontarget
  t.-t.-n. ratio
  t.-t.-n. ratio for myocardial imaging
Tarlov cyst
TARP
  total atrial refractory period
Tarrant position
tarsal
  t. arch
  t. bone
  t. canal
  t. coalition
  t. cyst
  t. joint
  t. ligament

  t. navicular
  t. plate
  t. sinus
  t. tunnel
  t. tunnel syndrome
tarsoepiphysial aclasis
tarsometatarsal
  t. angle
  t. articulation
  t. joint
  t. ligament
tartrate
  thorium t.
task
  block motor t.
task-rest pattern
taurodontism
TAUS
  transabdominal ultrasound
Taussig-Bing
  T.-B. anomaly
  T.-B. congenital malformation of heart
  T.-B. syndrome
Taussig-Snellen-Alberts syndrome
tautography
taut pericardial effusion
TAV
  transcutaneous aortovelography
Taveras injector
Tawara atrioventricular node
Taxus Express stent
Taylor
  T. position
  T. type dysplasia
Taylor-Blackwood mechanism
TB
  tuberculosis
  HIV-related TB
TBI
  tracheobronchial injury
  traumatic brain injury
TBNA
  transbronchial needle aspiration
TBT
  transcervical balloon tuboplasty
TBV
  total brain volume
TBW
  total body water
TC
  thoracic circumference
Tc
  technetium
^{99m}Tc, Tc-99m
  technetium-99m
    ^{99m}Tc aggregated albumin imaging agent

^{99m}Tc albumin colloid imaging agent
^{99m}Tc albumin microspheres imaging agent
^{99m}Tc biciromab imaging agent
^{99m}Tc bicisate imaging agent
^{99m}Tc Ceretec
^{99m}Tc Ceretec bind
^{99m}Tc depreotide
^{99m}Tc depreotide scintigraphy
^{99m}Tc dimer captosuccinic acid imaging agent
^{99m}Tc disofenin imaging agent
^{99m}Tc ECD
^{99m}Tc ethyl cysteinate dimer (EDC)
^{99m}Tc exametazime imaging agent
^{99m}Tc furifosmin imaging agent
^{99m}Tc-galactosyl human serum albumin imaging agent
^{99m}Tc glucarate imaging agent
^{99m}Tc gluceptate imaging agent
^{99m}Tc glucoheptanoate
^{99m}Tc glucoheptanoate scintimammography
^{99m}Tc GSA imaging agent
^{99m}Tc hexamethylpropylene amine oxime
^{99m}Tc HIG scintigraphy
^{99m}Tc HMPAO
^{99m}Tc HMPAO hyperfixation
^{99m}Tc HMPAO-labeled leukocyte total-body scan
^{99m}Tc HMPAO uptake
^{99m}Tc HSA
^{99m}Tc human polyclonal immunoglobulin G scintigraphy
^{99m}Tc human serum albumin imaging agent
^{99m}Tc human serum albumin scintigraphy
^{99m}Tc lidofenin imaging agent
^{99m}Tc MAA
^{99m}Tc MAA rhinoscintigraphy
^{99m}Tc MDP skeletal scintigram
^{99m}Tc MDP uptake
^{99m}Tc mebrofenin imaging agent
^{99m}Tc medronate imaging agent
^{99m}Tc mertiatide imaging agent
^{99m}Tc microaggregated albumin imaging agent
^{99m}Tc Myoview myocardial perfusion imaging

^{99m}Tc oxidronate imaging agent
^{99m}Tc pentetate calcium trisodium imaging agent
^{99m}Tc pentetate sodium imaging agent
^{99m}Tc pertechnetate thyroid
^{99m}Tc phosphate
^{99m}Tc polyphosphate compound radiopharmaceutical
^{99m}Tc polyphosphate imaging agent
^{99m}Tc pyrophosphate
^{99m}Tc pyrophosphate imaging agent
^{99m}Tc red blood cell SPECT
^{99m}Tc sestamibi
^{99m}Tc sestamibi imaging agent
^{99m}Tc sodium pertechnetate imaging agent
^{99m}Tc succimer imaging agent
^{99m}Tc sulfur colloid
^{99m}Tc sulfur colloid imaging agent
^{99m}Tc teboroxime imaging agent
^{99m}Tc tetrofosmin imaging agent
^{99m}Tc (V) DMSA
^{99m}Tc (V) DMSA scanning
^{99m}Tc WBC scan

TCA
    tentorium cerebelli attachment
    transcondylar axis
TCAT
    transmission computer-assisted tomography
TCBF
    total cerebral blood flow
TCC
    transitional cell carcinoma
TCCS
    transcranial color-coded duplex sonography
TCD
    transcranial Doppler
    transverse cerebellar diameter
        TCD measurement
        TCD sonography
        TCD ultrasound
        TCD velocity
TCD100M digital transcranial Doppler system
TCD-detectable turbulence
^{99m}Tc-depreotide
^{99m}Tc-DMSA
    technetium-99m dimercaptosuccinic acid
        ^{99m}Tc-DMSA scintigraphy

NOTES

^{99m}Tc-DTPA
technetium-99m diethylenetriamine pentaacetic acid
^{99m}Tc-ECD
technetium-99m ethyl cysteinate dimer
^{99m}Tc-ECD radiopharmaceutical
T-cell
T-c. acute lymphoblastic leukemia
T-c. lymphoblastic lymphoma
T-c. neoplasm
T4-cell
T-cell-type acute lymphoblastic leukemia
^{99m}Tc-ethyl cysteinate dimer
TCF
time correlation function
^{99m}Tc-galactosyl human serum albumin imaging agent
TcHIDA
^{99m}Tc-HMPAO
^{99m}Tc-HMPAO cerebral perfusion SPECT imaging
^{99m}Tc-HMPAO radiopharmaceutical
^{99m}Tc-HMPAO radiotracer
^{99m}Tc-HMPAO SPECT
^{99m}Tc-iminodiacetic acid derivative radiopharmaceutical
^{99m}Tc-labeled
technetium-99m-labeled
^{99m}Tc-labeled anti-E-selectin Fab fragment
^{99m}Tc-labeled antigranulocyte antibody
^{99m}Tc-labeled cerebral perfusion imaging agent
^{99m}Tc-labeled denatured autologous RBC imaging
^{99m}Tc-labeled iminodiacetic acid
^{99m}Tc-labeled ligand
^{99m}Tc-labeled macroaggregated albumin scan
^{99m}Tc-labeled octreotide
^{99m}Tc-labeled phosphate analog
^{99m}Tc-labeled RBC
^{99m}Tc-labeled red blood cell scintigraphy
^{99m}Tc-labeled somatostatin
^{99m}Tc-labeled WBC
^{99m}Tc-labeled white blood cell scintigraphy
Tc-99m (*var. of* ^{99m}Tc)
^{99m}Tc-MAG3
technetium-99m mercapto-acetyl-glycyl-glycyl-glycine
^{99m}Tc-MAG3 radiopharmaceutical
^{99m}Tc-methoxyisobutylisonitrile scintigraphy

^{99m}Tc-MIBI
technetium-99m methoxyisobutylisonitrile
^{99m}Tc-MIBI radiopharmaceutical
^{99m}Tc-N-NOEt neutral myocardial perfusion imaging agent
TcO$_4$
technetium-99m pertechnetate
TcO$_4$ MIBI subtraction scintigraphy
TcO$_4$ thyroid scan
T-configuration
TCP/IP
transmission control protocol/Internet protocol
tcPO$_2$
transcutaneous oxygen pressure measurement
^{99m}Tc-PYP
technetium-99m-pyrophosphate
^{99m}Tc-PYP scintigraphy
^{99m}Tc-RBC
technetium-99m-red blood cell
denatured ^{99m}Tc-RBC
heat-damaged ^{99m}Tc-RBC
TCS
tethered cord syndrome
total calcium score
TCT900S helical CT scanner
^{99m}Tc-tagged RBC
TD
transition delay
trigger delay
TDD
teardrop distance
TDE
2-dimensional echocardiography
TDE-derived epsilon p and epsilon m
TDLU
terminal ductal lobular unit
TDMS
Trex digital mammography system
TE
echo delay time
echo time
thromboembolic
time delay between excitation and echo maximum
tracheoesophageal
TE fistula
teacup
t. breast calcification
t. fracture
teacup-shaped calcification
Teale amputation
tear
anular t.
attritional t.
Bateman classification of full-thickness t.'s

bowstring t.
bucket-handle meniscus t.
buttonhole t.
cleavage t.
complete t.
concentric anular t.
degenerative horizontal cleavage t.
dural t.
entry t.
esophageal t.
fishtail t.
flap t.
full-thickness t.
high-grade partial t.
iatrogenic dural t.
interstitial meniscal t.
intimal t.
intrasubstance cleavage t.
Johnson-Jahss classification of
  posterior tibial tendon t.
ligament t.
Mallory-Weiss esophageal t.
Mallory-Weiss mucosal t.
meniscus t.
mesenteric t.
micro t.
parrot-beak labral t.
parrot-beak meniscus t.
partial bursal surface t.
partial thickness split t.
peripheral meniscocapsular t.
posterior longitudinal ligament t.
quadriceps tendon t.
radial anular t.
radial split t.
rectal t.
rotator cuff t.
serosal t.
SLAP t.
stellate t.
superimposed acute partial t.
superior labral anterior to
  posterior t.
tendon t. (types I–IV)
teres minor tendon t.
tibial tendon t.
transverse anular t.
traumatic aortic t.
tricorn bucket-handle t.
vertical split nondetached t.

teardrop
  t. appearance

t. bladder
t. burst fracture
t. distance (TDD)
t. figure
t. heart
t. pelvic anatomy
t. ventriculomegaly

teardrop-shaped
  t.-s. flexion-compression fracture
  t.-s. lesion

tearing
  plaque t.

teat
  pyloric t.

teboroxime
  t. cardiac scan
  t. imaging agent
  t. resting washout (TRW)

TEC-2100 postioning laser
Technegas
TechneLite scan
Techneplex imaging agent
TechneScan
  T. Gluceptate
  T. HDP, MAA, MAG3, PYP
    imaging agent
  T. HIDA
  T. MDP
  T. Sulfur Colloid

technetium (Tc)
  t. albumin study
  hydrolyzed t.
  t. imaging agent
  t. polyphosphonate
  t. stannous pyrophosphate
  t. stannous pyrophosphate imaging

^{99m}technetium L-ethyl cysteinate dimer
technetium-99m (^{99m}Tc, Tc-99m)
  t.-99m albumin microsphere
  t.-99m antibody labeling
  t.-99m anti-CEA Fab murine
    monoclonal antibody imaging
  t.-99m antimony trisulfide colloid
  t.-99m antimyosin Fab fragment
  t.-99m depreotide
  t.-99m dextran
  t.-99m diethylenetriamine pentaacetic
    acid (^{99m}Tc-DTPA)
  t.-99m dimercaptosuccinic acid
    (^{99m}Tc-DMSA)
  t.-99m disofenin
  t.-99m DMSA, DTPA

NOTES

technetium-99m *(continued)*
    t.-99m DTPA aerosol
    t.-99m ethyl cysteinate dimer (^{99m}Tc-ECD)
    t.-99m etidronate
    t.-99m ferpentetate
    t.-99m generator
    t.-99m heat-denatured erythrocyte
    t.-99m heat-denatured RBC splenic scintigraphy
    t.-99m hepatoiminodiacetic acid scan
    t.-99m Hepatolite
    t.-99m hexamethylpropylene amine oxime
    t.-99m HMPAO mixed leukocyte LeukoScan
    t.-99m human albumin microsphere
    t.-99m human immune globulin
    t.-99m IDA analog
    t.-99m Infecton imaging
    t.-99m iron-ascorbate-DTPA
    t.-99m isonitriles radiopharmaceutical
    t.-99m leukocyte
    t.-99m MAG3 renography
    t.-99m mercapto-acetyl-glycyl-glycyl-glycine (^{99m}Tc-MAG3)
    t.-99m mercaptoacetyltriglycine
    t.-99m mertiatide
    t.-99m methoxyisobutylisonitrile (^{99m}Tc-MIBI)
    t.-99m methoxyisobutylisonitrile scintimammography
    t.-99m minimicroaggregated albumin
    t.-99m minimicroaggregated albumin colloid
    t.-99m nanocolloid
    t.-99m pertechnetate (TcO$_4$)
    t.-99m pertechnetate GI bleed
    t.-99m pertechnetate sodium
    t.-99m phytate scan
    t.-99m PIPIDA
    t.-99m pyrophosphate (^{99m}Tc-PYP)
    t.-99m pyrophosphate imaging
    t.-99m red blood cell (^{99m}Tc-RBC)
    sestamibi t.-99m
    t.-99m sestamibi dual-phase technique
    t.-99m sestamibi parathyroid
    t.-99m siboroxime
    t.-99m somatostatin analog SPECT
    t.-99m sulfur colloid GI bleed
    t.-99m tetrofosmin exercise-rest SPECT myocardial perfusion imaging
    t.-99m (V) DMSA scintigraphy
    t.-99m venography
technetium-99m-labeled (^{99m}Tc-labeled)

technetium-sulfur colloid
technetium-tagged
    t.-t. Cardiolite
    t.-t. RBC labeling
    t.-t. red blood cell
technetium-thallium subtraction imaging
technical
    RODEO imaging t.
Technicare
    T. camera
    T. Delta 2020 scanner
technique
    acquisition t.
    add-on t.
    adiabatic fast scanning t.
    advanced life support t.'s
    AEC t.
    afterloading t.
    air-gap t.
    algebraic reconstruction t. (ART)
    Amplatz t.
    antialiasing t.
    antiradial t.
    array spatial sensitivity encoding t. (ASSET)
    automatic vessel tracking t.
    autoradiographic t.
    axial multiplanar reformation t.
    background subtraction t.
    balanced-gradient t.
    2-balloon t.
    balloon-retriever t.
    bayesian t.
    best-guess t.
    black blood t.
    blended beam t.
    BLS t.'s
    bolus chase t.
    bolus chase imaging t.
    bougienage t.
    brain surface matching t.
    bread loaf t.
    breast mammographic t.
    breath-hold t.
    broad-use linear acquisition speed-up t. (BLAST)
    Brown-Roberts-Wells t.
    bull's eye t.
    cardiovascular imaging t.
    catheter-based intervention t.
    catheter-securing t.
    cerebral flow image t.
    chase bolus imaging t.
    chemical shift imaging t.
    chemical shift selective suppression t.
    chromatographic-fluorometric t.
    CLEAR t.
    coaxial sheath t.

computer subtraction t.
concentric circle t.
continuous suture graft inclusion t. (CSGIT)
contralateral subtraction t.
contrast-enhanced CT with saline flush t.
coronal oblique t.
Cr-chromate-labeled red cell t.
cress-correlation t.
Cr-labeled red blood cell t.
cross-correlation t.
cut-film t.
2D t.
3D t.
deblurring t.
deconvolution t.
dephase-rephase magnitude subtraction t.
depth-pulse t.
destructive interference t.
3D gradient echo acquisition t.
digital subtraction t.
discographic t.
2D multiplanar reformatted t.
DNA microinjection t.
double-contrast t.
double-freeze t.
double-umbrella t.
double-wire atherectomy t.
3D postprocessing t.
drip infusion t.
driven equilibrium Fourier transform t.
2D time-of-flight t.
dual-isotope subtraction t.
3D volume t.
3D volume-rendering t.
dye injection t.
dynamic bolus tracking t.
echo-tagging t.
ejection fraction by first-pass t.
Eklund t.
elephant trunk t.
endofluoroscopic t.
endovascular t.
enzyme-multiplied immunoassay t.
EPISTAR perfusion t.
equilibrium radionuclide angiocardiography t.
esophageal balloon t.
exclusion-HPLC t.

extended-field-of view t. (EFOV)
external looping t.
FAST t.
fast-FLAIR t.
Fast Imaging Employing Steady-State Acquisition t.
fat-suppressed T2-weighted FSE t.
fat suppression t.
4-field t.
field-fitting t.
FIESTA imaging t.
first-pass t.
FLAK t.
flow cytometry t.
flow mapping t.
fluoroscopic pushing t.
fluoroscopic road-mapping t.
Fourier-acquired steady state t.
Fourier imaging t.
FRODO t.
FSPGR t.
full-column t.
gadolinium-enhanced venographic t.
gated inflow t.
graded compression sonography t.
gradient-echo cine t.
gradient-echo recall t.
grasping t.
GRE t.
grid t.
Grüntzig PTCA t.
guidewire exchange t.
half-Fourier 3-dimensional t.
half-Fourier transformation t.
half-wedged field t.
Hampton t.
hanging-block t.
HARC-C wavelet compression t.
helical t.
high-kV t.
high-resolution bone algorithm t.
hybridization-subtraction t.
hybrid subtraction t.
image-guided injection t.
immersion t.
inhalation t.
integrated parallel acquisition t. (iPAT)
intercomparison measurement t.
interleaved phase contrast t.
intraoperative scanning t.
intravascular MRI catheter-based t.

T

NOTES

technique *(continued)*

inverse radiotherapy t.
inversion-recovery t.
Judkins t.
jugular t.
kinematic MR t.
kissing atherectomy t.
kissing-balloon t.
Klein t.
large-core t.
loading t.
localization t.
low-angle shot t.
low-dose film mammographic t.
low-dose screen-film t.
magnetic resonance hydrographic t.
magnetization transfer t.
mammographic t.
mammography t.
Markov chain Monte Carlo t.
Monte Carlo t.
motion artifact suppression t.
 (MAST)
moving table t.
MPGR t.
MP-RAGE t.
MR colonographic t.
MSCT t.
multiline scanning t.
multimodal image fusion t.
multiphasic multislice MRI t.
multiphasic multislice spin-echo
 imaging t.
multislice spin-echo t.
navigator echo motion correction t.
2-needle biopsy t.
nonaxial beam t.
noncoplanar arc t.
noncoplanar arch t.
noncoplanar beam t.
noninvasive t.
PACE t.
packing, extraction, and
 calculation t.
Papillon t.
partial flip-angle fast-scan t.
partial Fourier t.
partial saturation t.
PEI 1-shot t.
PEI 2-shot t.
percutaneous retrograde
 transfemoral t.
percutaneous transluminal coronary
 recanalization t.
perfusion measurement t.
pinhole t.
3-point Dixon t.
point-resolved spectroscopy
 localization t.

presaturation t.
pressure-controlled intermittent
 coronary occlusion t.
pressure half-time t.
projection-reconstruction t.
PROPELLER t.
PROPELLER FSE t.
pulsed-gradient spin-echo t.
pulse-echo t.
pulse-spray t.
quantitative imaging t.
radial t.
radiopharmaceutical volume-
 dilution t.
radiotracer t.
rapid pull-through t. (RPT)
rapid scan t.
rapid thoracic compression t.
RARE t.
ray casting t.
recanalization t.
region of interest imaging t.
reimplantation t.
relaxation enhancement t.
remodeling t.
respiratory triggered fast SE t.
road-mapping t.
robust registration t.
rotational therapy t.
sandwich t.
saturation recovery t.
scanning t.
scintillation counting t.
screening t.
Seldinger percutaneous t.
self-reversed parallel wire
 balloon t.
semiquantitative t.
sequential extraction-radiotracer t.
serial cut film t.
SHARP fat saturation t.
silhouette t.
single-field hyperthermia t.
single fill/void t.
single-needle biopsy t.
single-sample t.
single-shot imaging t.
single-slice eight-echo t.
SL t.
sliding thin-slab minimum intensity
 projection t.
Sones cineangiography t.
SPAMM t.
spin-echo t.
spin-label t.
spin-lock imaging t.
spiral echo-planar t.
spiral scanning t.
split-course t.

SPOP t.
stacked-foil t.
2-step t.
step-and-shoot t.
stereotactic automated t.
stimulated echo-tagging t.
STIR t.
storage phosphor-based t.
streptavidin peroxidase t.
subclavian turndown t.
subtraction t.
supervoltage t.
surface matching t.
Swiss roll t.
tandem t.
tardus-parvus t.
technetium-99m sestamibi dual-
  phase t.
Tesla system imaging t.
test bolus t.
time-of-flight t.
tissue characterization t.
tourniquet t.
transcatheter t.
transgluteal CT-guided t.
trephine t.
triple pass t.
trocar-cannula t.
turbo spin-echo t.
upgated t.
ureteral compression t.
in vivo t.
volume rendering t.
volumetric mapping t.
WakiTrak LS t.
water-suppression t.
wedged-pair t.
Welin t.
white-matter imaging t.
woggle t.
xeroradiographic t.

technology
acoustic response t.
adaptive focusing t. (AFT)
amorphous silicon filmless digital
  x-ray detection t.
ARTMA virtual patient t.
CellSeek t.
computer automated scan t.
  (CAST)
fused image t.
noncontact imaging t.

PASV valve t.
radiologic t.
SieScape imaging t.
single breath-hold dynamic
  subtraction CT with multidetector
  row helical t.
slip-ring t.
Toshiba Aplio xV tissue Doppler
  and contrast imaging t.
ultrasound imaging t.
Technovit 7210 VLC contact glue
Techtides
Tecmag
  T. Libra-S16 system
  T. Libra-S16 system scanner
tectal
  t. beaking
  t. cyst
  t. glioma
  t. lesion
  t. plate
tectocerebellar dysraphia
tectoral ligament
tectospinal tract
tectum, pl. **tecta**
  t. commissure
TED
  thromboembolic disease
TEDE
  total effective dose equivalent
Tedlar bag
TEE
  transesophageal echocardiography
teeth
  connate t.
  floating t.
  Hutchinson t.
  incisor t.
  milk t.
  molar t.
  premolar t.
  primary t.
  secondary t.
  supernumerary t.
  wisdom t.
TEF
  tracheoesophageal fistula
Teflon
  T. catheter
  T. dilator
  T. fascial dilator
  T. probe

NOTES

Teflon-coated guidewire
tegmental tract
tegmentum
    t. of brainstem
    medullary t.
    midbrain t.
    t. of pons
    pontine t.
tegmen tympani
TEGwire ST system
Teichholz
    T. ejection fraction
    T. equation
    T. equation for left ventricular
      volume
TEK
    total exchangeable potassium
T1EL
    type I endoleak
T2EL
    type II endoleak
tela choroidea
telangiectasia
    ataxia t.
    t. brain capillary
    capillary t.
    hemorrhagic hereditary t.
    Osler-Weber-Rendu t.
    pulmonary t.
    Sturge-Weber t.
telangiectasis
    bilateral juxtafoveal t.
telangiectatic
    t. angioma
    t. carcinoma
    t. fibroma
    t. lesion
    t. osteogenic sarcoma
    t. osteosarcoma
    t. vessel
telangiectaticum
Telebrix contrast medium
telecobalt therapy
telecollaboration surgery
telecord
telecurietherapy
telefluoroscopy
telemammography
telemetry
telencephalic
    t. malformation
    t. ventriculofugal artery
telencephalon
TelePACS
Telepaque imaging agent
teleradiogram
teleradiography
teleradiology
    diagnostic t.

    referral t.
    t. videoconferencing
teleradium therapy
teleroentgenogram
teleroentgenography
teleroentgentherapy
telescopic
    t. aerial dilator
    t. bougie set
teletherapy
    C-60 t.
    t. radiotherapy
Telocin diagnostic ultrasound system
telognosis
telomere repeat amplification protocol
Telos radiographic stress device
Temno II cutting needle
temp
    T. Tip drainage catheter
    T. Tip ureteral stent
temperature (T)
    t. distribution measurement
    firing t.
    mean perfusate t.
    Neel t.
    t. sensor
    variable t. (VT)
template
    deformable t.
    t. irradiation
    Syed t.
    Syed-Neblett t.
Tempofilter vena cava filter
temporal (T)
    t. aliasing
    t. artery
    t. artery tap maneuver
    t. average intensity
    t. bone
    t. bone anatomy
    t. bone fracture
    t. bone sclerosis
    t. bone tomogram
    t. bone tumor
    t. canal
    t. diameter
    t. filter
    t. fossa
    t. granulomatous arteritis
    t. gyrus
    t. horn
    t. horn atrophy
    t. horn of lateral ventricle
    t. instability artifact
    t. isthmus
    t. limb of the anterior commissure
    t. lobe
    t. lobe epilepsy (TLE)
    t. lobe herniation

t. lobe infarct
t. lobe lesion
t. lobe tumor
t. meningioma
t. orientation
t. peak (TP)
t. peak intensity
t. peritumoral enhancement
t. phase delay
t. plane
t. pole
t. predominance
t. process
t. pulse
t. resolution
t. sawtooth pattern
t. smoothing
t. space infection
t. sulcus
t. suture
temporalis muscle
temporally
temporal peritumoral enhancement
temporal pulse
temporary
t. atrial pacing wire
t. interstitial implant
t. pacing catheter
temporoinsular astrocytoma
temporomalar suture
temporomandibular
t. joint (TMJ)
t. joint arthrography
t. joint destruction
t. joint disc
t. joint osteolysis
t. ligament
temporooccipital
t. artery
t. glioma
t. junction
temporoparietooccipital junction
temporopontine tract
temporozygomatic suture
TENa
total exchangeable sodium
Tenckhoff catheter
tenderness
skin-rolling scapular t.
tendineae
ruptured chordae t.
tendines (*pl. of* tendo)

tendinitis, tendonitis
calcific t.
popliteal t.
tendinopathy
patellar t.
tendinous
t. attachment
t. band
t. insertion
t. part of epicranius muscle
t. raphe
tendo, pl. **tendines**
t. Achilles
t. calcaneus
tendo-Achilles bursa
tendon
abductor digiti quinti t.
abductor hallucis t.
abductor pollicis brevis t.
abductor pollicis longus t.
accessory communicating t.
Achilles t.
adductor hallucis t.
adductor pollicis brevis t.
adherent profundus t.
anchoring t.
anterior tibial t.
t. aponeurosis
aponeurotic t.
t. attenuation
attrition rupture of t.
biceps brachialis t.
biceps brachii t.
biceps femoris t.
bicipital t.
bifid biceps t.
boomerang t.
bowing of t.
brachialis t.
brachial plexus t.
brachioradialis t.
brevis t.
calcaneal t.
carpi radialis brevis t.
carpi radialis longus t.
central perineal t.
common t.
conjoined t.
coronary t.
cricoesophageal t.
digital extensor t.
digital flexor t.

NOTES

959

tendon (*continued*)
elbow extensor t.
extensor carpi radialis brevis t.
extensor carpi radialis longus t.
extensor carpi ulnaris t.
extensor digiti minimi t.
extensor digiti quinti t.
extensor digitorum brevis t.
extensor digitorum communis t.
extensor digitorum longus t.
extensor hallucis longus t.
extensor indicis proprius t.
extensor pollicis brevis t.
extensor pollicis longus t.
extensor quinti t.
flexor carpi radialis t.
flexor carpi ulnaris t.
flexor digitorum communis t.
flexor digitorum longus t.
flexor digitorum profundus t.
flexor digitorum sublimis t.
flexor digitorum superficialis t.
flexor hallucis brevis t.
flexor hallucis longus t.
flexor pollicis brevis t.
flexor pollicis longus t.
flexor profundus t.
flexor sublimis t.
gastrocnemius t.
gastrocnemius-soleus t.
Golgi t.
goose foot t.
gracilis t.
hamstring t.
t. of Hector
heel t.
hilus of t.
iliopsoas t.
t. inflammation
infrapatellar t.
infraspinatus t.
interosseous t.
t. irregularity
t. laceration
long head of biceps t. (LHBT)
longitudinal split biceps t.
longitudinal tear of the brevis t.
lumbrical t.
membranaceous t.
midpatellar t.
t. nodularity
t. nodule
obturator internus t.
palmaris longus t.
patellar t.
patelloquadriceps t.
peroneal brevis t.
peroneal longus t.
peroneus brevis t.

peroneus longus t.
peroneus tertius t.
plantaris t.
t. plate
pollicis longus t.
popliteal t.
popliteus t.
posterior tibial t. (PTT)
profundus t.
pronator teres t.
proprius t.
quadriceps t.
rectus femoris t.
rider's t.
t. rupture
sartorius t.
semimembranosus t.
semitendinosus t.
t. sheath
t. sheath giant cell tumor
t. sheath space infection
t. sheath stenosis
t. sheath thickening
t. shortening
t. sling
slip of t.
slipped t.
split anterior tibial t. (SPLATT)
sublimis t.
t. subluxation
subscapularis t.
superficialis t.
superficial palmaris longus t.
supraspinatus t.
t. tear (types I–IV)
thumb extensor t.
thumb flexor t.
tibial t.
tibialis anterior t.
tibialis posterior t.
t. tissue
toe extensor t.
triceps brachii t.
t. of Zinn
tendonitis (*var. of* tendinitis)
tendonosis, tendinosis
tendon-to-bone attachment
tendosynovial sarcoma
tenesmus
tennis
t. elbow
t. leg
t. shoulder
t. toe
tenocyte hyperplasia
tenodesis
band t.
tenography
tenonavicular

tenosynovial osteochondromatosis
tenosynovitis
    flexor t.
    LHBT t.
    peroneal t.
    stenosing t.
    tibialis posterior t.
    tuberculous t.
tense fontanelle
tensile
    t. force
    t. injury
tension
    t. collar
    t. cyst
    diffusion t. (DT)
    t. endothorax
    epicardial t.
    t. fracture
    intraventricular systolic t.
    t. pneumothorax
tension-time index (TTI)
tensor
    diffusion t. (DT)
    t. diffusion-weighted MR image
    t. fasciae femoris
    t. fasciae latae
    t. fasciae suralis
    t. tympani
    t. veli palatini
    t. veli palatini muscle
tented up
tenth-value layer
tenting
    baseline t.
    t. of diaphragm
    t. of hemidiaphragm
tentorial
    t. edge
    t. meningioma
    t. notch herniation
    t. ridge
    t. traversal
tentorium
    t. cerebelli
    t. cerebelli attachment (TCA)
    t. cerebelli lesion
    t. keyhole configuration
TER
    thermal enhancement ratio

time of formation of RF spin-echo when
    adjusted to be different from gradient
    spin-echo
terahertz
    t. ray
    t. wave
TeraRecon software
teratoblastoma of ovary
teratocarcinoma
    mediastinum t.
    t. of ovary
    pineal gland t.
teratogenic effect
teratogenicity of contrast agent
teratoid
    t. mediastinum
    t. tumor
teratoma, pl. **teratomata**
    atypical brain t.
    benign t.
    cardiac t.
    CNS t.
    cystic t.
    embryonal ovary t.
    immature ovarian t.
    malignant t.
    mature mediastinum t.
    mature ovarian cystic t.
    mediastinum t.
    neck t.
    orbital t.
    ovarian systic t.
    pineal t.
    solid ovarian t.
    spinal t.
    suprasellar atypical t.
    testicular t.
teratomatous mass
teres
    ligamentum t.
    t. major
    t. minor
    t. minor tendon tear
    pronator t. (PT)
terminad
terminal
    t. air sac
    t. airspace
    t. aorta
    t. bile duct
    t. bronchiole
    t. carcinoma

T

NOTES

terminal *(continued)*
t. cistern
t. crest
t. ductal lobular unit (TDLU)
t. edema
t. head
t. ileitis
t. ileum
t. inversion
t. pneumonia
t. reservoir syndrome
t. segment of posterior cerebral artery
t. synostosis
t. thrombosis
t. tuft
t. tuft resorption
t. ventricle
t. web
terminale
fatty filum t.
filum t.
os t.
persistent ossiculum t.
tight filum t.
terminalis
cistern of lamina t.
terminatio, pl. **terminationes**
termination
early-phase t.
late-phase t.
t. site
underdrive t.
terminus
duodenal t.
intrapapillary t.
rostral t.
terrestrial radiation
territory
posterior circulation t.
Terry Thomas sign
tertiary
t. collimation
t. hyperparathyroidism (tHPT)
t. hypothyroidism
t. sequestrum
t. syphilis
t. wave
Terumo
T. guidewire
T. Pinnacle R/OII radiopaque marker introducer sheath
Tesla
T. field
T. magnetic resonance imager
T. superconductive magnet unit
T. system
T. system imaging technique
Teslascan

tessellated
test *(See* testing)
abduction stress t.
acetazolamide vasodilator t.
Alcock t.
aluminum ion breakthrough t.
attached proton t. (APT)
axial manual traction t.
t. balloon occlusion
balloon occlusion tolerance t.
Barlow hip instability t.
bicycle exercise stress t.
t. bolus
bolus challenge t.
t. bolus technique
chlormerodrin accumulation t.
^{14}C lactose breath t.
coin t.
colorimetric t.
conglutinating complement absorption t.
contraction stress t. (CST)
costoclavicular t.
Dicopac t.
dipyridamole handgrip t.
duplex screening t.
dye reduction spot t.
exercise tolerance t. (ETT)
false-negative t.
false-positive t.
fat absorption t.
fetal stress t.
film screen contact t.
flat-hand t.
gallbladder function t.
gastrointestinal protein loss t.
Heaf t.
t. injection
internal carotid balloon t.
intrinsic field uniformity t.
Kruskal-Wallis t.
Leclercq t.
Linsman water t.
log-rank t.
lung connectivity t.
McMurray t.
t. meal
Mecholyl t.
molybdenum-99 breakthrough t.
Moschcowitz t.
Müller t.
NMR LipoProfile t.
nonstress t. (NST)
nonstress fetal t.
O'Connor finger dexterity t.
Ortolani t.
Osteo-Gram bone density t.
pelvic steal t.
perchlorate washout t.

peritoneal-venous shunt patency t.
positive washout t.
pulmonary function t.
quadriceps femoris tendon reflex t.
radioactive renogram t.
radioimmunoprecipitation t.
radioiodine t.
radioisotope renogram t.
RAILL t.
Seidlitz powder t.
sestamibi ^{99m}Tc with dipyridamole stress t.
Sharp-Purser t.
Shirmer t.
Smith orthogonal hole t.
sniff t.
Spearman rank t.
spinning-top t.
star-cancellation t. (SCT)
stop t.
Triboulet t.
triple-marker screening t.
t. tube structure
ultrasound t.
ultrasound dilution t.
ureteral perfusion t.
USP XX t.
vasodilatory hemodynamic stress t.
washout t.
Wetzel t.
Whitaker t.
Whitfield t.
Wilcoxon signed-rank t.
Yergason t.

testes (*pl. of* testis)
testicle
undescended t.
testicular
t. abscess
t. adrenal rest tissue
t. appendage torsion
t. artery
t. artery avulsion
t. carcinoma
t. choriocarcinoma
t. cyst
t. cystic lesion
t. degeneration
t. ectopia
t. feminization
t. gland
t. infarct

t. ischemia
t. metastasis
t. microlithiasis
t. parenchyma
t. posttraumatic edema
t. relapse
t. rupture
t. seminoma
t. stromal cell tumor
t. teratoma
t. torsion appendage
t. trauma
t. tubular adenoma
t. vein
t. vein embolization
t. venography
testiculoma
t. ovarii
testing (*See* test)
bronchial provocation t.
constant-load treadmill t.
Doppler ultrasound segmental blood pressure t.
nuclear gated blood pool t.
perimetry t.
pyrogen t.
radiation sensitivity t.
testis, pl. **testes**
appendix t.
burned-out tumor of t.
t. carcinoma
dilated rete t.
t. dysfunction
t. dysplasia
echo-poor t.
ectopic t.
efferent ductule of t.
t. fracture
t. germ cell tumor
hypoechoic t.
infarcted t.
maldescended t.
malpositioned t.
mediastinum t.
occult primary tumor of t.
rete t.
retractile t.
torsed t.
torsion of t.
tubular ectasia of rete t.
undescended t.
test-retest precision

NOTES

963

Tesuloid
tethered
> t. cord syndrome (TCS)
> t. small bowel fold
> t. spinal cord

tethering
tetraazacyclododecanetetraacetic acid (DOTA)
tetrabromophenolphthalein sodium
tetrad
> Fallot t.

tetradecyl sulfate
tetradiploid tumor
tetrahedron chest
tetrahydrobiopterin
tetrahydrouridine
tetraiodophenolphthalein
> t. contrast medium
> t. sodium

tetralogy
> t. of Fallot (TOF)
> pink t.

tetraphocomelia
tetraploid tumor
tetrasodium-meso-tetra
> manganese tetrasodium-meso-t. (Mn-TPPS$_4$)

tetrasodium pyrophosphate (TSPP)
tetrofosmin
Teutleben ligament
texaphyrin
> gadolinium t. (Gd-Tex)

textiloma
texture
> echo t.
> ground-glass t.
> inhomogeneous echo t.
> t. mapping
> peripheral t.
> t. slice

TFA
> thigh-foot angle
> tibiofemoral angle

T1-FAST
T-fastener
> T-f. delivery needle
> T-f. device

TFC
> threaded fusion cage
> triangular fibrocartilage

TFCC
> triangular fibrocartilaginous complex

TFD
> target-film distance

T1FS
> T1-weighted fat-suppressed image

TGA
> transposition of great artery

TGC
> time gain compensation

TGG
> thalamogeniculate group

THAD
> transient hepatic attenuation difference

thalamectomy
thalami (*pl. of* thalamus)
thalamic
> t. edema
> t. fracture
> t. fracture of calcaneus
> t. glioma
> t. hemorrhage
> t. infarct
> t. lesion
> t. plane
> t. syndrome of Dejérine-Roussy
> t. vein

thalamic-hypothalamic mass
thalamocaudate artery
thalamogeniculate
> t. artery
> t. group (TGG)

thalamoperforating
> t. artery
> t. branch

thalamostriate vein
thalamotegmental involvement
thalamotomy
> anterior t.
> dorsomedial t.
> parafascicular t.

thalamus, pl. thalami
> intralaminar t.
> pulvinar of t.

thallium
> t. 201 (^{201}Tl)
> t. debris
> t. imaging agent
> t. myocardial perfusion imaging
> t. myocardial scan
> t. myocardial scan with SPECT imaging
> t. perfusion scintigraphy
> t. redistribution phase
> t. rest-redistribution imaging
> t. scintography imaging
> t. single-photon emission computed tomography scan
> t. SPECT score
> t. stress imaging

thallium-201
> t.-201 chloride
> t.-201 imaging
> t.-201 myocardial scintigraphy
> t.-201 scan
> t.-201 single-photon emission CT
> t.-201 uptake and distribution

thallium-activated
>   t.-a. sodium iodide
>   t.-a. sodium iodine detector

thallium-to-scalp ratio
thallous chloride imaging agent
Thal-Quick chest tube
thanatophoric
>   t. dwarfism
>   t. dysplasia

Thayer-Doisy unit
THC
>   transhepatic cholangiogram

THC:YAG laser
thebesian
>   t. circulation
>   t. foramen
>   t. valve
>   t. vein

theca, pl. **thecae**
>   t. externa
>   t. interna

theca-cell ovarian tumor
thecal
>   t. abscess
>   t. sac
>   t. whitlow

theca-lutein ovarian cyst
The Closer arterial puncture site closure device
thecoma of ovary
Theile
>   T. canal
>   T. muscle

thenar
>   t. eminence
>   t. muscle
>   t. space
>   t. space abscess

theophylline attenuation
theorem
>   Bayes t.
>   Nyquist sampling t.
>   Stokes t.

theory
>   Bohr t.
>   crystal field t.
>   Culiner t.
>   density matrix t.
>   electron t.
>   Fourier optical t.
>   t. of fuzzy connectedness
>   fuzzy set t.

>   Kubelka-Munk t.
>   Planck quantum t.
>   quantum t.
>   slider crank t.

therapeutic
>   t. amniocentesis
>   t. angiography
>   t. barium enema
>   t. cardiac catheterization
>   t. chemoembolization
>   t. cordocentesis
>   t. embolus
>   t. external radiation
>   t. gain factor
>   t. index
>   t. intervention
>   t. pneumothorax
>   t. radiology
>   t. range
>   ray t.
>   t. response
>   t. thrombosis

therapeutic cardiac catheterization
therapist
>   enterostomal t.

therapy (*See* radiotherapy)
>   ablative laser t.
>   adjunctive t.
>   adjuvant t.
>   aggressive tissue-protective t.
>   antiestrogen radiologic t.
>   antitubercular t.
>   arc t.
>   beam t.
>   beta-ray ophthalmic plaque t.
>   boost t.
>   briscment t.
>   cardiac shock wave t. (CSWT)
>   catheter-directed thrombolytic t.
>   Chaoul t.
>   compartmental radioimmunoglobulin t.
>   computer-controlled conformal radiation t. (CCRT)
>   concomitant boost radiation t.
>   conformal neutron and photon radiation t.
>   conformal radiation t. (CRT)
>   contact radiation t.
>   continuous hyperfractionated accelerated radiation t.

NOTES

therapy *(continued)*

conventionally fractionated stereotactic radiation t.
coronary radiation t. (CRT)
craniospinal axis radiation t.
cross-fire radiation t.
3D conformal radiation t.
deep roentgen ray t.
dynamic conformal t.
dynamic radiation t.
electron arc t.
electron beam t.
embolization transcatheter t.
endocrine ablative t.
endolaser venous t. (ELVT)
enzyme replacement t.
enzyme supplementation t.
Exogen 2000+ noninvasive ultrasound t.
extended-field irradiation t.
external beam radiation t. (EBRT)
external x-ray t.
eye-view 3D conformal radiation t.
fast-neutron radiation t.
4-fiber t.
fibrinolytic t.
first-line t.
Fletcher-Suit system for radium t.
fluoroscopy-guided subarachnoid phenol block t.
fractionated external beam radiation t.
fractionated stereotactic radiation t.
fragmentation t.
gallstone dissolution t.
gamma ray t.
gamma-ribbon radiation t.
gene t.
grid t.
hadron t.
half-body radiation t.
heavy particle t.
high-dose t.
high-dose-rate intracavitary radiation t.
high-voltage roentgen t.
hyperfractionated accelerated radiation t. (HART)
hypofractionated radiation t.
hysterectomy and radiation t.
^{131}I t.
I-B1 radiolabeled antibody injection radiation t.
image-guided t.
image-guided radiation t. (IGRT)
indicator dilution t.
induction t.
infusion transcatheter t.
intensity-modulated arc t.

intensity-modulated radiation t. (IMRT)
interferential current t.
internal radiation t.
interstitial radiation t.
interstitial radioactive colloid t.
interstitial radium t.
intraarterial t.
intraarticular radiopharmaceutical t.
intracavitary radiation t.
intracavitary radioactive colloid t.
intracoronary radiation t. (ICRT)
intracoronary thrombolytic t.
intradiscal electrothermal t. (IDET)
intraoperative radiation t.
intraoperative red light t. (IRLT)
intravascular radiopharmaceutical t.
^{192}Ir seed t.
large-field radiation t.
lens-sparing external beam radiation t. (LSRT)
light t.
low-intensity laser t. (LILT)
MammoSite Radiation T.
megavolt t.
megavoltage grid t.
megavoltage radiation t.
megavoltage x-ray t.
microwave t.
microwave coagulation t.
MRI-guided periradicular nerve root infiltration t.
multimodality t.
neoadjuvant hormonal t.
neodymium:YAG laser t.
neuraxis radiation t.
neutron t.
neutron/gamma transmission t.
nonsurgical ablative t.
ocular radiation t. (ORT)
orthovoltage radiation t.
palliative radiation t.
pamidronate t.
partial-brain radiation t.
particle-beam radiation t.
percutaneous ethanol injection t.
percutaneous microwave coagulation t.
percutaneous transcatheter t.
peroral cone radiation t.
photodynamic t. (PDT)
photon-neutron mixed-beam radiation t.
PhotoPoint photodynamic t.
plesiocurie t.
postmenopausal estrogen t.
postorchiectomy paraaortic radiation t.
proton t.

pulsed dye laser t.
PUVA t.
radiation t. (RT)
radiofrequency ablation t.
radionuclide t.
radiopharmaceutical t.
radium beam t.
reperfusion t.
reprogramming t.
rotation t.
salvage t.
samarium-153 ethyl-
  enediaminetetramethylenephosphonic
  acid t.
selective internal radiation t.
  (SIRT)
short-distance radiation t.
sonodynamic t.
split-course hyperfractionated
  radiation t.
stereotactic radiation t.
stereotaxically guided interstitial
  laser t.
systemic adjuvant t.
telecobalt t.
teleradium t.
thrombolytic t.
tiered t.
timed-sequential t.
total androgen suppression t.
transcatheter t.
triple t. (TT)
triple-H t.
ultra-early thrombolytic t.
ultrasound ablative t.
ultrasound-guided percutaneous
  microwave coagulation t.
updraft t.
upper mantle radiation t.
virus-directed enzyme/prodrug t.
virus-mediated gene t.
whole-body radiation t.
whole-brain radiation t. (WBRT)
wide-field radiation t. (WFRT)
x-ray t.
Y-90 silicate t.
yttrium-90 silicate t.
t. zone
TheraSeed
  T. imaging agent
  T. seeding
TheraSphere

thermal
  t. ablation
  t. bioeffect
  t. compression
  t. conductivity
  t. convection pattern
  t. diffusion
  t. dosimetry system
  t. effect
  t. energy
  t. enhancement ratio (TER)
  t. equilibrium
  t. hot spot
  t. insult
  t. modeling
  t. neutron
  t. noise
  t. occlusion
  t. radiation
  t. relaxation time
  t. shape memory
  t. spectrum
  t. treatment parameter
Thermex
  Direx T.
thermistor plethysmography
thermoactinomyces vulgaris (TV)
thermocoagulation
thermodilution
  t. cardiac output
  t. catheter
  t. ejection fraction
  t. method of cardiac output
    measurement
  t. stroke volume
thermodynamics
thermogram
thermograph
  continuous scan t.
thermography
  blood vessel t.
  infrared t.
  laser-induced t. (LITT)
  liquid crystal t. (LCT)
  liquid crystal contact t.
thermoluminescence dosimetry
thermoluminescent
  t. dosimeter (TLD)
  t. dosimeter rod
thermometer
  aural t.
  disposable t.

NOTES

T

thermometer *(continued)*
    electronic t.
    glass t.
    tympanic membrane t.
thermometry
    invasive t.
    MRI t.
    noninvasive t.
thermomostography
thermonic emission
thermonuclear reaction
thermophilic actinomycetes
thermoplacentography
thermoradiosensitization
Thermo-Spheres
thermotherapy
    laser-induced t. (LITT)
    laser-induced interstitial t. (LITT)
    MR-guided laser-induced t.
    MRI-guided laser-induced
      interstitial t.
thermotolerance
Thermo-Treatment
    High Frequency Induced T.-T.
    (HiTT)
thermovision
thesaurosis
THI
    tissue harmonic imaging
    THI echocardiography
thick
    t. bone
    t. echo
    t. rind sclerosis
    t. slab 3D multiplanar reformatted
      image
thickened
    t. airway wall
    t. aortic valve
    t. bladder
    t. bladder wall
    t. bowel loop
    t. duodenal fold
    t. esophageal fold
    t. gallbladder wall
    t. gastric fold
    t. heel pad
    t. hypoechoic tissue
    t. irregular endometrium
    t. irregular small bowel fold
      dilatation
    t. nodular irregular small bowel
      fold
    t. septum
    t. sinus
    t. smooth small bowel fold
      dilatation
    t. stomach fold
    t. straight small bowel fold

thickening
    anterior joint capsule t.
    antral mucosal t.
    aortic valve t.
    aortic wall t.
    apical pleural t.
    asbestos-related pleural t.
    beaded septal t.
    breast skin t.
    bronchial wall t.
    capsular t.
    cecal t.
    circumferential t.
    diffuse gallbladder wall t.
    diffuse intimal t.
    diffuse pleural t.
    disproportionate upper septal t.
    facial t.
    focal cecal apical t.
    focal gallbladder wall t.
    focal intimal t.
    t. fraction
    fusiform t.
    gastric wall t.
    heel pad t.
    inner table t.
    interlobular septal t.
    interstitial t.
    intimal t.
    intralobular interstitial t.
    irregular gallbladder wall t.
    joint capsule t.
    ligamentous t.
    ligamentum flavum t.
    mediastinal t.
    minimal interstitial t.
    mottled t.
    mucosal t.
    mural t.
    myocardial t.
    nuchal skin t.
    optic excrescentic t.
    optic nerve fusiform t.
    outer table t.
    partial t.
    peribronchial t.
    pleural t.
    postlumpectomy skin t.
    rindlike t.
    sawtoothlike t.
    scrotal wall t.
    septal t.
    skin t.
    small bowel wall t.
    submucosal t.
    synovial t.
    tendon sheath t.
    trabecular t.
    urinary bladder wall t.

valve t.
wall t.

thickness
antropyloric muscle t. (APT)
arterial wall t.
bladder wall t.
effective section t.
endometrial t.
full t.
image slice t.
increased skull t.
interventricular septal t. (IVST)
intimal-medial t. (IMT)
patellar cartilage t.
posterior wall t. (PWT)
postmenopausal endometrial t.
preacinar arterial wall t.
septal wall t.
slab t.
slice t.
strut t.
subcutaneous quadriceps fat t.
  (SQFT)
urethral t. (UT)
ventricular free wall t.
wall t.

thickness-diameter of ventricle ratio
thick-septa collimator
thick-slice imaging
thick-walled
t.-w. cyst
t.-w. gallbladder
t.-w. ventricle

thigh
t. bone
t. muscle
t. muscle cross-section
t. splint

thigh-foot angle (TFA)
thin
t. border
t. cylindrical uniform field volume
t. fibrous cap
t. film analysis
t. linear structure
t. section
t. skull

thin-collimation
t.-c. image
t.-c. imaging

thin-cut axial CT image

thin-film transistor array
thinned
t. cartilage
t. myocardium

thinning
apical t.
cortical t.
parietal bone t.
pulmonary interstitial t.
white matter t.

thin-plate spine
ThinPRep Imaging system
thin-section
t.-s. axial image
t.-s. CT
t.-s. dual phase multidetector row
  computed tomography

thin-septa collimator
thin-slab
t.-s. coronal acquisition
t.-s. minimum intensity projection

thin-slice
t.-s. CT
t.-s. imaging

thin-walled
t.-w. atrium
t.-w. catheter
t.-w. cyst
t.-w. gallbladder
t.-w. guiding needle
t.-w. lung cavity

thiol
t. augmentation
t. modification

thiosemicarbazide
third
t. branchial arch
t. cardiac mogul
t. inflow
t. intercondylar tubercle of Parsons
t. portion of duodenum
t. projection of Chausse
t. ventricle
t. ventricle of cerebrum
t. ventricle tumor
t. ventricular hemangioblastoma

third-degree
t.-d. AV block
t.-d. heart block

third-order chorda
third-space sequestration

T

NOTES

third-trimester
    t.-t. gestational dating
    t.-t. placenta
Thom method
**Thompson-Epstein femoral fracture
   classification**
Thompson ligament
Thomson scattering
thoracentesis
    misplaced t.
thoraces (*pl. of* thorax)
thoracic (T)
    t. adenopathy
    t. angiography
    t. aorta
    t. aortic aneurysm
    t. aortic coarctation
    t. aortic dissection
    t. arch aortography
    t. asymmetry
    t. bone
    t. cage configuration
    t. cavity
    t. circumference (TC)
    t. crush
    t. deformity
    t. disc
    t. disc herniation
    t. duct
    t. duct-cutaneous fistula
    t. duct cyst
    t. duct imaging
    t. duct ligation
    t. duct route
    t. dysplasia
    t. empyema
    t. esophagus
    t. gas volume
    t. gibbus
    t. index
    t. inlet
    t. inlet lesion
    t. inlet soft tissue
    t. inlet syndrome
    t. joint
    t. kidney
    t. kyphosis
    t. lordosis
    t. lymphatics
    t. myelography
    t. OPLL
    t. outlet
    t. outlet stenosis (TOS)
    t. outlet syndrome (TOS)
    t. paraganglioma
    t. plane
    t. pulsion diverticulum
    t. root sleeve
    t. root sleeve diverticulum

    t. scoliosis
    t. sonography
    t. spinal cord
    t. spinal neoplasm
    t. spine
    t. spine anatomy
    t. spine curve
    t. spine fracture
    t. splenosis
    t. stomach
    t. vent
    t. vertebra
    t. view
    t. wall
thoracis
    skeleton t.
thoracoabdominal
    t. aorta
    t. aortic aneurysm
    t. diaphragm
    t. duplication
    t. gradient
    t. venous collateral circulation
    t. wall
thoracoacromial artery
thoracodorsal artery
thoracoepigastric vein
thoracofemoral conversion
thoracolumbar
    t. burst fracture
    t. fascia
    t. junction fracture
    t. kyphosis
    t. scoliosis
    t. spine
    t. spine column
    t. vertebral disc
thoracoomphalopagus
thoracopagus twins
thoracoplasty
Thoracoport
thoracoscope
    Boutin t.
    Storz t.
thoracoscopic poudrage
thoracoscopy
    video-assisted t. (VAT)
thoracostomy
    tube t.
    t. tube
thoracotomy
Thoramat
Thoravision selenium x-ray detector
thorax, pl. **thoraces**
    t. articulation
    asymmetric t.
    bell-shaped t.
    bony t.
    cylindrical t.

squared-off t.
symmetric t.
Thoreau filter
Thorel
T. bundle
T. pathway
thorium
t. compound
t. dioxide granuloma
t. dioxide imaging agent
t. emanation
radioactive t.
t. tartrate
t. X
thorium-201 SPECT scan
thorn ulcer
thorny bone radiation
Thorotrast
T. accumulation
T. imaging agent
thorotrastosis
Thorpe plastic lens
tHPT
tertiary hyperparathyroidism
thread-and-streaks
t.-a.-s. sign
t.-a.-s. vascular channel
threaded fusion cage (TFC)
threatened vessel closure
threshold
above-selected t. (AST)
alpha t.
attenuation t.
t. body
CACS t.
cell-dose t.
count-density t.
detection t.
t. dose
erythema t.
t. erythema dose
t. of Firooznia
fracture t.
malignancy t.
mask t.
seizure t.
signal-to-noise t.
ultrasound t.
thresholding
t. algorithm
diffusion anisotropy t.

gray-level t.
t. method
thrombectomy
adjunctive mechanical t.
t. device
mechanical t.
percutaneous mechanical t. (PMT)
Thrombex PMT system
thrombi (*pl. of* thrombus)
thrombin
t. formation
human t.
thrombin-activatable fibrinolysis inhibitor (TAFI)
thromboangiitis obliterans
thromboaspiration
thrombocythemia
thrombocytopenia-absent radius syndrome
thromboelastogram
thromboelastograph
thromboelastography
thromboembolic (TE)
t. disease (TED)
t. lung disease
t. pontine infarct
t. stroke
thromboembolism
aortic t.
chronic lung t.
mesenteric t. (MTE)
paraneoplastic t.
Prolyse in acute cerebral t. (PROACT)
pulmonary t.
thromboembolization
catheter-induced t.
deep venous t.
pulmonary t.
venous t.
thromboembolus
thrombogenic coil
thrombokinesis
thrombolysis
brachiocephalic artery t.
t. in brain ischemia flow grade
catheter-directed extremity t.
clot removal by laser t.
intracerebral t.
mechanical t.
T. in Myocardial Infarct (TIMI)

NOTES

T

thrombolysis *(continued)*
    pharmacomechanical t.
    venous t.
thrombolytic therapy
thrombopathy
thrombopenia
thrombophlebitis
    breast t.
    cerebral t.
    venography-related t.
thromboplastinogen
thromboresistance
ThromboScan
    T. imaging
    T. molecular recognition unit
    T. MRU
thrombosed
    t. filter-bearing inferior vena cava
    t. giant vertebral artery aneurysm
    t. intraaortic artery
thrombosis, pl. **thromboses**
    abdominal aorta t.
    acute renal vein t.
    aortic t.
    aortoiliac t.
    arterial t.
    ascending medullary vein t.
    atrial t.
    atrophic t.
    axillary vein traumatic t.
    axillosubclavian vein t.
    calf vein t.
    capsular t.
    cardiac t.
    catheter-induced subclavian vein t.
    central splanchnic venous t.
      (CSVT)
    cerebral venous t.
    cerebral venous sinus t. (CVST)
    chronic renal vein t.
    coronary t.
    cortical vein t.
    deep venous t. (DVT)
    dural venous sinus t.
    effort t.
    femoropopliteal t.
    hepatic artery t.
    hepatic vein t.
    iliofemoral t.
    infective t.
    intentional reversible t.
    intervillous placental t.
    intraarterial t.
    intracranial sinus t.
    intravascular t.
    jugular vein t.
    large-vessel t.
    luminal t.
    mesenteric arterial t.

    mesenteric venous t.
    native kidney renal vein t.
    necrotizing t.
    ovarian vein t.
    pelvic vein t.
    pericatheter t.
    portal vein t. (PVT)
    portomesenteric venous t.
    portosplenic t.
    postangioplasty mural t.
    primary subclavian-axillary vein t.
    pulmonary t.
    renal artery transplant t.
    renal vein t. (RVT)
    renal vein transplant t.
    sagittal t.
    secondary central venous t.
    septic t.
    shunt t.
    sinus t.
    splenic vein t.
    SSS t.
    stent t.
    subacute renal vein t.
    subclavian vein t.
    subclavian vessel t.
    superior ophthalmic vein t.
    superior sagittal sinus t.
    syndrome of impending t.
    terminal t.
    therapeutic t.
    transverse sinus t.
    upper extremity venous t. (UEVT)
    vein graft t.
    venous sinus t.
thrombospondin
thrombostasis
Thrombotest
thrombotic
    t. aneurysm
    t. endocarditis
    t. infarct
    t. microangiopathy
    t. obstruction
    t. occlusion
    t. pulmonary artery (TPA)
thrombus, pl. **thrombi**
    adherent t.
    anechoic t.
    ball-valve t.
    blood plate t.
    t. calcification
    calcified t.
    coral t.
    echogenic intraluminal t.
    t. embolus
    t. extension
    t. formation
    iliocaval t.

intraaneurysmal t.
intraarterial t.
intraatrial t.
intracardiac t.
intraluminal t.
intramural t.
intravascular tumor t.
laminated intraluminal t.
laser desiccation of t.
mobile t.
mural t.
t. nidus
obstructive t.
occlusive arterial t.
organized t.
pedunculated t.
percutaneous dissolution of t.
pericatheter t.
peroneal t.
platelet-rich t.
primary t.
t. remodeling
tibial obliterative t.
traumatic t.
tumor t.
ultrasonic lysis of t.

through
endoluminal fly t.

through-and-through
t.-a.-t. fracture
t.-a.-t. guidewire
t.-a.-t. injury

through-plane flow
through-sound transmission
through-the-scope
through-transfer imaging
through-transmission
thrower's
t. elbow
t. fracture

throwing arm injury
thrush breast heart
thrusting ventricle
thulium thumbprinting
thumb
adducted t.
adductor sweep of t.
basal joint of t.
base of t.
bowler's t.
cortical t.
t. extensor tendon

t. flexor tendon
floating t.
gamekeeper's t.
hitch-hiker's t.
hypoplastic t.
pouce t.
skier's t.
triphalangeal t.
t. web

thumb-in-palm deformity
thumbprint appearance
thumbprinting
t. appearance of the colon
gastric t.
thulium t.

thump
wall t.

Thurston
T. Holland fracture
T. Holland sign

thymectomy
thymic
t. agenesis
t. carcinoid
t. carcinoma
t. cyst
t. dysplasia
t. enlargement
t. hyperplasia
t. index
t. lymphoma
t. mass
t. neoplasm
t. sail sign
t. shadow

thymidine
t. labeling index (TLI)
t. phosphorylase (TP)
t. suicide study
tritiated t. (TT)

thymion
thymokesis
thymokinetic
thymolipoma
thymoma
benign t.
t. of heart
malignant t.
noninvasive t.

thymotoxic
thymus
congenital absence of t.

NOTES

T

thymus *(continued)*
    diffuse enlargement of the t.
    ectopic t.
    t. gland
    mass t.
    solid lesion t.
    t. weight
ThyRex timer
thyroarytenoid
thyrocardiac disease
thyrocervical
    t. trunk
    t. trunk of subclavian artery
thyroepiglottic ligament
thyroglossal
    t. duct
    t. duct cyst
    t. duct remnant
thyrohyoid ligament
thyroid
    t. abscess
    t. acropachy
    t. adenoma
    t. adenoma calcification
    t. adenoma nodule
    t. artery
    t. capsule
    t. carcinoma
    t. cartilage
    cold nodule t.
    t. colloid nodule
    t. cyst
    t. cystadenoma
    cystic area t.
    t. degeneration
    discordant nodule t.
    t. disease
    t. dysgenesis
    t. eminence
    t. follicle
    t. gland
    t. gland inflammation
    t. goiter
    t. hyperplasia
    t. insufficiency
    intrathoracic t.
    iodine-123, -131 t.
    t. isthmus
    lingual t.
    t. lobe
    t. lymph node
    t. lymphoma
    t. mass
    multinodular t.
    t. orbitopathy
    t. organification defect
    t. psammoma body
    t. radioiodine treatment
    t. radioiodine uptake

    retrosternal t.
    t. scintigraphy
    t. shield
    t. stimulation scan
    t. storm
    t. stunning
    substernal t.
    t. suppression scan
    ^{99m}Tc pertechnetate t.
    t. trapping defect
    t. ultrasonography imaging
    t. uptake measurement
    t. whole-body scan
thyroidal lymph node scintigraphy
thyroiditis
    acute suppurative t.
    chronic lymphocytic t.
    de Quervain t.
    Hashimoto t.
    painless t.
    Riedel t.
    subacute t.
    suppurative t.
thyroid shield
thyrotoxicosis medicamentosa
thyrotroph cell adenoma
thyroxine (T$_4$)
TI
    inversion time
    time following inversion pulse
    tricuspid incompetence
    tricuspid insufficiency
TIA
    transient ischemic attack
    carotid distribution TIA
    crescendo TIA
    ipsilateral hemispheric carotid TIA
tibarius
    torsus t.
tibia, pl. **tibiae**
    anterior bowing t.
    t. bone
    t. bone marrow development
    focal fibrocartilaginous dysplasia
      of t.
    malleolus tibiae
    posteromedial t.
    proximal t.
    repetitive anterior subluxation of
      the t.
    t. vara
tibial
    t. artery
    t. artery disease
    t. bending fracture
    t. collateral ligament
    t. collateral ligament bursa
    t. condyle
    t. condyle fracture

t. crest
t. diaphysial fracture
t. epiphysis
t. flare
t. hallux sesamoid
t. intercondylar eminence
t. medullary canal
t. node
t. obliterative thrombus
t. open fracture
t. pilon fracture
t. plafond
t. plafond fracture
t. plateau
t. plateau depression
t. plateau fracture
t. pseudoarthrosis
t. sesamoid bone
t. sesamoid ligament
t. sesamoid position
t. shaft fracture
t. spine
t. tendon
t. tendon tear
t. torsion
t. translation
t. triplane fracture
t. tubercle
t. tubercle ossification center
t. tubercle prominence
t. tuberosity
t. tuberosity fracture
t. varus
t. vein

tibialis
t. anterior
t. anterior tendon
t. posterior
t. posterior tendon
t. posterior tenosynovitis
t. sign

tibiocalcaneal
t. angle
t. fusion
t. joint complex
t. ligament

tibiofemoral
t. angle (TFA)
t. joint dislocation

tibiofibular
t. articulation
t. diastasis

t. fracture
t. joint
t. ligament
t. syndesmosis
t. synostosis

tibioligamentous fascicle
tibionavicular ligament
tibioperoneal
t. occlusive disease
t. runoff system
t. trunk

tibiotalar
t. angle
t. joint
t. rotation

tibiotalocalcaneal fusion
tibiotarsal dislocation
TIC
time intensity curve
TICA
traumatic intracranial aneurysm
tidal
t. inspiratory flow volume
t. wave of carotid arterial pulse
tiered therapy
tie sternum
Tietze syndrome
TIFF
tag image file format
tight
t. dural sac
t. filum terminale
t. filum terminale syndrome
t. lesion
t. spinal canal
tigroid
t. demyelination
t. pattern
Tikhonov regularization
tile mode display
Tillaux-Chaput fracture
Tillaux fracture
Tillaux-Kleiger fracture
tilt
bent-knee pelvic t.
caudal t.
gantry t.
infundibular t.
lunate t.
palmar t.
patellar t.
t. table

NOTES

tilt (*continued*)
  valgus t.
  varus t.
  volar t.
tilted
  t. optimized nonsaturating excitation (TONE)
  t. sacrum
tilting-disc valve
time
  acceleration t. (AT)
  acquisition t.
  activated partial thromboplastin t.
  arm-lung t.
  asymmetric appearance t.
  atrial activation t.
  atrioventricular t.
  bolus arrival t. (BAT)
  calculated clearance t.
  capillary filling t.
  carotid ejection t.
  cerebral circulation t.
  chromoscopy t.
  circulation t. (CT)
  colonic transit t.
  concentration times t. (C × T)
  t. constant
  conventional ultrashort echo t. (CUTE)
  corrected sinus node recovery t.
  correlation t.
  t. correlation function (TCF)
  t. course fracture scintigraphy
  cycle t.
  data acquisition t.
  dead t.
  decay t.
  deceleration t.
  t. delay between excitation and echo maximum (TE)
  delayed transit t.
  delta pressure/delta t. (dP/dt)
  diastolic perfusion t.
  diffusion t.
  t. domain
  echo t. (TE)
  echo delay t. (TE)
  echo train echo t. (T_E)
  effective transverse relation t.
  efficient relaxation t.
  ejection t. (ET)
  emptying t.
  esophageal transit t.
  fat and long T_2 suppressed ultrashort echo t. (FLUTE)
  fat-suppressed ultrashort echo t. (FUTE)
  fixing t.
  fluoroscopy t.

  t. following inversion pulse (TI)
  t. of formation of RF spin-echo when adjusted to be different from gradient spin-echo (TER)
  t. gain compensation (TGC)
  gantry rotation t.
  gastric transit t.
  image-acquisition t.
  image-reconstruction t.
  imaging t.
  increased left ventricular ejection t.
  t. intensity curve (TIC)
  interpulse t.
  inversion t. (TI)
  ischemic t.
  isovolumetric contraction t.
  isovolumic relaxation t. (IVRT)
  lattice relaxation t.
  left ventricular ejection t. (LVET)
  left ventricular fast filling t.
  left ventricular slow filling t.
  longitudinal recovery t.
  longitudinal relaxation t.
  long ultrashort T2-suppressed echo t. (LUTE)
  maximum inflation t.
  mean circulating t.
  mean circulation t. (MCT)
  mean examination t.
  mean pulmonary transit t. (MTT)
  mean transit t. (MTT)
  membrane closure t.
  t. motion (TM)
  myocardial contrast appearance t. (MCAT)
  [23]Na MR imaging with short echo t.
  t. to peak (TTP)
  perfusion t.
  phasing-in t.
  t. to PME (tPME)
  t. point
  prolonged ejection t.
  proton spin-lattice relaxation t.
  pulse reappearance t.
  pulse repetition t.
  pulse transit t. (PTT)
  pyelographic appearance t.
  radionuclide esophageal dead t.
  ramp t.
  reaction recovery t.
  receiver dead t.
  recovery t. (RT)
  regional mean transit t. (rMTT)
  relaxation t.
  repetition t. (RT)
  resolving t.
  retinocortical t.
  right ventricle-to-ear t.

rise t.
rotational correlation t.
scan t.
sequence t.
short T1 relaxation t.
sinuatrial conduction t. (SACT)
sinus node recovery t. (SNRT)
small bowel transit t.
sojourn t.
spin-lattice relaxation t.
spin-spin relaxation t.
systolic acceleration t.
systolic upstroke t.
thermal relaxation t.
transit t.
transverse relaxation t.
trigger delay t.
TR repetition t.
T1, T2 relaxation t.
tumor sojourn t.
ultrashort echo t. (UTE)
t. velocity integral
venous filling t. (VFT)
venous refill t. (VRT)
venous return t.
ventricular activation t. (VAT)
ventricular isovolumic relaxation t.

time-action analysis
time-activity curve
time-adaptive SENSE (TSENSE)
time-attenuation curve
time-averaged flow
time-compensated gain
timed
t. bolus delivery
t. imaging
time-density curve
time-dependent
t.-d. metabolic cascade
t.-d. xenon concentration
timed-sequential therapy
time-efficient T2 relaxometry
time-insensitive
time-lapse quantitative computed
  tomography lymphography
time-of-flight (TOF)
2-dimensional t.-o.-f. (2D TOF)
t.-o.-f. echo-planar imaging
t.-o.-f. effect
t.-o.-f. enhancement
t.-o.-f. flow measurement

t.-o.-f. magnetic resonance
  angiography (TOF-MRA)
t.-o.-f. method
t.-o.-f. PET imaging system
t.-o.-f. signal loss
t.-o.-f. technique
time-out
ventriculoatrial t.-o.
time-proportional phase incrementation
  (TPPI)
timer
ThyRex t.
time-resolved
t.-r. CE MRA
t.-r. imaging by automatic data
  segmentation (TRIADS)
t.-r. imaging of contrast kinetics
  (TRICKS)
time-sensitive
time-to-distant failure
time-to-local failure
time-to-peak (TTP)
t.-t.-p. activity
t.-t.-p. contrast (TPC)
t.-t.-p. filling rate (TPFR)
t.-t.-p. intensity (TTP)
t.-t.-p. value
time-to-treatment
t.-t.-t. bias
t.-t.-t. failure (TTF)
time-varied
t.-v. gain (TVG)
t.-v. gain control
time-varying magnetic field
time-velocity measurement
time-weighted average
TIMI
Thrombolysis in Myocardial Infarct
timing
bolus t.
gradient t.
t. parameter
tin (Sn)
t. 113 (^{113}Sn)
t. oxide inhalation
t. sulfide
t. with indium 113m
Tinel sign
tines
tiny ventricle
tip
active needle t.

NOTES

tip *(continued)*
    t. angle
    catheter t.
    conus t.
    t. deflector
    t. dispersion characteristic
    hockey-stick appearance of
      catheter t.
    mitral valve leaflet t.
    occipital t.
    petrous t.
    pole t.
    radiopaque distal t.
    rectal t.
    t. of spleen
    t. trauma
    valve t.
tip-deflecting guidewire
TIPS
    transjugular intrahepatic portosystemic
     shunt
      elective TIPS
      TIPS failure
      TIPS imaging
TIRP
    transcatheter intravascular ring platform
tissue
    aberrant t.
    abnormal t.
    t. adhesive
    adipose t.
    adventitial t.
    aerated t.
    anisotropic t.
    apical t.
    areolar connective t.
    bony t.
    breast t.
    bronchus-associated lymphoid t.
     (BALT)
    cancellous t.
    t. capsule
    cartilaginous t.
    cavernous t.
    t. characterization
    t. characterization technique
    chondroid t.
    chorionic t.
    collagenous t.
    t. conductivity
    connective t.
    t. contrast
    t. cooling
    cortical t.
    crushed t.
    dartoic t.
    dead t.
    t. deficit compensator
    degenerated t.

dense connective t.
t. density
destruction of t.
devitalized t.
disc t.
t. Doppler imaging
ectopic endometrial t.
ectopic thyroid t.
edematous t.
engorged t.
escape of air into lung
  connective t.
extraadrenal chromaffin t.
extralobular connective t.
exuberant granulation t.
fast exchange-soft t.
fatty prostatic t.
fetal lymphoid t.
t. of fetus
fibroadipose t.
fibroareolar t.
fibrocartilaginous t.
fibrocollagenous connective t.
fibrofatty breast t.
fibroglandular t.
fibromuscular t.
fibrosing t.
fibrotic t.
fibrous connective t.
fibrous scar t.
fibrovascular t.
t. flow
gangrenous t.
gastrointestinal-associated
  lymphoid t.
gelatinous t.
granulation t.
grumous t.
gut-associated lymphoid t. (GALT)
t. harmonic imaging (THI)
t. harmonic sonography
hyalinized fibrocollagenous t.
hyperplastic t.
hypertrophic t.
hypervascular granulation t.
hypoechoic t.
t. imprint
indurated t.
t. inhomogeneity factor
interlobular t.
interstitial t.
intertrabecular soft t.
intralobular connective t.
island of t.
t. island
isointense soft t.
isotropic t.
joint t.
late effect of normal t. (LENT)

lipomatous t.
loose mesenchymal t.
lymphatic t.
lymph node t.
lymphoid t.
lymphoreticular t.
mammary t.
t. mass
mediastinal thyroid t.
mesenchymal t.
mesenteric t.
t. migration
mucosa-associated lymphoid t.
  (MALT)
muscle t.
necrotic t.
neoplastic t.
neural crest t.
nodal t.
noncontractile scar t.
noncritical soft t.
nonviable t.
osseous tumor of soft t.
osteocartilaginous t.
t. outflow valve
t. oxygenation
paraffin-embedded t.
paratracheal soft t.
paravaginal soft t.
parenchymal t.
passively congested lung t.
t. perfusion
periarticular t.
peribronchial connective t.
perilobular connective t.
peritumoral t.
t. plasminogen activator (tPA)
t. plate
postcricoid soft t.
postoperative scar t.
postpharyngeal soft t.
preepiglottic soft t.
prevertebral soft t. (PVST)
proliferation of fibrous t.
regeneration of t.
regular connective t.
t. relaxometry
residual ductal t.
reticular connective t.
retrodiscal t.
retropharyngeal soft t.
retrosternal soft t.

retrotracheal soft t.
revascularized t.
scar t.
t. sequela
t. signature
t. slice
slow exchange soft t.
soft t.
t. space
stippled soft t.
stringlike bands of fibrous t.
subadventitial t.
subcutaneous connective t.
suppressed t.
swollen t.
sympathetic nervous t.
syngeneic t.
synovial t.
taenia t.
target t.
tendon t.
testicular adrenal rest t.
thickened hypoechoic t.
thoracic inlet soft t.
t. tolerance dose (TTD)
t. tolerance to radiation
tongue of t.
tuberculosis granulation t.
underlying t.
vascular t.
vascularized granulation t.
t. veil
ventricular soft t.
t. viability
visceral adipose t. (VAT)
t. water content
t. weighting factor
white cottonlike fibrous t.
2-tissue
3-tissue
tissue-air
  t.-a. interface
  t.-a. ratio (TAR)
tissue-based T2 relaxation
tissue-equivalent detector
tissue-maximum ratio (TMR)
tissue-phantom ratio (TPR)
tissue-specific imaging agent
tissue-type plasminogen activator
titanate
  barium t.

NOTES

titanium
    t. compound
    t. dioxide
    t. Greenfield filter
    t. plate
    t. Vortex Port system
Titterington position
TIV
    total intracranial volume
TJLB
    transjugular liver biopsy
TKA
    total knee arthroplasty
Tl-201
    Cardiolite Tl-201
    Tl-201 chloride
^{201}Tl
    thallium 201
    LDD-gated SPECT with ^{201}Tl
TLA
    translumbar aortography
    TLA needle
TLB
    transjugular liver biopsy
TLD
    thermoluminescent dosimeter
    tumor lethal dose
    TLD rod
TLE
    temporal lobe epilepsy
    refractory TLE
TLI
    thymidine labeling index
TM
    time motion
    TM ultrasound
TMA
    transmetatarsal amputation
    true metatarsus adductus
TME
    trapezium-metacarpal eburnation
    TME ratio
TMJ
    temporomandibular joint
TMR
    tissue-maximum ratio
    topical magnetic resonance
    transmyocardial revascularization
Tmx-2000 BPH thermotherapt thermotherapy system
TN
    true negative
to-and-fro flow
tobacco
    t. heart
    t. nodule
tocolysis
tocopherol (T)

alpha t.
    gamma t. (gamma-T, γ-T)
TOCU
    transoral carotid ultrasonography
        TOCU for internal carotid artery stenosis
Todani
    T. classification
    T. type cyst
Todaro triangle
Todd cirrhosis
toddler's fracture
TODE
    total organ dose equivalent
Tod muscle
toe
    base of t.
    t. extensor tendon
    Morton t.
    overriding t.
    tennis t.
TOF
    tetralogy of Fallot
    time-of-flight
    2D TOF
        2-dimensional time-of-flight
    TOF imaging
    TOF signal loss
TOF-MRA
    time-of-flight magnetic resonance angiography
Toldt
    white line of T.
tolerance
    drug t.
    Fletcher rule of irradiation t.
    irradiation t.
    narrow gating t.
Tolosa-Hunt syndrome
tombstone
    t. pelvis
    t. pelvis configuration
Tomocat imaging agent
tomogram
    blurred-image t.
    coned panoramic t.
    plain t.
    sagittal t.
    single-slice long-axis t.
    stacked t.
    temporal bone t.
tomograph
    Heidelberg retina t. II (HRT II)
tomographic
    t. cut
    t. imaging
    t. modality
    t. multiplane scanner
    t. section

t. skull immobilizer
t. slice
t. view
tomography (*See* CT, PET, PETT, SPECT)
  automated computed axial t. (ACAT)
  axial transverse t.
  bone computed t.
  cardiac-gated quantitative computed t.
  ^{11}C-methionine positron emission t. (MET-PET)
  coincidence detection positron emission t.
  computed t. (CT)
  computed transmission t.
  computerized axial t. (CAT)
  computerized cranial t.
  computerized transverse axial t. (CTAT)
  contrast-enhanced computed t.
  contrast enhanced computed t. (CECT)
  conventional t.
  cranial computed t. (CCT)
  digital axial t. (DAT)
  direct imaging of local gradients by group echo selection t. (DIGGEST)
  dual-phase helical computed t. (DHCT)
  dynamic computed t. (DCT)
  dynamic computerized t.
  electrical impedance t. (EIT)
  electrocardiogram-gated t.
  electrocardiogram-gated high-speed X-ray computed t.
  electron-beam t. (EBT)
  electron beam t.
  electron-beam computed t. (EBCT)
  emission t.
  emission computed t. (ECT)
  emission computer-assisted t.
  emission computerized axial t. (ECAT)
  endoscopic optical coherence t. (EOCT)
  exercise thallium-201 t.
  expiratory computed t.
  FDG positron emission t.

  ^{18}F-fluorodeoxyglucose positron emission t. (^{18}FDG-PET)
  flow mode ultrafast computed t.
  fluoride ion-positron emission t. (F-18-PET)
  fluorine-18 fluorodeoxyglucose-positron emission t.
  fluorodeoxyglucose positron emission t. (FDG-PET)
  focal plane t.
  focused appendix computed t. (FACT)
  gated single-photon emission-computed t. (GSPECT)
  helical biphasic computed t.
  high-resolution computed t. (HRCT)
  high-resolution 3D microcomputed t.
  high spatial resolution cine computed t. (HSRCCT)
  high-temporal-resolution cine computed t. (HTRCCT)
  H2 150-positron emission t.
  hypercycloidal t.
  hypocycloidal t.
  indirect computed t.
  intravascular contrast-enhanced computed t.
  kidney t.
  lateral t.
  limited-slice computed t.
  linear t.
  longitudinal section t.
  magnetic resonance t. (MRT)
  metrizamide-assisted computed t. (CTMM)
  microcomputed t.
  multidetector computed t.
  multidetector-row helical computed t.
  multiphasic perfusion computed t.
  multiphasic renal computerized t.
  multislice computed t.
  myocardial perfusion t.
  nonenhanced computed t. (NECT)
  nuclear magnetic resonance t.
  optic coherence t. (OCT)
  panoramic t.
  peripheral quantitative computed t. (pQCT)
  2-phase helical computed t.
  plesiosectional t.

NOTES

tomography *(continued)*
polycycloidal t.
polydirectional t.
positron emission t. (PET)
positron emission transaxial t. (PETT)
positron emission transverse t. (PETT)
process t. (PT)
quantitative computed t. (QCT)
quantitative contrast-enhanced computed t. (QECT)
radionuclide emission t.
rapid acquisition computed t.
rapid computed t.
rectilinear t.
reformatted computed t.
rotational t.
sellar t.
simultaneous multifilm t.
single-detector computed t. (SDCT)
single-photon emission t. (SPET)
single-photon emission-computed t. (SPECT)
skip t.
spiral computed t. (SCT)
spiral x-ray computed t. (SVCT, SXCT)
thin-section dual phase multidetector row computed t.
transmission computed t.
transmission computer-assisted t. (TCAT)
transversal t.
trispiral t.
tuned aperture computed t. (TACT)
ultrafast computed t. (UFCT)
ultrafast CT electron beam t.
ultrasonic t.
ultrasound computed t. (UCT)
ultrasound diffraction t.
volumetric computed t.
water-contrast computed t.
whole-body computed t.
wide-angle t.
xenon computed t. (XeCT)
xenon-enhanced computed t.
x-ray computed t. (XCT)
Tomolex tomographic system
Tomomatic
T. five-slice SPECT imaging system
T. three-slice SPECT imaging system
T. two-slice SPECT imaging system
tomomyelography

Tomoscan
T. AVEU spiral CT scanner
T. SR 7000 scanner
tomoscintigraphy
tomoscopy
tomosynthesis
circular t.
digital t.
TomoTherapy Hi-ART system
TomTec
TONE
tilted optimized nonsaturating excitation TONE sequence
tone
440-Hz t.
vascular t.
tongue
t. carcinoma
t. fasciculation
t. fracture
t. stud artifact
t. of tissue
venous malformation of the t.
tongue-shaped villus
tongue-type intraarticular fracture
tonically contracted sphincter
tonography
carotid compression t.
tonometric blood pressure monitor
tonsil
adenoid t.
buried t.
t. carcinoma
cerebellar t.
eustachian t.
faucial t.
lingual t.
pharyngeal t.
t. of torus tubarius
tubal t.
tonsillar
t. carcinoma
t. ectopia
t. herniation
t. pillar
tonus
arterial t.
too few sulci
tool
Quant-X color quantification imaging t.
surgical anatomy visualization and navigation t.'s (SAVANT)
tooth
fibroosteoma of t.
toothed vertebra
toothpaste shadow
top
Bicor T.

t. of carotid T occlusion
t. normal limits of size
Topaz CO₂ laser
tophaceous gout
tophus, pl. **tophi**
t. formation
gouty t.
topical
t. magnetic resonance (TMR)
t. water-soluble contrast medium
topodermatography
topogram
topographic
t. identification
t. measurement
topography
arterial t.
balloon t.
ocular globe t.
scintigraphic balloon t.
vessel t.
x-ray t.
torch
saline t.
Torcon blue catheter
torcula
torcular herophili
torcular-lambdoid inversion
tori (*pl. of* torus)
Tornado coil
torn meniscotibial ligament
Tornwaldt
T. bursitis
T. cyst
torque (T)
t. control guidewire
high t.
t. stress
torqueable guidewire
Torre syndrome
torr pressure
torsed
t. ovarian mass
t. testis
torsion
t. abnormality
acute testicular t.
adnexal t.
t. alignment
chronic testicular t.
t. deformity
external tibial t.

extravaginal testicular t.
t. fracture
t. of fracture fragment
gallbladder t.
t. impaction force
internal tibial t. (ITT)
internal tibiofibular t.
intravaginal t.
lung t.
missed testicular t.
ovarian t.
spermatic cord t.
splenic t.
t. stress
subacute testicular t.
testicular appendage t.
t. of testis
tibial t.
t. wedge nonunion
torso phased-array coil (TPΛC)
torsus tibarius
torticollis
tortuosity
t. of cervical vessel
elongation and t.
t. of ureter
vessel t.
tortuous
t. aorta
t. aortic arch
t. emptying
t. esophagus
t. vein
t. vein dilatation
t. vessel
toruloma
torus, pl. **tori**
t. fracture
t. hyperplasia
t. mandibularis
t. pylorus
t. tubarius
TOS
thoracic outlet stenosis
thoracic outlet syndrome
Toshiba
T. Aplio xV tissue Doppler and contrast imaging technology
T. Aspire continuous imaging
T. GGA 9300 camera
T. MR scanner
T. 900S helical CT scanner

NOTES

T

983

Toshiba *(continued)*
    T. 900S/XII scanner
    T. TCT-80 CT scanner
    T. Xpress SX helical CT scanner
    T. X-Vigor scanner
    T. Xvision scanner
TOSS
    total suppression of sideband
total
    t. ablation
    t. androgen suppression therapy
    t. anomalous pulmonary venous connection
    t. anomalous pulmonary venous drainage (TAPVD)
    t. anomalous pulmonary venous return (TAPVR)
    t. artificial heart
    t. atrial refractory period (TARP)
    t. body scan imaging
    t. body scanning
    t. body water (TBW)
    t. brain volume (TBV)
    t. calcium score (TCS)
    t. cerebral blood flow (TCBF)
    t. condylar depression fracture
    t. effective dose equivalent (TEDE)
    t. exchangeable potassium (TEK)
    t. exchangeable sodium (TENa)
    t. image noise
    t. intracranial volume (TIV)
    t. knee arthroplasty (TKA)
    t. knee implant
    t. lesion
    t. lung capacity
    t. lymphoid irradiation
    t. necrosis
    t. occlusion
    t. organ dose equivalent (TODE)
    t. peripheral resistance (TPR)
    t. placenta previa
    t. pulmonary resistance (TPR)
    t. radiation dose
    T. Recall digital imaging system
    t. reference air kerma (TRAK)
    t. resorption
    t. saturation recovery (TSR)
    t. stroke volume (TSV)
    t. suppression of sideband (TOSS)
totipotential stem cell
toto
    in t.
touch prep
Touraine-Solente-Golé syndrome
tourniquet
    caval t.
    t. technique
tourniquet-directed approach
towering cerebellum

Towne
    T. position
    T. projection
    T. view
toxic
    t. adenoma
    t. cardiomyopathy
    t. cirrhosis
    t. leukoencephalopathy
    t. lung disease
    t. megacolon
    t. multinodular goiter
    t. nodular goiter
    t. nodule
    t. pneumonia
    t. synovitis
toxicity
    bone marrow t.
    dose-limiting t.
    radiation-induced pulmonary t.
toxin
    bacterial t.
toxoabscess
toxoplasmosis
    cerebral t.
    CNS t.
    t. encephalitis
Toynbee muscle
TP
    temporal peak
    thymidine phosphorylase
    true positive
TPA
    thrombotic pulmonary artery
tPA
    tissue plasminogen activator
TPAC
    torso phased-array coil
TPBS
    3-phase bone scintigraphy
TPC
    time-to-peak contrast
TPFR
    time-to-peak filling rate
tPME
    time to PME
T-portagram
TPPI
    time-proportional phase incrementation
TPR
    tissue-phantom ratio
    total peripheral resistance
    total pulmonary resistance
TPWBBI
    3-phase whole-body bone imaging
TR
    time-to-repetition
      TR repetition time

ultralong TR
variable TE, TR
trabecula, pl. **trabeculae**
bony t.
septomarginal t.
trabecular
t. architecture
t. bone
t. bone detail
t. bone resorption
t. carcinoma
t. degeneration
t. destruction
t. disruption
t. fracture
t. microfracture
t. osteoma
t. pattern
t. thickening
t. weakening
trabeculated
t. atrium
t. bone
t. bone lesion
t. osteolysis
t. outline
trabeculation
endocardial t.
trabeculectomy
argon laser t. (ATL)
trabeculoplasty
trace
t. amount of radiopharmaceutical
t. edema
t. element distribution
t. map
tracer
t. abnormality
t. accumulation
t. activity
t. bolus
t. concentration equation
delayed transport of t.
deposition of t.
diffusible t.
t. dose
focal pooling of t.
gold-195m t.
t. horseradish peroxidase
T. microcatheter
^{13}N ammonia radioactive t.
neutron-rich biomedical t.

patchy distribution of t.
t. principle
radioactive t.
radiopharmaceutical t.
shunted t.
static rCBF t.
t. study
tantalum t.
transependymal uptake of t.
tumor-specific t.
t. uptake
trachea, pl. **tracheae**
anular ligament of t.
carina of t.
carrot shaped t.
intrathoracic t.
lunate-shaped t.
napkin-ring t.
saber-sheath t.
scabbard t.
tracheal
t. anastomosis
t. aspiration
t. band
t. B button
t. bifurcation
t. bifurcation angle
t. bronchus
t. caliber
t. cartilage
t. deviation
t. displacement
t. diverticulosis
t. fracture
t. granuloma
t. lumen
t. lymph node
t. mass effect
t. narrowing
t. ring
t. shift
t. stenosis
t. stricture
t. stripe
t. triangle
t. tube
t. tumor
t. wall stripe
tracheobiliary fistula
tracheobronchial
t. angle
t. fistula

NOTES

tracheobronchial *(continued)*
   t. foreign body
   t. hypersensitivity
   t. injury (TBI)
   t. lymph node
   t. mucosal necrosis
   t. papillomatosis
   t. rupture
   t. stenting
   t. tree
tracheobronchoesophageal fistula
tracheobronchography
   CT t.
tracheobronchomalacia
   acquired t.
tracheobronchomegaly
   congenital t.
tracheobronchopathia
  osteochondroplastica
tracheobronchoscopy
   CT-based virual t.
tracheocele
tracheoesophageal (TE)
   t. fistula (TEF)
   t. junction
   t. voicing
tracheomalacia
   congenital t.
tracheopathia
   t. osteochondroplastica
   t. osteoplastica
tracheostomy tube
tracing
   carotid pulse t.
   electrocardiogram t.
   pulmonary capillary wedge t.
   ray t.
   vessel t.
track
   t. cone length
   deep white matter t.
   t. dilatation
   t. etching
   ionization t.
   nephrostomy t.
   t. of pin
   t. valve
trackability
tracker
   T. 10 catheter
   T. Excel catheter
   T. 10 microcatheter
tracking
   abnormal t.
   anterior t.
   automatic peak t. (APT)
   bolus t.
   brain fiber t.
   focal spot t.

   t. limit
   magnetic bolus t.
   magnetic resonance needle t.
   MR imaging-guided endovascular
     device t.
   periportal t.
   presaturation bolus t.
   real-time biplanar needle t.
   real-time magnetic resonance
     imaging t.
   SureStart contrast t.
   vessel t.

tract
   aerodigestive t.
   alimentary t.
   anterior corticospinal t.
   anterior spinocerebellar t.
   anterior spinothalamic t.
   apple-peel appearance of GI t.
   ascending t.
   atriofascicular t.
   atrio-His bypass t.
   atrioventricular nodal bypass t.
   biliary t.
   brainstem pyramidal t.
   bronchial t.
   bulbar t.
   carcinoid GI t.
   central tegmental t. (CTT)
   cerebellar t.
   corticobulbar t. (CBT)
   corticopontine t.
   corticorubral t.
   corticospinal t. (CST)
   cuneocerebellar t.
   dentatothalamic t.
   dermal sinus t.
   descending t.
   digestive t.
   dorsal spinocerebellar t.
   dorsolateral t.
   extrapyramidal t.
   fascial t.
   fasiculoventricular bypass t.
   fetal urogenital t.
   fistulous t.
   flow t.
   frontopontine t.
   frontotemporal t.
   gastrointestinal t.
   geniculocalcarine t.
   genital t.
   genitourinary t.
   GI t.
   hepatic outflow t.
   hypothalamohypophysial t.
   ileal inflow t.
   iliotibial t.
   intermediolateral t.

intersegmental t.
intestinal t.
intrahepatic biliary t.
lateral corticospinal t.
lateral lemniscus t.
lateral spinothalamic t.
left ventricular outflow t. (LVOT)
Lissauer t.
long t.
lower t.
mesencephalic t.
motor t.
nucleus of solitary t.
occipitopontine t.
olfactory t.
outflow t.
pancreaticobiliary t.
pilonidal t.
posterior spinocerebellar t.
pyramidal t.
respiratory t.
reticulospinal t.
right ventricular outflow t. (RVOT)
seminal t.
sensory t.
sinus t.
spinocerebellar t.
spinoreticular t.
spinothalamic t.
tectospinal t.
tegmental t.
temporopontine t.
trigeminothalamic t.
upper aerodigestive t.
upper gastrointestinal t.
urinary t.
urogenital t.
ventral spinocerebellar t.
ventral spinothalamic t.
ventricular outflow t.
vestibulospinal t.

traction
t. anchor
breast t.
bronchiectasis t.
t. bronchiolectasis
t. diverticulum
t. epiphysis
t. exostosis
t. fracture
t. spur
tractogram

tractography
tractotomy
stereotactic t.
tragus
train
echo t.
spin-echo t.
trainer
virtual endoscopic surgery t.
(VEST)
trajectory
k-space t.
stack-of-spirals t.
TRAK
total reference air kerma
Trak Back pullback device
TRAM
transverse rectus abdominis
myocutaneous
TRAM flap
tramline
t. cortical calcification
t. effect in liver
t. shadow
trampoline fracture
tram-track
t.-t. appearance
t.-t. ductus arteriosus calcification
t.-t. gyral calcification
t.-t. pattern
t.-t. renal cortical necrosis
calcification
t.-t. streaming
transabdominal
t. catheterization of thoracic duct
t. cholangiography
t. color Doppler sonography
t. imaging
t. left lateral retroperitoneal
maneuver
t. pneumoperitoneum
t. scanning
t. sonogram
t. ultrasound (TAUS)
t. ultrasound scan
transanular patch reconstruction
transaortic
t. radiofrequency ablation
t. systolic gradient
transapical endocardial ablation
transarterial chemoembolization (TACE)

T

NOTES

transaxial
  t. annihilation photon pair
  t. CT scan
  t. fat-saturated 3D image
  t. imaging
  t. joint scan
  t. maximum-intensity projection
  t. PET scan
  t. scan plane
  t. slice
  t. thoracic inlet
transaxillary lateral view
transbrachial arch aortogram
transbronchial
  t. lung biopsy
  t. needle aspiration (TBNA)
transcaphoid fracture
transcapitate fracture
transcarpal amputation
transcatheter
  t. ablation
  t. arterial chemoembolization
    (TACE)
  t. arterial embolization (TAE)
  t. filter placement
  t. hepatic arterial
    chemoembolization
  t. intravascular ring platform
    (TIRP)
  t. oily chemoembolization
  radiofrequency modification t.
  t. stent-graft treatment
  t. technique
  t. therapy
transcerebral medullary vein
transcervical
  t. balloon tuboplasty (TBT)
  t. catheterization of fallopian tube
    imaging
  t. fallopian tube recanalization
  t. femoral fracture
transchondral talar fracture
transcondylar
  t. amputation
  t. axis (TCA)
  t. fracture
  t. line
transcoronal STIR image
transcortical
transcranial
  t. color-coded Doppler
  t. color-coded Doppler sonography
  t. color-coded duplex sonography
    (TCCS)
  t. color-coded duplex ultrasound
  t. color-coded sonography
  t. Doppler (TCD)
  t. Doppler ultrasound
  t. Doppler velocity

  t. examination
  t. lateral view
  t. real-time color Doppler imaging
  t. real-time color-flow Doppler
    sonography
transcutaneous
  t. angiogenesis gene delivery
  t. aortovelography (TAV)
  t. broadband sector transducer
  t. crush injury
  t. electrical nerve stimulator
  t. extraction catheter atherectomy
  t. oxygen pressure measurement
    ($tcPO_2$)
transducer
  Acuson linear array t.
  Acuson V5M multiplane
    transesophageal
    echocardiographic t.
  Acuson 128XP t.
  Aloka SSD-1700 t.
  anular array t.
  ART t.
  t. beam pattern
  biopsy t.
  biplanar t.
  broadband t.
  catheter-borne sector t.
  diffracting Doppler t.
  electronic linear array t.
  end-fire t.
  end-viewing t.
  epicardial Doppler flow sector t.
  Gaeltec catheter-tip pressure t.
  Gould Statham pressure t.
  high-frequency t.
  high-resolution linear array t.
  linear array t.
  Logic 700 MR t.
  magnetic resonance imaging-guided
    focused ultrasound sector t.
  7.5-MHz linear t.
  12- to 5-MHz linear array t.
  2.5-, 5-MHz sector t.
  Millar catheter-tip t.
  M-mode sector t.
  Mountain View t.
  MRI-guided focused ultrasound t.
  multiplanar t.
  phased-array t.
  piezoelectric t.
  PSH-25GT transcranial imaging t.
  puncture t.
  rectal multiplane t.
  sector t.
  signal t.
  transcutaneous broadband sector t.
  transesophageal t.
  Ultramark 8 t.

ultrasound t.
V510B Biplane TEE t.
V5M Multiplane t.
transducer-skin interface
transducer-tipped catheter
transduction
signal t.
transduodenal
t. endoscopic decompression
t. endosonography
t. fiberscopic duct injection
transdural fistula
transection (*var. of* transsection)
Transend steerable guidewire
transependymal uptake of tracer
transepiphysial fracture
transesophageal
t. Doppler color flow imaging
t. echocardiography (TEE)
t. echocardiography probe
t. transducer
transethmoidal encephalocele
transfascial spread
transfemoral
t. arteriography
t. cerebral angiography
transfer
energy t.
Fourier t.
gradient echo MR with
  magnetization t.
His-Haas muscle t.
t. imaging
interhemispheric t.
inversion t.
t. lesion
linear energy t. (LET)
magnetization t. (MT)
quantitative magnetization t.
rapid image t.
saturation t.
selective population t. (SPT)
sliding board t.
ultrafast video t.
ultrasound guidance during
  embryo t.
transferrin
indium t.
transfibular fusion
transfixing screw
transforaminal
t. examination

t. insonation
t. window
transform
automated Hough t.
cosine t.
2D Fourier t.
2-dimensional Fourier t. (2DFT)
3-dimensional Fourier t. (3DFT)
discrete cosine t. (DCT)
discrete Fourier t. (DFT)
driven equilibrium Fourier t.
fast Fourier t. (FFT)
fast inversion-recovery Fourier t.
  (FIRFT)
Fourier t. (FT)
Hough t. (HT)
t. imaging
inverse Fourier t. (IFT)
partially relaxed Fourier t. (PRFT)
water eliminated Fourier t. (WEFT)
wavelet t.
transformation
blastic t.
cavernous portal vein t.
t. constant
enthesopathic t.
Fourier discrete t.
hemorrhagic t.
malignant t.
t. matrix
nuclear magnetic resonance
  Fourier t.
photo t.
rho° t.
vascular t.
t. zone
transformer (t)
closed core t.
Coolidge t.
distribution t.
doughnut t.
t. equation
filament t.
high-voltage t.
t. law
t. loss
ratio t.
real-time chirp Z t.
step-down t.
step-up t.
transfusional iron overload

T

NOTES

transgastric
    t. echocardiographic view
    t. endosonography
transgluteal CT-guided technique
transgression
    cortical t.
transhamate fracture
transhepatic
    t. biliary stent
    t. catheter
    t. cholangiogram (THC)
    t. drainage
    t. portography
    t. variceal embolization
transhiatal esophagectomy
transient
    t. AV block
    t. bone marrow edema
    t. bone marrow edema syndrome
    t. cavitation
    t. cerebral ischemia
    t. chyle leak
    t. equilibrium
    t. gallbladder hydrops
    t. hepatic attenuation difference
    (THAD)
    t. hiatal hernia
    t. intussusception
    t. ischemic attack (TIA)
    t. ischemic carotid insufficiency
    t. left ventricular dilatation
    t. myocardial ischemia
    t. osteoporosis of hip
    t. perfusion defect
    t. peritumoral enhancement
    t. pleural effusion
    t. punctate cortical hyperintensities
    on T1-weighted image
    t. regional osteoporosis
    t. shunt obstruction
    t. sinus arrest
    t. symmetric pulmonary infiltrate
    t. synovitis
    t. synovitis of hip
    t. tachypnea
    t. tricuspid regurgitation
transiliac fracture
transillumination
    t. of head
    multispectral diffuse t.
transit
    biliary-to-bowel t.
    bolus t.
    delayed small bowel t.
    impaired tubular t.
    parenchymal t.
    t. scintigraphy
    small bowel delayed t.
    t. time

    tubular t.
    t. volume
transition
    allowed beta t.
    beta t.
    t. delay (TD)
    t. electron
    isobaric t.
    isomeric t.
    t. metal
    t. ureteral cell carcinoma
    t. zone
transitional
    t. cell carcinoma (TCC)
    t. cell neoplasm
    t. kidney cell carcinoma
    t. meningioma
    t. rhythm
    t. urethral cell papilloma
    t. urinary bladder cell carcinoma
    t. vertebra
    t. zone fissure
transjugular
    t. cholangiogram
    t. intrahepatic portosystemic shunt
    (TIPS)
    t. intrahepatic portosystemic shunt
    gradient
    t. intrahepatic portosystemic shunt
    imaging
    t. liver biopsy (TJLB, TLB)
    t. portography
    t. portosystemic stent shunt
    placement
    t. venography
translation
    condylar t.
    parallel mean t.
    perpendicular mean t.
    radioulnar proximodistal t.
    tibial t.
translational
    t. diffusion
    t. motion
translation-invariant filter
translesional gradient
translocation
    t. of coronary artery
    robertsonian t.
translucency
    first-trimester nuchal t.
    nuchal t.
translucent
    t. depression
    t. silicone tube
translumbar
    t. amputation
    t. aortic route

t. aortography (TLA)
t. aortography needle
transluminal
t. aortic endograft implantation
t. atherectomy
t. balloon angioplasty
carotid and vertebral artery t. (CAVATAS)
t. coronary artery angioplasty complex
t. dilatation
t. endarterectomy
t. endograft implantation
t. endografting
t. endovascular stent-graft placement
transluminally placed stented graft
transmalleolar
t. ankle
t. axis-thigh angle
transmantle dysplasia
transmedial plane
transmesenteric plication
transmetallation assessment
transmetatarsal amputation (TMA)
transmetatarsal-thigh angle
transmissible venereal tumor
transmission
airborne t.
t. block
t. computed tomography
t. computer-assisted tomography (TCAT)
t. control protocol/Internet protocol (TCP/IP)
t. data
direct-contact t.
t. dosimetry
t. electron microscopic study
indirect-contract t.
t. scan
sound t.
through-sound t.
transmission-based precautions
transmitral
t. flow
t. gradient
transmit-receive coil
transmitter coil
transmural
t. colitis
t. fibrosis
t. inflammation

t. invasion
t. match
t. myocardial infarct
t. necrosis
t. steal
transmyocardial
t. perfusion pressure
t. revascularization (TMR)
transnasally
transonic
Transonics
T. flow probe
T. system
transoral carotid ultrasonography (TOCU)
transorally
transorbital window
transosseous venography
transpapillary placement
transparent rendering
transpedicular
t. decompression
t. vertebroplasty
transperineal
t. implant
t. ultrasonography
t. ultrasound
transphysial bone bridge
transplant
allogeneic bone marrow t.
allogeneic peripheral cell t.
antigen-modulated mini-stem-cell t.
arteriovenous fistula t.
autologous bone marrow t.
bone marrow t.
cadaveric renal t.
enteric-drained pancreas t.
heart t.
heart-lung t.
hepatic t.
kidney t.
kidney-pancreas t.
liver t.
lung t.
marrow t.
organ t.
pancreas t.
renal t.
solid organ t. (SOT)
syngeneic bone marrow t.
tandem t.

NOTES

T

transplantation
    adult-to-adult liver t.
    autologous stem-cell t.
    living donor liver t.
    orthotopic liver t.
    split-liver t.
transplutonium radioisotope
transporionic axis
transport
    forward t.
    iodide t.
    Monte Carlo photon t. (MCPT)
    reverse t.
transporter
    dopamine t.
    vesicular amine t.
transposed
    t. adnexa
    t. aorta
transposition
    atrial t.
    carotid-subclavian t.
    t. cipher
    t. complex
    congenitally corrected t.
    gastric t.
    t. of great artery (TGA)
    great vessel t.
    t. of great vessel
    inferior vena cava t.
    t. of inferior vena cava
    Jatene t.
    t. of ovary
    subfascial t.
    ventricular t.
transpulmonary pressure (Ptp)
transpulmonic gradient
transpyloric plane
transradial styloid perilunate dislocation
transradiancy
transradiant
    t. air
    t. zone
transrectal
    t. echography
    t. sonography
    t. ultrasound (TRUS)
    t. ultrasound-guided biopsy of the
      prostate
transrenal ureteric occlusion
transsacral fracture
**TransScan TS2000 electrical impedance
  breast scanning system**
transscaphoid
    t. dislocation fracture
    t. perilunate dislocation
transscapular view
transsection, transection
    aortic t.

    spinal cord t.
    t. of spinal cord
    traumatic aortic t.
transseptal
    t. angiocardiography
    t. angiography
    t. perforation
    t. radiofrequency ablation
    t. sheath
transsphincteric anal fistula
transstenotic gradient
transsyndesmotic screw fixation
transtemporal
    t. insonation
    t. window
transtentorial herniation
transtentorially
transthoracic
    t. 3-dimensional echocardiography
    t. esophagectomy
    t. imaging
    t. lateral view
    t. needle aspiration biopsy
      (TTNAB)
    t. projection
    t. ultrasound
    t. view
transthyretin
transtracheal aspiration
transtricuspid valve diastolic gradient
transtriquetral fracture
transtubercular plane (TTP)
transudate
transudation of fluid
transudative
    t. pericardial fluid
    t. pleural effusion
transumbilical plane (TUP)
transureteroureterostomy
transurethral
    t. incision of prostate
    t. needle ablation (TUNA)
    t. resection (TUR)
    t. resection of bladder
    t. resection of prostate (TURP)
    t. ultrasound-guided laser-induced
      prostatectomy (TULIP)
transvaginal
    t. cone
    t. echography
    t. hysterosonography (TVHS)
    t. implant
    t. oocyte retrieval
    t. sonography (TVS)
    t. ultrasound (TVUS)
    t. ultrasound-guided drainage
transvalvular pressure gradient
transvenous
    t. digital subtraction angiography

t. implantation
t. occlusion
transversalis fascia
transversal tomography
transversarium
foramen t.
transverse
t. acoustic wave
t. anular tear
t. aortic arch
t. atlantal ligament
t. band
t. breath-hold gradient-echo cine magnetic resonance imaging
t. carpal ligament
t. cerebellar diameter (TCD)
t. cervical ligament
t. colon
t. colon carcinoma
t. colon loop
t. comminuted fracture
t. cord lesion
t. costal facet
t. cranial area
t. crural ligament
t. diameter between ischia
t. ECD brain SPECT image
t. esophageal fold
t. genicular ligament
t. heart
t. humeral ligament
t. hypoplasia
t. intertarsal ligament
t. lie
t. ligament of atlas
t. lucent metaphysial line
t. magnetization
t. maxillary fracture
t. mesocolon
t. metacarpal ligament
t. metatarsal ligament
t. myelitis
t. orientation
t. oval pelvis
t. pelvic diameter
t. pericardial sinus
t. perineal ligament
t. plane
t. plane alignment
t. plane force
t. plane vectorcardiography
t. presentation

t. process
t. process fracture
t. process of vertebra
t. rectus abdominis myocutaneous (TRAM)
t. relaxation
t. relaxation of proton spin
t. relaxation rate
t. relaxation time
t. relaxivity (R2)
t. ridge
t. scan
t. section
t. section imaging
t. sinus thrombosis
t. slice
t. suture of Krause
t. tarsal joint
t. temporal gyrus
t. testicular ectopia
t. tibiofibular ligament
t. ultrasound
t. view
transversely oriented endplate compression fracture
transverse/neutral view
transverse-plane PET image
transversum
septum t.
transversus
t. abdominis muscle
situs t.
transvesical oocyte retrieval
Transwell membrane
trap
duodenum water t.
metastable t.
suction polyp t.
TrapEase
T. inferior vena cava filter
T. permanent IVC filter
T. vena cava filter
trapeziometacarpal joint
trapezioscaphoid joint
trapeziotrapezoid joint
trapezium, pl. **trapezia**
t. bone
t. fracture
trapezium-metacarpal
t.-m. eburnation (TME)
t.-m. eburnation ratio
trapezius muscle

NOTES

T

trapezoid
- t. body
- t. bone
- t. bone of Henle
- t. bone of Lyser
- t. ligament

trapping
- air t.
- t. of aneurysm
- gas t.
- t. of radioisotope
- t. thyroid defect

Traube
- T. heart
- T. sign

trauma
- abdominal blunt t.
- acoustic t.
- asphyxial renal t.
- balloon-related t.
- bladder contusion t.
- blunt chest t.
- blunt gastrointestinal t.
- blunt pancreatic t.
- cardiothoracic t.
- carotid artery dissection t.
- chest wall t.
- eye t.
- focused abdominal sonography for t. (FAST)
- gallbladder t.
- genitourinary tract t.
- GI tract t.
- head t.
- hepatic t.
- high-energy t.
- hypovolemia t.
- kidney t.
- ligamentous t.
- liver t.
- multiple t.
- t. oblique
- ocular t.
- osseous t.
- pancreatic t.
- pelvic vascular t.
- penetrating t.
- t. register image
- renal t.
- splenic t.
- sustentacular t.
- testicular t.
- tip t.
- urethral t.
- urinary bladder t.
- vascular t.
- vessel t.

traumatic
- t. amputation

- t. aortic disruption
- t. aortic injury (TAI)
- t. aortic pseudoaneurysm
- t. aortic rupture
- t. aortic tear
- t. aortic transsection
- t. arthritis
- t. avulsion
- t. bone cyst
- t. bone survey
- t. brain injury (TBI)
- t. clinodactyly
- t. degeneration
- t. diaphragmatic hernia
- t. dislocation
- t. emphysema
- t. fat necrosis
- t. head injury
- t. infarct
- t. intracranial aneurysm (TICA)
- t. lipid cyst
- t. lung cyst
- t. meningeal hemorrhage
- t. meningocele
- t. osteoarthritis
- t. pneumatocele
- t. pneumomediastinum
- t. pneumonia
- t. pneumothorax
- t. rupture of diaphragm (TRD)
- t. spondylolisthesis
- t. spondylolysis
- t. syrinx
- t. thrombus
- t. tricuspid incompetence

traumatogenic occlusion
traversal
- k-space t.
- tentorial t.

traverse
traversing the fracture
TRAX catheter
t-ray
tray
- Müller t.

TRC
- tanned red cell

TRD
- traumatic rupture of diaphragm
- penetrating TRD

Treacher Collins syndrome
treatment
- allocation of t.
- cobalt-60 gamma knife radiosurgical t.
- cross-fire t.
- early endovascular t.
- endovenous laser t. (EVLT)
- t. energy

equivalent t.
ferromagnetic microembolization t.
fibrinolytic t.
intensity-modulated radiotherapy t.
(IMRT)
interstitial hyperthermia t.
intracavitary hyperthermia t.
iodine-131 antiferritin t.
low-energy radiofrequency
conduction hyperthermia t.
microwave hyperthermia t.
microwave nonsurgical t.
percutaneous tumor t.
t. planning system
t. port
refractory to t.
Sonographic Planning of
Oncology T. (SPOT)
superficial hyperthermia t.
thyroid radioiodine t.
transcatheter stent-graft t.
ultrasound hyperthermia t.

tree

airway t.
arterial t.
t. artifact
bile t.
biliary t.
bronchial t.
coronary artery t.
hepatobiliary t.
iliocaval t.
intrahepatic biliary t.
lower extremity arterial t.
tracheobronchial t.

tree-barking kidney
tree-in-bud

t.-i.-b. bronchiole
t.-i.-b. opacity
t.-i.-b. pattern
t.-i.-b. sign

tree-in-winter bile duct appearance
treelike airway structure
tree-shaped spot
trefoil

t. appearance
t. deformity

Treitz

T. fossa
T. hernia
ligament of T.
T. muscle

Trendelenburg

T. position
T. radiograph

trephine technique
treppe phenomenon
Trerotola thrombectomy device
Trevor disease
Trex digital mammography system
(TDMS)
triad

acute compression t.
Beck t.
Carney t.
Charcot t.
Currarino t.
Cushing t.
Garland t.
Kartagener t.
O'Donoghue unhappy t.
Osler t.
portal t.
Rigler t.
Saint t.
T. SPECT imaging system
wall-echo shadow t.
Whipple t.

TRIADS

time-resolved imaging by automatic data
segmentation

trial

carotid revascularization
endarterectomy stent t.
CAVATAS t.
Malmo mammographic screening t.
PROACT I, II t.
randomized clinical t. (RCT)
SONIA t.
Strokes Outcome and Neuroimaging
of Intracranial Atherosclerosis t.
WASID t.

triamine
triangle

aponeurotic t.
auricular t.
axillary t.
Bolton t.
Bryant t.
Burger scalene t.
Calot t.
t. of Capener
cardiohepatic t.
carotid t.

T

NOTES

triangle *(continued)*
    cephalic t.
    cervical t.
    clavipectoral t.
    Codman t.
    t. configuration
    crural t.
    cysticohepatic t.
    deltoideopectoral t.
    digastric t.
    Einthoven t.
    facial t.
    femoral t.
    Garland t.
    Gerhardt t.
    Grynfeltt t.
    Henke t.
    Hesselbach t.
    iliofemoral t.
    inguinal t.
    insular t.
    internal jugular t.
    Kager t.
    Koch t.
    Korányi-Grocco t.
    Labbé t.
    t. of Laimer
    Langenbeck t.
    Lesgaft t.
    Livingston t.
    lumbocostoabdominal t.
    mandibular t.
    mesenteric t.
    paramedian t.
    Pawlik t.
    posterior cervical t.
    Raider t.
    Rauchfuss t.
    scalene t.
    Scarpa t.
    submandibular t.
    supraclavicular t.
    sylvian t.
    Todaro t.
    tracheal t.
    urogenital t.
    vertebrocostal t.
    Ward t.
triangular
    t. area of dullness
    t. bone
    t. defect
    t. disc
    t. external ankle fixation
    t. fibrocartilage (TFC)
    t. fibrocartilaginous complex (TFCC)
    t. fontanelle
    t. ligament

    t. muscle
    t. ridge
triangulation method
triatrial heart
triatriatum
    cor t.
Triboulet test
tributary
    t. collateral
    extrahepatic portal vein t.
    large venous t.
tricarboxylic acid cycle
triceps
    t. brachii
    t. brachii tendon
trichinous embolus
trichloroacetic acid
trichobezoar
trichoptysis
trichorhinophalangeal (TRP)
TRICKS
    time-resolved imaging of contrast kinetics
    TRICKS method
tricompartmental chondromalacia of the knee
tricorn bucket-handle tear
tricuspid
    t. aortic valve
    t. incompetence (TI)
    t. insufficiency (TI)
    t. orifice
    t. orifice regurgitation
    t. stenosis
    t. valve (TV)
    t. valve anomaly
    t. valve anulus
    t. valve area
    t. valve atresia
    t. valve closure
    t. valve cusp
    t. valve deformity
    t. valve dysplasia
    t. valve flow
    t. valve gradient
    t. valve prolapse
    t. valve regurgitation
    t. valve strut
    t. vertebra
tricyclic
trident
    t. hand
    t. pelvis
Tridrate bowel preparation
trifascicular block
trifid
    t. precordial motion
    t. stomach
triflanged nail

trifurcation
  t. of artery
  patency t.
  popliteal artery t.
trigeminal
  t. cavernous fistula
  t. cavity
  t. cistern
  t. ganglion
  t. hemangioma
  t. nerve anatomy
  t. pattern
  t. rhizotomy
  t. schwannoma
  t. trigeminy
  t. trigonal hypertrophy
trigeminothalamic tract
trigeminy
  trigeminal t.
  ventricular t.
trigger
  t. delay (TD)
  t. delay time
  ECG t.
  electrocardiogram t.
  t. finger
  t. finger deformity
  respiratory t.
triggered
  t. pacing mode
  respiratory t.
triggered-flow mode
triggering
  clectrocardiograph t.
  fluoroscopic t.
  navigator echo-based real-time
    respiratory gating and t.
  respiratory t.
trigona (*pl. of* trigonum)
trigonal
  t. hypertrophy
  t. muscle
  t. process
trigone
  angles of t.
  t. of bladder
  collateral t.
  deltoideopectoral t.
  fibrous t.
  Henke t.
  hypertrophied t.
  hypoglossal t.

  inguinal t.
  lateral ventricle t.
  Lieutaud t.
  Pawlik t.
  t. of ventricle
  vertebrocostal t.
trigonocephaly
trigonum, pl. **trigona**
  t. calcis
  os t.
  unfused os t.
triiodinated imaging agent
triiodobenzoic
  t. acid
  t. acid contrast medium
triiodothyronine
trilaminar appearance
trilateral retinoblastoma
trilayer appearance
trileaflet aortic valve
trilinear interpolation
trilobate
trilobed
trilobulation
trilocular heart
trilogy of Fallot
trimalleolar ankle fracture
triode tube
triolein
  iodine-131 t.
Trionix
  T. camera
  T. scanner
  T. SPECT
Trionix-Triad camera
Triosil contrast medium
tripartite duodenal carcinoma
triphalangeal
  t. thumb
  t. thumb deformity
triphasic
  t. spiral CT
  t. waveform
Triphasix generator
triphenyltetrazolium chloride (TTC)
triphosphate
  adenosine t.
  arabinsylguanosine t.
  cyclic guanosine t.
  nucleoside t. (NTP)
triplanar fracture
triplane fracture

NOTES

T

triple
> t. label
> t. match
> t. pass technique
> t. signal pattern
> t. therapy (TT)
> t. track sign

triple-bubble sign
triple-dose
> t.-d. gadolinium-enhanced MR imaging without MT
> t.-d. gadolinium imaging

triple-head gamma camera
triple-H therapy
triple-leaf collimator
triple-marker screening test
triple-peak cerebellum configuration
triple-phase
> t.-p. bone scan
> t.-p. bone scan imaging

triple-resonance NMR probe circuit
triplet
> t. gestation
> ghost reduction by equalized acquisition t.'s (GREAT)

triple-voiding
> t.-v. cystogram
> t.-v. cystography

triplex
> t. mode Doppler sonography
> t. scanning

tripod
> t. fracture
> t. position

tripoint bullet
Tripter
> Direx T.

triquetral
> t. bone
> t. fracture
> t. impingement

triquetrohamate
> t. helicoid slope
> t. joint
> t. ligament

triquetrolunate dislocation
triquetropisiform articulation
triquetroscaphoid
> t. fascicle
> t. ligament

triquetrotrapezoid fascicle
triquetrum
triradiate cartilage
trisacryl gelatin microsphere
tris-acryl gelatin microsphere (TAGM)
trisodium
> gadofosveset t.
> mangafodipir t. (MnDPDP)

trisomic fetus

trisomy
> t. D, E syndrome
> t. 8 syndrome

TriSpan
> T. aneurysm neck-bride device
> T. detachable coil

trispiral tomography
tristimulus
> t. value
> t. value flip

tritiated
> t. thymidine (TT)
> t. thymidine labeling index

tritium
triton tumor
trocar-cannula technique
trochanter
> greater t.
> lesser t.

trochanteric
> t. bursa
> t. bursitis
> t. flare
> t. spine

trochlea, pl. **trochleae**
> peroneal t.

trochlear
> t. defect
> t. groove
> t. nerve
> t. nerve neoplasm
> t. notch
> t. process

trochleocapitellar groove
troika
> aponeurotic t.

Troisier
> T. node
> T. sign

troland
Trolard
> vein of T.

trolley-track sign
TRON 3 VACI cardiac imaging system
Tronzo intertrochanteric fracture classification
trophedema
trophic
> t. fracture
> t. lesion

trophoblastic
> t. material
> t. ring

tropical
> t. pancreatitis
> t. ulcer osteoma

tropic ulcer
tropism
> facet t.

tropolone
tropomyosin
trough
- t. line
- t. sign
- t. of venous pulse
- X t.
- Y t.

trousers
- military antishock t. (MAST)

Trousseau
- T. sign
- T. syndrome

TRP
- trichorhinophalangeal

TR-TE
- repetition time to echo time ratio
- long TR-TE
- short TR-TE

true
- t. aortic aneurysm
- t. apex (TA)
- t. back muscle
- t. channel
- t. conjugate measurement
- t. dynamic joint imaging
- t. event
- t. fast imaging and steady progression (FISP)
- t. fast imaging with steady-state precession (TrueFISP)
- t. heart aneurysm
- t. hermaphroditism
- t. histiocytic lymphoma
- t. intersex
- t. lateral view
- t. lumen
- t. metatarsus adductus (TMA)
- t. mitral stenosis
- t. negative (TN)
- t. pelvis
- t. porencephaly
- t. positive (TP)
- t. rib
- t. suture
- t. umbilical cord knot
- t. ventricular aneurysm
- t. vertebra
- t. vocal cord

TrueFISP
- true fast imaging with steady-state precession
- blood-to-myocardium contrast of T.

trueFISP MRI
true-negative
- t.-n. lesion
- t.-n. mammogram

true-positive result
TruFill n-BCA surgical glue
Trümmerfeld
- T. line
- T. zone

trumpet-like pelvocaliceal system
truncal
- t. artery
- t. instability
- t. renal artery stenosis
- t. rhabdomyosarcoma
- t. valve

truncated
- t. arch index
- t. atrial appendage
- t. NMR probe

truncation
- t. band artifact
- t. phenomenon

truncus arteriosus
trunk
- aortopulmonary t.
- arterial brachiocephalic t.
- atrioventricular t.
- bifurcation of t.
- brachiocephalic t.
- bronchomediastinal lymph t.
- celiac t.
- celiomesenteric t.
- cordlike t.
- costocervical t.
- dilated pulmonary t.
- joints of t.
- lumbosacral t.
- lymphatic t.
- meningohypophysial t.
- nerve t.
- neuromeningeal t.
- posterior vagal t.
- pulmonary t.
- sinus of pulmonary t.
- thyrocervical t.
- tibioperoneal t.

NOTES

T

trunk (*continued*)
    twin t.
    vagal t.
Trunkey fracture classification
TruPulse CO$_2$ laser
TRUS
    transrectal ultrasound
TRW
    teboroxime resting washout
TS
    tuberous sclerosis
T-Scan 2000
T-score measurement of bone mineral density
TSD
    target-skin distance
TSE
    turbo spin-echo
        TSE image
        single shot TSE (SShTSE)
TSENSE
    time-adaptive SENSE
TSE-relaxometry
T-shaped
    T-s. fracture
    T-s. uterus
TSPP
    tetrasodium pyrophosphate
        TSPP imaging
TSR
    total saturation recovery
T-stage
TS2000 TransScan 2000
TSV
    total stroke volume
TT
    triple therapy
    tritiated thymidine
TTC
    triphenyltetrazolium chloride
    T-tube cholangiogram
TTD
    tissue tolerance dose
TTF
    time-to-treatment failure
TTI
    tension-time index
TTNAB
    transthoracic needle aspiration biopsy
TTP
    time to peak
    time-to-peak intensity
    time-to-peak value
    transtubercular plane
TTTS
    twin-to-twin transfusion syndrome
T-tube
    T-t. cholangiogram (TTC)
    T-t. cholangiography

    French T-t.
    T-t. stent
tubal
    t. canal
    t. fimbrial opening
    t. insufflation
    t. mass
    t. obstruction
    t. occlusion
    t. pregnancy
    t. ring
    t. tonsil
tubarius
    tonsil of torus t.
    torus t.
tube
    Angio-Seal carrier t.
    angled pleural t.
    anode t.
    anteroposterior t.
    apically directed chest t.
    atretic t.
    auditory t.
    bilateral pleural t.
    blocked shunt t.
    bronchial t.
    calyx t.
    Cantor t.
    capillary t.
    carrier t.
    cathode ray t. (CRT)
    Celestin t.
    Chaoul voltage x-ray t.
    chest t.
    collecting t.
    Coolidge x-ray t.
    corneal t.
    Crookes t.
    cuffed endotracheal t.
    t. current
    t. decompression
    decompression t.
    Dennis t.
    t. device
    dialysis t.
    digestive t.
    discharge t.
    Dotter t.
    t. drainage
    electron multiplier t.
    endobronchial t.
    endotracheal t.
    eustachian t.
    fallopian t.
    feeding t.
    fenestrated t.
    field emission t.
    fMR t.
    Frederick-Miller t.

functional MR t.
gastrostomy t.
Geiger-Müller t.
t. geometry module
glow modular t.
Harris t.
Herring t.
high-heat-capacity x-ray t.
hot cathode x-ray t.
image intensifier t.
interstitial afterloading nylon t.
intestinal t.
J-shaped t.
large-caliber t.
Lenard ray t.
Lester Jones bypass t.
Levine t.
mediastinal t.
metallic distal end of t.
MIC gastroenteric t.
MIC jejunal t.
MIC-Key low profile transgastric-
   jejunal feeding t.
microfocal direct magnification in
   vitro x-ray t.
MIC transgastric jejunal feeding t.
Miller-Abbott t.
Minnesota t.
Miser t.
molybdenum target t.
Moss gastrostomy t.
muscular t.
nasoenteric t.
nasogastric (NG) t.
nasojejunal feeding t.
nasotracheal t.
neural t.
Newvicon camera t.
Nutriflex t.
obstructed shunt t.
Olshevsky t.
oroendotracheal t.
orogastric t.
Orthicon t.
overcouch t.
pharyngotympanic t.
photomultiplier t. (PMT)
pickup t.
pleural t.
polyethylene t.
t. position rotation
pull-type gastrostomy t.

rectifier t.
right-angle chest t.
roentgen t.
rotating anode t.
Salem sump t.
self-quenched counter t.
Sengstaken-Blakemore t.
separator t.
Shiner radiopaque t.
shunt t.
solid-phase extraction t.
SRO 2550 x-ray t.
stomach t.
straight chest t.
suction t.
sump t.
Thal-Quick chest t.
thoracostomy t.
t. thoracostomy
tracheal t.
tracheostomy t.
translucent silicone t.
triode t.
uterine t.
vacuum t.
valve t.
Vidicon camera t.
t. voltage waveform
Westergren t.
x-ray t.

tuber

brain t.
t. cincreum
t. cinereum hamartoma
cortical t.

tubercle

accessory t.
acoustic t.
adductor t.
amygdaloid t.
articular t.
auricular t.
calcaneal t.
carotid t.
Chaput t.
conoid t.
corniculate t.
costal t.
crown t.
cuneiform t.
darwinian t.
dental t.

NOTES

tubercle (*continued*)
    dissection t.
    dorsal t.
    epiglottic t.
    fibrous t.
    genial t.
    Gerdy t.
    Ghon t.
    greater t.
    iliac t.
    intercondylar t.
    jugular t.
    lesser t.
    Lister t.
    Lower t.
    t. of Morgagni
    noncaseating t.
    Parsons t.
    peroneal t.
    prominent t.
    pubic t.
    rib t.
    Rolando t.
    scalene t.
    supraglenoid t.
    tibial t.
    ulnar t.
tubercula (*pl. of* tuberculum)
tuberculate
tuberculated
tuberculation
tuberculin syringe
tuberculoid
tuberculoma
    brain t.
    calcified myocardial t.
    intracranial t.
    intraparenchymal t.
    lung t.
tuberculosis (TB)
    acinar t.
    adrenal t.
    airway t.
    anorectal t.
    anthrocotic t.
    atypical t.
    basal t.
    bone t.
    cavitary t.
    cestodic t.
    t. cutis indurativa
    t. cutis lichenoides
    t. cutis miliaris disseminata
    cystic t.
    Delmege sign of t.
    disseminated t.
    endobronchial t.
    extrapulmonary t.
    exudative t.

    fibroproductive t.
    fulminant t.
    genitourinary t.
    GI tract t.
    t. granulation tissue
    GU tract t.
    hematogenous t.
    inhalation t.
    t. lichenoides
    meningeal t.
    mesenteric t.
    t. miliaris disseminata
    miliary pulmonary t.
    multidrug-resistant t.
    neural t.
    open t.
    postprimary pulmonary t.
    primary pulmonary t.
    progressive primary t.
    pulmonary t.
    reactivation t.
    recrudescent t.
    renal t.
    Schick sign of t.
    skeletal t.
    spinal t.
    stable-state t.
    t. verrucosa cutis
tuberculous
    t. arthritis
    t. bone
    t. bronchiectasis
    t. bronchopneumonia
    t. cystitis
    t. dactylitis
    t. effusion
    t. empyema
    t. granuloma
    t. infiltrate
    t. lesion
    t. mediastinal adenopathy
    t. nodule
    t. osteomyelitis
    t. peritonitis
    t. pneumonia
    t. pneumothorax
    t. salpingitis
    t. spondylitis
    t. tenosynovitis
tuberculum, pl. **tubercula**
    t. sella
    t. sellae meningioma
tuberosis
tuberositas
tuberosity
    bicipital t.
    calcaneal t.
    coracoid t.
    costal t.

deltoid t.
femoral t.
greater t.
iliac t.
infraglenoid t.
ischial t.
lesser t.
navicular t.
omental t.
radial t.
tibial t.
ulnar t.
unguicular t.
tuberous sclerosis (TS)
tubing (*See* tube)
tuboabdominal pregnancy
tubogram
T t.
tuboligamentary pregnancy
tuboovarian
t. abscess
t. mass
t. pregnancy
tuboplasty
balloon t.
transcervical balloon t. (TBT)
ultrasound transcervical t.
tuboreticular structure
tubotympanic canal
tubouterine pregnancy
tubular
t. aneurysm
t. aortic hypoplasia
t. bone
t. breast carcinoma
t. bronchiectasis
t. cavity
t. dilatation
t. dysgenesis
t. ectasia
t. ectasia of rete testis
t. fertility index
t. fluid-density adnexal mass
t. function
t. gas pattern
t. hiatal hernia
t. kidney secretion
t. lesion
t. lung density
t. magnet
t. necrosis
t. nephrogram

t. opacity
t. polyp
t. signal void
t. stenosis
t. structure
t. transit
t. ventricle
t. wire mesh
tubule
collecting t.
connecting t.
convoluted t.
dentinal t.
discharging t.
distal convoluted t.
proximal convoluted t.
renal t.
seminiferous t.
straight t.
tubuloacinar
tubulointerstitial nephritis
tubulovillous
t. colon adenoma
t. polyp
Tuffier inferior ligament
tuft
t. fracture
osteolysis t.
osteosclerosis t.
penciling of terminal t.
silk t.
terminal t.
ungual t.
vascular t.
tug
lateral t.
tularemic pneumonia
TULIP
transurethral ultrasound-guided laser-
induced prostatectomy
tulip
t. bulb aorta
t. sheath
tumefactive
t. biliary sludge
t. multiple sclerosis
t. sludge
tumeur d'emblée mycosis fungoides
tumor
abdominal wall desmoid t.
t. ablation
Abrikosov t.

NOTES

tumor (continued)
acidophilic pituitary t.
acinic cell t.
acoustic nerve sheath t.
ACTH-producing t.
acute splenic t.
adenoid t.
adenomatoid odontogenic t.
adipose t.
adrenal t.
adrenocortical t.
amelanotic t.
ameloblastic adenomatoid t.
ampulla t.
amyloid t.
anaplastic t.
androgen-producing t.
angiogenesis t.
angiomatoid t.
aortic body t.
apple-core t.
Askin thoracopulmonary
  neuroepithelial t.
astrocytic t.
astroglial t.
Azzopardi t.
ball-valve t.
basiocciput t.
B-cell t.
t. bed
Bednar t.
benign congenital Wilms t.
benign duodenal t.
benign fibrous bone t.
benign lung t.
benign lymphoepithelial parotid t.
benign ovarian t.
benign small bowel t.
benign teratoid mediastinum t.
benign urethral t.
biphasic breast t.
bladder t.
t. blood supply
blood vessel t.
t. blush
t. blush on angiography
bone t.
bone-forming bone t.
t. boundary
brain t.
Braun t.
breast phyllode t.
Brenner t.
bright-signal-intensity t.
bronchial carcinoid t.
Brooke t.
brown t.
bulky t.
t. burden

burned-out t.
Buschke-Löwenstein t.
calcified amorphous t.
t. capillary permeability
t. capsule
carcinoid t.
cardiac t.
carotid body t.
cartilage-containing giant cell t.
cartilage-forming bone t.
cartilaginous soft-tissue t.
catecholamine-producing t.
cavernous t.
cell t.
t. cell-host bone relationship
cellular t.
central nervous system t.
cerebellopontine angle t.
cervical t.
chondrogenic t.
chondroid-origin t.
chromaffin t.
t. cleavage plane
clivus meningioma t.
CNS ghost t.
CNS multifocal t.
Codman t.
collision t.
colloid cystic t.
congenital cardiac t.
connective tissue fibrous t.
cranial nerve sheath t.
cystic t.
deep t.
deep-seated t.
t. defect
Denys-Drash t.
dermal duct t.
dermoid t.
desmoid t.
desmoplastic small round-cell t.
  (DSRCT)
destructive t.
discrete t.
t. dormancy
drug-resistant t.
ductectatic mucinous t.
dumbbell t.
duodenum malignant t.
dysembryoplastic neuroepithelial t.
  (DNET)
echogenic t.
eighth nerve t.
t. embolus
embryonic t., embryonal tumor
endobronchial t.
endocrine t.
endodermal sinus ovarian t.
endodermal sinus testis t.

endolymphatic sac t.
endometrioid t.
t. entity
epidermoid t.
epithelial t.
Erdheim t.
t. erosion
esophageal t.
essential t.
estrogen-producing t.
Ewing t.
t. extension
t. extirpation
extraaxial t.
extracompartmental t.
extradural t.
extrahepatic primary malignant t.
extramedullary t.
extratesticular t.
exuberant t.
fatty soft tissue t.
fecal t.
feign t.
feminizing adrenal t.
fetal mesenchymal t.
fibroid t.
fibrous connective tissue t.
finger of t.
flocculonodular t.
focal t.
focus of t.
fourth ventricle t.
friable t.
frontal lobe t.
fungating t.
galeal extension of t.
ganglion cell t.
gastroesophageal junction t.
gastrointestinal fibrous t. (GIFT)
gastrointestinal glial/schwannoma t.
 (GIGT)
gastrointestinal leiomyogenic t.
 (GILT)
gastrointestinal stromal t. (GIST)
gestational trophoblastic t.
giant cell t.
Glazunov t.
glial brain t.
globular t.
glomus body t.
glomus bone t.
glomus jugulare t.

glomus jugulotympanicum t.
glomus neck t.
Godwin t.
gonadal stromal t.
granulosa-theca cell t.
Grawitz t.
gross t.
Gubler t.
heart t.
hepatic t.
high-grade t.
highly vascular t.
hilar t.
Hodgkin t.
hourglass t.
HPV16-associated t.
HPV18-associated t.
hypervascular pancreatic t.
hypodiploid t.
hypoechogenic t.
hypoechoic solid t.
hypopharyngeal t.
hypothalamus t.
t. hypoxia
t. imaging
t. implant
incomplete t.
t. inflammation
inflammatory myofibroblastic t.
infratentorial Lindau t.
infundibular t.
t. of infundibulum
inoperable brain t.
intestinal carcinoid t.
intraaxial brain t.
intracavitary extension of t.
intracerebral t.
intracompartmental t.
intracranial t.
intraductal mucin-producing t.
intraductal papillary mucinous t.
 (IPMT)
intradural extramedullary t.
intradural intramedullary t.
intramedullary spinal cord t.
intramural t.
intraosseous desmoid t.
intraparenchymal lung t.
intrasellar t.
intraspinal t.
intraventricular brain t.
invasive malignant sheath t.

NOTES

tumor *(continued)*
islet cell t.
jugular bulb t.
juxtaglomerular t.
Klatskin t.
Krukenberg t.
Leydig cell t. (LCT)
lipogenic t.
lipomatous t.
t. of liver scar
lobulated t.
localized pleura t.
locally invasive t.
low-signal-intensity t.
lung t.
lymphocyte-rich t.
lymphoepithelial parotid t.
lymphoid t.
main t.
malignant duodenal t.
malignant mediastinum teratoid t.
malignant ovarian germ cell t.
malignant ovarian teratoma t.
malignant small bowel t.
t. margin
t. marker
masculinizing t.
t. mass
t. matrix
mediastinal teratoid t.
melanotic neuroectodermal t.
meningeal cell t.
mesenchymal t.
metastatic myocardial t.
metasynchronous t.
microcystic pancreatic t.
micropapillary t.
mucinous t.
mucinous ovarian t.
mucosal esophageal t.
müllerian mucinous borderline t.
multicentric carcinoid t.
multifocal brain t.
musculoskeletal t.
napkin-ring anular t.
neck germ-cell t.
t. necrosis
necrotic t.
t. neovascularity
t. neovasculature
nerve root t.
nerve sheath t.
neural origin bone t.
neuroectodermal t.
neuroendocrine t.
neurogenic t.
neuroglial t.
neuronal cell origin t.
t. nidus

nonechogenic t.
nonfunctioning islet cell t.
nonneoplastic t.
nonseminomatous germ cell t.
occult phosphaturic mesenchymal t.
odontogenic t.
optic complex t.
oral cavity t.
orbital childhood t.
osteoblastic t.
osteocartilaginous t.
t. osteoid
osteoid-origin t.
ovarian mesonephroid t.
ovary germ cell t.
Pancoast t.
pancreatic islet cell t.
papillary t.
paracardiac t.
parasellar dermoid t.
parasympathetic ganglia t.
paratesticular t.
parathyroid t.
parotid t.
paucilocular t.
pearly CNS t.
pediatric primary brain t.
pediatric solid t.
pedunculated vesical t.
Pepper t.
periampullary duodenal t.
perineural fibroblastoma t.
peripheral neuroectodermal t.
peritoneum desmoid t.
phantom breast t.
phantom lung t.
phosphaturic t.
phosphaturic-inducing t.
phyllode t.
pilar t.
pilocytic t.
Pindborg t.
pineal germ-cell t.
pineal gland t.
pineal parenchymal t.
pineal region t.
pituitary t.
placenta t.
pontine angle t.
poorly circumscribed t.
poorly differentiated t.
posterior fossa t.
Pott puffy t.
pregnancy t.
primary benign liver t.
primary implanted t.
primary intracranial germ cell t.
primary malignant liver t.
primary renal t.

primitive neuroectodermal t. (PNET)
primitive neuroepithelial t.
prolapsed t.
pseudomalignant t.
pseudoorbital t.
pulmonary t.
radiation-associated papillary t.
radiation-induced peripheral nerve t.
radiosensitive t.
Rathke pouch t.
Recklinghausen t.
t. recurrence
refractory t.
renal t.
renin-secreting t.
Response Evaluation Criteria in Solid T.'s (RECIST)
reticuloendothelial t.
retinal anlage t.
retroperitoneal t.
rhabdoid t.
round bone-cell t.
round-cell t.
Rous t.
sacral bone t.
sacrococcygeal remnant t.
sand t.
scannable t.
Schmincke t.
Schwann t.
scirrhous t.
Scully t.
secondary ovarian t.
t. seeding
seminomatous t.
serous t.
serous ovarian t.
Sertoli cell t. (SCT)
Sertoli-Leydig cell t.
sessile t.
t. shrinkage
t. signature
sinonasal t.
skull-base t.
small adrenal t.
small bowel benign t.
small bowel malignant t.
smooth muscle t.
t. sojourn time
solid and cystic pancreatic t.
solid ovarian t.

solid primary t.
solid pseudopapillary t.
solitary pleura t.
sphenoid ridge t.
t. spheroid
spinal axis t.
spinal cord t.
sporadic t.
spread of t.
squamous odontogenic t.
t. staining
t. stalk
sternocleidomastoid t.
stromal cell t.
subastrocytic t.
subcortical t.
subcutaneous t.
submucosal colon t.
submucosal esophageal t.
subserosal t.
subungual glomus t.
sugar t.
superior pulmonary sulcus t.
suprasellar extension of t.
supratentorial brain t.
supratentorial primitive neuroectodermal t.
t. of surface epithelium
surface ovarian epithelium t.
sympathetic ganglia t.
synovitis t.
temporal bone t.
temporal lobe t.
tendon sheath giant cell t.
teratoid t.
testicular stromal cell t.
testis germ cell t.
tetradiploid t.
tetraploid t.
theca-cell ovarian t.
third ventricle t.
t. thrombus
tracheal t.
transmissible venereal t.
triton t.
turban t.
ulcerative t.
umbilical t.
unilocular t.
urethral t.
urinary bladder t.
uroepithelial t.

T

NOTES

tumor (*continued*)
    vaginal t.
    vanishing lung t.
    t. vascularity
    t. vascularization
    vascular origin bone t.
    vasoactive intestinal polypeptide t.
      (VIPoma)
    ventricular t.
    vertebral body bone t.
    villous t.
    t. volume
    t. volumetry
    von Hippel retina t.
    Warthin t.
    well-circumscribed t.
    well-differentiated polycystic
      Wilms t.
    Wharton t.
    yolk sac ovary t.
    Zollinger-Ellison t.
tumoral
    t. calcification
    t. calcinosis
    t. callus
    t. fat
    t. invasion
tumor-angiogenesis factor
tumor-associated tissue eosinophilia
tumor-bearing bone
tumorigenesis
    mammary t.
tumorigenic
tumorlet
tumorlike
    t. lesion
    t. shadow
tumor-mimicking breast lesion
tumorous
tumor-related spontaneous bleed
tumor-specific tracer
tumor-to-gray matter ratio
tumor-to-normal brain ratio
tumor-to-white matter ratio
TUNA
    transurethral needle ablation
tuned aperture computed tomography
   (TACT)
tungstate
    calcium t.
tungsten (W)
    t. 188 (^{188}W)
    t. anode
    t. carbide pneumoconiosis
    T. eye shield
    t. powder
    T. syringe shield
    t. target

tungstosilicates
tunica, pl. **tunicae**
    t. albuginea
    t. albuginea cyst
    t. intima
    t. medium
    t. propria
    t. vaginalis
tunicary
tunicate
tunnel
    aortic-left ventricular t.
    baffled t.
    carpal t.
    cross-trigonal t.
    cubital t.
    fibroosseous t.
    intramural t.
    t. projection
    t. radiograph
    retropancreatic t.
    retroperitoneal t.
    t. subaortic stenosis
    subcutaneous t.
    subsartorial t.
    t. subvalvular aortic stenosis
    tarsal t.
    t. view
tunneled catheter
Tuohy aortography needle
Tuohy-Borst
    T.-B. adaptor
    T.-B. introducer
TUP
    transumbilical plane
TUR
    transurethral resection
turban tumor
turbidimetric detection
turbinate
    t. bone
    nasal t.
    paradoxic middle t.
turbo
    t. fast low-angle shot
      (turboFLASH)
    t. gradient-refocused echo
      (turboGRE)
    t. inversion recovery sequence
    t. IR sequence
    t. pulse sequence
    t. SE sequence
    t. short tau inversion recovery
    t. short tau/TI inversion recovery
    t. spin-echo (TSE)
    t. spin-echo technique
    t. spin-echo T2-weighted sequence
turboFLAIR imaging

turboFLASH
turbo fast low-angle shot
turboFLASH imaging
turboFLASH sequence
turboGRE
turbo gradient-refocused echo
turboSTIR image
turbulence
TCD-detectable t.
turbulent
t. blood flow
t. intraluminal flow
t. signal
turcica
sella t.
Turcot syndrome
turn
insufficient cochlear t.
turned-up pulp deformity
Turner
T. marginal gyrus
T. syndrome
turnover
bone t.
erythrocyte iron t.
plasma iron t.
red blood cell iron t.
TURP
transurethral resection of prostate
turret exostosis
turricephaly
Turyn sign
T2USA
Diomed 630 PDT laser model
T2USA
tutamen
TV
thermoactinomyces vulgaris
tricuspid valve
TVG
time-varied gain
TVHS
transvaginal hysterosonography
TVS
transvaginal sonography
TVUS
transvaginal ultrasound
T-wave
asymmetric negative T-w.
T1-weighted
T1-w. acquisition
T1-w. axial image

T1-w. axial image with fat
saturation
T1-w. axial localizer
T1-w. conventional spin-echo
T1-w. coronal fat-suppressed fast
spin-echo sequence
T1-w. coronal image
T1-w. coronal imaging
T1-w. FAST
T1-w. fat-suppressed gadolinium-
enhanced SE image
T1-w. fat-suppressed image (T1FS)
T1-w. gadolinium-enhanced SE
image
T1-w. image (T1WI)
T1-w. magnetic resonance
T1-w. sagittal imaging
T1-w. spin echo
T1-w. study
T2-weighted
T2-w. axial image
T2-w. combination sequence
T2-w. fast spin-echo coronal
oblique
T2-w. fat-saturated sequence
T2-w. image (T2WI)
T2-w. pulse sequence
T2-w. sagittal oblique image
T2-w. scan
T2-w. shortening
T2-w. signal
T2-w. spin-echo image
T2-w. spin-echo sequence
T2-w. turbo SE image
T1WI
T1-weighted image
T2WI
T2-weighted image
twiddler's syndrome
twig
t. of artery
cutaneous t.
muscular t.
twin
conjoined t.
craniopagus t.
dichorionic-diamniotic t.
discordant t.
dizygotic t.
donor t.
t. ectopic pregnancy
t. embolization syndrome

NOTES

twin *(continued)*
    fraternal t.
    ischiopagus t.
    monochorionic-monoamniotic t.
    monozygotic t.
    omphalopagus t.
    t. peak sign
    perfused t.
    t. pregnancy discordant growth
    pygopagus t.
    thoracopagus t.
    t. trunk
    vanishing t.'s
twin-beam CT
twining
    t. line
    T. position
    t. recess
    T. view
twinkling artifact
twin-peaked pulse
twin-reversed arterial perfusion sequence
twin-to-twin transfusion syndrome (TTTS)
twist
    myocardial t.
twisted
    t. ankle
    t. body habitus
    t. ribbonlike rib
    t. small bowel ribbon appearance
twister gradient
twist-release coil
tylectomy
tylosis, pl. **tyloses**
    t. palmaris et plantaris
tympani
    tegmen t.
    tensor t.
tympanic
    t. bone
    t. cavity
    t. membrane thermometer
    t. plexus
tympanic membrane thermometer
tympanicum
    glomus t.

tympanography
tympanosclerosis
type
    t. A carotid cavernous fistula
    t. A–C right ventricular hypertrophy
    centrocytelike t.
    collagen defect t. I, II
    diffuse fibrosis t.
    t. 1, 2 endoleak
    glutaric aciduria t. I, II
    t. I endoleak (T1EL)
    t. II collagen C-telopeptide
    t. II endoleak (T2EL)
    t. III endoleak
    enhancement pattern t. I–IV
    t. I, II muscle fiber
    t. II (infracristal) ventricular septal defect
    IPMT of branch duct t.
    t. I (supracristal) ventricular septal defect
    t. IV endoleak
    t. IV (muscular) ventricular septal defect
    MPS t.'s I–IV
    mucopolysaccharidosis t.'s I–IV
    neurofibromatosis t. 1 (NF1)
    neurofibromatosis t. 2 (NF2)
    odontoid fracture t.'s I–III
    pleomorphic t.
    portal vein anomaly t. I–V
    reticular t.
    sonographic hip t.
type-B aortic dissection
type-MHRE/72
typhoid
    t. nodule
    t. pleurisy
typhus nodule
typical
    t. cobblestone pattern
    t. medullary carcinoma
tyropanoate sodium
Tyropaque imaging agent
tyrosinase
tyrphostin radiotracer for PET
T-zone lymphoma

U
    unit
    uranium
U-1100 UV-Vis spectrophotometer
U1-NA cephalometric measurement
UA
    umbilical artery
    uterine artery
        UA to OA anastomosis
        UA velocimetry
UAE
    uterine artery embolization
UAL
    ultrasound-assisted lipoplasty
ubiquinone
UBIS 5000 ultrasound bone sonometer
UBM
    ultrasound backscatter microscopy
    ultrasound biomicroscopy
        UBM imaging
UBO
    unidentified bright object
UC
    ulcerative colitis
UCG
    ultrasonic cardiogram
UCL
    ulnar collateral ligament
UCLA
    University of California Los Angeles
        UCLA imaging protocol
        UCLA pouch
U-clips
        nitinol U-c.
UCT
    ultrasound computed tomography
UE
    angle electron
    upper extremity
UES
    upper esophageal sphincter
UEVT
    upper extremity venous thrombosis
UFCT
    ultrafast computed tomography
UFE
    uterine fibroid embolization
U-fiber damage
UGI
    upper gastrointestinal
Uhl
        U. anomaly
        U. disease
UHMM
    ultra-high magnification mammography

Uhthoff sign
UI
    urethral inclination
UIP
    usual interstitial pneumonia
    usual interstitial pneumonia of Liebow
UIQ
    upper inner quadrant
UL
    upper lobe
    urethral length
ulcer
        acid peptic u.
        active duodenal u.
        acute peptic u.
        anastomotic u.
        anterior wall antral u.
        antral u.
        aortic penetrating u.
        aphthoid u.
        aphthous stomach u.
        apical duodenal u.
        arteriolar ischemic u.
        atheromatous u.
        atherosclerotic aortic u.
        Barrett u.
        u. base
        bear's claw u.
        benign gastric u.
        bleeding u.
        bulbar peptic u.
        channel pyloric u.
        chronic peptic u.
        collar-button u.
        colonic u.
        u. crater
        craterlike u.
        Cruveilhier u.
        Curling u.
        Cushing u.
        Cushing-Rokitansky u.
        decubitus u.
        u. disease
        duodenal u.
        esophageal u.
        flask-shaped u.
        focal u.
        frontier u.
        gastric u. (GU)
        gastrointestinal u.
        giant duodenal u.
        giant peptic u.
        greater curvature u.
        healed gastric u.
        healing u.

ulcer *(continued)*
    Hunner u.
    hypertensive ischemic u.
    indolent radiation-induced rectal u.
    intestinal u.
    intractable u.
    ischemic u.
    jejunal u.
    juxtapyloric u.
    kissing u.
    Kocher dilatation u.
    lesser curvature u.
    linear u.
    malignant gastric u.
    marginal u.
    Martorell hypertensive u.
    minute bleeding u.
    mucosal u.
    multiple small bowel u.'s
    necrotic u.
    u. osteoma
    patchy colonic u.
    penetrating aortic u.
    penetrating atherosclerotic u. (PAU)
    peptic u.
    perforated u.
    u. perforation
    phagedenic u.
    postbulbar u.
    postsurgical recurrent u.
    prepyloric u.
    punched-out u.
    punctate u.
    puncture u.
    pyloric channel u.
    radiation-induced u.
    rake u.
    recurrent u.
    rodent u.
    Rokitansky-Cushing u.
    round u.
    ruptured u.
    Saemisch u.
    secondary u.
    serpiginous u.
    sloughing u.
    small bowel multiple u.
    solitary rectal u.
    stasis u.
    stercoral u.
    stomach u.
    stress u.
    subatheromatous u.
    thorn u.
    tropic u.
    urinary u.
    venous u.
    V-shaped u.
    u. with heaped-up edges

ulcerated
    u. atheromatous plaque
    u. carotid artery plaque
ulcerating
    u. adenocarcinoma
    u. granuloma of pudenda
ulcerative
    u. colitis (UC)
    u. esophageal carcinoma
    u. jejunitis
    u. jejunoileitis
    u. lesion
    u. lymphoma
    u. tumor
ULDR
    ultra-low dose rate
ulegyria
Ullmann line
ulna, pl. **ulnae**
    capitulum ulnae
    coronoid of u.
    fetal biometry u.
    sigmoid cavity of u.
ulnar
    u. bone
    u. bursa
    u. chondromalacia
    u. collateral ligament (UCL)
    u. deviation
    u. deviation view
    u. digital artery
    u. drift deformity
    u. extensor
    u. facing of metacarpal head
    u. fracture
    u. groove
    u. hand
    u. head
    u. impaction syndrome
    u. inclination
    u. nerve entrapment
    u. nerve lesion
    u. notch
    u. ridge
    u. sesamoid bone
    u. styloid
    u. styloid process
    u. styloid process index (USPI)
    u. sulcus
    u. traction spurring
    u. translocation of carpus
    u. tubercle
    u. tuberosity
    u. tunnel syndrome
    u. variance
ulnaris
    extensor carpi u. (ECU)
    flexor carpi u.
ulnocarpal ligament

ulnolunate
  u. impaction syndrome
  u. impingement
  u. ligament
ulnotriquetral
  u. distance
  u. ligament
ULP
  ultra-low profile
ULQ
  upper left quadrant
ultimobranchial pouch
ultra
  u. ICE 9F/9 MHz catheter
  U. Tag kit
  U. Vision Rapid screen
UltraCision ultrasonic knife
Ultracranio T
ultra-early thrombolytic therapy
UltraEase ultrasound pad
ultrafast
  u. computed tomography (UFCT)
  u. computed tomography scanner
  u. contrast-enhanced MRA
  u. CT
  u. CT electron beam tomography
  u. CT imaging
  u. 3D MR digital subtraction
  angiography
  u. FLASH 2D sequence
  u. MRI
  u. video transfer
ultrafiltration
UltraFine Erbium laser system
Ultraflex stent
Ultra-Fluid
  70–50% Lipiodol U.-F.
ultra-high
  u.-h. magnification
  u.-h. magnification mammography
  (UHMM)
ultra-high-resolution, parallel-hole
  collimator
UltraICE catheter
Ultraject prefilled syringe
ultralong TR
ultra-low
  u.-l. dose rate (ULDR)
  u.-l. profile (ULP)
Ultramark
  ATL U. 8, 9
  U. 9 HDI ultrasound

  U. 9 scanner
  U. 8 transducer
  U. 4 ultrasound
UltraPACS diagnostic imaging system
UltraPulse CO$_2$ laser
ultrascan
  B-mode u.
Ultraseed brachytherapy
ultrashort
  u. echo time (UTE)
  u. method
ultrashort echo time (UTE)
ultrasmall superparamagnetic iron oxide
  (USPIO)
UltraSoft
  2/3-cm U. GDC
  2/6-cm U. GDC
  U. GDC
ultrasonic
  u. aortography
  u. aspiration
  u. assessment
  u. assessment of injury
  u. atherolysis
  u. attenuation
  u. cardiogram (UCG)
  u. cardiography
  u. cephalometry
  u. guidance
  u. hysterography
  u. hysterosalpingography
  u. lithotripsy
  u. lithotripter cannula
  u. lysis
  u. lysis of thrombus
  u. pachymetry
  u. probe
  u. tomographic image
  u. tomographic imaging
  u. tomography
  u. wave
ultrasonically activated scalpel
ultrasonogram
ultrasonographic
  u. echo
  u. finding
  u. modeling
ultrasonographically guided injection
ultrasonography (US) (*See* ultrasound)
  axillary u.
  compression u.
  endovascular u.

U

NOTES

ultrasonography *(continued)*
    infant cranial Doppler u.
    intracaval endovascular u.
    intraductal u.
    intraportal endovascular u. (IPEUS)
    laparoscopic contact u. (LCU)
    periorbital directional Doppler u.
    pulsed wave Doppler u.
    real-time u.
    rectal endoscopic u.
    transoral carotid u. (TOCU)
    transperineal u.
    venous u.
    vertebrobasilar transcranial color-
      coded duplex u.
ultrasonometer
    QUS-2 calcaneal u.
ultrasonometry
ultrasound (US)
    abdominal u.
    u. ablative therapy
    ACM u.
    Acuson 128 Doppler u.
    ADR Ultramark 4 u.
    AI 5200 diagnostic u.
    Aloka linear u.
    Aloka sector u.
    A-scan u.
    u. augmented mammography
    automated cardiac flow
      measurement u.
    u. backscatter microscopy (UBM)
    u. backscatter microscopy imaging
    u. biomicroscopy (UBM)
    BladderScan u.
    B-mode u.
    breast u.
    Bruel-Kjaer u.
    carotid duplex u.
    color-coded duplex u.
    color-coded real-time u.
    color Doppler u. (CDUS)
    color duplex u.
    color power transcranial Doppler u.
    u. computed tomography (UCT)
    contact B-scan u.
    contrast-enhanced u.
    cranial u.
    CT-guided u.
    1D u.
    2D B-mode u.
    3D freehand u.
    u. diagnosis
    diagnostic range u.
    u. diagnostic yield
    Diasonics u.
    diathermy u.
    u. diffraction tomography
    u. dilution

    u. dilution test
    Doppler u.
    duplex u. (DU)
    duplex B-mode u.
    duplex carotid u.
    duplex Doppler u.
    duplex-pulsed Doppler u.
    u. echocardiography
    EchoGen-enhanced u.
    u. echogenicity
    endoanal u.
    endorectal u. (ERU, ERUS, EUS)
    endoscopic u. (EUS)
    endovaginal u. (EVUS)
    endovascular u.
    "entertainment" u.
    FDI u.
    fetal u.
    FloWire Doppler u.
    focused u.
    freehand interventional u.
    full bladder u.
    gallbladder u.
    gastrointestinal endoscopic u.
    u. gel
    graded compression u.
    gray-scale u.
    gray-scale endorectal u.
    u. guidance during embryo transfer
    Hewlett-Packard u.
    high-frequency Doppler u.
    high-frequency therapeutic u.
    high-intensity focus u.
    high-intensity focused u. (HIFU)
    high-resolution u.
    Hitachi u.
    u. hyperthermia treatment
    hypoechoic area of u.
    u. imaging technology
    immersion B-scan u.
    intracoronary u. (ICUS)
    intraluminal u. (ILUS)
    intraoperative u. (IOUS)
    intrarectal u.
    intravascular u. (IVUS)
    Irex Exemplar u.
    laparoscopic u. (LapUS, LUS)
    laparoscopic intracorporeal u.
      (LICU)
    level I obstetric u.
    limitation of u.
    low frequency u. (LFUS)
    low-intensity pulsed u.
    M-mode u.
    u. monitoring
    multiplanar endorectal u.
    neonatal adrenal u.
    neonatal transfontanellar brain u.
    Neurosector u.

Nicolet Elite Doppler u.
noninvasive u.
obstetric u.
Olympus endoscopic u.
u. pad
pancreaticobiliary u.
pelvic u.
photoacoustic u.
power Doppler u.
PowerVision u.
u. probe
ProSound SSD-5500 u.
pulsed Doppler u.
pulsed therapeutic low-intensity u.
pulse-inversion harmonic u.
real-time scan u.
renal u.
RT 6800 u.
RT 3200 Advantage u.
sagittal u.
SieScape u.
Sonicator portable u.
Sonolayer model SSA-270A u.
SonoSite digital u.
SonoSite hand-carried u.
SonoSite iLook 24 u.
SonoSite MicroMaxx laptop u.
SonoSite 180Plus u.
SonoSite Titan u.
spectral u.
u. stethoscope
suprapubic transabdominal u.
u. system
TCD u.
u. test
u. threshold
TM u.
transabdominal u. (TAUS)
u. transcervical tuboplasty
transcranial color-coded duplex u.
transcranial Doppler u.
u. transducer
transperineal u.
transrectal u. (TRUS)
transthoracic u.
transvaginal u. (TVUS)
transverse u.
Ultramark 4 u.
Ultramark 9 HDI u.
u. venography
Vingmed u.
ultrasound-assisted lipoplasty (UAL)

ultrasound-based strain rate and strain imaging
ultrasound-guided
u.-g. anterior subcostal liver biopsy
celiac plexus neurolysis, endoscopic u.-g.
u.-g. compression
u.-g. core biopsy
u.-g. cyst aspiration
u.-g. large core-needle biopsy
u.-g. methotrexate injection
u.-g. nephrostomy puncture
u.-g. percutaneous cholecystostomy
u.-g. percutaneous interstitial laser ablation
u.-g. percutaneous microwave coagulation therapy
u.-g. pseudoaneurysm compression
u.-g. reduction of a spigelian hernia
u.-g. stereotactic biopsy
u.-g. transthoracic needle aspiration
u.-g. vacuum-assisted biopsy
UltraSTAR computer-based ultrasound reporting system
ultrastructural abnormality
UltraSure DTR-one imaging ultrasound system
UltraTag RBC
Ultrathane Amplatz ureteral stent
ultratherm
Ultrathin Diamond balloon
ultraviolet
u. A, B, C
extravital u.
u. fluorescent dosimeter
intravital u.
u. lamp
psoralen and u. A (PUVA)
u. radiation
u. ray
u. spectrophotometry
u. spectrum
u. (UV) irradiation
Ultravist 150, 240, 300, 370 contrast agent
Umbau zone
umbilical
u. artery (UA)
u. artery velocimetry
u. canal
u. cord

U

NOTES

umbilical (*continued*)
  u. cord anatomy
  u. cord angiomyxoma
  u. cord cyst
  u. cord edema
  u. cord hemangioma
  u. cord hematoma
  u. cord lesion
  u. cord pseudocyst
  u. fissure
  u. granuloma
  u. hernia
  u. ligament
  u. mass
  u. plane
  u. portography
  u. ring
  u. tumor
  u. vein
  u. vein varix
umbilicovesical fascia
umbilicus
umbo, pl. **umbones**
  u. membranae tympani
  u. membranae tympanicae
umbonate
UMC-I microwave delivery system
UM 4 real-time sector scanner
unattached fraction
unbalanced hemivertebra
uncal
  u. gyrus
  u. herniation
  u. herniation syndrome
uncalcified pleural plaque
uncertainty principle
unciform bone
uncinate
  u. aura
  u. gyrus
  u. process
  u. process fracture
  u. process mass
  u. process of pancreas
uncoiling
  u. ascending aorta
  u. descending aorta
  u. of the great vessels
uncommitted metaphysial lesion
uncompensated rotary scoliosis
uncomplicated
  u. myocardial infarct
  u. myoma
  u. pneumothorax
  u. supraclavicular stenosis
uncoupled spin
uncoupler
  mitochondrial u.

uncovering
  lateral meniscal u.
uncovertebral
  u. joint
  u. spur
uncus
  arachnoid of u.
  u. of temporal lobe
undefined lymphoma
undepressed skull fracture
"undercalling" disease
undercorrection
underdamping
underdetection
underdrainage
underdrive
  u. mode
  u. termination
underexposed image
under-filled submentovertical projection
underinflation
  lung u.
underloading
  ventricular u.
underlying
  u. disorder
  u. tissue
underperfusion
under-scan
  u.-s. method
  u.-s. method projection
undersurface
  u. of liver
  u. of patella
underventilated lung
underventilation
undescended
  u. testicle
  u. testis
undifferentiated
  u. liver sarcoma
  u. nasopharyngeal carcinoma
  u. non-Hodgkin lymphoma
undifferentiation
undisplaced fracture
Undritz anomaly
undulant impulse
undulating
  u. contour
  u. course
unenhanced
  u. magnetic resonance imaging
    scan
  u. MR imaging
unequal pulmonary blood flow
uneven
  u. air expansion
  u. exposure

u. recruitment of alveolar
populations
u. ventilation
unfavorable neutron-to-proton ratio
unfolding
incomplete u.
unfused
u. os trigonum
u. physis
ungual
u. fibroma
u. tuft
unguicular tuberosity
uniaxial
unibasal
unicaliceal kidney
unicameral
u. bone cyst
u. brain
unicentral
unicentric angiofollicular lymph node
hyperplasia
unicollis
unicommissural aortic valve
unicondylar fracture
unicornis unicollis uterus
unicornous
unicornuate uterus
unicoronal synostosis
unicortical screw
unicuspid
u. aortic valve stenosis
u. with aortic valve
unicusp with central raphe
unidentified bright object (UBO)
unidirectional
u. airflow
u. block
u. current
u. lead configuration
unidirectional airflow
unifascicular block
unifocal
unifocalization
uniform
u. attenuation coefficient
u. distribution
u. loading
u. phantom scan
u. sensitivity
u. TR excitation
u. uptake

uniformity
differential u.
extrinsic field u.
field u.
image u.
intervertebral disc space u.
intrinsic field u.
scintillation camera field u.
SPECT u.
uniformly hyperechoic
Uni-Fuse infusion catheter
uniglandular
unigravida
unilateral
u. adrenal mass
u. bronchogram
u. carotid stenosis
u. consolidation
u. diaphragmatic elevation
u. facet dislocation
u. facet subluxation
u. fetal chest mass
u. flow restriction
u. fracture
u. fragmentation
u. hallux valgus
u. hydrocephalus
u. hyperlucent lung
u. hypertrophy
u. interfacetal dislocation
u. intrafacetal dislocation
u. kidney mass
u. large smooth kidney
u. lesion
u. lobar emphysema
u. locked facet injury
u. lung perfusion
u. megalencephaly
u. mesial temporal sclerosis
u. occlusion
u. ossification
u. overinflation
u. pleural effusion
u. pulmonary agenesis
u. pulmonary edema
u. Raynaud phenomenon
u. small kidney
unilobar
unilobular cirrhosis
unilocular
u. cyst
u. cystic lesion

U

NOTES

1017

unilocular (*continued*)
   u. disc
   u. osteolysis
   u. tumor
   u. well-demarcated bone defect
     expansile lesion
unimalleolar fracture
uninfected infarct
uninhibited bladder
union
   bony u.
   delayed fracture u.
   faulty u.
   fibrous u.
   u. of fracture fragment
   nonbony u.
   osseous u.
   secondary u.
   solid bony u.
unipapillary kidney
unipara
unipediculate approach
unipennate muscle
uniphasic imaging agent
unipolar pacing mode
unirhinal phantosmia
uniseptate
unit (U)
   adapted standard mammography u.
   add-on stereotactic u.
   AdvanTeq II TENS u.
   Angström u.
   Aspen sonography u.
   atomic mass u. (amu)
   Bart abdominoperipheral
     angiography u.
   Behnken u.
   Bethesda u.
   BICAP u.
   biplane DSA u.
   British thermal u.
   burst-forming u.
   C-arm portable x-ray u.
   cobalt 60 beam therapy u.
   colony-forming u.
   Cox sterilizer and incinerator u.
   CT u.
   Dent-X intraoral x-ray u.
   depicted Hounsfield u.
   dry heat sterilizer and
     incinerator u.
   Eclipse TENS u.
   electromagnetic u. (emu)
   EMI u.
   gamma u.
   gray u.
   Gyroscan ACS-NT MR u.
   Hampson u.

   heat u. (HU)
   Hercules 7000 mobile x-ray u.
   Holzknecht u. (H)
   Hounsfield u. (H, HU)
   Hounsfield calcium density
     measurement u.
   Intelect Legend Combo stimulator
     and ultrasound u.
   International Commission on
     Radiation U.'s (ICRU)
   JACE-Stim electrotherapy u.
   Kienböck u. (X)
   Leksell gamma u.
   linear accelerator u.
   MAGNETOM Espree open MRI u.
   MAGNETOM Vision MR u.
   Mammotest u.
   Maxima II TENS u.
   molecular recognition u. (MRU)
   monitor u.
   Multistar angiographic u.
   musculotendinous u.
   Odelca camera u.
   Optiplanimat automated u.
   Orbix x-ray u.
   Orthopantomograph-panoramic digital
     radiography u.
   ostiomeatal u.
   photodisplay u.
   Picker Eclipse MR u.
   pilosebaceous u.
   Plasma 1000 ICP-AES u.
   pressor u.
   quantum u.
   u. of radioactivity
   reflectometer tuning u.
   roentgen u. (RU)
   rutherford u.
   Sheffield gamma u.
   Siemens SOMATOM nonhelical u.
   sonography u.
   Sonos 2000 ultrasound u.
   Surgitron portable radiosurgical u.
   Symphony MR u.
   terminal ductal lobular u. (TDLU)
   Tesla superconductive magnet u.
   Thayer-Doisy u.
   ThromboScan molecular
     recognition u.
   1.5T Signa MR u.
   video display u. (VDU)
   u. of wavelength
   whole-body u.
   Wood u.
   X u.
   x-ray u.
uniting canal
univentricular heart

university
U. of California Los Angeles (UCLA)
U. of Florida linear accelerator
U. of Florida staging system
Univision echocardiographic system
Unix/X11 workstation
unknown
u. primary
u. primary site
unleveling
pelvic u.
unloading
bone u.
unmitigated
unmodulated radiofrequency current
unmyelinated nerve fiber
unneurulated neural placode
unopacified bowel loop
unopposed image
unossified cartilage
unpaired
u. parietal branch
u. visceral branch
unplicated sheath
unraveling
digital u.
unresectable
u. colorectal carcinoma
u. lesion
unresolved pneumonia
unroofed coronary sinus syndrome
unruptured follicle
unsaturated
u. compound
u. spin
unsegmented vertebral bar
unsharp
u. masking
u. mask-type contrast
unsharpness
absorption u.
geometric u.
motion u.
system u.
unshunted hydrocephalus
unstable
u. fracture
u. joint
u. lesion
unsuppressed
u. examination

u. imaging
u. water signal
untethered
untransformed nadir
ununited fracture
unusual
u. fetal lie
u. interstitial pneumonitis
u. marrow distribution
u. occurrence report (UOR)
unwinding of aorta
unwrapping
Dixon method of phase u.
UOQ
upper outer quadrant
UOR
unusual occurrence report
up
ramp u.
tented u.
UP7 film
uPACS picture archiving system
updraft therapy
upfront delay
upgated technique
uphill varix
UPJ
ureteropelvic junction
UPJ obstruction
upper
u. aerodigestive tract
u. airway obstruction
u. esophageal sphincter (UES)
u. extremity (UE)
u. extremity venous thrombosis (UEVT)
u. gastrointestinal (UGI)
u. gastrointestinal endoscopy
u. gastrointestinal hemorrhage
u. gastrointestinal series
u. gastrointestinal tract
u. GI with small bowel follow-through
u. inner quadrant (UIQ)
u. jaw bone
u. left quadrant (ULQ)
u. limits of normal
u. lobe (UL)
u. lobe vein prominence
u. lung disease
u. lung field
u. mantle radiation therapy

U

NOTES

upper *(continued)*
- u. moiety ureter
- u. motor neuron
- u. motor neuron lesion
- u. outer quadrant (UOQ)
- u. pole
- u. pole collecting system
- u. pole moiety
- u. pole of ureter
- u. pulmonary lobe atelectasis
- u. rate interval
- u. respiratory tract disease
- u. right quadrant (URQ)
- u. sternal border
- u. thoracic esophagus
- u. thoracic spine fracture

upregulated AQP4 expression

upregulation
- radiation-induced u.

upright
- u. chest film
- u. compression spot film
- u. position
- u. postvoid view

UPSC
- uterine papillary serous carcinoma

upscanning

upside-down stomach

up-sloping curve of kidney

upstairs-downstairs heart

upstream blood

upstroke
- carotid pulse u.
- u. phase of cardiac action potential
- weak carotid u.

uptake
- absence of u.
- absent radiotracer u.
- asymmetric limb u.
- bilateral diffuse increased u.
- bilateral reduction of tracer u.
- u. in bone marrow
- cell preparation bone marrow u.
- contrast u.
- decreased thyroid radiotracer u.
- diffuse lung u.
- dye u.
- u. and excretion
- extracardiac focal u.
- extracerebral soft tissue u.
- extraosseous u.
- extraskeletal u.
- ^{18}F 2-deoxyglucose u.
- FDG u.
- fluorescein u.
- focal decreased radiotracer u.
- focal pulmonary u.
- Ga-67 u.
- gallium u.

- hepatocyte tracer u.
- heterogeneous u.
- incidental lung u.
- increased isotope u.
- increased thyroid u.
- increased tracer u.
- intense u.
- iodine u.
- isotope u.
- laryngeal musculature fluorodeoxyglucose u.
- localized u.
- mediastinal u.
- metabolic tracer u.
- mottled hepatic u.
- mottled liver u.
- muscle u.
- myocardial u.
- ^{13}N ammonia u.
- near-normal radiotracer u.
- normal variant of Ga-67 u.
- observed maximal u.
- predicted maximal u.
- progressive u.
- prominent u.
- radioactive iodine u. (RAIU)
- u. of radioactive material
- radioiodine u.
- radioisotope u.
- u. of radionuclide
- radiopharmaceutical u.
- radiotracer u.
- u. ratio (UR)
- regional tracer u.
- u. and retention
- symmetric pattern of radiotracer u.
- T4 u.
- ^{99m}Tc HMPAO u.
- ^{99m}Tc MDP u.
- thyroid radioiodine u.
- tracer u.
- uniform u.
- variable u.
- V-like pattern of u.

uptilted cardiac apex

upward
- u. and backward dislocation
- u. lens dislocation
- u. retraction

UR
- uptake ratio

urachal
- u. abnormality
- u. anomaly
- u. carcinoma
- u. cyst
- u. diverticulum
- u. ligament
- u. sinus

urachus
 patent u.
uracil
uranium (U)
 u. imaging agent
²³⁵uranium, uranium 235
urate
 u. arthropathy
 u. calculus
 u. nephropathy
urceiform
urceolate
uremic amaurosis
ureter
 atonic u.
 beaded u.
 bifid u.
 champagne glass u.
 circumcaval u.
 u. cobra head
 cobra-head u.
 corkscrew u.
 curlicue u.
 u. deviation
 u. diameter
 dilatation of u.
 dilated u.
 ectopic u.
 extravesical intrasphincteric
  ectopic u.
 hockey-stick appearance of u.
 hood-shaped u.
 intestinal u.
 intramural portion of distal u.
 intravesical u.
 J-hook deformity of distal u.
 J-shaped u.
 kinked u.
 lower moiety u.
 lower pole u.
 moderately dilated u.
 notching u.
 orthotopic u.
 pipestem u.
 postcaval u.
 redundant u.
 retrocaval u.
 retroiliac u.
 rigid u.
 saddle peristalsis u.
 sawtooth u.
 seesaw peristalsis u.

 spring onion u.
 straight u.
 tortuosity of u.
 upper moiety u.
 upper pole of u.
ureteral
 u. achalasia
 u. adenomyosis
 u. bud
 u. bud bifurcation
 u. calculus
 u. carcinoma
 u. compression technique
 u. dilatation
 u. distention
 u. division
 u. duplication
 u. endometriosis
 u. filling
 u. filling defect
 u. fistula
 u. jet
 u. notching
 u. occlusion
 u. orifice
 u. perforation
 u. perfusion test
 u. reflux study
 u. renal transplant obstruction
 u. seesaw peristalsis
 u. spindle
 u. stasis
 u. stenosis
 u. stenting
 u. stone
 u. stricture
ureterectasis
ureteric
 u. clipping
 u. jet
 u. kinking
ureteritis cystica
ureterocele
 ectopic u.
 orthotopic u.
 pyoureter ectopic u.
 simple u.
ureterocutaneous fistula
ureterocystography
ureteroenteral anastomotic stricture
ureterogram
 retrograde u.

NOTES

U

ureterography
    bulb u.
    retrograde u.
ureterohydronephrosis
ureteroileostomy
ureterointestinal fistula
ureterolysis
ureteroneocystostomy
ureteropelvic
    u. junction (UPJ)
    u. junction obstruction
ureteroperitoneal fistula
ureteropyelogram
    retrograde u.
ureteropyelography
ureteropyelostomy
ureterorenal junction
ureterorenoscopy
ureteroscope
    solid-rod u.
ureteroscopy
ureterostomy
ureteroureteral anastomosis
ureterovaginal fistula
ureterovesical
    u. junction
    u. junction obstruction
urethra
    angle of inclination of u.
    anterior u.
    bulbous u.
    cavernous u.
    female u.
    male u.
    membranous u.
    pendulous u.
    penile u.
    posterior u.
    prostatic u. (PU)
    ragged u.
    spinning-top u.
urethral
    u. amyloidosis
    u. angle
    u. atresia
    u. calculus
    u. crest
    u. diverticulum
    u. gland
    u. groove
    u. inclination (UI)
    u. length (UL)
    u. metallic stent
    u. obstruction
    u. orifice
    u. papilla
    u. ridge
    u. straddle injury
    u. stricture

    u. syndrome
    u. thickness (UT)
    u. trauma
    u. tumor
    u. uterus
    u. valve
    u. warming
urethritis
urethrocystogram
urethrocystography
    u. imaging
    retrograde u.
    voiding u.
urethrocystometry
urethrogram
    normal fold u.
    retrograde u. (RUG)
urethrography
urethroplasty
    prostatic u.
    retrograde transurethral prostatic u.
urethroscopy
urethrotome
urethrotomy
    internal u.
urethrovaginal fistula
urethrovesical angle (UVA)
uric
    u. acid calculus
    u. acid nephropathy
urinary
    u. bladder adenocarcinoma
    u. bladder atony
    u. bladder calculus
    u. bladder capacity
    u. bladder contusion
    u. bladder diverticulum
    u. bladder exstrophy
    u. bladder extrinsic mass
    u. bladder fundus
    u. bladder hemangioma
    u. bladder leiomyoma
    u. bladder lymphoma
    u. bladder rupture
    u. bladder stone
    u. bladder trauma
    u. bladder tumor
    u. bladder wall calcification
    u. bladder wall mass
    u. bladder wall thickening
    u. blunt trauma bladder
    u. conduit
    u. diversion
    u. excretion
    u. excretory route
    u. extravasation
    u. fistula
    u. glucosyl-galactosyl-pyridinoline
    u. obstruction

u. stasis
u. stent
u. tract
u. tract anomaly
u. tract calculus
u. tract fibroepithelioma
u. tract gas
u. ulcer
urine
u. ascites
postvoid residual u.
radiopaque u.
residual u.
retained u.
urinoma
urinothorax
uriposia
urodynamic pressure-flow study
uroepithelial
u. malignancy
u. tumor
urogenital
u. canal
u. diaphragm
u. embryology
u. malignancy
u. sinus
u. tract
u. triangle
urografin imaging agent
urogram
constant infusion excretory u.
diuresis u.
excretory u.
retrograde u. (RU)
urographic density
urography
antegrade u.
ascending u.
cystoscopic u.
descending u.
diuretic radionuclide u.
drip infusion u.
excretion u.
excretory u. (EU)
excretory urethrogram drip
infusion u.
u. imaging
intravenous u. (IVU)
magnetic resonance u. (MRU)
oral u.

percutaneous antegrade u.
retrograde u.
urokinase
catheter-directed u.
u. imaging agent
urokymography
Urolase
U. fiber laser
U. fiber laser ablation
urolithiasis
Uromiro contrast medium
uropathy
chronic obstructive u.
obstructive u.
uroradiologic procedure
uroradiology
Uroselectan
urostealith calculus
urothelial
u. carcinoma
u. striation
urothelium
Urovision
Urovist
U. Cysto imaging agent
U. Meglumine Diu/CT imaging
agent
U. Sodium 300 imaging agent
URQ
upper right quadrant
urticate
urtication
US
ultrasonography
ultrasound
USCI
U. PET balloon
U. probe
U. Probe balloon-on-a-wire
dilatation system
useful beam
useful-beam radiation
USPI
ulnar styloid process index
USPIO
ultrasmall superparamagnetic iron oxide
USPIO imaging agent
USP XX test
usual
u. interstitial pneumonia (UIP)

NOTES

usual *(continued)*
    u. interstitial pneumonia of Liebow (UIP)
    u. interstitial pneumonitis
UT
    urethral thickness
UTE
    ultrashort echo time
uteri (*pl. of* uterus)
uteric fold
uterine
    u. adenomyosis
    u. agenesis
    u. anatomy
    u. artery (UA)
    u. artery embolization (UAE)
    u. artery pseudoaneurysm
    u. artery waveform
    u. blood volume flow
    u. body
    u. canal
    u. cavity
    u. cervical ganglion
    u. cervix
    u. cervix carcinoma
    u. cirsoid aneurysm
    u. contraction
    u. corpus carcinoma
    u. didelphia
    u. didelphys
    u. duplication anomaly
    u. fibroid
    u. fibroid embolization (UFE)
    u. fibroid polyp
    u. fundus
    u. horn
    u. hypoplasia
    u. insufficiency
    u. isthmus
    u. leiomyoma
    u. ligament
    u. mass
    u. myoma
    u. myometrium
    u. opacity
    u. papillary serous carcinoma (UPSC)
    u. retroflexion
    u. sarcoma metastasis
    u. size
    u. synechia
    u. tube
    u. venography
    u. wry neck
utero
    fetal death in u.
    fetal echocardiography in u.
    in u.
uteroabdominal pregnancy

uterocervical canal
uterogram
uterography
uteropelvic
uteroplacental
    u. circulation
    u. insufficiency
uterosacral ligament
uterosalpingogram
uterosalpingography
uterotubal pregnancy
uterotubography
uterovaginal
    u. canal
    u. plexus
uterovesical
    u. fossa
    u. junction
    u. ligament
    u. pouch
uterus, pl. **uteri**
    adenocarcinoma of u.
    anteflexed u.
    anteverted u.
    aplastic u.
    arcuate u.
    u. arcuatus
    bicameral u.
    bicornis u.
    bicornuate u.
    biforate u.
    bilocular u.
    bipartite u.
    bleeding u.
    body of u.
    cervix uteri
    cochleate u.
    cornu of u.
    corpus uteri
    Couvelaire u.
    didelphic u.
    double u.
    double-mouthed u.
    duplex u.
    empty u.
    enlargement of u.
    fetal u.
    fibroid u.
    fundus uteri
    gas gangrene of u.
    gravid u.
    heart-shaped u.
    horn of u.
    infantile u.
    isthmus of u.
    large-for-dates u.
    nonpregnant horn of bicornuate u.
    outer border of u.
    pear-shaped u.

pregnant u.
prostatic u.
pubescent u.
retroflexed u.
retroverted u.
ribbon u.
round ligament of u.
saddle-shaped u.
u. subseptus
T-shaped u.
unicornis unicollis u.
unicornuate u.
urethral u.

utilization
radioiron red cell u.

utricle
large u.

utriculosaccular canal
utriculus prostaticus
U-tube stent
UVA
urethrovesical angle
uveitis
granulomatous u.
uviometer
uvioresistant
uviosensitive
uvula, pl. **uvuli**
u. of bladder
cerebellar u.
musculus u.
u. palatina
uvulopalatoplasty
laser-assisted u. (LAUP)

NOTES

U

V
   lung volume
   vanadium
   ventricular
      V pattern
      V peak of jugular venous pulse
      V sync
V4
   fourth ventricle
V18
      V18 Control Wire guidewire
      V18 guidewire
      V18 micro guidewire
v
   volt
V510B Biplane TEE transducer
V5M Multiplane transducer
VA
   alveolar ventilation
   ventriculoatrial
   vertebral artery
   virtual angioscopy
      VA shunt
va
   volt-ampere
VABES
   vasoablative endothelial sarcoma
Vac-Lok patient immobilization system
VACTERL
   vertebral, anal, cardiac, tracheal,
   esophageal, renal, limb
      VACTERL spectrum
      VACTERL syndrome
vacuolated
vacuole
vacuolization
vacuum
   v. arthrography
   v. cassette system
   v. cleft
   v. disc phenomenon
   v. extraction
   facet joint v.
   v. tube
vacuum-assisted
   v.-a. biopsy
   v.-a. core biopsy
   v.-a. imaging-guided biopsy
vagale
   glomus v.
vagal trunk
vagatomy effect
vagi (*pl. of* vagus)
vagina, pl. **vaginae**
   anterior fornix of v.

   azygos artery of v.
   double v.
   vestibule of v.
vaginal
   v. agenesis
   v. canal
   v. carcinoma
   v. code irradiation
   v. cuff
   v. cylinder
   v. endosonography
   v. fistula
   v. fornix
   v. fundus
   v. intraepithelial neoplasm
   v. ligament
   v. malignant melanoma
   v. orifice
   v. plexus
   v. tumor
   v. wall
vaginalis
   portio v.
   processus v.
   tunica v.
   vestigium processus v.
vaginitis emphysematosa
vaginogram
vaginography
   barium v.
vaginoperineoplasty
vagotomy
vagus, pl. **vagi**
   v. nerve
   v. nerve stimulated functional
      magnetic resonance imaging
      (VNS-fMRI)
   v. nerve stimulation (VNS)
   v. nerve stimulation-synchronized
      blood oxygen level-dependent
      functional MRI
Valdini method
valence
   v. band
   v. bond
   electron v.
   ionic polar v.
valgus
   adolescent hallux v.
   anatomic genu v.
   v. angulation
   bilateral hallux v.
   v. carrying angle
   cubitus v.
   v. deviation

V

valgus *(continued)*
    digitus v.
    v. foot
    hallux v. (HV)
    v. heel deformity
    hindfoot v.
    v. index
    metatarsus v.
    pes malleus v.
    v. stress
    talipes v.
    v. tilt
    unilateral hallux v.
valgus-external rotation injury
vallecula, pl. **valleculae**
    v. cerebelli
vallecular
    v. dysphagia
    v. narrowing
valley-to-peak dose rate
Valsalva
    coronary sinus of V.
    V. maneuver
    V. muscle
    sinus of V.
valsalviana
    dysphagia v.
value
    ADCav v.
    attenuation v.
    bright pixel v.
    comparative v.
    CT attenuation v.
    dark pixel v.
    echo-train v.
    v. flip
    negative predictive v.
    pixel v.
    positive predictive v. (PPV)
    S v.
    soft tissue attenuation v.
    standard uptake v. (SUV)
    time-to-peak v. (TTP)
    tristimulus v.
    T1, T2 v.
    velocity encoding v. (VENC)
    venous blood gas v.
valve
    absent v.
    afferent nipple v.
    Ahmed glaucoma v.
    anterior semilunar v.
    v. anulus
    aortic v. (AoV)
    aortocoronary v.
    v. area
    artificial cardiac v.
    atrioventricular nodal v.
    v. attenuation

    ball-occluder v.
    ball-type v.
    Bauhin v.
    Beall v.
    bicommissural aortic v.
    bicuspid aortic v.
    bicuspid atrioventricular v.
    bileaflet v.
    billowing mitral v.
    biological tissue v.
    Björk-Shiley heart v.
    blunting of v.
    Braunwald-Cutter v.
    Bunsen-type v.
    calcified aortic v.
    capillary v.
    Carbomedics v.
    cardiac v.
    caval v.
    C-C heart v.
    central caged ball occluder v.
    central caged disc occluder v.
    v. cinefluoroscopy
    cleft mitral v.
    v. closure
    Codman Medos programmable v.
    v. commissure
    competent ileocecal v.
    composite aortic v.
    conduit v.
    congenital absence of pulmonary v.
    congenital anomaly of mitral v.
      (CAMV)
    convexoconcave heart v.
    coronary sinus v.
    v. cusp
    v. dehiscence
    v. diameter
    disc-type v.
    doming of v.
    dysplastic pulmonary v.
    early opening of v.
    eccentric monocuspid disc v.
    echo-dense v.
    ectatic aortic v.
    efferent nipple v.
    E-to-F slope of v.
    eustachian v.
    failed v.
    fibroelastoma of heart v.
    fishmouth configuration of
      mitral v.
    flail mitral v.
    flaplike v.
    floppy mitral v.
    flow-controlled v.
    foramen ovale v.
    frenulum of v.
    globular v.

gradient across v.
Harken v.
heart v.
v. of Heister
hockey-stick deformity of
  tricuspid v.
v. of Houston
hypoplastic v.
ileocecal v.
incompetent ileocecal v.
v. leaflet
leaky v.
low-profile mitral v.
lymphatic v.
v. malformation
mechanical v.
Medos Hakim programmable v.
midsystolic buckling of mitral v.
miniaturized mitral v.
mitral v.
monocusp v.
monocuspid tilting disc v.
M-shaped pattern of mitral v.
mural leaflet of mitral v.
narrowed v.
native aortic v.
v. of navicular fossa
neoaortic v.
nonfunctioning heart v.
notching of pulmonic v.
Omniscience v.
v. opening slope
v. outflow strut
parachute deformity of mitral v.
PASV v.
v. plane
v. pocket
posterior urethral v. (PUV)
premature mid diastolic closure of
  mitral v.
preservation of native aortic v.
pressure-activated safety v. (PASV)
programmable ventricular shunt v.
v. prolapse
prolapse of aortic v.
prolapsed mitral v. (PMV)
prosthetic heart v.
prosthetic mitral v.
pullback across aortic v.
pulmonary v.
pulmonic v. (PV)
pyloric v.

quadricuspid aortic v.
quadricuspid pulmonary v.
rectal v.
regurgitant v.
v. replacement
retrograde blood flow across v.
rheumatic heart v.
v. ring
Rosenmüller v.
rotating hemostatic v.
saillike tricuspid v.
semilunar v.
shunt v.
sigmoid v.
Smelloff-Cutter v.
Sophy programmable v.
spiral v.
spongiosa of mitral v.
stenosed aortic v.
stenotic tricuspid v.
stentless porcine aortic v.
stent-mounted allograft v.
stent-mounted heterograft v.
synthetic v.
systolic anterior motion of
  mitral v.
thebesian v.
thickened aortic v.
v. thickening
tilting-disc v.
v. tip
tissue outflow v.
track v.
tricuspid v. (TV)
tricuspid aortic v.
trileaflet aortic v.
truncal v.
v. tube
unicommissural aortic v.
unicuspid with aortic v.
urethral v.
v. vegetation
venous v.
Vieussens v.
v. wrapping
xenograft v.
4-valve-tube rectification
valviform
valvoplasty, valvuloplasty
  balloon mitral v.
valvotome
  spade-shaped v.

NOTES

valvotomy
    balloon v.
valvula, pl. **valvulae**
valvular
    v. aortic insufficiency
    v. aortic stenosis
    v. apparatus
    v. atresia
    v. cardiac defect
    v. damage
    v. disease (VD)
    v. dysfunction
    v. efficiency
    v. heart disease
    v. incompetence
    v. leaflet calcification
    v. opening
    v. orifice
    v. pneumothorax
    v. pulmonic stenosis
    v. regurgitant lesion
    v. regurgitation (VR)
    v. scarring
    v. sclerosis
valvuloplasty (*var. of* valvoplasty)
van
    V. Aman pulmonary pigtail
      catheter
    v. Buchem disease
    v. Buchem syndrome
    V. de Graaf generator
    V. der Hoeve syndrome
    V. Nuys Prognostic Index for
      DCIS
    V. Rosen view
    V. Sonnenberg chest drain set
    V. Sonnenberg sump catheter
vanadium (V)
vanishing
    v. bone disease
    v. lung syndrome
    v. lung tumor
    v. testes syndrome
    v. twins
Vanzetti sign
vaporization
    plaque v.
Vaquez disease
vara
    adolescent tibia v.
    Blount tibia v.
    congenital tibia v.
    coxa v.
    epiphysial coxa v.
    infantile tibia v.
    tibia v.
variability
    anatomic v.
    beat-to-beat v.

    interpretive v.
    intertumoral v.
    intratumoral v.
    peak flow v.
variable
    v. cerebral dysplasia
    v. density SMASH (VD-auto-
      SMASH)
    v. energy
    v. flip-angle excitation
    v. intensity
    v. projection (VARPRO)
    quantitative exercise thallium-201 v.
    v. response rate
    v. segment
    v. stiffness guidewire
    v. temperature (VT)
    v. TE, TR
    v. tube current
    v. tube potential
    v. uptake
variable-angle
    v.-a. gamma camera
    v.-a. spinning (VAS)
    v.-a. uniform signal excitation
      (VUSE)
Varian
    V. accelerator
    V. Associates 11.7-T, 51-mm bore
      spectrometer
    V. brachytherapy system
    V. CT scanner
    V. LINAC
    V. MLC system
    V. NMR spectrometer
variance
    Hulten v.
    v. image
    negative ulnar v.
    neutral ulnar v.
    positive ulnar v.
    ulnar v.
variant
    anatomic bile duct v.
    blastic v.
    congenital mediastinal arterial v.
    v. Creutzfeldt-Jacob disease (vCJD)
    Dandy-Walker v.
    electrocardiographic v.
    fibrosarcoma v.
    Heidenhain v.
    high-riding v.
    labral v.
    mediastinal arterial v.
    normal v.
    ossification v.
    pancreaticobiliary function v.
variation
    anatomic v.

area/hemidiameter v.
B$_O$ field v.
biologic v.
circadian v.
coefficient of v. (c.v.)
v. in density
exposure v.
field v.
interobserver v.
intraobserver v.
low interobserver v.
normal anatomic v.
observer v.
positional v.
pulse width v.
surface dose v.
view-to-view v.

Varibar
V. contrast agent
V. honey barium sulfate
V. nectar barium sulfate
V. oral contrast agent
V. pudding barium sulfate
V. thin honey barium sulfate
V. thin liquid barium sulfate

varication
variceal
v. column
v. decompression
v. hemorrhage
v. sclerosis
v. wall

varices (*pl. of* varix)
ectopic v.
gastric v.

varicocele
idiopathic v.

varicography
varicoid esophageal carcinoma
varicose
v. aneurysm
v. bronchiectasis
v. vein

varicosity
paraovarian v.
reticular v.'s

variegated pattern
variocele tumor of breast
varioliform erosion
VariTone
Varivas loop graft
varix, pl. **varices**

v. of aneurysm
arterial v.
arteriovenous v.
colonic v.
Dagradi classification of
esophageal v.
downhill v.
duodenal v.
ectopic v.
esophageal v.
gastric v.
intraaxial v.
lung v.
Okuda transhepatic obliteration
of v.
orbital v.
paraesophageal v.
pericholedochal v.
pulmonary v.
ruptured pelvic v.
saphenous v.
stomach v.
sublingual v.
umbilical vein v.
uphill v.

VARPRO
variable projection
varum
genu v.
varus
v. angulation
cubitus v.
v. deformity
v. deviation
digitus v.
v. foot
hallux v.
v. heel
mechanical genu v.
v. metatarsophalangeal angle
metatarsus v.
pes v.
rearfoot v.
v. rerotation
v. stress
v. stress laxity
subtalar v.
talipes v.
tibial v.
v. tilt

V

NOTES

varus-valgus
    v.-v. instability
    v.-v. plane
varying degrees of obliquity
VAS
    variable-angle spinning
    vestibular aqueduct syndrome
vas, pl. **vasa**
    v. deferens
vascular
    v. abdominal calcification
    v. abnormality
    v. access device
    v. access safety kit
    v. and airway modeling
    v. anomaly
    v. assessment
    v. band
    v. bed
    v. blood
    v. blood pool
    v. blush
    v. bone
    v. brachytherapy
    v. brain occlusion
    v. bud
    v. bundle
    v. bypass graft
    v. catastrophe
    v. cell adhesion molecule-1
    (VCAM-1)
    v. channel
    v. cirrhosis
    v. colon ectasia
    v. compartment
    v. compromise
    v. congestion
    v. contour
    v. cord damage
    v. encasement
    v. esophageal compression
    v. fibrous polyp
    v. flask
    v. flow imaging
    v. goiter
    v. groove
    v. hamartoma
    v. hemangioma
    v. hemostatic device (VHD)
    v. hydraulic conductivity
    v. hydraulics
    v. impedance
    v. insufficiency
    v. insult
    v. invasion
    v. jejunization
    v. kidney anatomy
    v. leak syndrome
    v. leiomyoma

    v. lesion
    v. lumen
    v. malformation
    v. marking
    v. MR contrast enhancement
    v. myxoma
    v. necrosis
    v. network
    v. obstruction
    v. occlusive disease
    v. origin bone tumor
    v. patency
    v. pedicle
    v. perforation
    v. phase
    v. plexus
    v. protrusion
    v. pterygoid attachment
    v. redistribution
    v. reflection
    v. renal anatomy
    v. reserve
    v. ring
    v. sarcoma
    v. sclerosis
    v. segmentation
    v. segmentation and extraction
    v. shadow
    v. sheath
    v. sling
    v. smooth muscle
    v. space of placenta
    v. spasm
    v. stasis
    v. stent
    v. stroma
    v. structure
    v. supply
    v. systemic resistance
    v. tissue
    v. tone
    v. tracheal compression
    v. transformation
    v. trauma
    v. tuft
    v. villous atrophy
    v. wall
    v. xenograft
    v. zone
vascularity
    decreased pulmonary v.
    femoral head v.
    increased pulmonary v.
    moyamoya v.
    overcirculation v.
    pulmonary v.
    sunburst brain v.
    tumor v.

vascularization
  hand v.
  tumor v.
vascularized granulation tissue
vasculature
  cardiac v.
  cerebral v.
  depiction of v.
  extracranial cerebral v.
  increased pulmonary v.
  interlobular v.
  peripheral v.
  pruned appearance of pulmonary v.
  pulmonary v.
  splanchnic v.
vasculitic lesion
vasculitis
  mesenteric v. (MV)
vasculopathy
  lenticulostriate v. (LSV)
vasoablative endothelial sarcoma (VABES)
vasoactive
  v. intestinal polypeptide tumor (VIPoma)
  v. response
vasoconstriction
  hypoxic pulmonary v.
  peripheral circulatory v.
  peripheral cutaneous v.
  pulmonary arteriolar v.
  spontaneous transient v.
  systemic arterial v.
vasoconstrictor response
vasodepressor response
vasodilating agent
vasodilation
  breakthrough v.
vasodilator administration
vasodilatory
  v. capacity
  v. effect
  v. hemodynamic stress test
  v. response
vasoepididymography
vasogenic
  v. edema
  v. impotence
  v. shock
vasography
vasomotor
  v. change

  v. reaction
  v. symptom
vasoocclusive angiotherapy (VAT)
vasoreactivity
  cerebral v.
  pulmonary v.
vasoregulation
vasorelaxation of epicardial vessel
vasorum
  aortic vasa v.
  vasa v.
VasoSeal
  V. closure device
  V. diagnostic device
  V. Elite
  V. elite vascular closure
  V. ES, VHD arterial puncture site closure device
  V. therapeutic device
vasospasm
  catheter-induced v.
  cerebral v.
  primary v.
vasospastic vessel
vasovagal reaction
VasoView balloon dissection system
vastus
  v. intermedius
  v. lateralis
  v. medialis
  v. medialis advancement (VMΛ)
  v. medialis muscle
VAT
  vasoocclusive angiotherapy
  ventricular activation time
  video-assisted thoracoscopy
  visceral adipose tissue
VATER
  vertebral, anal, tracheal, esophageal, renal
  VATER association
  VATER complex
Vater
  ampulla of V.
  V. diverticulum
  V. duct
  V. fold
  papilla of V.
vaterian segment
vault
  cranial v.
  plantar v.
  rectal v.

V

NOTES

Vaxcel
> V. peripherally inserted catheter
> V. PICC

VAX 4100 system

VB
> virtual bronchoscopy

Vbeam
> V. pulsed dye laser
> V. pulsed dye laser system

VBI
> vertebrobasilar insufficiency

VBR
> ventricle-brain ratio

VC
> vital capacity

VCA
> vertical-center-anterior

VCAM-1
> vascular cell adhesion molecule-1

VCB
> ventricular capture beat

VCE
> vein contrast enhancer

VCF
> ventricular contractility function
> vertebral compression fracture

VCG
> vectorcardiogram

vCJD
> variant Creutzfeldt-Jacob disease
>   pulvinar sign of vCJD

VCMG
> videocystometrography

VCU, VCUG
> voiding cystourethrogram
> voiding cystourethrography

VCUG
> vesicoureterogram
> voiding cystourethrogram

VD
> valvular disease

Vd
> apparent volume of distribution

VD-auto-SMASH
> variable density SMASH

VDI
> venous distensibility index

(V)-dimer captosuccinic acid (DMSA)

VDS
> ventral derotating spinal
>   VDS implant

VDU
> video display unit

VE
> voluntary effort

VEA
> ventricular ectopic activity

VEB
> ventricular ectopic beat

VEC
> velocity-encoded cine
> velocity-encoded cine imaging

VEC-MR
> velocity-encoded cine magnetic
> resonance

vectocardiogram
vectocardiography
vector
> bulk magnetization v.
> expression v.
> v. loop
> v. loop vectorcardiography
> macroscopic magnetization v.
> mean cardiac v.
> net magnetization v.
> nonviral v.
> QRS v.
> v. quantitization
> spin v.
> v. subtraction
> T v.

vectorcardiogram (VCG)
vectorcardiography
> Frank v.
> frontal plane v.
> v. imaging
> sagittal plane v.
> spatial v.
> transverse plane v.
> vector loop v.

vegetation
> dendritic v.
> friable v.
> heart valve v.
> valve v.

vegetative lesion
veil
> tissue v.

veiling glare
vein
> absent peripheral v.
> accessory cephalic v.
> accessory hemiazygos v.
> accessory hepatic v.
> accessory saphenous v.
> accessory vertebral v.
> accompanying v.
> adrenal v.
> anal v.
> anastomotic v.
> aneurysmal v.
> angular v.
> anonymous v.
> antebrachial v.
> antecubital v.
> anterior cardiac v.
> anterior internal vertebral v.
>   (AIVV)

anterior jugular v.
anterior terminal v. (ATV)
aplasia of deep v.
appendicular v.
aqueous v.
arciform v.
arcuate v.
arterial v.
v., artery, nerve
ascending lumbar v.
auditory v.
auricular v.
autogenous v.
axillary v.
azygos v.
basal placenta v.
basilic v.
basivertebral v.
blind percutaneous puncture of
  subclavian v.
Boyd perforating v.
brachial v.
brachiocephalic v.
brain bridging v.
branches of v.
bronchial v.
bulb of v.
Burrow v.
cannulated central v.
capacious v.
capillary v.
cardiac v.
cardinal v.
carotid v.
caudate v.
cavernous transfer of portal v.
cavernous transformation of
  portal v.
central v.
cephalic v.
cerebral v.
cervical v.
choroid v.
chronic insufficiency of v.
ciliary v.
circumaortic left renal v.
circumflex v.
colic v.
common basal v.
common cardinal v.
common facial v.
common femoral v.

communicating v.
companion v.
condylar emissary v.
congenital stenosis of pulmonary v.
conjunctival v.
v. contrast enhancer (VCE)
coronary v.
cortical v.
costoaxillary v.
cutaneous v.
cystic v.
deep v.
dense abdominal v.'s
digital v.
v. dilatation
dilated collateral v.
diploic v.
distended v.
dorsal penile v.
dorsispinal v.
dual popliteal v.
duodenal v.
embryonal v.
embryonic umbilical v.
emissary v.
engorged v.
epigastric v.
episcleral v.
esophageal v.
ethmoidal v.
external jugular v. (EJV)
external pudendal v.
extirpation of saphenous v.
extradural vertebral plexus of v.
facial v.
familial varicose v.
feeder v.
femoral v.
fibular v.
flat neck v.
frontal v.
v. of Galen malformation
gastric v.
gastroepiploic v.
v. graft
v. graft occlusion
v. graft stenosis
v. graft thrombosis
great cardiac v.
greater saphenous v.
harvested v.
hemiazygos v.

V

NOTES

vein *(continued)*

hemispheric v.
hepatic v.
ileocolic v.
iliac v.
iliofemoral v.
inferior mesenteric v.
inferior ophthalmic v.
inferior pulmonary v.
inferior rectal v.
inferior thyroid v.
v. inflammation
infradiaphragmatic v.
innominate v.
intercostal v.
internal cerebral v. (ICV)
internal jugular v. (IJV)
internal thoracic v.
intraforaminal v.
intrahepatic umbilical v.
v. intussusception
jugular v.
Labbé v.
labial v.
leaking v.
left hepatic v. (LHV)
left pulmonary v. (LPV)
left retroaortic renal v.
lesser saphenous v.
lobe of azygos v.
marginal v.
Marshall v.
median antebrachial v.
mediastinal v.
medullary v.
meningeal v.
mesencephalic v.
mesenteric v.
middle cardiac v.
middle hepatic v. (MHV)
middle rectal v.
v. nodularity
oblique v.
ophthalmic v.
orbital varix ophthalmic v.
ovarian v.
palmar cutaneous v.
pancreatic v.
parathyroid v.
paraumbilical v.
parent v.
v. patency
patency and valvular reflux of
  deep v.
penile v.
perforating v.
pericallosal v.
pericardiacophrenic v.
pericardial v.

perithyroid v.
peroneal v.
petrosal v.
pontomesencephalic v.
popliteal v.
portal v.
posterior auricular v.
posterior cardinal v.
posterior interventricular v.
posterior tibial v.
precentral cerebellar v.
prepyloric v.
pudendal v.
pulmonary v.
pulsating v.
quadrigeminal v.
ranine v.
renal v.
retroaortic renal v.
Retzius v.
reversed greater saphenous v.
right hepatic v. (RHV)
right pulmonary v. (RPV)
saphenous v.
Sappey inferior v.
sausaging of v.
Schlesinger v.
Schwartz test for patency of deep
  saphenous v.'s
scimitar v.
scrotal v.
segmental v.
septal v.
Servelle v.
simultaneous acquisition of artery
  and v. (SAAV)
single popliteal v.
sludging of retinal v.
small cardiac v.
small saphenous v.
soleal v.
spermatic v.
splenic v.
v. stone
striate v.
subcardinal v.
subclavian v.
subclavian-innominate v.
subcutaneous v.
subependymal v.
superficial femoral v.
superficial pedal v.
superior intercostal v.
superior mesenteric v. (SMV)
superior ophthalmic v.
superior pulmonary v.
superior rectal v.
supracardinal v.
systemic v.

testicular v.
thalamic v.
thalamostriate v.
thebesian v.
thoracoepigastric v.
tibial v.
tortuous v.
transcerebral medullary v.
v. of Trolard
umbilical v.
v. valve wrapping
varicose v.
vermian v.
vertebral v.
vela (*pl. of* velum)
velamentous
    v. insertion
    v. insertion of cord
    v. placenta
velamentum
velar
Velcro strap immobilizer
veliform
vellus
velocimetry
    laser Doppler v.
    UA v.
    umbilical artery v.
velocity
    acoustic v.
    angular v.
    v. artifact
    blood flow v.
    v. calculation
    carotid v.
    closing v.
    v. compensation
    coronary blood flow v. (CBFV)
    decreased closing v.
    diastolic regurgitant v.
    v. distribution function (F(v))
    v. encoding on brain MR
      angiography
    v. encoding value (VENC)
    fiber-shortening v.
    flow v.
    forward v.
    v. gradient
    high v.
    v. imaging
    impact v.
    intrasac spectral Doppler flow v.

main portal vein peak v. (MPPv)
v. mapping
maximal transaortic jet v.
mean aortic flow v.
mean posterior wall v.
mean pulmonary flow v.
midshunt peak v. (MSPv)
mitral inflow v.
modal v.
muzzle v.
neurologic sequelae
peak aortic flow v.
peak early diastolic filling v.
peak late diastolic filling v.
peak pulmonary flow v.
peak regurgitant flow v.
peak systolic v. (PSV)
peak transmitted v.
portal vein v.
v. profile
regurgitant v.
retrograde blood v.
v. spectrum
TCD v.
transcranial Doppler v.
v. waveform (VWF)
velocity-compensating gradient pulse
velocity-density imaging
velocity-encoded
    v.-e. cine (VEC)
    v.-e. cine imaging (VEC)
    v.-e. cine magnetic resonance
     (VEC-MR)
    v.-e. cine MRI
    v.-e. cine MR imaging
    v.-e. color Doppler signal
    v.-e. color Doppler sonography
    v.-e. image
    v.-e. sequence
velocity-evaluation phantom
velocity-induced phase shift
velocity-time graph
velolaryngeal endoscopy
velopharyngeal
    v. closure
    v. insufficiency
velopharynx
Velpeau
    V. axillary view
    V. deformity
velum, pl. **vela**
vena, pl. **venae**

NOTES

vena (*continued*)
   v. cava
   v. cava anomaly
   v. caval filter
   v. comitans
venacavagram
venacavography
   inferior v. (IVCV)
venae (*pl. of* vena)
Vena Tech
   V. T. LGM filter
   V. T. LGM vena cava filter
   V. T. low-profile filter
   V. T. LP vena cava filter
VENC
   velocity encoding value
venereum
   lymphogranuloma v.
venetian blind artifact
venoarterial cannulation
venobiliary fistula
venocavogram, venacavogram
venodilator
venofibrosis
venogram
   magnetic resonance v. (MRV)
   renal v.
venography
   adrenal v.
   antegrade v.
   ascending contrast v.
   cerebral CT v.
   contrast v.
   conventional v.
   CT pulmonary v. (CTPV)
   descending v.
   digital free hepatic v.
   direct v.
   direct spiral computed
    tomography v.
   epidural v.
   extradural v.
   free hepatic v.
   gonadal v.
   hepatic v.
   iliac v.
   v. imaging
   impedance v.
   intraosseous v.
   isotope v.
   limb v.
   lower extremity CT v. (LE-CTV)
   lower limb v.
   magnetic resonance v. (MRV)
   neuro phase-contrast v.
   ovarian v.
   peripheral v.
   portal v.
   radionuclear v.

   radionuclide v.
   renal v.
   selective v.
   spermatic v.
   splenic portal v.
   splenoportal v.
   subtraction v.
   technetium-99m v.
   testicular v.
   transjugular v.
   transosseous v.
   ultrasound v.
   uterine v.
   vertebral v.
   wedged hepatic v.
venography-related
   v.-r. air embolism
   v.-r. arrhythmia
   v.-r. thrombophlebitis
venolobar syndrome
venolymphatic
Venoscope
   Landry vein light V.
venospasm
venostasis
venosum
   foramen v.
venosus
   ductus v.
   sinus v.
venotomy
venous
   v. access device
   v. anatomy
   v. aneurysm
   v. angiocardiography
   v. angioma
   v. angioplasty
   v. anomaly
   v. aortography
   v. avulsion
   v. backflow
   v. blood
   v. blood gas value
   v. brain angiography
   v. brain angle
   v. bypass graft
   v. calcification
   v. cannulation
   v. capillary
   v. circulation
   v. collateral
   v. contamination
   v. decompression
   v. defect
   v. distensibility index (VDI)
   v. distention
   v. Doppler examination
   v. drainage

v. edema
v. embolism
v. filling time (VFT)
v. fistulogram
v. groove
v. heart congestion
v. hemangioma
v. hemorrhage
v. hyperemia
v. hypertension
v. imaging
v. infarct
v. injection
v. insufficiency
v. interposition graft
v. intraplacental lake
v. intravasation
v. intussusception
v. junction
v. ligament
v. malformation of the tongue
v. motion
v. neck angle
v. network
v. obstruction
v. occlusion
v. occlusive disease
v. overlay
v. oxygen content
v. phase
v. plethysmography
v. plexus
v. pooling
v. pouch
v. pressure
v. refill time (VRT)
v. return
v. return time
right subclavian central v. (RSCVP)
v. scan
v. sclerosis
v. segment
v. sheath
v. sinus
v. sinus flow void
v. sinus thrombosis
v. skull lake
v. spasm
v. stasis
v. statis syndrome
v. stenting

systemic v.
v. thromboembolic disease (VTED)
v. thromboembolization
v. thrombolysis
v. thrombosis embolus
v. thrombotic disease
v. ulcer
v. ultrasonography
v. valve
v. vascular malformation
v. ventricle
v. waveform
v. web
venovenous cannulation
vent
pulmonary arterial v.
thoracic v.
ventilation
airway pressure release v.
alveolar v. (VA)
v. defect
high-minute v.
v. image
v. lung scan
mask v.
maximal voluntary v. (MVV)
mechanical v.
minute v.
partial liquid v.
v. pneumonitis
pulmonary perfusion and v.
v. radionuclide
reduced alveolar v.
regional v.
v. scintigraphy
v. scintigraphy equilibrium phase
v. study
uneven v.
volume-controlled inverse ratio v.
volume-cycled v.
ventilation-perfusion (V/Q)
v.-p. defect
v.-p. imaging
impaired v.-p.
v.-p. inequality
v.-p. lung scan
v.-p. mismatch
v.-p. pulmonary scintigraphy
v.-p. ratio
ventilator
babyPAC v.
SLE 2000 v.

V

NOTES

ventilatory
- v. capacity-demand imbalance
- v. dysfunction
- v. effort
- v. failure

venting of heart

ventosa
- spina v.

ventrad

ventral
- v. aorta
- v. aspect
- v. branch
- v. bridge
- v. cochlear nucleus
- v. decubitus position
- v. derotating spinal (VDS)
- v. derotating spinal implant
- v. duct of Wirsung
- v. epidural abscess
- v. epidural fat
- v. hernia
- v. hernia defect
- v. horn
- v. mesentery
- v. muscle
- v. occipitotemporal (visual) cortex (VOTC)
- v. pancreas
- v. pancreatic anlage
- v. pancreatic bud
- v. pontine infarct
- v. primary ramus
- v. root
- v. sacrococcygeal ligament
- v. sacroiliac ligament
- v. spinocerebellar tract
- v. spinothalamic tract
- v. surface
- v. venous pressure line

ventralward

ventricle
- absent v.
- akinetic left v.
- aortic vestibule of v.
- Arantius v.
- atrialized v.
- augmented filling of right v.
- auxiliary v.
- backrush of blood into left v.
- ballooned floor of v.
- v. batwing appearance
- batwing configuration of v.
- bulb of occipital horn of lateral v.
- bulb of posterior horn of lateral v.
- cephalic v.
- cerebral v.
- colloid cyst of third v.

- compensatory enlargement of v.
- dilatation of v.
- dilated v.
- double-inlet left v.
- double-inlet single v.
- double-outlet both v.'s (DOBV)
- double-outlet left v. (DOLV)
- double-outlet right v. (DORV)
- dual v.
- v. effacement
- elongation of v.
- enlargement of v.
- fifth v.
- floor of v.
- fourth v. (V4)
- fractional shortening of left v.
- frontal horn of lateral v.
- Galen v.
- high-riding third v.
- hourglass v.
- hyperdynamic fourth v.
- hypokinetic left v.
- hypoplastic heart v.
- hypoplastic left v.
- hypoplastic right v.
- v. impedance adapter
- inflow tract of left v.
- ipsilateral lateral v.
- laryngeal v.
- v. of larynx
- lateral v.
- left v.
- loculated v.
- Morgagni v.
- morphologic left v.
- native v.
- outflow of v.
- papilloma of fourth v.
- parchment right v.
- partial obliteration of lateral v.
- pineal v.
- primitive v.
- right v.
- roof of fourth v.
- v. root
- rudimentary v.
- shift of v.
- single v.
- sixth v.
- slit v.
- Sylvius v.
- temporal horn of lateral v.
- terminal v.
- thick-walled v.
- third v.
- thrusting v.
- tiny v.
- trigone of v.
- tubular v.

venous v.
Verga v.
ventricle-brain ratio (VBR)
1-ventricle heart
ventricose
ventricular (V)
v. aberration
v. activation time (VAT)
v. apex
v. aqueduct
v. assist device
v. atresia
v. atrium
v. block
v. branch
v. canal
v. capture beat (VCB)
v. catheter blockage
v. cavity
v. cineangiogram
v. cleft
v. contractility function (VCF)
v. contraction pattern
v. decompensation
v. depression
v. disproportion
v. D-loop
v. drainage
v. dysfunction
v. dysplasia
v. echo
v. ectopic activity (VEA)
v. ectopic beat (VEB)
v. effective refractory period
(VERP)
v. ejection fraction
v. electrical instability
v. encasement
v. end-diastolic volume
v. endomyocardial biopsy
v. enlargement
v. escape mechanism
v. failure
v. filling
v. free wall
v. free wall rupture
v. free wall thickness
v. function curve
v. function equilibrium image
v. function parameter
v. gradient
v. horn

v. hypertrophy
v. index (VI)
v. intracerebral hemorrhage
v. inversion
v. irritability
v. isovolumic relaxation time
v. left-handedness
v. ligament
v. loop
v. mass
v. muscle necrosis
v. myocardium
v. myxoma
v. obstruction
v. outflow tract
v. outlet
v. output
v. paroxysmal tachycardia
v. perforation
v. preexcitation
v. premature beat (VPB)
v. premature complex (VPC)
v. premature contraction (VPC)
v. premature contraction couplet
v. premature depolarization (VPD)
v. pressure
v. pseudoperfusion beat
v. rate
v. repolarization
v. reserve
v. response
v. rhythm
v. right-handedness
v. segmental contraction
v. septal aneurysm
v. septal defect (VSD)
v. septal rupture
v. septal summit
v. septum (VS)
v. shift
v. size
v. soft tissue
v. space
v. span
v. standstill
v. stiffness
v. synchrony
v. system
v. systole
v. transposition
v. trigeminy
v. tumor

V

NOTES

ventricular *(continued)*
- v. underloading
- v. view
- v. wall dilatation
- v. wall motion
- v. wall motion echocardiography

ventricularization of pressure
ventriculoarterial
- v. conduit
- v. connection

ventriculoatrial (VA)
- v. block
- v. conduction
- v. interval
- v. shunt
- v. time-out

ventriculocele
ventriculocisternostomy
ventriculofugal artery
ventriculogmegaly
ventriculogram
- axial left anterior oblique v.
- bicycle exercise radionuclide v.
- biplane v.
- cine left v.
- contrast v.
- digital subtraction v.
- dipyridamole thallium v.
- exercise radionuclide v.
- gated blood pool v.
- gated nuclear v.
- gated radionuclide v.
- intraoperative v.
- iohexol CT v.
- left v. (LVG)
- left anterior oblique projection v.
- metrizamide v.
- radionuclide v. (RNV, RVG)
- retrograde left v.
- right anterior oblique position v.
- xenon-133 v.

ventriculography
- bubble v.
- cardiac v.
- v. catheter
- cerebral v.
- first-pass radionuclide v.
- isotope v.

ventriculoinfundibular fold
ventriculomegaly
- ex vacuo v.
- fetal v.
- teardrop v.

ventriculoperitoneal (VP)
- v. diversion
- v. shunt

ventriculoradial dysplasia
ventriculostomy

ventriculotomy
- map-guided partial endocardial v.

ventriculus cordis
ventricumbent
ventriduct
ventriduction
ventriflexion
ventrimesal
ventrimeson
ventrodorsad
ventrodorsal
ventroinguinal
ventrolateral
ventromedial hypothalamic hamartoma
ventromedian
ventroposterior
ventrose
VentTrak monitoring system
Venturi effect
venule
- high endothelial v.
- postcapillary v.

venulitis
- cutaneous necrotizing v.

vera
- vertebra v.

verae
- costae v.

Verga
- V. lacrimal groove
- V. ventricle

vergae
- septum cavum v.

verge
- anal v.

vergence
- downward v.

Verluma diagnostic imaging agent
vermetoid
vermian
- v. agenesis
- v. hypoplasia
- v. medulloblastoma
- v. pseudotumor
- v. vein

vermian-cerebellar hypoplasia
vermicular
- v. appendage
- v. appendix

vermiform
- v. appendix
- v. process

verminous aneurysm
vermis
- cerebellar v.
- folium v.
- v. hypoplasia

vermography
vernal edema

Verner-Morrison syndrome
Verneuil canal
vernix membrane
Verocay body
VERP
    ventricular effective refractory period
verruciform
verruciformis
verrucose
verrucosus
    nevus v.
verrucous
    v. carcinoma
    v. hemangioma
Versadopp ultrasonic Doppler probe
VersaLight laser
VersaPulse holmium laser
Versatome
    V. D8 Perioperative Doppler
     System
    V. laser
verse
    inclination v.
versive motor
vertebra, pl. **vertebrae**
    abdominal v.
    accordion v.
    anterior scalloping of v.
    articular process of v.
    basilar v.
    beaked v.
    block v.
    body of v.
    bone-within-bone v.
    bony projection from v.
    bullet-shaped v.
    butterfly v.
    butterfly-wing v.
    caudal v.
    cervical v.
    cleft v.
    coccygeal v.
    codfish v.
    coin-on-edge v.
    coronal cleft v.
    cranial v.
    v. dentata
    displaced v.
    dorsal v.
    facet surface of v.
    false v.
    fishmouth v.

fishtail v.
focal subluxation of vertebrae
fractured v.
fused vertebrae
great terminal v.
honeycomb v.
hooked v.
hourglass v.
H-shaped v.
ivory v.
last normal v. (LNV)
limbus v.
v. lumbales
lumbar v. (L)
v. magnum
mature v.
midbody of v.
movable v.
non-rib-bearing v.
notched v.
odontoid v.
pedicle of v.
picture frame v.
v. plana
posterior scalloping of v.
primitive v.
prominent v.
rib-bearing v.
rugger jersey v.
sacral v.
sandwich v.
saucerization of v.
solitary collapsed v.
v. spuriae
sternal v.
subluxed v.
tail v.
thoracic v.
toothed v.
transitional v.
transverse process of v.
tricuspid v.
true v.
v. vera
wedge-shaped v.
vertebral
    v., anal, cardiac, tracheal,
     esophageal, renal, limb
     (VACTERL)
    v., anal, tracheal, esophageal, renal
     (VATER)
    v. angiography

V

NOTES

vertebral *(continued)*
    v. ankylosis
    v. arch
    v. arch ligament ossification
    v. arterial dissection
    v. arteriography
    v. artery (VA)
    v. artery fenestration
    v. artery of Henry
    v. artery occlusion
    v. artery segment V0-V4
    v. artery stenosis
    v. artery syndrome
    v. artery system
    v. articular sinus
    v. body alignment
    v. body bone tumor
    v. body collapse
    v. body endplate
    v. body fracture
    v. body height
    v. body index
    v. body line
    v. body margin
    v. body marrow signal intensity
    v. body ossification center
    v. body overgrowth
    v. body plate
    v. body ratio method
    v. body retrolisthesis
    v. body retropulsion
    v. body shape
    v. body size
    v. border abnormality
    v. canal
    v. chordoma
    v. column
    v. compression fracture (VCF)
    v. cross-section
    v. disc
    v. disc interspace
    v. endplate abnormality
    v. epiphysitis
    v. expansile lesion
    v. foramen
    v. fusion
    v. groove
    v. hemangioma
    v. hyperostosis
    v. lamina
    v. osteochondrosis
    v. osteomyelitis
    v. part of diaphragm
    v. plana fracture
    v. process
    v. rib
    v. scalloping
    v. segmentation anomaly

    v. spine
    v. steal phenomenon
    v. stripe
    v. vein
    v. venography
    v. venous plexus
    v. wedge compression fracture
    v. wedging
vertebrobasilar
    v. artery
    v. artery occlusion
    v. artery syndrome
    v. circulation
    v. complex
    v. disease
    v. distribution stroke
    v. dolichoectasia
    v. insufficiency (VBI)
    v. ischemia
    v. occlusion
    v. system
    v. transcranial color-coded duplex
      ultrasonography
vertebrocostal
    v. rib
    v. triangle
    v. trigone
vertebrojugular fistula
vertebromammary diameter
vertebropelvic ligament
vertebrophrenic angle
vertebroplasty
    percutaneous v.
    transpedicular v.
vertebrospinous process
vertebrosternal rib
vertebrovertebral fistula
vertex, pl. **vertices**
    v. of bony cranium
    V. camera
    v. corneae
    v. cranii
    v. cranii ossei
    cube v.
    v. presentation
vertical
    v. axis
    v. diameter
    v. heart
    v. long-axis slice
    v. muscle
    v. partial laryngectomy
    v. plane
    posterior temporal v. (PTV)
    v. ray
    v. shear fracture
    v. split nondetached tear
    v. synchronization pulse

v. talus
v. talus foot deformity
vertical-center-anterior (VCA)
v.-c.-a. angle
verticalis
vertical-long axis
vertices (*pl. of* vertex)
verticillate
verticomental
verticosubmental
v. position
v. projection
v. view
vertigo/orthostatic dysregulation
vertigraphy
VERT software
vesalian bone
vesalianum of vertebral body
Vesalius
foramen of V.
vesical
v. distention
v. diverticulum
v. fascia
v. fistula
v. injury
v. neck
v. outlet obstruction
v. stone formation
v. venous plexus
vesicancy
vesicant
vesicatory
vesicle
acoustic v.
acrosomal v.
air v.
allantoic v.
auditory v.
brain region v.
v. calculus
cerebral v.
cervical v.
encephalic v.
graafian v.
grapelike v.
malpighian v.
metanephric v.
pulmonary v.
seminal v.
synaptic v.
vesicocolic fistula

vesicorectal
vesicosacral ligament
vesicoumbilical ligament
vesicoureteral
v. reflux (VUR)
v. scintigraphy
vesicoureteric reflux
vesicoureterogram (VCUG)
vesicourethral
v. angle
v. canal
vesicouterine
v. ligament
v. pouch
vesicovaginal fistula
vesicula
vesicular
v. amine transporter
v. block
v. bronchiolitis
v. emphyscma
v. lymph node
v. pattern
vesiculogram
vesiculography
v. imaging
seminal v.
vesiculosa appendix
vessel, pl. **vessels**
abdominal great v.
aberrant v.
absorbent v.
afferent lymph v.
angiographically occult v.
anomalous v.
antegrade filling of v.
arcuate v.
atraumatic occlusion of v.
axillary v.
beading of v.
blood v.
brachiocephalic v.
bronchial v.
v. caliber
capillary v.
cephalized v.
cerebral blood v.
chyle v.
chyliferous v.
circumflex v.
codominant v.
collateral v.

NOTES

V

vessel *(continued)*
  collecting v.
  commencement of v.
  complex of v.
  contralateral v.
  corkscrew v.
  coursing v.
  cranial v.
  cross-pelvic collateral v.
  culprit v.
  curved v.
  v. cutoff of contrast material
  deep lymphatic v.
  v. diameter
  diminutive v.
  disease-free v.
  displacement of brain v.
  v. displacement brain infection
  distal runoff v.
  dominant v.
  eccentric v.
  efferent lymph v.
  end-on v.
  enlarged pulmonary v.
  extracranial v.
  feeding v.
  femoropopliteal v.
  fenestrated v.
  v. filling
  gastroepiploic v.
  great v.
  hairpin v.
  heart and great vessels
  hilar v.
  ileocolic v.
  iliac v.
  uncoiling of the great vessels
  increased prominence of
    pulmonary v.
  infrapopliteal v.
  in-plane v.
  intercostal v.
  interlobular v.
  internal pudendal v.
  intimal attachment of diseased v.
  intracranial v.
  intradural v.
  kidney v.
  lacteal v.
  lenticulostriate v.
  v. loop
  lymphatic v.
  lymphocapillary v.
  mesenteric v.
  mesocolonic v.
  minute v.
  musculophrenic v.
  native v.
  nondominant v.

  occipital v.
  v. occlusion
  origin of v.
  parent v.
  patency of v.
  patent v.
  pelvic collateral v.
  penile v.
  perforator v.
  perfusate v.
  pericallosal v.
  peripelvic collateral v.
  peripheral v.
  peroneal v.
  pial v.
  plump v.
  pole of v.
  portosystemic collateral v.
  posterior lumbar v.
  proximal and distal portion of v.
  pulmonary v.
  radicular v.
  reduced prominence of
    pulmonary v.
  renal hilar v.
  v. reshaping by angioplasty
  retroesophageal v.
  retroperitoneal lymphatic v.
  retrotracheal v.
  v. runoff
  v. rupture
  splanchnic v.
  splenic v.
  subclavian v.
  superficial lymphatic v.
  superior gluteal v.
  takeoff of v.
  telangiectatic v.
  v. topography
  v. tortuosity
  tortuosity of cervical v.
  tortuous v.
  v. tracing
  v. tracking
  transposition of great v.
  v. trauma
  vasorelaxation of epicardial v.
  vasospastic v.
  vestigial v.
  v. wall abnormality
  Windkessel v.
  wraparound v.

2-vessel
  2-v. runoff
  2-v. umbilical cord

3-vessel
  3-v. coronary disease
  3-v. multiple projection biplane
    angiography

3-v. runoff
3-v. umbilical cord
4-vessel
4-v. arteriography
4-v. cerebral angiography
4-v. multiple projection biplane angiography
VEST
virtual endoscopic surgery trainer
VEST system
vest
Bremer AirFlo V.
halo v.
immobilizing v.
vestibula (*pl. of* vestibulum)
vestibular
v. apparatus
v. aqueduct
v. aqueduct syndrome (VAS)
v. canal
v. division of eighth cranial nerve
v. ganglion
v. labyrinth
v. ligament
v. schwannoma
v. window
vestibule
anatomic esophageal v.
esophageal v.
inner ear v.
large v.
laryngeal v.
v. of larynx
v. of vagina
vestibulocochlear nerve
vestibulogenic
vestibulospinal tract
vestibulum, pl. **vestibula**
vestige
coccygeal v.
vestigial
v. commissure
v. fold
v. left sinuatrial node
v. vessel
vestigium, pl. **vestigia**
v. processus vaginalis
V-Flex Plus stent
VFT
venous filling time

VHD
vascular hemostatic device
VHD closure device
VHL
von Hippel-Lindau
VI
ventricular index
Viabahn
V. covered stent
V. endoprosthesis
Viabil
V. biliary endoprosthesis
V. stent
viability
myocardial tissue v.
tissue v.
viable
v. fetus
v. myocardium
vial
multidose v.
reaction v.
VIATORR
V. Endoprosthesis
V. transjugular intrahepatic portosystemic shunt stent graft
Viatronix Virtual Colonoscopy system
VIA 7991 ventricle impedance adapter
VIBE
volumetric interpolated breath-hold examination
VIBE sequence
vibex, pl. **vibices**
vibrating-reed electrometer
vibration
v. frequency
lattice v.
molecular v.
vibratory motion
Vibrio
vibroacoustography
vicarious contrast excretion
Victoreen dosimeter
Vidar scanner
video
v. barium swallow
v. cystourethrography
v. densitometer
v. digital gastrointestinal radiography
v. display camera
v. display unit (VDU)

NOTES

video *(continued)*
    v. electroencephalography
      monitoring
    v. pill camera
    v. proctogram
    v. signal generator
videoangiography
    digital v.
video-assisted thoracoscopy (VAT)
videoconferencing
    teleradiology v.
videocystometrography (VCMG)
videodensitometric
videodensitometry
videodensity curve
videofluoroscopic imaging
videofluoroscopy
    spinal v.
videognosis
videolaseroscopy
videometry
videomicroscopy
videoradiography
video-rate two-photon laser scanning
    microscope
videotape study
videothoracoscopy
vidian
    v. artery
    v. canal
    v. nerve
vidicon
Vidicon camera tube
Vieussens
    ansa of V.
    V. anulus
    circle of V.
    isthmus of V.
    limbus of V.
    V. loop
    ring of V.
    V. valve
view *(See viewing)*
    abdominal v.
    afferent v.
    air-contrast v.
    Alexander v.
    amputated-foot v.
    angiographic system for unlimited
      rolling field-of-v.'s (angioSURF)
    angled craniocaudal v.
    anterior feet v.
    anterior-posterior, posterior-
      anterior v.
    anteroposterior v.
    apical lordotic v.
    apical and subcostal 4-
      chambered v.
    AP inversion stress vagina v.

AP supine portable v.
Arcelin v.
axial sesamoid v.
axillary tail v.
ball catcher v.
basal short-axis v.
base v.
baseline v.
beam's eye v. (BEV)
Beath v.
bicipital groove v.
biplane orthogonal v.
bird's eye v.
v. box
Broden v.
brow-down skull v.
brow-up skull v.
Bucky v.
bull's eye v.
Caldwell v.
Caldwell occipitofrontal v.
cardiac long axis v.
cardiac short axis v.
carpal tunnel v.
Carter-Rowe v.
caudal v.
caudocranial tangential v.
cephalic tilt v.
cerebellar v.
cervical spine dens v.
4-chamber apical v.
Chamberlain-Towne v.
change-of-angle v.
Chassard-Lapiné v.
Chausse v.
Chaussier v.
chest v.
cine v.
cineradiographic v.
classic carpal tunnel v.
clenched fist v.
Cleopatra v.
closed-mouth v.
close-up v.
coalition v.
comparison v.
coned-down v.
coned-down compression v.
cone spot compression v.
contact lateral v.
coronal bending v.
coronal reconstruction v.
couch v.
cranial angled v.
craniocaudal v.
cross-table lateral v. (CTLV)
decubitus v.
3D endoluminal v.
dens v.

dorsal v.
dorsiflexion v.
dorsoplantar v.
Dunlop-Shands v.
efferent v.
Eklund v.
endoluminal v.
en face v.
equilibrium v.
erect v.
exaggerated craniocaudal v.
expiration v.
expiratory v.
extended field of v.
extension v.
external rotation v.
fan-shaped v.
fast spin-echo v.
FCS v.
femoral v.
Ferguson v.
fetal echocardiographic v.
field of v. (FOV)
first-pass v.
Fleckinger v.
flexion and extension v.'s
fluoroscopic v.
follow-through v.
frogleg lateral v.
frontal v.
Fuchs odontoid v.
full cervical spine v.
full column v.
full length v.
Garth v.
gated v.
Granger v.
Grashey shoulder v.
great vessel v.
half-axial v.
Hampton v.
Harris v.
Harris-Beath axial hindfoot v.
heavily penetrated v.
Heinig v.
hemiaxial v.
hepatoclavicular v.
hip-to-ankle v.
Hobb v.
Hughston v.
ice-pick v.
infrapatellar v.

inspiration and expiration v.'s
inspiratory v.
v. insufficiency artifact
internal and external rotation v.'s
intraoperative v.
inversion ankle stress v.
Jones v.
Jude pelvic v.
Judet v.
knee v.
KUB v.
kyphotic v.
large field of v. (LFV)
lateral anterior drawer stress v.
lateral bending v.
lateral decubitus v.
lateral extension v.
lateral flexion v.
lateral oblique v.
lateral tilt stress ankle v.
lateromedial oblique v.
Laurin x-ray v.
Law v.
Lawrence v.
left anterior oblique v.
limited v.
long axial oblique v.
long axis parasternal v.
longitudinal ultrasound v.
lordotic v.
Low-Beers v.
lumbar spine v.
magnification v.
Mayer v.
medial oblique v.
mediolateral v.
mediolateral oblique v.
Merchant v.
v. microtomography
mortise v.
MPR v.
multiplanar reformatting v.
navicular v.
Neer lateral v.
Neer transscapular v.
nonforeshortened angiographic v.
nonstanding lateral oblique v.
nonweightbearing v.
normal anteroposterior v.
notch v.
oblique v.
occipital v.

NOTES

view *(continued)*

odontoid v.
open-mouth odontoid v.
optimally positioned v.
orthogonal v.
outlet v.
overcouch v.
overhead oblique v.
Owen v.
panoramic v.
Panorex v.
pantomographic v.
parallax v.
parasternal long-axis v.
parasternal short-axis v.
patellar skyline v.
pelvic v.
v. per segment (VPS)
Pillar v.
plain v.
planar v.
2-plane v.
plantar axial v.
plantar flexion stress v.
plumbline v.
portable v.
posterior skull v.
posteroanterior v.
posterooblique v.
postevacuation v.
postoperative v.
postreduction v.
postvoid v.
preliminary v.
preoperative v.
prereduction v.
profile ray v.
prone angled v.
prone lateral v.
push-pull ankle stress v.
push-pull hip v.
ray-sum v.
rear endoluminal v.
reconstruction v.
rectangular field of v.
recumbent v.
replacing oblique v.
retroflexed v.
retromammary space v.
Rhese v.
rib v.
right anterior oblique v.
right lateral decubitus v.
right ventricular inflow v.
Rokus v.
rolled v.
room's eye v. (REV)
rotated craniocaudal v.
routine magnification v.

Rumstrom v.
sagittal and coronal
  reconstruction v.
sagittal magnetization transfer v.
Schatzki v.
Schüller v.
scottie dog v.
scout v.
selective coronary arteriography v.
semiupright v.
serendipity v.
v. shadow projection
  microtomographic system
short axis parasternal v.
single-breath v.
sitting-up v.
ski jump v.
skyline v.
spider x-ray v.
spot compression v.
standing dorsoplantar v.
standing false profile v.
standing lateral v.
standing postvoid v.
standing weight-bearing v.
static v.
steep left anterior oblique v.
Stenver v.
stereoscopic v.
sternal v.
stress Broden v.
stress eversion v.
stress inversion v.
Stryker notch v.
subcostal 4-chamber v.
subcostal long-axis v.
subcostal short-axis v.
submaxillary v.
submental vertex v.
submentovertical v.
subscapular echocardiographic v.
subtalar v.
subxiphoid v.
sunrise v.
sunset v.
superoinferior v.
supine full v.
suprasternal notch v.
swimmer's v.
tangential scapular v.
thoracic v.
tomographic v.
Towne v.
transaxillary lateral v.
transcranial lateral v.
transgastric echocardiographic v.
transscapular v.
transthoracic v.
transthoracic lateral v.

transverse v.
transverse/neutral v.
true lateral v.
tunnel v.
Twining v.
ulnar deviation v.
upright postvoid v.
Van Rosen v.
Velpeau axillary v.
ventricular v.
verticosubmental v.
virtual endoscopic v.
von Rosen v.
washout v.
Waters v.
weeping willow v.
weightbearing dorsoplantar v.
West Point v.
White leg-length v.
whole-body imaging with
  magnified v.'s
x-ray v.
Zanca v.

2-view
2-v. chest x-ray
2-v. film-screen mammography
4-view
4-v. chest x-ray
4-v. wrist survey
5-view chest x-ray
viewbox
v. luminance
virtual reality v.
viewer
dedicated v.
Mammo Mask dedicated v.
viewing
cine-based v.
film-based v.
fly-through v.
group v.
PVR fly-through v.
V. Wand
ViewMax software
view-to-view variation
vignetting
vigorous achalasia
Villaret-Mackenzie syndrome
villoglandular polyp
villotubular adenoma
villous
v. adenoma

v. atrophy
v. carcinoma
v. frond
v. hypertrophy
v. papilloma
v. placenta
v. proliferation
v. stomach polyp
v. tumor
villus, pl. **villi**
anchoring v.
arachnoid v.
atrophic v.
duodenal v.
fingerlike v.
floating v.
gallbladder v.
hydropic v.
intestinal v.
leaflike v.
placental v.
ridged-convoluted v.
tongue-shaped v.
vinculum breve
Vingmed
V. CFM ultrasound system
V. ultrasound
violation
articular cartilage v.
violin-string appearance
VIPoma
vasoactive intestinal polypeptide tumor
viral
v. esophagitis
v. infusion
v. particle
v. pleuritis
v. vector delivery
Virchow
V. gland
V. hydatid
V. law of skull growth
V. metastasis
V. plane
V. psammoma
V. sentinel node
Virchow-Robin
V.-R. perivascular space
V.-R. space of brain
V.-R. space dilatation
Virchow-Troisier node

V

NOTES

virtual
    v. angioscopy (VA)
    v. array
    v. arterial endoscopy
    v. bone biopsy
    v. bronchoscopy (VB)
    v. colonoscopy
    V. CT colonography
    v. cystoscopy
    v. endoscope
    v. endoscopic surgery trainer
      (VEST)
    v. endoscopic view
    v. enteroscopy
    v. fly-through
    v. reality flexible cystoscopy
    v. reality imaging
    v. reality simulator
    v. reality viewbox
    v. retinal display system
Virtuoso
    V. imaging system
    V. portable 3D imaging system
virulent atherosclerosis
virus
    herpes simplex v. (HSV)
    herpes simplex v. 1 (HSV1)
    human immunodeficiency v. (HIV)
virus-directed enzyme/prodrug therapy
virus-mediated gene therapy
viscera (*pl. of* viscus)
visceral
    v. adipose tissue (VAT)
    v. angiography
    v. angiomatosis
    v. aortography
    v. arteriography
    v. artery
    v. catheter
    v. edema
    v. embolus
    v. heterotaxia
    v. layer
    v. lesion
    v. lymph node
    v. muscle
    v. pelvic fascia
    v. pericardial calcification
    v. pericardium
    v. peritoneum
    v. pleura
    v. pleurisy
    v. situs solitus
    v. skeleton
    v. space
    v. surface of liver
viscerocranium
    cartilaginous v.
    membranous v.

viscerography
visceromegaly
visceroparietal
visceroperitoneal
visceropleural
visceroptosis
viscerosomatic
viscid
viscosity coefficient
viscous
viscus, pl. **viscera**
    abdominal v.
    abdominopelvic v.
    hollow v.
    intraabdominal v.
    intraperitoneal v.
    mediastinal v.
    pelvic v.
    perforated hollow v.
    retroperitoneal v.
    ruptured hollow v.
    solid v.
    strangulated v.
VISI
    volar intercalated segment instability
    VISI deformity
visibility of the foramen magnum
visible
    v. anterior motion
    v. peristalsis
vision
    V. camera
    V. high-performance gradient
      system
    V. MR imaging system
    stereoscopic v.
    V. Ten V-scan scanner
    V. 1.5 T Siemens MRI scanner
Visipaque 270, 320 contrast agent
Vistaflex balloon-expanded stent
Vistec x-ray detectable sponge
visual
    v. cortex
    v. inspection
    v. laser ablation of prostate
      (VLAP)
    v. object agnosia
    v. shimmering
    v. word form area (VWFA)
visualization
    breakthrough v.
    delayed v.
    direct v.
    double-contrast v.
    endoluminal v.
    genital v.
    inadequate v.
    intraoperative x-ray v.
    needle v.

object-based v.
optimal v.
poor v.
scene-based v.
selective v.
suboptimal v.
volume mode v.
v. of the Z line
visualized
suboptimally v.
Visulas Nd:YAG laser
VISX
V. excimer laser
V. Star 3 excimer laser
V. Star S2 excimer laser
V. Star S2 excimer laser system
V. WaveScan Wavefront System
vita glass
vital capacity (VC)
vitelline
v. duct
v. fistula
Viterbi decoding
Vitesse Cos laser
Vitrea
V. 2 computer workstation
V. 2 3D CT angiographic software
V. 3D imaging
V. 3D system
V. workstation v. 1.1, 1.2
vitreous
v. hemorrhage
v. lymphoma
primary v.
vivo
DAI in v.
hydrolysis in v.
in v.
measurement in v.
micron-resolution retinal image
in v.
water diffusion in v.
Vladimiroff-Mikulicz amputation
VLAP
visual laser ablation of prostate
V-like pattern of uptake
VMA
vastus medialis advancement
VMO
vastus medialis obliquus

VNS
vagus nerve stimulation
VNS epoch
VNS-fMRI
vagus nerve stimulated functional
magnetic resonance imaging
VNS-synchronized BOLD fMRI
VNUS
VNUS closure system
VNUS radiofrequency generator
vocal
v. cord
v. cord carcinoma
v. cord paralysis
v. ligament
v. muscle
vocalis muscle
Vogele-Bale-Hohner head holder
Vogt
V. bone-free projection
V. cephalosyndactyly
VOI
volume of interest
voicing
tracheoesophageal v.
void
color v.
v. determination
flow v.
serpentine signal v.
signal v.
tubular signal v.
venous sinus flow v.
voiding
v. cystogram
v. cystourethrogram (VCU, VCUG)
v. cystourethrography (VCU,
VCUG)
v. sequence
v. study
v. urethrocystography
volar
v. angulation
v. capsule
v. carpal ligament
v. dislocation
v. inclination
v. intercalated segment instability
(VISI)
v. plate
v. radiocarpal ligament disruption
v. rim

NOTES

volar *(continued)*
    v. rim distal radial fracture
    v. tilt
    v. wrist
volar-flexed intercalated segment instability
volarward
Volkmann
    V. canal
    V. deformity
    V. fracture
    V. ischemic contracture
volt (v)
    billion electron v. (BEV)
    electron v. (eV, ev)
    kiloelectron v. (keV, kev)
    million electron v. (MeV)
Volta effect
voltage
    v. amplifier
    operating v.
    pulse v.
    ripple v.
volt-ampere (va)
volume
    v. acquisition
    adaptive cardio v. (ACV)
    adequate stroke v.
    alveolar v.
    amnionic fluid v.
    amygdala v.
    v. analysis
    aortic flow v.
    aqueductal CSF stroke v.
    articular cartilage v.
    Arvidsson dimension-length method for ventricular v.
    atomic v.
    atrial emptying v.
    augmented stroke v.
    v. averaging
    back stroke v.
    bladder v.
    blood v.
    brain v.
    capillary blood v.
    cardiac v.
    caudate v.
    cavity v.
    central blood v.
    cerebellar v.
    cerebral blood v. (CBV)
    cerebrospinal fluid v.
    chamber v.
    circulating blood v.
    circulation v.
    clinical target v. (CTV)
    closing v.
    v. coil

3D v.
decreased stroke v.
decreased tidal v.
determination of lung v.
diastolic atrial v.
diminished lung v.
Dodge area-length method for ventricular v.
v. element
end-diastolic v.
end-expiratory lung v.
endocardial v.
end-systolic v. (ESV)
end systolic pressure to end systolic v.
end-systolic residual v.
epicardial v.
v. estimation
expiratory reserve v. (ERV)
extracellular fluid v.
fetal aortic flow v.
flow v.
fluid v.
forced expiratory v.
forward stroke v. (FSV)
fractional moving blood v.
fractional vascular v.
gas v.
gland v.
gross tumor v. (GTV)
heart stroke v.
heart-to-thorax v.
hippocampal v.
v. histogram
image v.
v. imaging
v. implant calculation
increased extracellular fluid v.
inspiratory reserve v. (IRV)
v. of interest (VOI)
interstitial lung disease with increased lung v.
intracranial v.
ipsilateral lung v.
left atrial maximal v.
left ventricular chamber v.
left ventricular end-diastolic v.
left ventricular inflow v. (LVIV)
left ventricular maximal v.
left ventricular outflow v. (LVOV)
left ventricular stroke v.
v. loss
low lung v.
lung v. (V)
mean corpuscular v.
minimal v.
minute v.
v. mode
v. mode visualization

molar v.
ovarian v.
v. overload
patient v.
pericardial reserve v.
ping-pong heart v.
planning target v. (PTV)
plasma v.
postvoid residual urine v.
prism method for ventricular v.
pulmonary blood v. (PBV)
pyloric v.
pyramid method for ventricular v.
quantitative amniotic fluid v.
radioactivity per v.
radionuclide stroke v.
reduced lung v.
reduced plasma v.
reduced stroke v.
regional cerebral blood v. (rCBV)
v. regulation
regurgitant stroke v. (RSV)
relative cerebral blood v. (rCBV)
v. rendered mode
v. rendering (VR)
v. rendering of helical CT data
v. rendering technique
residual v. (RV)
respiratory v.
right ventricular end-diastolic v.
 (RVEDV)
right ventricular end-systolic v.
 (RVESV)
right ventricular stroke v.
scan v.
v. score
sensitive v.
Simpson rule method for
 ventricular v.
slice v.
stroke v. (SV)
supratentorial v.
systolic atrial v.
Teichholz equation for left
 ventricular v.
thermodilution stroke v.
thin cylindrical uniform field v.
thoracic gas v.
tidal inspiratory flow v.
total brain v. (TBV)
total intracranial v. (TIV)
total stroke v. (TSV)

transit v.
tumor v.
ventricular end-diastolic v.
voxel v.
whole-brain parenchymal v.
volume-controlled inverse ratio
 ventilation
volume-cycled ventilation
volume-mode EBCT
volume-ratio method
volume-rendered
 v.-r. CT colonography
 v.-r. 3D image
 v.-r. MR angiogram
volume-selective excitation
volumetric
 v. acquisition
 v. analysis
 v. computed tomography
 v. data set
 v. expiratory HRCT
 v. function
 v. image
 v. image data
 v. imaging
 v. interpolated breath-hold
  examination (VIBE)
 v. interstitial hyperthermia
 v. magnetic resonance brain
  mapping
 v. mapping technique
 v. minimally invasive stereotaxis
 v. multiplexed transmission
  holography
 v. resampling
 v. scan
volumetry
 CT-aided v.
 3D ultrasound v.
 hippocampal magnetic resonance v.
 tumor v.
 v. of ventilated airspace
voluming artifact
voluntary
 v. effort (VE)
 v. muscle
Voluson ultrasound system
volute
volvulus
 cecal v.
 colonic v.
 gastric v.

V

NOTES

volvulus (*continued*)
    mesenteroaxial v.
    midgut v.
    organoaxial v.
    sigmoid colon v.
    small bowel v.
    stomach v.
Volz wrist
vomer bone
vomerine canal
vomerorostral canal
vomerovaginal canal
von
    v. Hippel-Lindau (VHL)
    v. Hippel-Lindau syndrome
    v. Hippel retina tumor
    v. Meyenburg complex
    prefrontal bone of v. Bardeleben
    v. Recklinghausen disease
    v. Rosen view
    v. Willebrand disease
Voorhoeve disease
vortex, pl. **vortices**
    v. coccygeus
    v. cordis
    V. port system
vorticity
VortXX coil
Vostal radial fracture classification
VOTC
    ventral occipitotemporal (visual) cortex
Voxar Plug n View 3D imager
voxel
    adjacent v.
    v. array
    cubic v.
    v. element
    v. gradient
    isotropic v.
    v. localization
    proton brain exam-single v.
      (PROBE-SV)
    seed v.
    v. size
    spectroscopic v.
    v. volume
Voxel-Man software
VoxelView
    V. software
    V. system
Voxgram multiple-exposure holography
VP
    ventriculoperitoneal
    VP shunt
VPB
    ventricular premature beat
VPC
    ventricular premature complex
    ventricular premature contraction

VPD
    ventricular premature depolarization
VPS
    view per segment
V/Q
    ventilation-perfusion
      V/Q imaging
      V/Q lung segment scan
      V/Q mismatch
VR
    valvular regurgitation
    volume rendering
Vrolik disease
VRT
    venous refill time
VS
    ventricular septum
VScore with AutoGate cardiac imaging
VSD
    ventricular septal defect
V-shaped
    V-s. fracture
    V-s. ulcer
V-sign of Naclerio
VT
    variable temperature
      VT multinuclear spectrometer
VTED
    venous thromboembolic disease
vulgaris
    thermoactinomyces v. (TV)
vulva, pl. **vulvae**
    preinvasive disease of cervix,
      vagina, and v.
    synechia vulvae
vulvar
    v. adenoid cystic adenocarcinoma
    v. carcinoma
    v. intraepithelial neoplasm
    v. malignancy
vulvectomy
    radical v.
vulvouterine canal
vulvovaginal carcinoma
VUR
    vesicoureteral reflux
VUSE
    variable-angle uniform signal excitation
V0-V4
    vertebral artery segment V0-V4
V-wave pressure
VWF
    velocity waveform
    Doppler VWF
VWFA
    visual word form area

W
 tungsten
  W ray
¹⁸⁸W
 tungsten 188
w
 watt
Waardenburg syndrome
Waddell sign
wafer
 w. of endocardium
 Gliadel w.
waferlike appearance
wafer-shaped injury
Wagner line
Wagstaffe fracture
waist
 w. in balloon
 cardiac w.
 w. immobilizer
waistlike constriction
waiter's tip palsy
WakiTrak
 wide aperture kinematic table with
  isotropic resolution
 WakiTrak LS technique
Walcher position
Waldeyer
 W. fascia
 W. fossa
 W. ring
 W. ring lesion
 W. ring lymphoma
Walker
 W. carcinoma
 W. carcinosarcoma
 W. magnet
Walker-Walburg syndrome
walking
 w. pneumonia
 w. saturation band
walking-stick appearance
wall
 aneurysmal w.
 anterior abdominal w.
 anterolateral abdominal w.
 apical w.
 arterial w.
 axial w.
 bladder w.
 body w.
 bowel w.
 bullous edema of bladder w.
 w. calcification
 capillary w.

 carotid w.
 cavity w.
 chest w.
 cystic w.
 dorsal abdominal w.
 fetal abdominal w.
 w. filter
 friable w.
 full-thickness button of aortic w.
 gallbladder w.
 w. hypokinesis
 inferior w.
 inferoapical w.
 intestinal w.
 left anterior chest wall w.
 left ventricular w. (LVW)
 left ventricular free w. (LVFW)
 left ventricular posterior w.
  (LVPW)
 linear focus within cyst w.
 luminal w.
 midabdominal w.
 w. motion
 w. motion abnormality (WMA)
 w. motion imaging
 w. motion score
 w. motion score index
 w. motion study
 multiple bull's eye lesions
  bowel w.
 myocardial w.
 nasal cavity w.
 orbital w.
 paraumbilical anterior abdominal w.
 pelvic w.
 posterior w. (PW)
 posterior abdominal w.
 posterior free w.
 posterolateral w.
 septal w.
 w. shear stress
 stomach w.
 thickened airway w.
 thickened bladder w.
 thickened gallbladder w.
 w. thickening
 w. thickness
 thoracic w.
 thoracoabdominal w.
 w. thump
 vaginal w.
 variceal w.
 vascular w.
 ventricular free w.

W

wall-echo
>   w.-e. shadow (WES)
>   w.-e. shadow triad

walled-off abscess

Wallenberg lateral medullary syndrome

wallerian degeneration

Wallgraft
>   W. cobalt-based alloy balloon-
>   expandable stent
>   W. covered stent
>   W. endoprosthesis
>   W. endoprosthesis stent-graft

Wallstent
>   W. biliary endoprosthesis
>   W. Iliac RP self-expanding stent
>   Magic S/P W.
>   8 × 50-mm self-expanding
>   Easy W.
>   W. RP self-expanding stent
>   W. stent

Walt Disney dwarfism

Walther
>   W. fracture
>   W. oblique ligament

Waltman loop

wand
>   programmer w.
>   Viewing W.

wandering
>   w. gallbladder
>   w. goiter
>   w. heart
>   w. kidney
>   w. liver
>   w. spleen

Wang applicator

Wang-Binford edge detector

Warburg
>   W. disease
>   W. effect

Ward triangle

warfarin
>   w. embryopathy
>   w. sodium

**Warfarin-Aspirin Symptomatic
  Intracranial Disease (WASID)**

warming
>   urethral w.

warm nodule

Wartenberg sign

Warthin tumor

washboard effect

wash-in
>   w.-i. effect
>   w.-i. phase

wash-in/wash-out study

washout
>   contrast medium w.
>   w. curve

>   delayed w.
>   differential w.
>   w. effect
>   w. gradient
>   kidney w.
>   w. kinetics
>   lung w.
>   MIBG w.
>   nitrogen w.
>   w. phase
>   w. phase ventilation scan
>   w. pyelography
>   rapid tracer w.
>   w. study
>   teboroxime resting w. (TRW)
>   w. test
>   w. view

WASID
>   Warfarin-Aspirin Symptomatic
>   Intracranial Disease
>   WASID trial

wasp-tail deformity

**Wassel classification of thumb
  polydactyly**

wastage
>   pregnancy w.

wasting
>   cerebral salt w.
>   muscle fiber w.

Watanabe discoid meniscus classification

watch
>   Yperwatch gamma control w.

water
>   w. bolus
>   coexistent intravoxel fat and w.
>   w. density
>   w. density area
>   w. density line
>   diffusion characteristics of w.
>   w. diffusion in vivo
>   doped w.
>   w. eliminated Fourier transform
>   (WEFT)
>   glucose w.
>   heavy w.
>   intracellular w.
>   ion-bound w.
>   w. on brain
>   oxygen-supersaturated w.
>   w. path
>   w. path scan
>   w. perfusable tissue index
>   polar-bound w.
>   w. range
>   w. retention
>   w. seal
>   w. selective spin-echo imaging
>   w. signal on magnetic resonance
>   imaging scan

structured w.
w. suppression pulse sequence
total body w. (TBW)
water-bottle
w.-b. configuration
w.-b. heart
water-contrast computed tomography
water-density mass
waterfall
w. appearance
w. hilum
w. stomach
water-infusion catheter
water-like signal intensity
Waters
W. position
W. positioner
W. projection
W. view
W. view radiograph
water-sealed drainage
watershed
w. area
w. brain infarct
w. mechanism
w. zone in brain
water-soluble
w.-s. contrast enema
w.-s. contrast esophageal swallow
w.-s. contrast medium (WSCM)
w.-s. iodinated imaging agent
w.-s. myelography
w.-s. nonionic imaging agent
Waterston
W. groove
W. shunt
Waterston-Cooley shunt
water-suppressed proton spectrum
water-suppression technique
water-trap stomach
**Watson-Jones tibial tubercle avulsion
fracture classification**
watt (w)
wave
abdominal fluid w.
acoustic w.
aperiodic w.
circular polarization w.
constant tilt w.
continuous w. (CW)
electromagnetic w.
energy w.

w. of excitation
extracorporeal shock w.
fluid w.
longitudinal acoustic w.
motion-sensitive spin-echo sequence
mechanical w.'s
peristaltic w.
pressure w.
primary peristaltic w.
pulsed w.
radiofrequency w.
rapid filling w. (RFW)
reference w.
secondary w.
sine w.
slice excitation w. (SEW)
slow filling w.
sound w.
square w.
standing w.
systolic S w.
terahertz w.
tertiary w.
transverse acoustic w.
ultrasonic w.
waveform
apiculate w.
arterial w.
cerebrospinal fluid flow w.
dampened w.
Doppler spectral w.
flow velocity w.
w. generator
gradient w.
low-resistance spectral w.
parvus et tardus w.
pressure w.
pulsed Doppler w.
pulse volume w.
segmental bronchus renal artery w.
sinusoidal w.
spectral w.
tardus-parvus w.
triphasic w.
tube voltage w.
uterine artery w.
velocity w. (VWF)
venous w.
wavelength (Λ)
Compton w.
de Broglie w.
double-echo Broglie W.

NOTES

W

wavelength *(continued)*
    energy w.
    readout w.
    unit of w.
wavelet
    w. compression
    w. encoding
    w. scalar quantization (WSQ)
    w. subband
    w. transform
wavelet-encoded magnetic resonance imaging
WaveWire angioplasty guidewire
wax phantom
waxy liver
3-way stopcock
WBC
    white blood cell
    ^{111}In WBCs
    In-111 oxine WBCs
    radiolabeled WBCs
    ^{99m}Tc-labeled WBC
WBR
    whole-body radiation
WBRT
    whole-brain radiation therapy
    whole-brain radiotherapy
weak
    w. carotid upstroke
    w. signal
weakened artery
weakening
    trabecular w.
weakness
    respiratory muscle w.
    structural w.
wear-and-tear degeneration
web
    antral w.
    w. contracture
    duodenal w.
    esophageal w.
    fibrous w.
    finger w.
    hepatic w.
    intestinal w.
    laryngeal w.
    lateral w.
    postcricoid w.
    terminal w.
    thumb w.
    venous w.
webbed
    w. finger
    w. neck
    w. penis
Weber C fracture
Weber-Christian mesentery
weblike appearance

wedge
    w. arteriography
    w. bond
    w. compression fracture
    45-degree spinal w.
    55-degree tomography w.
    dynamic w.
    w. factor
    w. filter
    w. flexion-compression fracture
    w. fracture of spine
    w. hepatic venous pressure (WHVP)
    w. isodose angle
    matchline w.
    mediastinal w.
    w. pressure
    w. resection
    step w.
wedged hepatic venography
wedged-pair
    w.-p. beam
    w.-p. technique
wedge-shaped
    w.-s. defect
    w.-s. density
    w.-s. infarct
    w.-s. lesion
    w.-s. lobe
    w.-s. mass
    w.-s. support
    w.-s. vertebra
    w.-s. zone
wedging
    anterior w.
    w. deformity
    keystone w.
    vertebral w.
    w. of vertebral interspace
week
    gestational w.
weeping willow view
WEFT
    water eliminated Fourier transform
Wegener granulomatosis
Wegner
    W. line
    W. sign
Weibel-Palade body
weight
    body w.
    estimated fetal w. (EFW)
    fetal w.
    normal spleen w.
    thymus w.
weightbearing
    w. acetabular dome
    w. axis
    w. bone

w. dorsoplantar view
w. film
w. joint
w. rotational injury
w. surface
weighted
spin density w.
w. spin-echo column
weighted-CT-dose index
weighting
exponential w.
human visual sensitivity w.
multislice spiral w.
Weill-Marchesani syndrome
Weill sign
Weil syndrome
Weiner spatially varying filter
Weiss sign
Weitbrecht
W. cord
W. foramen
W. ligament
Welcher basal angle
Welcker angle
weld
callus w.
welder's lung
welding
laser w.
Welin technique
well-circumscribed
w.-c. breast mass
w.-c. lesion
w.-c. neoplasm
w.-c. tumor
well counter
well-defined
w.-d. appearance
w.-d. border
w.-d. lesion
w.-d. mass
well-demarcated scar
well-differentiated
w.-d. adenoma
w.-d. astrocytoma
w.-d. polycystic Wilms tumor
well-inflated lung
well-preserved ejection fraction
96-well scanning fluorometer
well-type ionization chamber
Wenckebach
W. AV block

W. cardioptosis
W. phenomenon
Werdnig-Hoffmann disease
Wermer syndrome
Werner
W. classification
W. classification (thyroid eye disease)
W. syndrome
Wernicke area
Wernicke-Korsakoff syndrome
Wertheim hysterectomy
WES
wall-echo shadow
west
W. lacuna skull
W. Point view
W. syndrome
zones 1–4 of W.
Westcott needle
West-Engstler skull
Westergren tube
Westermark sign
western boot in open fracture
Westphal-Strümpell disease
Westphal zone
wet
w. bowel preparation
w. brain
w. laser imaging
w. lung
w. lung syndrome
w. pleurisy
w. reading
w. stomach
w. swallow
Wetzel test
WFRT
wide-field radiation therapy
Wharton
W. duct
W. gland
W. tumor
wheal
Wheatstone bridge
wheelchair artifact
W3000 helical CT
whiplash injury
Whipple
W. disease
W. operation

W

NOTES

Whipple *(continued)*
  W. procedure
  W. triad
whirlpool
  w. appearance
  w. sign
whirl sign
whistling deformity
Whitacre spinal needle
Whitaker test
white
  w. asbestos
  black and w. (BW)
  w. blood cell (WBC)
  w. blood cell imaging
  w. blood cell with indium-111
    scintigraphy
  w. branching linear pattern
  w. cerebellum sign
  w. commissure of spinal cord
  w. cottonlike fibrous tissue
  w. echo writing
  w. epidermoid
  w. epithelium
  W. leg-length view
  w. light pattern projector
  w. line
  w. line of Toldt
  w. lung
  w. masking
  w. matter
  w. matter abnormality
  w. matter commissure
  w. matter demyelination
  w. matter diffusivity
  w. matter disease
  w. matter edema
  w. matter hypodensity
  w. matter infarct
  w. matter lambda
  w. matter lesion
  w. matter shearing injury
  w. matter signal hyperintensity
  w. matter thinning
  w. matter tract direction
  w. metastasis
  w. noise artifact
  w. pneumonia
  w. point
  w. radiation
  w. shuttering
  w. star breast lesion
Whitehead deformity
white-matter imaging technique
white-out
Whitfield test
whitlow
  herpetic w.

  melanotic w.
  thecal w.
WHO
  World Health Organization
  WHO classification
whole-body
  w.-b. bone scan
  w.-b. compact MR system
  w.-b. computed tomography
  w.-b. counter
  w.-b. counting
  w.-b. dose monitoring
  w.-b. echo-planar MR imaging
  w.-b. ^{29}FDG scanning
  w.-b. imaging with magnified
    views
  w.-b. inflammatory response
  w.-b. irradiation
  w.-b. nuclear physical examination
  w.-b. PET scan
  w.-b. radiation (WBR)
  w.-b. radiation therapy
  w.-b. radiotherapy
  w.-b. scan imaging
  w.-b. screening examination
  w.-b. sweep
  w.-b. 1.5 Tesla scanner
  4T w.-b. GI Signa MRI scanner
  w.-b. thallium imaging
  w.-b. 3T MRI system scanner
  w.-b. transmission scan
  w.-b. 1.5-T Siemens Vision scanner
  w.-b. unit
whole-brain
  w.-b. acquisition
  w.-b. irradiation
  w.-b. magnetization transfer
    measurement
  w.-b. parenchymal volume
  w.-b. radiation therapy (WBRT)
  w.-b. radiotherapy (WBRT)
whole-breast sonography
whole-lung opacity
whole-volume coil
Wholey steerable guidewire
whorl
  coccygeal w.
whorled appearance
whorling
WHVP
  wedge hepatic venous pressure
Wiberg
  W. angle
  CE angle of W.
  center-edge angle of W.
  W. patellar types classification
Wickham-Miller nephroscope
Widal syndrome

wide
- w. aperture kinematic table with isotropic resolution (WakiTrak)
- w. caliber
- w. field lesion
- w. latitude film
- w. rib
- w. suture
- w. tortuous aorta
- w. window setting

wide-angle tomography
wide-based, blunt-ended, right-sided, atrial appendage
wide-beam scanning
wide-field radiation therapy (WFRT)
widely patent
wide-mouth sac
wide-neck carotid cavernous aneurysm
widened
- w. anterior meningeal index
- w. cardiac silhouette
- w. collecting system
- w. duodenal sweep
- w. heart shadow
- w. joint space
- w. mediastinum
- w. optic canal
- w. sacroiliac joint
- w. sulcus
- w. superior orbital fissure
- w. sweep duodenum
- w. symphysis pubis
- w. teardrop distance
- w. thoracic outlet

widening
- acute mediastinal w.
- ankle mortise w.
- w. of aorta
- crural cistern w.
- growth plate w.
- infundibulum w.
- interpedicular distance w.
- interspinous w.
- joint w.
- mediastinal w.
- sacroiliac joint w.
- scapholunate w.

widespread
- w. hyperattenuating mediastinal adenopathy
- w. metastasis

width
- aryepiglottic fold w.
- collimated slice w.
- collimation w.
- contrast window w.
- intracranial w. (ICW)
- isodose w.
- line w.
- metatarsal head w. (MHW)
- prevertebral w.
- pulse w. (PW)
- radial w.
- spectral w.
- window w.

Wiedemann-Beckwith syndrome
Wiener
- W. MRI filter
- W. spectrum

Wigby-Taylor position
Wigle scale for ventricular hypertrophy
Wilcoxon signed-rank test
Wilkie syndrome
Wilkins radial fracture classification
Williams-Beuren syndrome
Williams-Campbell syndrome
Williams syndrome
Willis
- W. antrum
- arterial circle of W.
- artery of W.
- circle of W.
- W. pouch

willisii
- chordae w.

willow fracture
Wilson
- W. block
- W. cloud chamber
- W. disease
- W. fracture
- W. muscle

Wilson-Mikity syndrome
Wiltze angle
Wimberger
- W. ring
- W. sign

Winchester disc
windblown deformity
winding
- wire w.
- Y w.
- zero-pitch solenoidal w.

NOTES

W

Windkessel vessel
window
  acoustic w.
  acquisition w.
  aortic w.
  aortopulmonary w.
  apical w.
  beryllium mammography x-ray
    tube w.
  biologic w.
  bone w.
  brain w.
  w. center
  coincidence-resolving w.
  cortical w.
  CT bone w.
  cycle-length w.
  w. ductus
  w. efficiency
  energy w.
  esophageal w.
  gastric w.
  w. level
  localization w.
  lung w.
  mediastinal w.
  oval w.
  parasternal w.
  pericardial w.
  w. period
  pulmonary parenchymal w.
  radiation w.
  sampling w.
  short acquisition w.
  soft tissue w.
  spectral w.
  subcostal w.
  subdural w.
  suprasternal w.
  transforaminal w.
  transorbital w.
  transtemporal w.
  vestibular w.
  w. width
  xenon energy w.
windowed balloon
windowing
  intensity w.
window/level setting
windsock
  w. aneurysm
  w. appearance
  w. appearance of duodenum
  w. diverticulum
  w. sign
windswept
  w. deformity
  w. hand
  w. pelvis

windup injury
wine
  w. glass
  w. glass appearance
  w. glass pelvis
  w. glass shape
wing
  absent greater sphenoid w.
  champagne glass iliac w.
  greater sphenoid w.
  iliac w.
  sphenoid w.
  w. of sphenoid bone
winged
  w. configuration
  w. scapula
winging
  scapular w.
Winiwarter-Buerger disease
Winquist-Hansen femoral fracture
  classification
Winslow
  foramen of W.
  W. ligament
Winston-Lutz for LINAC-based
  radiosurgery
Winter-King-Moe scoliosis
wire (*See* guidewire)
  w. fixation
  heavy-duty standard exchange w.
  0.0015-inch platinum w.
  0.00175-inch platinum w.
  ^{192}Ir w.
  iridium w.
  J-tipped w.
  K-w.
  Kirschner w. (K-wire)
  w. localization
  pacemaker w.
  Rosen w.
  standard exchange w.
  sternotomy w.
  super-stiff glide w.
  temporary atrial pacing w.
  w. winding
wire-fixation buckle
wireless
  w. capsule endoscopy
  w. handheld Web pad
wire-loop lesion
wire-related defect
wiring
  intraosseous w.
Wirsung
  W. dilatation
  W. duct
  ventral duct of W.
wisdom teeth
Wiseman classification

Wishart-Lee-Abbott NF2
wispy connection
withdrawal pressure
within-slice filtering process
within-view motion
Wits measurement
WMA
    wall motion abnormality
woggle
    w. device
    w. technique
Wolf
    W. method
    W. Piezolith 2200 lithotripter
Wolfe
    W. breast carcinoma classification
    W. DY, NI, P1, P2 pattern
    W. mammographic parenchymal
    pattern
Wolff-Chaikoff effect
wolffian
    w. cyst
    w. duct
    w. duct carcinoma
Wolff law
Wolff-Parkinson-White syndrome
Wolf-Hirschhorn syndrome
Wolfram syndrome
Wolin meniscoid lesion
Wolman xanthomatosis
womb stone
Wood
    W. lamp
    W. light
    W. unit
    W. unit index
    W. units index of resistance
wooden shoe configuration
woody mass
wool
    w. coil
    w. tail
work
    left ventricular stroke w. (LVSW)
    myocardial w.
    right ventricular stroke w. (RVSW)
working
    w. film
    W. Formulation classification
    w. sheath
workstation
    AccuView computer w.

    Advantage W. 3.1
    Alpha 21064 microprocessor w.
    DIMAQ integrated ultrasound w.
    eNTEGRA w.
    freestanding w.
    Fuji QA 771 w.
    image processing w.
    imaging w.
    ISG medical imaging w.
    MacSpect real-time NMR w.
    MagicView w.
    Navigator computer w.
    Octane postprocessing w.
    PACS w.
    Pegasys w.
    postprocessing w.
    POWERstation LNX w.
    RADstation radiology w.
    Renaissance 3D w.
    Shebele physician reporting w.
    stacked-metaphor w.
    Sun w.
    Unix/X11 w.
    Vitrea 2 computer w.
    Vitrea w. v. 1.1, 1.2
world
    W. Health Organization (WHO)
    W. Health Organization
    classification
worm aneurysm
wormian bone
wormy appearance
wound
    w. dehiscence
    exit w.
    gunshot w. (GSW)
    high-velocity gunshot w.
    missile w.
    penetrating w.
    perforating w.
    stag w.
    surgical w.
woven bone
wrap
    aneurysmal w.
    aortic w.
    no frequency w.
wraparound
    w. ghosting artifact
    w. vessel

W

NOTES

wrapped
    w. aneurysmal sac
    w. artifact
wrapping
    valve w.
    vein valve w.
Wratten 6B filter
wrenched knee
wrestler's elbow
wrinkle artifact
wrinkled pleura
wrinkler muscle
Wrisberg
    W. cardiac ganglion
    intermediate nerve of W.
    W. ligament
    ligaments of Henry and W.
wrist
    w. capsule
    w. dislocation
    w. extensor compartment

gymnast's w.
w. joint
palmar w.
w. quadrature phased-array surface coil
SLAC w.
w. triquetrum bone
volar w.
Volz w.
wristdrop
writing
    black echo w.
    white echo w.
WSCM
    water-soluble contrast medium
W-shaped ileal pouch
WSQ
    wavelet scalar quantization
Wyburn-Mason
    W.-M. arteriovenous malformation
    W.-M. syndrome

X
Kienböck unit
magnification
xanthosine
X axis
X gradient
syndrome X
X trough
X unit

x
7x. 40 mm percutaneous
transluminal angioplasty balloon
8x. 8-pixel block

Xanar 20 Ambulase CO₂ laser
xanthelasma
xanthic calculus
xanthoastrocytoma
pleomorphic x. (PXA)
xanthogranuloma
bone x.
juvenile x.
xanthogranulomatous
x. cholecystitis
x. pyelonephritis
xanthoma, pl. **xanthomata**
Achilles tendon x.
gastric x.
malignant fibrous x.
x. tuberosum simplex
xanthomatosis
cerebrotendinous x.
primary familial x.
Wolman x.
xanthomatous
x. granuloma
x. pseudotumor
xanthosarcoma
xanthosine (X)
X-band Linac
X-CBF
cerebral xenon-enhanced blood flow
XCCL
exaggerated craniocaudal lateral
XCT
x-ray computed tomography
Xe
xenon
¹³³Xe
xenon 133
¹²⁷Xe
xenon 127
¹²⁹Xe
xenon 129
X-Echo-Speed
Signa Horizon X.-E.-S.

XeCl
xenon chloride
XeCl excimer
XeCl laser
XeCT
xenon computed tomography
Xenetix 250, 300, 350 contrast medium
xenograft
bovine heart x.
porcine heart x.
x. valve
vascular x.
xenon (Xe)
x. 127 (¹²⁷Xe)
x. 129 (¹²⁹Xe)
x. 133 (¹³³Xe)
x. arch photocoagulator
x. arc lamp
x. chloride (XeCl)
x. computed tomography (XeCT)
x. CT measurement
x. CT scanning
x. energy window
x. imaging agent
x. trap system
x. washout study
xenon-133
x. SPECT imaging
x. ventriculogram
xenon-chloride laser (XeCl laser)
xenon-enhanced
x.-e. computed tomography
x.-e. CT
xenotransplantation
xerogram
xerography
xeromammogram
chest wall lateral x.
xeromammography
xeroradiogram
xeroradiograph
xeroradiographic
x. selenium plate
x. technique
xeroradiography
xerosialography
xerotomography
x-height
Xillix
X. LIFE-GI fluorescence endoscopy
system
X. LIFE-Lung fluorescence
endoscopy system
Ximatron simulator

X

XIP
    x-ray in plaster
xiphicostal ligament
xiphisternal joint
xiphogus
xiphoid
    x. angle
    x. appendix
    x. bone
    x. cartilage
    x. ligament
    x. process
xiphopubic area
xiphosternalis
    synchondrosis x.
x-irradiation
XKnife stereotactic radiosurgery system
XL
    inductive reactance
X-linked
XOP
    x-ray out of plaster
Xplorer
    X. 1000 digital imaging system
    X. imaging system
X-Prep bowel preparation
X-Press suture-mediated closure device
Xpress/SW helical CT scanner
Xpress/SX helical CT scanner
XRA
    x-ray arteriography
x-radiation
x-ray
    x-r. arteriography (XRA)
    x-r. attenuation
    baseline chest x-r.
    x-r. beam
    x-r. beam size
    x-r. burn
    cast-off x-r. (COX)
    characteristic x-r.
    chest x-r. (CXR)
    x-r. computed tomography (XCT)
    x-r. crystallography
    x-r. detector
    x-r. diffraction
    x-r. diffraction analysis
    x-r. dosimetry
    x-r. energy
    E sign on x-r.

    x-r. film
    x-r. generator
    x-r. image
    inside-out x-r.
    Jude pelvic x-r.
    x-r. mammography
    x-r. microscope
    mobile mass x-r. (MMR)
    monochromatic x-r.
    x-r. out of plaster (XOP)
    peripheral dual energy x-r.
     (pDEXA)
    x-r. in plaster (XIP)
    portable x-r.
    postreduction x-r.
    prereduction x-r.
    scanning-beam digital x-r. (SBDX)
    x-r. shadow projection
     microtomographic system
    x-r. spectrometer
    x-r. spectrum
    x-r. therapy
    x-r. thickness gauge
    x-r. tomographic microscope (XTM)
    x-r. topography
    x-r. tube
    x-r. tube housing
    x-r. tube rating chart
    x-r. unit
    x-r. view
    2-view chest x-r.
    4-view chest x-r.
    5-view chest x-r.
x-shaped guidewire
X-terminal
XTM
    x-ray tomographic microscope
XTRAC laser
XT radiopaque coronary stent
X-Vigor
    X-V. CT scanner
    X-V. scanner
X-wave pressure
XY
    XY plane
    XY syndrome
xylenol orange imaging agent
xylol pulse indicator
X, Y, and Z coordinates for target lesion

Y

yttrium
Y axis
Y bone plate
Y cartilage
Y configuration
Y fracture
Y trough
Y winding

^{50}Y, Y-50
yttrium-50

^{90}Y, Y-90
yttrium-90
^{90}Y microsphere

YAG

yttrium-aluminum-garnet
YAG laser

Yaglazr system

Yakolev

Yb

ytterbium

yellow

zinc, y. (ZY)

yellow cartilage

yellow-out

Yergason test

yield

y. comparison
diagnostic y.
low y.
ultrasound diagnostic y.

yin-yang, ying-yang

y.-y. appearance
y.-y. sign

Y-jaws

YLF

yttrium lithium fluoride

Y-line

yoke

yolk

y. sac (YS)

y. sac diameter
y. sac ovary tumor
y. stalk

Young syndrome

yo-yo

y.-y. esophageal peristalsis
y.-y. ureteral peristalsis

Yperwatch gamma control watch

YS

yolk sac

Y-shaped

Y-s. acetabulum
Y-s. distortion
Y-s. ligament

Y-T fracture

ytterbium (Yb)

y. pentetate sodium

ytterbium-169 DTPA

ytterbium-90 microsphere

yttrium (Y)

ferritin-labeled y.
y. lithium fluoride (YLF)
y. radioactive source

yttrium-50 (^{50}Y, Y-50)

yttrium-90 (^{90}Y, Y-90)

y. microsphere
y. silicate therapy

yttrium-aluminum-garnet (YAG)

contrast transesophageal
echocardiography:y.-a.-g.
(CTE:YAG)
y.-a.-g. laser

yttrium-90-labeled

Y-tube

Yueh centesis needle

Yuge

oculosubcutaneous syndrome of Y.

Yunis-Varon syndrome

Y-wave pressure

Z

Z axis
Z axis field
Z band
Z gradient
Z line
Zaglas ligament
Zahn
Z. anomaly
pocket of Z.
Zanca view
Zanelli position
ZA-stent Nitinol self-expandable stent
Z-dependent CT
zebra
z. stripe appearance
z. stripe artifact
z. stripe image
z. stripe pattern
Zeeman hamiltonian function
Zeiss
Z. EndoLive endoscope
Z. Visulas 690s laser
Zellballen
Zellweger syndrome
Zener diode
Zenith
Z. AAA endovascular graft
Z. stainless steel self-expandable
stent
Zenker
Z. degeneration
Z. diverticulum
Z. necrosis
Z. pouch
zeolite pneumoconiosis
zero
z. exposure
z. filling
z. line
z. net flow
z. padding
z. phase
z. reference level
z. time of the x-ray apparatus
zero-field splitting
zero-fill
z.-f. artifact
z.-f. interpolation (ZIP)
zero-filling interpolation scheme
zero-pitch solenoidal winding
ZeroRad MRI scan
zeroth moment
ZES
Zollinger-Ellison syndrome

zetacrit
Zetafuge
zeugmatography
Fourier transformation z.
rotating-frame z.
zeugopodium
Zeus system
Z-filtering
z-flying focal spot
Zickel supercondylar nail
Zielke derotation level
Zieve syndrome
zigzag stent
Zilver
Z. self-expanding stent
Z. stent
Zilverstent
Zimmerman
Z. arch
Z. cell
Zimmermann elementary particle
Zimmer method
zinc (Zn)
z. 65 (^{65}Zn, Zn-65)
irradiated z.
z., yellow (ZY)
Zinn
Z. anulus
Z. ligament
tendon of Z.
Z-interpolation algorithm
ZIP
zero-fill interpolation
zipper artifact
zirconium (Zr)
z. granuloma
z. with niobium 95
Zlatkin grading system
Z-line of esophagus
ZMC
zygomatic complex
zygomaticomaxillary complex
zygomaxillary complex
ZMC fracture
Z-MED balloon catheter
Z-MIVE
cis-11beta-methoxy-17alpha-iodovinyl-
estradiol
^{123}I-labeled Z-MIVE
Zn
zinc
^{65}Zn, Zn-65
zinc 65

Z

Zollinger-Ellison
    Z.-E. syndrome (ZES)
    Z.-E. tumor
zona, pl. **zonae**
    z. fasciculata
    z. glomerulosa
    z. orbicularis
    z. reticularis
zonal
    z. gastritis
    z. prostate anatomy
    z. sampling
    z. uterine anatomy
zonary
zone
    air-trapping z.
    arrhythmogenic border z.
    basal z.
    bilaminar z.
    border z.
    clear z.
    convergence z.
    cross-sectional z.
    detection z.
    dorsal root entry z. (DREZ)
    echo-free central z.
    entry z.
    epileptogenic z.
    esophageal transition z.
    focal z. (FZ)
    focal high-intensity z.
    z. focusing
    fracture z.
    Fraunhofer z.
    Fresnel z.
    high-intensity z. (HIZ)
    high-signal-intensity z.
    hypoechogenic retroplacental
      myometrial z.
    hypoechoic z.
    hypovascular z.
    ischemic z.
    junctional z.
    lipid z.
    Looser transformation z.
    lung z.
    marginal z.
    midlung z.
    z. of partial preservation (ZPP)
    patchy z.
    penumbra z.
    posterior root entry z.
    prostatic transition z.
    pyramidal hemorrhagic z.
    Rolando z.
    root entry z.
    root exit z. (REZ)
    rough z.
    z. of slow conduction

    sonolucent z.
    therapy z.
    transformation z.
    transition z.
    transradiant z.
    Trümmerfeld z.
    Umbau z.
    vascular z.
    wedge-shaped z.
    z.'s 1–4 of West
    Westphal z.
zonifugal
zonipetal
zonogram
zonography
    stereoscopic z.
zonoskeleton
zonula ciliaris
zoonosis
    respiratory z.
Z-point pressure
ZPP
    zone of partial preservation
Zr
    zirconium
Z-score in bone mineral density
    measurement
Z-stent
    Gianturco Z.-s.
    Gianturco biliary Z.-s.
Zuckerguss
Zuckerkandl
    Z. body
    Z. convolution
    Z. fascia
    Z. organ
Zurich growth centile diagram
Zuska disease
zwitterion
ZY
    zinc, yellow
    ZY plane
zygal
zygapophysial
    z. articulation
    z. joint
zygapophysis
    z. inferior
    z. superior
zygoma
zygomatic
    z. arch
    z. bone
    z. complex (ZMC)
    z. process
zygomaticofacial
    z. canal
    z. foramen
zygomaticofrontal suture

zygomaticomalar
  z. area
  z. reconstruction
zygomaticomaxillary
  z. complex (ZMC)
  z. fracture

zygomaticotemporal
  z. canal
  z. suture
zygomaxillary
  z. complex (ZMC)

NOTES

Contents: The Appendices

Appendix 1
Anatomical Illustrations

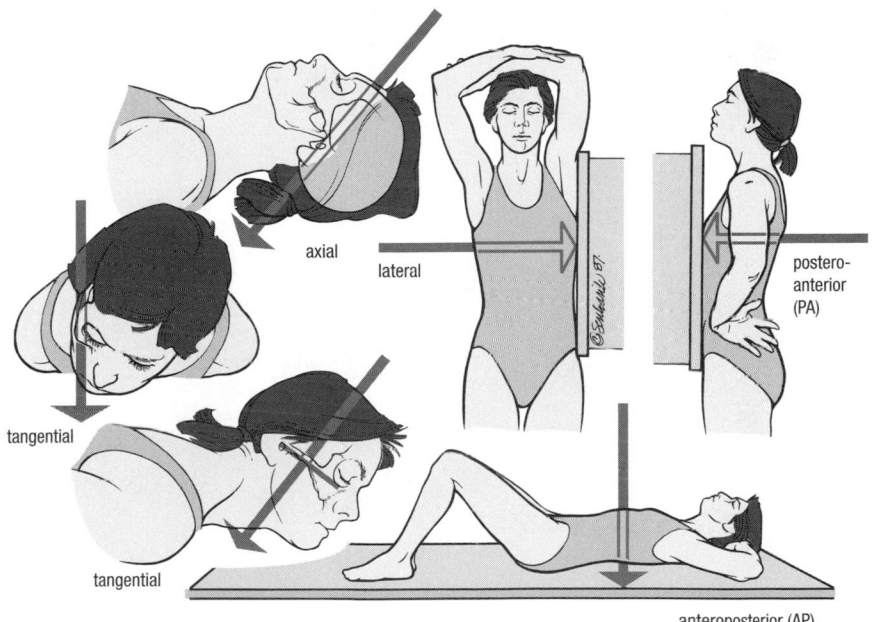

axial

lateral

postero-anterior (PA)

tangential

tangential

anteroposterior (AP)

radiographic projections: x-rays pass through body parts with the denser structures absorbing more x-rays, resulting in the lighter areas on the radiograph

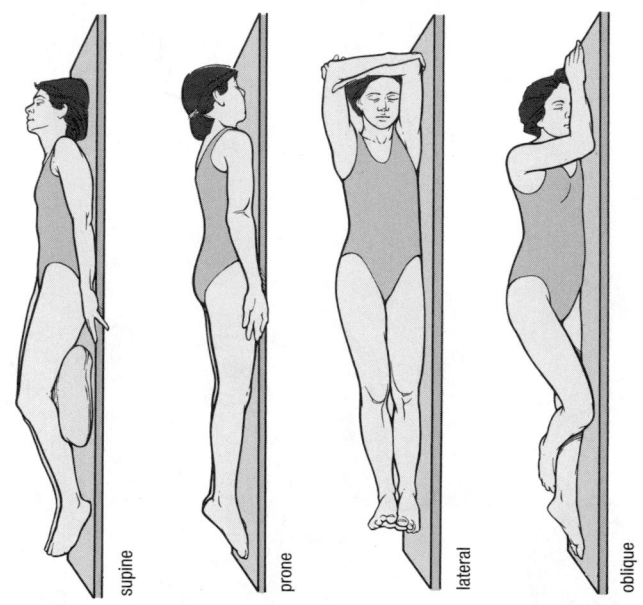

supine

prone

lateral

oblique

patient positions

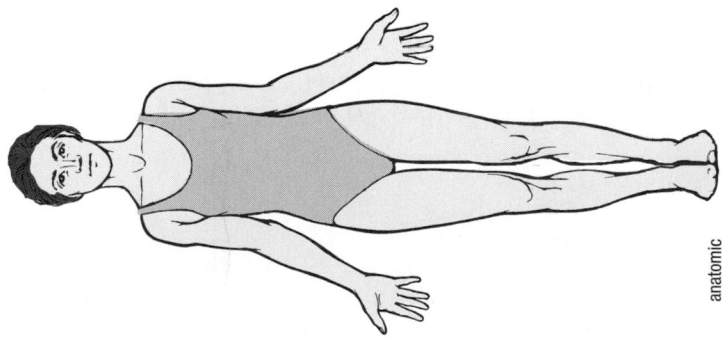

anatomic

Anatomical Illustrations

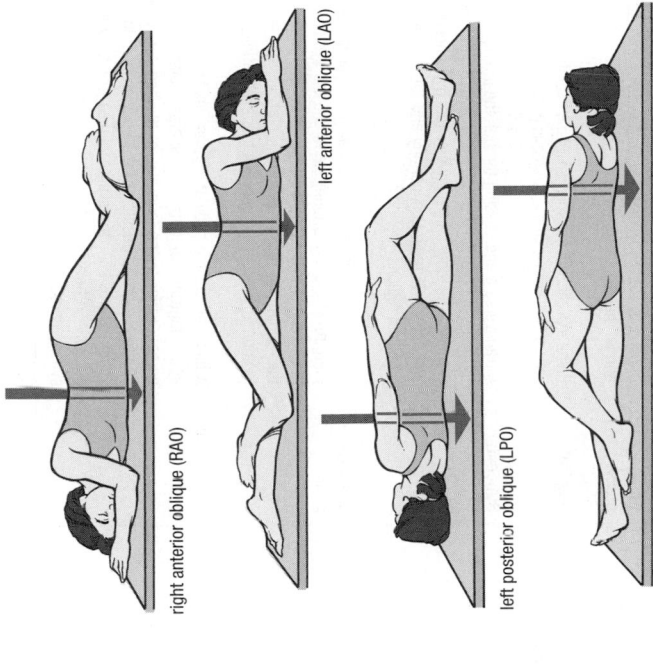

right anterior oblique (RAO)

left anterior oblique (LAO)

left posterior oblique (LPO)

right posterior oblique (RPO)

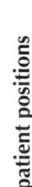

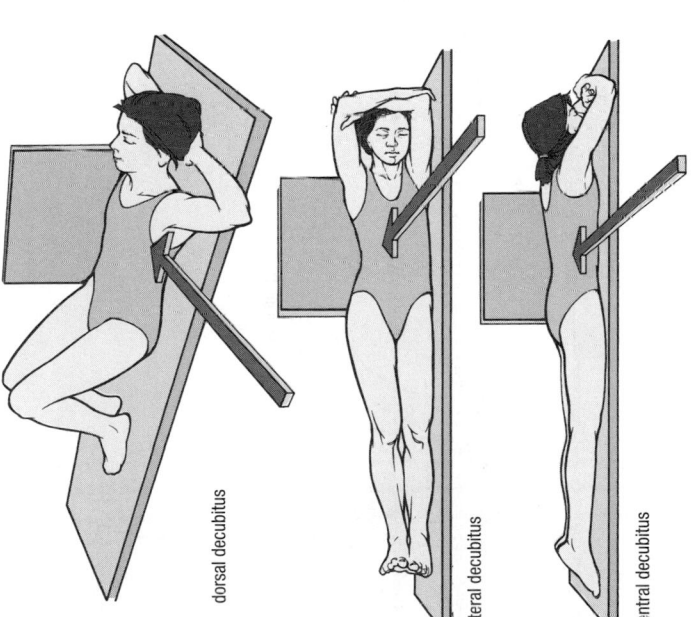

dorsal decubitus

lateral decubitus

ventral decubitus

patient positions

A3

Anatomic Planes

Frontal (coronal) plane: A vertical plane at right angles to a sagittal plane, dividing the body into anterior and posterior portions, or any plane parallel to the central coronal plane.

Longitudinal plane: Running lengthwise; in the direction of the long axis of the body or any of its parts.

Median (midsagittal) plane: A plane vertical in the anatomic position, through the midline of the body that divides the body into right and left halves.

Sagittal plane: Plane parallel to the median plane; sagittal planes are vertical planes in the anatomic position.

Subcostal plane: A transverse plane passing through the inferior limits of the costal margin, i.e., the tenth costal cartilages; it marks the boundary between the hypochondriac and epigastric regions superiorly and the lateral and umbilical regions inferiorly.

Transpyloric plane: A transverse plane midway between the superior margins of the manubrium sterni and the symphysis pubis; the pylorus may be located on this plane in the supine or prone positions, but in the erect (anatomic) position it descends to the lower level.

Transverse plane: A plane across the body at right angles to the frontal and sagittal planes; transverse planes are perpendicular to the long axis of the body or limbs, regardless of the position of the body or limb; in the anatomic position, transverse planes are horizontal planes; otherwise the two terms are not synonymous.

transverse plane
transpyloric plane (9th costal cartilage)
subcostal plane (10th costal cartilage)
transverse plane
median plane
sagittal planes
frontal planes

terms of relationship, anatomic planes

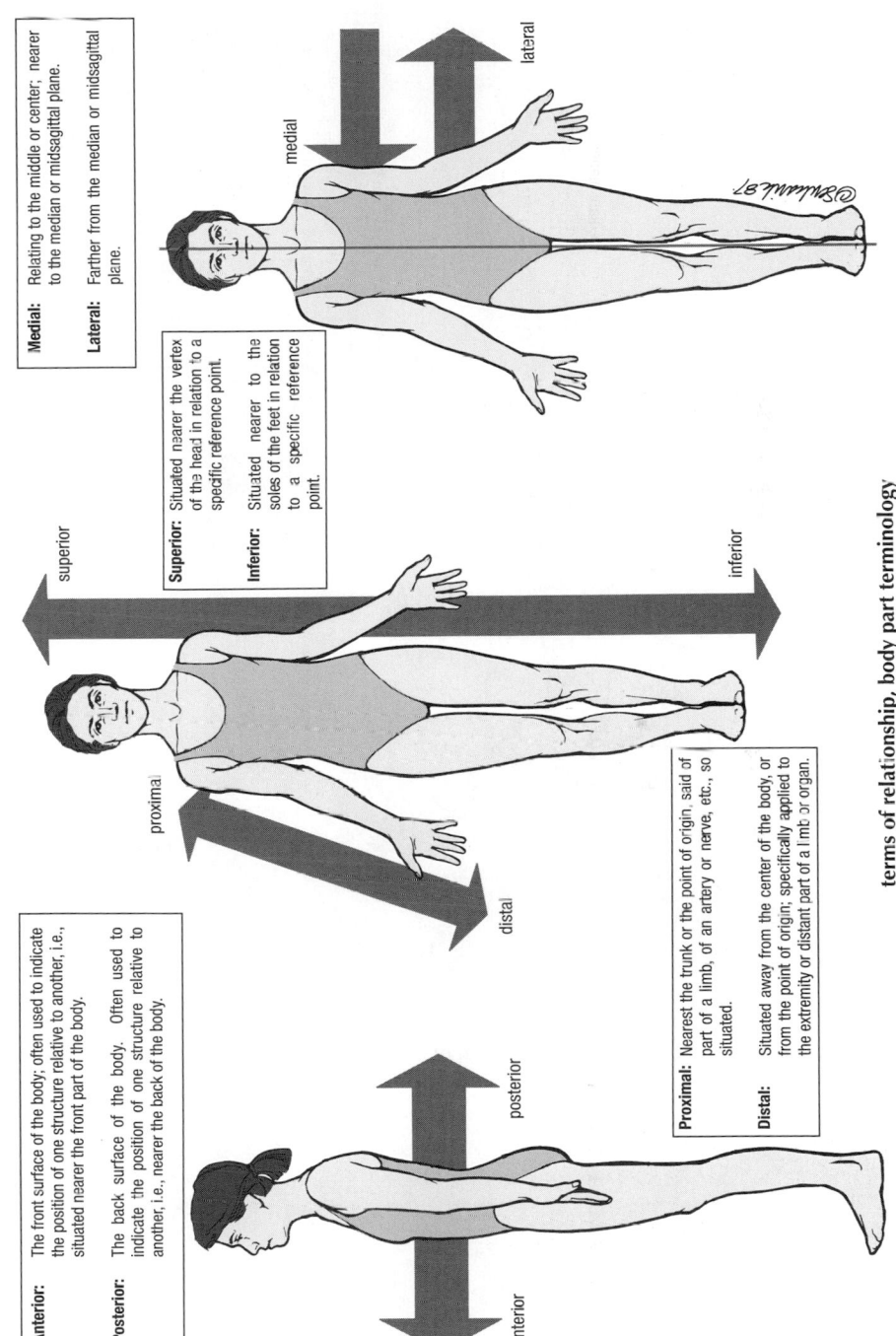

Medial: Relating to the middle or center; nearer to the median or midsagittal plane.

Lateral: Farther from the median or midsagittal plane.

medial

lateral

Superior: Situated nearer the vertex of the head in relation to a specific reference point.

Inferior: Situated nearer to the soles of the feet in relation to a specific reference point.

superior

inferior

proximal

distal

Proximal: Nearest the trunk or the point of origin, said of part of a limb, of an artery or nerve, etc., so situated.

Distal: Situated away from the center of the body, or from the point of origin; specifically applied to the extremity or distant part of a limb or organ.

Anterior: The front surface of the body; often used to indicate the position of one structure relative to another, i.e., situated nearer the front part of the body.

Posterior: The back surface of the body. Often used to indicate the position of one structure relative to another, i.e., nearer the back of the body.

posterior

anterior

terms of relationship, body part terminology

A5

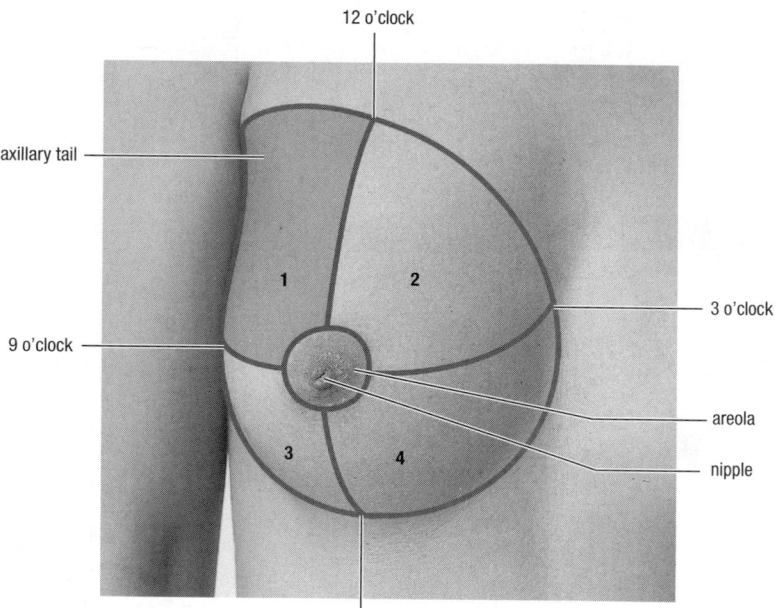

quadrants of the right breast: (1) upper outer (50% of cancerous breast tumors are found in the quadrant), (2) upper inner, (3) lower outer, (4) lower inner

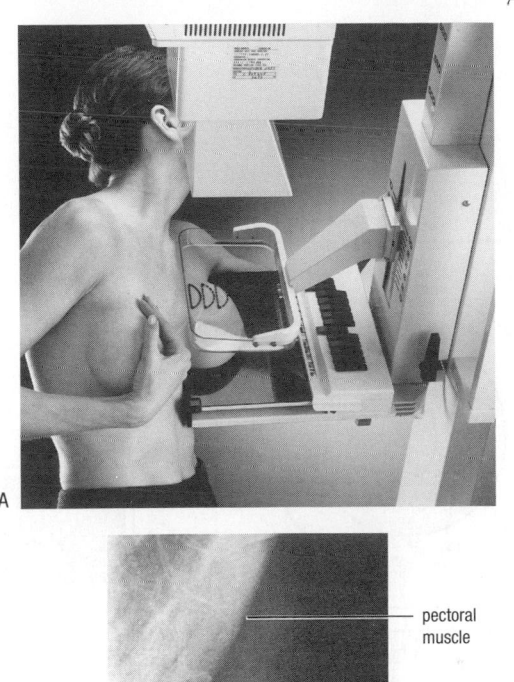

A

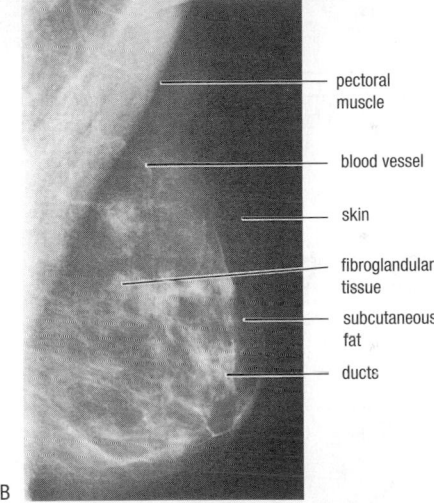

pectoral muscle

blood vessel

skin

fibroglandular tissue

subcutaneous fat

ducts

B

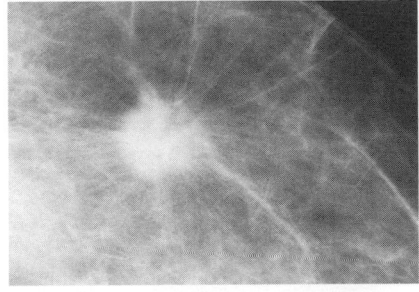

C

mammography: (A) patient positioning for a mediolateral oblique (MLO) view, (B) normal mammogram of left breast, (C) infiltrating duct carcinoma

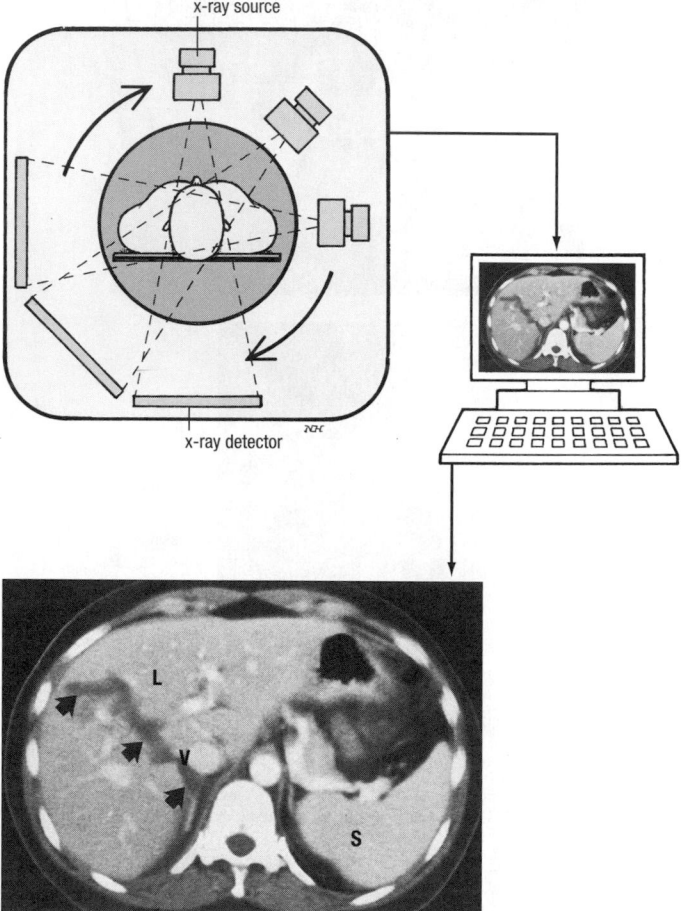

CT scan: patient involved in a motor vehicle accident demonstrates a jagged laceration (arrows) extending from posterior to inferior vena cava (V) through right lobe of the liver (L); (S), spleen

computed tomography (CT): a radiologic procedure using a scanner to examine the body site by taking a series of cross-sectional images one slice at a time in a full-circle rotation; a computer then calculates and converts the rates of absorption and density of the x-rays into a picture on a screen

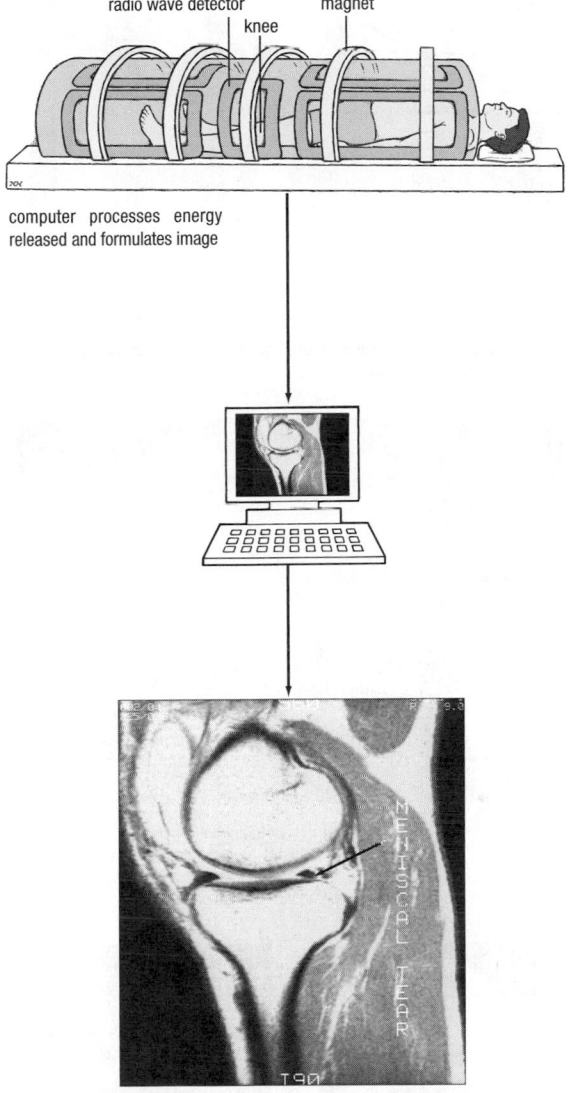

radio wave detector   magnet
              knee

computer processes energy
released and formulates image

magnetic resonance image of knee (lateral
view): torn meniscus

magnetic resonance imaging (MRI): a nonionizing (non-x-ray) technique using magnetic fields and
radiofrequency waves to visualize anatomic structures; it is useful in detecting joint, tendon, and
vertebral disorders; the patient is positioned within a magnetic field as radio wave signals are con-
ducted through the selected body part; energy is absorbed by tissues and then released

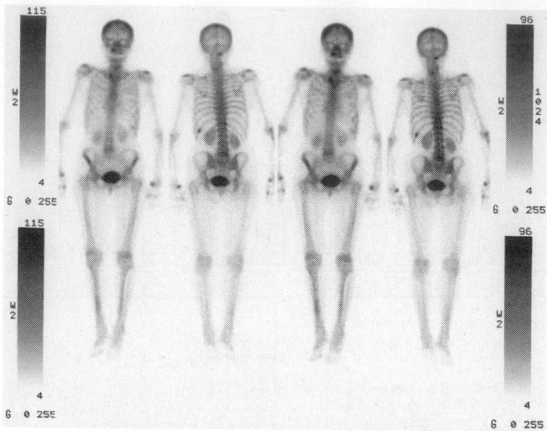

full-body bone scan: nuclear scan of bone tissue to detect abnormalities such as tumors and malignancies

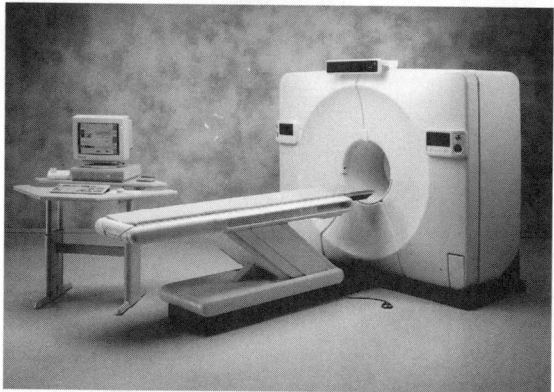

positron emission tomography (PET): combination of nuclear medicine and computed tomography produces images of brain anatomy and corresponding physiology, and is used to study conditions and diseases, including stroke, Alzheimer disease, epilepsy, and metabolic brain disorders

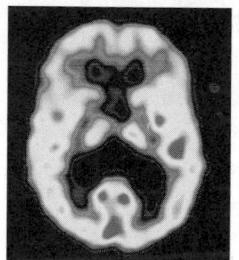 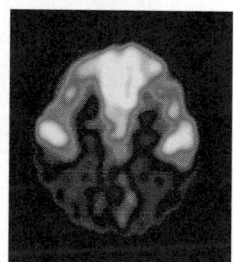

PET scan: (A) normal brain, (B) Alzheimer disease

nuclear medicine imaging: a diagnostic technique using injected or ingested radioactive isotopes and a gamma camera for determining size, shape, location, and function of various body parts

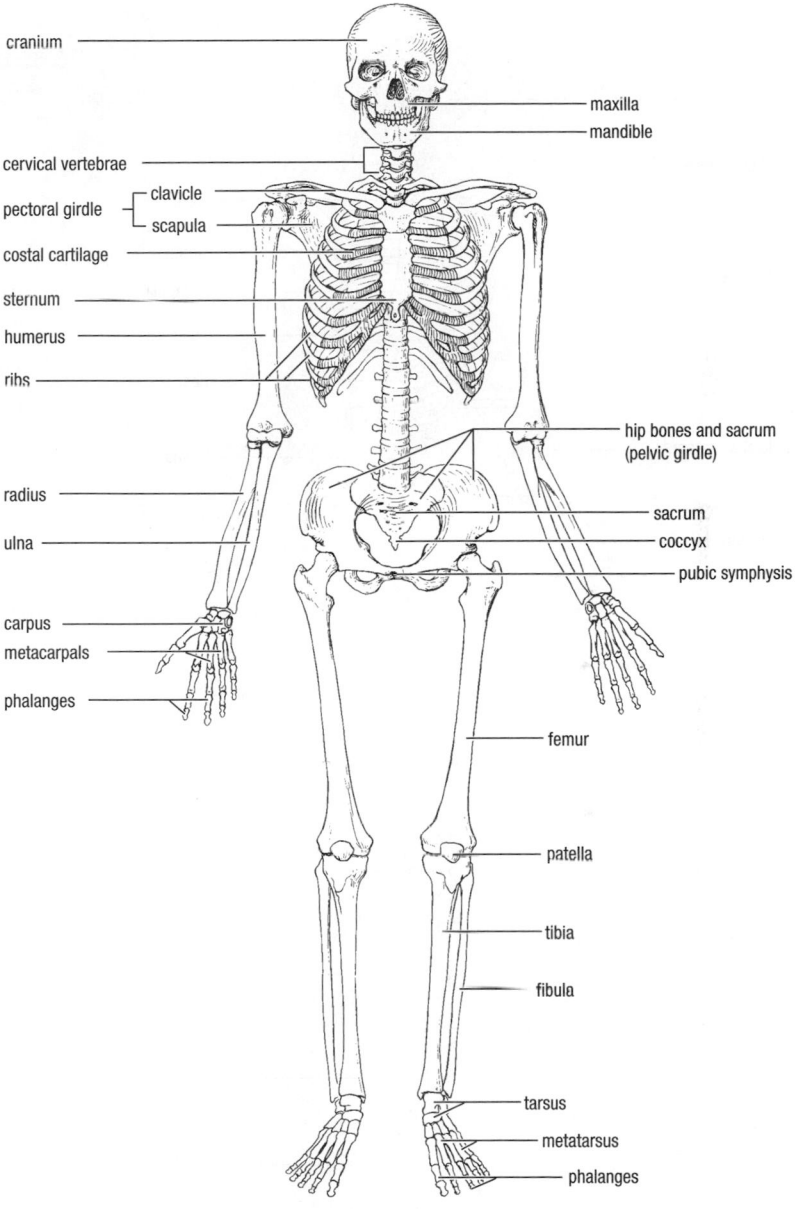

cranium

maxilla

mandible

cervical vertebrae

pectoral girdle — clavicle
— scapula

costal cartilage

sternum

humerus

ribs

hip bones and sacrum
(pelvic girdle)

radius

sacrum

ulna

coccyx

pubic symphysis

carpus

metacarpals

phalanges

femur

patella

tibia

fibula

tarsus

metatarsus

phalanges

skeleton, adult, anterior view

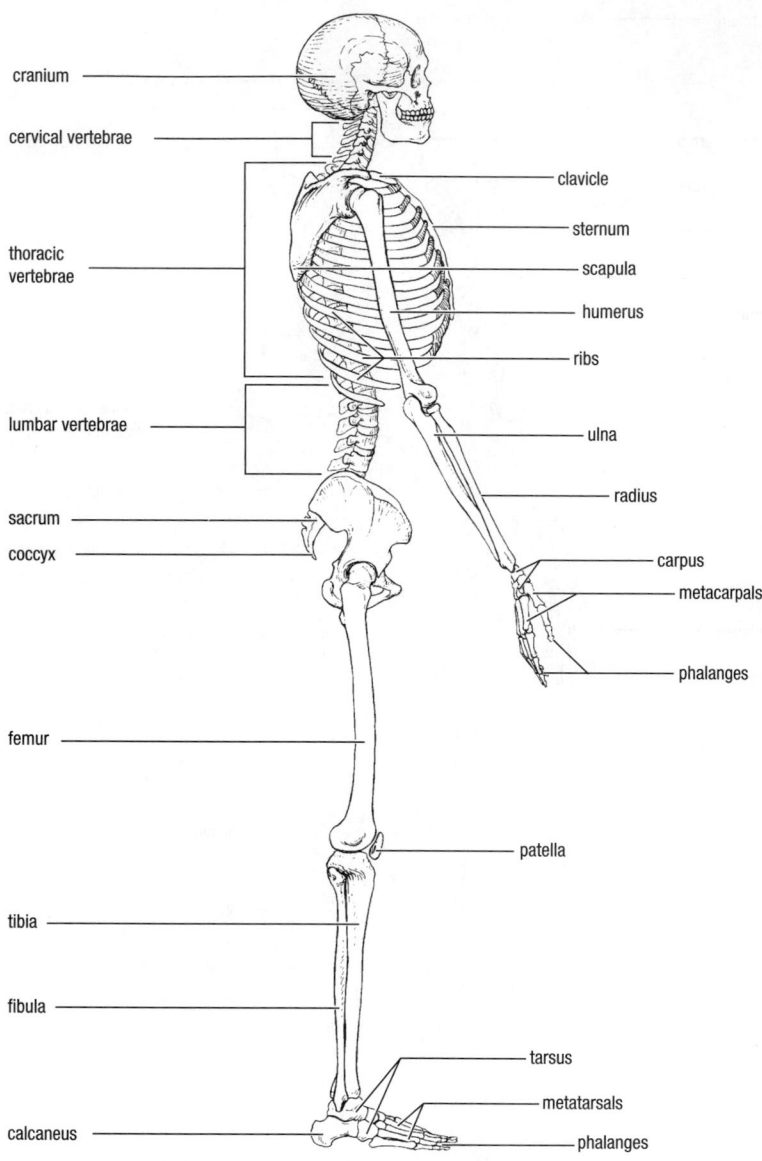

cranium

cervical vertebrae

clavicle

sternum

thoracic
vertebrae

scapula

humerus

ribs

lumbar vertebrae

ulna

radius

sacrum

coccyx

carpus

metacarpals

phalanges

femur

patella

tibia

fibula

tarsus

metatarsals

calcaneus

phalanges

skeleton, adult, lateral view

Anatomical Illustrations

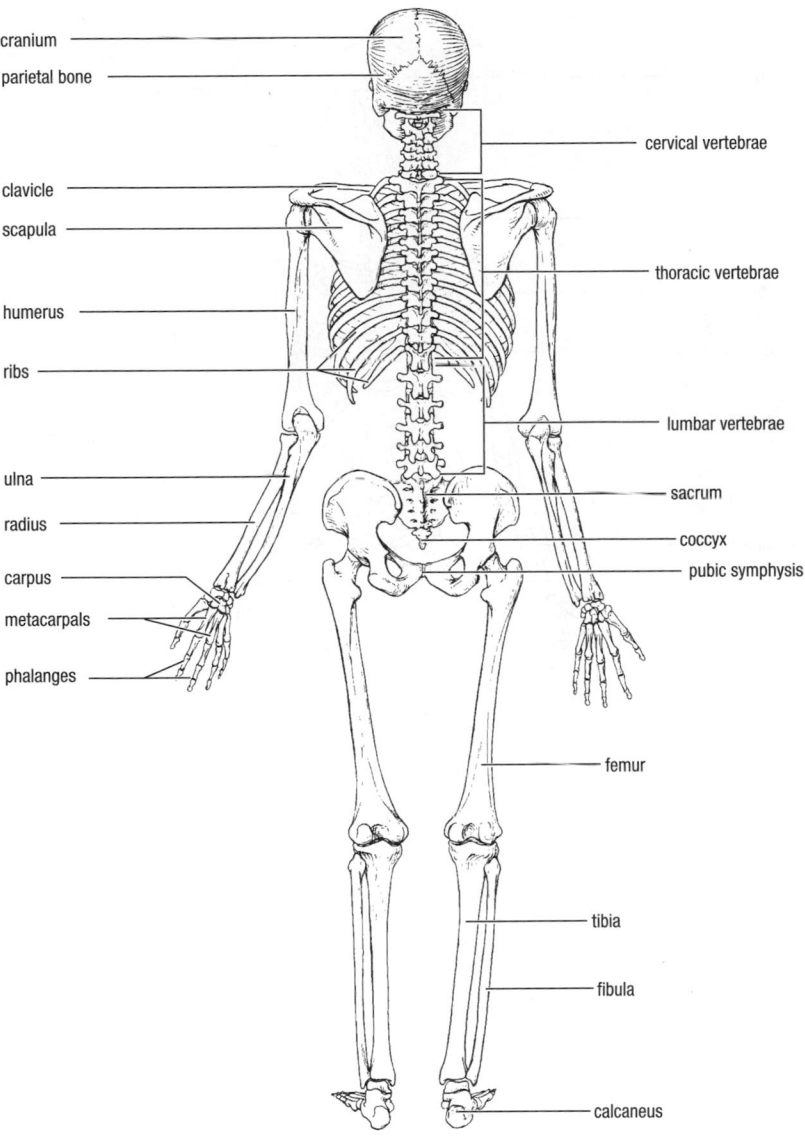

cranium
parietal bone
cervical vertebrae
clavicle
scapula
thoracic vertebrae
humerus
ribs
lumbar vertebrae
ulna
sacrum
radius
coccyx
carpus
pubic symphysis
metacarpals
phalanges
femur
tibia
fibula
calcaneus

skeleton, adult, posterior view

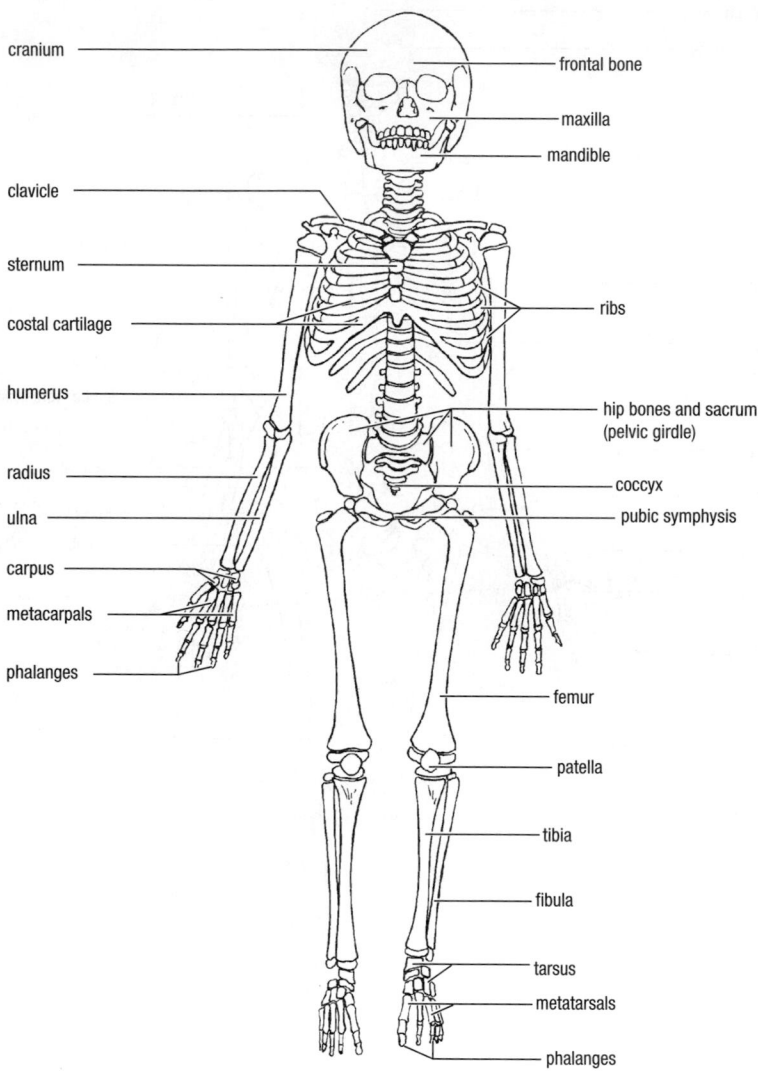

cranium ——————————

frontal bone

maxilla

mandible

clavicle ——————————

sternum ——————————

costal cartilage ——————

ribs

humerus ——————————

hip bones and sacrum
(pelvic girdle)

radius ——————————

coccyx

ulna ——————————

pubic symphysis

carpus ——————————

metacarpals ——————

phalanges ——————————

femur

patella

tibia

fibula

tarsus

metatarsals

phalanges

skeleton, child, anterior view

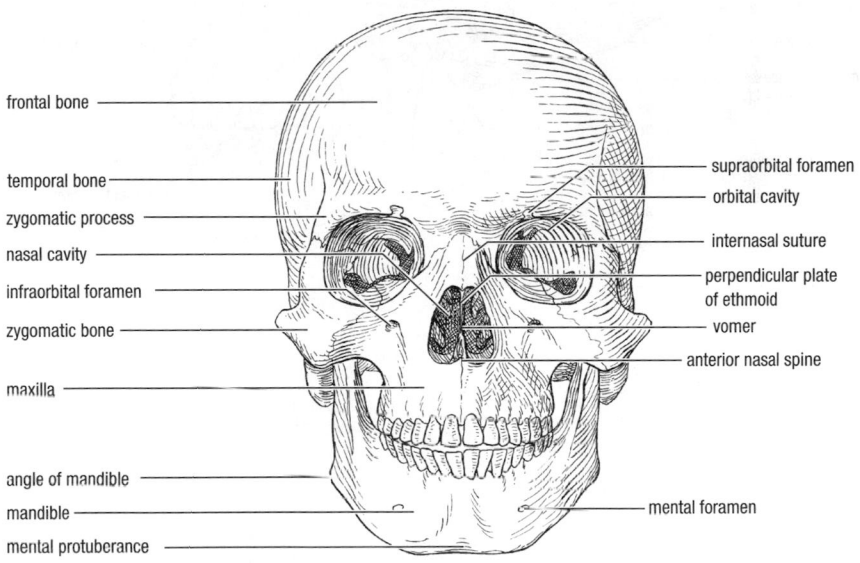

frontal bone

temporal bone

zygomatic process

nasal cavity

infraorbital foramen

zygomatic bone

maxilla

angle of mandible

mandible

mental protuberance

supraorbital foramen

orbital cavity

internasal suture

perpendicular plate
of ethmoid

vomer

anterior nasal spine

mental foramen

skull, frontal view

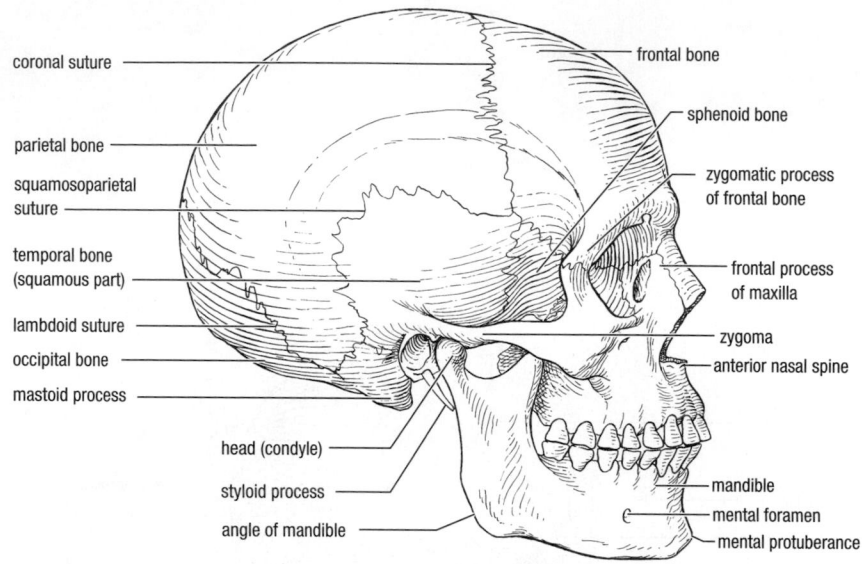

coronal suture

parietal bone

squamosoparietal
suture

temporal bone
(squamous part)

lambdoid suture

occipital bone

mastoid process

head (condyle)

styloid process

angle of mandible

frontal bone

sphenoid bone

zygomatic process
of frontal bone

frontal process
of maxilla

zygoma

anterior nasal spine

mandible

mental foramen

mental protuberance

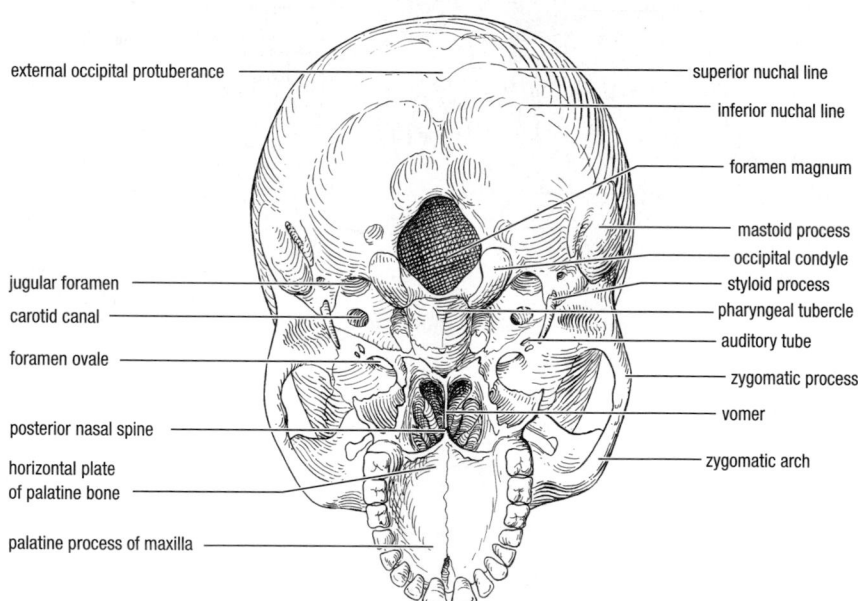

external occipital protuberance

jugular foramen

carotid canal

foramen ovale

posterior nasal spine

horizontal plate
of palatine bone

palatine process of maxilla

superior nuchal line

inferior nuchal line

foramen magnum

mastoid process

occipital condyle

styloid process

pharyngeal tubercle

auditory tube

zygomatic process

vomer

zygomatic arch

skull, lateral (top) and inferior (bottom) views

Anatomical Illustrations

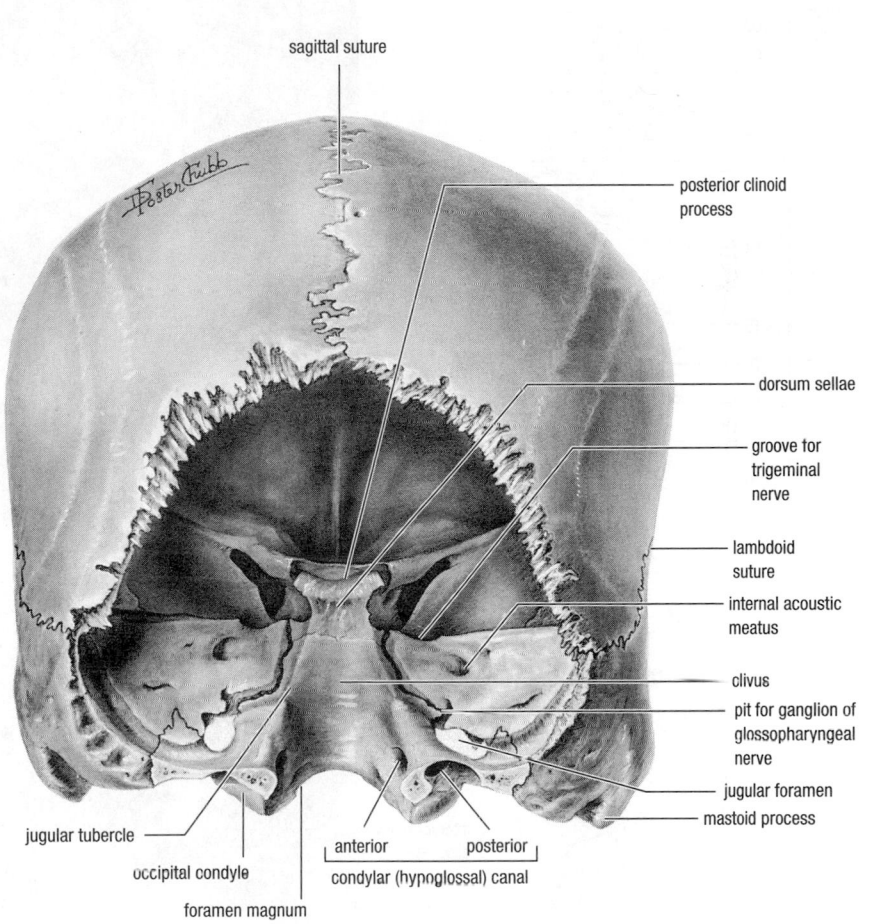

sagittal suture

posterior clinoid process

dorsum sellae

groove for trigeminal nerve

lambdoid suture

internal acoustic meatus

clivus

pit for ganglion of glossopharyngeal nerve

jugular foramen

mastoid process

jugular tubercle

occipital condyle

anterior   posterior

condylar (hypoglossal) canal

foramen magnum

skull: bony features of posterior cranial fossa

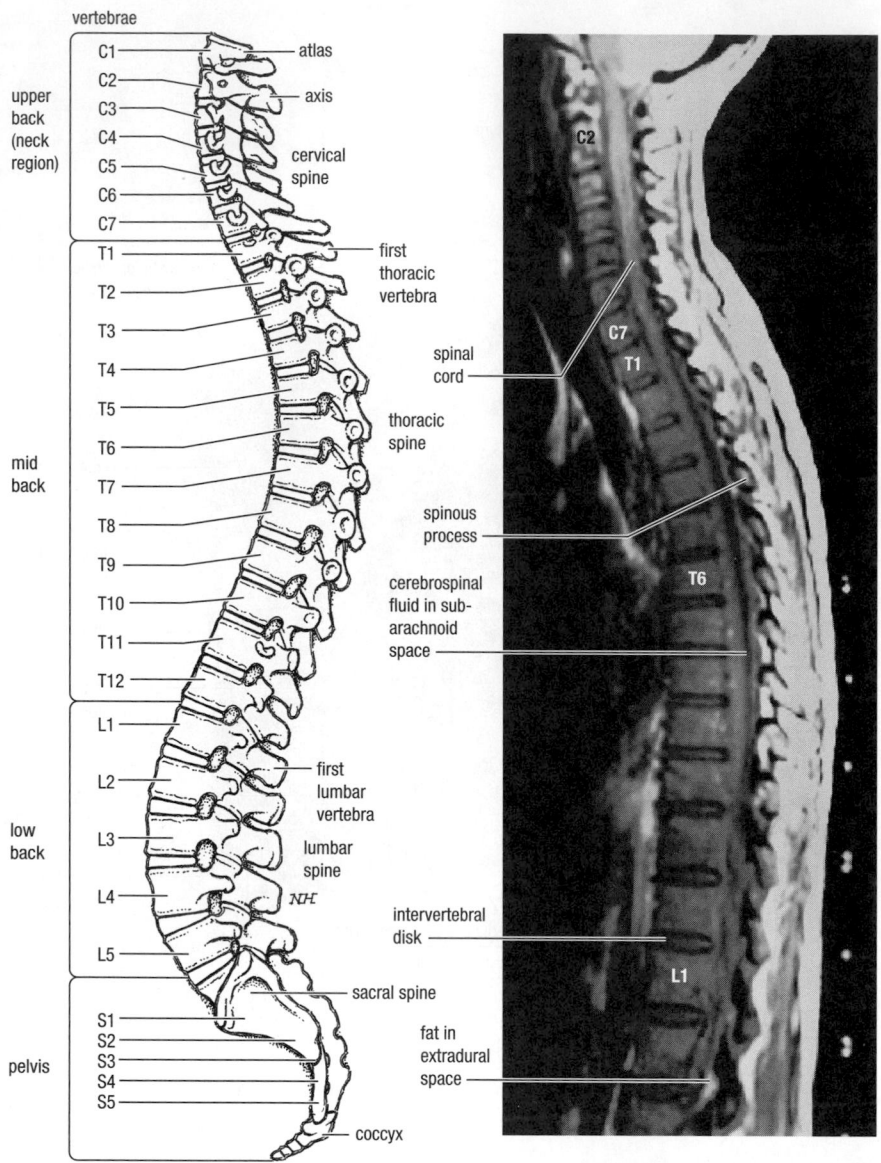

vertebral column, lateral view (radiograph courtesy of Dr. D. Salonen, University of Toronto, Toronto, Ontario, Canada)

Anatomical Illustrations

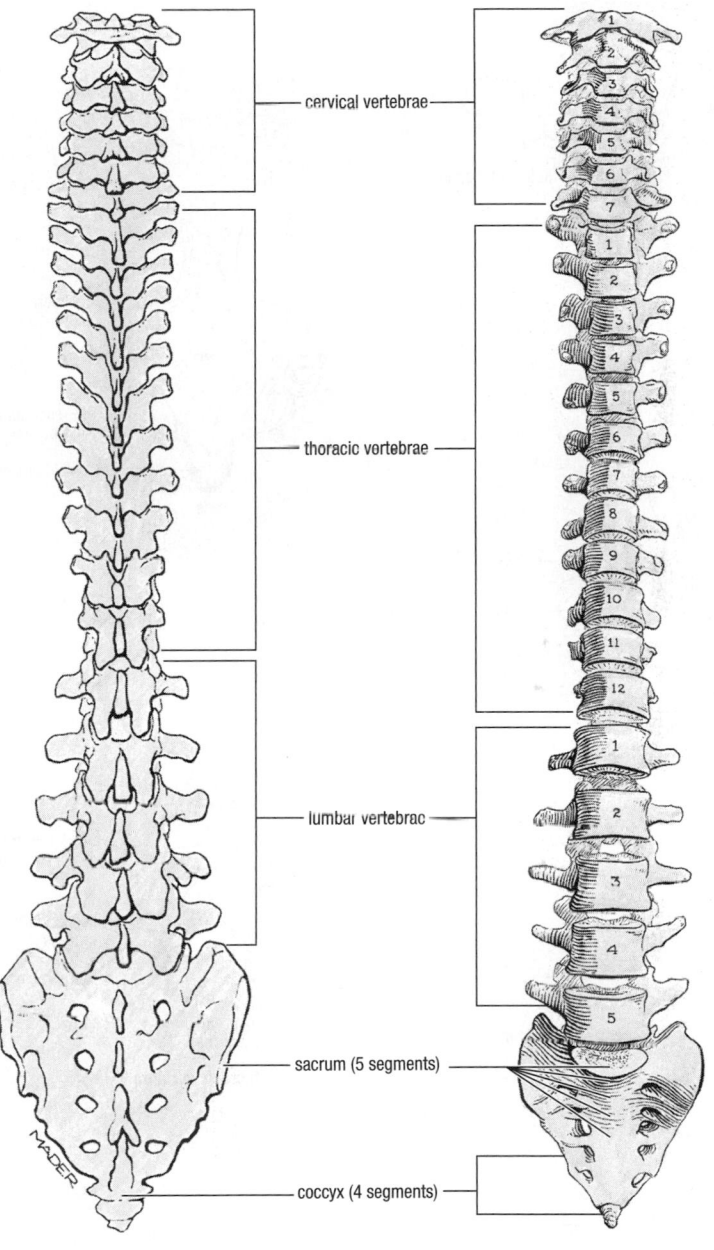

cervical vertebrae

thoracic vertebrae

lumbar vertebrae

sacrum (5 segments)

coccyx (4 segments)

vertebral column, posterior (left) and anterior (right) views

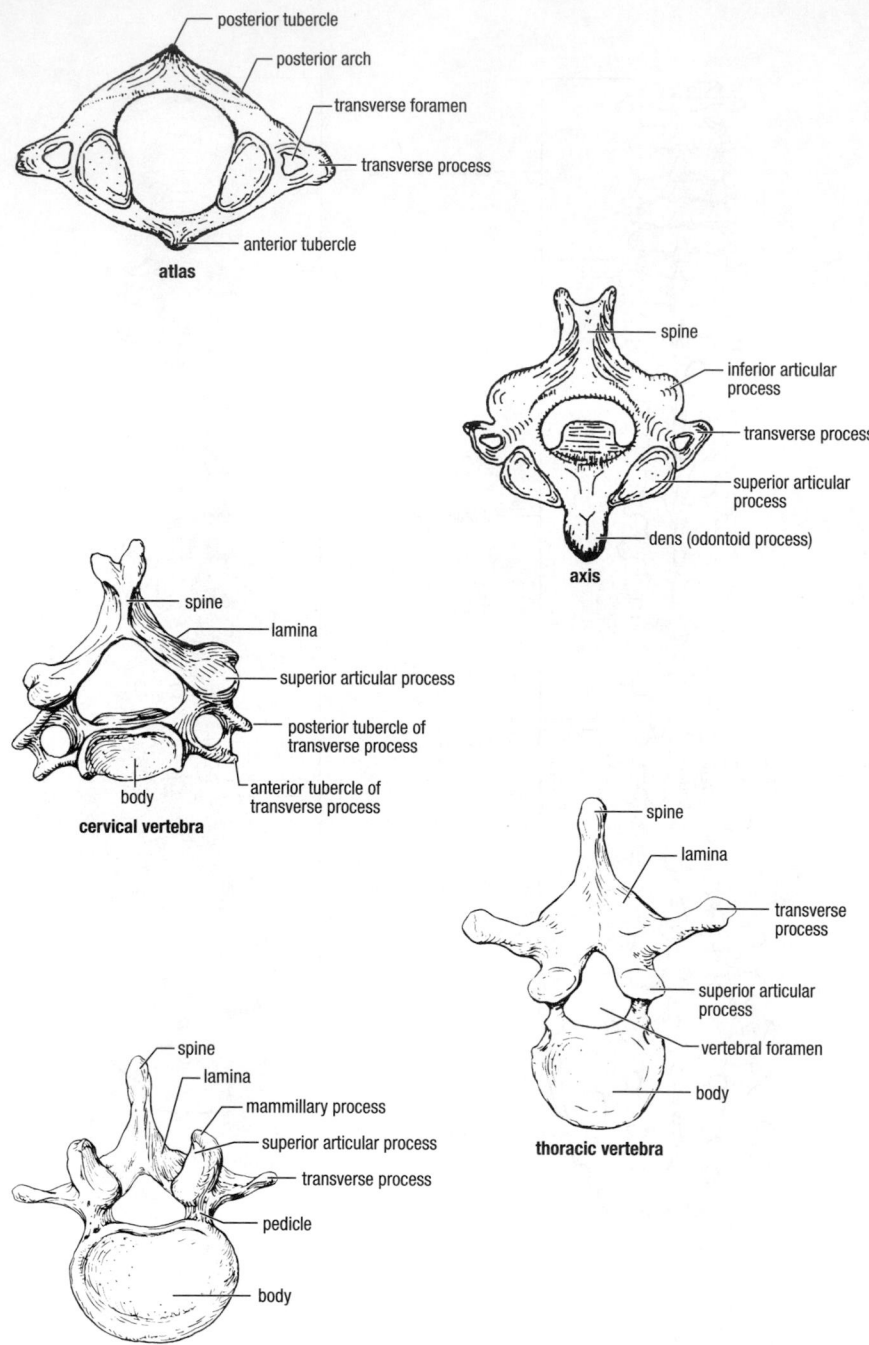

posterior tubercle

posterior arch

transverse foramen

transverse process

anterior tubercle

atlas

spine

inferior articular process

transverse process

superior articular process

dens (odontoid process)

axis

spine

lamina

superior articular process

posterior tubercle of transverse process

anterior tubercle of transverse process

body

cervical vertebra

spine

lamina

transverse process

superior articular process

vertebral foramen

body

thoracic vertebra

spine

lamina

mammillary process

superior articular process

transverse process

pedicle

body

typical atlas, axis, cervical, thoracic, and lumbar vertebrae

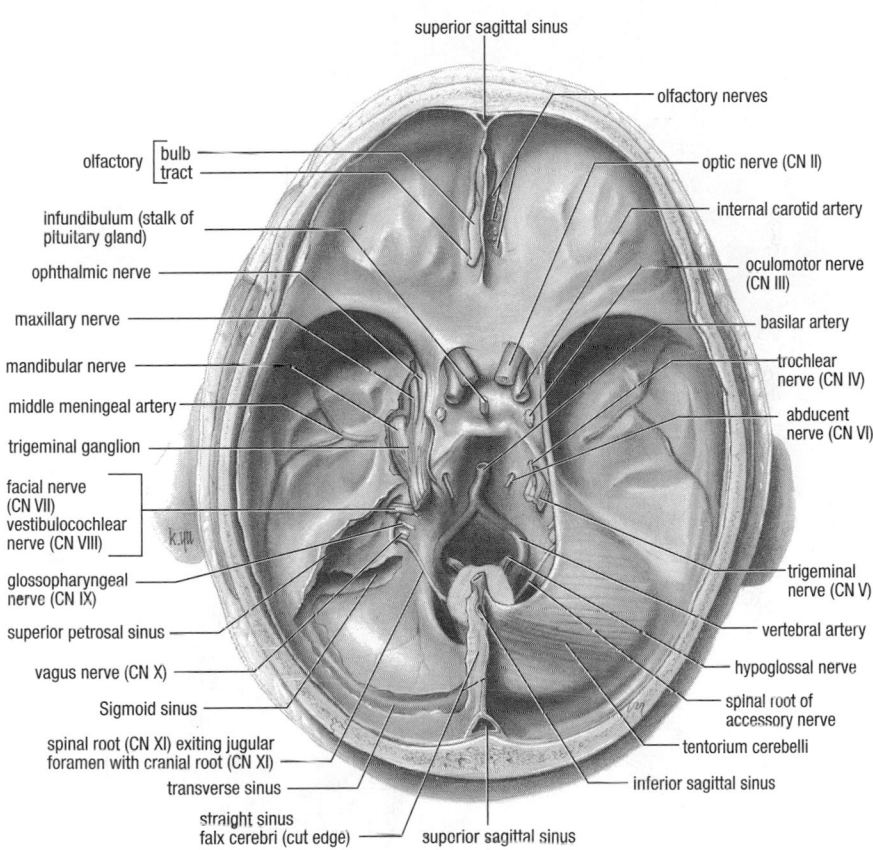

superior sagittal sinus

olfactory nerves

olfactory [bulb
　　　　　 tract

optic nerve (CN II)

internal carotid artery

infundibulum (stalk of
pituitary gland)

oculomotor nerve
(CN III)

ophthalmic nerve

maxillary nerve

basilar artery

mandibular nerve

trochlear
nerve (CN IV)

middle meningeal artery

abducent
nerve (CN VI)

trigeminal ganglion

facial nerve
(CN VII)
vestibulocochlear
nerve (CN VIII)

trigeminal
nerve (CN V)

glossopharyngeal
nerve (CN IX)

superior petrosal sinus

vertebral artery

vagus nerve (CN X)

hypoglossal nerve

Sigmoid sinus

spinal root of
accessory nerve

spinal root (CN XI) exiting jugular
foramen with cranial root (CN XI)

tentorium cerebelli

transverse sinus

inferior sagittal sinus

straight sinus
falx cerebri (cut edge)

superior sagittal sinus

nerves and vessels of the interior base of the skull, superior view

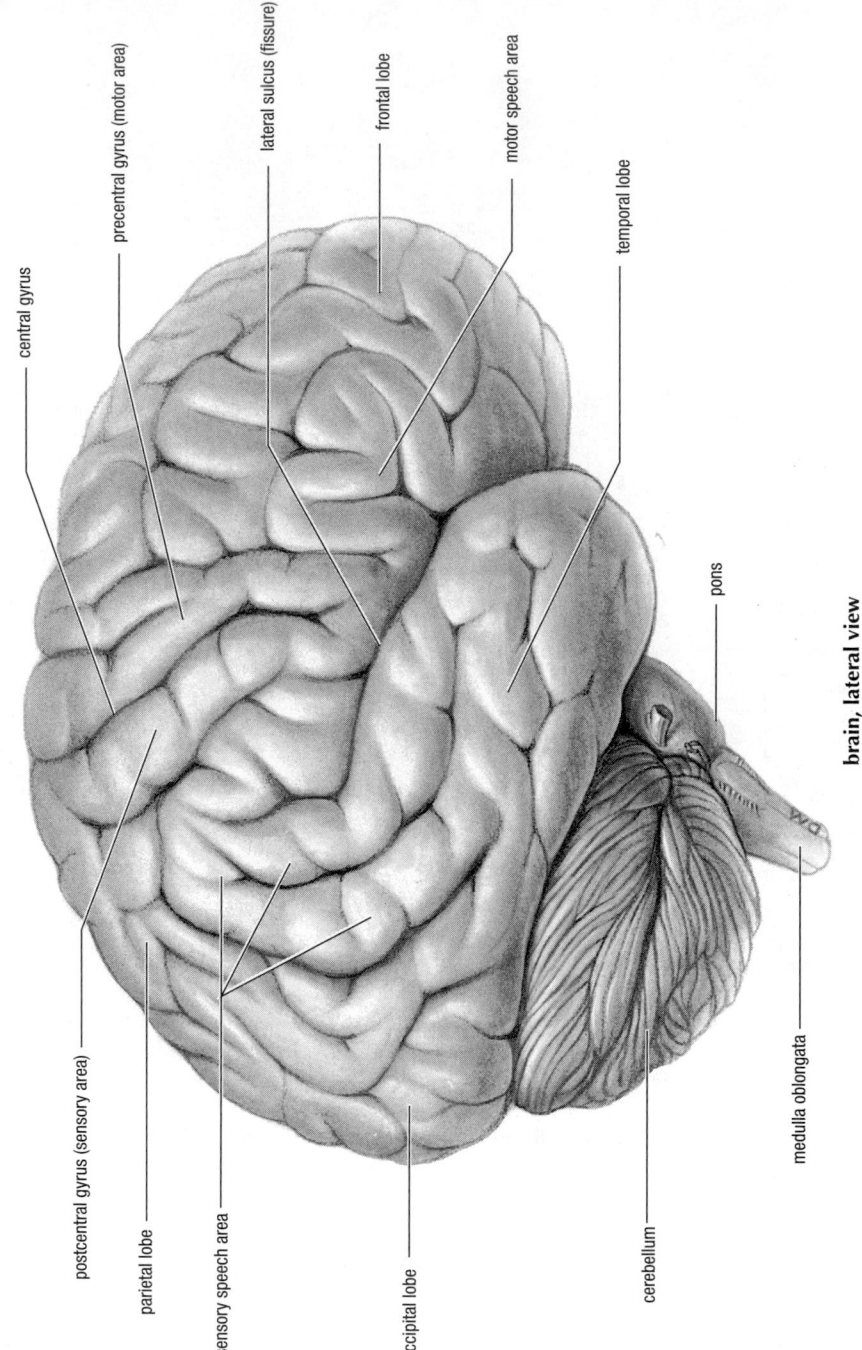

central gyrus

precentral gyrus (motor area)

lateral sulcus (fissure)

frontal lobe

motor speech area

temporal lobe

pons

postcentral gyrus (sensory area)

parietal lobe

sensory speech area

occipital lobe

cerebellum

medulla oblongata

brain, lateral view

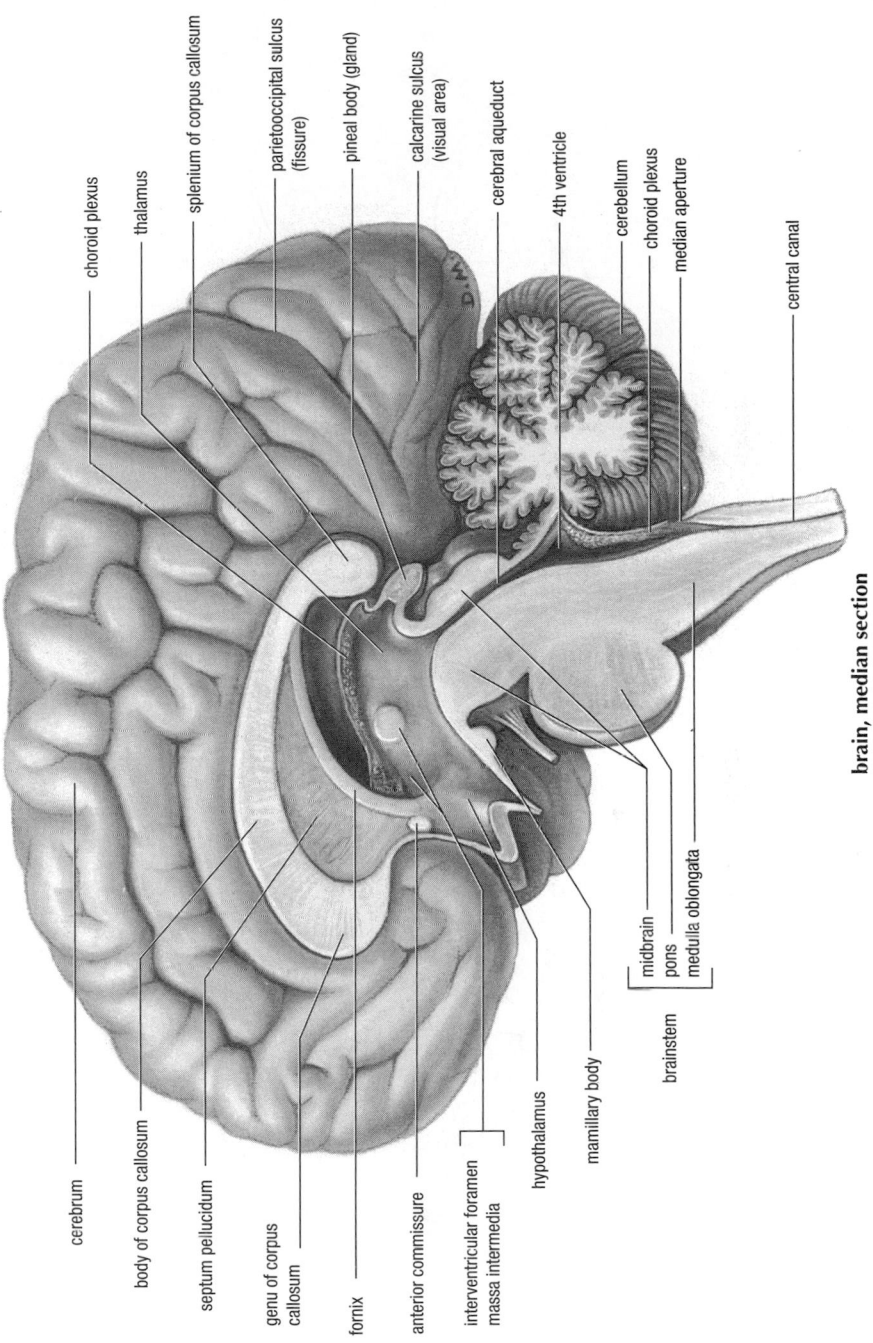

brain, median section

Labels:
- choroid plexus
- thalamus
- splenium of corpus callosum
- parietooccipital sulcus (fissure)
- pineal body (gland)
- calcarine sulcus (visual area)
- cerebral aqueduct
- 4th ventricle
- cerebellum
- choroid plexus
- median aperture
- central canal
- cerebrum
- body of corpus callosum
- septum pellucidum
- genu of corpus callosum
- fornix
- anterior commissure
- interventricular foramen
- massa intermedia
- hypothalamus
- mamillary body
- midbrain
- pons
- medulla oblongata
- brainstem

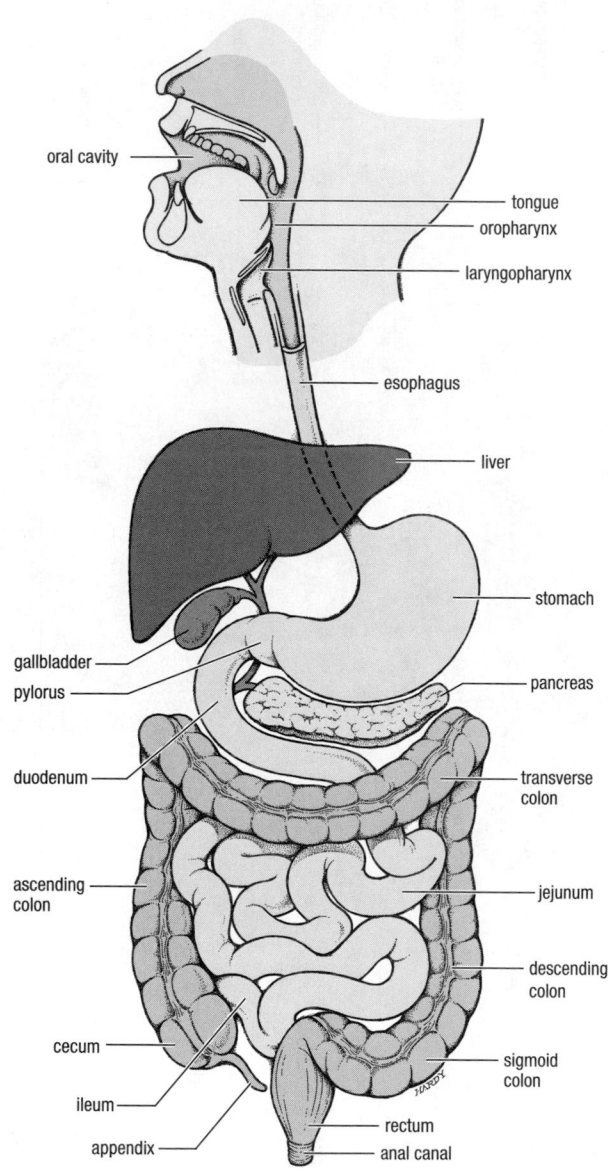

oral cavity

tongue

oropharynx

laryngopharynx

esophagus

liver

stomach

gallbladder

pylorus

pancreas

duodenum

transverse colon

ascending colon

jejunum

descending colon

cecum

ileum

sigmoid colon

appendix

rectum

anal canal

digestive system and adjacent organs

Contrast Media, Imaging Agents, and Related Substances

[11]Cu-TETA octreotide
5-iodo-2-deoxyuridine (IUdR)
acetrizoate
AcuTect
Adenoscan
Altropane
AMI 121
AMI 227
amidotrizoic acid
Amipaque
Amiscan
Anatrast
Angiografin
AngioMARK
Apomate
arcitumomab
Baricon
barium sulfate
Barobag enema kit
Baro-Cat
Baros effervescent granules
Barosperse
benzamide
benzoic acid
Biliscopin
Biloptin
bismuth
calcium 45 (^{45}Ca)
calcium 47 (^{47}Ca)
calcium ipodate
carbon 11 (^{11}C)
carbon-11-labeled cocaine
carbon-11-labeled fatty acids
carbon-11 acetate
carbon-11 butanol

carbon-11 carfentanil
carbon-11 flumazenil
carbon-11 N-methyl-spiperone
carbon-11 nomifensine
carbon-11 raclopride
carbon-11 thymidine
CardioGen-82
Cardiolite
Cardiotec
CEA-Scan
CEA-Tc 99m (^{99m}Tc CEA)
CentoRx
Ceretec
cerium
cesium chloride
CheeTah
Cholebrine
Choletec
Cholografin
Cholografin Meglumine
Cholografin-Dilute
Chromitope Sodium
chromium
Clariscan
Cobatope-57
Combidex
Conray 30, 43, 60, 400
copper
copper 64 (^{64}Cu)
cyanocobalamin
Cysto-Conray
Cysto-Conray II
Cystografin
Cystografin Dilute
d,1-HMPAO
Definity
deuterium

dextrose 5% in water
Diaginol
diatrizoate
diatrizoate meglumine
diatrizoate sodium
diatrizoic acid
diazepam
diethylenetriaminepentaacetic acid (DTPA)
Digibar 190
Digital HD
Dionosil
Dionosil Oily
dobutamine
dodecafluoropentane (DDFP)
Dopascan
dysprosium
EchoGen
Echovist
Enecat CT enema
EneMark rectal marker kit
Enhancer
Entero Vu
Entrobar
Entrocel
EntroEase
Entrokit
Eovist
Esopho-Cat
ethiodized oil
Ethiodol
etidronate disodium
Evans blue
exametazime
E-Z-AC
E-Z-Cat
E-Z-Cat Dry

E-Z-HD
E-Z-Paque
E-Z-Paste
F-18 fluoro-2-deoxyglu-
cose
F-18 sodium fluoride
Feridex IV
feruglose
ferumoxsil
Fibrimage
Flo-Coat
fluorine
fluorine-18-dihydrox-
yphenylalanine (^{18}F-
DOPA)
fluorodeoxyglucose
(FDG)
FS-069
furosemide
gadobenate dimeglumine
(Gd-BOPTA)
gadobenic acid
gadobutrol
gadodiamide (Gd-DTPA-
BMA)
gadolinium (Gd)
gadolinium chelate
gadolinium oxide
gadopentetate dimeglu-
mine (Gd-DTPA)
gadoterate meglumine
(Gd-DOTA)
gadoteridol (Gd-D03A)
gadoversetamide
gadoxetic acid (Gd-EOB-
DTPA)
galactose
gallium
Gastrografin
GastroMARK
Gastromiro
Gastrovist
Gd-DTPA with mannitol

Glofil-125
glucagon
glucarate
HD 200 Plus
HD 85
Hepatolite
Hexabrix
Hippuran
holmium
human serum albumin
(HSA)
hydrogen peroxide
hyoscine butylbromide
Hypaque Meglumine
Hypaque Sodium
Hypaque-76
Hypaque-Cysto
Imagent GI
Imavist
ImmuRAIT
indium 111 (^{111}In)
indium-111 pentetreotide
Indium-Oxine
indocyanine green (ICG)
Intropaste
iobitridol
iocetamic acid
iodamide
iodide
iodine-123 MIBG
iodine-131 MIBG
iodipamide
iodipamide meglumine
iodixanol
iodized oil
iodohippurate sodium I-
123
iodohippurate sodium I-
131
iodopyracet
Iodotope
ioglunide
iohexol

Iomeron 150, 250, 300,
350
iopamidol
iopanoate
iopanoic acid
iophendylate
iopromide
iothalamate
iothalamate meglumine
iothalamate sodium
iothalamic acid
iotrolan
iotroxamide
ioversol
ioxaglate
ioxaglate meglumine
ioxaglate sodium
ioxaglic acid
ioxilan
ioxithalamate
ipodate
ipodate sodium
iridium
iridium 192 (^{192}Ir)
Isopaque
isosulfan blue
Isovue
Isovue Multipack-250,
-300, -370
Isovue-200, -250, -300,
-370
Isovue-M 200, 300
Kinevac
LeukoScan
LeuTech
Levovist
Lipiodol
Liqui-Coat HD
Liquid Barosperse
L-tyrosine
Lymphazurin
LymphoScan
macroaggregated albumin

Macrotec
magnesium
magnetite albumin
Magnevist
mangafodipir trisodium
manganese chloride
mannitol and saline
MD-76R
MD-Gastroview
MDP-Bracco
Medebar Plus
Medescan
meglumine
meglumine diatrizoate
meglumine iocarmate
meglumine iodipamide
meglumine iothalamate
meglumine iotroxate
Metastron
methyl methacrylate
methylglucamine
metrizamide
metrizoate
Micropaque
mineral oil
Miraluma
MS-325
Multihance
Myoscint
Myoview
naloxone
NeoSpect
NeoTect
Neurolite
nicotinamide
nimodipine
Niopam
nitrogen-13 ammonia
nofetumomab
OctreoScan
octreotide
Omnipaque 140, 180, 240, 300, 350

Omniscan
OncoScint CR/OV
OncoSeed
OptiMARK
Optiray 160, 240, 300, 320, 350
Optison
Oragrafin Calcium
Oragrafin Sodium
Oxilan
palladium
Pantopaque
pentagastrin
pentetreotide
peppermint oil
Perchloracap
perflubron
perfluorocarbon
Persantine
pertechnetate
phosphoric acid
phosphorus
Phosphotec
Polibar
Polibar Plus
potassium
potassium perchlorate
Prepcat
Prohance
propyliodone
ProstaScint
Quadramet
radiopaque polyvinyl chloride
RAPID strand
Readi-Cat
Readi-Cat 2
recombinant thyrotropin
Reno-60
Renocal-76
Reno-DIP
Renografin-60
Reno-M 30

Reno-M Dip
Renovist
Renovist II
Renovue-65
Renovue-Dip
rhenium
RIGScan CR49
rubidium chloride
Rubratope-57
samarium
samarium-153 ethylenediamine tetramethylene phosphoric acid (^{153}Sm-EDTMP)
satumomab pendetide
Scan C
selenium
sestamibi
Sethotope
sincalide
Sinografin
Sitzmarks
sodium
sodium bicarbonate
sodium chloride
sodium diatrizoate
sodium iodide
sodium iodipamide
sodium iodohippurate
sodium iothalamate
sodium ipodate
sodium meglumine ioxaglate
sodium methiodal
sodium metrizoate
sodium pertechnetate
sodium tartrate
sodium tyropanoate
Sol-O-Pake
Solu-Biloptin
Solutrast
somatostatin
Sonazoid

A27

SonoRx
SonoVue
sorbitol
sprodiamide
strontium
sucrose polyester
sulfobromophthalein
sulfur colloid
tantalum
tantalum 178 (^{178}Ta)
teboroxime
Techneplex
TechneScan HDP, MAA,
  MAG3, PYP
technetium 99m (^{99m}Tc)
technetium stannous py-
  rophosphate (TSPP)
technetium-99m albumin
technetium-99m albumin
  aggregated
technetium-99m albumin
  colloid
technetium-99m albumin
  microspheres
technetium-99m bi-
  ciromab
technetium-99m bicisate
technetium-99m de-
  preotide
technetium-99m dimer-
  captosuccinic acid
technetium-99m disofenin
technetium-99m exam-
  etazime
technetium-99m furifos-
  min
technetium-99m galacto-
  syl human serum albu-
  min
technetium-99m glucarate
technetium-99m glucep-
  tate

technetium-99m hepa-
  toiminodiacetic acid
  (Tc-HIDA)
technetium-99m Hepato-
  lite
technetium-99m human
  serum albumin
technetium-99m lidofenin
technetium-99m
  macroaggregated albu-
  min
technetium-99m MAG 3
technetium-99m mebro-
  fenin
technetium-99m
  medronate
technetium-99m merti-
  atide
technetium-99m N-para-
  isopropyl-acetanilide-
  iminodiacetic acid (Tc-
  PIPIDA)
technetium-99m ox-
  idronate
technetium-99m pentetate
technetium-99m pentetate
  calcium trisodium
technetium-99m pertech-
  netate sodium
technetium-99m
  polyphosphate
technetium-99m py-
  rophosphate
technetium-99m ses-
  tamibi
technetium-99m siborox-
  ime
technetium-99m sodium
technetium-99m sodium
  pertechnetate
technetium-99m succimer
technetium-99m sulfur
  colloid

technetium-99m teborox-
  ime
technetium-99m tetrofos-
  min
Telebrix
Telepaque
Teslascan
tetrabromophenolph-
  thalein
tetraiodophenolphthalein
thallium 201
thallous chloride
TheraSeed
thorium dioxide
Thorotrast
Tomocat
Tomocat 1000
Tonojug
Tonopaque
Top-Cat
triiodobenzoic acid
Triosil
tyropanoate
Ultra-R
UltraTag
Ultravist 150, 240, 300,
  370
uranium
Urografin
Uromiro
Urovist Cysto
Urovist Meglumine
Urovist Sodium 300
UroVysion
Varibar
Verluma
Visipaque 270, 320
Xenetix 250, 300, 350
xenon
xylenol orange

Common Radiation Oncology Terms

abscopal effect
absolute dose
absorbed dose
accelerator
acute exposure
adjacent field
adjuvant therapy
afterloading technique
algorithm
alloy
alpha cradle immobilization device
alpha particle
amygdaloid complex
angle
antiemetic
applicator
Aquaplast immobilization device
arc
arc therapy
asymmetric collimation
attenuation
backpointer
backscatter
beam film
beam modifier
beam quality
beam shaping
beam's eye view
Becquerel (Bq)
belly board
beta particle
beta plaque
beta radiation
betatron
bite block
block
bolus
boost
brachytherapy
Bragg peak

breast board
breast bridge
Bremsstrahlung x-ray
buildup region
calcification
calculation
calipers
cast
catheter
centigray (cGy)
central axis
central axis depth dose
central plane
Cerrobend
cesium
cesium teletherapy unit
cesium 137 (^{137}Cs, Cs-137)
chemoradiotherapy
chemotherapy regimen
Clinac linear accelerator
clinical target volume (CTV)
cobalt teletherapy unit
cobalt 60 (^{60}Co, Co-60)
cobalt-60 teletherapy
cold spot
collimator
collimator angle
collimator leaf
compensator
composite plan
computer assisted tomography (CT, CAT)
coned down
conformal radiation therapy (CRT)
conformal radiotherapy
contact therapy
contour
contour preparation
conventional therapy
convergence

coplanar beam arrangement
couch angle
couch kick
craniospinal irradiation
CT simulator
curative intent care
curative radiotherapy
curie (Ci)
cyclotron
decay
Delclos applicator
depth dose
desquamation
digitally composited radiograph (DCR)
digitally reconstructed radiograph
  (DRR)
diode
divergence
divergent beams
dose calculation
dose distribution
dose escalation
dose-volume histograms
dosimetrist
dosimetry
dwell position
dynamic multileaf collimator (DMLC)
dynamic wedge
electromagnetic radiation
electron
electron beam radiation therapy
electron cone
Ellis filter
entrance port
equal weighting
extended distance
external beam radiation therapy (EBRT,
  XRT)
external radiation
eye shield
facial mask
field arrangement
field block

field weighting
film digitizer
filter
Fletcher-Suit applicator
fluid-attenuated inversion recovery
  (FLAIR)
fluorodeoxyglucose positron emission
  tomography (FDG PET)
fraction
fractionated external beam radiation
  therapy
fractionation
frontocentral
gamma knife
gamma radiation
gamma ray
gantry
gap
gap calculation
geometry
gold 198 (^{198}Au, Au-198)
Gray (Gy)
gross tumor volume (GTV)
half beam block
half-life
half-value layer (HVL)
half-value thickness
hand block
headrest (sizes range from A to F)
Heyman capsule
high dose
high dose rate (HDR)
high linear energy transfer (LET) radiation
high-dose-rate remote afterloading machine
high-dose-rate remote brachytherapy
high-dose-rate remote radiation therapy
high-energy proton therapy
hindbrain
hot spot
hyperfractionated radiation
hyperfractionation

hyperthermia
hypofractionated radiation
image fusion
immobilization device
immunotherapy
implant
implant radiation
independent collimator
informed consent
intensity modulated radiation therapy (IMRT)
interaortocaval lymphadenopathy
internal radiation
interpeduncular cistern
interstitial brachytherapy
interstitial implant
interstitial radiation therapy
intracavitary irradiation
intracavitary radiation
intracavitary therapy
intracavity brachytherapy
intraluminal implant
intraoperative radiation therapy
inverse square law
iodine 125 (^{125}I, I-125)
ionization chamber
iridium
iridium 192 (^{192}Ir, Ir-192)
irradiated volume
irregular fields
isocenter
isocentric
isodose curve
isodose distribution
isodose plan
isotherm
isotope
Karnofsky Performance Status (KPS)
kilovolt (kV)
laser
laser alignment system
LD 50/30
lead

lesion length
lethal dose (LD)
linear accelerator (LINAC)
linear energy transfer (LET)
localization film
local-regional
low dose rate (LDR)
lucite filter
lumen
magnetic resonance imaging (MR, MRI)
mantle field
megavoltage (MeV)
megavolts (MV)
minimum target dose
missing tissue compensator
mold
monitor unit (MU)
monoclonal antibody
mucositis
multileaf collimator (MLC)
multiplanar reconstruction
neutron
neutron beam therapy
noncoplanar beam arrangements
nuclide
oblique
off-axis factor
orthogonal pair
orthovoltage x-ray therapy
ovoid
oxygen enhancement ratio (OER)
palladium
palliation
palliative intent care
paraaortic field
parallel opposed fields
parenchymal hyperlucency
particle beam
particle beam treatment
penumbra
percentage depth dose (PDD)
perimesencephalic cistern

Common Radiation
Oncology Terms

permanent implant
permanent interstitial implant seed
phosphorus 32
photon
photon beam radiation therapy
pin and arc
piriform sinus
planning target volume (PTV)
point calculation
port
port film
portal
portal imaging
positron emission tomography (PET)
prescription point
primary beam
prostate seed implant
proton
proton beam therapy
pterygoid process
punctate foci
radiation absorbed dose (RAD)
radiation biology
radiation field
radiation physics
radiation portal
radiation therapy
radiation therapy planning (RTP)
radiation therapy technologist (RTT)
radiation treatment planning (RTP)
radiobiology
radiocolloid
radioimmunotherapy (RIT)
radioiodine seeds (I-125)
radiolabeled antibodies
radionuclide
radioprotector, radiation protector
radioresistance
radiosensitivity
radiosensitizer
radiotherapy
radium
radium implant

radium 226
radon
Red Journal (International Journal of
    Radiation Oncology/Biology/Physics)
reference depth
relative biological effect (RBE)
remote brachytherapy
removable implant
ribbon
roentgen (R)
Roentgen Equivalent Man (REM)
rotational therapy
separation
sestamibi
shield
short tau inversion recovery (STIR) im-
    age
simulated annealing
simulation
simulator
single-photon emission computed to-
    mography (SPECT) imaging
skin sparing
source axis distance (SAD)
source film distance (SFD)
source-to-skin distance (SSD)
source surface distance (SSD)
spiculated margin
split course
stereotactic external-beam radiation
stereotactic head frame
stereotactic injection
stereotactic radiation therapy
stereotactic radiosurgery (SRS)
stereotactic radiotherapy (SRT)
stereotaxic radiosurgery
stereotaxis
strontium 89 (^{89}Sr, Sr-89)
strontium 90 (^{90}Sr, Sr-90)
superficial machine
superficial therapy
supervoltage range
supervoltage therapy

surface mold
systemic radiation therapy
T1 fat-saturated
tandem
target localization
tattoo
teletherapy
testicular shield
thermoluminescent dosimeter (TLD)
thermoplastic
three-dimensional conformal radiation therapy (3DRT)
three-dimensional radiotherapy treatment planning (3DRTP)
tolerance dose
total body irradiation (TBI)
total skin electron (TSE) irradiation
treatment beam
treatment field

treatment plan
treatment time
tumor localization
tumor volume
tungsten
two-dimensional radiotherapy treatment planning (2DRTP)
unequal weighting
unsealed internal radiation therapy
vaginal cylinder
verification film
volumetric calculation
Von de Graaf generator
wedge
wedge filter
wing board
X-knife
x-ray
x-ray therapy

AIR CONTRAST BARIUM ENEMA

PROCEDURE: Barium was allowed to fill the cecum in a retrograde manner under fluoroscopic control. Using a double-contrast technique, multiple films were obtained. Several diverticula were visualized. The sigmoid was somewhat laterally displaced to the left. There also appeared to be elevation of the small bowel. A diffuse soft tissue density was seen in the lower abdomen. No mucosal ulcerations or polypoid lesions could be identified.

IMPRESSIONS: Air-contrast barium enema shows displacement of the bowel, suggestive of pelvic mass. The possibility of an enlarged bladder should be considered. No evidence of polypoid lesions or masses seen within the visualized colon.

BILATERAL MAMMOGRAPHY

FINDINGS: Bilateral mammographic examination demonstrates atrophic breasts. There are moderate fibrocystic disease changes centrally in each breast, generally symmetrical. There is moderate ductal hyperplasia in the subareolar regions on each side. No dominant mass lesion is seen. No abnormal calcifications are detected. The skin and subcutaneous fat appear smooth. Vascularity appears normal.

IMPRESSIONS: Atrophic breasts with moderate fibrocystic disease and moderate ductal hyperplasia. No evidence of malignant mass lesion seen.

The above findings place this patient at a higher risk for breast cancer. Annual mammography is strongly recommended.

CHEST MRI

REASON FOR STUDY: An MRI was requested in this patient who has a possible left hilar mass on CT scanning. However, on CT imaging it was difficult to differentiate between a mass lesion and a pulmonary vein; therefore, an MRI was performed.

TECHNIQUE: Cardiac and respiratory compensation was used. T1- and T2-weighted images were obtained.

FINDINGS: There is a 4-cm soft tissue density mass in the left hilum adjacent to the left pulmonary artery. The mass becomes bright on T2-weighted imaging. It is not consistent with a vessel and by MRI criteria definitely represents a soft tissue mass. No other lesions or abnormalities are seen throughout the mediastinum.

IMPRESSION: Metastatic lesion, left hilum.

CT OF LARYNX

PROCEDURE: Preliminary scout views were performed. Multiple axial sections were obtained with infusion with respiration as well as during Valsalva maneuver.

There is an air-filled dilated saccule on the left consistent with an internal laryngocele. This does deflate when the patient is in quiet respiration. The laryngocele measures 1.3 x 3 cm in size. No other soft tissue or bony abnormalities are detected throughout the pharynx and neck. Clinical correlation is recommended.

IMPRESSION: Findings of an air-filled dilated saccule of the laryngeal ventricle on the left. This is consistent with an internal laryngocele measuring 1.3 x 3 cm in size.

LEFT TIBIA, STATUS POST FIXATION

FINDINGS: X-ray demonstrates drainage tubes have been removed from the area of the left knee. The plate and screws are still present in the distal tibia. The bone is fixed in anatomic position and alignment. Skin clips are still present.

IMPRESSION: Internal fixation left distal femoral fracture, stable.

MR ARTHROGRAM, LEFT SHOULDER

CLINICAL INFORMATION: Rule out labral tear.

TECHNIQUE: Sagittal, axial, and coronal T1 fat-saturated, coronal T2 fat-saturated views of the left shoulder were performed after interarticular instillation of gadolinium.

FINDINGS: There is deep undercutting of the superior labrum directed slightly laterally into the base of the biceps tendon. This probably constitutes a SLAP II type tear. Glenoid articular cartilage is normal. Superior, middle, and inferior gleno-humeral ligaments are normal. No rotator cuff tear is seen. There is no fluid in the subacromial-subdeltoid bursa.

IMPRESSION: Deep undercutting of the superior labrum extending posterior to the biceps tendon and also slightly directed laterally into the base of the biceps tendon. This probably constitutes superior labrum anterior and posterior II tear.

MRI OF THE HIPS

HISTORY: This patient is status post right hip dislocation with fracture of the superior portion of the right femoral head several months ago. She now returns due to hip pain.

PROCEDURE: An MRI is performed to rule out avascular necrosis of the right hip. T1- and T2-weighted images were obtained in the coronal and sagittal planes.

FINDINGS: There is a low-intensity line along the medial portion of the right femoral head, consistent with avascular necrosis. The location of this is somewhat unusual for avascular necrosis, as this is usually seen along the superior aspect of the femoral head. There is minimal irregularity along the superior aspect of the right femoral head, but this corresponds to the site of previous fracture and therefore is not likely to represent avascular necrosis in this area.

IMPRESSIONS
1. Avascular necrosis of the right femoral head.
2. Status post fracture of the superior portion of the right femoral head.

PELVIC SONOGRAM

CLINICAL INFORMATION: Possible ectopic pregnancy, positive pregnancy test, left adnexal tenderness.

The uterus is normal in size and architecture. No intrauterine pregnancy is identified. The endometrial echo appears normal. There is fluid in a tubular structure in the left adnexal area, probably fluid in the fallopian tube. No other adnexal masses or cysts are visualized on either side. No free fluid visible in the cul-de-sac.

IMPRESSIONS: No intrauterine pregnancy is demonstrated. There appears to be some fluid in the left fallopian tube. Recommend clinical correlation.

PORTABLE CHEST

REASON FOR STUDY: A supine AP chest study at 1445 hours on the day of bypass surgery is compared with the study performed earlier on this date.

FINDINGS: The hemidiaphragms remain smooth and the costophrenic angles are clear. Thoracotomy tubes are present in the lower anterior hemithorax on either side. The lungs appear generally clear and well expanded. Vascularity appears normal. A CVP line is in place on the left. The mediastinum is slightly widened. The cardiac silhouette appears normal in size and configuration. The bony thorax is unchanged.

IMPRESSION: Stable chest, status post bypass surgery.

RIGHT HIP TOMOGRAMS

Tomography demonstrates incomplete filling in of a major fracture zone involving the right proximal femur, as previously noted.

The intramedullary fixation device is seen to project outside the superior and lateral cortical margins of the right femoral neck. This is likely at least 1 cm; however, a precise measurement cannot be accurately obtained because of the superimposed metallic device on the femoral neck. A 1.2-cm medial displacement of the major distal fracture fragment persists. Moderate varus deformity is also persistent.

Three additional partially threaded metallic pins are noted. The most lateral pin involves an avulsed greater trochanteric fracture fragment. The other 2 pins are positioned at the level of the femoral neck and head.

IMPRESSIONS
1. Comminuted proximal right femoral diaphyseal fracture with medial displacement of the major distal fracture fragment and persistence of moderate varus deformity.
2. Projection of the major intramedullary fixation device outside of the margins of the superior and lateral aspects of the femoral neck.
3. Incomplete filling in of fracture line.

THORACIC SPINE WITH CONED-DOWN VIEW, T9 TO L1

FINDINGS: Degenerative spurs are demonstrated on the right at T8-9 and T9-10. There is an old healed fracture of the left 10th rib posteriorly near the spine. The vertebral bodies appear intact without destructive lesions. The pedicles are intact.

IMPRESSIONS: No destructive lesions are identified. The increased uptake seen on bone scan could be explained by the degenerative changes and the old, healed rib fracture.

UPPER GI SERIES

Preliminary views of the abdomen reveal spurring of the articular surface of the left femoral head. There is narrowing of the left hip joint medially. There are areas of increased density with interspersed lucency in the left femoral head, suggestive of avascular necrosis. Degenerative changes with spurring are seen involving the superior aspect of the right sacroiliac joint.

There is prompt initiation of the swallowing mechanism. Esophageal dysmotility is evidenced. Tertiary contractions are seen in the middle and distal thirds of the thoracic esophagus. Gastroesophageal reflux is present. A 3-cm filling defect is seen in the body of the stomach that could represent a polyp. There is deformity of the distal portion of the gastric antrum. An active ulcer crater is present in the pyloric channel, and there is associated deformity of the base of duodenal bulb. A duodenal sweep is normal.

IMPRESSIONS
1. Esophageal dysmotility and evidence of gastroesophageal reflux. No evidence of esophagitis present.
2. Active ulcer crater, posterior aspect of pyloric channel. Associated deformity of the gastric antrum and base of duodenal bulb.

Common Terms by Procedure

AIR CONTRAST BARIUM ENEMA
abdomen
air-contrast barium enema
barium
bladder
cecum
colon
displacement
diverticula
double-contrast technique
fluoroscopic
mucosal ulceration
pelvic mass
polypoid lesion
retrograde
sigmoid

BILATERAL MAMMOGRAPHY
atrophic breast
calcification
ductal hyperplasia
fibrocystic disease
mass lesion
subareolar region
subcutaneous fat
vascularity

CHEST MRI
cardiac compensation
hilar mass
hilum
mass lesion
mediastinum
metastatic lesion
pulmonary artery
pulmonary vein
respiratory compensation
soft tissue mass

T1-weighted image
T2-weighted image
vessel

CT OF LARYNX
air-filled
axial section
bony abnormality
infusion
laryngeal ventricle
laryngocele
neck
pharynx
respiration
saccule
scout view
soft tissue abnormality
Valsalva maneuver

LEFT TIBIA, STATUS POST FIXATION
alignment
anatomic position
distal femoral fracture
distal tibia
drainage tube
internal fixation
plate and screw
x-ray

MR ARTHROGRAM, LEFT SHOULDER
articular cartilage
axial
biceps tendon
coronal
fat-saturated view
gadolinium
glenohumeral ligament
glenoid

Common Terms by Procedure

instillation
interarticular
labral tear
rotator cuff tear
sagittal
SLAP tear
subacromial-subdeltoid bursa
superior labrum
T1
T2

MRI OF THE HIPS
avascular necrosis
coronal plane
femoral head
fracture
hip dislocation
low-intensity line
sagittal plane
superior aspect
T1-weighted image
T2-weighted image

PELVIC SONOGRAM
adnexal
architecture
cul-de-sac
cyst
ectopic pregnancy
endometrial echo
fallopian tube
fluid
intrauterine pregnancy
mass
tubular structure
uterus

PORTABLE CHEST
AP
bony thorax
bypass
cardiac silhouette
configuration

costophrenic angle
CVP
hemidiaphragm
hemithorax
lung
mediastinum
supine
thoracotomy tube
vascularity

RIGHT HIP TOMOGRAMS
cortical margin
diaphyseal fracture
displacement
femoral head
femoral neck
femur
fracture
fracture fragment
fracture line
fracture zone
greater trochanter
intramedullary fixation device
pin
projection
tomography
varus deformity

THORACIC SPINE WITH CONED-DOWN VIEW, T9 TO L1
bone scan
degenerative
degenerative spur
destructive lesion
fracture
pedicle
rib
spine
uptake
vertebral body

UPPER GI SERIES
abdomen
articular surface
avascular necrosis
contraction
deformity
degenerative
density
duodenal bulb
duodenal sweep
esophageal dysmotility
esophagitis
femoral head

filling defect
gastric antrum
gastroesophageal reflux
hip
lucency
polyp
pyloric channel
sacroiliac joint
spurring
swallowing mechanism
tertiary
thoracic esophagus
ulcer crater

Common Terms by Procedure

Common Breast Imaging Terms

90-degree lateral view
abscess
accessory nipple
acinar space
adenocarcinoma
adenoma
adrenocortical tumor
amorphous calcification
androgen
anechoic
angiolipoma
angioma
angiosarcoma
anterior compression view
artifact
aspiration
ataxia-telangiectasia
atypical ductal hyperplasia (ADH)
automated gun-needle device
axial resolution
axillary adenopathy
axillary dissection
axillary lymph node
axillary lymphadenopathy
bacterial mastitis
beam intensity
benign
biopsy
biopsy change
biopsy marker
branch pattern
bullet
calcification
callback
capsular calcification
cassette
change-of-angel view
chest wall
circumscribed mass
cleavage view

comedo mastitis
complex cystic mass
complex sclerosing lesion (CSL)
compression paddle
computed tomography (CT)
computer-aided detection
computerized axial tomography (CAT)
contrast resolution
core
coupling gel
craniocaudal (CC) view
cross-liked silicone gel
cryptorchism
curvilinear lucency
cyst
Dacron central line cuff
dendritic gynecomastia
density
dermatofibrosarcoma protuberans
diabetic mastopathy
diagnostic imaging
diffuse change
digital mammography
dilated lymphatic channel
dilated vasculature
dimpling
Doppler ultrasound
double spot compression
double spot compression magnification
   view
draining sinus
duct cannulation
duct ectasia
ductal calcification
ductal carcinoma in situ (DCIS)
ductal lavage
ductography
dynamic range
dystrophic calcification
ecchymosis

echogenicity
edema
egg shell
electromagnetic field radiation
elevation resolution
epithelial hyperplasia
exaggerated craniocaudal view (XCCL)
extensive intraductal component (EIC)
extramammary metastasis
fat necrosis
fat-containing lesion
fatty lobulation
fenestrated alphanumeric
fibroadenolipoma
fibroadenoma
fibrous mastopathy
filariasis
filling defect
fine-needle aspiration (FNA)
floating echo
focal fibrosis
focal parenchymal asymmetry
focal zone
follicular center cell
follicular center cell lymphoma
geometric unsharpness
giant cell arteritis
global area
granulomatous disease
grid malfunction
gross finding
gun-needle device
gurgling
gurgling cyst
halo sign
hamartoma
hematoma
Hickman catheter Dacron cuff
high-grade
histiocytoid feature
histoplasmosis
hyalinized
hyperechoic

hypoechoic band
hypoechoic mass
imaging-guided biopsy
inframammary fold (IMF)
internal echo
intracystic
intracystic calcification
invasive ductal carcinoma
ipsilateral axilla
kilovoltage
kyphosis
labeling
lactational
lactiferous
lateral resolution
lateral tug
leiomyosarcoma
Lexan
lexicon
linear
lipoma
lobular carcinoma in situ (LCIS)
low-grade
lumpectomy site
lymphatic channel
magnetic resonance imaging (MRI)
magnification view
malignant
mammogram
mammography
mammography guided wire localization
margin
mass
matrix determination
mediolateral oblique (MLO) view
metastasis
metastatic pattern
microcyst
microlobulated
milk of calcium
milliamperage output
mishandling crimp
mixed-density mass

moderately differentiated
motion
mucinous feature
multicentric cancer
needle biopsy
needle-wire system
negative-density artifact
neurofibroma
nipple ring
oil cyst
opacified
orthogonal ultrasound
orthogonal view
outlining mole
outlining mole crevice
outlining skin lesion
pancake
pancake breast
papilloma
parenchyma
peak kilovoltage
peau d'orange
pectoral muscle
pectoralis minor muscle
positron emission tomography (PET)
phantom image
photocell positioning
phyllodes tumor
pleomorphic liposarcoma
pneumocystogram
pneumocystography
poor contrast
poorly differentiated
popcorn calcification
popcorn-like
posterior nipple line
posterior nipple line (PNL)
postlumpectomy fluid collection
psammoma body
pseudoangiomatous stromal hyperplasia
  (PASH)
pseudolesion
punctate calcification

radial scar
radiolucent
radiopathologic concordance
retroglandular fat
reverberation artifact
rim
rodlike
rolled view
round mass
scanning technique
scatter radiation
scintimammography
screening mammography
sebaceous cyst
sentinel lymph node
septation
shadowing
skin fold
skin fold simulating
skin mass
smudgy
spatial resolution
specular echo
spiculated mass
spicule
spot compression view
spot tangential view
standoff pad
stereotactic-guided biopsy
sternalis muscle
subject contrast
suboptimal contrast
synchronous lesion
talc
tissue-air interface
touch prep
trabecular marking
transducer orientation
triangulation
tubular
tumor sojourn time
tumor-marking clip
ultrasound

ultrasound-guided biopsy
ultrasound-guided core biopsy
underexposed image
uneven exposure
upside-down cassette
vacuum-assisted imaging-guided biopsy

vascular lesion
water-density mass
well differentiated
wire localization
x-ray attenuation

Common Radiographic Imaging Techniques

angiography

Angiography is accomplished by passing a catheter through an artery to the area of the body being investigated. A contrast material is injected into the vessels highlighting them, and x-rays are taken. The procedure is used to determine if blood vessels, including those in the brain, heart, kidneys, and other parts of the body, are diseased, enlarged, blocked, narrowed, or otherwise abnormal.

computed tomography (CT)

The CT scan is also referred to as a CAT scan (computerized axial tomography). CT scans can image both hard and soft tissues, including bones, organs, muscles, and tumors. Three-D images are generated by computer graphics software using x-ray data obtained from multiple cross-sections of an area in any given plane.

magnetic resonance imaging (MRI)

MRIs align the magnetic nuclei of a patient. Radiofrequency pulses are then used to produce signals that are converted into 3-dimensional tomographic images of any given plane.

mammography

Mammography uses low-dose x-rays to examine the breasts to enable early detection of breast cancers and other breast diseases. The screening mammogram is a tool capable of detecting breast cancers up to 2 years before they can be felt by self-examination or by a physician. Diagnostic mammograms are used to evaluate abnormal or suspicious areas of the breast, such as lumps found by the patient or physician.

myelography

Myelography is used to visualize the spinal column and its contents. A contrast media is used to help identify spinal lesions resulting from disease or trauma.

positron emission tomography (PET)

The PET scan is a diagnostic tool used to obtain physiologic images through the detection of radiation from the emission of positrons, tiny particles emitted from a radioactive substance administered to the patient. The level of organ or tissue function can be determined by interpreting the degree of brightness and/or colors on the PET images.

ultrasonography (Doppler ultrasound)

Diagnostic Doppler ultrasound detects movement of blood cells and other moving structures in the body, measuring both direction and speed of movement. By measuring changes in frequency of the echoes reflected from moving structures, arteries and veins can be viewed in motion. Ultrasound is also widely used for fetal monitoring.

X-rays

X-rays utilize high-energy radiation to produce images to assist in the diagnosis of diseases and structural abnormalities in the body. High-dose x-rays are used to treat cancer.